Critical Care Medicine: The Essentials

FOURTH EDITION

Critical Care Medicine: The Essentials

FOURTH EDITION

John J. Marini, MD

Director of Physiological and Translational Research
HealthPartners Research Foundation
Professor of Medicine
University of Minnesota
Minneapolis/St. Paul, Minnesota (USA)

Arthur P. Wheeler, MD

Director, Medical Intensive Care Unit
Associate Professor of Medicine
Director, Vanderbilt Clinical Coordinating Center
Division of Allergy, Pulmonary and Critical Care
Vanderbilt University
Nashville, Tennessee (USA)

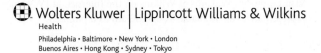

Philadelphia • Baltimore • New York • London
Buenos Aires • Hong Kong • Sydney • Tokyo

Acquisitions Editor: Frances DeStefano
Product Manager: Nicole Dernoski
Production Manager: Bridgett Dougherty
Senior Manufacturing Manager: Benjamin Rivera
Marketing Manager: Angela Panetta
Design Coordinator: Doug Smock
Production Service: SPi Technologies

© 2010 by LIPPINCOTT WILLIAMS & WILKINS, a WOLTERS KLUWER business
530 Walnut Street
Philadelphia, PA 19106 USA
LWW.com

Printed in China

Library of Congress Cataloging-in-Publication Data
Marini, John J.
   Critical care medicine : the essentials / John J. Marini, Arthur P. Wheeler. — 4th ed.
      p. ; cm.
   Includes bibliographical references and index.
   ISBN 978–0–7817–9839–6
  1. Critical care medicine—Handbooks, manuals, etc. 2. Surgical intensive care—Handbooks, manuals, etc.
I. Wheeler, Arthur P. II. Title.
   [DNLM: 1. Critical Care—methods. 2. Emergencies. 3. Intensive Care—methods. WX 218 M339c 2010]
   RC86.8.M386   2010
   616.02'8—dc22

                                             2009030607

To purchase additional copies of this book, call our customer service department at (800) 638-3030 or fax orders to (301) 223-2320. International customers should call (301) 223-2300.

Visit Lippincott Williams & Wilkins on the Internet: at LWW.com. Lippincott Williams & Wilkins customer service representatives are available from 8:30 am to 6 pm, EST.

10 9 8 7 6 5 4 3 2

RRS1009

To my students, residents, fellows, and colleagues—here and abroad—who inspire and educate me on many levels within and outside the sphere of critical care medicine.

John J. Marini

To my sons Aaron and Eric, now grown men, continued sources of wonder, inspiration, and great pride, and to my steadfast love, Lisa.

Arthur P. Wheeler

Preface

Critical care is a high-stakes activity—both from outcome and cost perspectives. What should a young intensivist be taught? Our worlds of medical education and practice continue to change quickly. While electronic retrieval of patient information and scientific literature is of immeasurable help, electronically facilitated submission, peer review, and production methods have accelerated publication turnover. Pressures to shorten time in hospital and improve documentation tug the team toward the computer and away from the patient, placing strains on face-to-face communications among doctor, patient, family, and nurse. Because of mandated and pragmatic changes in practice, there has been a dramatic shift in care from a "one doctor–one patient" relationship to one in which there are frequent personnel changes. The chances for error in this new system are magnified. Simultaneously, older patients with chronic multisystem dysfunction and attendant complex problems account for a growing fraction of those admitted. While practicing on the cutting edge of intensive care medicine has always been challenging, there now seems more to know and too much to keep track of. We do not seem to be winning the race.

Another trend seems clear. In this exciting age of molecular medicine, mastery of bedside examination and physiology has been de-emphasized. Simultaneously, clinical research has shifted from exploration of problems confronted at the bedside to large population-based interventional trials. When well done (and we are getting better at them), these studies hold considerable value and often help decide initial "best practice" for many patients. Yet, clinical trials will never inform all decisions, and it is incumbent upon the practitioner to know when clinical research does not apply to the patient at hand and to recognize when the initial plan suggested by trial results needs modification. Physicians who apply "best practice" to the individual cannot rely only on protocols and the latest guidelines. Recommendations come into and drop out of favor,

but physiologic principles and fundamentals of critical care change very little. Because problems are complex and treatment decisions interwoven, well-honed analytical skills are indispensable. Management must be guided by informed judgment, applying the best information presently known based on core physiological principles and patient response.

Cardiorespiratory physiology forms the logical base for interpreting vital observations and delivering effective critical care. Committed to short loop feedback and "mid-course" corrections, the intensivist should be aware of population-based studies but not enslaved to them. Likewise, it is important to realize that treatments that improve physiological endpoints do not always translate into improved patient outcomes and that failure of a patient to respond as expected to a given treatment does not invalidate that intervention for future patients. Add to these traits those of cost consciousness, empathy, and effective communication, and you are well positioned to deliver cost-effective care in our demanding practice environment.

Multiauthored books—even the best of them—have chapters of varying style and quality that are often lightly edited. We believe that a book intended for comprehension is best written with a single voice and purpose. After nearly 25 years and four editions working together, we feel free to comment freely, quibble, complain, and edit each other's work.

As in preceding editions, we have tried to extract what seem to be those grounding bits of knowledge that have shaped and reshaped our own approach to daily practice. We titled this book "The Essentials" when it was first written, but admit that our own tips and tricks—useful pearls that we think give insight to practice—have been sprinkled liberally throughout. We practice in widely separated hospitals and our research interests involve different types of problems and methods. This diversity helps keep perspective on what is "essential"—or at least interesting to know. This book was written to be read primarily for durable understanding; it is not intended for quick lookup on-the-fly. It is not a book of quick facts, bullet points, check lists, options, or directions. It would be difficult to find a white coat pocket big enough to carry it along on rounds. Depth of treatment has not been surrendered in our attempt to be clear and concise.

The field of critical care and the authors, both once young, have now matured. Fortunately, we remain committed to caring for the sickest patients, discovering new ways to thwart disease, and passing on what we know to the next generation who eventually will care for us. Many principles guiding surgery and medicine are now time-tested and more or less interchangeable. For the fourth edition, we have streamlined the book's organization with this in mind. We have examined and updated the content of each chapter, added and changed illustrations, and in a few cases, discarded what no longer fits. Mostly, however, we fine-tuned and built upon a solid core. This really is no surprise—physiologically based principles endure. It is gratifying that most of what we wrote three editions ago still seems accurate—and never more relevant.

John J. Marini
Arthur P. Wheeler

Acknowledgments

Of all the paragraphs in this book, this one is among the most difficult to write. Perhaps it is because so many have helped me reach this point—some by their inspiring mentorship, some by spirited collaboration, some by invaluable support, and some by enduring friendship. I hope that those closest to me already know the depth of my gratitude. A special few who shaped my earliest years in academic medicine have given me far more than I have yet given back. The debts I owe to Len Hudson and Bruce Culver cannot easily be repaid. By their clear examples they showed me how to combine love for applied physiology, scientific discovery, and education, while never forgetting that the first priority of medicine is to advance patient welfare.

"Each wave owes the essence of its line only to the withdrawal of the preceding one."
—Andre Gide

John J. Marini

More than two decades after the first edition, I appreciate more than ever the help of all the people who nurtured me along the way. My parent's sacrifice and delusional view of my talents and my teachers caring instruction resulted in achievement beyond my ability. My father's insistence on hard work, loyalty, and honesty is the core of my life and practice. Inquisitive students taught me almost as much as the bright, devoted nurses I work with. Wonderful friends, especially the one I married, keep me sane, happy, in my place, and remind me of what is important. Finally, I thank all the patients and their families who teach us grace and courage even when losing their battles with critical illness.

Arthur P. Wheeler

The authors gratefully acknowledge the collaboration of the following authors on this 4th edition: David Dries on the revision of Chapter 35 and Shailesh Shetty on the revision of Chapter 21.

John J. Marini
Arthur P. Wheeler

Contents

Section II. Medical and Surgical Crises

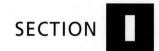
Techniques and Methods in Critical Care

Hemodynamics

1 Because of differences in wall thickness and ejection impedance, the two sides of the heart differ in structure and sensitivity to preload and afterload. The normal right ventricle is relatively sensitive to changes in its loading conditions. When failing or decompensated, both ventricles are preload insensitive and afterload sensitive.

2 Right ventricle afterload is influenced by hypoxemia and acidosis, especially when the capillary bed is diminished and the vascular smooth musculature is hypertrophied, as in chronic lung disease. The ejection impedance of the left ventricle is conditioned primarily by vascular tone, wall thickness, and ventricular volume, except when there is an outflow tract narrowing or aortic valve dysfunction.

3 Regulating cardiac output to metabolic need requires appropriate values for average heart rate and stroke volume. *Either* or both may be the root cause of failing to do so.

4 Even when systolic function is well preserved, impaired ventricular distensibility and failure of the diseased ventricle to relax in diastole can produce pulmonary vascular congestion and "flash pulmonary edema." Echocardiographic diastolic dysfunction often precedes heart failure and commonly develops against the background of systemic hypertension, ischemia, or other diseases that reduce left ventricular compliance.

5 The relationship of cardiac output to filling pressure can be equally well described by the traditional Frank–Starling relationship or by the venous return curve. The driving pressure for venous return is the difference between mean systemic pressure (the average vascular pressure in the systemic circuit) and right atrial pressure. Venous resistance is conditioned by vascular tone and by anatomic factors influenced by lung expansion. At a given cardiac output, mean systemic pressure is determined by venous tone and degree of vascular filling.

6 Radiographic evidence of acute heart failure includes perivascular cuffing, a widening of the vascular pedicle, blurring of the hilar vasculature, and diffuse infiltrates that spare the costophrenic angles. These infiltrates tend to lack air bronchograms and are usually unaccompanied by an acute change in heart size. Chronic congestive heart failure is typified by Kerley B lines, dilated cardiac chambers, and increased cardiac dimensions.

7 The key directives in managing cor pulmonale are to maintain adequate right ventricle filling, to reverse hypoxemia and acidosis, to establish a coordinated cardiac rhythm, to reduce oxygen demand, to avoid both overdistention and derecruitment of lung tissue, and to treat the underlying illness.

8 Pericardial tamponade presents clinically with venous congestion, hypotension, narrow pulse pressure, distant heart sounds, and equalized pressures in the left and right atria. Diastolic pressures in both ventricles are similar to those of the atria.

■ CHARACTERISTICS OF NORMAL AND ABNORMAL CIRCULATION

Anatomy

Cardiac Anatomy

The circulatory and respiratory systems are tightly interdependent in their primary function of delivering appropriate quantities of oxygenated blood to metabolizing tissues. The physician's ability to deal with hemodynamic dysfunction requires a well-developed understanding of the anatomy and control of the circulation under normal and abnormal conditions. The bloodstream's interface with the airspace (the alveoli) divides the circulatory path into two functionally distinct limbs—right, or pulmonary, and left, or systemic. Except during congestive

TABLE 1.1 RIGHT VERSUS LEFT HEART PROPERTIES

	RIGHT HEART		LEFT HEART	
	NORMAL	FAILING	NORMAL	FAILING[a]
Preload sensitivity	+++	+	++	+
Afterload sensitivity	++	+++	+	+++
Contractility	++	+	+++	++
Effect of: Afterload	±	+++	±	++
Pleural pressure	±	± to +	+	++
pH	++	+++	±	±
Hypoxemia	++	++++	±	±
Response to inotropic and vasoactive drugs	NA	++	NA	++++

[a]Not including aortic valve disease.

1 failure, the atria serve primarily as reservoirs for blood collection, rather than as key pumping elements. The right ventricle (RV) is structured differently than its left-sided counterpart (Table 1-1). Because of the low resistance of the pulmonary vascular bed, the normal RV generates mean pressures only one seventh as great as those of the left side while driving the same output. Consequently, the free wall of the RV is normally thin, preload sensitive, and poorly adapted to an acute increase of afterload. The thicker left ventricle (LV) must generate sufficient pressure to drive flow through a much greater and widely fluctuating vascular resistance. Because the RV and LV share the interventricular septum, circumferential muscle fibers, and the pericardial space, their interdependence has important functional consequences. For example, when the RV swells in response to increased afterload, the LV becomes functionally less distensible and left atrial pressure tends to increase. At the same time, the shared muscle fibers allow the LV to assist in generating the increased need for RV and pulmonary arterial pressures. Ventricular interdependence is enhanced by processes that crowd their shared pericardial fossa: high lung volumes, high heart volumes, and pericardial effusion.

Coronary Circulation

The heart is nourished by the coronary arteries, and its venous outflow drains into the coronary sinus that opens into the right atrium. The right coronary artery emerges anteriorly from the aorta, distributing to the RV, to the sinus and atrioventricular (AV) nodes, and to the posterior and inferior surfaces of the LV. The left coronary system (circumflex and left anterior descending arteries) nourishes the interventricular septum, the conduction system below the AV node, and the anterior and lateral walls of the LV. If the heart were to relax completely, the difference between mean arterial pressure (MAP) and coronary sinus pressure would drive flow through the coronary circulation. However, because aortic pressure varies continuously and because the tension within the myocardium that surrounds the coronary vessels influences the *effective* downstream pressure, perfusion varies with the phases of the cardiac cycle. The LV is perfused most actively in early diastole—not when aortic pressure is at its maximum but when myocardial tension is least. The LV myocardial pressure is highest close to the endocardium and lowest near the epicardium. Hence, under stress, the endocardium is more likely to experience ischemia.

Coronary blood flow normally parallels the metabolic activity of the myocardium. Because changes in heart rate are accomplished chiefly by shortening or lengthening diastole, tachycardia reduces the time available for diastolic perfusion while increasing the heart's need for oxygen. This potential reduction in mean coronary flow is normally overridden by vasodilatation. However, coronary disease prevents full expression of such compensation. During bradycardia, longer periods of time are available for diastolic perfusion and metabolic needs are less. However, diastolic myocardial fiber tension rises as the heart expands, and marked bradycardia may lower both mean arterial and coronary perfusion pressures.

Vascular Anatomy

Left Side

Between heartbeats, the continuous flow of blood from the heart to the periphery is maintained by the recoil of elastic vessels that were distended during systole. Arterioles serve as the primary resistive elements, and by adjusting their caliber, these small vessels regulate tissue blood flow and aid in the control of arterial pressure. The true capacitance vessels of the circulation are the venules and small veins. At any one time, only a small percentage of the total capacitance bed is recruited or distended. The precise distribution of the circulating blood volume among various tissue beds is governed by metabolic or functional requirements and gated by arteriolar vasoconstriction.

Right Side

2 In the low-pressure pulmonary circuit, relatively few structural differences distinguish normal arteries from veins. The pulmonary capillary meshwork, however, is even more luxuriant than in the periphery. Apart from innate anatomy, blood flow distribution is influenced by gravity, alveolar pressure, regional pleural pressures, oxygen tension, pH, circulating mediators, and chemical stimuli (e.g., nitric oxide).

Circulatory Control

Determinants of Cardiac Output

3 When averaged over time, cardiac output (product of heart rate and stroke volume) must match the metabolic requirements. In a real sense, metabolic activity regulates the cardiac output of a healthy individual; insufficient cardiac output activates inefficient anaerobic metabolism that cannot be sustained indefinitely. Agitation, anxiety, pain, shivering, fever, and increased breathing workload intensify systemic O_2 demands. In the critical care setting, matching output to demand is often achieved with the help of sedative, analgesic, antipyretic, inotropic, or vasoactive agents. It is important to remember that increasing or decreasing cardiac output can reflect shifting O_2 demands, rather than a change in ventricular loading conditions or response to therapeutic intervention.

Although the precise mechanism that links output to metabolism remains uncertain, the primary determinants of stroke volume are well defined: precontractile fiber stretch in diastole (preload), the tension developed by the muscle fibers during

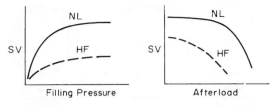

■ **FIGURE 1-1** Stroke volume (SV) response of normal (NL) and failing heart (HF) to loading conditions. Impaired hearts are abnormally sensitive to afterload, but show blunted responses to preload augmentation.

systolic contraction (afterload), and the forcefulness of muscular contraction under constant loading conditions (contractility) (Fig. 1-1). Factors governing these determinants, as well as their normal values, differ for the two ventricles, even though over time the *average* stroke volume of both ventricles must be equivalent.

Determinants of Stroke Volume—General Concepts

Preload

According to the Frank–Starling principle, muscle fiber stretch at end-diastole influences the vigor of cardiac contraction. The tendency of ejected volume to increase as the transmural filling pressure rises normally constitutes an important adaptive mechanism that enables moment-by-moment adjustments to changing venous return. During heart failure, the Starling curve flattens, and the ventricle becomes preload insensitive—higher filling pressures become necessary to achieve a similar output. Although preload parallels end-diastolic ventricular volume, myocardial remodeling can gradually modify the relationship between absolute chamber volume and preload. Therefore, muscle fiber stretch within a *chronically* dilated heart may not differ significantly from normal. End-diastolic volume is determined by ventricular compliance and by the pressure distending the ventricle (the transmural pressure). Transmural pressure is the difference between the intracavitary and juxtacardiac pressures. In comparison to the LV, the normal RV operates with a comparatively steep relationship between transmural pressure and ventricular volume. A poorly compliant ventricle, or one surrounded by increased intrathoracic or pericardial pressure, requires a higher intracavitary pressure to achieve any specified end-diastolic volume and degree of precontractile fiber stretch (Fig. 1-2). The cost of higher filling pressure may be impaired myocardial perfusion or

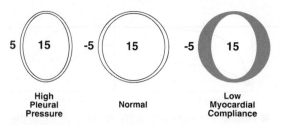

■ FIGURE 1-2 Concept of transmural pressure. The muscle fiber tensions that determine preload and afterload are developed by pressure differences across the ventricle. For example, in diastole, a measured intracavitary pressure of 15 mm Hg may correspond to a large or small chamber volume and myocardial fiber tension, depending on the compliance of the ventricle and its surrounding pressure.

pulmonary edema. Functional ventricular stiffening can result from myocardial disease, pericardial tethering, or extrinsic compression of the heart (Table 1-2). The precise position of the ventricle on the Starling curve is difficult to determine. However, studies of animals and normal human subjects suggest that there is little preload reserve in the supine position, and that, once supine, further increases in cardiac output are met primarily by increases in heart rate and/or ejection fraction. Thus, the Frank–Starling mechanism may be of most importance during hypovolemia and in the upright position.

Diastolic Dysfunction

4 Diastole is usually considered a passive process in which transmural pressure distends elastic heart muscle. In normal individuals and many patients with heart disease, this approximation is more or less accurate. However, diastole is more properly considered an energy-dependent active process. (In fact, in some instances, more myocardial oxygen may be consumed in diastole than in systole.) Failure of the heart muscle to relax at a normal rate (secondary to ischemia, long-standing hypertension, or hypertrophic myopathy) can cause

sufficient functional stiffening to produce pulmonary edema despite preserved systolic function. As defined by echocardiography, many apparently normally functioning elderly adults have abnormal patterns of cardiac relaxation. Perhaps one third or more of adult patients with congestive heart failure (CHF) develop symptoms on this basis, with the incidence increasing markedly with advancing age. Key echocardiographic features of diastolic dysfunction are described in Chapter 2. Diastolic dysfunction often precedes systolic dysfunction and should be considered an early warning sign of deterioration. Although diastolic and systolic impairments often coexist, the diastolic dysfunction syndrome is an especially likely explanation when signs of pulmonary congestion predominate over those of systemic perfusion. In all patients with diastolic dysfunction, the early rapid filling phase of ventricular diastole is slowed, and the extent of ventricular filling becomes more heavily influenced by terminal-phase atrial contraction. Sudden loss of the atrial "kick" often precipitates congestive symptoms. "Flash pulmonary edema" is often the consequence of sudden diastolic dysfunction resulting from ischemia, tachycardia, or atrial fibrillation. Diastolic dysfunction should be suspected when congestive symptoms develop despite normal systolic function in predisposed patients. Confirmation requires ancillary testing by echocardiography, Doppler ultrasound, radionuclide angiography, contrast ventriculography, or other imaging method. With all techniques, attention must be focused on diastole, particularly during the phase of rapid filling. In most institutions, echocardiography has become the method of choice for critically ill patients due to its convenience and reliability. Indicators of mitral valve function such as deceleration time, early diastolic (E) to late diastolic (A) wave velocity ratio, and isovolume relaxation time are helpful. Signals of the required clarity are often impossible to obtain,

TABLE 1-2 REDUCED DIASTOLIC COMPLIANCE		
MYOCARDIAL THICKENING OR DYSFUNCTION	**PERICARDIAL DISEASE**	**EXTRINSIC COMPRESSION**
Ischemia/infarction	Tamponade	PEEP/Hyperinflation
Hypertension	Constriction	Tension pneumothorax
Infiltration		RV dilation
Congenital defect		LV crowding
Valvular dysfunction		Impaired chest wall compliance

however, in the critically ill patient, particularly with transthoracic (as opposed to transesophageal) imaging. Regarding treatment, control of blood pressure, heart rate, and ischemia are the essential objectives. Diuretics are indicated to relieve congestive symptoms. Calcium channel blockers (e.g., verapamil, diltiazem, nifedipine) have been demonstrated to be useful in animal studies and in humans with hypertrophic cardiomyopathy. Selective β-blockers (e.g., metoprolol, carvedilol) can help reduce tachycardia, lower blood pressure, and promote long-term remodeling, but must be chosen wisely and used with extreme caution when significant systolic dysfunction, conduction system disturbance, or bronchospasm coexist. Predictably, inotropes do not improve the diastolic function.

Afterload

Although afterload is often equated with elevations of blood pressure or vascular resistance, it is better defined as the muscular tension that must be developed during systole per unit of blood flow. As such, the systolic wall stress is affected by blood pressure, wall thickness, and ventricular volume. In the normal heart, moderate changes in afterload are usually countered by increases in contractility, preload, or heart rate, so that forward output is usually little affected. Heart size remains small, and filling pressures do not rise excessively. However, once preload reserves have been exhausted, raising afterload

can profoundly depress cardiac output if contractile force and/or heart rate do not compensate. Just as the relationship between preload and stroke volume rises more steeply for the right than for the LV, so too is the normal RV more sensitive than the left to changes in afterloading (Fig. 1-1). The dilated chambers of a *failing* heart—both right and left—are inherently afterload sensitive (Fig. 1-1). Cardiomegaly and mitral regurgitation are clinical findings that help identify potential candidates for afterload reduction. Quantitative assessment of ejection impedance can be made by determining pulmonary (PVR) and systemic vascular resistance (SVR). These indices, the quotients of driving pressure and cardiac output across their respective beds, are calculated as if the blood flow fulfilled the assumptions of Poiseuille's law. Because cardiac output must be interpreted relative to body size, both indices have a wide range of normal values. Although SVR rising in response to adrenergic tone or drug treatment helps support the upstream arterial pressure that perfuses critical tissue beds when cardiac output falls (e.g., kidney), elevating vascular resistance may impair downstream capillary filling in others. Moreover, in aggregate, vascular impedance may rise sufficiently to compromise cardiac output. Judicious reduction of arterial vessel tone may then allow cardiac output to improve and vital organ perfusion to increase, while maintaining an acceptable blood pressure. Chamber diameter also impacts afterload. In a dilated chamber, higher systolic fiber

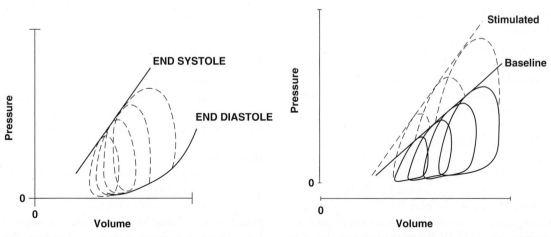

■ **FIGURE 1-3** Transmural ventricular pressure volume loops. **Left:** Four complete cardiac cycles are represented for different states of ventricular filling. The end-diastolic pressure volume relationship (EDPVR) defines the Frank–Starling curve. During each cycle, there are sequential stages of diastolic filling, isovolumic contraction, active systolic ejection, and isovolumic relaxation. The end-systolic pressure volume relationship (ESPVR) correlates well with contractility. **Right:** As the myocardium is stimulated by catecholamines, the slope of the ESPVR increases, resulting in a greater pressure and ejection fraction during systole for any degree of diastolic filling.

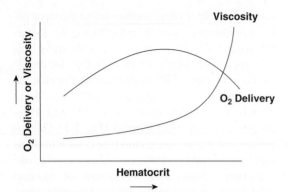

■ **FIGURE 1-4** Hypothetical relationship of O_2 delivery to hematocrit and viscosity. As hematocrit rises, O_2 delivery increases up to the point at which increasing viscosity slows the transit of oxygenated blood through the tissues and/or impairs cardiac output. The precise value of hematocrit at which O_2 delivery peaks is a function of circulating blood volume, shifting to lower values in the setting of volume contraction.

tension must be generated to produce a given intracavitary pressure, especially in fibers on the periphery. Thus, a diuretic or selective venodilator (nitroglycerine) may reduce afterload as well as preload. Apart from vessel length and diameter, blood viscosity is an important determinant of rheology and effective afterload. Blood viscosity rises nonlinearly with hematocrit. With increasing hematocrit, crowded erythrocytes pass more sluggishly through tissues and effective O_2 transport eventually reaches a maximum, the value of which depends on circulating blood volume relative to vascular capacity (Fig. 1-4). Individual tissues appear to have different tolerances to changes in hematocrit and different optimal values for oxygen extraction. Viscosity may also rise dramatically in the settings of hypothermia or hyperproteinemia.

Pleural Pressure and Afterload

Systolic pressure is a marker of the highest intracavitary pressure developed by contracting muscle fibers. The intracavitary pressure is a result of muscular forces and the regional pleural pressure that surrounds the heart. Variations in pleural pressure may significantly alter afterload and therefore, the function of the compromised LV. Although multifactorial in origin, the paradoxical pulse observed during acute asthma results in part from inspiratory afterloading of the LV. When the pressure that surrounds the heart declines, greater muscle fiber tension must be developed to generate a given intracavitary and systemic blood pressure during systole. Such alterations of ventricular loading conditions

help explain why vigorous breathing efforts impair the function of the ischemic or failing heart.

Right ventricular (RV) afterload tends to rise nonlinearly with increasing lung volume. The pulmonary vascular pressure–flow relationship may differ slightly for positive versus negative pressure breathing. However, the RV afterload corresponding to any given lung volume is not greatly influenced by changes of pleural pressure, because the vessel that accepts its outflow (the pulmonary artery) is subjected to similar variations in pressure.

Contractility

Many stimuli compete to influence the contractile state of the myocardium. Sympathetic impulses, circulating catecholamines, acid–base and electrolyte disturbances, ischemia, anoxia, and chemodepressants (drugs, mediators, or toxins) or hormones (e.g., high dose insulin) may influence ventricular performance, independent of changes in preload or afterload. Contractility is sometimes impaired transiently after blunt cardiac trauma, or when ischemic myocardium is reperfused (e.g., after cardiopulmonary resuscitation, angioplasty, or lysis of coronary thrombosis). Such "stunned myocardium" may stage a complete recovery after several days of transient dysfunction. No physical sign reliably reflects altered contractility. An S_3 gallop, narrow pulse pressure, and poorly audible heart tones suggest impaired contractility, but these signs are difficult to quantify and are influenced by myocardial compliance, intravascular volume status, and vascular tone. Radionuclide ventriculograms and echocardiography provide excellent noninvasive means of determining ventricular size and basal contractile properties of the LV, but are not well suited to continuous monitoring. The commonly used "ejection fraction" is influenced greatly by the loading conditions of the heart. Moreover, two-dimensional echocardiographic images may misrepresent three-dimensional changes in chamber geometry.

Heart Rate

Changes in the rate of the healthy heart result from the interplay between the two divisions of the autonomic nervous system. Ordinarily, parasympathetic tone predominates. (When both divisions of the autonomic nervous system are blocked, the intrinsic heart rate of young adults rises from approx. 70 to 105 beats/min.) The heart's ability to respond to an increased demand for output is largely determined by its capacity to raise the heart rate appropriately. Pathological bradycardias often depress cardiac output and O_2 delivery, especially when a diseased or failing ventricle is unable to call upon a preload reserve. Relative bradycardia is often observed in the clinical setting—a "normal" heart rate is not appropriate for a stressed patient with high O_2 demands or impaired myocardium. Because two key determinants of oxygen delivery are affected, bradycardia induced by hypoxemia profoundly depresses O_2 delivery and may rapidly precipitate circulatory collapse. Marked increases in heart rate may also lead to circulatory depression when they cause myocardial ischemia, or when reduced diastolic filling time or loss of atrial contraction impair ventricular preload. (Good examples include mitral stenosis and diastolic dysfunction.) As a general rule, sinus heart rates exceeding (220 – age)/min reduce cardiac output and myocardial perfusion, even in the absence of ischemic disease or loss of atrial contraction. (To illustrate, sinus-driven heart rate should not exceed 150/min in a 70-year-old patient.)

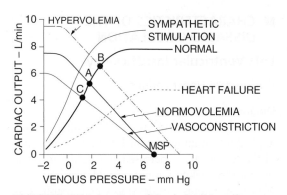

■ **FIGURE 1-5** Interaction of Frank–Starling and venous return (VR) curves. With normal heart function, observed cardiac output is determined by such vascular factors as filling status (A → B) and vasoconstriction (C). Sympathetic stimulation and heart failure have opposing effects on the Starling curve and cardiac output. The mean systemic pressure (MSP) driving venous return is a hypothetical point determined by extrapolating the venous return curve to the venous pressure axis where all cardiac output ceases. Note that VR improves linearly as CVP falls—up to the point at which central vessels collapse.

Peripheral Circulation

Vascular tone is integral to cardiac output regulation—the heart cannot pump what it fails to receive in venous return, and vasoconstriction is a key determinant of afterload. In fact, control of cardiac output may be viewed strictly from a vascular perspective (Fig. 1-5). Under steady-state conditions, venous return is proportional to the quotient of venous driving pressure and resistance. Under most circumstances, the downstream pressure for venous return is right atrial pressure. The upstream pressure driving venous return, the mean systemic pressure (P_{MS}), is the volume-weighted average of pressures throughout the entire systemic vascular network. Because a much larger fraction of the total circulating volume is contained on the venous side of the circulation, P_{MS} is much closer to the right atrial pressure (P_{RA}) than to MAP. Were the P_{RA} to rise suddenly to equal the P_{MS}, all blood flow would stop. Indeed, in an experimental setting, P_{MS} can be determined by synchronously clamping the aorta and vena cava to stop flow and opening a wide-bore communication between them. Mean systemic pressure is influenced by the circulating blood volume and vascular capacitance, which in turn is a function of vascular tone. Thus, P_{MS} rises under conditions of hypervolemia, polycythemia, and right-sided CHF; it declines during abrupt vasodilation, sepsis, hemorrhage, and diuresis. Up to a

certain point, lowering P_{RA} while preserving P_{MS} increases driving pressure and improves venous return. However, when P_{RA} is reduced below the surrounding tissue pressure, the thin-walled vena cava collapses near the thoracic inlet. Effective downstream pressure for venous return then becomes the pressure just upstream to the point of collapse, rather than the P_{RA}.

At any given moment, the cardiac output is determined by the intersection of the venous return curve and the Starling curve. In the analysis of a depressed cardiac output, both aspects of circulatory control must be scrutinized. For example, when positive end-expiratory pressure (PEEP) is applied, P_{RA} rises, inhibiting the venous return. However, P_{MS} rises simultaneously and compensatory vascular reflexes are called into action to reduce the venous capacitance and expand the circulating volume. Therefore, unlike patients with depressed vascular reflexes or hypovolemia, most healthy individuals do not experience a reduction of cardiac output under the influence of moderate PEEP. Although an increase in venous resistance can also reduce the venous return, it is uncommon for the venous resistance to increase without an offsetting change in P_{MS}. However, positional compression of the inferior vena cava by an intra-abdominal mass (e.g., during advanced pregnancy) may account for postural changes in cardiac output in such patients.

■ CHARACTERISTICS OF THE DISEASED CIRCULATION

Left Ventricular Insufficiency

Congestive Heart Failure

Diagnostics

The term "heart failure" (or CHF) is often loosely applied to conditions in which the filling pressures of the left heart are increased sufficiently to cause dyspnea or weakness at rest or mild exertion. Congestive symptoms can develop when systolic cardiac function is preserved (volume overload, renal insufficiency, diastolic dysfunction, RV encroachment, and pericardial effusion), as well as during myocardial failure itself. Unlike the normal LV, which is relatively sensitive to changes in its preload and insensitive to changes in its afterload, the failing LV has the opposite characteristics (see Fig. 1-1). Changes in afterload can therefore make a major difference in LV systolic performance, whereas preload manipulation usually elicits little benefit, unless it reduces afterload indirectly by shrinking chamber volume and wall tension. Wide QRS complexes characterize the ventricular asynchrony of bundle branch block, and in certain patients, resynchronization by biventricular pacing may improve left ventricular (LV) filling time, reduce mitral regurgitation, and lessen septal dyskinesis. Radiographic evidence of acute heart failure includes perivascular cuffing, a widened vascular pedicle, blurring of the hilar vasculature, and diffuse infiltrates that tend to spare the costophrenic angles. Unlike pneumonia and acute respiratory distress syndrome (ARDS), these infiltrates tend to lack air bronchograms and are usually unaccompanied by an acute change in heart size. Chronic CHF is typified by Kerley B lines, dilated cardiac chambers, and increased cardiac dimensions.

The increased stretching of myocardial tissue in response to ventricular overload promotes the release of two endogenous natriuretic peptides: atrial natriuretic peptide (ANP) and B-type natriuretic peptide (BNP). Cardiac natriuretic peptides can lower excessive levels of angiotensin II, aldosterone, and endothelin I (another endogenous vasoconstrictive peptide) thus inducing a variety of beneficial effects—arterial and venous vasodilation, enhanced diuresis, and inhibition of sodium reabsorption.

ANP is stored within granules in the atria and ventricles, so even a minor amount of cardiac muscle stretch, such as that resulting from routine exercise, can cause an efflux of this peptide into the circulation. BNP, by contrast, is synthesized within the ventricles, and only minimal amounts are stored in granules. Instead, BNP is synthesized de novo, or as needed, in response to left ventricular wall elongation secondary to myocardial stress (e.g., volume overload). Thus, the BNP compensatory response to myocardial injury is highly specific to ventricular dysfunction or distention. BNP levels consistently rise above their normal values in patients with CHF. The properties of BNP point to a potentially important role for this peptide, not only as a diagnostic tool in CHF, but also as a treatment option in certain patients. BNP measurements can provide information critical to rapidly identifying the patients having CHF, diagnosing its severity, and gauging long-term outcomes in these patients, especially when other diagnostic assessments are ambiguous.

When faced with a patient who appears to have pulmonary venous congestion, a number of key questions should be asked in determining its etiology.

1. **Is forward output adequate to perfuse vital tissues?** When perfusion is severely impaired, consideration should be given to mechanical ventilation and invasive hemodynamic monitoring, especially in the setting of coexisting pulmonary venous congestion and lactic acidosis. Reducing tissue O_2 demand and correcting disturbances in oxygen content, serum pH, electrolyte balance, and ventricular loading conditions are of prime importance. Inotropic or vasopressor therapy may be indicated for hypotension, whereas hypertensive patients and those with a highly elevated SVR may benefit from vasodilators.

2. **Is there evidence of systolic dysfunction?** Adequate perfusion does not necessarily imply intact systolic function—forward output may be maintained at the cost of high preloading pressures and pulmonary vascular congestion. If perfusion is adequate and systolic function of cardiac valves and myocardium remains intact, the patient may simply be volume overloaded or manifesting diastolic dysfunction. Echocardiography helps greatly in this assessment.

3. **What is the LV size?** LV chamber dilation usually indicates a chronic process—most commonly long-standing ischemic heart disease, cardiomyopathy, or LV diastolic overload (aortic or mitral valvular insufficiency). Therapy in

such cases should be directed at optimizing afterload (with systemic vasodilators) or at improving myocardial oxygen supply (coronary vasodilators). If there is excessive inspiratory effort, mechanical ventilation can reduce both O_2 demand and left ventricular afterload by raising inspiratory and mean pleural pressures. If left ventricular cavity size is normal, mitral stenosis, tamponade, constrictive pericarditis, acute myocardial infarction, hypertrophic cardiomyopathy, or diastolic dysfunction should be suspected. Left ventricular wall hypertrophy, myocardial infiltration, or interdependence with a swollen RV may limit stroke volume and cardiac output, despite normal contractility. A distended left atrium sometimes provides a clue in such cases.

4. **Does the LV show global or regional hypokinesis?** Regional hypokinesis/dyskinesis suggests localized disease (e.g., ischemia or infarction). Echocardiography and precordial electrocardiography (ECG) are instrumental in this assessment. Generalized hypokinesis of a heart with normal chamber size often reflects the stunned myocardium of trauma, diffuse ischemia, drug overdose, toxin ingestion, or posttachycardia dysfunction.

5. **Is there evidence for valvular dysfunction?** Aortic stenosis may depress cardiac output by causing excessive afterload, myocardial ischemia, or hypertrophic impairment of ventricular filling. Mitral regurgitation impairs forward output and produces congestive symptoms by allowing retrograde venting of the ejected volume. Acute chamber enlargement (regardless of cause) may worsen congestive symptoms by producing transient mitral regurgitation due to papillary muscle dysfunction or mitral ring dilation.

6. **Is there evidence for increased pulmonary vascular permeability or hypoalbuminemia?** The tendency to form pulmonary edema relates not only to hydrostatic pressure, but also to the plasma oncotic pressure and pulmonary capillary permeability. Hence, edema may form at a relatively low pulmonary venous pressure if oncotic pressure is reduced or the microvascular endothelium is leaky. Conversely, the lungs may remain dry despite high left heart filling pressures when enlarged lymphatic drainage channels with greater capacity have had time to develop (e.g., mitral stenosis). Kerley lines are the radiographic signatures of lymphatic dilation.

The physical examination should be directed toward the detection of hypoperfusion (reduced mental status, oliguria) and compensatory vasoconstriction (reduced skin temperature, prolonged capillary filling time, etc.). Rales are often difficult to detect in bedridden patients who breathe shallowly and in those receiving mechanical ventilatory support. Auscultation of dependent regions is mandatory. The chest X-ray (CXR) provides key information regarding heart size, vascular distribution, pulmonary infiltrates, and pleural effusions. Computed tomography is informative in questionable cases—especially when the chest wall interferes with CXR interpretation. Echocardiography and radionuclide ventriculography provide important information regarding chamber size, contractility, diastolic filling, valvular function, P_{RA}, pericardial volume, and filling status of the central pulmonary veins. Although transesophageal echocardiography is not always feasible to perform, the detail it provides is generally superior to its transthoracic counterpart, especially in patients with obstructive lung disease or massive obesity.

Therapeutics

As a general rule, the therapy of CHF should be geared to documented pathophysiology. Reversal of abrupt-onset tachycardias and arrhythmias is frequently the key to relieving congestion, especially in patients with valve dysfunction, or stiff or ischemic hearts. Whereas diuretics help in most cases, inotropic and vasoactive agents should be reserved for documented disorders of myocardial function refractory to adjustments of filling pressure, pH, and electrolytes. Angiotensin-converting enzyme (ACE) inhibitors (e.g., captopril, enalapril) and/or systemic vasodilators should be used when an elevated SVR and/or valvular insufficiency are documented in the setting of adequate preload and blood pressure. Nitrates may aid cardiac ischemia but can precipitate hypotension in patients with borderline or inadequate filling pressures. New-onset atrial or ventricular arrhythmias or conduction disturbances (e.g., atrial fibrillation, atrial flutter, heart block) should be treated aggressively if they reduce forward output or cause pulmonary edema.

Although calcium channel blockers can benefit congestive failure by controlling hypertension, slowing tachycardia, or reversing coronary spasm, they should only be used in well-selected patients; these agents depress cardiac contractility and may impair conduction. In similar fashion, β-blockers reduce myocardial oxygen consumption by decreasing the heart rate and contractility, but have the potential to precipitate CHF, conduction system disturbances, or bronchospasm. β-Adrenergic blockade should be reserved for cases of documented ischemia or other firm indications (e.g., thyroid storm, delirium tremens, uncontrolled supraventricular tachycardia). They should *not* be considered first-line measures in other acute forms of CHF.

Nesiritide, hBNP, a 32-amino acid recombinant human BNP, represents a unique treatment for acutely decompensated CHF (ADHF) and was the first drug introduced in its class. hBNP has been approved for the IV treatment of patients with ADHF who have dyspnea at rest or with minimal exertion. hBNP has been shown to exert potent vasodilatory effects and to effect significant diuresis and natriuresis in patients with severe CHF. In patients with ADHF, hBNP also has been shown to significantly decrease plasma norepinephrine and aldosterone levels, as well as cardiac preload and vascular resistance, without stimulating the changes in heart rate seen with inotropic agents. When added to standard therapy in the treatment of ADHF, hBNP improves hemodynamic function to a significantly greater extent than nitroglycerin (see Chapter 3). Its use has become somewhat controversial, however, as it may cause profound hypotension, bradycardia, and renal dysfunction in some patients.

Another promising class of noncatecholamine-based agents is the calcium sensitizers. The initial representative of this category is levosemendan, a drug yet to be deployed on a wide scale (see Chapter 3).

Right Ventricular Dysfunction

Certain disease conditions account for the great majority of acute problems arising primarily from RV dysfunction: RV ischemia and infarction; cor pulmonale complicating parenchymal, vascular, or hypoventilatory hypoxemic lung diseases (e.g., sleep apnea); and ARDS.

Right Ventricular Infarction

The RV receives the majority of its blood supply from the right coronary artery. It is not surprising, therefore, that RV infarction complicates as many as 30% of inferior myocardial infarctions, as well as a much smaller percentage of anterior infarctions. The diagnosis should be suspected when there are signs of systemic venous hypertension, an unimpressive or clear CXR, and evidence of ST segment elevation or Q waves over the right precordium (V_4R). A suggestive enzyme profile confirms the diagnosis. In the initial phase of management, RV infarctions typically demand aggressive administration of intravenous fluids to sustain optimal blood pressure and cardiac output. The LV may be required to take up the work of pumping blood through both the systemic circuit (directly) and the pulmonary circuit (indirectly), using ventricular interdependence. Dilatation of the RV and fluid loading tighten these linkages by crowding the two ventricles within the pericardial sac, stretching shared circumferential muscle fibers, and shifting the mobile interventricular septum. Recovery from, accommodation to, or compensation for RV infarction tends to occur over several days. If cardiac output can be supported during this interval, the outlook for patients without other cardiopulmonary diseases is generally good. Prognosis depends not only on the size of the infarction, but also on the presence or absence of increased PVR.

Cor Pulmonale

Pathogenesis

In its purest form, *cor pulmonale* (see Chapter 21) is defined as hypertrophy, dilatation, or failure of the RV in response to excessive PVR. By definition, this term excludes cardiomyopathy or secondary changes in RV function resulting from pulmonary venous hypertension or LV failure. Three reinforcing causes of pulmonary hypertension are a restricted capillary bed, alveolar hypoxia, and acidosis. Although extensive obliteration, constriction, or compression of the capillary bed may be the underlying cause, increased cardiac output and superimposed hypoxemia or acidosis may dramatically elevate pulmonary arterial pressure (P_{PA}). The normal RV cannot sustain adequate forward output at mean pulmonary arterial pressures that exceed approximately 35 mm Hg. Given sufficient time, however, the RV wall can thicken sufficiently to generate pressures that rival those in the systemic circuit. Arterial smooth muscle also hypertrophies over time, intensifying the response to alveolar hypoxemia and pharmacologic vasoconstrictors. Most diffuse pulmonary insults can raise the PVR enough to decompensate an already compromised RV. Massive pulmonary embolism is the most common cause of acute cor pulmonale in a patient without prior cardiopulmonary abnormality. In mechanically ventilated patients, lung overdistention with attendant capillary compression may markedly accentuate RV loading.

Chronic cor pulmonale can result from severe lung disease of virtually any etiology (especially those that obliterate pulmonary capillaries and induce chronic hypoxemia). Acutely decompensated cor pulmonale occurs frequently in patients with chronic obstructive pulmonary disease (COPD). In such patients, RV afterload can fall dramatically with correction of bronchospasm, hypoxemia, and acidosis. Since about one half of the normal pulmonary capillary bed can be obstructed without raising the resting mean P_{PA} significantly above the normal range, pulmonary hypertension in a normoxemic person at rest usually signifies an important reduction in the number of patent pulmonary capillaries. After the capillary reserve has been exhausted, P_{PA} varies markedly with cardiac output. Thus, elevations of pulmonary arterial pressure often signify variations in cardiac output, rather than worsening of lung pathology.

Diagnosis
The measurement of central venous pressure (CVP), pulmonary artery occlusion ("wedge") pressure (P_w), and the computation of PVR help separate right from left heart disease. Echocardiography is an invaluable diagnostic adjunct, often allowing estimation of pulmonary arterial pressure as well as providing detailed anatomical information regarding the dimensions and functions of the two ventricles. The physical findings of acute cor pulmonale are those of pulmonary hypertension: hypoperfusion, RV gallop, and a loud P_2. Pulsatile hepatomegaly, systemic venous congestion, and edema strongly implicate RV failure. Deep breathing may accentuate these right heart findings, as inspiratory increases of blood flow returning to the thorax raise P_{PA} and stress the compromised RV. Hepatomegaly, a palpable P_2, and a right parasternal lift usually indicate severe subacute or chronic pulmonary hypertension. Unfortunately, many of these signs are difficult to elicit in patients with hyperinflated or noisy lungs.

Ancillary Diagnostic Tests
Radiographic signs of pulmonary arterial hypertension include dilated, sharply tapering central pulmonary arteries with peripheral vascular "pruning." Although precise measurements are often difficult to make, a right lower lobar artery dimension greater than 18 mm diameter (on the standard PA film) or main pulmonary arteries greater than 25 mm in diameter (judged on lateral) strongly suggest subacute or chronic pulmonary hypertension. Overall heart size may appear normal until disease is advanced, especially in patients with hyperinflation. Encroachment of the RV on the retrosternal airspace in the lateral view is an early but nonspecific sign.

The contrast-enhanced CT scan of the thorax may confirm RV dilatation. Catheter-based techniques allow computation of RV volume and/or RV ejection fraction. Beat-by-beat analysis of the thermodilution temperature profile allows both to be assessed, whereas a double indicator (dye/thermodilution) method permits determination of these indices as well as central blood volume, stroke work, lung water, and others.

ECG criteria for RV hypertrophy are insensitive and nonspecific. In acute cor pulmonale, changes characteristic of hypertrophy are lacking. P pulmonale and a progressive decrease in the R/S ratio across the precordium are sensitive but nonspecific signs. Conversely, the S_1, Q_3, T_3 pattern, right axis deviation greater than 110 degrees, R/S ratio in V_5 or V_6 less than 1.0, and a QR pattern in V_1 are relatively specific but insensitive signs. Radionuclide ventriculography and echocardiography help document RV and LV functions noninvasively. In patients with true cor pulmonale, LV systolic function should remain unaffected.

Management of Acute Cor Pulmonale
The key directives in managing cor pulmonale are to maintain adequate RV filling and perfusion pressure, to reverse hypoxemia and acidosis, to establish a coordinated cardiac rhythm, and to treat the underlying illness. The majority of patients with decompensated COPD and cor pulmonale have a reversible hypoxemic component. Although oxygen must be administered cautiously, patients with CO_2 retention should not be denied O_2 therapy. Acidosis markedly accentuates the effect of hypoxemia on PVR, whereas hypercarbia without acidosis exerts less effect. This should be borne in mind when deciding the need for buffering pH in permissive hypercapnia. Bronchospasm, infection, and retained secretions must be addressed. When extreme polycythemia complicates chronic hypoxemia, careful lowering of the hematocrit to approximately 55% may significantly reduce blood viscosity, decrease RV afterload, and improve myocardial perfusion. To improve viscosity, it may be advisable to rewarm a hypothermic patient.

The effects of digitalis, inotropes, and diuretics in acute cor pulmonale are variable; these drugs should be employed cautiously. Gentle diuresis helps relieve symptomatic congestion of the lower extremities, gut, and portal circulation. Diuresis may reduce RV distention and myocardial tension, improving its afterload and perfusion. Any depression of cardiac output resulting from diuresis may also cause a secondary reduction of P_{PA}. In patients requiring RV distention and ventricular interdependence to sustain adequate stroke volume, vigorous diuresis or phlebotomy may have adverse consequences. Central vascular pressures, therefore, should be carefully monitored. The effects of cardiotonic agents in the treatment of acute cor pulmonale are also unpredictable. Digitalis has only a small inotropic effect on the performance of a non-hypertrophied RV, but may be valuable in chronic cor pulmonale and for controlling heart rate in atrial fibrillation without depressing myocardial function. Inotropes such as dopamine and dobutamine can improve left ventricular function and boost the perfusion pressure of the RV. Furthermore, because the ventricles share the septum and circumferential muscle fibers, it is likely that improved left ventricular contraction benefits the RV through systolic ventricular interdependence. Arrhythmias induced by such agents, however, may disrupt the AV coordination that is so vital to effective RV filling and performance.

For a minority of patients, calcium channel blockers (e.g., nifedipine, diltiazem, amlodipine) reduce PVR and boost cardiac output by decreasing RV afterload. This effect, however, is highly variable; these drugs may also reduce depressed myocardial function or reduce coronary perfusion pressure. Evaluation of response is best conducted cautiously during formal cardiac catheterization before they are prescribed. For patients with a clearly reversible component to the pulmonary hypertension, inhaled nitric oxide (or aerosolized prostacyclin [Flolan]) may prove to be a useful bridge to definitive therapy or physiologic adaptation. Unfortunately, tolerance to nitric oxide gradually develops and in itself does not provide a long-term solution. For patients with severe ongoing pulmonary hypertension, anticoagulation is thought advisable. Several therapies recently released into clinical practice hold promise for some patients with reactive pulmonary vasculature. These include epoprostenol and its analog treprostinil (Remodulin), bosentan (Tracleer), and sildenafil (Viagra) and their derivatives.

Acute Respiratory Failure

Mechanisms of Circulatory Impairment in ARDS

Although cardiac output usually increases in the early stage of ARDS, in response to the precipitating stress or to compensate for hypoxemia, this is less often true when the illness is far advanced. The performance of one or both ventricles may deteriorate as the lung disease worsens, compounding the problem of inadequate tissue O_2 delivery. The cardiac dysfunction that accompanies advanced respiratory failure is incompletely understood. Effective preload may be reduced by PEEP, third spacing, capillary leakage, and myocardial stiffening secondary to ischemia or catecholamine stimulation. Contractility of either ventricle may be impaired by hypotension, ischemia, electrolyte abnormalities, or cardiodepressant factors released during sepsis, injury, or other inflammatory condition. Compression, obliteration, and hypoxic vasoconstriction of the pulmonary vasculature impede ejection of the afterload-sensitive RV, a low pressure–high capacity pump. Increased wall tension also tends to diminish RV perfusion. Severe pulmonary hypertension is an ominous sign in the later stages of ARDS.

Assessing Perfusion Adequacy

The assessment of perfusion adequacy in ARDS is addressed in detail elsewhere (see "Oxygenation Failure," Chapter 24). However, a few points deserve emphasis. Individual organs vary widely with regard to O_2 demand, completeness of O_2 extraction, and adaptability to ischemia or hypoxia. Cerebral and cardiac tissues are especially vulnerable to anoxia. In these organs, the O_2 requirement per gram of tissue is high, O_2 stores are minimal, and O_2 extraction is relatively complete—even under normal circumstances. Subtle changes in mental status may be the first indication of hypoxemia, but the multiplicity of potential causes (e.g., early sepsis, dehydration, anxiety, sleep deprivation, drug effects) renders disorientation and lethargy difficult to interpret. Although cool, moist skin often provides a valuable clue to inadequate vital organ perfusion, vasopressors and disorders of vasoregulation common to the critically ill patient reduce the utility of this finding.

The normal kidney provides a window on the adequacy of vital organ perfusion through variation of its urine output, pH, and electrolyte composition. Adequate urine volume and sodium and bicarbonate excretion suggest sufficient renal blood flow when the kidneys are normally functioning. Unfortunately, rather than reflecting the adequacy of perfusion, variations in urine volume and alterations of urine composition are often due to drug effects, diurnal variations, and or glomerular or tubular dysfunction. As sustained hypoperfusion activates anaerobic metabolic pathways, arterial pH and bicarbonate concentrations decline and lactic acid levels rise, widening the anion gap. Although adequacy of cardiac output can seldom be determined unequivocally by any single calculated index, analysis of the O_2 contents of arterial and mixed venous blood is valuable when addressing questions of tissue O_2 supply and utilization. In recent years, near infrared spectrophotometry, gastric mucosal pH and sublingual PCO_2 have been investigated as markers of insufficient O_2 delivery to vital organs. Despite the potential value of such indices, inadequacy of systemic O_2 delivery is perhaps best judged from a battery of indicators, including the clinical examination of perfusion-sensitive organ systems (urine output and composition, mental status, ECG, etc.), the cardiac index, SVR, the presence or absence of anion gap acidosis, lactate, the mixed venous oxygen saturation (SvO_2), and the calculated O_2 extraction.

Improving Perfusion Adequacy in ARDS

Apart from efforts to improve cardiac output and arterial O_2 content (e.g., packed cell transfusion, inotropic, or vasoactive drugs), tissue oxygenation and perfusion may be enhanced by reducing metabolic demand. Metabolic needs (and perfusion requirements) may be reduced strikingly by controlling sepsis and fever, alleviating anxiety and agitation, and providing assistance (O_2, bronchodilators, ventilatory support) to reduce the work of breathing. Therapy directed at improving cardiac output in the setting of ARDS should be guided by assessing the heart rate, contractility, and the loading conditions of each ventricle independently. Minor elevations of pulmonary venous pressure exacerbate edema, necessitating higher

levels of PEEP, mean airway pressure, and supplemental O_2. Attempts should be made to reduce RV afterload by correcting hypoxemia and acidosis. Although a certain minimum level of PEEP must be maintained in the early phase of ARDS to avoid ventilator-induced lung damage, unnecessary elevations of mean airway pressure may overdistend patent lung units, thereby compressing alveolar capillaries and accentuating the impedance to RV ejection.

Pericardial Constriction and Tamponade

The pericardium normally supports the heart, shields it from damage or infection, enhances diastolic ventricular coupling, and prevents excessive acute dilatation of the heart. In the intensive care unit (ICU), three types of pericardial disease are noteworthy: acute pericarditis, pericardial tamponade, and constrictive pericarditis.

Acute Pericarditis

Acute pericardial inflammation arises from diverse causes (Table 1-3). The characteristic complaint is chest pain, eased by sitting and leaning forward and aggravated by supine positioning, coughing, deep inspiration, or swallowing. Dyspnea, referred shoulder pain, and sensations of chest or abdominal pressure are frequent. Unless muffled by effusion, pericarditis can usually be detected on physical examination by a single or multicomponent friction rub. The rub is often evanescent or recurrent, best heard with the patient leaning forward and easily confused with the crunch of pneumomediastinum, a pleural rub, coarse rhonchi, or an artifact of the stethoscope moving against the skin. Early ECG changes include ST segment elevation, which, unlike the pattern in acute myocardial infarction, is concave upward and typically present in all leads except V_1. The reciprocal depression pattern of regional infarction is absent. Initially, the T waves are upright in leads with

TABLE 1-3   CAUSES OF PERICARDITIS

INFECTIONS	DISSECTING ANEURYSM	MALIGNANCY
Viral	Rheumatologic diseases	Trauma
TB	Dresslers syndrome	Uremia
Bacterial	Anticoagulation	Radiation
Fungal	Myocardial infarction	Drugs

ST segment elevation—another distinction from acute infarction. Depression of the PR segment occurs commonly early in acute pericarditis. The ST segments return to baseline within several days, and the T waves flatten. Unlike the situation that accompanies acute myocardial infarction, ST segments usually normalize before the T waves invert. Eventually, T waves normalize—a process that may require weeks or months. Management of uncomplicated pericarditis (without tamponade) includes careful monitoring, treatment of the underlying cause, and judicious use of nonsteroidal anti-inflammatory agents for selected cases. Occasionally, pericarditis is complicated by hydraulic cardiac compression (tamponade) or the development of a constricting pericardial sac.

Pericardial Tamponade

Although pericardial fluid tends to reduce pain and discomfort by buffering the friction between the heart and pericardium, the rapid accumulation of pericardial fluid may compress the heart, resulting in tamponade (see Chapter 3). At least 250 mL of fluid must collect before an obviously enlarged heart shadow is noted on the chest roentgenogram; a normal or unchanged chest film does not exclude the presence of a hemodynamically important effusion. Effusions that cause tamponade can be circumferential, asymmetrical, or loculated. In the supine patient, small unloculated effusions pool posteriorly. Common settings include post-op from thoracic surgery, chest trauma, and catheterization or endovascular instrumentation (e.g., misplaced guidewires and/or central venous catheters). Tamponade physiology classically results in a triad of low arterial pressure, elevated neck veins, and a quiet precordium, and in its extreme form can produce pulseless electrical activity (PEA). Recumbency intensifies dyspnea, while sitting upright tends to relieve it. Although tamponade is properly considered a diagnosis founded on history and physical examination, massive obesity interferes with making a confident diagnosis from physical signs alone. Low QRS complex voltage and some degree of electrical variation are sometimes observed on the ECG tracing, but these classical findings are not reliable. (The ECG does help, however, in ruling out other diagnostic possibilities.) Arterial pressure tracings disclose exaggerated reductions of systolic pressure, a shared characteristic of the conditions that tend to mimic it. These include tension pneumothorax, severe gas trapping (auto-PEEP), massive pulmonary embolism, and cardiogenic shock. Echocardiography helps confirm the diagnosis of tamponade, serving as an invaluable bedside aid in distinguishing among these differential possibilities. Right atrial collapse in the face of distended central veins is a *sensitive* indicator, but RV collapse is more *specific*.

As fluid accumulates, nonspecific ECG findings include reduced QRS voltage and T wave flattening. In this setting, electrical alternans suggests the presence of massive effusion and tamponade. Although echocardiographic quantification of effusion size is imprecise, it is the most rapid and widely used technique. Large pericardial effusions (>350 mL) give rise to anterior echo-free spaces and exaggerated cardiac swinging motions. Diastolic collapse of right heart chambers suggests a critical degree of fluid accumulation and tamponade. Alternative diagnostic techniques include the CT scan with intravenous contrast and the MRI scan (when feasible).

Physiology of Pericardial Tamponade

Acute pericardial tamponade is a hemodynamic crisis characterized by increased intracardiac pressures, limitation of ventricular filling throughout diastole, and reduction of stroke volume. Normally, intrapericardial pressure is similar to intrapleural pressure, but less than either right or left ventricular diastolic pressures. Rapid accumulation of pericardial fluid causes sufficient pressure within the sac to compress and equalize right and left atrial pressures, reducing maximal diastolic dimensions and stroke volume. Reflex increases in heart rate and adrenergic tone initially maintain cardiac output. In this setting, any process that quickly reduces venous return or causes bradycardia (e.g., hypoxemia, β-blockade) can precipitate shock.

Tamponade alters the dynamics of systemic venous return and cardiac filling (Fig. 1-6). As cardiac volume transiently decreases during ejection, pericardial pressure falls, resulting in a prominent X descent on the venous pressure tracing. Tamponade attenuates the normal early diastolic surge of ventricular filling and abolishes the Y descent (its representation on the venous pressure tracing). Pulsus paradoxus, a result of exaggerated normal physiology, may develop simultaneously. Inspiration is normally accompanied by an increase in the diastolic dimensions of the RV and a small decrease in LV volume. These changes reduce LV ejection volume and systolic pressure (<10 mm Hg) during early inspiration.

Pericardial tamponade accentuates this normal fluctuation to produce pulsus paradoxus. With an arterial line in place, paradoxical pulse is easily quantified by noting the respiratory variation of systolic pressure during the end-inspiratory and end-expiratory phases of the ventilatory cycle. Paradoxical pulse can also be detected in traditional fashion by lowering the cuff pressure of a sphygmomanometer slowly from a point 20 mm Hg above systolic pressure until the Korotkoff sounds are heard equally well throughout both inspiration and expiration. The "paradox" is the difference between the pressure at which systolic sound is first audible and the point at which the systolic sound is heard consistently throughout the respiratory cycle. Pulsus paradoxus and certain other hemodynamic manifestations of pericardial tamponade depend on inspiratory augmentation of systemic venous return; as the RV swells, it restricts left ventricular chamber volume. Paradox may be absent in pericardial tamponade if underlying ·heart disease markedly elevates left ventricular diastolic pressure or if the LV fills by a mechanism independent of respiratory variation (e.g., aortic regurgitation). It may be hard to detect in the presence of tachycardia or arrhythmia.

Clinical Manifestations of Pericardial Tamponade

Reduced systemic arterial pressure and pulse volume, systemic venous congestion, and a small, quiet heart comprise the classic presentation of pericardial tamponade. However, other disorders, including obstructive pulmonary disease, restrictive cardiomyopathy, RV infarction, massive pulmonary embolism, and constrictive pericarditis, may also present with systemic venous distention, pulsus paradoxus, and clear lungs. Hyperactivity of the adrenergic nervous system is evidenced by tachycardia and cold, clammy extremities. The most common physical findings are jugular venous distention and pulsus paradoxus. However, tachypnea may render these signs difficult to elicit. Orthopnea that is not explained by neuromuscular weakness, obstructive lung disease, or pulmonary edema warrants strong consideration of tamponade.

Laboratory Evaluation

No feature of the CXR is diagnostic of pericardial tamponade. Electrical (QRS) alternans on the ECG in a patient with a known pericardial effusion is suggestive, but not definitive evidence. Electrical alternans may also occur with constrictive pericarditis, tension pneumothorax, severe myocardial dysfunction, and after myocardial infarction. Adjunctive studies are needed to confirm tamponade physiology. Apart from demonstrating pericardial fluid, the echocardiogram can provide additional clues to pericardial tamponade. These include reduction of the "E to F" slope, brisk posterior motion of the intraventricular septum during inspiration, RV diastolic collapse, prominent "swinging" of the heart, and exaggerated inspiratory increases and expiratory decreases in RV size. Yet, however suggestive they may be, the findings of a single echocardiographic study cannot predict the presence or severity of pericardial tamponade. Cardiac catheterization confirms the diagnosis, quantifies the magnitude of hemodynamic compromise, and uncovers coexisting hemodynamic problems. Catheterization typically demonstrates an elevated P_{RA} with a prominent systolic X descent and diminutive or absent Y descent (Fig. 1-6). There is elevation and diastolic equilibration of intrapericardial, RV, and left ventricular pressures ("equalization"). RV diastolic pressures lack the "dip and plateau" configuration characteristic of constrictive pericarditis. Because the pressure–volume curve of the distended and liquid-filled pericardial sac is very steep, aspirating 50 to 100 mL of fluid usually leads to a striking reduction in intrapericardial pressure and dramatic improvements of systemic arterial pressure and cardiac output. Pericardiocentesis lowers the diastolic pressures in the pericardium, right atrium, RV, and LV and reestablishes normal pressure gradients.

Management

In pericardial tamponade, it is essential to maintain adequate filling pressure and heart rate. Peripheral vascular tone must be maintained with pressors, if needed. Volume depletion (e.g., excessive diuresis),

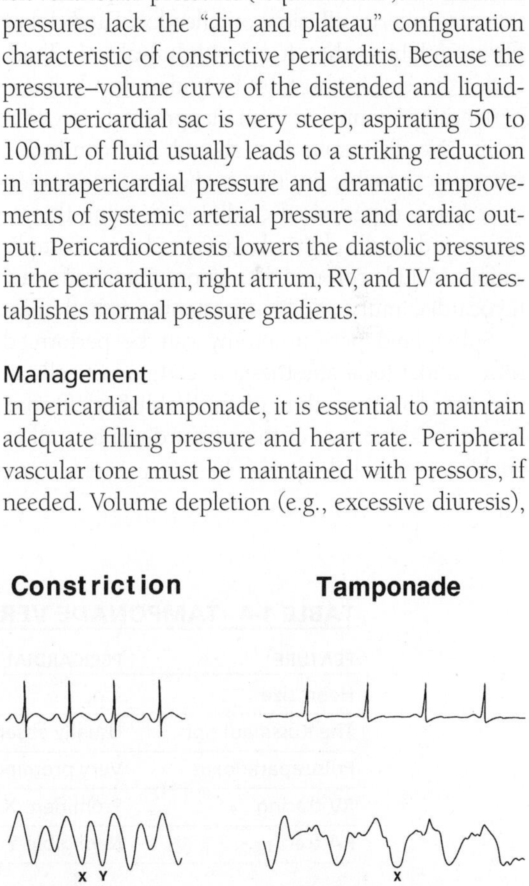

Constriction   **Tamponade**

■ **FIGURE 1-6** Contrast of pericardial constriction and tamponade as reflected in CVP tracings. Unlike the venous pressure tracing of constriction, the "Y descent" is attenuated in tamponade because early diastolic filling is impaired. The systolic "X descent" is well preserved in both conditions.

hypoxemia, and β-blockade (and other causes of bradycardia) can be life-threatening. As a general rule, fluids should be "wide open," and sinus tachycardia—a compensatory response—left untreated. Intubation of the airway must not be performed unnecessarily and when delay is not prudent, performed only with extreme caution. Positive pressure can further reduce cardiac filling, and vasodilation may drop the central pressures needed for compensation. Pericardial fluid can be evacuated by one of three methods: needle pericardiocentesis, pericardiotomy via a subxiphoid window (often under local anesthesia), or pericardiectomy. During pericardiocentesis, the probability of success and the safety of the procedure relate directly to the size of the pericardial effusion. Whereas partial drainage of a massive pericardial effusion may be lifesaving, aspiration of a small pericardial effusion (<200 mL) that is freely mobile within the pericardial sac may be only marginally helpful. A significant hemodynamic effect is also unusual in the absence of a documented anterior effusion, or when loculated clot or fibrin inhibits the free withdrawal of fluid. Pericardiocentesis must not be undertaken by inexperienced personnel or in an inappropriate environment. Needle aspiration should be conducted whenever possible in the cardiac catheterization suite by an experienced cardiologist, using fluoroscopic and needle electrode ECG guidance. Complications include coronary laceration, pneumothorax, myocardial injury, and life-threatening arrhythmias.

Subxiphoid pericardiotomy can be performed safely under local anesthesia in certain critically ill patients. This procedure often establishes effective continuous drainage of the pericardium as well as enables pericardial biopsy. In many cases, open surgical drainage may be required to definitively relieve pressure. Regardless of drainage method, successful relief of tamponade is documented by the fall of intrapericardial pressure to normal, the reduction of elevated P_{RA}, separation of right from left heart filling pressures, augmentation of cardiac output, and disappearance of pulsus paradoxus. After drainage, the majority of patients should be closely monitored for at least 24 h in the ICU for evidence of recurrent tamponade. Persistent elevation and equilibration of right and left ventricular diastolic pressures after pericardiocentesis or subxiphoid pericardiotomy suggests a component of pericardial constriction. Pericardiectomy may be required in patients with a component of constriction and in those who experience recurrent tamponade despite repeated needle or subxiphoid drainage.

Constrictive Pericarditis

Constrictive pericarditis results from a confining pericardial shell that prevents adequate chamber filling. Although both constriction and tamponade are characterized by elevation and equilibration of right and left ventricular diastolic pressures, they can be differentiated by several key hemodynamic features (Table 1-4). Constrictive pericarditis limits filling primarily in late diastole, whereas tamponade affects filling throughout. In chronic constrictive pericarditis, an "M" or "W" contour may be formed by prominent dips in *both* systolic (X descent) and diastolic (Y descent) pressures. The Y descent is diminutive in tamponade. Whereas constrictive pericarditis may sometimes demonstrate atrial pressure changes reminiscent of

TABLE 1-4   TAMPONADE VERSUS CONSTRICTION

FEATURE	PERICARDIAL TAMPONADE	CONSTRICTIVE PERICARDITIS
Heart size	↑ or ↑↑	↔ to ↑↑
The Kussmaul sign	Usually absent	Usually present
Pulsus paradoxus	Very prominent	May be absent
RV tracing	Prominent X descent	Dip and plateau
RA tracing	Negligible Y descent	M or W contour
		Prominent Y descent
Pericardial fluid	Always present	May be present
ECG	Often reduced amplitude Alternans possible	Low QRS T wave depression

tamponade, the RV pressure contour usually shows a prominent "dip and plateau" ("square root") configuration. Pericardial constriction can be mimicked by restrictive or ischemic cardiomyopathy: in both conditions, RV and left ventricular diastolic pressures are elevated, SV and cardiac output are depressed, left ventricular end-diastolic volume is normal or decreased, and end-diastolic filling is impaired. However, restrictive cardiomyopathy is more likely when marked RV systolic hypertension is present and left ventricular diastolic pressure exceeds RV diastolic pressure by more than 5 mm Hg. Differentiation between these two entities, however, may require an exploratory thoracotomy. Constrictive pericarditis should be suspected in patients with right-sided congestive symptoms. Supportive (but nondiagnostic) clinical features of constriction include a history of prior cardiothoracic trauma, acute pericarditis, or mediastinal radiation. Physical examination may reveal an early diastolic sound (knock) or mild cardiac enlargement. The Kussmaul sign (inspiratory augmentation of the venous pulse wave) is characteristic, but pulsus paradoxus is not. As already mentioned, the RV tracing demonstrates a prominent "dip and plateau" waveform, and the venous or RA waveform shows a prominent Y descent. Common ECG findings include low QRS voltage, generalized T wave flattening or inversion, and an atrial abnormality suggestive of P mitrale. Because constrictive pericarditis tends to progress inexorably, surgical intervention is eventually required if the patient is an otherwise appropriate candidate. Hemodynamic and symptomatic improvement is evident in some patients immediately after operation; in others, however, improvement may be delayed for weeks or months.

■ **SUGGESTED READINGS**

Chatterjee K, Rame JE. Systolic heart failure: Chronic and acute syndromes. *Crit Care Med.* 2008;36(Suppl. 1):S44–S51.

den Uil CA, Klijn E, Lagrand WK, et al. The microcirculation in health and critical disease. *Prog Cardiovasc Dis.* 2008;51(2):161–170.

Gaasch WH, Zile MR. Left ventricular diastolic dysfunction and diastolic heart failure. *Annu Rev Med.* 2004;55:373–394.

Goldstein JA. Cardiac tamponade, constrictive pericarditis, and restrictive cardiomyopathy. *Curr Probl Cardiol.* 2004;29(9):503–567.

Salem R, Vallee F, Rusca M, et al. Hemodynamic monitoring by echocardiography in the ICU: The role of the new echo techniques. *Curr Opin Crit Care.* 2008;14(5):561–568.

Shabetai R. Pericardial effusion: Haemodynamic spectrum. *Heart (British Cardiac Society).* 2004;90(3):255–256.

Sheehan F, Redington A. The right ventricle: Anatomy, physiology and clinical imaging. *Heart.* 2008;94(11):1510–1515.

Hemodynamic Monitoring

KEY POINTS

1 Arterial blood pressure monitoring is an invaluable aid to the management of patients with hemodynamic instability, respiratory compromise, or brain injury and should be strongly considered in those who are in need of frequent BP or arterial blood gas assessment. It is always wise to compare readings obtained from an arterial line with those of a cuff pressure (preferably in more than one limb), and to do so whenever the monitored number disagrees with the clinical impression. Certain modern instruments allow online assessment of arterial blood gases and pH as well as provide reliable data for hemodynamic evaluation.

2 Before using hemodynamic information derived from catheter measurements, the transducer system must be accurately zeroed and calibrated. The dynamic pressure response of the catheter–transducer system should be checked by the rapid flush technique ("snaptest").

3 As opposed to a damped pulmonary artery tracing, a true wedge pressure is significantly less pulsatile and has a value lower than the mean pulmonary artery pressure.

4 All pulmonary artery pressures are influenced to varying degrees by fluctuations in pleural pressure. Respiratory fluctuations of pleural pressure are conditioned by the alveolar pressure transmission fraction: $C_l/(C_l + C_w)$. Major respiratory efforts may cause the end-expiratory wedge pressure value to exceed the relaxed value. During active breathing, the mean, nadir, and postparalysis wedge pressures reflect left ventricle filling and pulmonary vascular pressures better than the traditional end-expiratory wedge pressure.

5 It is always hazardous to infer the status of a dynamic system from a single number. The monitored "challenge" is a key maneuver in determining hemodynamic reserves. This may involve reversible noninvasive maneuvers (e.g., a change of positive end-expiratory pressure, measurement of respiratory pulse pressure variation, leg lifting) or rapid fluid bolusing. During a rigorous fluid challenge, the clinician notes symptoms, physical signs, cardiac output, blood pressure, wedge pressures, and/or pulmonary artery pressure in response to a fluid bolus. A notable improvement in key target variables (cardiac output, systemic blood pressure) without the development of symptoms or excessive cardiac filling pressures encourages an increase in the rate of fluid administration.

6 The complete hemodynamic profile should include sampling of mixed-venous (or less desirably, central venous) blood, a comparison of central venous and pulmonary artery wedge pressures, and calculations of systemic vascular resistance and pulmonary vascular resistance. Without such information, adequacy of cardiac output and mechanisms of hemodynamic impairment are often difficult to determine.

7 Echocardiogram provides vital data that compliment catheterization and physical examination. Wall motion abnormalities, ventricular contractility, chamber dimensions, dynamics of the central veins, diastolic properties, and valve functioning are well evaluated by this noninvasive method. Pulmonary artery pressure estimation is often possible. Although the *relative* importance of the pulmonary artery catheter has faded as echocardiogram and other minimally invasive hemodynamic monitoring techniques have been perfected for bedside use, the Pulmonary Artery (Swan Ganz) catheter remains an excellent option for well-selected patients whose clinicians understand the physiologic data stream it provides.

■ ARTERIAL BLOOD PRESSURE MONITORING

Noninvasive Arterial Pressure Monitoring

Sphygmomanometer pressures are notoriously inaccurate when cuff width is less than two thirds of arm circumference. Spurious elevations of blood pressure (BP) occur when measurements are made with an inappropriately narrow cuff and when arteriosclerosis prevents the brachial artery from collapsing under pressure. Conversely, because tight proximal occlusions can artifactually lower the BP, BP should initially be checked in both arms. As noted, it is always wise to compare readings obtained from an arterial line with a cuff pressure periodically and whenever the monitored number disagrees with the clinical impression. In many hypotensive patients with low cardiac output (CO), the "muffle" and disappearance points of diastolic pressure are poorly audible. In shock, all Korotkoff sounds may be lost. In this setting, Doppler ultrasonography may detect systolic pressures below the audible range.

The Arterial Pressure Waveform

Normally, mean arterial pressure (MAP) is similar in all large arterial vessels of a supine subject; there is only a slight pressure gradient between aortic and radial vessels. Posture-related hydrostatic increases of pressure are shared equally between arteries and veins, so that perfusion pressure is little affected. Although MAP is largely the same throughout the arterial tree, waveform contours differ with the caliber of the arterial vessel in question. Peak systolic pressure actually rises in the periphery due to wave reflection. When a vessel is totally occluded by a monitoring catheter, wave reflection may amplify pressure fluctuations to produce sharp spikes of systolic arterial pressure (to over 300 mm Hg in some cases) (Fig. 2-1). The ability of any specific

gradient between arterial and venous pressures to perfuse tissue depends directly on the resistance of the vascular bed. An MAP of 60 mm Hg may produce luxuriant flow through dilated vascular beds, whereas an MAP of 100 mm Hg may be inadequate during accelerated hypertension.

Depending on the shape of the arterial pressure waveform, the peak systolic (P_S) and nadir diastolic (P_D) pressures contribute to varying degrees to MAP. At normal heart rates (60 to 100 beats/min), $MAP \approx P_D + 1/3 (P_S - P_D)$. During tachycardia, P_S contributes relatively more, and during bradycardia, relatively less. Because its duration is generally longer, the diastolic pressure is the most important contributor to MAP.

Arterial Waveform Analysis for Cardiac Output Estimation

It is important to remember that pressure imperfectly indexes flow: unlike pressure, flow is largely continuous, not pulsatile. However, though not appropriate for patients with irregular rhythms and shock states, monitoring devices that analyze the shape of the arterial pressure waveform do a creditable job during sinus rhythm of tracking and trending the CO within their limitations. Their value is seriously compromised by atrial fibrillation and other chaotic arrhythmias.

Simplified Functional Hemodynamic Monitoring

Useful classification of hemodynamic compromise can be attempted using a few simple bedside observations that determine mean arterial pressure and index stroke volume. The arterial pressure waveform is central to such an analysis in that it provides the mean arterial pressure and the stroke volume variation of respiration that indexes the sufficiency of intravascular volume (Fig. 2-2). A >10% change of pulse pressure with passive respiration

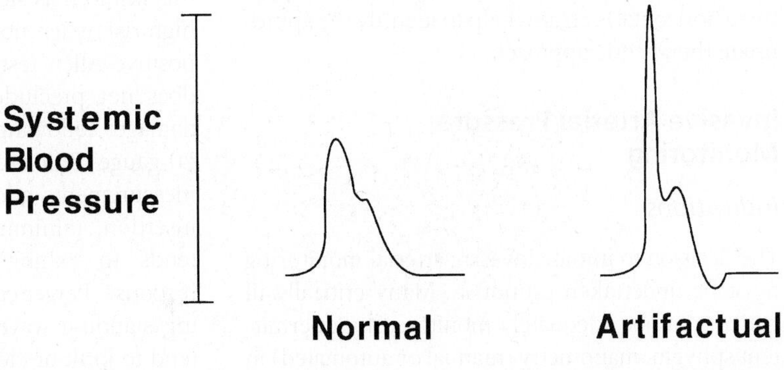

■ **FIGURE 2-1** Artifactual elevation of systolic arterial pressure. An underdamped arterial pressure tracing amplified by reflection within an occluded artery may exaggerate the systolic pressure as well as any mean pressure computed from the raw "systolic" and diastolic pressure values.

Systemic Blood Pressure

Normal   **Artifactual**

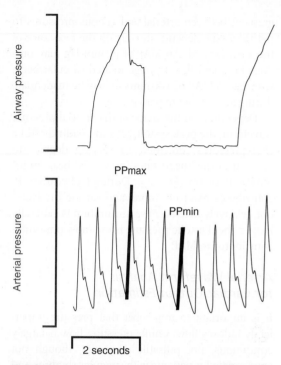

■ **FIGURE 2-2** Changes in pulse pressure variation with respiration in a passively ventilated subject. The relatively large difference in pulse pressure during different phases of the ventilation cycle suggests relative underfilling of the vasculature.

suggests the need for additional preload. $PPV(\%) = 100 \times [PPmax - PPmin]/[PPmax + PPmin/2]$. It must be borne in mind, however, that arrhythmias and active breathing negate the value of pulse pressure variation. With this proviso, combining an evaluation of mean arterial pressure and variation of pulse pressure can yield an insight into the type of therapy indicated. A low mean arterial pressure combined with a low stroke volume (as indicated by wide pulse pressure variation) strongly suggests hemorrhage, heart failure, or tamponade. A low MAP combined with negligible pulse pressure variation is more compatible with sepsis. The responses of these indices to a reversible volume challenge intervention (such as lifting the legs with the upper torso horizontal) can also help to identify the appropriate therapeutic approach.

Invasive Arterial Pressure Monitoring

Indications

The decision to initiate invasive arterial monitoring must be undertaken cautiously. Many critically ill patients can be adequately monitored by intermittent sphygmomanometry (manual or automated) in combination with the physical exam. Patients with hemodynamic instability or shock, malignant hypertension, or failure to oxygenate are most likely to benefit from arterial cannulation. A well-adjusted catheter system provides accurate pressure information necessary for hemodynamic monitoring and facilitates blood sampling, often obviating the need for venipuncture.

Although convenient and usually reliable, indwelling arterial catheters occasionally give misleading information—especially when the radial artery has been cannulated for an extended time. Errors are most likely to arise in patients who are elderly, are hypotensive, or have underlying vascular disease. Attempts should be made at least once daily to confirm the line pressure by sphygmomanometry. This is especially important in patients receiving vasoactive drugs regulated by radial line pressures. Consideration should be given to measuring femoral pressure when the cuff-derived value and clinical impression disagree seriously with the recorded value (generally in the direction of indicating greater pressure than the catheter records).

Complications

Serious complications can arise due to local hemorrhage, infection, and thrombosis. For this reason, the radial artery of the nondominant arm should be used whenever possible. Although common, regional thrombosis of the radial artery seldom results in tissue-damaging ischemia; digital embolization is the greater hazard. Large catheter size, low CO, preexisting arteriopathy, absence of collateral perfusion, and vasopressors increase the risk (artery caliber tends to parallel the wrist size).

The Allen test is performed by raising the wrist well above the heart level and compressing the radial and ulnar arteries simultaneously for 10s, blanching the capillary bed. When the ulnar artery is then released, flushing should occur within a few seconds. Not all patients in shock can be tested in this fashion, as sluggish flow may falsely suggest a high risk when none exists. Conversely, although a positive Allen test (see following) is reassuring, it does not preclude the development of ischemic damage following radial artery thrombosis. A 20-gauge Teflon catheter is preferred for arterial measurements and sampling because it facilitates insertion, minimizes the risk of thrombosis, and tends to exhibit the best dynamic frequency response. Larger catheters occlude the vessel, creating standing waves while smaller-gauge catheters tend to kink or clot off. Rarely, the arterial catheter may erode the vessel wall to cause aneurysm, localized hematoma, compressive neuropathy, or arteriovenous fistula. Although local colonization is very common, serious soft tissue infections are rare during percutaneous cannulation if the puncture site is kept sterile, the catheter is used for only a few days, and precautions are taken during blood sampling to preserve sterility. Femoral catheters and "cutdowns" are most likely to infect. The radial artery is not an appropriate site for injection of any drug. Intra-arterial injections of certain drugs, particularly calcium channel blockers and vasopressors, can cause ischemic necrosis of the hand, a functionally devastating injury. Prolonged, high pressure flushing can potentially drive clot or gas bubbles retrograde to produce cerebral embolism.

■ DATA FROM VASCULAR CATHETERS

In a certain sense, concern for the performance or stability of the cardiorespiratory system helps define the need for intensive care. Reliable data relevant to the heart and vasculature are instrumental in diagnosing problems, in selecting and regulating therapy, and in timing interventions. Yet, interpreting the complex relationships among vascular pressures and flows is often complicated by spontaneous fluctuations in metabolism and by variations of the respiratory pressures that influence them. Relatively few clinicians become expert in data interpretation. Balloon flotation pulmonary artery (PA) catheters have been relegated to a secondary status with the recognition that echocardiography (ECHO), noninvasive CO monitoring (e.g., arterial waveform analyzers), and information from central venous pressure (CVP) catheters—conventional and specially modified— suffice for many purposes. Yet, the PA catheter provides data of clinical value that cannot be obtained otherwise (e.g., pulmonary venous pressure and true mixed venous oxygen saturation). Moreover, because the PA catheter incorporates the CVP and requires similar insertion principles, it serves as an appropriate focal point for our discussion.

Inserting the Balloon Flotation Catheter

Although detailed descriptions of insertion technique for the balloon flotation catheter are available elsewhere, a few points are worth emphasizing here. In patients with bleeding disorders, the physician should select a site conducive to applying direct pressure. As opposed to the subclavian and femoral sites, the internal jugular approach tends to be the simplest and least fraught with complications. The right side provides more direct and reliable access to the superior vena cava (SVC) than the left, but either approach can be used effectively. For puncture of the internal jugular or subclavian veins, insertion must be accomplished with the patient supine or, preferably, in the Trendelenburg position to ensure vessel distention and minimize the risk of air embolism. In a dyspneic patient with orthopnea, this may require prior sedation and endotracheal intubation. If intubation is not an option, the femoral or brachial approach should be considered.

Difficult Insertion and Placement

Problems that occur during placement are generally of two types: (a) difficulty entering the central veins of the thorax and (b) difficulty directing the catheter tip into the PA. Both types of problem can be mastered only by gaining sufficient direct experience. With regard to central vein entry, placement of the introducer/sheath assembly is the crucial step. Ultrasonic imaging with a purpose-designed instrument is a valuable aid in locating the vein, monitoring the puncture, and avoiding complications. Sheath insertion must be gentle and never forced. The stab incision made to facilitate the puncture must be sufficiently long and deep to allow easy passage of the easily collapsible and damaged sheath over the introducer. Apart from anatomic aberrations (e.g., prior vascular trauma or clotting), common reasons for difficulty encountered in floating the catheter tip to proper position include low CO, severe pulmonary hypertension with right ventricular (RV) overload and tricuspid regurgitation, and massive RV enlargement. The balloon should always be inflated cautiously and must fill easily without the need for force. If blood does not draw easily through the sheath assembly, concern is raised for extravascular placement. No catheter or sheath placed via the right internal jugular should cross the midsternal line on a well-centered routine pulmonary arterial chest film. While pulsatile blood flow raises the possibility of inadvertent arterial cannulation, it should be kept in mind that the jugular vein lies in close proximity to the innominate and carotid arteries. Therefore, patients with well-filled central veins as well as those with tricuspid regurgitation may exhibit impressively pulsatile blood flow from a well-placed CVP catheter.

When the catheter is inserted via the right internal jugular vein, the balloon is inflated approximately 15 cm from the point of neck entry. Patients vary with regard to the dimensions of their vascular anatomy, but as a rule of thumb, the catheter tip should not require advancement by more than 20 cm beyond its current position before encountering the next vascular compartment (Fig. 2-2). In other words, an SVC tracing should be evident within 20 cm of skin entry, and the RV should be entered within 40 cm. The PA should be encountered within the first 60 cm of tip advancement (often considerably less). Coiling within the RV and misdirection of the catheter should be suspected after 45 to 50 cm has been advanced without securing an appropriate PA waveform. To facilitate placement, the patient can be repositioned (e.g., lateral decubitus or Fowler's) in an attempt to establish favorable balloon orientation and blood streaming for balloon flotation. Fluoroscopy can be a helpful adjunct in difficult cases and is especially worthwhile to consider before attempting an insertion of a PA catheter from a femoral site, which tends to present more placement problems than brachial, subclavian, or jugular punctures.

Interpreting Data from the Pulmonary Artery Catheter

The balloon flotation catheter allows acquisition of three types of primary data: (a) central venous, PA, and balloon-occluded (wedge) pressures; (b) intermittent or continuous CO determinations; and (c) sampling of mixed-venous or postalveolar capillary blood. This information can be used in its primary form or can be manipulated to provide useful indices of fluid volume status, right and left ventricular (LV) performance and loading conditions, or tissue perfusion (Table 2-1). Specially modified fiberoptic CVP catheters provide O_2 saturation data from the SVC in addition to CVP.

In recent years, justifiable concern has been raised that PA catheters often impair rather than improve the outcome of critical illness. An influential retrospective analysis of a large database published in the mid-1990s suggested that patients of equivalent severity were more likely to die when a catheter was used than when it was not. The data did not substantiate the suspicion that the instrument itself produced lethal illness by sepsis, balloon rupture of a pulmonary vessel, or other specific mechanism. Apprehension regarding its use was reinforced, however, by studies conducted in North America and Europe that revealed how inexpertly the data from the catheter were interpreted by critical care specialists. Although a general consensus has since emerged that PA catheters often provide important, therapy-guiding information, there is also agreement that the potential for iatrogenic injury is considerable and that numerous concepts of cardiopulmonary physiology must be mastered to interpret its data effectively. A recent NIH ARDS-net trial of fluids and catheter strategies demonstrated no survival benefit or harm with use of the PA catheter.

Pulmonary Vascular Pressures

Measurement of Pulmonary Vascular Pressures

Used in conjunction with the CO, the PA and wedge pressures yield important diagnostic information regarding intravascular filling, the tendency for pulmonary edema formation, the status of the pulmonary vasculature, and the vigor of LV contraction. This time-honored technique, although currently under assault from less-invasive methods and nowadays less commonly employed, often provides data of great value in assessing the relative function of the ventricles and the hydrostatic contribution of left heart failure and central vascular pressures to lung edema.

System Requirements for Accurate Pressure Measurement

Static Requirements

Zeroing Accurate recording of intravascular pressure requires error-free measurement of static pressure and faithful tracking of an undulating (dynamic) waveform. Attention must be paid to the technical details of data acquisition to avoid error. For wedge pressure recording, for example, an uninterrupted fluid column must extend from the left atrium (LA) through the catheter lumen to the flexible diaphragm of an electromechanical transducer. The transducer membrane deforms in response to pressure exerted by the fluid column

---

TABLE 2-1 HEMODYNAMIC DATA PROVIDED BY THE PA CATHETER[a]

DIRECT	DERIVED[a]
Cardiac output	Vascular resistance
Mixed-venous	Pulmonary
oxygen saturation	Systemic
Vascular pressures	Stroke-work index
Right atrium	Arteriovenous O_2
Right ventricle	content difference
Pulmonary artery	
Balloon occlusion (wedge)	

[a]Partial listing.

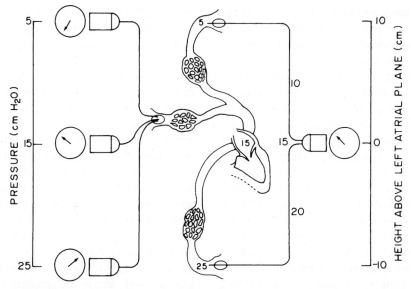

■ **FIGURE 2-3** Zeroing the transducer. The transducer must not be moved from its original position after the display has been adjusted to record zero pressure with the liquid-filled system exposed to atmospheric pressure at the LA level. After zeroing, a hydrostatic column influences the recorded value when the transducer is lifted or lowered from its original position **(left)**. Conversely, when the transducer remains at the "zeroed" position **(right)**, movement of the catheter tip makes no difference to the pressure recorded, provided that a continuous column of fluid extends from the LA through the catheter to the transducer dome.

and generates proportional electrical signals for amplification and display. Because this segment of the system is fluid filled, the vertical distance separating the LA from the transducer exerts a hydrostatic pressure against the sensor that adds to or subtracts from the actual (LA) pressure (Fig. 2-3). To eliminate bias from positioning, the transducer is placed at the LA level. The display is then adjusted to read zero pressure when the dome is closed to the patient and opened to the atmosphere. Neither the transducer level relative to the LA nor the zero offset adjustment can be changed without a new "rezeroing" procedure. A similar caution to assure accuracy of positioning and zeroing applies to systemic arterial pressure monitoring. Sudden changes of systemic pressures are sometimes explained by movement of the transducer in relation to its originally zeroed position.

Calibration   Once the transducer is balanced (zeroed) to the LA level, the system must be accurately calibrated. With most modern systems, this can be accomplished automatically by the electronic processing equipment itself. In older systems, a known pressure is manually applied to the transducer membrane to complete the calibration. This is easily accomplished by creating an open water column (above the zeroed transducer) of known height, using the connecting tubing that

links the transducer and the fluid-filled catheter. Because the electronic display expresses pressure in mm Hg, whereas the calibrating pressure is applied in cm H_2O, an appropriate conversion must be made: 1.34 cm $H_2O = 1$ mm Hg (or 0.7 mm Hg = 1 cm H_2O). A stopcock is closed to the patient, opened to atmosphere at the LA level, and lifted a known vertical distance. The electronics are then adjusted to display the pressure actually applied by the water column. This calibration can be quickly accomplished before insertion by raising the distal tip of the fluid-filled catheter (on line to the zeroed transducer) a known distance above the mid LA. Although automated electronic calibration is integral to many bedside monitors currently in use, these more basic procedures just discussed should be performed whenever utmost accuracy is required or the monitor's output is in doubt.

As a final check that the zeroed and calibrated system is ready to record, the operator should shake the catheter tip through a substantial vertical range and observe the amplitude of the sinusoidal response on the monitor.

Dynamic Requirements   Whatever the components and linkages, a well-calibrated system measures the static vascular pressure rather accurately, unless the catheter itself becomes kinked or occluded. However, to track dynamic pressures faithfully, the liquid-filled portions of the system must have appropriate frequency-response characteristics. These properties are the natural resonant frequency of the system and its degree of damping. Without an appropriate frequency response, the system may exaggerate or attenuate important subcomponents of complex pressure waveforms. An improperly tuned system often generates erroneous systolic and diastolic pressure values and may not allow differentiation between distorted PA and wedge pressure tracings. Moreover, partially occluded catheters connected to "continuous flush" devices can falsely elevate mean pressures as well. Air bubbles, loose or damaged fittings, inefficient coupling of disposable transducer domes to the sensing membrane, and excessively lengthy or compliant connecting tubing reduce the system's natural resonant frequency, blunting its ability to respond. Damping is produced by air bubbles, defective stopcocks, clot or protein debris within the catheter, impingement of the catheter tip against a vessel wall, and long, narrow, or kinked catheter tubing. Prior to insertion, vertically whipping the catheter tip can give a simple, qualitative indication of frequency response. After insertion, a simple check for adequate frequency response can be conducted using the rapid flush device of the catheter system ("snap test") (Fig. 2-4). During the rapid flush, a sustained pulse of high pressure is temporarily applied to the transducer membrane. When the flush is suddenly terminated, pressure abruptly falls. Immediately upon sudden release, the tracing from a responsive system should overshoot (plunge below) its normal baseline and briefly (<1 s) oscillate before recovering a crisp, well-defined PA waveform. A poorly tuned system fails to overshoot or oscillate and recovers to a damped configuration after a noticeable delay.

Accurately calibrated strip-chart or frozen screen records of pulmonary vascular pressure should be examined frequently, particularly when serious diagnostic or therapeutic questions arise. Pressures must be referenced consistently to the same point in the respiratory cycle. For the wedge pressure, this is preferably at end expiration, except during very vigorous breathing when the mean value of the wedge may better reflect average transmural pressure. Influenced by fluctuations of intrathoracic pressure, electronically processed digital displays of "systolic, diastolic, and mean" pressures may be misleading, particularly during forceful or chaotic breathing. The strip-chart and frozen calibrated screen recordings allow the clinician to adjust for the influence of ventilatory effort. The simultaneous recording of pulmonary wedge pressure (P_w), together with airway or (preferably) esophageal pressure, greatly facilitates interpretation.

Types of Pressure Measurement

Although there is an understandable tendency to concentrate on the PA and wedge pressures, the experienced clinician recognizes that RV dysfunction often contributes to hemodynamic compromise during critical illness and, therefore, carefully assesses its loading and performance characteristics as well. Indeed, with current catheter technology, preload, afterload, and contractility can be more directly and completely monitored for the RV than for the LV.

Central Venous Pressure   CVP catheters serve a wide variety of clinical purposes. Since the first clinical use of the PA catheter, many physicians have considered these lines primarily as secure and predictable routes for infusing drugs, nutrients, and volume expanders; the "triple lumen" central catheters are invaluable for this purpose.

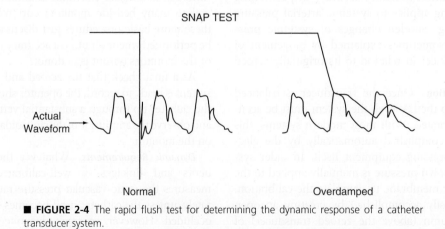

SNAP TEST

Actual Waveform →

Normal

Overdamped

■ **FIGURE 2-4** The rapid flush test for determining the dynamic response of a catheter transducer system.

Yet, by whatever means it is acquired, the CVP tracing should not be ignored for the hemodynamic data it provides. In the supine position, the mean CVP is virtually identical to the mean RA pressure, which reflects the status of RV preload. When considered together with RV compliance and pleural pressure, mean CVP serves to index the preload of the RV. A comparison of the central venous and wedge pressures proves helpful in diagnosing RV infarction and cor pulmonale. Furthermore, the contour of the CVP tracing can indicate tricuspid regurgitation caused by RV overload, suggest pericardial restriction and tamponade, or detect the cannon waves of AV block. The sawtooth pressure waves characteristic of atrial flutter can sometimes be detected on the CVP tracing when the surface electrocardiogram is inconclusive. In the absence of lung or heart disease, CVP serves well to indicate the degree of circulatory filling (e.g., during acute GI hemorrhage). Sudden and disproportionate elevations of CVP with respect to wedge pressure accompany pulmonary embolism with clot or air, RV infarction, or acute lung disorders (bronchospasm, aspiration, pneumothorax). CVP is a primary component of the systemic vascular resistance (SVR) calculation. Superior vena caval O_2 saturation, which correlates well with (but slightly exceeds) the mixed venous value, may be very helpful in monitoring the efficacy of resuscitation from hypotension and shock. Modified fiberoptic (spectrophotometric) CVP catheters can provide this information continuously.

Interpreted in conjunction with the wedge pressure, CVP can be used to estimate fluctuations in transmural filling pressure. Because the SVC is a flaccid structure embedded in the pleural space, fluctuations in CVP crudely reflect changes in intrapleural and pericardial pressures. It has been suggested that the CVP tracks changes in pleural pressure well enough that the transmission fraction of alveolar pressure to the pleural space can be computed under passive inflation conditions as follows:

$$\text{Transmission fraction} = (\text{CVP}_{EI} - \text{CVP}_{EE})/(P_{PLAT} - P_{EX})$$

where CVP_{EI} and CVP_{EE} are the end-inspiratory and end-expiratory values of CVP, and P_{PLAT} and P_{EX} are the corresponding static airway pressures recorded during occluded airway (stopped flow) maneuvers. Although the wedge pressure can theoretically be used in this way, it is a less reliable indicator of changes in pleural pressure. For example, respiratory fluctuations in P_w (and estimated transmission fraction) may be exaggerated under non–zone-III conditions (see following).

Pulmonary Artery Pressure   The RV generates the systolic PA pressure (P_{PA}) in forcing the CO through the pulmonary vascular network against resistance. Because the difference between mean arterial and venous pressures drives the flow, P_{PA} can be made to rise by increasing the downstream venous pressure (as in LV failure), CO, or the flow resistance (as in primary lung diseases). With its large capillary reserve, the normal pulmonary vascular bed offers little resistance to runoff. Consequently, pulmonary artery diastolic pressure (P_{PAD}) seldom exceeds LA pressure by more than a few mm Hg, even when flow is increased. Obliteration of pulmonary vascular channels, however, increases resistance, obligating a larger gradient of pressure. Under these conditions, P_{PAD} may substantially exceed the pressure within pulmonary veins and LA. Just as importantly, the lack of recruitable vasculature reduces the compliance reserve that normally buffers P_{PA} against fluctuations in CO. Consequently, major variations in P_{PA} often attend changes in output or vascular tone, making P_{PAD} an unreliable index of LV filling in serious lung disorders. The pulmonary vascular network is designed to accept large (5- to 10-fold) variations in CO without building sufficient pressure across the delicate endothelial membrane to cause interstitial fluid accumulation and alveolar flooding. Therefore, the RV normally develops only enough power to pump against modest impedance. As a rule, the normal RV cannot sustain acute loading to mean pressures greater than 35 mm Hg without decompensation. Over long periods, however, as during a protracted course of acute respiratory distress syndrome (ARDS), the RV strengthens and P_{PA} builds. Indeed, the height to which P_{PA} is forced to rise may be a useful prognostic index, correlating inversely with outcome. Given adequate time to adapt to massively increased afterload, systemic levels of arterial pressure can be sustained. Once the pulmonary vascular reserve is exhausted, an additional obliteration or narrowing by embolism, hypoxia, acidosis, or infusion of vasoactive drugs may evoke a marked pulmonary pressor response. Such elevations of hydrostatic pressure may cause fluid leakage, even across precapillary and postcapillary vessels. It is certainly possible, therefore, that hydrostatic pulmonary edema can form even when LA and pulmonary venous pressures (reflected by the wedge) remain within the normal range, especially if the serum oncotic pressure is low.

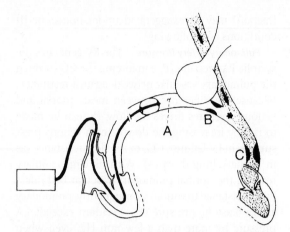

■ FIGURE 2-5 Definition of a wedge pressure (P_w). The P_w, measured at point *A*, is nearly identical to the pressure at the junction of static and flowing venous blood (*). P_w will not be influenced by partial occlusions of the static column (*B*) that extends from the catheter tip to the junction. However, obstructions (*C*) downstream from the junction point dissipate pressure, causing P_w to significantly exceed mean P_{LA}. Although generally located in a large pulmonary vein, the junction point may reside in a small pulmonary venule in certain disease states.

Pulmonary Arterial Occlusion (Wedge) Pressure
Balloon inflation encourages the catheter tip to migrate from a main PA into a smaller-caliber vessel, where it impacts and wedges. With the distal catheter orifice isolated from P_{PA}, fluid motion stops along the microvascular channels served by the occluded artery (Fig. 2-5). Because no resistive pressure drop occurs along this newly created static column, the pressure at the catheter tip equilibrates with the pressure at the downstream junction ("j" point) of flowing and nonflowing venous blood. It is believed that this junction normally occurs in a vessel of a size similar to that of the occluded artery—that is, in a large vein. Pulmonary wedge pressure, therefore, provides a low-range estimate of the mean hydrostatic pressure within the more proximal fluid-exchanging vessels. When resistance in the small veins is high, P_w may not accurately reflect the true tendency for edema formation. Pulmonary capillary pressure is seriously underestimated when mean P_{PA} substantially exceeds P_w. As a crude approximation, the pressure relevant to fluid filtration across the pulmonary vessels generally exceeds P_w by about 40% of the difference between the mean PA and wedge pressures (Fig. 2-6).

The validity of the P_w measurement rests on the assumption that the occlusion of a major vessel by the balloon does not reduce the total blood flow through the lungs. This is not always a good assumption when the pulmonary vascular reserve is limited—as after pneumonectomy. In these circumstances, balloon inflation can detrimentally afterload the RV, potentially reducing pulmonary blood flow and P_w during the measurement. Because large pulmonary veins are inherently low-resistance vessels, P_w usually deviates little from P_{LA}. Mean P_{LA}, in turn, closely approximates left-ventricular end-diastolic pressure (P_{LVED}) in the absence of mitral valvular obstruction or incompetence or markedly reduced ventricular compliance. Because P_{LVED} is the intravascular pressure component that determines preload, P_w not only provides a low-range estimate of the hydrostatic pressure in the pulmonary venous circuit but also gives some indication of presystolic LV fiber stretch when interpreted in conjunction with an estimate of extramural pleural pressure (e.g., by esophageal balloon).

Obtaining a Valid Wedge Pressure   Unfortunately, a number of technical and physiologic factors encourage errors of data acquisition as well as misinterpretation of recorded values (Table 2-2). The validity of P_w as a measure of pulmonary venous pressure depends on the existence of open vascular

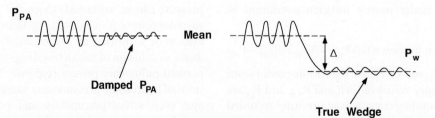

■ FIGURE 2-6 Distinguishing a damped PA pressure (P_{PA}) tracing from a true wedge pressure (P_w) during balloon inflation. The mean pressure of a damped P_{PA} tracing should approximate that of the undamped P_{PA} waveform recorded with the balloon deflated **(left)**. A true wedge pressure is distinguished by a mean pressure that is substantially lower than that of the P_{PA} **(right)**.

TABLE 2-2 CHECKLIST FOR VERIFYING THE POSITION OF PA CATHETER

	ZONE III	ZONE I OR II
Respiratory variation of P_w	$<\frac{1}{2}\Delta P_{alv}$	$>\frac{1}{2}\Delta P_{alv}$
P_w contour	Cardiac ripple	Unnaturally smooth
Catheter tip location	LA level or below	Above LA level
PEEP trial	$\Delta P_w < \frac{1}{2}\Delta PEEP$	$\Delta P_w > \frac{1}{2}\Delta PEEP$
P_{PAD} vs. P_w	$P_{PAD} > P_w$	$P_{PAD} < P_w$

channels connecting the LA with the transducer. However, microvessels exposed to interstitial and alveolar pressures separate the catheter tip from the downstream "j" point. Because these vessels are collapsible, the interrelation between alveolar gas and fluid pressures governs the patency of the vascular pathway.

Zoning Conceptually, the upright lung can be divided into three zones, viewing the pulmonary vascular network as a variable (Starling) resistor vulnerable to external compression by alveolar pressure (Fig. 2-7). These zones theoretically extend

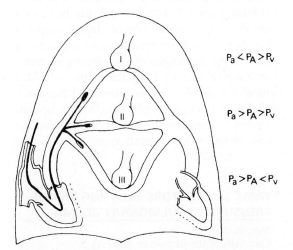

■ FIGURE 2-7 Perfusion zones of the lung and their influence on the recorded wedge pressure. Ascending vertically in the lung, arterial (P_{PA}) and pulmonary venous (P_{PV}) pressures decline relative to alveolar pressure (P_A), which remains uniform throughout the lung. In both zones I and II, P_A exceeds P_{PV} during balloon occlusion, collapsing alveolar vessels. Wedge pressure provides a valid measure of pulmonary venous pressure only when a continuous fluid column connects the catheter tip with the LA (e.g., zone III).

vertically because regional vascular pressures within the lung are affected by gravity, unlike the uniform gas pressure within the alveoli. In zone I, near the apex of the upright lung, alveolar pressure exceeds both P_{PA} and pulmonary venous pressure, flattens alveolar capillaries, and stops the flow. In zone II, alveolar pressure is intermediate between P_{PA} and pulmonary venous pressure, so flow in this region is determined by the arterial–alveolar pressure gradient. In zone III, near the lung base, alveolar pressure is less than either vein or artery pressure and does not influence the flow. Inflation of the catheter balloon isolates downstream alveoli from P_{PA}. To sense pressure at the "j" point, the catheter tip must communicate with the pulmonary veins via a channel whose vascular pressure exceeds alveolar pressure. Intuitively, it would seem that only in zone III could patent vascular channels remain open to connect the catheter lumen and the LA. Outside zone III, alveolar pressure would exceed pulmonary venous pressure, collapsing the capillaries in those regions and forcing P_w to track fluctuations in alveolar pressure, rather than P_{LA}. Although conceptually valid, it is now clear that this simple schema does not always apply. If a portion of the capillary bed in communication with the occluded catheter tip extends below the LA reference level, the hydrostatic column extending down to those vessels will raise their intraluminal pressures sufficiently to maintain a patent channel, even when the tip of the catheter lies at the level of zone II. Alveolar pressure will not collapse these lowermost vessels until it exceeds P_{LA} plus this hydrostatic pressure (often 5 to 10 cm H_2O). Moreover, zone III conditions tend to be reestablished at end exhalation, even if alveolar distension collapses the capillary bed at the higher lung volumes prevailing during the remainder of the tidal respiratory cycle. Thus, "zoning" is not usually a problem with positive end-expiratory pressure (PEEP) up to 10 cm H_2O, even in patients with nearly normal lungs. This problem seldom occurs so long as the catheter tip lies at or below the level of the LA—its usual position. Furthermore, densely infiltrated or flooded alveoli may protect the patency of vascular channels, despite an unfavorable relationship between pulmonary venous pressure and the pressure within gas-filled alveoli. Shunted blood is not exposed to aerated alveoli. When a zoning artifact does arise, lateral decubitus positioning can be used to place the catheter tip in a dependent position relative to the LA, effectively converting the wedged region from zone II to zone III.

During spontaneous breathing in the supine position, the great majority of lung vessels normally remain in zone III throughout the respiratory cycle. The extent of zones I and II will increase when alveolar pressure rises relative to pulmonary venous pressure, as during hypovolemia or during the inspiratory portion of a positive pressure breath. Because PEEP both augments alveolar pressure and reduces venous return, its application tends to diminish the span of the zone III region. Catheter tip positioning in a vertical plane higher than the LA further increases the likelihood of zoning artifacts. A catheter wedged outside zone III will show marked respiratory variation and an unnaturally smooth waveform. In the absence of overt RV overload and failure, the respiratory fluctuation in P_w—influenced by alveolar pressure—will substantially exceed that of the CVP. Although a marked rise in P_w during the respiratory cycle suggests zone III positioning, a valid P_w may still be restored at end exhalation, as already noted. However, a change in end-expiratory P_w greater than one half of an applied change in PEEP strongly suggests that end-expiratory P_w reflects alveolar, not LA, pressure.

Overwedging   Even when the catheter tip is well-positioned, asymmetrical balloon inflation or transverse orientation of the catheter axis relative to that of the vessel lumen can artifactually elevate P_w (overwedging) by isolating the catheter tip from the vascular lumen. Often, the catheter is too peripheral. When this occurs, the blind pocket of fluid bounded by the balloon and vascular wall continues to receive inflow from the continuous flushing system, forcing an elevation of the recorded pressure baseline. The overwedged P_w eventually exceeds mean P_{PA}, an event without logical physiologic interpretation. Such a pressure gradient situation would imply retrograde flow. Under these circumstances, the balloon should be deflated and the catheter gently flushed and repositioned, if necessary.

Wedge Pressure as a Measure of Hydrostatic Filtration Pressure   The pressure within the large pulmonary veins, the presumed "j" point, has long been regarded as a good reflection of the mean pressure within the fluid filtering vessels. It was once believed that the small capillaries were the only vessels to conduct significant fluid exchange with the interstitium and that very little pressure drop occurred beyond the capillary level. However, both assumptions now appear doubtful; extra-alveolar vessels clearly participate actively in fluid exchange. Furthermore, as much as 40% of the pulmonary vascular resistance (PVR) can be attributed to the capillaries and small veins. It is therefore likely that P_w seriously underestimates the mean filtration pressure under certain conditions. Pulmonary veno-occlusive disease, for example, characteristically causes pulmonary edema in the face of a normal P_w. Such discrepancies may help to account for hydrostatic edema occurring in the face of normal wedge pressure and presumably intact vascular endothelium. Furthermore, the "j" point may sometimes occur in a small vein (for example, when an underinflated catheter tip wedges within a small PA). Under these circumstances, considerable resistance may be interposed between the "j" point and the LA, leading to a discrepancy between these two pressures. A $P_w - P_{LA}$ discrepancy has been reported to develop in the setting of endotoxemia or sepsis, conditions known to be associated with pulmonary venous constriction.

When P_w is used to estimate the hydrostatic contribution to edema formation, five additional factors should be considered: chronicity of the pathologic process, extravascular pressure, mean PA pressure, plasma oncotic pressure, and endothelial permeability (Table 2-3) (Fig. 2-8). Over time, compensatory mechanisms for evacuation of interstitial fluid (e.g., improved lymphatic drainage) may allow high pulmonary venous pressure without frank edema. For example, P_w can be chronically elevated in mitral valvular disease despite a clear chest X-ray. Extramural pressure undoubtedly varies along the length of the filtering segment. For example, recruited capillaries are imbedded within the alveoli whereas derecruited capillaries and larger fluid-permeable vessels may be surrounded by pressure similar to (or lower than) the mean pleural value. Normal interstitial pressures

---

TABLE 2-3   FACTORS RELATING WEDGE PRESSURE TO PULMONARY EDEMA

Magnitude of P_w
Chronicity of the pathologic process
Diameter of wedged vessel
Plasma oncotic pressure
Pulmonary vascular permeability
Mean $P_{PA} - P_w$ pressure difference
Cardiac output
Pulmonary vascular resistance
   Arteriolar
   Venular

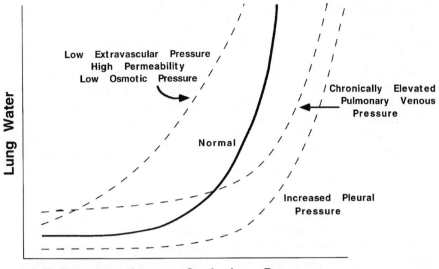

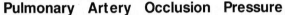

■ **FIGURE 2-8** Relationship of lung water to PA occlusion pressure for a variety of clinical conditions. Normally, the curve relating lung water to PA occlusion pressure (P_w) demonstrates a sharp upward inflection as P_w exceeds 20 to 25 mm Hg. Leakage is enhanced by high vascular permeability (e.g., ARDS), low serum osmotic pressure, and low extravascular pressure (as during forceful inspiratory effort). Conversely, a high P_w may be well tolerated without excessive lung water accumulation if pleural pressure is increased or if pulmonary venous pressure is chronically elevated.

also vary somewhat across the horizontal plane extending from the hilum to the lateral aspect of the visceral pleura. Moreover, the heterogeneous mechanics of the diseased lung undoubtedly intensify such regional variations, and the magnitude of these variations must fluctuate dramatically in different phases of the tidal ventilatory cycle. Because the hydrostatic gradient across the fluid-exchanging vessels is the difference between intravascular pressure (estimated by P_w) and extravascular pressure, pulmonary edema can form at a normal P_w if the interstitial pressure is sufficiently reduced by markedly negative pleural pressures (for example, during acute re-expansion edema, asthma, or strangulation). Very negative interstitial pressures can be produced locally during the normal ventilation cycle when there is persistent regional microatelectasis adjacent to freely expanding alveoli. Conversely, edema may not form at high pleural pressures (PEEP, auto-PEEP), despite marked elevations of P_w. Therefore, it is wise to interpret P_w in light of possible alterations of intrathoracic and interstitial pressures. One rational but imprecise method is to approximate the change in interstitial pressure to be the change in pleural pressure, measured or estimated at the same point in the respiratory cycle.

An important role for plasma oncotic pressure is predicted by the classical Starling equation that describes transvascular fluid exchange. Capillary oncotic pressure is reduced by the hypoproteinemia of cirrhosis, malnutrition, nephrosis, or the administration of excessive crystalloid. When the ratio of plasma/interstitial protein concentration falls, pulmonary edema forms at a lower transvascular pressure, especially when the lung is acutely injured. Gross edema formation is unusual when the serum colloid osmotic pressure exceeds P_w by greater than 4 mm Hg, but is increasingly likely at lower values. Although clearly contributory in many settings, reduced plasma oncotic pressure alone rarely explains edema in the face of normal hydrostatic pressures and an intact capillary membrane.

As already noted, endothelial permeability is a major factor governing the influence of P_w on lung water accumulation. Unlike the curve relating P_w to edema formation when permeability is normal, the steep relationship between these variables exhibits no distinct inflection pressure when permeability is increased. Thus, there does not appear to be a "safe range" of rising P_w values over which accelerated edemagenesis can be completely avoided; when the lung is injured, even small changes in P_w greatly influence the tendency for alveolar flooding.

Wedge Pressure as a Measure of Left Ventricular Preload When afterload and contractility are held constant, end-diastolic muscle fiber length (preload) determines the stroke volume. Over brief periods, fiber length parallels ventricular volume, and diastolic ventricular volume is a joint function of myocardial distensibility (compliance) and the net transmural ("inside" minus "outside") pressure stretching the ventricle. Just as extravascular pressure must be considered when judging the hydrostatic tendency for fluid filtration, transmural pressure is the effective force distending the heart. The intracavitary pressure at end-diastole (P_{LVED}) pushes the ventricle outward from within and is helped or hindered by the extramural pressure surrounding the heart (approximated by pleural pressure). Mean LA pressure (P_{LA}) closely approximates P_{LVED}, except at high filling pressures ($P_{LVED} > 20\,mm\,Hg$) or in the presence of mitral valve obstruction. In this upper range, atrial systole may boost P_{LVED} significantly above P_{LA}. In theory, the "a" wave of the LA tracing reflects the presystolic pressure generated by atrial contraction, which may considerably exceed the mean value when the ventricle is stiff. In practice, however, the low-fidelity P_w tracing does not allow for such distinctions. As a close estimate of mean P_{LA}, P_w is used clinically to judge the intracavitary filling pressure of the LV and thereby to monitor preload.

The other pressure determinant of precontractile fiber stretch, pleural pressure (P_{pl}), varies continuously throughout the respiratory cycle. Pulmonary wedge pressure must be interpreted cautiously, with attention directed toward the fluctuations in P_{pl}, which influence its transmural value. Although P_{pl} is seldom measured directly, changes in P_{pl} can be measured noninvasively with an esophageal balloon catheter. When the signal quality of the esophageal pressure (P_{es}) has been validated (e.g., by recording equivalent pressure deflections during spontaneous efforts against a transiently occluded airway), referencing P_w to esophageal pressure provides an acceptable monitor of changes in LV transmural pressure under most conditions, independent of P_{pl} fluctuation. Under the influence of mediastinal weight, the balloon senses only local pressure and measures neither absolute global pleural pressure nor the mean pressure that surrounds the entire LV. The fiber length achieved by any specific transmural pressure depends on ventricular compliance. Unfortunately, ventricular compliance

is rarely known with precision and can change abruptly. The LV and RV are made interdependent by sharing muscle fibers, the septum, and the pericardial sac. Thus, the LV can stiffen when the RV distends in response to changes in PVR or volume loading. Ischemia, inotropic drugs, and circulating catecholamines can also produce abrupt but reversible reductions in diastolic compliance. Shrinkage of RV chamber size, relief of ischemia, removal of adrenergic stimulation, and the administration of nitroglycerin or nitroprusside produce the opposite (muscle relaxing) effects.

A balloon flotation PA catheter is now available to track RV volume and ejection fraction by thermodilution. Reliable double indicator dilution (thermodilution/dye) systems for tracking central blood volume and lung water have also been developed that appear capable of rendering information of potential clinical and research value. The impact of both innovations on medical practice, however, remains modest.

Compensating for Elevated Pleural Pressure

Positive End-Expiratory Pressure Regardless of **4** the mode of chest inflation, end exhalation often provides a convenient reference point for P_w interpretation because during quiet breathing, P_{pl} normally returns to its resting baseline at that time. End-expiratory P_{pl} can exceed its normal value when the expiratory musculature actively contracts, tension pneumothorax is present, or elevated airway pressure at end exhalation increases lung volume (PEEP, auto-PEEP). If PEEP is intentionally applied and exhalation is passive, the relationship between the compliances of the lung (C_l) and chest wall (C_{cw}) determines the resulting elevation in pleural pressure:

$$\Delta P_{pl} = \Delta PEEP \times [C_l/(C_l + C_{cw})].$$

In the patient with normal lungs and chest wall, end-expiratory P_{pl} increases by approximately one half of the applied PEEP during passive inflation because C_l and C_{cw} are similar over the tidal volume range. However, under conditions of reduced lung compliance and normal chest wall compliance (e.g., many cases of ARDS), the "transmitted" fraction may be one quarter of the PEEP value or even less. Thus, if a PEEP of $14\,cm\,H_2O$ ($10\,mm$ Hg) is applied to the airways of a patient with ARDS, both P_{pl} and P_w at end exhalation should increase by approximately $2.5\,mm$ Hg. As discussed following, these simple rules of thumb cannot be applied during active expiratory efforts. Some clinicians seek to avoid confusion by transiently discontinuing PEEP and measuring P_w under conditions of ambient end-expiratory pressure. Because venous return usually increases when PEEP is interrupted, a low P_w measured off PEEP should indicate that intravascular filling pressures on PEEP are not excessive. Nonetheless, hemodynamic conditions often change rapidly and unpredictably after PEEP discontinuation, and a P_w in the middle or high range is of questionable value. When auto-PEEP is present, total PEEP, and therefore P_w, may not change noticeably after PEEP disconnection unless the next ventilatory breath is also delayed. Lengthy discontinuation of PEEP may also cause oxygenation to deteriorate significantly in some patients with severe lung injury or edema. A "recruiting maneuver" may be needed afterward to restore airway patency.

The lowest (nadir) wedge pressure obtained within 1 to 3 s of ventilator disconnection has been shown experimentally to reflect the transmural P_w that occurs on PEEP. It is believed that any tendency for increasing venous return during disconnection does not affect pressures in the pulmonary vasculature for several seconds. This principle is less likely to apply when the lung slowly deflates, as during dynamic hyperinflation in severe airflow obstruction. Although this technique has not been adequately validated in the clinical setting, its simplicity and theoretical rationale are attractive for use in well-selected patients.

Auto-PEEP (Intrinsic PEEP)   When insufficient time is allowed between the ventilatory cycles for the chest to deflate to its relaxed volume, airflow continues across critically narrowed airways throughout exhalation, driven by an alveolar pressure higher than airway opening pressure. This results in an occult "auto-PEEP" (intrinsic PEEP) effect at the alveolar level. Auto-PEEP is most likely to occur in patients with airflow obstruction who require high minute volumes, but because the endotracheal tube and exhalation valve are highly resistive elements, it can also develop at any time minute ventilation is significantly elevated—even in normal subjects. Inverse ratio ventilation and high frequency ventilation are other settings in which high levels of auto-PEEP can be encountered. Compliant lungs and stiff chest walls (e.g., obesity, burns, abdominal surgery, ascites) transmit a high percentage of alveolar pressure to the pleural space, producing large fractional increases in P_{pl} and P_w. In the setting of severe airflow obstruction, this is often half or more of the auto-PEEP value. Unless accounted for, auto-PEEP encourages overestimation of intravascular volume and inappropriate therapy. Although unmeasured during normal ventilator operation, the auto-PEEP level is detectable by the simple bedside maneuver of expiratory port occlusion at the end of passive exhalation (Fig. 2-9).

Active Exhalation   Active exhalation and chaotic breathing present other difficult problems in the interpretation of the wedge pressure. For spontaneously breathing patients with airflow obstruction, expiratory effort adds to the recorded auto-PEEP value. Vigorous expiratory muscle contraction often elevates end-expiratory P_{pl} during acute respiratory distress of any etiology. Large respiratory fluctuations of P_w (>10 mm Hg) should alert the clinician to this possibility. When the respiratory variation of P_w exceeds 10 mm Hg, the end-expiratory P_w exceeds the postparalysis value in direct (almost 1 for 1) proportion to the respiratory variation observed. During active breathing, the mean wedge pressure averaged over the entire tidal cycle

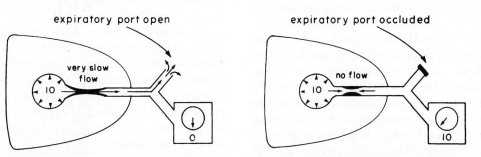

■ **FIGURE 2-9** The auto-PEEP effect and its measurement. In the presence of severe airflow obstruction and high ventilation requirements, alveolar pressure at end exhalation remains elevated as flow continues throughout expiration, driven by the recoil pressure of the hyperexpanded lung **(left)**. Transiently stopping flow at end exhalation equalizes pressure throughout the lung and ventilator circuit **(right)**. Occult alveolar pressure is then detectable by the ventilator.

may be a better indicator of the true ventricular filling pressure than the end-expiratory P_w when a reliable estimate of pleural pressure is not available. In theory, the effect of vigorous breathing can be overcome by simultaneously recording P_{es} or by giving short-acting muscle relaxants during the measurement. Silencing respiratory efforts, however, dramatically alters hemodynamic status and may mask any diastolic dysfunction that occurs under the stress (and increased LV afterload) of vigorous breathing. It does, however, give some indication of whether diuresis is indicated. A high P_w under passive conditions suggests the potential for hydrostatic edema during active breathing. Even when transmural P_w can be computed with certainty, effective preload is difficult to estimate without the knowledge of the myocardial pressure–volume relationship.

5   **Principle of Functional Monitoring**   It is always hazardous to infer the status of a dynamic system from a single number. The monitored "challenge" is a key maneuver in determining hemodynamic reserves and should be conducted using information from as many monitoring methods as are readily available—physical examination, vital signs, ECHO, as well as directly monitored intravascular pressures and flows. Challenging may involve reversible noninvasive maneuvers (e.g., PEEP, measurement of pulse pressure variation of BP with the respiratory cycle, or leg lifting), rapid fluid bolusing or diuresis, and/or inotrope administration.

The Fluid Challenge   Uncertainty concerning LV compliance is a major reason why absolute P_w values do not track LV volume or preload accurately in the setting of critical illness. Except when the calculated transmural P_w is very high or very low, decisions regarding fluid therapy of a patient in an oxygenation or perfusion crisis are often best made by an empirical trial of rapid volume loading (a fluid challenge). Pulmonary wedge pressure, systemic BP, CO, heart rate, and the physical examination are monitored before and after a rapid infusion of physiologic saline or colloid. A fluid bolus (250 to 500 mL) is administered over 5 to 20 min, depending on the suspected cardiovascular fragility of the patient. If hemodynamic variables improve with little change in the measured P_w, administration of additional volume is prudent. Conversely, marked increases of heart rate or P_w (>5 to 7 mm Hg), together with marginal improvement in BP and CO, indicate that increasing the rate of volume infusion risks pulmonary edema with little hemodynamic benefit.

Cardiac Output Determination

Measurement

Fick Principle   In its simplest form, the primary basis for CO determination, the Fick principle, can be explained as follows. The quantity of any marker contained within a static volume is the product of that volume and its concentration. Classically, a dye detectable by spectrophotometry (e.g., indocyanine or "cardio" green) that binds to plasma protein has been used as the indicator. In a dynamic system into which a marker is continuously added and lost, the introduction rate of the marker is the product of flow rate and its concentration difference across the region of loss. In the steady state, no net addition or loss of the marker occurs. For example, if arterial oxygen is being consumed by the body and replenished by the lungs at equal rates, the $\dot{V}O_2$ is the product of CO and the O_2 concentration difference between systemic arterial and mixed venous (PA) blood. Therefore, if the O_2 consumption rate is known or readily estimated, determining the O_2 contents in systemic and PA blood samples allows calculation of the flow rate (CO). Under non–steady-state conditions, however, these calculations can be wildly erroneous.

Thermodilution   A similar principle applies during determinations of CO by thermodilution, where the marker that is injected and dissipated is thermal deficit, or "cold," and its rate of disappearance as it is diluted by the warm venous blood is an indication of blood flow. Although all PA catheters can provide a sample of mixed-venous blood for use in an oxygen-Fick determination, thermodilution capability allows more convenient, repeatable, and precise measurement of forward blood flow. A sensitive, rapidly responding thermistor bonded to the catheter tip continuously senses temperature, altering its electrical resistance in response to thermal changes within PA blood. As a side benefit, the thermistor provides a highly reliable, continuous readout of core body temperature. When a bolus of cooler, room temperature fluid enters the right atrium (RA), it mixes with warm venous blood returning from the periphery. The churning action of the RV homogenizes the two fluids, and the thermistor records the dynamic thermal curve generated when the mixture washes past the proximal PA. The relationship linking output to temperature is the Stewart–Hamilton formula:

$$\dot{Q} = V\,(T_B - T_I)\,K_1\,K_2/\!\int T_B\,(t)\,dt$$

where $\dot{Q}$ = CO; V = injected volume; T_B = blood temperature; T_I = injectate temperature; $T_B(t)dt$ = change in blood temperature as a function of time; and K_1 and K_2 are computational constants. The components of the numerator are either known constants (V, K_1, K_2) or measured values (T_B, T_I). The denominator is the area beneath the time–temperature curve, derived by computer integration of the thermistor signal. When close attention is paid to the method of data acquisition, thermodilution CO values compare favorably with those obtained by the steady-state O_2 Fick method and by dye dilution.

Technical Considerations and Potential Errors

Thermistor Position   Except for a few rather obvious exceptions, most technical errors in CO determination result in overestimation of the true value. To generate a valid estimate of output, the thermistor should sample a well-mixed cold charge of known strength and must lie freely within the lumen of the central PA. Impaction against a vessel wall or encapsulation by clot tends to insulate the thermistor from the cool stream, falsely elevating the reported value. A P_{PA} waveform that appears damped or wedged may indicate malpositioning and potential problems. It is a good clinical practice to inspect the temperature–time profile periodically, especially when the value conflicts with the rest of the clinical picture, extreme variability is encountered among serial estimates, or another question of temperature accuracy exists. A valid curve shows a rapid early descent to a trough value, smoothly returning to baseline within 10 to 15 s of injection. Distorted curves should alert the clinician to inadequate blending of injectate with blood, thermistor contact with the wall of the vessel, abnormal respiratory patterns, and arrhythmias or abrupt changes in heart rate. Information from irregular curves should be discarded.

Injectate Volume and Temperature   Icing the injectate accentuates the thermal difference between marker and blood, increasing the signal strength. Although icing theoretically enhances output accuracy and reproducibility, the excellent sensitivity of the thermistor/computer systems currently available allows the use of room temperature injectates without appreciable loss of accuracy. Room temperature injectates do not require the 45-min equilibration period necessary to complete cooling, maintenance of proper injectate temperature is facilitated, and errors induced by rewarming during handling are minimized. Although 10-mL injectate volumes are often used with room temperature injectates, 5-mL volumes (with

appropriate computer adjustment) can be used with acceptable results when frequent measurements introduce a significant danger of volume overload. Seriously hypothermic patients, however, require the larger volume for an acceptable signal-to-background ratio. Whatever volume is chosen for injection, syringes should be filled carefully; variation in injected volume contributes significantly to measurement error. The crystalloid fluid chosen for injection—saline or dextrose—does not materially influence the output calculation. When completed within 4 s, the speed of injection has little influence on outcome; automated, gas-powered injectors offer no convincing advantage over manual technique.

Respiratory Variation   The temperature of PA blood tends to vary throughout the respiratory cycle, particularly during mechanical ventilation. Although it has been suggested that injection be timed to begin consistently at a single point in the ventilatory cycle, the need for this practice is controversial. One logical compromise is to obtain at least three injections spaced equally along the respiratory cycle, averaging the results.

Catheter–Computer Mismatch   Coefficients vary widely with the volume and temperature of the injectate and the type of catheter used. Mismatching should be suspected when measured CO does not fit well with the clinical picture, particularly when catheters of varied manufacture are used with the same computer.

Tricuspid Regurgitation   The computer integrates the volume under the temperature–time curve assuming unidirectional flow, no loss of signal amplitude, and no delay in signal detection. Tricuspid regurgitation, which occurs very commonly in acute cardiopulmonary disorders, can violate one or more of these assumptions, leading either to overestimation or underestimation of the true value. Such artifacts should be suspected when the value seems discordant with the remainder of the database or when there is a sudden and otherwise unexplained change in measured output.

Anatomical Variation   Thermodilution values for CO are usually accurate when computational constants are correctly entered, the catheter is well positioned, and appropriate injection technique is utilized. However, such non–operator-dependent variables as intracardiac shunting, incompetence of the tricuspid valve, and thermistor malfunction due to thermal shielding by wall contact or clot may compromise validity. Errors can also result from inadvertent augmentation of the cold charge by concomitant rapid administration of intravenous fluids near the RA.

Ejection Fraction, Ventricular Volume, and "Continuous" Cardiac Output Determinations Historically, the episodic injection of cool liquid has been used to implement thermodilution technique. When a modified PA catheter is fitted with a rapid-response thermistor and electrodes for sensing and gating beat-to-beat changes in temperature, good estimates for RV ejection fraction (RVEF) can be made. With estimates for CO, stroke volume, and RVEF in hand, RV volume can then be calculated. Some authors consider the latter to be a more reliable indicator of preload status and fluid responsiveness than pressure-based measures, but this remains controversial.

Another thermal-based approach is to inject small quantities of heat at the RA/RV level using a resistance element. Blood temperature is monitored near the catheter tip a short distance downstream. This method serves as the basis for near-continuous measurement of CO, RV stroke volume, and chamber volume estimation. Data from these instruments appear to agree well with those from conventional thermodilution techniques.

Minimally Invasive Nonthermal Methods for Cardiac Output Determination Although thermodilution remains well entrenched as the standard for CO estimation, needs often arise for gathering such data without invasive catheterization. Several interesting methods that do not require central vascular access have been recently introduced into practice: noninvasive expired carbon dioxide analysis, lithium dilution, esophageal Doppler, pulse contour analysis, and thoracic electrical bioimpedance all have physiologic rationales and limitations for applications in intensive care (Table 2-4). The expired CO_2 method tracks the rate of CO_2 excretion during partial rebreathing, which is proportional to the pulmonary blood flow and the product of the arteriovenous difference in CO_2 content. Estimates for VCO_2 and for arterial CO_2 content can be made from the exhaled gas profile, and rebreathing eliminates the need for mixed-venous CO_2 content measurement. At the present time, this method requires an intubated patient under approximately steady-state metabolic conditions. Its accuracy is questionable when PCO_2 is not linearly related to content ($PaCO_2 < 30$ mm Hg) and in settings where seriously diseased lungs generate a large right- to-left shunt fraction.

CO by lithium dilution requires venous injection of lithium chloride and peripheral measurement of its concentration in a small sample of arterial blood. Such values appear to correlate well with traditional thermodilution estimates. Pulse contour analysis is based on the concept that the arterial pulse waveform is influenced by stroke volume, which can be estimated as the integral of the end-diastolic to end-systolic pressure divided by the aortic impedance. The latter requires knowledge of CO determined by another method (e.g., lithium dilution). Once calibrated, however, pulse contour analysis tracks CO changes with acceptable accuracy. Thoracic electrical bioimpedance, the least interventional of any of these methods, measures the resistance of the thorax to a high-frequency, very low magnitude current applied using multiple thoracic electrodes. Because impedance is inversely proportional to fluid content, changes in CO are reflected as changes in conductivity. This method is influenced by fluid content unrelated to CO and, therefore, is not sufficiently accurate for absolute CO determinations in the severely ill. Arterial pulse contour analysis is another useful flow monitoring technology that is gaining adherents for some critical care applications. Unfortunately, its sensitivity is impaired in low flow and arrhythmic states. Finally, esophageal Doppler methodology requires placement of a Doppler probe in close proximity to the descending aorta, where it can assess aortic cross-sectional area and blood flow velocity. Multiple estimates and approximations are needed, and though it is likely to give good trending information, its accuracy for absolute CO determinations and its long-term reliability remain questionable for applications in critical care.

Conceptual Advantages and Limitations of Noninvasive Cardiac Output Measurements CO is of utmost value in classifying patients with regard to cardiac compromise and in assessing responses to therapy. In mildly to moderately ill patients, noninvasive measurements are acceptably accurate and may serve each purpose admirably if they are combined with other information gathered from the physical examination, clinical laboratory, ECHO, and measurements of central venous oxygen saturation (see following). For certain purposes (e.g., qualitatively following the response to vasoactive

---

TABLE 2-4 MINIMALLY INVASIVE CARDIAC OUTPUT DETERMINATION

- Expired CO_2 (modified Fick) analysis
- Lithium dilution
- Esophageal Doppler
- Arterial pulse contour analysis
- Thoracic bio-impedance

agents or fluid loading), trending data may be helpful even when precision is compromised by serious illness or refusal of the patient to undergo invasive instrumentation. Yet, in most seriously ill patients, these methods do not substitute for a well-functioning PA catheter, which offers the more complete and accurate set of data needed to acquire an integrated picture of the patient's hemodynamic status.

Clinical Interpretation of Cardiac Output   Important diagnostic information can often be obtained regarding the functional status of the heart and the vasculature by combining measures of CO and ventricular filling pressure. The fluid challenge is particularly helpful for this purpose. However, CO must be interpreted in relation to the mass and the metabolism of the patient. A CO of 3 L/min may suffice for the needs of a hypothermic, cachectic 40-kg patient, but the same CO may be associated with a circulatory crisis in a previously healthy 100-kg burn victim. The cardiac index (CI, CO/surface area) attempts to adjust for variations in tissue mass. Body surface area (BSA) can be determined from standard nomograms or can be approximated by this regression equation:

$$BSA = 0.202 \times wt^{0.425} \times ht^{0.725}$$

where BSA is expressed in square meters, weight (wt) in kilograms, and height (ht) in meters. Used alone, however, even the CI is of limited help in assessing perfusion adequacy. Over a broad range, any given value for CI may be associated with luxuriant, barely adequate, or suboptimal tissue O_2 transport, depending on hemoglobin concentration, metabolic requirements, and blood flow distribution. Measures of urine output and metabolic acid production (anion gap, serum lactate) together with indices of tissue O_2 utilization (e.g., O_2 extraction) provide better guides of perfusion adequacy.

Indices of Vascular Resistance   The CO measurement can be used in conjunction with pulmonary and systemic pressure measurements to compute the vascular resistance values needed to gauge ventricular afterload and diagnose the etiology of a hypotensive crisis. These indices of vascular resistance complement the mean systemic BP in guiding vasodilator and vasopressor therapy. PVR and SVR are crude indices, calculated as if blood flow fulfilled the assumptions of Poiseuille's law for laminar flow:

$$PVR = (P_{\overline{PA}} - P_w)/CO \text{ and } SVR = (MAP - P_{RA})/CO$$

where CO = cardiac output, MAP = mean systemic arterial pressure, $P_{\overline{PA}}$ = mean PA pressure, and P_{RA} = mean right atrial pressure.

Although PVR and SVR are commonly used in the clinical setting, vascular resistance calculations should preferably be referenced to BSA, using the CI (instead of CO). The resulting values, the systemic (SVRI) and pulmonary (PVRI) indices, avoid the misleading variations of the raw parameters with body size. Significant elevations of PVRI virtually always indicate underlying lung pathology, reflecting the interplay of constrictive and occlusive forces on a compromised pulmonary capillary bed. Unfortunately, however, the complex relation between PVR and CO often confounds physiologic interpretation. Changes in the PVRI should be evaluated with full awareness that the PVRI is output dependent. In computing PVR, keep in mind that when the pulmonary vascular bed is compromised, resistance may vary as a function of blood flow. In fact, the magnitude of PVR, as well as its response to an intentional change in CO, may serve as a useful prognostic index in such acute lung diseases as ARDS (Fig. 2-10). Failure of PVR to rise in response to a boost in CO suggests ample reserve; a sharp increase in PVR that parallels CO indicates extensive obliteration of the pulmonary vascular bed. SVR may rise homeostatically to high values in support of suboptimal CO, helping to maintain an appropriate perfusion pressure across vital capillary beds. However, an excessive elevation of SVR can impair the performance of weakened LV. It should be kept firmly in mind that an error in CO might dramatically alter the computations of vascular resistance and thereby misdirect classification or management of the clinical problem.

Oxygen Delivery   CO data find one of their most useful applications in the management of hypoxemia. Because tissues attempt to extract the amount of oxygen required to maintain aerobic metabolism, the mixed-venous O_2 tension falls when O_2 delivery (the product of CO and arterial O_2 content) becomes insufficient for tissue needs. If the fraction of venous blood shunted past the lung remains unchanged, arterial O_2 tension may fall precipitously as this abnormally desaturated blood is blended with postcapillary blood from better ventilated lung units. Thus, depressed CO values may contribute to hypoxemia, and variations in CO may sometimes explain the otherwise puzzling changes in arterial O_2 tension. As a primary determinant of O_2 delivery, CO measurements often prove helpful during selection of the appropriate

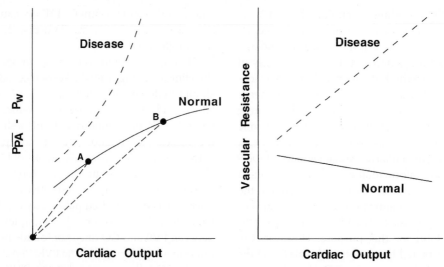

■ **FIGURE 2-10** Relationship of CO to the pressure difference driving the flow across the pulmonary vasculature ($P_{\overline{PA}} - P_w$) and PVR. The relationship of $P_{\overline{PA}} - P_w$ to CO does not pass through the origin so that computed values of PVR (the slope of this relationship) appear to fall as CO rises in normal subjects. In disease, the relationship of driving pressure to flow is highly curvilinear, and, therefore, PVR may appear unchanged or rising. Calculating PVR on the basis of *changes* in ($P_{\overline{PA}} - P_w$) and CO helps to eliminate these interpretive difficulties.

PEEP level for the patient with life-threatening hypoxemia. Depression of venous return coincident with PEEP application may nullify any beneficial effect of improved pulmonary gas exchange on tissue O_2 delivery (see Chapter 9).

A rational goal of resuscitative therapy of severe sepsis and shock is to restore balance between oxygen delivery and demand. Boosting CO is fundamental to such an approach. Aggressive goal-oriented resuscitation in the earliest phase of management appears to improve mortality, whereas the literature is inconclusive as to which patients in other clinical settings benefit from raising CO to normal or (when possible) to supranormal values. Whatever the value of such strategies, the Swan–Ganz catheter enables sampling of three useful measures: CO, RA, and mixed venous oxygen saturations.

Sampling of Central Venous and Mixed-Venous Blood

Oxygen Supply and Demand

6 Analysis of mixed-venous blood provides valuable information in evaluating the oxygen supply–demand axis. Blood flow to individual organs (e.g., the kidneys) is not precisely governed by metabolic rate, so venous O_2 content varies widely among sites. Normally, blood from the inferior vena cava (IVC) is more fully saturated than is blood from the

SVC. During shock states, however, the converse is often true. Samples drawn from either of these central vessels or from the incompletely blended pool within the RA are not entirely representative of the true mixed-venous value. Blood withdrawn from the proximal PA, however, has been blended in the RV and is therefore more appropriate for analysis. Care should be taken to withdraw blood slowly, with the balloon deflated and the catheter tip positioned in the proximal PA. Otherwise, contamination from the postcapillary region may artifactually increase the oxygen content.

Although it is generally acknowledged that the saturation of blood withdrawn from the SVC will differ somewhat from the mixed-venous value, the differences are not usually great, and the need to access the PA has been questioned when trending is the key concern and early resuscitation with adequate fluid volumes is the priority. For example, using repeated (or continuously recorded) saturations from a CVP catheter may allow timely assessment of fluid resuscitation adequacy under emergent circumstances, as in severe sepsis and shock. Even though its value has been documented in the latter condition, it remains debatable whether this approach offers parallel benefit in other resuscitation settings.

The value of mixed-venous blood analysis is best understood in the framework of tissue O_2

demand–supply dynamics. Briefly, the product of CO and arterial oxygen content defines the overall rate of O_2 delivery. Each organ receives a variable percentage of the total amount, a flow that may be luxuriant, just adequate, or insufficient to satisfy its aerobic metabolic demand. The O_2 tension (PvO_2) and saturation (SvO_2) of the venous effluent reflect the balance between supply and need. When flow does not rise to meet increased tissue demands, more O_2 is extracted from each milliliter of capillary blood, and PvO_2 and SvO_2 fall. Conversely, when the O_2 transport/demand ratio increases, the arteriovenous oxygen difference narrows and PvO_2 and SvO_2 rise. PvO_2 and SvO_2 may not reflect serious perfusion deficits if arterial blood is anatomically or functionally shunted past metabolizing tissue. For example, in cirrhosis, cyanide poisoning, or the early phases of sepsis, nonnutritive flow may cause SvO_2 to be normal or high, despite serious tissue hypoxia. Because of these distribution and utilization pitfalls, it is always wise to compute the anion gap and monitor lactate simultaneously. Low venous O_2 tensions, when sustained, more reliably signal anemia or an impending perfusion crisis. Reduced flow and diminished arterial O_2 concentration (due to reductions in SaO_2 or hemoglobin) depress the effective O_2 transport, encouraging lower values for PvO_2 and SvO_2.

Uses and Limits of Mixed-Venous O_2 Saturation

The mixed-venous oxygen saturation correlates with survival in acute myocardial infarction, acute respiratory failure, and shock. As O_2 delivery is reduced from the normal level without a matching change in O_2 demand, tissues initially compensate by maintaining oxygen consumption ($\dot{V}O_2$) at the expense of a falling SvO_2 (Fig. 2-11) (i.e., from tissue oxygen extraction ratio: $SaO_2 - SvO_2/SaO_2$). However, beyond a certain critical value of O_2 delivery, the O_2 extraction mechanism reaches the limits of compensation, SvO_2 stabilizes, and $\dot{V}O_2$ becomes delivery dependent. Once this critical value is reached, SvO_2 becomes an insensitive monitor of changes in perfusion. Such delivery dependence has been demonstrated both in experimental animal models of acute lung injury and in certain clinical settings. Below this critical value of O_2 delivery, anaerobic metabolism must supplement aerobic mechanism. The SvO_2 at which this limit

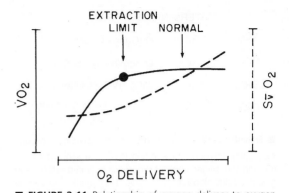

■ **FIGURE 2-11** Relationship of oxygen delivery to oxygen consumption ($\dot{V}O_2$) and to the saturation of mixed-venous blood ($S\bar{v}O_2$). As oxygen delivery is reduced from the normal value (e.g., by reducing CO), all the metabolic demands remain unchanged. Increased extraction can initially maintain oxygen consumption at the cost of a falling $S\bar{v}O_2$. At some critical level of oxygen delivery, the limits of extraction are reached, forcing $\dot{V}O_2$ to become delivery dependent.

occurs varies, depending on whether the delivery was reduced by anemia, arterial hypoxemia, or falling CO.

Despite the importance of PvO_2 as a global indicator of end-capillary tissue O_2 tension, PvO_2 can vary with alterations in the affinity of hemoglobin for O_2, even when O_2 content remains stable. Therefore, direct assessment of SvO_2 is the preferred index for clinically evaluating the oxygen-perfusion axis; estimation of SvO_2 from PvO_2, pH, and temperature is fraught with error due to the steepness of the O_2 tension–saturation relationship. Traditionally, SvO_2 has been determined on individual blood samples analyzed by laboratory instruments that measure SaO_2 by transmission oximetry (co-oximeter) or O_2 content by fuel cell determination. The application of fiberoptic reflectance oximetry to the balloon flotation catheter has enabled continuous bedside monitoring of SvO_2. O_2 saturation rises when blood is withdrawn past the wedged fiberoptic tip, facilitating the distinction between wedged and damped P_{PA} tracings. This feature may also help avoid tissue infarction consequent to inadvertent distal migration of the catheter. Continuous measurement of SvO_2 also speeds the process of determining the optimal PEEP level because alterations in net tissue O_2 flux are made quickly apparent.

Changes in SvO_2 have no unique interpretation and must be viewed in light of the variables that determine O_2 transport and demand—the amount

DETERMINANTS OF $S\bar{v}O_2$

$$\dot{V}O_2 \quad = \quad \dot{Q}\,(C_aO_2 - C_{\bar{v}}O_2)$$

$$\dot{V}O_2 \quad \alpha \quad \dot{Q}\,Hgb\,(SaO_2 - S\bar{v}O_2)$$

$$S\bar{v}O_2 \quad \alpha \quad SaO_2 - (\dot{V}O_2/\dot{Q}Hgb)$$

$$S\bar{v}O_2 \quad \alpha \quad SaO_2 - \left(\frac{O_2\,Consumption}{O_2\,Delivery}\right)$$

■ **FIGURE 2-12** Determinants of mixed-venous oxygen saturation. Oxygen consumption ($\dot{V}O_2$) is a product of CO ($\dot{Q}$) and the oxygen content difference between arterial and mixed-venous blood ($C_AO_2 - S\bar{v}O_2$). Hemoglobin concentration (Hgb) and saturation (SaO_2, $S\bar{v}O_2$) determine the blood oxygen content. Therefore, the saturation of mixed-venous blood ($S\bar{v}O_2$) is determined by four interacting variables: a decrease in $S\bar{v}O_2$ can be caused by reductions in SaO_2, $\dot{Q}$, or Hgb or by an increase in $\dot{V}O_2$. Changes in any one of these determinants can be nullified by an offsetting change in another. For example, if metabolism changes, $\dot{V}O_2$ and $\dot{Q}$ can fall or rise in proportion to one another, leaving $S\bar{v}O_2$ unchanged.

and distribution of CO, hemoglobin concentration and function, arterial O_2 tension, and metabolic rate. Although a change in SvO_2 does not indicate which of the multiple factors comprising the Fick equation is responsible, integration of SvO_2 with clinical observations, blood gas information, and CO data often establishes an early, if presumptive, diagnosis (Fig. 2-12). Declining values for SvO_2 and CO, together with unchanging PaO_2, imply hemodynamic deterioration, whereas a rising CO with a falling SvO_2 are consistent with increased metabolic demand or acute loss of circulating blood. Initial experience with the fiberoptic catheter as an online monitor has underscored the rapidity with which SvO_2 responds to transient changes in metabolism or altered O_2 delivery. Sensitivity to such changes is undoubtedly enhanced when the heart is unable to raise its output sufficiently in response to stress. Then, SvO_2 must reflect altered arterial oxygenation or increased O_2 demand, undampened by the buffering effect of cardiac compensation. Such wide fluctuations may help explain why SaO_2 often varies markedly in the absence of convincing clinical improvement or deterioration. From initial clinical experience, it appears that SvO_2 often falls in advance of detectable changes in the primary hemodynamic variables, and a downward trend may alert the clinician to intervene. A decline in SvO_2 may be the first indication of occult bleeding,

incipient pump failure, or impending cardiac arrest. Conversely, an increasing SvO_2 may signal the onset of sepsis. A growing literature documents rapid and convincing changes in SvO_2 accompanying drug therapy (vasopressors, vasodilators, sedatives), intravascular volume manipulation (diuresis, fluid infusion, transfusion), position shifts, and ventilatory changes. Although fiberoptic oximetry has a distinct physiologic rationale and appears to be a useful adjunct to PA catheterization, the clinical value of these instruments is still debated.

Gastric Mucosal pH

In recent years, there has been waning enthusiasm for monitoring the pH of the gastric mucosa (gastric tonometry) as an indicator of hypoperfusion. Unlike skeletal muscle, the intestinal tract tolerates hypoxemia poorly, so the gastric mucosal pH may provide an index of oxygenation in a region of the body that is among the first to initiate anaerobiosis during hypoperfusion and the last to restore normal perfusion after resuscitation. When conditions are favorable, equilibration appears to be established between luminal and mucosal PCO_2. When bicarbonate concentrations are known, intramucosal pH can therefore be calculated from the tonometrically measured PCO_2 of the saline within the balloon. These assumptions cannot be made with confidence, however, if acid enters and bicarbonate refluxes from the duodenum, the patient receives enteral feeding that refluxes into the stomach, or the stomach is continuously aspirated by a sump tube.

Despite its considerable potential as a sentinel index of dysoxic stress, however, its widespread use cannot be recommended. Appropriate interpretation, limitations, and relative advantages of this technique over more standard management practices for assessing perfusion adequacy are still being investigated and debated.

Complications of the Pulmonary Artery Catheter

Apart from any harm caused by errors in the acquisition or interpretation of data, the complications of PA catheterization arise during insertion, during manipulation of the catheter, and as a result of its residence within the central vascular structures (Table 2-5).

TABLE 2-5 COMPLICATIONS OF THE PULMONARY ARTERY CATHETER

COMPLICATION	CAUSE	PREVENTION
Arrhythmia	Catheter coiling or excess catheter in RV	ECG monitoring
	Catheter tip reentry into RV from PA	Follow the "rule of 20s"
		Expedient catheter passage
	Hypoxemia, coronary ischemia, electrolyte disturbances	Reverse hypoxemia, electrolyte disturbances
		Prophylaxis vs. ischemia
Complete heart block	Preexisting left bundle branch block	Temporary pacer on standby
Catheter malpositioning		
Extracardiac	Forceful insertion	Advance only with caution
		Consider fluoroscopy
Catheter knotting	Excessive catheter length	Follow the "rule of 20s"
	Extensive manipulation	Do not insert >15 cm into the PA
	Dilated heart	Consider fluoroscopy in difficult cases
		Inflate balloon fully during insertion
Catheter fragmentation and meteorism	Forceful insertion or removal	Avoid forceful catheter insertion or withdrawal
	Withdrawal across needle	Follow recommended instructions for insertion
	Cutting catheters for wire exchanges	Avoid cutting catheter during exchanges
Pulmonary infarction	Persistent wedging of a distally positioned catheter	Wedge with maximal balloon volume (1.25–1.5 mL)
	Prolonged balloon occlusion	Maintain catheter tip in the main PA
		Maintain balloon occlusion for a maximum of 15 s
		Catheter withdrawal if persistent wedge or damped PA tracing
		Recheck tracings carefully 30–60 min after insertion and after patient repositioning
		Ensure balloon deflation post wedging
PA rupture	Catheter advancement with uninflated balloon	Advance catheter only with balloon inflated
	Balloon inflation and distal PA	Slowly inflate to wedge position only with continuous PA monitoring
	Eccentric balloon inflation	Stop inflation immediately when PA pressure rises or falls significantly during occlusion
	Balloon inflation with liquid	Limit wedge measurement to 15 s
	Pulmonary hypertension	Do not flush distal lumen when wedged
		Maintain catheter in central PA
		Position catheter to accept >1.25 mL for wedge
		Inflate balloon only with air
		Minimize the number of wedge pressures attempted

(continued)

TABLE 2-5 COMPLICATIONS OF THE PULMONARY ARTERY CATHETER *(Continued)*

COMPLICATION	CAUSE	PREVENTION
Thrombosis	Predisposition to clotting	Continuous flush
		Limited duration of catheter placement
Vascular infection	Prolonged catheterization (>72–96 h)	Remove catheter when no longer needed
		Strict attention to sterile technique
		Frequent inspection of insertion site
		Remove catheter if persistent fever or bacteremia detected

Insertion-Related Complications

Catheter-Related Arrhythmias

Premature atrial and ventricular contractions commonly occur during insertion of the Swan–Ganz catheter, especially when the patient is predisposed to them. Failure to inflate the balloon adequately, slow passage of the catheter through the heart, and insertion of an excessive length of catheter are likely contributors. Special caution should be exercised if the patient is hypoxemic or has an electrolyte disturbance at the time of instrumentation. Complete heart block has been reported to follow the insertion of the PA catheter in patients with preexisting conductor system disease, as transient right bundle branch block occurs commonly during this procedure. Although the risk is probably not as great as once feared, it is advisable to have a temporary pacemaker available prior to inserting the catheter in a patient with preexisting left bundle branch block.

Catheter Malpositioning

Experience is the most important determinant of successful catheter placement. Although often difficult and time consuming, vascular access should never require forceful insertion. The clinician must be thoroughly familiar with the pressure tracings that arise from the various cardiovascular structures encountered and be aware of departures from the "rule of progressive 20s" (see Fig. 2-2).

Knotting and Fragmentation

Catheter knotting can occur, especially when the catheter is extensively manipulated, an excessive length is inserted, the heart is dilated, or the balloon is not inflated during passage. Knotting is most likely to be detected upon attempted catheter withdrawal. The same is true for catheter fragmentation and meteorism (embolization of catheter fragments). Care to avoid forceful insertion or removal, withdrawal of the catheter through a needle, and cutting of the catheter during wire exchanges will generally prevent this serious complication.

Pulmonary Infarction

Pulmonary infarction is distressingly common. Persistent wedging of the catheter tip and the dislodgement of clot formed on the catheter are the most likely explanations. Infarction occurs rarely when the catheter is well positioned (tip within the main PA) and the balloon requires its maximum volume (1.25 to 1.5 mL) for inflation to the wedge position.

Pulmonary Artery Rupture

PA rupture can cause fatal hemoptysis. Several factors predispose PA perforation: advanced age, hypothermia, and pulmonary hypertension. Women are disproportionately represented. Overinflation of a catheter balloon in a small PA is the most likely mechanism. Therefore, the balloon should never be inflated abruptly, and inflation should be stopped immediately when there is evidence either of the approach to the wedge position or of overwedging. Advancing the catheter tip without balloon inflation should never be undertaken.

Although a variety of therapeutic measures have been suggested, such as the application of PEEP, deliberate balloon inflation, and positioning with the catheter with its tip side down, their efficacy is not proven. Maintenance of the airway and support of the circulation are the first priorities as for any patient with severe hemoptysis. It seems prudent not to deflate the balloon until definitive therapy is imminent.

Complications Related to Long-Term Catheterization

Thrombosis

Although thrombosis about the catheter at its insertion site or at various points along the catheter occurs very commonly, serious consequences are not commonly encountered. Yet, thrombosis at or near the insertion site may result in subclavian vein thrombosis, superior vena caval syndrome, or internal jugular vein occlusion. The indwelling catheter may also result in platelet consumption, pulmonary emboli, or right-sided valvular damage. These complications seldom rise to the level of clinical significance in most patients.

Infection

Any indwelling catheter may produce serious infection. The PA occlusion catheter is no exception. With strict attention to sterile insertion technique, meticulous care of all catheter lines, stopcocks, transducers, and infusions should be taken; most PA catheters can be used for more than 72 h without serious infectious complications. The incidence of infection tends to rise thereafter. If the local site looks uninflamed and the patient remains afebrile, a catheter can remain in place for 5 days or more without serious risk. Many practitioners, however, change PA catheters at approximately 96 h, but there is no set standard in this regard.

Whenever the patient is febrile or septic, blood cultures should be obtained and the catheter removed if it appears to be the most likely source. Assuming that the local site does not appear infected, some practitioners insert a fresh PA catheter without changing the site of insertion. This practice, however, is controversial. Should the local site appear suspicious, the introducer must be removed along with the catheter, and a fresh site is selected—assuming that the catheter is still required.

■ ECHOCARDIOGRAPHY, RADIONUCLIDE VENTRICULOGRAPHY, AND OTHER IMAGING TECHNIQUES

Neither ECHO nor radionuclide ventriculography (RVG) provides continuous information and therefore cannot properly be considered true monitoring techniques. Yet, each has an important place in characterizing the nature of cardiac pathology in the intensive care unit (ICU). These methods allow the physician to answer specific diagnostic questions and to categorize the overall structure and performance of the heart as well as to estimate chamber dimensions. In a sense, they can be considered complementary to central venous, pulmonary and systemic and arterial monitoring.

Echocardiography

General Principles

ECHO provides a valuable bedside method for the noninvasive assessment of cardiac function. The ECHO probe both emits a high frequency (1 to 10 MHz), rapidly pulsed ultrasonic signal and receives its acoustic reflection. These data are then integrated to form an interpretable image. Appropriate contrast agents often enhance the sonic differentiation of anatomic structure. Three different ECHO techniques have been introduced into clinical practice: (a) M-mode, which provides a one-dimensional (1D) view of the heart; (b) real-time or sector scanning, in which a two-dimensional (2D), dynamic view is produced; and (c) Doppler ECHO, a technique to quantify blood flow velocity and direction and estimate intravascular pressures. The ejection fraction and wall motion symmetry of the LV can be adequately approximated, but RV performance is less reliably assessed because of its irregular (noncylindrical) geometry. Color kinesis (color flow) aids in regional wall motion assessment and in determining reflux across valvular structures. Transesophageal echocardiography (TEE) provides very high resolution images of previously difficult-to-examine regions of the heart and has given good cardiac images in patients in whom transthoracic (surface) ECHO is severely limited (e.g., obese, hyperinflated). ECHO is noninvasive, inexpensive, rapidly performed, and diagnostic in a wide variety of valvular, myocardial, and pericardial disorders. Ambiguity, limited resolution, and interpreter error are its most important limitations. Inferences regarding

7

three-dimensional (3D) structures (e.g., ejection fraction) are made from data collected in 2D format. Because the ultrasound signal is attenuated by fat and reflected by air-tissue boundaries, transthoracic ECHO is of limited value in patients with obesity or obstructive lung disease. Chest wall deformities, dressings, and occlusive coverings often prevent optimal transducer positioning. TEE may require ventilatory support in patients with cardiorespiratory failure. Skilled technical support and an experienced interpreter are essential for optimal results.

Types of Echocardiogram

M-Mode Echocardiography

M-mode ECHO provides a 1D "ice pick" view through the heart, forming images from sound reflected along the narrow axis of the beam. M-mode examines the movements of a well-defined tissue core over time. It is well suited to detecting subtleties of motion, such as those needed to detect the severity and significance of impaired ventricular relaxation ("diastolic dysfunction"). Broad structures lying perpendicular to the ECHO axis reflect the acoustic beam efficiently and are well delineated. The anterior and posterior ventricular walls, intraventricular septum, aortic root, and valve leaflets (particularly the anterior mitral valve) are represented clearly. Conversely, the pulmonic and tricuspid valves are more difficult to visualize; thickening, vegetations, or abnormal motions of the aortic and mitral valve are frequently detected whereas those of the pulmonic or tricuspid valves are often missed. Because only a single axis or view can be obtained at any particular instant, M-mode is distinctly inferior to real-time 2D ECHO for detecting valve or wall motion abnormalities. M-mode usually allows accurate measurement of isolated chamber dimensions, but its narrow sampling window may not accurately reflect the anatomy of the entire atrium or ventricle. Similarly, loculated pericardial effusions, pleural fluid collections contiguous to the pericardial surface, and small intraventricular defects may be missed entirely.

Two-Dimensional Echocardiography

2D (real-time) ECHO is the best technique for examining ventricular wall and valve motion. Because 2D ECHO provides a wider field of view than M-mode, any process localized to a segment of the pericardium or myocardium is better seen (e.g., loculated pericardial fluid, small ventricular septal defects, and small LV aneurysms). Diastolic as well

as systolic performance of the left heart (and to a lesser extent, the right heart) can be evaluated. Color-flow Doppler units allow qualitative assessment of the directionality of blood flow across valves—a vital advantage when assessing valvular performance. 2D ECHO is an invaluable technique for assessing the *relative* performance of the two ventricles, and when a regurgitant tricuspid leak is present, as it very often is when the RV is abnormally overloaded, the PA pressure can often be accurately estimated. Emergency echocardiographic assessment can be invaluable when doubt exists concerning the cause of abrupt-onset hypotension and/or cardiac arrest. Massively dilated RV and central PA, for example, may provide an important clue to pulmonary embolism as the cause and may prompt the use of thrombolytics. Collapsibility of the IVC (during spontaneous breathing) and/or of the SVC during the inspiratory phase of positive-pressure ventilation correlates well with the responsiveness to a fluid challenge.

Intravenous optisonic contrast improves the chamber definition and allows the determination of anatomy with sufficient precision to identify septal defects (as will agitated saline). The regional wall motion abnormalities of recent or remote myocardial infarction are well defined. Chamber dimensions and wall thickness are readily assessed. Ischemic and infarcted areas contract with less vigor and are rather easily detected, allowing the ECHO to functionally image the heart during pharmacologic stress testing. Superior resolution and the ability to delineate valve motion make 2D ECHO superior to M-mode ultrasound for examining right-sided cardiac valves and for detecting mitral prolapse and vegetations. 2D ECHO is also the preferred technique for calculation of valve area. In recent years, the value of ECHO in assessing the relative filling of the central circulation has been emphasized.

Transesophageal Echocardiography

TEE uses a miniature ultrasound transducer inserted into the esophagus via an endoscope to obtain high-resolution echocardiographic images. Although TEE is limited by the need to perform endoscopy, it frequently reveals the details of valvular motion, diastolic left heart function, chordae abnormalities, and small valvular vegetations missed by surface ECHO. TEE imaging is an accurate means of diagnosing aortic dissection, atherosclerosis, and aortic trauma. It is more reliable than transthoracic 2D ECHO for this purpose. TEE also offers advantages in patients with a body habitus that prevents surface echocardiographic imaging, most notably patients with obesity and hyperinflation of the chest.

Doppler Echocardiography and Aortic Flow Estimation

Doppler ECHO deduces velocity of moving blood by interpreting changes in the frequency of reflected sound waves. Either M-mode or 2D ECHO can be used in conjunction with Doppler technology to estimate CO or flow across a valvular orifice. Once valve area is determined and blood velocity is known, flow may be calculated. In many (but certainly not all) patients—those with detectable tricuspid regurgitation—PA pressure can also be estimated. Thus, Doppler potentially provides a means for estimating CO noninvasively. Pressures in various cardiac chambers may also be inferred from Doppler flow estimates. Finally, as already noted, color-flow Doppler helps to detect the regurgitant jets of blood characteristic of valvular insufficiency and abnormal communications between structures (e.g., atrial septal defect).

Esophageal Doppler *monitoring* of aortic blood flow has been investigated and perfected over the course of more than three decades as a means by which to track changes in CO by interrogating the descending aorta. Miniaturized probes that are intended for continuous use at the bedside are now commercially available. Whatever their limitations for precise quantitation of CO may be (see earlier discussion), their ease of use—even by nurses and other relatively untrained operators—holds significant promise as a noninvasive means for detecting and promptly addressing hemodynamic deterioration.

Specific Diagnostic Problems

Intravascular Volume and Cardiac Filling

Certain 2D ECHO findings reliably indicate relative overdistention of the RV (e.g., D-shaped septum), whereas others such as ventricular walls that touch during systole or inspiratory collapse of the IVC reflect serious volume depletion.

Investigation of Pericardial Effusion and Tamponade

Investigation of pericardial effusion and tamponade is a common use of ECHO in the ICU. Although optimal studies may detect effusions of 25 to 50 mL, delineation of such small pericardial effusions can be fraught with difficulty, especially when pleural effusions coexist. Normally, the epicardium and pericardium are closely apposed, with only slight separation occasionally seen in systole. Accumulated pericardial fluid separates these two structures throughout both phases of the cardiac cycle. Small amounts of fluid in the pericardial sac pool posteriorly in supine patients can be easily missed. 2D is superior to M-mode ECHO for detecting small amounts of pericardial fluid. In such cases, visualizing the LA may be revealing. Pericardial fluid rarely accumulates behind the LA for anatomic reasons. When larger effusions accumulate, diagnosis becomes much easier, as fluid collects anteriorly as well as posteriorly in the pericardial space. When pericardial effusions become very large, the heart may swing to and fro within the sac, producing artifactual wall motion and apparent abnormalities of mitral and tricuspid valve function. The diagnosis of pericardial effusion is commonly missed by ECHO when there is fibroadhesive pericardial disease, simultaneous pleural effusion, or massive LA enlargement. The diagnosis of tamponade is a clinical one that cannot be made solely by ECHO criteria. Tamponade physiology may be suspected, however, when a large pericardial effusion is present or when the RA or ventricular cavities show intermittent collapse. Evidence of decreased flow through the mitral valve during inspiration and relatively enlarged RV dimensions are also suggestive.

Paradoxical Embolism

ECHO may also be used in the ICU to detect intracardiac shunts in patients with refractory hypoxemia or suspected paradoxical embolism. In such cases, the contrast injected is either an ECHO dense dye or (more commonly) an intravenous fluid containing microbubbles (e.g., agitated saline, sonicated 5% human albumin). In such testing, the acoustic contrast agent is introduced by vein while the ECHO transducer probes the left heart chambers. If a right-to-left cardiac shunt is present, there is prompt appearance of acoustic noise in the LA or ventricle shortly after injection. The legs are preferentially used for such injections because RA streaming patterns favor crossing of the contrast material into the left heart. Although this "bubble" technique has relatively high specificity for right-to-left shunt, it lacks the sensitivity of angiographic dye injections. The sensitivity of TEE substantially exceeds that of surface techniques for detection of intracardiac shunts.

■ NUCLEAR CARDIOLOGY

With the rise of cardiac catheterization, interventional angiography, MRI, multidimensional CT scanning, and increasingly sophisticated ECHO, nuclear medicine techniques now hold a very limited and progressively tenuous place for imaging the heart in critically ill patients. Planar and Spect images obtained after Technetium-99m (Cardiolite) and stress challenge with adenosire or dobutamine may detect areas of reversible cardiac ischemia or acute myocardial infarction (Chapter 21). RVG uses radio-labeled red blood cells to define the boundaries of the heart and to track the changes in its volume. Images may be obtained immediately after injection (single-pass scanning) or, more frequently, after a period of equilibration (gated ventriculography MUGA). In gated ventriculography, multiple images are acquired at various phases of the cardiac cycle by coupling the detector to an ECG trigger. Comparing ventricular volume (count density) during diastole and systole allows calculation of the relative change in ventricular volume resulting from ventricular contraction—the ejection fraction. Ventricular size, contour, and segmental wall motion may also be assessed. Unfortunately, RVG does not visualize the atria or details of valvular anatomy. RVG proves useful in patients who demonstrate changes in ejection fraction or wall motion during ischemia induced by exercise or provocative pharmacologic agents (e.g., dobutamine); ischemic myocardium becomes dysfunctional and occasionally paradoxic in its motion. ECG-gated RVG studies require a relatively regular ventricular rhythm for computerized data collection. Therefore, patients with atrial fibrillation or frequent premature atrial or ventricular beats are poor candidates for this study. In most instances, RVG must also be performed outside the ICU, necessitating patient transport. Finally, dramatically improved ECHO imaging now relegates RVG to a minor place in ICU diagnosis.

■ SUGGESTED READINGS

Chaney JC, Derdak S. Minimally invasive hemodynamic monitoring for the intensivist: Current and emerging technology. *Crit Care Med.* 2002;30(10):2338–2345.

Cousins TR, O'Donnell JM. Arterial cannulation: A critical review. *AANA J.* 2004;72(4):267–271.

Hadian H, Pinsky MR. Functional hemodynamic monitoring. *Curr Opin Crit Care.* 2007;13:318–323.

Magder S. Clinical usefulness of respiratory variations in arterial pressure. *Am J Respir Crit Care Med.* 2004;169:151–155.

Michard F. Changes in arterial pressure during mechanical ventilation. *Anesthesiology.* 2005;103:419–428.

O'Quin R, Marini JJ. Pulmonary occlusion pressure: Clinical physiology, measurement, and interpretation. *Am Rev Respir Dis.* 1983;128: 319–326.

Pinsky MR, Payen D, eds. *Functional Hemodynamic Monitoring in the Intensive Care Unit. Update in Intensive Care and Emergency Medicine Series.* Vol. 42. New York: Springer-Verlag; 2005.

Preisman S, Kogan S, Berkenstadt H, et al. Predicting fluid responsiveness in patients undergoing cardiac surgery: Functional haemodynamic parameters including the Respiratory Systolic Variation Test and static preload indicators. *Br J Anaesth.* 2005;95:746–755.

The National Heart, Lung, and Blood Institute Acute Respiratory Distress Syndrome (ARDS) Clinical Trials Network. Pulmonary-artery versus central venous catheter to guide treatment of acute lung injury. *N Engl J Med.* 2006;354:2213–2224.

Vincent JL, Pinsky MR, Sprung CL, et al. The pulmonary artery catheter: In medio virtus. *Crit Care Med.* 2008;36(11):3093–3096.

Support of the Failing Circulation

KEY POINTS

1 Circulatory insufficiency and shock result from inadequate perfusion relative to tissue demands. Although certain physical and laboratory parameters may be suggestive, shock is defined by overt dysfunction of key vital organs—not by parameters that selectively reflect either oxygen supply or demand.

2 Attention to the *demand* side of the perfusion imbalance is a potent and often overlooked means of reversing the pathophysiology of shock.

3 Early goal-oriented intervention may be crucial in deciding outcome.

4 Three basic mechanisms may cause or contribute to circulatory insufficiency: pump failure, insufficient vascular tone (vasoplegia), and hypovolemia. Heart rate and rhythm as well as the determinants of stroke volume (preload, contractility, and afterload) should be considered independently for their potential to contribute to cardiovascular dysfunction.

5 The parameters that characterize heart function must be scaled to body size; any specific value of cardiac output oxygen consumption, or vascular resistance may take on different significance for large and small patients.

6 During shock, the respiratory muscles may outstrip the heart's ability to deliver adequate blood flow to them. Mechanical support may relieve the ventilatory burden, thereby increasing the blood flow available to other marginally perfused organs.

7 Repeated examination of mental status, urine output, and skin perfusion provides information essential in guiding therapy. Invasive monitoring with arterial and pulmonary artery catheters, in conjunction with the fluid challenge, provide the data necessary to wisely select vasoactive agents and regulate the rates of volume and drug infusion.

8 Adequate circulatory volume must be ensured before vasopressors are used. The type of fluid should be selected by considering the need for blood, the nature of the fluid lost from the vascular space, the acuity of the problem, the urgency of reversal, the financial cost, and the potential risk of the product to the patient.

9 Most (but not all) vasoactive agents used to support the circulation are catecholamine derivatives with α, $\beta 1$, or $\beta 2$ activity, in varying proportions. The relative intensity of each effect may vary with dosage.

10 Mechanical interventions (ventilatory support, positive end-expiratory pressure, aortic balloon pumping) may be needed to reduce afterload or modify preload. Once initiated, these interventions should be maintained only as long as necessary but should be withdrawn cautiously.

■ PHYSIOLOGY OF THE FAILING CIRCULATION

Circulatory Insufficiency

Circulatory insufficiency and shock reflect **1** inadequate perfusion relative to tissue demands. Although certain physical and laboratory parameters may be suggestive, shock is defined by overt dysfunction of vital organ systems—not uniquely by such "supply side" parameters as blood pressure (BP) or cardiac output (CO) or by such "demand side" parameters as oxygen consumption ($\dot{V}O_2$). What might be considered a normal CO in a healthy patient at rest may inadequately perfuse the tissue beds of a critically ill patient. The prime objective of circulatory support, therefore, is to maintain near-optimal vital organ perfusion, as reflected in mental status, urinary output, and systemic pH, at acceptable cardiac filling pressures.

2 Organ perfusion is governed by driving pressure and vascular resistance. Ordinarily, an adequate pressure gradient is present, and vasomotor tone regulates individual organ perfusion in proportion to metabolic demand. Under resting conditions, only a small percentage of all vascular channels are fully open. However, when the available pressure fails to maintain adequate flow despite optimized vasodilation (e.g., during a cardiovascular crisis or hypovolemia) or when defective vasoregulation fails to maintain perfusion pressure or flow distribution (e.g., during sepsis), vital tissues are not adequately nourished to maintain all normal cellular functions. The vascular beds of different organs vary in the extent to which they can compensate for deprivation of normal regional blood flow and/or drop in circulatory pressure. Certain conditions, such as sepsis, may interfere with these delicate vasomotor controls. The shock syndrome may be initiated when these compensatory mechanisms reach their limits. Once shock physiology is under way, vasoactive mediators and products of inflammation, some with myocardial depressant properties, may be released into the circulation system to perpetuate the circulatory crisis. Even with appropriate treatment, mortality exceeds 50% for septic shock and for cardiogenic shock unaddressed by coronary reperfusion.

Determinants of Cardiac Output

Although attention usually is focused on the pump that energizes the circulation (the heart), vascular compliance and tone are potentially of equal importance. Thus, whereas the Frank–Starling relationship offers a useful if somewhat restricted perspective on circulatory kinetics, CO can be viewed equally well as a function of the effective pressure gradient driving blood from the periphery back to the heart and the resistance to venous return. The average upstream peripheral force driving venous return, the mean systemic pressure (MSP), is the equilibrium pressure that would exist throughout the vasculature if the heart abruptly stopped pumping. Because of the large capacitance of the venous relative to the arterial bed, MSP (normally 7 to 10 mm Hg) lies much closer in value to the central venous pressure (CVP) than to mean arterial pressure (MAP). MSP is influenced by both blood volume and vascular tone. Early in many shock states, aggressive filling of the vasculature is often required to compensate for the vasoplegia that otherwise would cause MSP to fall. Capacitance beds must be filled before vessel tone and MSP can rise to

adequate levels. (Vigorous early resuscitation of **3** the intravascular compartment helps account for the reported success of "goal-directed therapy.") The downstream back pressure to venous return is right atrial pressure (P_{RA}). If MSP fails to rise sufficiently to compensate for an increase in P_{RA}, CO falls. Indeed, the relationship between CO and P_{RA} is linear for any fixed value of MSP, and the slope of this relationship is influenced by the resistance to venous return. The tendency of the vena cava to collapse limits the extent to which effective driving pressure ($MSP - P_{RA}$) can be increased by reducing P_{RA} (Fig. 3-1). The actual CO observed at any moment is defined by the intersection of Starling and venous return curves. Thus, both pump factors (heart rate [HR], loading conditions, and contractility) and circuit factors (intravascular volume, vessel tone) influence circulatory performance. Three basic mechanisms may cause or contribute to circulatory failure: (a) pump failure, **4** (b) failure of vascular tone, and (c) hypovolemia.

Pump Failure

Heart Rate

CO, the product of heart rate (HR) and stroke volume (SV), can be depressed by abnormalities of either variable (see Chapter 1). To meet metabolic demand, isolated abnormalities of either SV or HR can be offset by adjustments in the other cofactor over a wide range. Both extremes of HR may cause CO to fall to shock levels. During sinus rhythm,

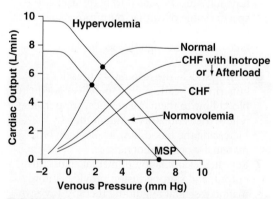

■ **FIGURE 3-1** Regulation of CO. CO is determined by the intersection of the Frank–Starling and venous return curves. Venous return, which is driven by the difference between MSP and CVP, tends to improve as CVP falls, until the point at which venous pressure is insufficient to prevent vessel collapse (*arrow*). For the same venous return curve, the failing heart reduces its output, despite a higher filling pressure. CO can be maintained at a nearly normal level by increasing intravascular volume and/or using an inotrope or afterload reducer.

the maximal sustainable physiologic HR can be estimated as (HR_{max} = 220 – age). HRs that exceed this value may compromise CO and myocardial perfusion, even in healthy individuals. When the heart is noncompliant or compromised by coronary insufficiency, CO may fall at much lower HRs. Furthermore, the loss of atrial contraction that accompanies many tachyarrhythmias (i.e., atrial fibrillation) may depress CO on this basis alone.

In the intensive care unit (ICU), hypoxemia, enhanced vagal tone, and high-grade conduction block caused by intrinsic heart disease or pharmacologic agents are key mechanisms causing marked bradycardia. The normally compliant and contractile ventricle can adapt to physiologic or pathologic depressions in HR via the Starling mechanism; for example, young, well-conditioned athletes often maintain resting HRs less than 40 beats/min. However, patients with impaired myocardial contractility or effective compliance (e.g., ischemia, diastolic dysfunction, pericardial disease) may suffer marked depressions in CO and BP when HRs fall into the low normal range (<50 beats/min). This is especially true when the normally coordinated activation sequence is compromised or metabolic demands are high. Because bradycardia lengthens diastole as a proportion of total cycle time, MAP sinks closer to the diastolic value as HR slows. Perfusion of the heart and other key organs may suffer. It must be remembered that the appropriate physiologic response to hypovolemia is sinus tachycardia; hypotension suspected on the basis of massive gastrointestinal (GI) hemorrhage, therefore, should be accompanied by a compensatory tachycardia. A normal HR in this setting implicates an erroneous diagnosis or superimposed vagal, drug, or pathologic explanations.

Stroke Volume—Loading Properties and Contractility

SV is determined by end-diastolic volume and ejection fraction (see Chapter 1). End-diastolic volume, in turn, is the product of transmural filling pressure and myocardial compliance. As discussed in Chapter 1, SV and CO are often well preserved despite florid cardiogenic pulmonary edema. The myocardial hypertrophy of chronic hypertension or aortic stenosis, or the functional ischemia of coronary disease can result in symptomatic diastolic dysfunction. In such cases, control of hypertension and relief of ischemia and/or CO demand accelerate recovery and help prevent symptomatic recurrence.

Foremost among the primary depressants of contractility and ejection fraction during critical illness are (a) acute ischemia; (b) extensive myocardial necrosis; (c) humoral mediators (collectively known as "myocardial depressant factors") released during inflammation and trauma; and (d) drugs that impair contractility (e.g., certain β-blockers, calcium channel blockers, and antiarrhythmics—most notably of the type Ia class). Cardiogenic shock consequent to acute myocardial infarction implies cumulative tissue losses exceeding 40% of the total myocardial mass.

Structural defects, such as papillary muscle rupture or post infarction ventriculoseptal defect (VSD), may compromise CO on a mechanical basis, even when there has been subcritical myocardial damage. Because the output of a failing heart is influenced by the impedance to ventricular ejection (afterload), increased vascular tone may improve BP at the expense of tissue perfusion. Patients with "tight" aortic stenosis are especially sensitive to changes in preload and contractility.

To scale for metabolic needs, the CO must be referenced to body surface area. The resulting quotient, the cardiac index (CI), attempts to take the mass of metabolizing tissue into account (normal >2.5 L/min/m^2). CO adequacy can be judged only with respect to metabolic demands. Under some circumstances, even a normal CI may be insufficient for vital organ support. Such "high-output" cardiac failure can be precipitated by fever, anemia, thiamine deficiency, thyrotoxicosis, and arteriovenous shunting. Patients with extensive burns, severe sepsis, or cirrhosis also may have vastly higher CO requirements than the average resting patient.

Failure of Vascular Tone

Because organ perfusion depends on the gradient of pressure and the resistance to flow through the tissue bed, failure of vasomotor tone and/or distributive control may produce the shock syndrome, even when the CI is maintained within the normal range. Early sepsis provides a common example of maldistributive shock, characterized by reduced afterload and normal or elevated CO and $\dot{V}O_2$, despite undernourished vital tissue beds. General and spinal anesthesia, autonomic failure resulting from acute spinal cord injury, and certain drugs may also produce generalized, nonselective vasodilation that leads to underperfusion of critical organs. The inability to produce sufficient glucocorticoid (cortisone), a common deficiency in critical illness (relative adrenal insufficiency), suppresses both vasomotor tone and myocardial contractility.

The therapy of shock states often focuses on maintaining a targeted BP. This is an appropriate orientation, considering that the cerebral and coronary vasculatures (and to a lesser extent that of the kidney) are critically dependent on their perfusion gradients and relatively unaffected by the drug-induced vasoconstriction experienced elsewhere. It must be emphasized that adequate BP and adequate flow are not synonymous; vasoactive drugs may cause intense ischemia of "nonvital" beds (gut, muscle, skin), occasionally with serious consequences for overall outcome.

Although moderate acidosis is generally well tolerated, severe metabolic acidosis may aggravate the shock state by causing myocardial depression, catecholamine resistance, increased right ventricular afterload, and potentially irreversible precapillary arteriolar dilation. Selective arteriolar dilation produces direct cellular injury and massive transudation of fluid into the extracellular space. Adrenal insufficiency and (less commonly) myxedema are two frequently overlooked endocrine problems that may contribute to vasomotor insufficiency and circulatory failure.

Hypovolemia

Although inadequacy of circulating blood volume is in itself a primary cause of circulatory failure, a *relative* deficiency of intravascular volume often contributes cause in the setting of impaired pump function or reduced vascular tone (e.g., sepsis). Primary hypovolemic shock develops during hemorrhage or when extensive extracellular volume losses result from burns, pancreatitis, vomiting, diarrhea, anaphylaxis, hypoproteinemia, or multiple traumas. Right ventricular infarction and pericardial disease mimic hypovolemia despite systemic venous congestion and/or normal wedge pressure because they impair left ventricular (LV) compliance.

Cardiodepression and Electrolyte Disturbances

Contractility of myocardium and vascular smooth muscle can be adversely influenced by nonphysiologic concentrations of key electrolytes, especially when several disorders are encountered simultaneously. Hypermagnesemia and hyponatremia occasionally are the primary causes of difficulty but usually serve a secondary role. The most frequent underlying causes of cardiovascular depression are hyperkalemia and deficiency of ionized calcium. An approach to the diagnosis and management of these disorders is provided in Chapter 13.

Pharmacologic Effects

Although all antihypertensive drugs may evoke hypotension, two commonly used classes of therapeutic agents—calcium channel blockers and β-blockers—directly interfere with cardiac function and may either exacerbate congestive heart failure (CHF) or encourage cardiovascular collapse. The appropriate response to excessive calcium channel blockade is to administer sufficient calcium to counter the drug's adverse effect; either the chloride or gluconate salt can be given as a bolus. Calcium chloride can be administered by continuous infusion as well. Catechol-based vasopressors and inotropes are indicated in addressing hypotension, but all may prove ineffective until calcium channel blockade is overcome. High dose insulin (1–10 u/kg/hour) has shown promise in both emergency and experimental toxicology environments when glucose and potassium are kept within normal limits.

β Blockade

Through their actions on myocardial contractility, HR, bronchodilation, alveolar liquid clearance, and peripheral vasodilation, stimulation of one or more subtypes of β receptor is of fundamental importance to the recovery of the acutely compromised circulation. By influencing these properties, β-blocking drugs have unquestioned utility in managing a range of cardiovascular problems arising in the acute care setting, including ischemic cardiovascular disease, tachycardia, hyperthyroidism, aortic dissection, and acute hypertensive crisis. Whereas the use of well-selected β-blocking drugs is appropriate to the management of specific disorders that require such intervention, they should be withheld from the care of acutely ill patients in the absence of firm and specific indications (acute myocardial ischemia, symptomatic tachyarrhythmia, etc.). Currently, β-blocking drugs are frequently used in the outpatient setting not only for hypertension, but also to address diastolic dysfunction or chronic CHF (where they may help structural adaptation or remodeling). This practice, although partially justified by outcome studies of selective β-blockers in large populations, may backfire during periods of stress (e.g., sepsis, myocardial infarction, dietary indiscretion), especially in the elderly. The β-blocking drug already "on board" then accentuates

TABLE 3-1 POTENTIALLY ADVERSE ACTIONS OF β BLOCKADE

Impaired cardiac contractility
Limitation of compensatory HR
Bronchospasm
Impaired pulmonary edema clearance

hypotension or contributes to "flash pulmonary edema" by interfering with the compensatory mechanisms of these patients with compromised cardiovascular reserve (Table 3-1). Certain long-acting, nonselective, and inexpensive β-blockers (e.g., atenolol) are especially problematic in that native drug and/or active metabolites are renally excreted and therefore accumulate during prerenal azotemia. The approach to managing life-threatening β receptor blockade is similar to that just described for calcium channel blockade: high dose insulin may be considered if β-stimulants, vasopressin and glucagon prove inadequate to reverse shock.

Effect of Shock on Organ Function

The closely autoregulated central nervous system of the healthy subject can tolerate marked reductions in MAP (to 50 to 60 mm Hg) without sustaining irreversible tissue damage. However, cerebrocortical functions are among the first to be impaired as shock develops.

As a rule, serious reductions of MAP are tolerated poorly by the GI tract. Early in shock, the gut suffers marked reductions in flow. This flow reduction eventually impairs mucosal function and bowel integrity, occasionally to the point of frank ischemic necrosis. A reduction of gastric mucosal pH is among the first indications of inadequate gut perfusion. One popular paradigm suggests translocation of bacteria across the abnormally permeable gut mucosa and into the lymphatic system or bloodstream as the next step on the path to multisystem organ failure. Hepatic ischemia may elevate liver function tests, alter the metabolism of drugs, and impair removal of toxins, lactate, and coagulation products.

Shock often impairs the clotting system sufficiently to initiate disseminated intravascular coagulation (DIC). The stimulus is multifactorial, and the important contributing factors are vascular endothelial injury, cell death, and impaired hepatic clearance of fibrin degradation products (see Chapter 30). In response to hypotension, the kidneys secrete renin to retain sodium and water. Intense vasoconstriction of the afferent arterioles shunts blood from the cortex to the medulla, reducing glomerular filtration to a greater degree than total renal blood flow or CO. If profound or prolonged, underperfusion may culminate in acute tubular necrosis. Antidiuretic hormone released from the pituitary helps conserve water and may contribute to hyponatremia.

During protracted shock, the skeletal muscles may release sufficient quantities of myoglobin into the circulation to impair renal tubular function (rhabdomyolysis). The hyperpnea that accompanies profound hypotension requires the respiratory muscles to consume large quantities of oxygen, outstripping the heart's ability to deliver adequate flow to them, and ventilatory failure may result. Intubation and mechanical ventilation during circulatory shock decrease respiratory muscle O_2 consumption, thereby increasing the blood flow available to other critical organs. Thus, in the vigorously breathing patient, mechanical ventilation often improves circulatory homeostasis.

Evaluation of Perfusion Adequacy

The history, physical examination, laboratory tests, and ancillary tests form the core of the evaluation process of the patient with circulatory inadequacy (Table 3-2). The clinician should rapidly undertake a targeted history, with review of prior vital signs and recent events and/or interventions that led to the shock state. Special attention is paid to preexisting illness and the medication listing.

TABLE 3-2 VITAL DATABASE IN HYPOTENSIVE STATES

CLINICAL HISTORY
Past medical history and baseline vital signs
Recent interventions and events

PHYSICAL EXAMINATION
Vital signs
Urine output
Skin temperature and character
Capillary refill time
Neck veins/cardiac auscultation

LABORATORY TESTS
Arterial blood gases
Central venous O_2 saturation
Hemoglobin/hematocrit
Anion gap
Lactate
Brain natriuretic peptide (BNP)
Cortisol
Troponin

ANCILLARY INFORMATION
Radiographs chest and abdomen (when indicated)
Electrocardiogram
Echocardiogram

Key features of the physical examination include otherwise unexplained alterations of vital organ function (mental status, urine output); hypotension relative to the usual baseline; sluggish capillary refilling; and cool, clammy skin. Neck vein examination and cardiac auscultation are essential focus points, keeping alert for signs of isolated right ventricular failure. Electrocardiogram (and in most cases echocardiogram) should be obtained in shock that is not of obvious cause or that does not reverse easily. Laboratory tests that reflect cardiac dysfunction (troponin, brain natriuretic peptide [BNP]) and/or perfusion inadequacy (anion gap, lactate) are often worth repeating as therapy progresses. Relative adrenal insufficiency is common enough to warrant measurement of serum cortisol concentration and its response to stimulation, especially in those refractory to intravenous fluid and vasopressor resuscitation. Arterial blood gas and central venous oxygen saturation data are sufficiently valuable that insertion of catheters should be considered to provide for their serial monitoring.

7

■ THERAPY OF THE FAILING CIRCULATION

Goal-Directed Therapy

Because prolonged hypoperfusion leads to sustained organ failure and irreversibility, most experienced clinicians agree that shock should be reversed as quickly as feasible to safely do so. Early aggressive intervention to restore an effective circulation has become an accepted goal, even if the precise target at which to aim is debated. Two elements seem important: early intervention and restoration of adequate perfusion to vital organs. What measurable indicator to shoot for? Generally speaking, supranormal values for CO and oxygen delivery are neither easy to achieve nor needed. Restoring near-normal values for central venous O_2 saturation, however, currently is thought prudent, based on the persuasive results of an important prospective clinical trial. The central venous saturation reflects the ratio of O_2 delivery to consumption. Targeting a central venous saturation of >70% has been associated with higher survival than use of an MAP target. Unlike the mixed venous O_2 saturation, central venous sampling can be readily achieved via routine central lines as well as monitored continuously via specialized catheters. As a helpful but not infallible indicator of perfusion adequacy, central venous O_2 saturation should

be considered a valuable complement to routine arterial pressure monitoring.

Indications for Monitoring

Repeated examinations of mental status, urine output, and skin perfusion provide information essential in guiding therapy. MAP normally exceeds 90 mm Hg. Although no specific BP should be used as the sole endpoint of circulatory support, a MAP of 60 to 70 mm Hg is required for most patients to perfuse the heart, brain, and kidneys adequately; higher pressures are required in those with vascular disease and/or long-standing hypertension prior to presentation. The catch phrase for all types of quantified observation is *functional* monitoring. Absolute values for any hemodynamic parameter take a back seat to the response of the target variable to intervention.

Arterial and ventricular filling pressures should be monitored continuously when hypotension produces signs of vital organ dysfunction that are not readily reversed. For young patients without underlying heart or lung disease, a CVP catheter may suffice to monitor filling pressures. The central venous oxygen saturation is an overlooked and potentially valuable indicator of perfusion adequacy in the setting of hypovolemic or cardiogenic shock. When Doppler-aided echocardiography, CVP measurement, and radiographic imaging leave doubt as to appropriate management or the patient remains hemodynamically unstable, the placement of a pulmonary arterial catheter, which aids in accurate assessment of LV filling pressure, CO, and mixed venous oxygen saturation on an ongoing basis (see Chapter 2), may be considered. By enabling calculations of vascular resistance indices, pulmonary artery (PA) catheters can be helpful in diagnosing the etiology of shock and in guiding therapy. Although a PA catheter clearly is *not* indicated in all, it is of value in many circumstances, and most hypotensive patients requiring vasopressor support should be monitored invasively via arterial catheter. Severe peripheral vasoconstriction and the reduced pulse pressure of certain shock states make determination of systemic BP by standard cuff methods difficult and unreliable. Arterial catheterization allows frequent determinations of blood gases, effortless blood drawing when other sites prove difficult or are unavailable, and continuous assessment of BP. A bladder catheter also should be placed in patients with hypotension to monitor urine output as an index of renal perfusion and adequacy of O_2 delivery. Consideration should be given to

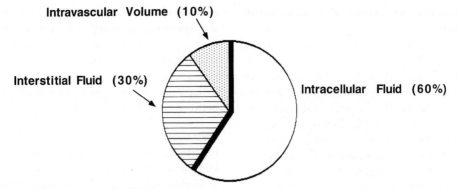

■ FIGURE 3-2 Body fluid distribution.

carefully measuring bladder pressure (an indicator of intra-abdominal pressure) when the possibility of an ongoing or developing abdominal compartment syndrome is entertained.

Fluid Therapy

Water normally constitutes about 60% of body weight. Of this total, approximately two thirds is intracellular and approximately one third is extracellular (Fig. 3-2). Of the extracellular fluid, one quarter is intravascular and three quarters is interstitial. Isotonic solutions (e.g., normal saline and Ringer's lactate) initially distribute only into the extracellular space, whereas the distributive space of hypotonic (or potentially hypotonic) fluids approximates that of total body water. Therefore, hypotonic fluids (e.g., one-half normal saline) or fluids subject to rapid metabolism of their osmotic components (e.g., D5W) only affect intravascular volume transiently (only one twelfth of the volume of D5W remains intravascular after dextrose metabolism). As a result of normal fluid partitioning, replacing a specific volume of lost plasma requires at least four times as much isotonic crystalloid and even more hypotonic fluid. Because two thirds of isotonic crystalloid enters the interstitial space within 60 min of its administration, edema should be expected after massive fluid resuscitation with crystalloid. Although the resulting tissue edema is generally thought to be well tolerated, the lungs as well as the peripheral tissues are affected. After rapid and massive resuscitation, a compartment syndrome can develop in an extremity or in the abdomen, especially in those who have undergone profound and sustained ischemia.

When first given, large volumes of fluid initially dilute the packed cell volume (PCV) and serum proteins. As fluid redistributes out of the vascular space, these values tend to return gradually toward their preinfusion baselines. The time required for this equilibration or "circulation dwell time" is brief for crystalloid. Redistribution begins within minutes and is completed within hours.

Hypotension complicated by renal insufficiency or anuria presents a difficult challenge that requires skillful management. Dialysis often is required for these patients to clear toxins, restore electrolyte balance, allow nutritional support, and offset metabolic acidosis. Early dialysis has been suggested (but not proven) to shorten the course to recovery and deserves consideration from the outset of anuria resistant to volume repletion and diuretics. Continuous venovenous or arteriovenous hemofiltration can be especially helpful when fluid overloading or acidosis complicates management, because it allows the gradual removal of sodium and water—a useful aid for oliguric patients who require frequent saline or bicarbonate infusions. Effective dialysis can be performed using similar methodology (see Chapter 29).

Use of the Fluid Challenge

Fluid challenge is instrumental for assessing the need for volume replacement in hypotensive patients. In fact, for most hypotensive patients without evidence of pulmonary edema, fluid administration is rarely an inappropriate first response. Although some patients respond transiently to simple leg elevation (the head and chest must be horizontal), such a quick and reversible translocation of volume is a "one time only" maneuver, is generally short lived, and only serves to indicate potential responsiveness to a volume infusion strategy. Another reversible challenge is to raise or lower the level of positive end-expiratory pressure (PEEP) in those in whom such maneuvers are not contraindicated. Wide respiratory variation of systolic BP or of pulse pressure during controlled ventilation is a helpful indicator (see Chapter 2) of intravascular volume need.

The keys to effective fluid challenge are (a) use crystalloid as the challenge fluid, (b) use a relatively large volume (500 to 1,000 mL) to maximize chances of detecting a significant hemodynamic effect, (c) infuse the fluid rapidly, and (d) closely monitor the patient's response. Because the majority of an isotonic fluid load diffuses into the interstitial space within hours, crystalloid infusions are a relatively "reversible" method for expanding the intravascular compartment. Large volumes of fluid are infused rapidly to maximize the hemodynamic impact before redistribution dissipates the preloading effects. Fluid challenge should not be performed without close monitoring by a clinical caregiver. To obtain meaningful information safely, it is important that physical examination, CVP (or wedge pressure), HR, and arterial pressure be monitored closely. A marked, sustained increase in filling pressure after fluid infusion signals that the heart is operating on the flat portion of the Starling curve, particularly if CO or MAP fails to rise. In such patients, further administration of intravascular fluid may overload the circulation, causing pulmonary edema. Conversely, if the fluid bolus causes small or transient increases in filling pressure that are accompanied by a substantial increase in MAP (and/or CO, when measured) and a stable or reduced HR, fluid administration is likely to benefit.

Selection of Fluids

8 Selection of intravenous fluid is controversial. One logical approach is to replace adequate quantities of the missing constituent. For example, blood replacement is rational to counter severe hemorrhage, whereas isotonic crystalloid is appropriate for the dehydrated patient with near-normal electrolytes. Because of the risks associated with infusions of blood products, and because maintenance of a normal hemoglobin concentration may not benefit perfusion or outcome, transfusions should be carefully considered and their use minimized. Blood is not essential for resuscitation unless there is acute blood loss, marked anemia that is poorly tolerated, and/or ongoing coagulopathy (see Chapter 14). The major difference between colloids and crystalloids resides in the tendency of the former to remain within the vascular space. Unlike saline, most infused colloids remain intravascular for many hours; it may require as much as five times more crystalloids than colloids to achieve equivalent intravascular volume expansion. However, colloids are expensive, frequently costing many times more than crystalloids to achieve similar volume expansion effects, and are associated with a minor allergic risk, and some impair coagulation. Published studies have not shown a consistent mortality difference between colloids and crystalloids in this setting.

Crystalloid

Physiologic "normal" saline is the preferred crystalloid for volume expansion, except in patients with hyperchloremic acidosis, a setting in which saline may worsen the problem. The concentrations of sodium and chloride in 0.9% saline are significantly higher than those in normal plasma (especially chloride), contributing to hypernatremia and hyperchloremia when infused in large quantities, which often give rise to metabolic "acidosis" as bicarbonate must decline to maintain electrical neutrality (see Chapter 12). Ringer's lactate, although a physiologically balanced fluid, has a slightly lower Na^+ concentration than normal saline; therefore, less infused volume remains intravascular. Additionally, it contains 4 mEq/L of K^+, which is undesirable for patients with renal failure, oliguria, and hyperkalemia. Although the lactate in Ringer's solution does not potentiate systemic lactic acidosis, its metabolism to bicarbonate occurs slowly in patients with shock or hepatic hypoperfusion. Hypertonic crystalloid (3%, 7.5%, 15% saline) has been used effectively for emergency resuscitation, and some investigators have infused hypertonic saline continuously over 24 h for ongoing hemodynamic support. The mechanism of action appears directly associated with volemia, as these solutions clearly help redistribute total body water into the extracellular compartment. Other putative actions of these hypertonic solutions include anti-inflammatory, endothelium-stabilizing, and antioxidant effects. Hypertonic saline risks the development of hypernatremia and hypervolemia, and its proper role in resuscitation continues to be debated.

Colloid Infusions

Albumin Albumin is available as a 5% (isotonic) or 25% (hypertonic) solution. Controversial and currently unconfirmed epidemiologic studies have suggested a poorly characterized higher mortality rate with albumin use. Undisputed is the fact that isotonic "salt poor" albumin contains up to 145 mEq/L of sodium. The 25% solution delivers relatively less salt per unit of colloid than its isotonic counterpart and, therefore, may offer an advantage in edematous patients. The oncotic effect of 1 g of albumin is to draw 18 g of H_2O into the vascular compartment. Because albumin leaks gradually from the intravascular space, its circulating half-life in many forms of shock is only about 16 h. Albumin must not be used as a nutritional supplement for hypoalbuminemic patients (e.g., nephrotic syndrome or hepatic failure). Exogenous albumin is catabolized rapidly or excreted in these conditions, negating its nutritional value and blunting its effect on volume expansion. In unusual circumstances (e.g., anabolism with preexisting hypoalbuminemia, cirrhosis with oliguria), the administration of albumin can raise intravascular oncotic pressure for extended periods and should be considered if pulmonary edema is present and refractory to diuretics. Although once a definite risk for transmitting certain viral infections, albumin is now heat treated, and donors are better screened, obviating this hazard. It contains no viable coagulation factors. Although albumin is clearly more costly and had been incriminated as a potential contributor to morbidity, a definitive Australian clinical trial comparing albumin and crystalloid as replacement fluids demonstrated no convincing advantage or hazard for either option.

Fresh Frozen Plasma   Fresh frozen plasma (FFP) provides another source of colloid protein. Because FFP carries a significant risk of allergic reaction and potentially risks infection, it should not be used solely for volume expansion. However, when hypovolemia and coagulopathy coexist, FFP may help reverse both. The usual FFP dosing range is 10 to 20 mL/kg, but the need is case dependent.

Dextran   Dextran, a mixture of heterogenous polysaccharides available as 40,000 or 70,000 molecular weight (MW) solutions, is now rarely used. Clearance of small MW fractions occurs rapidly through renal filtration, whereas larger molecules are taken up and metabolized by the reticuloendothelial system. The effect of dextran on circulatory volume is relatively brief, with only 20% to 30% remaining intravascular after 24 h. Dextran offers several potential advantages: it produces volume expansion greater than the volume infused, promotes "microvascular" flow by coating vessel walls and decreasing red cell–vessel wall interaction, and reduces serum viscosity.

Unfortunately, dextran also has important adverse characteristics. Reductions in platelet adherence and degranulation may incite bleeding, most often when doses exceed 1.5 g/kg/day. If urinary flow is sluggish, renal failure may occur

secondary to tubular obstruction. Minor allergic reactions are seen in approximately 5% of cases (patients with previous streptococcal or salmonella infections are predisposed). Fatal anaphylactic reactions occur rarely. The osmotic diuresis that follows dextran resuscitation may necessitate ongoing fluid replacement. Finally, dextran interferes with several common laboratory tests, occasionally producing false elevations of serum glucose, bilirubin, and protein concentrations. Dextran also mimics antibody-induced red cell agglutination, making cross-matching of blood more difficult.

Hydroxyethyl Starch   Hydroxyethyl starch (HES), a polysaccharide structurally similar to glycogen, is supplied as a mixture of MW fractions from 10,000 to 1,000,000. HES expands plasma volume in direct relationship to the amount infused. Small MW fractions of HES are cleared predominantly by the kidney, whereas reticuloendothelial cells metabolize larger MW fractions. HES is also degraded by serum alpha amylase. Trace amounts of intracorporeal HES have been detected more than 4 months after its administration. Prolonged or massive starch infusion may accumulate in phagocytes, resulting in unknown effects on immune function.

HES prolongs the partial thromboplastin time (PTT) modestly for most patients, but the mechanism is uncertain. HES also causes a transient decrease in platelet count and clot tensile strength. Intracerebral hemorrhage has been reported in intracorporeal HES recipients. Clotting abnormalities may be reversed with transfusions of FFP and platelets. Allergic reactions occur in less than 1% of patients receiving HES; anaphylactic reactions are extremely rare. HES may artifactually increase the sedimentation rate and often doubles the serum amylase. In a minority of patients, indirect bilirubin may be elevated spuriously by up to 1 mg/dL. HES and 5% albumin are similar in cost, and both are more expensive than dextran.

Given the associated trade-offs detailed, a 5:1 ratio of crystalloid to colloid is sometimes advocated because it provides more effective volume resuscitation than crystalloid alone at less cost than using colloid exclusively. A crystalloid-containing regimen also helps replete intracellular fluid losses.

Gelatins   Gelatins are polydisperse polypeptides produced by degradation of bovine collagen. Although gelatins were long considered not to influence blood coagulation other than by dilution, there is now increasing evidence that gelatins do influence platelet function and blood coagulation. Overall, gelatins appear to be without predictably

TABLE 3-3 INOTROPIC DRUGS[a]

	ADRENERGIC RECEPTOR ACTIVATION	RELATIVE EFFECTS IN MIDRANGE OF DOSAGE		
		INOTROPIC	CHRONOTROPIC	VASOCONSTRICTOR
Milrinone	0	+++	0	−
Dobutamine	$\alpha\beta1\beta2$	+++	+	− to +[a]
Dopamine	$\alpha\beta1\Delta$	+++	++	− to +[a]
Epinephrine	$\alpha\beta1\beta2$	+++	++	+++
Isoproterenol	$\beta1\beta2$	++++	++++	−
Methoxamine	α	0	0	++++
Norepinephrine	$\alpha\beta1$	+++	+++	++++
Phenylephrine	$\alpha\beta1$	+	0	++++
Vasopressin	0	+ or −	+ or −	+ to +++

[a]Effect dependent on dosage range.

adverse effects on kidney function. Well-controlled studies on the use of gelatins and their influence on renal function in the critically ill, however, are missing. Gelatins are not commonly available in North America, and their modest and short-lived effectiveness in expanding plasma volume has decreased the initial enthusiasm for this type of colloid worldwide.

In general, crystalloids appear to be just as effective as colloids in the majority of clinical settings, suggesting that the more expensive colloids are overused. However, specific patient populations, such as those with liver disease, those who have edema in conjunction with a low plasma oncotic pressure, and those at high risk of acute renal failure, may benefit from judicious colloid administration.

Vasoactive and Inotropic Drugs

General Principles

The primary goal of vasopressor therapy is to support vital organ perfusion—not to achieve any specific BP. Because vasoactive drugs are relatively ineffective in volume-depleted patients and are partially inhibited in the setting of severe acidosis, restoration of adequate circulating volume and reversal of profound acidosis (to pH > 7.10) are needed for maximal pressor effect. The potential utility of sodium bicarbonate should be kept in mind during prolonged resuscitation efforts. As already noted, glucocorticoid deficiency also blunts the impact of vasomotor agents. Moreover, vasopressors may be ineffective when serum concentrations of K^+, Mg^{2+}, or ionized Ca^{2+} are strikingly abnormal.

Making an optimal choice of vasopressor requires a clear understanding of the operative pathophysiology, an understanding of adrenergic receptor distribution and action, and a working knowledge of the pharmacologic alternatives. The vasopressor and inotropic drugs are classified by their tendencies to stimulate receptors with different physiologic actions. Alpha effects are vasoconstricting in the peripheral circulation. $\beta1$ receptor activation is both chronotropic and inotropic. $\beta2$ effects induce vasodilation and bronchodilation (Table 3-3). Dopaminergic (Δ) receptor activation increases renal blood flow, but these Δ effects are usually overwhelmed by the simultaneous α and β actions of the drugs available to elicit them. The ability to select the appropriate agent requires not only the knowledge of the drug's properties but also an assessment of the action required. For example, a tachycardic and hypotensive patient with warm extremities may respond best to a nearly pure α stimulator, such as phenylephrine, whereas a hypotensive patient who has cold, clammy extremities may respond better to dobutamine, a potent inotropic agent with modest vasodilating action and fewer tendencies for chronotropic stimulation than dopamine. For any given patient, optimal therapy may involve several vasoactive agents with complementary actions. It is worth considering, however, that certain drugs—notably dopamine—can stimulate both $\beta1$ and α adrenergic receptors preferentially, depending on dosage. Moreover, the sensitivity to any specific dosage varies widely among patients. For a volume-replete but hypotensive patient, the problem is either inadequate pump function or insufficient vascular tone. As a principle, it is desirable to titrate a single well-selected drug to effect (or toxicity) before it is abandoned or supplemented by additional agents. Whatever drug or drug combination is selected, its physiologic impact must be monitored appropriately (see Chapter 2). The ongoing need for these potent and potentially hazardous agents, as well as their dosage, must be reassessed frequently. Over time, patients tend to become "dependent" on these agents, so weaning rather than abrupt termination generally is the most prudent course.

Specific Agents

Potent vasoconstrictors (e.g., epinephrine, norepinephrine, phenylephrine, and dopamine) are best administered through a central line to avoid tissue necrosis resulting from extravasation.

Catecholamine Receptor Stimulators

Epinephrine   Epinephrine has balanced α and β agonist properties and serves as the standard to which all other vasopressors are compared. Epinephrine "coarsens" ventricular fibrillation and augments arterial tone during cardiac arrest. MAP, systemic vascular resistance (SVR), and CO are boosted in patients with an organized heart rhythm. Although epinephrine may prove effective when other vasoactive drugs fail (e.g., in anaphylactic shock), potential side effects include palpitations, arrhythmias, and angina caused by increased myocardial oxygen consumption. Concern has also been raised that epinephrine may contribute to splanchnic ischemia (concurrent administration of dobutamine may attenuate these effects). For patients with hypotension caused by ischemia-induced pump dysfunction, epinephrine may increase myocardial oxygen delivery to a greater degree than it increases myocardial oxygen consumption. Patients already taking β-blocking drugs may experience unopposed α effects when given a balanced α and β agonist such as epinephrine.

Norepinephrine   Norepinephrine (levarterenol) combines intense α with moderate $\beta 1$ activities. Its primary effect, therefore, is to vasoconstrict. Despite increases in SVR and LV afterload, CO usually remains stable or improves because of offsetting augmentation of HR and contractility. However, excessive increases in afterload induced by norepinephrine may reduce CO. Side effects include hypertension and increased myocardial oxygen consumption. Norepinephrine is often useful in the

early phases of septic shock, a condition in which CO is normal or elevated but SVR is reduced. Although the usual dosing range (0.5 to 20 μg/min) is generally effective, patients with refractory shock may require doses 10-fold higher to show adequate BP response. Such high doses do not appear to be associated with worsened side effects, but from present evidence, it is not clear whether they improve outcome. Norepinephrine frequently is combined with dobutamine, vasopressin, or other complementary pressor agent (such as milrinone) in the setting of refractory shock.

Isoproterenol   Isoproterenol has primarily $\beta 1$ (chronotropic and inotropic) actions but also possesses the $\beta 2$ properties of vasodilation and bronchodilation. Although now used only rarely, it will increase HR and CO in the setting of marked bradycardia (e.g., 3° atrioventricular [AV] block). Although now supplanted by effective antiarrhythmics, isoproterenol was formerly used to increase HR and shorten the QT interval in patients with arrhythmias resulting from QT prolongation (e.g., torsades de pointes). Increases in CO because of isoproterenol result primarily from increases in HR. MAP may actually fall, despite rising CO, as a result of peripheral vasodilation.

Neosynephrine   Neosynephrine (phenylephrine) is a pure α agonist that lacks cardiac stimulant properties. In high doses, increases in afterload resulting from neosynephrine may actually decrease CO. Neosynephrine is used to increase BP in the treatment of supraventricular tachycardias and currently sees some use in combination with intravenous nitroglycerin in patients with acute cardiac ischemia. Used together in that setting, they provide decreased preload and coronary vasodilation while maintaining arterial BP.

Dopamine   Dopamine is a naturally occurring precursor of norepinephrine with a spectrum of effects that varies with the infusion rate, clinical pathophysiology, and individual responsiveness. In normal subjects, very low infusion rates (1 to 2 μg/kg/min) theoretically improve renal blood flow, but the weight of current evidence indicates that any such effect is insignificant in the critically ill. At doses of 2 to 5 μg/kg/min, dopamine has primarily $\beta 1$ actions and very mild $\beta 2$ effects. At such doses, dopamine independently stimulates renal dopamine receptors, increasing renal blood flow, enhancing glomerular filtration rate (GFR), and promoting Na^+ excretion. Although the dopaminergic effects are not lost, α effects become more prominent at doses between 8 and 12 μg/kg/min. In still higher doses, dopamine possesses a pharmacologic profile much like that of norepinephrine. Dopamine increases the potential for tachycardia and arrhythmias, having a greater tendency for this unwanted side effect than dobutamine. Dopamine causes intense vasoconstriction and, if extravasated, may induce soft tissue necrosis—an effect antagonized by local infiltration of phentolamine.

Dobutamine   Dobutamine is an isoproterenol analog with primarily β1 actions. Dobutamine causes much less α stimulation than dopamine and less β2 activity than isoproterenol. Unlike isoproterenol, dobutamine boosts CO primarily by increasing SV rather than HR. Dobutamine is best suited to the treatment of low CO states in patients with a near-normal BP and good peripheral vascular tone. It is often given together with norepinephrine or phenylephrine, which helps offset its peripheral vasodilating effects. At commonly used doses, dobutamine is less likely than isoproterenol or dopamine to produce tachycardia, but mild increases in HR occur frequently, particularly in hypovolemic patients. Rarely, dobutamine increases AV conduction in patients with atrial fibrillation or flutter, leading to accelerated HR. In some patients with a very high baseline SVR, dobutamine may cause sufficient peripheral vasodilation to induce hypotension.

Noncatecholamine-Based Agents

Amrinone and Milrinone   Amrinone and milrinone are phosphodiesterase inhibitors with inotropic and vasodilating properties similar to dobutamine, but with even less tendency to cause arrhythmias. These agents have inotropic properties distinct from the catecholamines or digitalis glycosides. Amrinone is a positive inotrope and vasodilator that raises CO by increasing SV, not by increasing HR. Although useful in treating refractory heart failure, vasodilation not offset by a simultaneous α stimulator may give rise to limiting hypotension. While renal excretion provides the primary route of clearance, hepatic metabolism is significant. Therefore, the drug may accumulate in patients with either hepatic or renal failure. Increases in inotropic activity may aggravate outflow obstruction in hypertrophic cardiomyopathy. Increased ventricular rates have been reported during atrial fibrillation or flutter, but the chronotropic effect is generally less than that with any other currently available inotrope.

Thrombocytopenia occurs in a small minority of patients. High doses of amrinone given for long periods of time may elevate liver function tests or cause frank hepatic necrosis.

Vasopressin   Vasopressin, a weak vasoconstrictor in healthy normal subjects, has several applications in modern critical care practice. For many years this drug has been known to reduce portal pressure and has been used for that purpose in upper GI hemorrhage due to gastric and esophageal varices. More recently, it has shown to have additive effects when combined with a catecholamine-based vasoconstrictor (e.g., norepinephrine), particularly in the setting of refractory septic shock. Although not dramatically effective when used independently, vasopressin tends to boost urine output and improve other signs of shock when used as a secondary (supplemental) agent. Clinical trials suggest that its use be directed toward those in whom the catecholamine-based agents are insufficient to sustain an adequate perfusing pressure. Vasopressin should be considered a complement to—not replacement for—catechol vasopressors. In the setting of cardiopulmonary arrest secondary to ventricular fibrillation or pulseless ventricular tachycardia, the use of vasopressin as an alternative vasoconstrictor to the catecholamine-based agents has gained entry into current practice.

Glucocorticoids   The hypotensive consequences of acute adrenal crisis and have been known for the better part of a century. Only recently, however, has relative adrenal insufficiency (glucocorticoid levels inappropriate to severe stress) been recognized to complicate the course of critical illness, especially in patients with debilitating underlying diseases. Replacement of glucocorticoids may be crucial to reversing shock physiology in such patients. Unless extremely high or extremely low, a single measured cortisol level is not adequate to assess competence or reserve. Although a matter of some controversy, many experienced intensivists consider response to an adrenocorticotropic hormone (ACTH) analog (cosyntropin) necessary to justify its ongoing use. There also is general agreement that many patients in shock who remain hypotensive after fluid repletion and vasopressors will respond to "stress dose" glucocorticoids (preferably 200 to 300 mg of hydrocortisone, given in 3 or 4 divided doses per day over 3 to 7 days). Rapidity of resuscitation in response to steroids is supported by the results of large, recent clinical trials, whereas the impact on mortality has yet to be convincingly shown. Mineralocorticoid supplementation is not essential to the response, but is sometimes given as well. Because hydrocortisone acts relatively quickly and has such a high therapeutic index of benefit to risk, it seems reasonable to embark on such a regimen in virtually any patient with refractory shock, independently of the stimulation test results.

Glucagon and Insulin   The primary application of glucagon, which inhibits phosphodiesterase and improves myofibrillar calcium availablity, is in the treatment of *β*-blocker overdose. These patients may be desperately ill and in shock because of the negative inotropic and chronotropic effects of those agents. Atropine and isoproterenol are often helpful, but when ineffective or contraindicated, glucagon 0.5 to 5 mg initial bolus followed by a continuous infusion of 1 to 5 mg per h may be indicated. Glucose, insulin, potassium solutions have been used for many years in diverse settings and with variable results. Very recently, high-dose insulin (1 to 10 units/kg/h and with very closely monitored glucose and potassium blood concentrations) has been gaining strong support from animal and clinical experiments as a preferred therapy over glucagon or milrinone for overdoses of *β*-blocker, calcium channel blocker, or mixed ingestions with cardiotoxic properties arising from adrenergic, calcium and/or sodium channel blockade. (Tricyclic antidepressants and bupivicaine are examples of the latter.)

Other Drugs   In specific settings—for example, acute hyperkalemia and calcium channel blockade—calcium chloride may be invaluable. Furthermore, although not routinely indicated, it should be kept in mind that severe acidosis may limit catecholamine effectiveness; cautious administration of bicarbonate or alternative buffer (such as tromethamine [THAM]) may effectively serve as a vasopressor. (Raising pH is particularly effective in hyperkalemia.) Levosimendan, a calcium sensitizing agent now in clinical trials, has shown promise as a contraction-improving agent that may be superior to phosphodiesterase inhibitors (milrinone-like drugs) in the setting of cardiogenic shock. Finally, afterload-reducing agents (lisinopril or even nitroprusside) may sufficiently improve the ejection of a failing LV to improve perfusion of vital organs without compromising BP.

Mechanical Interventions and Devices

The output of the *failing* LV is sensitive to reductions in afterload (the fiber tension developed during systole) and relatively insensitive to reductions in precontractile fiber stretch or preload. Reducing the vigor of respiratory efforts may partially relieve the burden of the failing heart simply by decreasing its output requirements. Moreover, conversion to positive-pressure-assisted breathing raises the mean intrathoracic pressure, reducing the afterload to the LV without compromising its effective preload. For similar reasons, the application of PEEP can be an extremely helpful intervention in this setting.

Pacemakers can boost CO and reduce left atrial filling pressure when used on patients whose HR is inappropriately low relative to $\dot{V}O_2$. AV sequential pacemakers are perhaps most physiologic, the insertion of which requires special skills in the ICU setting. Pacemakers are discussed in greater detail in Chapter 4.

Fluids and vasoactive agents traditionally have been the primary options for support of failing circulation but, recently, mechanical devices have been developed and used on occasion for special indications. Artificial hearts and implanted left ventricular assist devices (LVAD) can provide temporary support options for patients with myocardial failure. Problems of infection, immobility, embolism, and cost have limited the use of implantable devices. Much more experience has accumulated with the intra-aortic balloon pump (IABP). This device is inserted in a retrograde fashion through the femoral artery into the descending aorta, above the renal arteries. Cycle-by-cycle diastolic inflation of the large tube-shaped aortic balloon augments both coronary artery and systemic perfusion pressures. Balloon deflation during systole reduces LV afterload, improving systemic perfusion. Ischemia of renal and peripheral arteries, cholesterol or gas embolism, stroke, coagulopathy, hemolysis, infection, and aortic dissection constitute major hazards. The IABP has been proven to be most useful in temporary support of patients with acute mitral insufficiency, ventricular septal defects, postsurgical and post-angiostent-related "stunning," or myocardial ischemia refractory to medical therapy (see Chapter 21). Gradual weaning from IABP usually is required and generally accomplished by reducing the ratio of balloon-assisted to unaided cardiac cycles. The IABP may be life sustaining for patients awaiting cardiac transplantation. For patients without appropriate physiology (aortic insufficiency, mitral stenosis, aortic dissection) or correctable mechanical defects, IABP and other ventricular assist devices are of unproven benefit and/or contraindicated.

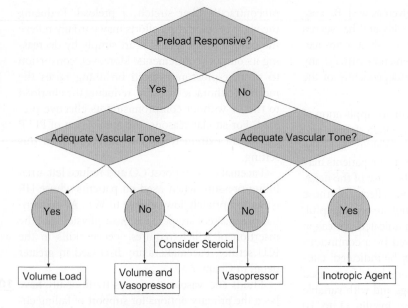

■ **FIGURE 3-3** Sequence for challenge-testing the components of the cardiovascular system in the setting of hypoperfusion. Ensuring adequate vascular filling and cardiac preloading should be considered a prerequisite for embarking on pharmacologic interventions directed toward the vasculature and myocardium.

A General Strategy for Managing Hemodynamic Instability

Faced with managing a hypotensive patient with suspected hypoperfusion due to insufficient cardiac priming or impaired vascular tone, it is important to have a consistent and logical approach to choosing interventions. Three important questions must be answered: (a) is pump performance impaired due to structural or functional causes (e.g., myocardial infarction or ischemia, arrhythmia)?; (b) is the problem one of insufficient preloading?; and (c) is vasomotor tone impaired? These questions usually need to be answered by *functional* testing—a therapeutic challenge to each physiologic component, approached in a defined sequence that begins with a test of preload adequacy and proceeds to pharmacologic interventions aimed at the vessels and heart, depending on response (Fig. 3-3).

■ CONGESTIVE HEART FAILURE

The physiology underlying management of CHF is detailed in Chapter 1. In essence, the common problem of these conditions relates to an imbalance between the hydrostatic pressure in the fluid-exchanging vessels of the lung (capillaries, small arterioles, and small venules) on one hand and the vascular oncotic forces and lymphatic drainage capacity on the other. Because neither lymphatic drainage nor vascular oncotic pressure can be improved easily or rapidly, clinical attention usually centers on reducing the left atrial pressure that regulates the filtering pressures upstream.

Causes

Left atrial pressure can rise for many reasons: reduced compliance of the left heart secondary to hypertrophy, ischemia, catecholamines, or interdependence with a swollen right ventricle (see diastolic dysfunction discussed previously); impaired contractility because of intrinsic myocardial disease, circulating depressant factors, or performance-impairing drugs; pathologically slow or inappropriately rapid HRs (requiring higher filling pressure to support SV or preventing adequate filling of the LV, respectively); conduction system disease and arrhythmias; or mitral valvular stenosis or insufficiency. Pulmonary congestion may be accompanied by adequate or insufficient forward output, depending on underlying cardiopathology and precipitating cause for the exacerbation.

Precipitants

For a predisposed patient, decompensation usually is brought on by excessive demands for CO relative to capacity to meet them (fever, increased work of breathing, physiologic stress); medication error or noncompliance; an adverse change in cardiac preload (renal insufficiency, overly zealous administration of intravascular volume, dietary indiscretion); a sudden augmentation of cardiac afterload (hypertension, ischemia, forceful inspiratory efforts); or alterations in myocardial compliance, heart rhythm, or contractility (electrolyte disturbances, ischemia, and sepsis are major offenders in this latter category).

Diagnosis

The key bedside indicators of pulmonary congestion are well known—new crackles, wheezes, and rhonchi; the appearance of an S_3 gallop; and, in many instances, distended neck veins, cool extremities, diaphoresis, and tachypnea. Alert patients almost always—but not invariably—experience exertional dyspnea and orthopnea. Hyponatremia and an elevated BUN/Cr ratio reflect prerenal perfusion inadequacy. Atrial and brain natriuretic peptides (ANP and BNP) are released in response to high ventricular filling pressures—whether induced by systolic or diastolic dysfunction. These peptides exert natriuretic, diuretic, and hypotensive effects (in part mediated through inhibition of the renin–angiotensin system) that may prove useful in both diagnosis and therapy (see following). BNP is more sensitive to aberrations of ventricular function and, therefore, is both more useful and widely used than ANP. Values of BNP less than 100 pg/mL argue strongly against heart failure or volume overload as the primary cause of dyspnea, whereas values that exceed 400 pg/mL are highly suggestive of contributions from those causes. Intermediate values suggest chronic LV dysfunction or *cor pulmonale*. Clearly, more than one cause for dyspnea may be present, so an elevated BNP level does *not* necessarily establish congestive failure as the primary cause. BNP is believed to be a useful monitor of CHF treatment effectiveness in the outpatient setting and has prognostic value in the setting of acute coronary syndrome. Interestingly, BNP levels may be helpful in gauging the adequacy of dialysis for intravascular volume regulation.

The chest radiograph often exhibits characteristic features: Kerley lines, blurred hilar structures, pleural effusions, a widened vascular pedicle, and diffuse, symmetrical infiltrates with spared costophrenic angles and without prominent air bronchograms. A balloon occlusion wedge pressure confirms an elevated pulmonary venous pressure that rises sharply after volume challenge. The echocardiogram usually provides evidence of a dilated left atrium, distended vena cava, impaired contractility, or diastolic dysfunction (see Chapter 2).

Management of Congestive Failure

The sitting position, supplemental oxygen, diuresis, afterload reduction, adequate sedation, and relief of an excessive breathing workload by continuous positive airway pressure (CPAP), biphasic airway pressure (Bi-PAP), or mechanical ventilation are fundamental to the care of patients with acute left heart failure. (Cor pulmonale is discussed in Chapter 1.) Opiates and nitrates may be useful in acute pulmonary edema (see below). With regard to diuretics, consideration should be given to the use of a furosemide or bumetanide drip to more closely observe and consistently regulate diuresis (rather than conventional boluses) for patients who are particularly fragile with regard to intravascular volume status and/or are refractory to bolus dosing. The addition of a thiazide diuretic (metoclopramide or chlorothiazide) may amplify the effect of the loop diuretics. Venous ultrafiltration can be extremely effective and well tolerated for removing fluid in patients without adequate urinary response to diuresis. These pump-driven circuits can remove up to 200 mL/fluid/h. For those with hypoproteinemia, the simultaneous administration of albumin not only increases intravascular volume and oncotic pressure, but also improves delivery of these loop diuretics to their primary site of action. Nesiritide may prove an effective (but expensive) agent in patients who are not effectively managed by diuretics and salt restriction (see following).

Precipitating causes must be identified and eliminated, if possible. Electrical cardioversion of rapid atrial arrhythmias and slowing of rapid atrial fibrillation with diltiazem, amiodarone, esmolol, metoprolol or digoxin may sometimes be indicated. Opiates (morphine, fentanyl) and nitrates have multiple therapeutic effects in carefully selected patients. Morphine relieves anxiety, thereby reducing O_2 consumption and doubles as a venodilator that reduces central vascular volume. Fentanyl is often used when repeated or continuously administered opiate effects are required in patients with renal insufficiency. Nitrates also increase venous capacitance, simultaneously dilating the coronary vasculature in patients with ischemic disease. Although short-acting β-blockers may clearly be helpful in treating patients with adequate systolic function and appropriate indications (e.g., rapid arrhythmia, ongoing ischemia, thyrotoxicosis), *extreme* caution should attend their use in the acute setting.

Vasoactive Drugs in CHF

Nitroprusside and hydralazine can be helpful when CHF is either caused or exacerbated by systemic hypertension. Angiotensin-converting enzyme (ACE) inhibitors reduce the ejection impedance of the afterload-sensitive LV and often prove fundamental to successful management. Although calcium channel blocking agents can also be used for this purpose, they also tend to suppress ventricular contractility. Verapamil is the greatest offender in this regard; nifedipine and nimodipine are better tolerated.

Cardiotonic Agents in CHF

Digoxin has served a time-honored but increasingly limited role in improving the contractility of a dilated heart. In the critical care unit, many practitioners reserve it for controlling HR in atrial fibrillation when other agents are less desirable because of their potential for adverse inotropic effects and the need is not immediate. As in treatment of overt shock, catecholamine-based inotropes such as dobutamine or dopamine are generally the agents of choice, unless their tendency to increase HR overcomes the inotropic benefit by reducing LV filling time or by inciting ischemia. Milrinone may be particularly useful in circumstances in which inotropy is desired but concomitant elevation of HR must be minimized. Occasionally, norepinephrine or phenylephrine helps to maintain coronary perfusion pressure and sustain forward output when hypotension accompanies failure. For patients with florid pulmonary edema, intubation and mechanical ventilation may be a key therapeutic intervention if CPAP and non-invasive ventilation by mask is not feasible or is poorly tolerated, acidosis is progressing, or hypoxemia and the work of breathing are severe.

Nesiritide

Nesiritide, a recombinant analog of human BNP that is given by intravenous infusion, may be an effective agent in the treatment of heart failure. The mechanism of action is debated, but it seems likely that it counterbalances vasoconstricting and antidiuretic neurohormones as well as promotes natriuresis. Nesiritide is worth considering when intravenous catecholamines are limited by side effects (such as tachycardia), when intravenous diuretic therapy is relatively ineffective, or when moderate renal dysfunction complicates severe CHF (without shock). Although nesiritide can be used for many days and then abruptly discontinued, its effects tend to persist for several days after the CHF exacerbation has resolved. The N-terminal fragment of the prohormone from which endogenous BNP is cleaved (N-pro-BNP) serves as an effective monitor of its activity.

■ SUGGESTED READINGS

Constanzo MR. Ultrafiltration in the management of heart failure. *Curr Opin Crit Care.* 2008;14:524–530.

Dellinger RP, Levy MM, Carlet JM, et al. Surviving sepsis campaign: International guidelines for management of severe sepsis and septic shock: 2008. *Intensive Care Med.* 2008;34(1):17–60.

Haddad F, Doyle R, Murphy DJ, et al. Right ventricular function in cardiovascular disease, Part II: Pathophysiology, clinical importance, and management of right ventricular failure. *Circulation.* 2008; 117(13):1717–1731.

Hollenberg SM. Vasopressor support in septic shock. *Chest.* 2007;132(5): 1678–1687.

Hollenberg SM, Terlink JR. Advances in congestive heart failure management in the ICU: Bench to bedside. *Crit Care Med.* 2008;36(1): S1–S139.

London JA, Sena MJ. Pharmacologic support of the failing heart. *Surg Clin North Am.* 2006;86(6):1503–1521.

Ng TM, Singh AK, Dasta JF, et al. Contemporary issues in the pharmacologic management of acute heart failure. *Crit Care Clin.* 2006;22: 199–219.

Pirracchio R, Ligearet D, Noveneau M, et al. The use of natriuretic peptides in the intensive care unit. *Curr Opin Crit Care.* 2008;14:536–542.

Reynolds HR, Hochman JS. Cardiogenic shock: Current concepts and improving outcomes. *Circulation.* 2008;117(5):686–697.

Rivers E, Nguyen B, Havstad S, et al. Early goal-directed therapy in the treatment of severe sepsis and septic shock. *N Engl J Med.* 2001; 345:1368–1377.

Vincent JL, Gerlach H. Fluid resuscitation in severe sepsis and septic shock: An evidence-based review. *Crit Care Med.* 2004;32(Suppl. 11):S451–S454.

Arrhythmias, Pacing, and Cardioversion

The treatment of arrhythmias has become less common and much simpler over the last two decades as a result of a series of important discoveries. For example, it was revealed that it is unnecessary to convert most patients with atrial fibrillation (A-fib) to sinus rhythm and the suppression of premature ventricular contractions (PVCs) does not improve outcomes. In addition, many of the drugs used for years to control ventricular arrhythmias were abandoned because they were found to increase mortality. The sophistication and effectiveness of implantable and transthoracic pacing systems dramatically improved. Radiofrequency ablation made many chronic troublesome arrhythmias curable, and for arrhythmias that cannot be cured, (e.g., genetic long QT syndrome, recurrent sudden death), implantable defibrillators have been lifesaving. Adenosine has been immensely helpful for diagnosis and therapy, and the role of amiodarone in the treatment was refined. Finally, the widespread application of rapid reperfusion strategies for acute coronary syndrome eliminated millions of periinfarction arrhythmias and probably as many arrhythmias from postinfarction heart failure. Despite these advances, the critical care physician must still be able to make an accurate diagnosis of an arrhythmia by rapidly interpreting an electrocardiogram (ECG) and provide appropriate emergency treatment.

■ COMPONENTS OF THE ELECTROCARDIOGRAM

The first step in evaluation of the ECG is to identify atrial activity (P waves) which is best seen in the inferior leads (II, III, and aVF). P wave shape should be examined for consistency; the pattern should be studied for evidence of atrial flutter or fibrillation and for the position and consistency of the P wave relative to the QRS complex. P wave inversion in limb lead II signifies retrograde atrial depolarization diagnostic of a nonsinus mechanism. After the atrial rhythm has been characterized, ventricular activity

(QRS complex) should be examined. If the QRS is narrow, ventricular depolarization most likely occurs in response to normal sequential atrioventricular (AV) conduction or at least is of supraventricular origin. A QRS complex (>0.12 s) suggests (a) ventricular origin, (b) an aberrantly conducted supraventricular beat, (c) a bypass pathway, or (d) supraventricular conduction delayed by a drug (e.g., tricyclic antidepressant) – electrolyte (e.g., hyperkalemia) abnormality. The QRS should be examined for regularity, rate, and the relationship to the P waves. If every QRS complex is not preceded by a P wave, some form of AV block, or A-fib or flutter, or ventricular tachycardia (VT), is likely. Because of the normal delays associated with AV nodal conduction, a QRS complex occurring less than 0.1 s after a P wave is unlikely to be related to it.

■ **GENERAL APPROACH TO ARRHYTHMIAS**

Acute arrhythmias are detrimental when they are symptomatic, reduce tissue perfusion, or increase myocardial oxygen demand. Chronic tachyarrhythmias can also be harmful by causing cardiomyopathy. In making management decisions, the patient's symptoms; adequacy of perfusion; the risks of treatment versus observation; and chronic-**1** ity of the problem must be considered. Tachyarrhythmias evoking unconsciousness, hypotension, pulmonary edema, or angina should be terminated immediately as should symptomatic bradycardia. Patients with isolated PVCs lacking evidence of heart failure or ischemia have an excellent prognosis without treatment. In such patients, drug suppression of the arrhythmia is unlikely to improve outcome, but is apt to produce untoward side effects. A past history of well-tolerated arrhythmia similar to the one currently present also suggests that rapid treatment is not necessary. Conversely, patients with myocardial ischemia and those with a history of malignant or degenerative arrhythmias should be treated aggressively. Arrhythmias are often exacerbated if not provoked **2** by electrolyte disturbances, mechanical irritation of the heart, drugs, and ischemia. Thus, hypokalemia or hyperkalemia, hypomagnesemia, alkalosis, anemia, and hypoxemia all exacerbate arrhythmic tendencies. Intracardiac catheters, pacemaker malfunction, digitalis, theophylline, and sympathomimetic agents (e.g., catecholamines, cocaine) can provoke a wide variety of arrhythmias

that cease upon their removal. It is also clear that several antiarrhythmic drugs (e.g., quinidine, sotalol, flecainide) can have serious proarrhythmic effects. Electrical instability is also heightened by ischemia. For example, hypotension reduces myocardial perfusion, whereas excess intravascular volume or high ventricular afterload can increase wall tension and oxygen demand.

Dealing with Uncertainty

Asymptomatic, or minimally symptomatic narrow complex tachyarrhythmias, and pulseless arrhythmias rarely present diagnostic or therapeutic dilemmas. By contrast, an unfamiliar arrhythmia, especially a wide complex tachycardia (WCT), in a patient with a moderate decrease in blood pressure or modest symptoms is often anxiety provoking. The first step when confronted with an unfamiliar arrhythmia is to confirm that it is real. Electrical artifacts may occur as a result of poor surface electrode contact or electromechanical devices such as aortic balloon or infusion pumps. Shivering, seizure activity, and tremors of Parkinson disease can produce ECG artifacts that may be confused with serious arrhythmias.

The most consternation is caused by monomorphic WCT not clearly of ventricular or supraventricular origin. To avoid mistakes under pressure, it is important to develop an approach to diagnosis and therapy in advance (Table 4-1). When patients are hemodynamically compromised, it is best to treat arrhythmias as if they were life threatening **3** and the vast majority of WCTs are ventricular.

TABLE 4-1 TREATMENT FOR REGULAR MONOMORPHIC WIDE COMPLEX TACHYCARDIA OF UNCERTAIN ORIGIN

(Pulseless or symptomatic hypotensive patients should receive immediate unsynchronized cardioversion.)

Lidocaine (1–1.5 mg/kg × 1 IV bolus)
↓
Repeat lidocaine (0.5–0.75 mg/kg IV q5–10min) (Maximum dose 3 mg/kg)
↓
Procainamide (20–30 mg/min) (Maximum 17 mg/kg IV load)
↓
Amiodarone (150 mg at 15 mg/min IV) (May repeat × 2–3 at 10-min intervals)
↓
If unresponsive, DC synchronized cardioversion

However, it is important to exclude the presence of high-grade AV block. (Infranodal escape rhythms must not be terminated before treating the underlying heart block.) Hence, patients with WCT in distress should receive either cardioversion or drug therapy for VT (e.g., amiodarone, lidocaine, procainamide) depending on clinical urgency. Traditionally, lidocaine was the drug of first choice, and failure to respond to it supports a diagnosis of supraventricular tachycardia (SVT) with aberrant conduction. (In this setting, procainamide and amiodarone are good choices because they will control many types of SVT and VT.) Although these drugs rarely help clarify the diagnosis, they often control the rhythm long enough to get expert advice or perform more sophisticated diagnostic maneuvers. In the patient failing a trial of lidocaine, adenosine may also be tried. (By transiently blocking the AV node, adenosine is very effective at slowing or terminating SVT.) In cases of WCT, verapamil or diltiazem is a suboptimal choice for empirical therapy because their cardiodepressant and vasodilating properties often further lower the blood pressure in the setting of VT, and SVTs utilizing a bypass tract can be accelerated. Similarly, adenosine is not a good choice if the patient is suspected to have a bypass tract. A discussion of the most common arrhythmias and their treatment follows.

■ TACHYARRHYTHMIAS

Sinus Tachycardia

Sinus tachycardia (ST) is the primary means of raising cardiac output in response to metabolic demands; thus, it is physiologic in the setting of exercise, fever, or hyperthyroidism. ST is also appropriate compensation for hypovolemia, limited stroke volume, reduced systemic vascular resistance, or reduced myocardial compliance. Anxiety, pain, and drugs (e.g., catecholamines, cocaine, theophylline) may also be responsible. Unless ST causes ischemia by increasing myocardial oxygen consumption, or precipitates pulmonary edema by shortening diastolic filling time in a patient with reduced ventricular compliance, it is simply a marker of illness. The best therapy for ST is to treat the underlying cause. In patients with symptomatic ischemia, β-blockade often proves helpful. However, β-blockers should be used cautiously in tachycardic patients with hypotension, acute infarction, or chronic congestive heart failure because ST often reflects incipient decompensation. Likewise, caution is indicated using β-blocker in patients with obstructive lung disease because of the risk of exacerbating bronchospasm.

Nonsinus Supraventricular Tachycardias

The nomenclature surrounding SVT is confusing but the concepts are simple. SVT usually results from a self-perpetuating reentry mechanism; much less commonly, SVT stems from rapid discharge of an ectopic atrial focus. Graphic examples of the most common forms of SVT are shown in Figure 4.1.

Reentrant Tachycardias Involving the AV Node

Reentrant SVTs occur when two potential transmission pathways have differing conduction speeds and refractory periods permitting a reverberating circuit to develop. This group of arrhythmias is classified by whether that circuit lies solely within the AV node or whether one limb of the circuit bypasses the AV node. By far the most common form is AV nodal reentrant tachycardia (AVNRT) in which a "micro-reentrant" pathway exists entirely

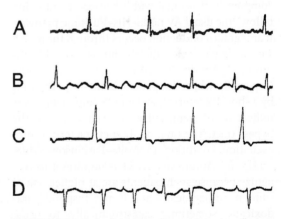

■ **FIGURE 4-1** Stylized electrocardiographic tracings illustrating the distinguishing features of the most common supraventricular arrhythmias. **Panel A** shows the irregular ventricular response and absence of well-defined P waves characteristic of A-fib. By contrast, **Panel B** illustrates the rapid inverted "sawtooth" atrial depolarizations of atrial flutter. Commonly a 2:1 ventricular response often results in a ventricular rate of 150 beats/min. **Panel C** shows the most common pattern of AVNRT in which an isoelectric baseline is punctuated by slightly irregular narrow complex ventricular depolarizations. Close examination reveals inverted monomorphic P waves buried in the QRS and T waves. **Panel D** illustrates the characteristic polymorphic P wave pattern of MAT.

within the AV node. Although sometimes confused with atrial flutter with 2:1 conduction, AVNRT can usually be identified by its isoelectric inter-QRS baseline and slightly irregular, narrow QRS, occurring at a rate 150 to 200 beats/min. QRS complexes frequently exhibit a rate-related, right-bundle branch block pattern that may simulate VT. (P waves are often buried in the QRS complex or T wave, producing a "pseudo-S wave.") When visible, P waves are frequently inverted in the inferior leads because atrial depolarization characteristically begins in the AV node located low in the right atrium and spreads cephalad. Unlike A-fib or flutter, in which the ventricular response slows to vagal stimulation or adenosine therapy, AVNRT either remains completely unaffected or stops abruptly.

The less common form of reentrant SVT is AV reentrant tachycardia (AVRT) in which ventricular rates are typically a bit faster (150 to 250 beats/min). AVRT is caused by a "macro-reentrant" circuit in which one conduction limb goes through the AV node and one limb bypasses it. AVRT is subclassified by the direction the current takes through the AV node. If antegrade conduction is through the AV node, it is termed "orthodromic." Unless there are rate-related conduction delays, in orthodromic AVRT the QRS complex is of normal width because conduction follows the usual AV-node–His–Purkinje pathway. If antegrade conduction occurs through the accessory or bypass tract, the rhythm is termed "antidromic." Antidromic AVRT may be identified (especially while the patient is in sinus rhythm) by a short PR interval, wider QRS, and delta waves indicative of ventricular preexcitation on the bypass tract. The rare, but best characterized preexcitation condition is Wolfe–Parkinson–White syndrome. Antidromic AVRT is important to recognize because such patients are at higher risk of sudden cardiac death, and it may respond paradoxically, sometimes catastrophically, to usual SVT treatments. Intra-SA node, or intra-atrial, reentrant rhythms may occur but will not be discussed further because they are rare.

Adenosine and vagal maneuvers like carotid sinus massage are valuable tools to distinguish reentrant SVTs from VT and from non-nodal-reentrant atrial arrhythmias like A-fib and flutter and ectopic atrial tachycardia. VT is unresponsive to vagal maneuvers, and if the rhythm is A-fib, only transient slowing of the ventricular rate is likely. If the rhythm is flutter, blocking the AV node will unmask the characteristic flutter waves but will not stop the atrial reentrant circuit.

SVTs are generally well tolerated and self-limited, often requiring no treatment with the possible exception of stopping exacerbating drugs (e.g., theophylline, catecholamines, and cocaine) and correcting electrolyte disorders. If treatment is needed, maneuvers or drugs that inhibit conduction through the AV node are highly effective. Massage of the nondominant carotid artery for 10 to 15 s, alone or in conjunction with the Valsalva maneuver, often interrupts AVNRT and AVRT. To avoid cerebral ischemia, both carotid arteries should not be compressed simultaneously, and vessels with bruits and those of patients with a history of stroke or transient ischemia should not be massaged. When mechanical maneuvers fail, drug intervention is indicated. Adenosine has supplanted calcium channel blockers (e.g., verapamil) as the initial therapy of choice for hemodynamically stable SVT. As a potent but short-lived AV node blocker, a 6 to 18 mg of IV (intravenously) adenosine dose terminates AVNRT and AVRT with a success rate equal to or greater than that of verapamil. Although very effective at stopping the original arrhythmia, up to 10% of patients with AVNRT and AVRT convert to A-fib. Adenosine does not terminate A-fib or flutter. Calcium channel blockers, like verapamil, represent second-line therapy but should be avoided when supraventricular origin is in doubt, hypotension is present, or a bypass tract is suspected. The nodal blocking effects may encourage atrial conduction over the bypass tract, and the vasodilating effects of calcium channel blockers may cause hypotension unless rhythm conversion occurs. If used, verapamil doses of 2.5 to 5 mg IV are usually adequate. (Comparable doses of diltiazem may be substituted, but nicardipine is less effective.) β-blockers like propranolol (0.5 to 1 mg every 5 min, up to a 4-mg total dose) or metoprolol may also be effective. If the patient's ability to tolerate β-blockade is uncertain, the short-acting esmolol can be tried. Digoxin has long been used in the treatment of AVNRT but often requires hours for effect, making it most useful in hemodynamically stable patients and in those requiring prophylaxis. By boosting systemic blood pressure, vasoconstrictive drugs (e.g., phenylephrine) may reflexly decrease AV-nodal conduction. However, vasopressors may precipitate cardiac or cerebrovascular complications and are therefore usually avoided. Cholinergic stimulants like neostigmine can increase nodal vagal tone thereby ending nodal

4

reentrant arrhythmias but have an unacceptable side effect profile. Because *all* of the reentrant circuit is in the AV node in AVNRT, it tends to be easily broken by AV-nodal blocking measures. Because just one limb of the conducting circuit passes through the AV node in AVRT, adenosine (or any other AV-nodal blocker) often stops the arrhythmia but there is a risk; blocking antegrade conduction through the AV node may promote very rapid conduction through a bypass tract with a very rapid, even life-threatening (VT or VF) response. This complication is most likely in patients who develop A-fib or flutter with a bypass tract.

Lidocaine has no effect on SVT. Type Ia antiarrhythmics (e.g., quinidine and procainamide) exert vagolytic effects and often worsen SVT by accelerating AV conduction unless nodal-blocking drugs are administered first. In refractory SVT, temporary overdrive atrial pacing may restore sinus rhythm and is easily done when an atrial pacer or pacing pulmonary artery catheter is already in place, as is common after cardiac surgery. Hemodynamically unstable SVT should be treated with low-energy (10 to 50 WS [watt-seconds]) synchronized cardioversion. An outline of therapy for SVT is presented in Table 4-2.

Primary Atrial Tachycardias

Ectopic Atrial Tachycardia

Ectopic atrial tachycardia can result from a single ectopic focus firing at a rapid rate, or more commonly from multiple rapidly discharging atrial foci.

The later mechanism is known as multifocal atrial tachycardia (MAT) and most often occurs in association with obstructive lung disease or metabolic crisis, but it also complicates left ventricular failure, coronary artery disease, diabetes, sepsis, and toxicity with digitalis, theophylline, and sympathomimetic drugs. Among patients with lung disease, hypoxemia, hypercapnia, acidosis, alkalosis, pulmonary hypertension, and β-agonist therapy have all have been identified as risk factors. When multiple P-wave morphologies are conducted at a normal ventricular rate, the condition is referred to as a "wandering atrial pacemaker." MAT is recognized by irregularly irregular QRS complexes of supraventricular origin, varying PR intervals, and the presence of at least three morphologically distinct P waveforms on an isoelectric baseline. (The less common unifocal atrial tachycardia has a single P wave morphology.) Comparable heart rates (100 to 180 beats/min) and beat-to-beat variation in PR and RR intervals often cause MAT to be confused with A-fib.

Because ectopic tachycardias do not depend on the AV node, measures to increase AV-nodal refractoriness are usually ineffective. Although β-blockers and calcium channel blockers may temporarily slow or convert MAT, the definitive treatment is to reverse the underlying cause. Correction of hypokalemia and supplementing magnesium, perhaps even if levels are within the normal range, can be helpful and is unlikely to be harmful unless renal insufficiency is present. ($MgSO_4$ given as 2 gm IV may slow the rate, if not convert the rhythm.) Verapamil

---

TABLE 4-2 TREATMENT PLAN FOR NARROW COMPLEX REGULAR TACHYCARDIA

If unstable, direct current synchronized cardioversion
↓
Vagal maneuvers
↓
Adenosine (6–18 mg rapid IV bolus)
(may repeat × 2)

SVT	Ectopic atrial tachycardia
Preserved LV function Metoprolol 5 mg IV (15 mg max.) Verapamil 2.5–5 mg IV	**Preserved LV function** Metoprolol 5 mg IV (15 mg max.) Verapamil 2.5–5 mg IV

Impaired LV function
Digoxin 0.125–0.25 mg
  IV q4–6h
Amiodarone 150 mg IV over
  15 min
	Impaired LV function
	Amiodarone 150 mg IV over
	  15 min
	(Cardioversion is ineffective)

(up to 20 mg), or diltiazem, can be useful by decreasing the frequency of the atrial impulses, not by blocking their entry to the ventricle. Unfortunately, verapamil commonly reduces blood pressure, an effect that to some extent can be ameliorated by pretreatment with calcium gluconate. β-blockade can also control the rate or less often abolish MAT, but has obvious limitations in a population of patients many of whom have lung disease. If β-blockers are used, short-acting agents (i.e., esmolol) or cardioselective blockers (i.e., metoprolol) make the most sense. Metoprolol, 5 mg IV every 10 min can be tried and if well tolerated, the patient can be converted to an oral dose of 50 to 100 mg once or twice daily. Neither cardioversion, digitalis, nor the antiarrhythmics lidocaine, quinidine, procainamide, and phenytoin benefit patients with MAT. The role of radiofrequency ablation for MAT is uncertain at this time. Whereas theophylline and β-agonists may occasionally precipitate MAT, their cautious use may improve underlying bronchospasm sufficiently to reverse the arrhythmia. In patients who demonstrate MAT in response to theophylline or β-agonists, corticosteroids or inhaled anticholinergics represent attractive alternative options for treating bronchospasm because they are not cardiostimulatory.

Atrial Fibrillation

A-fib is a common, (prevalence approx. 5% among patients >70 years) chaotic atrial rhythm in which no single ectopic pacemaker captures the entire atrium, hence there is no detectable P wave on ECG. New onset A-fib often complicates chest surgery, pulmonary embolism, valvular heart disease, obstructive lung disease, and hyperthyroidism. The irregular ventricular rhythm may be confused with MAT, frequent premature atrial contractions, ST, or atrial flutter with variable AV block. Because there is no organized atrial depolarization or contraction to facilitate left ventricular priming, cardiac output may fall significantly, especially in patients with impaired ventricular compliance. Although the atria may depolarize up to 400 times/min, the AV node rarely conducts impulses at rates higher than 180 to 200 beats/min. However, fever, sepsis, vagolytic drugs, and the presence of accessory conduction pathways may increase the ventricular response. On physical examination, A-fib is suggested by a fluctuating S1 (because of varying mitral valve position at the onset of ventricular systole) and a pulse deficit (because of occasional

systoles with low ejection volumes). There are three prominent risks of A-fib: hypoperfusion from too rapid a ventricular rate, systemic embolism from clot formation in the noncontractile atrium, and cardiomyopathy from chronic tachycardia.

Treatment is guided by ventricular rate, hemodynamic adequacy, baseline left ventricular function, duration of the rhythm, and presence of a nodal bypass tract. Acute hemodynamic compromise from a rapid ventricular rate (>150) mandates synchronized cardioversion (100 to 200 WS of monophasic energy or the biphasic equivalent). Occasionally, higher energy levels are required. (The longer the duration, the more resistant A-fib is to conversion.) Ventricular rates greater than 200 beats/min suggest accelerated conduction due to vagolytic drugs (e.g., type Ia antiarrhythmics) or presence of an accelerated conduction pathway. If the ventricular rate is less than 60 beats/min, drug effect (e.g., digitalis, β-blockers, calcium channel blockers) or conduction system disease should be suspected. In untreated patients with a slow ventricular response, electrical cardioversion, or nodal-blocking drugs may produce symptomatic bradycardia or even asystole; a risk that is sufficiently high that a temporary pacemaker should be inserted prior to attempting cardioversion.

There is no rush to correct chronic, hemodynamically stable A-fib. Before conversion is attempted, the likelihood of attaining and maintaining sinus rhythm should be assessed and the risk of systemic embolism should be considered. When left atrial diameter exceeds 4 cm, conversion to stable sinus rhythm is unlikely. Although many clinicians advocate at least one attempt at restoring sinus rhythm, most patients do quite well if anticoagulated and the resting ventricular rate is maintained less than 100 beats/min. Landmark trials indicate that restoration of sinus rhythm does not result in a significant reduction of the risk of embolization in the anticoagulated patient, but without anticoagulation the annual risk is substantially higher.

For hemodynamically stable A-fib, the first step in treatment is to slow the resting ventricular rate to ≤100 beats/min. If ventricular function is good, calcium channel or β-blockers are preferred rate-controlling agents. If ventricular function is impaired, digoxin is a better choice, although amiodarone and diltiazem can be used with caution. With digoxin alone or in combination with a β-blocker or calcium channel blocker, approximately 20% of patients with recent onset A-fib convert to sinus rhythm. Because drugs that block normal AV conduction can accelerate conduction over the bypass tract, calcium channel or β-blocking drugs or digitalis are recommended only if there is reasonable certainty that a nodal bypass tract does not exist. Amiodarone is perhaps the best initial therapy for both rate control and rhythm conversion if a nodal bypass tract is suspected.

If A-fib is of less than 48-h duration, the ventricular rate is controlled; and it is judged that there is a reasonable likelihood of sustaining sinus rhythm and there are two reasonable courses of action. One is to perform synchronized cardioversion using 100 to 200 WS shock. Cardioversion is highly effective initially but unfortunately, A-fib recurs in most patients unless pharmacologic inhibition is continued; therefore, it makes little sense to convert patients intolerant of suppressive medications. The alternative course of action is to use amiodarone, ibutilide, or procainamide to chemically convert A-fib to sinus rhythm. Of the available choices, amiodarone is highly effective but has several practical limitations: when given IV, approximately 25% of patients develop hypotension and chemical phlebitis is common. Amiodarone has significant β-blocking properties and increases plasma levels of digoxin; both of which can lead to significant bradycardia after rhythm conversion. In addition, amiodarone potentiates the effects of warfarin and routinely results in abnormal thyroid function tests. Finally, amiodarone can cause pulmonary toxicity, especially when used in high doses or for long periods of time. Procainamide is effective in approximately 40% of patients but is generally poorly tolerated long-term. Ibutilide's use is limited because the drug is only available parenterally and it rarely has a proarrhythmic effect, especially in patients with QT prolongation.

If A-fib has been present for more than 48 h, anticoagulation should be undertaken for 3 to 4 weeks before rhythm conversion so as to minimize the risk of embolization (unless atrial clot can be excluded with certainty using transesophageal echocardiography). After conversion, anticoagulation should be continued for another 3 to 4 weeks. For the patient in whom A-fib cannot be corrected, long-term anticoagulation is indicated to prevent systemic embolism and stroke. The annual incidence of stroke averages 1% for patients without mitral valve disease or heart failure but can be as high as 6% for patients with both risk factors.

Atrial Flutter

Atrial flutter (flutter) arises in a localized region of reentry outside the AV node or, less commonly, in a rapidly firing ectopic focus. Depolarization usually originates from low in the right atrium, producing inverted P waves in the inferior leads and upright P deflections in lead V1. Flutter frequently complicates pneumonia, exacerbations of chronic lung disease, and the postoperative course of thoracic surgery patients but seldom occurs following myocardial infarction (MI). Flutter is intrinsically unstable, often converting to A-fib spontaneously or in response to drug therapy. Because the flutter circuit does not involve the AV node, atrial rates are usually quite rapid (260 to 340 beats/min). The AV node cannot conduct impulses at such high rates, so the ventricular response is a fraction, typically ½ or ¼ of the atrial rate. Most commonly, 2:1 AV block leads to a regular ventricular rate of approximately 150 beats/min. The ventricular response can be slowed, but the rhythm is rarely terminated by vagal maneuvers. If there is uncertainty about the rhythm, administration of adenosine is almost always diagnostic, revealing the characteristic "sawtooth" atrial depolarizations. Examination of the jugular pulse or recording of a right atrial pressure tracing can sometimes reveal the diagnostic atrial "flutter" waves.

The treatment of flutter is the same as that for A-fib. With a success rate greater than 95%, electrical cardioversion is the most effective method of restoring sinus rhythm, even when low doses (50 to 100 WS) of energy are used. Overdrive atrial pacing also effectively terminates this rhythm. Because a high percentage of patients revert to flutter or A-fib after conversion, long-term rate or rhythm control using the same medications as outlined for A-fib is indicated.

Ventricular Extrasystoles

Ventricular extrasystoles are commonly associated with organic heart disease, ischemia, and drug toxicity. These autonomous discharges usually occur before the next expected sinus depolarization and are therefore termed PVCs. A PVC is recognized by an abnormally wide QRS complex accompanied by an ST segment and a T wave whose axes are directed opposite that of the QRS. "Electrically insulated" from the ventricles, the sinoatrial (SA) node continues to discharge independently during the PVC but usually fails to influence the ventricle. Occasionally, when the timing is conducive, a combined supraventricular/ventricular electrical impulse may form a "fusion beat." Because the SA node is not reset by the PVC, the first conducted sinus beat following the PVC appears only after a fully compensatory pause. (A PVC may be interpolated between two sinus beats without a compensatory pause in patients with bradycardia.) It is often difficult to distinguish PVCs from aberrantly conducted supraventricular beats. Factors favoring PVCs are listed in Table 4-3. Aberrantly conducted supraventricular beats (usually in a right bundle branch block configuration) often appear when a short RR interval follows a long RR interval in patients with A-fib or MAT. This "Ashman" phenomenon results from variable, rate-related recovery of the conduction system after depolarization. Occasionally, ventricular extrasystoles are not premature but delayed. These escape beats, usually occurring at a rate of 30 to 40 beats/min, function as a safety mechanism to produce ventricular contraction when normal sinus conduction fails. Ventricular extrasystoles that occur in succession at rates less than 40 beats/min are referred to as "idioventricular." A rate of 40 to 100 beats/min defines an "accelerated" idioventricular rhythm. For obvious reasons, ventricular escape beats should not be suppressed. The primary treatment of idioventricular rhythm is to increase the SA nodal rate with atropine, isoproterenol, or pacing.

The prognosis and treatment of PVCs depends on their cause and frequency. Most PVCs do not require treatment. Indeed, it is clear that pharmacologic suppression of isolated PVCs or minimally symptomatic complex ventricular ectopy in the postmyocardial infarction setting may be associated with a higher likelihood of sudden death. Although some patterns are clearly more dangerous than others, VT or ventricular fibrillation (VF) often develops without a "warning rhythm." Historically accepted indications for acute treatment of PVCs in the critically ill include (a) frequent (>5/min) or multifocal PVCs in the setting of cardiac ischemia, (b) VT or frequent PVCs causing angina or hypotension, or the once widely accepted but now more controversial, and (c) an "R on T" configuration (PVC interrupts ascending portion of preceding T wave). Common underlying causes of PVCs include ischemia, acidosis, hypoxemia, electrolyte disorders, drugs, and toxins. Surprisingly, "antiarrhythmic" agents have a relatively high frequency (approx. 20%) of worsening existing arrhythmias or causing new rhythm disturbances, the so-called proarrhythmic effect.

The vast majority of PVCs should be ignored, or treatment should be aimed at the underlying cause. Intravenous lidocaine is the drug of choice for PVCs requiring acute treatment. Amiodarone and procainamide are acceptable parenteral alternatives. Quinidine should not be used in the acute setting because it is sometimes harmful, is frequently ineffective, has a delayed onset of action, and is available only as an oral preparation.

Ventricular Tachycardia

VT is defined as three or more consecutive ventricular beats occurring at a rate greater than 100/min (commonly 140 to 220/min). Some clinicians prefer the more stringent definition of ten or more consecutive beats. The beats of VT are recognized by wide QRS complexes with T waves of opposite polarity. The ECG hallmark of VT is AV dissociation (a phenomenon resulting from the independent firing of the SA node and the ventricular focus). Mild beat-to-beat variation in the RR interval is usually present. VT is usually symptomatic and generally occurs in patients with underlying heart disease. "Primary" VT associated with transient myocardial ischemia carries little prognostic significance; however, late or secondary VT occurring several days after infarction is associated with a high likelihood of recurrence and a poor prognosis. The mechanism of VT is the rapid firing of an ectopic ventricular pacemaker or electrical reentry within the His–Purkinje network. Antecedent isolated PVCs are not consistently present but VT is usually often initiated by a PVC with

TABLE 4-3 CHARACTERISTICS FAVORING VENTRICULAR ARRHYTHMIAS OVER SUPRAVENTRICULAR ARRHYTHMIA WITH ABERRANT CONDUCTION

Rr' or qR in V1
Notched QRS complex with R > r'
QS in V6 or an R/S ratio in V6 < 1.0
QRS duration > 0.14 s
Fully compensatory pause
Fusion beats or capture beats
AV dissociation
Extreme left axis deviation (negative leads I and aVF)
Uniform depolarization rate

delayed linkage to the preceding QRS. Occasionally, retrograde atrial depolarization may occur. VT may take two distinct forms: *monomorphic*, in which all complexes appear similar; and *polymorphic*, in which the appearance of complexes changes, as does the QRS axis. Polymorphic VT is often associated with a prolonged baseline QT interval and when it has a sinusoidal appearance, it is termed *Torsades de pointes* ("the twisting of points"). Differentiating SVT from monomorphic VT can sometimes be difficult, particularly when supraventricular beats are aberrantly conducted or a bundle branch block is present. Varying S1 or cannon A waves in the jugular venous pulse suggest VT, as do capture or fusion beats observed on the ECG. The arrhythmia is usually supraventricular if regular, upright P waves occur at an appropriate time before each QRS complex. However, if an inverted P wave *follows* each QRS, VT or junctional tachycardia is more likely. In contrast to reentrant SVTs, VT fails to respond to vagal stimulation and adenosine. The ECG characteristics used to distinguish SVT from VT are helpful but not infallible (see Table 4-3).

Regardless of morphology, in the hemodynamically compromised patient, VT should be treated with synchronized cardioversion, beginning with 100 WS of monophasic energy or its biphasic equivalent, and then rapidly escalating the energy of the shock until effective. Therapy should include removal of potentially precipitating agents (Table 4-4) and correction of electrolyte abnormalities, especially hypokalemia and hypomagnesemia. Because it is has low toxicity, is inexpensive, and may help, it probably makes sense to administer 2 to 6 gm of IV $MgSO_4$ to most patients with VT, especially if polymorphic. (Caution is indicated in patients with renal failure.) Following cardioversion of VT to a stable rhythm, amiodarone, lidocaine, or procainamide is indicated to prevent recurrence. Polymorphic VT is a special case: effective therapy requires shortening the QT interval, usually by accelerating the sinus rate to more than 100 beats/min using atropine, isoproterenol, or ventricular pacing. If the patient with VT is hemodynamically stable, amiodarone, lidocaine, or procainamide may be used as primary therapy. In patients with recurrent VT or recurrent VF, electrophysiologist consultation and an ablation procedure or insertion of an implantable cardio-defibrillator should be considered. Unfortunately, effective drug therapy can be discovered for only a minority of patients with recurrent VT.

TABLE 4-4 DRUGS ASSOCIATED WITH *TORSADES DE POINTES*

PSYCHIATRIC MEDICATIONS	ANTIARRHYTHMICS
Amitriptyline	Bepridil
Chlorpromazine	Disopyramide
Droperidol	Dofetilide
Doxepin	Ibutilide
Fluvoxamine	Procainamide
Haloperidol	Sotalol
Imipramine	Quinidine
Nortriptyline	
Thioridazine	
Ziprasidone	

ANTIBIOTICS	MISCELLANEOUS
Fluoroquinolones	Terfenadine
Erythromycin	Astemizole
Clarithromycin	Cisapride
Pentamidine	Loratadine
Ketoconazole	Methadone
Itraconazole	Tacrolimus
Fluconazole	
Amantadine	

■ BRADYARRHYTHMIAS

Except when caused by intrinsic disease of the sinus mechanism or conduction system, bradycardia tends to reflect a noncardiac etiology, like high vagal tone, hypoxemia, hypothyroidism, or drug effect (particularly β-blockers, calcium channel blockers, or digoxin). Bradycardia is usually of little importance in patients with normally compliant hearts, adequate preload reserves, and the ability to peripherally vasoconstrict. However, if stroke volume cannot be increased (e.g., dehydration, pericardial disease, noncompliant myocardium, loss of atrial contraction, depressed contractility), bradycardia may precipitously lower the cardiac output and blood pressure.

Sinus Bradycardia

Bradycardia may be physiologic in the trained heart and when metabolic demands are reduced (e.g., hypothermia, hypothyroidism, starvation). Sinus bradycardia (SB) is characterized by normal P wave morphology and 1:1 AV conduction at a rate less than 60 beats/min. The association of SB with inferior and posterior MIs may be related to ischemia of nodal tissue and increased vagal tone. The vagotonic actions of morphine and β-blockers aggravate bradycardia in such patients. SB does not require treatment unless it causes hypotension, pulmonary edema, or angina, or it precipitates ventricular escape beats. However, SB may be a marker of other pathologic processes important to reverse (e.g., hypoxemia, visceral distention, pain, hypothyroidism). SB may be treated with atropine or catecholamine infusions, but both therapies have the potential to increase myocardial O_2 consumption in the setting of myocardial ischemia.

If initial doses of atropine (0.5 to 1 mg IV q 3 to 5 min) fail to raise heart rate to an acceptable level, external pacing or infusion of dopamine (5 to 20 μg/kg/min), epinephrine (2 to 10 μg/min), or isoproterenol (2 to 10 μg/min) should be tried. Among patients with SB resulting from β-blocker, calcium channel blocker, or digitalis intoxication, these treatments are often ineffective. Specific therapy with antibodies for digitalis intoxication, glucagon in β-blocker overdose, or $CaCl_2$ (1 to 3 g IV) in calcium channel blocker overdose may be effective. Although not studied in a systematic fashion, the simultaneous infusion of insulin, glucose, and potassium may accelerate heart rate in β-blocker and calcium channel blocker overdose and may improve contractility as well.

■ ATRIOVENTRICULAR BLOCK
First-Degree Atrioventricular Block

In first-degree AV block (1° AVB), AV nodal or infranodal conduction is slowed, prolonging the PR interval (>0.2 s). 1° AVB is usually physiologically unimportant, but it may signal drug toxicity or progressive conduction system disease, and in the ICU, it is usually a temporary phenomenon caused by increased vagal tone or medications. Isolated 1° AVB does not require therapy. However, pacing is indicated if 1° AVB accompanies right bundle branch block and left anterior fascicular block in the setting of a myocardial ischemia. Complete heart block often follows in such patients. Although external pacing may be effective, the more difficult to initiate, transvenous route usually proves more reliable in capturing the ventricle.

Second-Degree Atrioventricular Block

There are two forms of second-degree AV block (2° AVB), a condition in which some atrial impulses are conducted whereas others are blocked. Mobitz I (Wenkebach) conduction is characterized by sequential and progressive prolongation of the PR interval, culminating in periodic failure to transmit the atrial impulse. This pattern often repeats every three or four beats. (While the PR intervals of successive beats progressively lengthen, the RR intervals shorten.) The conduction blockage is almost always within the AV node and is most frequently the result of digitalis toxicity or intrinsic heart disease (e.g., infarction, myocarditis, or cardiac surgery). Because the right coronary artery supplies the AV node in most patients, Mobitz I block often accompanies inferior MI. In this setting, Mobitz I block is usually benign and self-limited with ventricular escape rates of 40 to 50 beats/min. Conversely, Mobitz I block complicating anterior infarction suggests extensive damage and a guarded prognosis. Although atropine or isoproterenol may be used to improve conduction, no treatment is usually required. Ventricular pacing is effective but rarely necessary.

Mobitz II AV block originates below the level of the AV node, in the His–Purkinje system predominately supplied by branches of the left anterior descending coronary artery. In contrast to Mobitz I block, the PR interval remains constant but atrial depolarizations are inconsistently conducted. The QRS complex may be prolonged if the His bundle is the site of blockade. Mobitz II block is usually not transient and, because it often progresses to symptomatic AV block of higher degree, almost always requires treatment. Mobitz II block with 2:1 conduction is difficult or impossible to separate from Mobitz I block in which every other P wave is nonconducted. (One helpful clue may be that QRS prolongation is more common in Mobitz II block.) Atropine fails to influence the infranodal site of blockade, making transvenous pacing necessary in most cases (see following).

Third-Degree Atrioventricular Block

During complete or third-degree AV block (3° AVB), the atria and ventricles fire independently, usually at different but regular rates. 3° AVB may result from degenerative myocardial disease or myocarditis, MI, or infiltration of the conducting system (e.g., sarcoidosis, amyloidosis). Toxic concentrations of digitalis and other drugs may also produce 3° AVB. On physical examination, AV dissociation produces a varying first heart sound and cannon A waves in the jugular venous pulse, the result of occasional simultaneous atrial and ventricular contractions. Blockage of the AV node itself produces a "narrow complex" junctional rhythm at a rate of 40 to 60 beats/min and usually results from MI. In most cases, it is transient and asymptomatic. On the other hand, infranodal AV block, a pattern associated with a wide QRS (>0.10 s), is almost always symptomatic because it tends to produce slower heart rates (30 to 45 beats/min). The inherent instability of pacemakers originating distal to the AV node renders infranodal 3° AVB worthy of treatment, regardless of rate. Immediate insertion of a transvenous pacemaker is indicated.

■ ANTIARRHYTHMIC DRUGS

Antiarrhythmic therapy is far from ideal because antiarrhythmics fail to suppress the rhythm disorder in approximately 50% of cases, and in many situations rhythm control does not improve outcome. Furthermore, antiarrhythmic drugs have a narrow therapeutic window with a high incidence of gastrointestinal and central nervous system side effects. Paradoxically, antiarrhythmic drugs exacerbate the underlying problem or cause new arrhythmias in as many as 20% of treated patients ("proarrhythmic" effects). Moreover, preoccupation with the drug management of physiologically insignificant arrhythmias may distract from addressing important problems (e.g., ischemia, electrolyte disturbance, heart failure, thyrotoxicosis, or drug intoxication). Normalizing arterial oxygenation, pH, potassium, and magnesium often improves or abolishes the arrhythmic tendency. In hypotensive or pulseless patients with tachyarrhythmias, electrical cardioversion (not pharmacotherapy) is the treatment. Synchronized cardioversion is the preferred method, except in VF where unsynchronized shock is used. Surprisingly, in the setting of ischemic heart disease, only β-blocking agents have convincingly reduced mortality and their beneficial effect is not likely related to arrhythmia suppression alone. A simplified version of a standard classification system for antiarrhythmic drugs is presented in Table 4-5, and an overview of drugs used in the treatment of symptomatic arrhythmias is presented in Table 4-6. For patients with sustained VT or recurrent VF, automatic implantable pacer/defibrillators have all but eliminated drug therapy, reducing annual mortality to 1% to 2%. Unfortunately, an invasive procedure is required for placement; the procedure is costly, and the sporadic, unexpected shocks it delivers can be psychologically disabling.

TABLE 4-5 CLASSIFICATION OF COMMONLY USED ANTIARRHYTHMICS

CLASS	MECHANISM OF ACTION	EXAMPLES
Ia	Depress conduction Accelerate repolarization	Quinidine Procainamide Disopyramide
Ib	Depress conduction Accelerate repolarization	Lidocaine Phenytoin Tocainide Mexiletine
Ic	Marked reduction in conduction	Flecainide Encainide
II	β-receptor blockade	Propranolol Esmolol Metoprolol
III	Repolarization prolonged	Amiodarone Bretylium Sotalol
IV	Block Ca^{2+} slow channels, decrease automaticity and nodal conduction	Verapamil Diltiazem Nicardipine

TABLE 4-6 TREATMENT OF SYMPTOMATIC ARRHYTHMIAS

ARRHYTHMIA	PRIMARY TREATMENT[a]	ALTERNATIVE OR SUPPLEMENTAL MEASURES	COMMENT
Atrial fibrillation/flutter	Cardioversion	Rate control with digoxin, diltiazem, esmolol, or amiodarone, procainamide	Inhibit recurrence with Ca^{2+} blocker or β-blocker
AV reentrant and AV nodal reentrant tachycardia	Vagal stimulation Adenosine	Ca^{2+} blocker, β-blocker, or Digoxin	Cardioversion if drugs fail or reversal urgent
Multifocal atrial tachycardia	Correction of metabolic or cardiopulmonary cause	Ca^{2+} blocker or β-blocker	Drugs slow the rate but rarely reestablish sinus mechanism
Bradycardia	Removal of offending medications, correction of hypoxemia		Hypoxemia and vagal reflexes are common precipitants
Supranodal	Atropine/oxygen	Catecholamine infusion	
Infranodal	Isoproterenol/pacing		
Ventricular premature contractions	Lidocaine	Procainamide	Treatment often unnecessary
Monomorphic ventricular tachycardia	Cardioversion	Lidocaine, procainamide, sotalol, amiodarone	
Polymorphic ventricular tachycardia	Cardioversion Iso proterenol	Magnesium, overdrive pacing	
Ventricular fibrillation	Cardioversion	Lidocaine	Success rate correlates inversely with duration
Digitoxic rhythms	Digitalis antibodies	Phenytoin, procainamide, lidocaine, KCl propranolol	

[a]Correction of hypoxemia, hypotension, disturbances of pH, and electrolytes (Ca^{2+}, Mg^{2+}, K^+) are key elements of therapy for all arrhythmias.

Specific Antiarrhythmic Drugs

Amiodarone

Amiodarone is a highly effective antiarrhythmic for a wide variety of supraventricular and ventricular rhythm disturbances. At one time, amiodarone was used in high doses only for refractory life-threatening ventricular arrhythmias, in large part because of its significant toxicities. Now, lower, less-toxic doses have been shown to be effective for a variety of supraventricular arrhythmias. For cardiac arrest, 300 mg given rapidly intravenously (is indicated. For serious ventricular arrhythmias, 150 mg given by rapid IV infusion over 15 min may be effective. For less-critical ventricular arrhythmias, a loading dose of 360 mg given as a 1-mg/min infusion is followed by an additional 540 mg given as a 0.5-g/min infusion. AVNRT, AVRT, A-fib and flutter are controlled in up to 70% of patients, and ventricular arrhythmias may be controlled almost as frequently. Amiodarone may be the most effective agent for controlling A-fib, but questions persist about its long-term safety, and many recipients discontinue therapy because of toxicity. The most common side effects are gastrointestinal and neurological; however, pulmonary toxicity is a well-recognized, potentially fatal complication. On its own, amiodarone may induce SA or AV nodal blockade as well as infranodal conduction system disorders. Unpredictable interactions can also occur with other antiarrhythmics. Amiodarone routinely increases plasma levels of digitalis, quinidine, procainamide, and flecainide and potentiates the anticoagulant effect of warfarin.

β-Adrenergic Blockers

A variety of β-adrenergic blocking drugs differing with respect to speed of onset, receptor selectivity, duration of action, and side effects is available. The prototype is propranolol, whose primary actions are shared by most members of the class. Propranolol, a nonspecific β-blocker, is a negative ionotrope and chronotrope that decreases the rate of SA node depolarization and conduction velocity. Although useful in states of catecholamine excess (e.g., pheochromocytoma, hyperthyroidism, cocaine toxicity), β-blockade may produce disastrous results in patients who depend on catecholamine stimulation for compensation. Such problems are likely to arise in patients with volume depletion, impaired cardiac contractility, or stroke volume limited by hypertrophy or constriction. Cardio selective β-blockers (e.g., metoprolol, carvedilol) may be somewhat better tolerated. Propranolol helps slow the rate in AVNRT, AVRT, A-fib, and flutter. The drug is a less than ideal choice for treating most ventricular arrhythmias, except when these are exacerbated by tachycardia or ischemia. In emergency situations, propranolol may be administered in IV doses of 0.5 to 1 mg every 10 min. Contraindications include severe bradycardia or high-grade AV block, advanced heart failure, obstructive lung diseases, or digitalis toxicity. β-blocking drugs may aggravate coronary spasm. When selecting a β-blocker, the desired duration of action should be a key consideration. The antiarrhythmic and antihypertensive effects of atenolol may last for 24 h. Conversely, the ultra-short action of esmolol may help in the acute management of supraventricular tachyarrhythmias without depressing myocardial function for protracted periods.

Calcium Channel Blockers

Calcium channel blockers, often convert AVNRT and AVRT to sinus rhythm and slow the ventricular response of A-fib and flutter, but rarely convert MAT, A-fib or flutter to sinus rhythm. Verapamil has the longest track record, and IV doses of 2.5 to 5 mg at 5- to 10-min intervals are usually promptly effective. Verapamil must be given with extreme caution; even with commonly used doses, high-grade AV block (occasionally asystole) may result. (Asystole is more common in VT than in SVT.) Because of its vasodilating effects, hypotension is common in the volume-depleted and elderly; however, this troublesome effect can often be avoided by pretreatment with intravenous calcium gluconate. Diltiazem is somewhat safer and more predictable in its actions.

Digitalis

The major use of digitalis is to slow AV conduction in A-fib and flutter, especially in patients with impaired ventricular function. In this role, it is usually given in 0.125- to 0.25-mg doses IV every 4 to 6 h until the ventricular response rate is less than 100/min. (The dose is titrated to the desired degree of AV block, with less regard for "therapeutic levels.") Nonetheless, levels above 3 ng/mL are poorly tolerated and usually not necessary. Heart block, increased myocardial irritability, gastrointestinal distress (nausea and vomiting), and central nervous system disturbances (confusion, visual aberrations) are the most common side effects.

Lidocaine

Lidocaine, a type II antiarrhythmic, effectively suppresses ventricular irritability but has little effect on supraventricular arrhythmias. In the setting of myocardial ischemia, it is probably more effective than procainamide for VT, with the reverse being true for nonischemia-related VT. Because a survival benefit has not been demonstrated and side effects are common, prophylactic therapy in myocardial ischemia is not recommended. Lidocaine distributes into multiple compartments; therefore, it requires several loading doses to achieve and maintain effective serum concentration. Loading is usually accomplished by giving two to three decremental doses (e.g., 100, 75, and 50 mg) spaced about 10 min apart. For similar reasons, a modified drug bolus should accompany increased infusion rates in the correction of an inadequate serum concentration. Lidocaine doses should be reduced in the elderly and in patients with heart failure, shock, or liver disease (see Chapter 15). No adjustment is needed for renal dysfunction, but patients should be closely monitored after institution or withdrawal of drugs interfering with the hepatic metabolism of lidocaine (e.g., cimetidine, propranolol). Neurological toxicity, including confusion, lethargy, and seizures, emerges with lidocaine levels greater than 5 mcg/mL. Lidocaine may also exacerbate the neuromuscular blocking effects of paralytic drugs. Hemodynamic effects are usually inconsequential but include mild depression of blood pressure and cardiac contractility. Because of its multicompartment distribution, lidocaine declines slowly (over 6 h) after abrupt termination, making tapering of the drug unnecessary.

Phenytoin

Phenytoin is a rarely used type II antiarrhythmic effective in treating digitalis-induced ventricular tachyarrhythmias. Phenytoin shortens the QT and PR intervals and increases AV block. Typical loading doses are 10 to 20 mg/kg, but they must be given slowly (<50 mg/min) as the rhythm is monitored. The drug and its solvent, propylene glycol, may provoke serious arrhythmias or hypotension during rapid administration. Phenytoin lowers blood pressure by decreasing cardiac output and systemic vascular resistance. Ataxia is the major toxicity, occurring at levels greater than 20 mg/dL. Phenytoin potentiates the effects of other drugs that are highly protein bound (e.g., warfarin).

Procainamide

Procainamide is a type Ia antiarrhythmic, in many ways similar to quinidine, useful for both supraventricular and ventricular arrhythmias. It effectively controls PVCs and VT and may convert supraventricular arrhythmias to sinus rhythm. Procainamide is more effective than lidocaine for nonischemia-related VT. Like other type Ia drugs, procainamide may accelerate the ventricular rate in A-fib or flutter unless conduction is slowed with digitalis or β-blockers or calcium channel blockers. In the average-sized patient, a total loading dose of 1 g is given by injecting sequential boluses of 100 mg every 5 min. When continuous therapy is required, loading may be followed by an infusion of 2 to 6 mg/min. Procainamide is a vasodilator and negative ionotrope, thereby decreasing blood pressure and contractility. Both the QRS and QT intervals of the ECG often increase modestly, and procainamide may precipitate *torsades de pointes*. Procainamide is less likely than quinidine to cause gastrointestinal distress but over long periods, can induce a lupus-like syndrome in as many as 20% of patients. A positive antinuclear antibody (ANA) develops in approximately 50% of all patients using the drug chronically, effects that are reversible with discontinuation of therapy. Rare cases of hemolysis or agranulocytosis have been reported.

Sotalol

Sotalol increases the action potential duration and has β-blocking properties and therefore is a reasonable drug to control AVNRT, and is moderately effective for A-fib and flutter. In contrast to other β-blockers and AV nodal blocking agents (e.g., digitalis, verapamil), sotalol can also influence AVRT, which utilizes an accessory pathway (e.g., Wolf–Parkinson–White syndrome). Sotalol is also one of the few agents demonstrated to decrease the frequency of sustained VT and VF and its associated mortality. Because of its QT prolonging effects, use in the setting of hypokalemia or hypomagnesemia or combination with other drugs known to prolong the QT interval is unwise. Sotalol's QT-prolonging actions can precipitate *torsades de pointes*, hence it should probably be initiated during ECG monitoring in a hospital.

■ ELECTRICAL CARDIOVERSION

External Cardioversion

Electrical shock terminates arrhythmias by simultaneously depolarizing the entire myocardium potentially allowing a stable pacemaker to emerge (see Chapter 20). Electrical cardioversion is indicated for pulseless or hypotensive tachyarrhythmias and VF. Synchronized cardioversion is the preferred method whenever an organized rhythm is present, but is superfluous for VF. Synchronization times the electrical discharge to occur slightly after the R wave (a "nonvulnerable" point in the cardiac cycle where shock is unlikely to induce VF). To trigger the discharge synchronization requires monitoring of an ECG lead that demonstrates a tall R wave (usually Lead I or II). Rarely, tall, steeply sloping T waves may trigger discharge at inappropriate times. If possible, patients undergoing elective cardioversion should take nothing by mouth for 8 h before the procedure, to minimize the risk of aspiration. Trained personnel should be present to monitor airway patency, ventilation, oxygenation, and level of sedation. Benzodiazepines, ultra-short acting barbiturates, propofol, or short-acting synthetic narcotics can produce sufficient sedation and amnesia for patient comfort. Hypoxemia, electrolyte disorders (especially hypokalemia and hypomagnesemia), and thyroid function should be corrected before the procedure elective synchronized cardioversion. Digitalis preparations should be withheld for 24 to 48 h before cardioversion to minimize risks of postcardioversion arrhythmias.

The appropriate dose of electricity depends on the underlying rhythm and if a monophasic or biphasic device is used. Unsuccessful attempts should be followed by subsequent shocks with incremental energy. Being relatively unstable, flutter may convert with as little as 5 J (WS), but the more stable A-fib may require 50 WS. Patients with reentrant SVT often require 50 to 100 WS, and VT often requires 200 WS for conversion. In patients with AVNRT and AVRT, electrical "fatigue" of the SA or AV nodes may delay recovery of normal conduction and automaticity. For this reason, the physician should be prepared to initiate transcutaneous pacing and immediately insert a temporary transvenous pacemaker. Adverse effects of cardioversion include skin burns and disorders of conduction and repolarization. The myocardium may be dysfunctional for a variable period afterward. Creatine phosphokinase (CPK), troponin, and lactic dehydrogenase (LDH) may rise slightly. The most dreaded complication of cardioversion is systemic embolization, a problem most commonly seen in nonanticoagulated patients with dilated cardiomyopathy, mitral stenosis, or chronic A-fib.

Implantable Defibrillators

The technology of implantable pacer/defibrillators (ICDs) is changing too rapidly to allow an enduring discussion of individual devices. Improved longevity, smaller size, better software, and the development of combined pacing/defibrillating devices have dramatically advanced the utility and popularity of these tools. It is clear that mortality can be reduced by insertion of an ICD in patients with impaired ventricular function and sustained VT compared to chemical antiarrhythmic therapy.

■ PACEMAKERS

Permanent Pacemakers

A complete discussion of the issues surrounding permanent pacemakers is well beyond the scope of this book, but the ICU physician must have a basic understanding of pacer terminology and be able to troubleshoot simple problems. Fortunately, standardized nomenclature has emerged to describe pacer functions (see Table 4-7). The most basic pacers can be described by the chamber(s) that is paced, the chamber(s) from which sensing takes place, and what effect a sensed patient depolarization has on the pacer. For example, a pacer that has ventricular pacing, ventricular sensing, and is inhibited by a spontaneous ventricular depolarization, would be termed a VVI pacer. Along the same lines, a DDD pacer has atrial and ventricular pacing and sensing leads. The atrial lead is stimulated first, and if a ventricular depolarization does not occur within the normally expected conduction time, then the ventricle is paced. Spontaneous atrial and ventricular signals are capable of inhibiting the pacing function. Sophisticated devices now are capable of detecting increased patient activity or breathing and accelerating the pacing rate, so-called rate modulation. In addition, complex pacers capable of coordinating atrial and ventricular contractions and simultaneous contraction of both ventricles improve long-term outcomes.

Regardless of the kind of permanent pacer present troubleshooting is usually straightforward and begins with a chest radiograph and 12-lead ECG. The chest film can demonstrate lead fracture or electrode migration. The ECG helps parse problems into those of sensing or pacing. The first step is to look for a pacer "spike" and see if it captures (i.e., chamber depolarization). The observation of capture at a reasonable rate all but rules out pacer malfunction. If there is capture but at an unsuitably slow rate, mechanical failure of the pacer (e.g., lead fracture, pulse generator malfunction) or oversensing are likely explanations. Oversensing, is pacer inhibition by inappropriate electrical signals such as those of other ECG components (e.g., T waves), external electromagnetic interference, or from

TABLE 4-7 GENERIC CODE FOR PACEMAKER DESIGNATIONS

		CATEGORY		
1 CHAMBER(S) PACED	2 CHAMBER(S) SENSED	3 RESPONSE TO SENSING	4 RATE MODULATION	5 MULTISITE PACING

0 = none
A = atrium
V = ventricle
D = dual atrium
     and ventricle
S = single atrium
     or ventricle
	0 = none
	A = atrium
	V = ventricle
	D = dual atrium
	     and ventricle
	S = single atrium
	     or ventricle
		0 = none
		T = triggered
		I = inhibited
		D = dual triggered
		     and inhibited
			0 = none
			R = rate modulation
				0 = none
				A = atrium
				V = ventricle
				D = dual atrium
				     and ventricle

muscle artifact. If the capture rate is too rapid, undersensing may be to blame. Undersensing occurs when the pacing generator fails to appropriately recognize cardiac electrical signals as a result of lead fracture, or changes in electrical transmission between the lead and the myocardium (e.g., myocardial infarct, fibrosis, electrolyte imbalance, drug intoxication). Failure to capture or pace is often a mechanical device failure, but is appropriate if the patient's intrinsic rhythm is sufficient to completely inhibit pacer output. Placing a magnet over the pacer will differentiate between oversensing and mechanical failure: In the former case the pacer will operate normally in an asynchronous mode, in the latter case the pacer continues to malfunction.

Temporary Pacemakers

Because temporary transvenous pacemakers are frequently inserted in the ICU, understanding their **6** use and associated problems is essential. Temporary pacemakers are indicated for (a) high-grade (especially symptomatic) AV block, (b) overdrive suppression of refractory atrial tachyarrhythmias, (c) suppression of *torsades de pointes* resulting from bradycardia, (d) sick sinus syndrome, and (e) control of postcardiac surgery arrhythmias. In emer**7** gent situations, noninvasive transthoracic pacing is worth trying but often fails to capture the ventricle. More likely to be successful is insertion of a transvenous pacing catheter. Effective temporary pacing requires that the catheter electrodes firmly contact the endocardium of the right ventricle. When optimally positioned, the pacer will sense the occurrence of native electrical discharges and achieve ventricular capture using a very low energy pulse. Although complex pacemakers capable of sequential AV pacing are available, these are rarely necessary in the ICU and often do not function properly when inserted emergently. A simple ventricular pacer will suffice in almost all cases.

Three basic kinds of pacing conductors are available: semistiff dedicated pacing "wires," balloon-tipped pacing catheters, and pacing-capable pulmonary artery catheters. All three are bipolar, that is, they contain both a distal cathode and proximal anode. (When electively inserting a pulmonary artery catheter in a patient with left bundle branch block, a pacing-capable catheter should be considered because insertion can rarely precipitate complete heart block.) The stiff pacing wires may

be the most difficult to place emergently, but once in place, are usually the most stable. By contrast, the easier-to-place, flow-directed balloon catheters are least stable.

Although the *right* internal jugular and *left* subclavian sites are the easiest access points, brachial or femoral veins can be used for pacer insertion. Fluoroscopic guidance can be helpful to properly position the catheter, but often cannot be arranged emergently. Therefore, in most cases the pacing lead is inserted using only ECG guidance. The ECG can be used in two ways to guide placement. For patients with an underlying rhythm, the distal electrode can be connected to the V1 lead of the ECG while standard limb leads are attached to the patient. The pacer is then slowly advanced, while continuously monitoring the ECG signal. While the catheter is in the superior vena cava, a small negative atrial deflection will be noted. If the catheter "bypasses" the heart, into the inferior vena cava, the atrial deflection becomes positive. If that happens the catheter needs to be withdrawn and readvanced. When the right ventricle is finally entered, a large ventricular signal will be sensed. Advancing the catheter further results in an "injury" current in the monitored lead when the ventricular wall is encountered. (These findings are most evident if simultaneous recording of one or two limb leads is performed.) The pacer is then disconnected from the ECG machine, and an attempt to pace the ventricle is made. In patients without a ventricular rhythm, the surface ECG is merely monitored as the pacing wire or catheter is blindly advanced toward the right ventricle with the pacing generator discharging in an asynchronous mode. When capture occurs, the ECG demonstrates a wide QRS ventricular depolarization.

To generate depolarizations the bipolar electrodes are connected to an external pacing generator. The simplest of these devices has three adjustments: discharge rate, output pacing current (in milliamps), and sensitivity (the electrical strength, in millivolts, of intrinsic cardiac current necessary to inhibit firing of the pacer). In asystolic patients, the pacing catheter should be inserted with the generator in the asynchronous mode, with a high output (5 to 10 mA) at a rate of approximately 100 beats/min. Using the highest output current maximizes the chance of capture and using a rate of 100 beats/min provides a sufficiently frequent spike to make it easily recognizable. In addition, a rate of 100 beats/min is almost always sufficient to generate an adequate cardiac output when capture occurs. Monitoring the surface ECG will initially reveal a narrow pacing "spike" until the catheter encounters the right ventricular wall. Upon capture, the ECG will show the typical bundle branch block pattern of depolarizations originating in the ventricle. Very rarely, the pacing electrode will lodge in the right atrium producing a normal narrow QRS complex.

After insertion, the generator should be adjusted to achieve three major goals: (a) a heart rate sufficient to meet cardiac output requirements, (b) minimize the pacing threshold (current necessary to achieve capture), and (c) adjust the sensitivity threshold to prevent simultaneous patient and pacer discharge. If spontaneous electrical activity is present, the pacer should usually be operated in the "demand" mode, discharging only when intrinsic activity is deficient. Initially, the sensitivity should be set on the lowest value (usually 1.5 mV) and then gradually increased until the pacer fails to sense the intrinsic beats. The point at which the pacer fails to recognize intrinsic electrical activity is the "sensitivity threshold." With regard to pacer output, to minimize endocardial injury, the minimum current necessary to capture the ventricle should be used. This "pacing threshold" is determined by reducing the output setting from the initial 5 to 10 mA range until the pacer fails to capture the ventricle. Ideally, capture can be achieved with outputs as low as 0.5 mA. Because a patient's sensitivity to pacing varies with a variety of factors, including catheter position, it is customary to set the output at a value two to three times the pacing threshold. Once pacing and sensitivity thresholds have been set, the rate can be adjusted to provide optimal cardiac output.

Several problems may occur with emergent temporary pacemaker placement. Although unusual, the pacing catheter can perforate the thin-walled right atrium or ventricle. Perforation can occur at the time of insertion but more commonly is delayed for hours to days after placement. Its detection is signaled by an increase in the pacing threshold or failure to capture. Electrical changes may be accompanied by chest or shoulder pain or the development of hiccups as the diaphragm is stimulated by the pacer. Physical exam at that time may reveal a new pericardial friction rub or tamponade; chest radiograph or echocardiogram confirms puncture by demonstrating a shifted electrode position or accumulated pericardial fluid. The pacer can provoke atrial and ventricular arrhythmias, especially if it is coiled in the ventricle or placed in the right ventricular outflow tract. Again, malposition can be detected by plain chest radiograph. As may occur with any indwelling catheter, infection or thrombosis may develop. Both risks relate predominately to the duration of the catheterization and sterility of insertion.

Because of the technical expertise and time necessary to insert an intravenous pacer, transcutaneous pacing technology has been developed. Although transcutaneous devices are less likely than transvenous devices to achieve ventricular capture, when they are effective, pacing can be achieved in seconds instead of minutes. Thus transcutaneous pacing is best viewed as a temporizing measure until transvenous pacing is achieved or the underlying cause of bradycardia is reversed.

Pacing with an external pacer is initiated by firmly applying the pacing/defibrillating pads to the chest with the negative electrode on the anterior chest wall at the left sternal border (V3 position). Ideally, the positive electrode is placed on the back between the spine and scapula directly opposite the negative pad. The pacing rate and output (mA) are variable but unlike internal pacers, the sensing threshold is typically not adjustable. Starting at an output of 5 mA and increasing the output at 5-mA intervals until capture is achieved or discomfort becomes intolerable is a reasonable strategy for the conscious bradycardic patient. For the unconscious patient, starting at a maximal output setting (typically 200 mA) until capture is achieved, then decreasing the output until capture is lost is a prudent strategy. When "electrical capture" is seen on the ECG, the patient's pulse and blood pressure should be checked to ensure adequate cardiac output. Setting the demand rate near 100 will almost always be sufficient to meet metabolic demands if capture is achieved.

External pacing has two major problems: failure to capture and pain. Obese patients, and those with pericardial effusion, severe emphysema, and those on mechanical ventilators, may be more difficult to pace. Improper position of the electrodes or poor skin–electrode contact can also lead to pacing failure. In addition, capture is less likely if begun long after the onset of bradycardia or asystole. Pain is a common problem for the conscious patient. Discomfort can be improved with simple sedatives and analgesics and by increasing the pulse duration.

■ SUGGESTED READINGS

Cannom DS, Prystowsky EN. Management of ventricular arrhythmias: Detection, drugs, and devices. *JAMA.* 1999;281(2):172–179.

Crespo EM, Kim J, Selzman KA. The use of implantable cardioverter defibrillators for the prevention of sudden cardiac death: A review of the evidence and implications. *Am J Med Sci.* 2005;329(5):238–246.

Fox DJ, Tischenko A, Krahn AD, et.al. Supraventricular tachycardia: Diagnosis and management. *Mayo Clin Proc.* 2008;83(12):1400–1411.

Investigators of the AVID Trial. A comparison of antiarrhythmic-drug therapy with implantable defibrillators in patients resuscitated from near-fatal ventricular arrhythmias. The Antiarrhythmics versus Implantable Defibrillators (AVID) Investigators. *N Engl J Med.* 1997;337(22):1576–1583.

Kaszala K, Huizar JF, Ellenbogen KA. Contemporary pacemakers: What the primary care physician needs to know. *Mayo Clin Proc.* 2008;83(10):1170–1186.

McNamara RL, Tamariz LJ, Segal JB, et al. Management of atrial fibrillation: Review of the evidence for the role of pharmacologic therapy, electrical cardioversion, and echocardiography. *Ann Intern Med.* 2003;139:1018–1033.

Morady F. Radio-frequency ablation as treatment for cardiac arrhythmias. *N Engl J Med.* 1999;340(7):534–544.

Zipes DP, Ackerman MJ, Mark Estes NA III, et al. Task force 7: Arrhythmias. *J Am Coll Cardiol.* 2005;45(8):1354–1363.

Respiratory Monitoring

KEY POINTS

1 Although pulse oximetry is an invaluable clinical tool, it provides a signal-averaged number, the output of which lags behind the actual physiologic value of interest. Pulse oximetry is influenced by extraneous rhythmic vibration, carbon monoxide, and methemoglobin. Even if the recorded pulse rate correlates exactly with an independently measured value, oximetry loses accuracy when true arterial saturation falls to less than 80%.

2 After a step change in ventilation, arterial carbon dioxide concentration approaches steady-state equilibrium less quickly than does the arterial oxygen tension because the storage reservoir of the body for CO_2 is far larger than that for O_2.

3 The compliance of the respiratory system is influenced by the number of patent alveolar units, by their elasticity, and by the characteristics of the surrounding chest wall. The static and dynamic pressure volume curves of the respiratory system can provide vital information unavailable through computation of simpler indices, such as tidal compliance.

4 The mechanics of breathing (resistance and compliance) are most easily assessed during passive inflation with a known constant flow, using an end-inspiratory pause. During active breathing, the mechanical properties of the lung can be assessed if pleural pressure is recorded using an esophageal balloon.

5 Auto-PEEP, usually a reflection of dynamic hyperinflation, contributes to the work of breathing and patient–ventilator asynchrony. Because auto-PEEP varies from site to site throughout the lungs of a diseased patient, the externally measured value may not accurately reflect the degree of

overdistention. In obstructive diseases (asthma, cronic obstructive lung disease), the end-inspiratory plateau pressure indicates the degree of hyperinflation better than does auto-PEEP itself.

6 The flow tracing can be used to detect (but not quantify) auto-PEEP, airway secretions, and poor coordination between the tidal rhythms of patient and ventilator. The zero-flow points of the flow tracing partition the ventilatory cycle into its inspiratory and expiratory phases. The airway pressure tracing complements the flow tracing, helping to detect and quantify the work of breathing.

7 As an index of mean lung and chest wall volumes, mean airway pressure recorded under passive conditions is an important determinant of arterial oxygenation, the back pressure to venous return, and the tendency for gas leakage after barotrauma. Mean airway pressure alone has limited value during active breathing and seriously underestimates mean alveolar pressure when expiratory pressure losses exceed inspiratory pressure losses.

8 The mechanical work of breathing is not synonymous with breathing effort. The pressure time index better indicates total ventilatory stress, correlating inversely with pump reserve.

9 Respiratory muscle dyssynchrony, elevations in the $P_{0.1}$, and an excessive frequency to tidal volume ratio are helpful indicators of respiratory muscle overload and incipient muscle fatigue.

10 Breathing pattern variability, the CO_2 challenged $P_{0.1}$, the ratio between spontaneous tidal volume and vital capacity, the frequency to tidal volume ratio, and the ratio between minute ventilation and maximum voluntary ventilation are helpful indicators of ventilatory reserve.

Data relevant to the output, efficiency, capacity, and reserve of the respiratory system guide appropriate management during cardiorespiratory failure. Monitoring techniques can be classified conveniently into those that characterize pulmonary and systemic exchange of respiratory gases, ventilatory capability, and respiratory mechanics (flow, pressures, and breathing workload).

■ MONITORING GAS EXCHANGE

Arterial Blood Gas Analysis

Analysis of arterial blood gases (ABG) provides data that are fundamental to the diagnosis of respiratory and metabolic disturbances and to assessing the effect of therapeutic interventions. Although certain inferences can be made from the blood gas data alone, full interpretation and appreciation of their implications for decision making require knowledge of the clinical context, serum electrolyte concentrations, and in certain settings, the serum albumin and lactate concentrations as well.

Arterial O_2 Tension and Saturation

The physiologic significance of hypoxemia depends on chronicity, compensatory mechanisms, hypoxic ventilatory response, and tolerance of vital organs most at risk—chiefly, the heart and brain. Clearly, a patient with critical coronary stenosis, acute cor pulmonale, or symptomatic cerebrovascular compromise should be kept fully saturated, as should patients with ongoing dyspnea, symptomatic circulatory inadequacy, or severe anemia. Conversely, maintaining less than full saturation may be appropriate for patients who depend chronically on moderate hypoxemia to allow CO_2 retention, for those with intact compensatory mechanisms, and for patients in whom full O_2 saturation can be achieved only at the expense of high fractions of inspired oxygen or ventilating pressure. Quite recently, devices intended to monitor *tissue* oxygenation and perfusion adequacy have been released for clinical use. Near infrared spectrophotometry and sub-lingual PCO_2 monitoring, for example, show considerable promise. Although theoretically appealing, the value of these instruments has yet to be determined.

In the absence of carbon monoxide, methemoglobin, or abnormal hemoglobin, arterial O_2 saturation can be estimated with acceptable accuracy from the PaO$_2$ and pH alone—at least near the upper plateau of the oxyhemoglobin relationship. If the arterial O_2 content is required, or if carboxyhemoglobin or methemoglobin concentrations are high, direct analysis by co-oximetry must be requested. (This is particularly important when analyzing mixed-venous O_2 saturations.) Whether to "temperature correct" the analyzed specimen is debatable, depending somewhat on the purpose to which such information is put. For example, temperature correction would seem appropriate if the oxygen-exchanging efficiency of the lung were the primary question, whereas the need to correct SaO$_2$ for temperature is more debatable when tissue O_2 *adequacy* is the concern. Individual hospital laboratories have different practices and reporting policies with regard to these issues.

Acid–Base Status, pH, and PaCO$_2$

Hydrogen ion concentration must be regulated carefully to preserve enzyme function. Normally, acids are generated by the hydration of CO_2 ("respiratory" acid) and by other processes of metabolism ("metabolic acids"—primarily phosphate, sulfate, and lactate). In disease states, hydrogen ion concentration can rise secondary to the production of excess lactate (ischemia, hypoxemia), generation of ketoacids (diabetes, starvation), ingestion of certain alcohols or drugs (e.g., metformin), or failure of the body to excrete or metabolize the generated load of hydrogen ion (ventilatory failure, kidney dysfunction, or liver disease). Occasionally, sufficient hydrogen or bicarbonate ion is lost in the urine or stool or is aspirated from the gastrointestinal tract to affect acid–base balance. To address such disorders, the clinician must understand the primary determinants of acid–base homeostasis and deftly interpret the pH, PaCO$_2$, and HCO$_3^-$ components of the blood gas report alongside the electrolyte profile (to calculate anion gap).

The body defends against radical changes in pH primarily by regulating its two pathways for eliminating acid: respiratory and renal. (A full discussion of acid–base principles is provided in Chapter 12.) The Henderson–Hasselbach equation for the bicarbonate buffer system relates pH to the concentrations of bicarbonate and PaCO$_2$:

$$pH = 6.1 + \log HCO_3^- /(0.03\ PaCO_2)$$

In this expression, knowledge of any two variables enables calculation of the third. In practice, PaCO$_2$

(lung excreted) and pH are measured, and HCO_3^- (kidney excreted) is estimated. Once formed, hydrogen ions are neutralized partially by combining with bicarbonate ion (producing CO_2) and by reversible oxidation of protein. The bicarbonate buffer system:

$$CO_2 + H_2O \leftrightarrow H_2CO_3 \leftrightarrow H^+ + HCO_3^-$$

generates CO_2 when H^+ is added to the extracellular fluid. The rising CO_2 and H^+ concentrations stimulate the respiratory center in an attempt to limit hypercapnia, effectively eliminating H^+ by driving the preceding equation leftward. Over time (generally several days are required), the healthy kidney will adapt to hypercapnia or hypocapnia by adjusting the bicarbonate level to help restore the Henderson–Hasselbach-defined 20:1 normal ratio between bicarbonate concentration and the product of $PaCO_2$ and its solubility coefficient (0.03). Respiratory compensation for metabolic disturbances is generally incomplete and occurs more reliably and vigorously in response to metabolic acidosis than to metabolic alkalosis.

Despite its functional importance, this bicarbonate buffer system is not the only one available—skeletal calcium and certain proteins, chiefly hemoglobin, also play a significant role. Thus, a rising $[H^+]$ is partially buffered by hemoglobin, as well as by HCO_3^-, giving rise to a generally small discrepancy between the difference in HCO_3^- relative to normal (24 mEq/dL) and the calculated base excess or deficit, which quantifies the magnitude of the metabolic disturbance or compensation. An acutely rising $PaCO_2$ tends to generate bicarbonate as a portion of the H^+ formed in the hydration of CO_2 that is buffered by hemoglobin; the opposite occurs during hyperventilation. Thus, even in the absence of renal activity, the acutely rising $PaCO_2$ of pure hypoventilation is accompanied by a gently rising $[HCO_3^-]$; an acutely falling $PaCO_2$ by a gently falling $[HCO_3^-]$.

Definitions

Acidosis and *alkalosis*—the underlying processes that contribute to the pH status—may be pathogenic or compensatory. The normal ranges for arterial pH and $PaCO_2$ are 7.38 to 7.44 and 35 to 45 mm Hg, respectively. A pH that exceeds 7.45 indicates *alkalemia*, generated by bicarbonate retention, hyperventilation relative to metabolic need, or both. A pH < 7.35 indicates *acidemia,* caused by metabolic or renal depletion of bicarbonate, hypoventilation relative to metabolic

need, or both. Venous blood varies in composition depending on the delivery/consumption characteristics of the sampled tissue bed. Mixed-venous gases, representing admixture from tissues throughout the body, generally have a PCO_2 that is 4 to 8 mm Hg higher and a pH that is 0.05 to 0.10 units lower than arterial gases. Occasionally, these arteriovenous discrepancies can be much wider, and in such cases, the venous value may more accurately reflect the acid–base status of vital tissue beds.

Interpretation

The ABG Provides the pH and allows the clinician to determine the relative contributions. Because compensation is never complete, the dominant underlying mechanism—acidosis or alkalosis—is suggested by the pH. Does a blood gas demonstrating a $PaCO_2$ of 32 mm Hg and an HCO_3^- of 16 mEq/L indicate respiratory alkalosis with renal compensation, or metabolic acidosis with respiratory compensation? A major clue is provided by the pH—acidemia would suggest that the fundamental problem is metabolic. Failure of the $PaCO_2$ to fall to the *expected* level would suggest a superimposed problem with ventilatory drive or ventilatory pump. Classically, "Winters' Formula" (following) predicts the respiratory compensation for an uncomplicated metabolic acidosis. Intensive care unit (ICU) clinicians must be alert for "triple" acid–base disorders in which two metabolic derangements with opposing influences on pH are in play. The anion gap calculation usually provides the key to appropriate interpretation.

Chronicity of the process can be judged by comparing the observed values of pH, bicarbonate, and base excess with those *expected* for acute hypercapnia or hypocapnia (see following). To place such information into proper perspective for diagnosis and management decisions, the clinician must take account of the clinical backdrop and examine the serum electrolytes and albumin for evidence of renal insufficiency, renal tubular dysfunction, and an anion gap that indicates the presence of such noncarbonic (metabolic) acids as lactate, ketoacids, and salicylate.

The Anion Gap

The anion gap is the difference between the serum sodium concentration and the sum of chloride and bicarbonate ions. Normally, the gap is 13 mEq or less—a reflection of the sulfates, phosphates, and other unmeasured negatively charged ions that correspond to kidney-excreted "mineral" acids. Because of the anionic nature of serum proteins, the calculated gap should be increased approximately by 2 to 2.5 mEq/L for each g/dL of hypoalbuminemia. Another useful bedside computation is the "Δ/Δ," the ratio of the anion gap to the bicarbonate gap. As lactic acidosis develops, the anion gap increases relatively more than the HCO_3^- falls because HCO_3^- has a wider volume of distribution. The ratio varies but averages approximately 1.5 in moderate lactic acidosis—less if the acuity is extreme and more as the severity worsens. Values less than 1 should prompt consideration of another source of H^+ excess, whereas a value greater than 2 suggests a concurrent metabolic alkalosis.

Rules for Compensation

As already noted, primary metabolic disturbances are incompletely compensated by changes in ventilation, and primary respiratory disturbances are partially offset by renal excretion or retention of bicarbonate. Knowledge of these expected compensations allows a judgment to be made regarding the nature and chronicity of the underlying processes.

Respiratory Compensation for Metabolic Disturbances A useful equation for predicting the $PaCO_2$ during a primary metabolic disturbance is as follows:

Metabolic Acidosis: (Winters' Formula)

Expected $PaCO_2 = 1.54 \times [HCO_3^-] + 8.36$ mm Hg

Metabolic Alkalosis:

Expected $PaCO_2 = 0.7 \times [HCO_3^-] + 20$ mm Hg

For example, if a measured HCO_3 were 16, the expected compensation would be $PaCO_2 = 1.5 \times [HCO_3^-] + 8 = 24 + 8 = 32$ mm Hg. Note that the pH would be less than 7.40, however, because the HCO_3^- to $(0.03 \times PaCO_2)$ ratio is $16/(0.03 \times 32) = 16/0.96 = 16.7 < 20$. If measured HCO_3^- were 36 mEq/L, the expected compensation would be $PaCO_2 = 0.7 \times [HCO_3^-] + 20$ mm Hg $= 0.7 \times (36) + 20 = 25.2 + 20 = 45$ mm Hg.

Metabolic Adjustments for Primary Respiratory Disturbances The kidney requires time to compensate for a sustained respiratory disturbance and adjusts more successfully to respiratory alkalosis than to respiratory acidosis. The following are simple rules for the HCO_3^- expected in the acute and chronic settings.

Acute Rule: $[HCO_3^-]$ rises 1 mEq/L for each 10 mm Hg rise in $PaCO_2$ above 40 mm Hg and falls 2 mEq/L for each 10 mm Hg fall in $PaCO_2$ below 40 mm Hg.

Chronic Rule: $[HCO_3^-]$ rises 4 mEq/L for each 10 mm Hg rise in $PaCO_2$ above 40 mm Hg and falls 3 mEq/L for each 10 mm Hg fall in $PaCO_2$ below 40 mm Hg.

Algorithm for Evaluating Blood Gas Data

A systematic approach to blood gas evaluation incorporates the elements of the foregoing discussion. The first priority is to verify the technical validity of the sample—errors in sampling, sample processing, analysis, and transcription occur commonly. (Is the sample characteristic of a venous rather than the intended arterial specimen? Are the pH, $PaCO_2$, and $[HCO_3^-]$ internally consistent? Does the $[HCO_3^-]$ correlate with the $[HCO_3^-]$ directly analyzed from venous blood? Is the PaO_2 reported physically *possible* given the FiO_2 administered?)

Although there is no best method for interpreting a technically valid report, one logical approach has the following steps:

1. Look at the arterial pH: A pH outside the normal range defines acidemia (<7.35) or alkalemia (>7.45).
2. Look at the $PaCO_2$: If $PaCO_2$ is less than 35 mm Hg, the patient has primary or compensatory respiratory alkalosis. If $PaCO_2$ is more than 45 mm Hg, the patient has primary or compensatory respiratory acidosis.
3. Look at the $[HCO_3^-]$ and compute the base excess, knowing that each 10 mm Hg rise in $PaCO_2$ generates 1 mEq/L of bicarbonate via protein buffers and each fall of 10 mm Hg depletes $[HCO_3^-]$ by a similar amount. Compute the difference between the adjusted $[HCO_3^-]$ and 24 as the base excess or deficit. If the base excess exceeds 2, the patient has a metabolic alkalotic disturbance—primary or secondary. A deficit exceeding 2 indicates a primary or compensatory metabolic acidosis.
4. Look at the serum electrolyte and albumin concentrations. Calculate the albumin-adjusted anion gap and the "Δ/Δ" for clues to the nature of metabolic derangements (see Chapter 12). A metabolic acidosis unaccompanied by an anion gap usually means renal tubular dysfunction, excessive administration of chloride in the form of "normal" saline, or gastrointestinal loss of bicarbonate.

5. Consider the clinical setting and make a judgment regarding the nature of the primary acid–base disturbance. As a general but not infallible rule, pH will be driven in the direction dictated by the primary variable—an alkalemia in conjunction with a low $PaCO_2$ is at least partially driven by a respiratory mechanism; acidemia in conjunction with a low $PaCO_2$ suggests that the respiratory alkalosis is compensatory.

6. Look for evidence of a mixed disorder (as opposed to a simple but compensated disturbance) by calculating the expected value of the variable not involved in the primary disturbance, using the rules given earlier. Acid–base disorders can be single (e.g., respiratory acidosis, with or without compensation), double (e.g., respiratory acidosis, metabolic alkalosis), or even triple (e.g., respiratory acidosis, metabolic alkalosis, and metabolic acidosis)—as indicated by an anion gap together with CO_2 retention and a disproportionately elevated HCO_3^-. Review the clinical data and electrolytes for clues to the clinical significance of the acid–base data.

Monitoring Oxygenation

The human eye is not adept at detecting or quantifying arterial hypoxemia. Although intimately linked, O_2 saturation and tension (partial pressure) provide complementary clinical data. PaO_2 reflects the maximal tension driving O_2 to the tissues, whereas saturation reflects O_2 content per gram of hemoglobin. Reflectance oximetry is used when a fiberoptic catheter continuously tracks oxygen saturation in the central venous, pulmonary arterial, or systemic arterial bloodstreams. Multichannel fiberoptic chemiluminescent catheter systems for continuously monitoring PaO_2, $PaCO_2$, and arterial pH have been introduced into the clinical practice several times over the past two decades, but durability has been a problem and the adoption rate has been slow. These can be quite useful, however, for tracking either rapidly changing clinical events or progress after a clinical intervention (e.g., ventilator adjustment).

Sensors of Muscle Oxygen Utilization

Arterial Pulse Oximetry

Transcutaneous photometric oximetry is useful for monitoring patients with marginal or fluctuating oxygen exchange. For patients supported by mechanical ventilation, transcutaneous oximetry continuously measures SaO_2, enabling rapid adjustment of FiO_2, mean airway pressure, and positive end-expiratory pressure (PEEP) and warning of arterial desaturation during weaning, sleeping, or changes of body position. As a general rule, *trends* in oximetry values are of greater significance than the absolute value of saturation, at least over the clinical saturation range usually encountered.

Technical Issues

Lightweight probes direct filtered light of several specific wavelengths onto the surface of the digit, nasal bridge, or earlobe. The relative absorption of these spectrophotometric beams as they pass through the tissue (which differs for O_2 saturated and desaturated blood) is converted into the appropriate saturation value by computer-stored algorithms. Phasic variations separate the incoming arterial component from venous and background absorption. Pulse oximetry probes do not require tissue heating because phasic changes in blood volume and optical density cue the instrument to the arterial component of the blood contained in the vascular bed. Most units also display pulse rate, and many display a simulated arterial waveform or some other visual indicator of pulse intensity. A tracing whose waveform baseline varies dramatically with ventilation strongly suggests variation of stroke output synchronous with the respiratory cycle—a condition typical for gas trapping and auto-PEEP (AP).

Oxygen saturation is not the only useful parameter that can be estimated noninvasively by spectrophotometry. Quite recently, widening of the optical wavelength spectrum and advanced signal processing algorithms have been developed to enable noninvasive monitoring of hemoglobin, carboxyhemoglobin, and methemoglobin concentrations. As the reliability of these measures is improved and validated for use in critical care, such technology promises to add considerably to early event detection.

The pulse rate should be "correlated" to the electrocardiogram (ECG) measured rate to assess signal quality. Good correlation does not ensure accuracy, but poor correlation of the heart rate displayed on the ECG and pulse oximeter calls the reported saturation value into question. With a good pulse signal, currently available instruments are quite accurate in their upper range (i.e., saturations >80%) but become less reliable as the patient desaturates or perfusion deteriorates. Even when accurate, pulse oximetry presents a signal-averaged, and therefore delayed, report. Poor perfusion and/or probe contact are the primary causes of an erroneous signal, and placement on a different digit, nose bridge, or earlobe may improve reliability.

Potential Artifacts

Routine ABG reports of saturation are calculated from the measured PaO_2 and pH. A direct determination of arterial blood saturation (preferably by co-oximetry) is the most definitive check. Motion artifact often is an important problem for patients who are not immobilized. Because detection of the "arterial" segment of the cycle depends on small phasic changes in the tissue volume, large-amplitude vibrations of other kinds that are unassociated with arterial pulsation can confuse the sampling algorithm—especially when the frequencies of the rhythmic vibration approximate the patient's own heart rate. When a patient has a rhythmic tremor (Parkinson disease, anxiety, agitation, seizures, essential tremor, shivering, etc.), tissue volumes can vary phasically in such a way as to invalidate the oximeter's output, which trends toward the default value. In the absence of any detected discrimination between the "baseline" and "arterial" absorption differences, many devices default to a recorded display of 85% to 88%. Rarely, when arterial perfusion is poor and venous pulsations are vigorous, the recorded value may be erroneously depressed.

Anemia and jaundice do not routinely affect the accuracy of pulse oximetry. Pulse oximetry values tend to be misleadingly high in some black patients, but by no means in all. (The existing literature conflicts on this point.) Carboxyhemoglobin and methemoglobin can produce falsely high saturation values, and specific nail polishes (particularly blue, green, or black) interfere with light transmission and absorbance, as do certain blood-borne dyes, such as indocyanine green and methylene blue. These tend to artifactually reduce the O_2 saturation reported.

Interpretation

Many practitioners do not fully understand the oxyhemoglobin dissociation relationship (Fig. 5-1) or the value and limitations of transmission oximetry. Over the clinically relevant range, the oxyhemoglobin dissociation curve is highly nonlinear, so a drop of a few percentage points in SaO_2 over the 95% to 100% interval reflects a much larger change in PaO_2 than does a similar decrement over the 80% to 85% interval. Pulse oximeters record the relative absorption of light by oxyhemoglobin

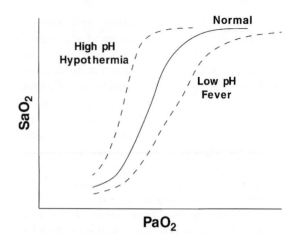

■ **FIGURE 5-1** Relationship of blood oxygen saturation (SaO_2) to blood oxygen tension (PaO_2). A normal curve has a sigmoidal shape, with the upper plateau of the relationship (90% saturation) reached at a PaO_2 of approximately 55 to 60 mm Hg. Alkalemia and hypothermia shift the curve up and to the left; acidemia and fever shift it down and to the right.

and deoxyhemoglobin. Therefore, for a fixed value of viable hemoglobin, the saturation parallels its relative O_2 content, but a high saturation guarantees neither its total O_2 content nor the adequacy of tissue O_2 delivery. For example, a patient may have a "full" SaO_2 after inhaling a high concentration of carbon monoxide, and yet directly measuring arterial oxygen *content* per deciliter of blood (by co-oximetry) may demonstrate profound arterial O_2 depletion. Moreover, a patient in circulatory shock may maintain a perfectly normal SaO_2 despite serious O_2 privation. Cyanide blocks the uptake of oxygen by the tissues, so O_2 consumption is low even as arterial and mixed-venous saturations are normal or increased. Arterial oxygen saturation also bears no direct relationship to the adequacy of ventilation; a patient breathing a high-inspired concentration of oxygen will maintain a nearly normal SaO_2 for extended periods in the face of a full respiratory arrest.

Other gas-measuring techniques (e.g., transcutaneous and transconjunctival measurements of O_2 and CO_2) have been used widely in neonatology to monitor tissue gas tensions, but traditional monitors have been generally less helpful for adults. These transcutaneous techniques require frequent calibration, excellent skin and electrode preparation to ensure gas transfer to the skin surface, and regular site changes to avoid burning the warmed patch of skin they monitor. More importantly, they are profoundly affected by inadequacy of perfusion and therefore track arterial gas tensions unreliably during many critical illnesses. Alert patients tolerate conjunctival probes poorly. Newer tissue oxygen sensors appear to hold considerably more promise.

Several methods now in active development have been used largely in a research setting but show considerable promise for clinical monitoring of microcirculatory function during circulatory failure. These include CO_2 measurements for sublingual, buccal, and subcutaneous microcirculatory CO_2 levels, as well as absorbance, reflectance, and near infrared spectroscopy (NIRS) for measuring microcirculatory hemoglobin saturation. NIRS can probe to considerable depth and has already found clinical application in the assessment of cerebrocortical viability. Orthogonal polarization spectral (OPS) imaging and sidestream dark field technology allow microscopic visualization of the deeper lying microcirculation and the flow of red blood cells in the microcirculation. Sublingual capnography combined with OPS imaging has been used to investigate the relationship between the microcirculation and metabolic status during resuscitation. Combinations of these technologies, which look at different functional compartments of regional microcirculations, can integratively probe the *distributive* alterations of oxygen transport during sepsis, septic shock, and therapy that are not provided by conventional monitoring of systemic hemodynamic and oxygen-derived variables.

O_2 Consumption

Although theoretically valuable for assessing nutritional requirements, adequacy of oxygen delivery, or response to hemodynamic interventions, total body oxygen consumption ($\dot{V}O_2$) is often difficult to measure accurately at the bedside—even in those receiving mechanical ventilation. Two primary methods are in general use: direct analysis of inspired and expired gases and the Fick method (computation of $\dot{V}O_2$ from the product of cardiac output [CO] and the difference in O_2 content between samples of arterial and mixed-venous blood). Neither method reflects average oxygen consumption when the patient's metabolic rate fluctuates during data collection. For some purposes, an estimate of CO_2 production—which is considerably more convenient to obtain—may serve to answer the question of interest (see following).

Delivery Dependence of $\dot{V}O_2$

Controversy has surrounded the concept of supply dependency of O_2 consumption for patients having sustained trauma, massive surgery, or sepsis. Failure to provide sufficient O_2 delivery may result in anaerobiosis, multisystem organ failure, and an adverse or fatal outcome. Moreover, it generally is agreed that prognosis in these conditions is somewhat better for critically ill patients in whom higher O_2 delivery is manifest. By inference, it has been suggested that in these settings, supranormal O_2 delivery is needed to satisfy the O_2 demands of certain vital organs. Prompt and vigorous resuscitation must be carried out, as patients who do not spontaneously generate sufficient O_2 delivery or who cannot extract O_2 effectively have a worse prognosis than other patients undergoing the same stress who do. Yet, it is highly questionable whether attempts to sustain O_2 delivery at supranormal values are well advised. Some data even suggest potential harm. Specific subgroups of surgical patients could, in fact, benefit; there are no tightly controlled data available to settle this question in either direction. Patients having sustained massive trauma or extensive surgery may represent a fundamentally different physiologic problem and respond more favorably than patients with medical crises such as sepsis. It now seems clear that targeting supranormal values for oxygen delivery confers no routine benefit for patients in the latter category. Without better evidence, therefore, maximizing $\dot{V}O_2$ cannot be accepted as the primary target variable for circulatory support.

Efficiency of Oxygen Exchange

Computing Alveolar Oxygen Tension

To judge the efficiency of pulmonary gas exchange, mean alveolar oxygen tension (PAO_2) must first be computed. The ideal PAO_2 is obtained from the modified alveolar gas equation:

$$PAO_2 = PIO_2 - (PaCO_2/R) + [(PaCO_2 \times FiO_2 \times (1 - R)/R)]$$

Here R is the respiratory exchange ratio and PIO_2 is the inspired oxygen tension adjusted for FiO_2 and water vapor pressure at body temperature (47 mm Hg at 37°C).

$$PIO_2 = (\text{barometric pressure} - 47) \times FiO_2$$

Under steady-state conditions, R normally varies from approximately 0.7 to 1.0, depending on the mix of metabolic fuels. When the same patient is monitored over time, R generally is assumed to be 0.8 or neglected entirely. Under most clinical conditions, the alveolar gas equation can be simplified to:

$$PAO_2 = PIO_2 - (1.25 \times PaCO_2)$$

For example, at sea level with a normally ventilated patient breathing room air:

$$\begin{aligned} PAO_2 &= 0.21 \times (760 - 47) - 1.25 \times (PaCO_2) \\ &= 150 - (1.25 \times 40) \\ &\cong 100 \, mm \, Hg \end{aligned}$$

Alveolar–Arterial Oxygen Tension Difference P(A–a)O$_2$

The difference between alveolar and arterial oxygen tensions, $P(A–a)O_2$, takes account of alveolar CO_2 tension and therefore eliminates hypercapnia from consideration as the sole cause of hypoxemia. However, although useful, a single value of $P(A–a)O_2$ does not characterize the efficiency of gas exchange across all FiO_2s—even in normal subjects. The $P(A–a)O_2$ in a young normal subject ranges from approximately 10 mm Hg (on room air) to approximately 100 mm Hg (on an FiO_2 of 1.0). (Breathing room air, the upper limit of normal approximates age/4 + 4 mm Hg.) Moreover, PAO_2 changes nonlinearly with respect to FiO_2 as the extent of $\dot{V}/\dot{Q}$ mismatch increases. When the $\dot{V}/\dot{Q}$ abnormality is severe and abnormally distributed among gas exchanging units, the PAO_2 may vary little with FiO_2 until high fractions of inspired oxygen are given (Fig. 5-2). Finally, the $P(A–a)O_2$ may be influenced by the fluctuations in venous oxygen content.

Venous Admixture and Shunt

Under normal circumstances, fluctuations in mixed-venous O_2 saturation (SvO_2) do not contribute significantly to hypoxemia. However, as ventilation/perfusion inequality or shunting develops, the O_2 content of mixed-venous blood (CvO_2) exerts an increasingly important effect on SaO_2. Measuring SvO_2 with a fiberoptic Swan–Ganz catheter enable venous admixture (Q_s/Q_t) to be computed with relative ease. In the steady state:

$$Q_s/Q_t = (CAO_2 - CaO_2)/(CAO_2 - C\bar{v}O_2)$$

where the oxygen content of alveolar capillary blood (CAO_2), arterial blood (CaO_2), or mixed-venous blood ($C\bar{v}O_2$), expressed in mL of O_2 per 100 mL of blood, equal the sum:

$$[0.003 \times PO_2] + [0.0138 \times (SO_2 \times Hgb)]$$

(In the latter equation, PO_2 [mm Hg] and SO_2 [%] refer to the oxygen tension and saturation of blood at the respective sites. Hemoglobin [Hgb] is expressed in gm/dL.) Like $P(A–a)O_2$, Q_s/Q_t is also influenced by variations in $\dot{V}/\dot{Q}$ mismatching and by fluctuations in SvO_2 and FiO_2. If Q_s/Q_t is abnormally high but all alveoli are patent, calculated admixture will diminish toward the normal physiologic value (approx. 5%) as FiO_2 increases. Conversely, if the Q_s/Q_t abnormality results from blood bypassing the patent alveoli through intrapulmonary communications or through an intracardiac defect, there will be no change in Q_s/Q_t as FiO_2 increases ("true" shunt).

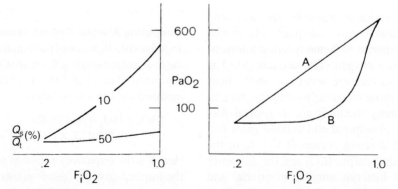

■ **FIGURE 5-2** Effect of true shunt (Q_s/Q_t; **left**) and ventilation/perfusion mismatching **(right)** on the relationship between arterial oxygen tension (PaO_2) and inspired oxygen fraction (FiO_2). Hypoxemia caused by true shunt is refractory to supplementary oxygen once the shunt fraction exceeds 30%. Similar reductions in PaO_2 caused by ventilation/perfusion mismatching respond to oxygen; however, the FiO_2 required to boost PaO_2 into an acceptable range depends on whether hypoxemia is caused by an extensive number of units with mildly abnormal ventilation/perfusion mismatching (*line A*) or by a smaller number of units with very low ventilation to perfusion ratios (*line B*).

Simplified Measures of Oxygen Exchange

Several pragmatic approaches have been taken to simplify bedside assessment of O_2 exchange efficiency. The first is to quantitate $P(A–a)O_2$ during the administration of pure O_2. After a suitable wash-in time (5 to 15 min, depending on the severity of the disease), pure shunt accounts for the entire $P(A–a)O_2$. Furthermore, if hemoglobin is fully saturated with O_2 dividing the $P(A–a)O_2$ by 20 approximates the shunt percentage (at FiO_2 = 1.0). As pure O_2 replaces alveolar nitrogen, some patent but poorly ventilated units may collapse—the process of "absorption atelectasis." Moreover, because shunt percentage is affected by changes in CO and mixed-venous O_2 saturation, these simplified measures may give a misleading impression of changes within the lung itself. Whatever its shortcomings, determining the shunt fraction is worthwhile because it alerts the clinician to consider nonparenchymal causes of hypoxemia (e.g., arteriovenous malformation, intracardiac right-to-left shunting). Furthermore, because PaO_2 shows little response to variations in FiO_2 at true shunt fractions greater than 25%, the clinician may be encouraged to reduce toxic and marginally effective concentrations of oxygen.

The PaO_2/FiO_2 (or "P/F") ratio is a convenient and widely used bedside index of oxygen exchange that attempts to adjust for fluctuating FiO_2. Although simple to calculate, this ratio is affected by changes in SvO_2 and does not remain equally sensitive across the entire range of FiO_2—especially when shunt is the major cause for admixture. Another easily calculated index of oxygen exchange properties, the PaO_2/PAO_2 (or "a/A") ratio, offers similar advantages and disadvantages as FiO_2 is varied. Like the P/F ratio, it is a useful bedside index that does not require blood sampling from the central circulation but loses reliability in proportion to the degree of shunting. Furthermore, in common with all measures that calculate an "ideal" PAO_2, even the a/A ratio can be misleading when fluctuations occur in the primary determinants of SvO_2 (hemoglobin and the balance between oxygen consumption and delivery).

None of the indices discussed thus far account for changes in the functional status of the lung that result from alterations in PEEP, AP, or other techniques for adjusting average lung volume (e.g., inverse ratio ventilation, lateral positioning, or prone positioning). If the objective is to categorize the severity of disease or to track the true O_2 exchanging status of the lung in the face of such interventions, the P/F ratio falls short. The *oxygenation index*, $PaO_2/(FiO_2 \times \text{mean } P_{AW})$, that takes the effects of PEEP and inspiratory time fraction into account has gained widespread popularity in neonatal and pediatric practice but has yet to catch hold in adult critical care. Although preferable, this index, too, is imperfect; mean airway pressure and FiO_2 bear complex and alinear relationships to PaO_2 when considered across their entire ranges.

Monitoring Carbon Dioxide and Ventilation

Kinetics and Estimates of Carbon Dioxide Production

Body stores of carbon dioxide are far greater than those for oxygen. When breathing room air, only approximately 1.5 L of O_2 is stored (much of it in the lungs) and some of this stored O_2 remains unavailable for release until life-threatening hypoxemia is underway. Although breathing pure O_2 can fill the alveolar compartment with an additional 2 to 3 L of oxygen (a safety factor during apnea or asphyxia), these O_2 reserves are still much less than the approximately 120 L of CO_2 normally stored in body tissues. Because of limited oxygen reserves, PaO_2 and tissue PO_2 change rapidly during apnea, at a rate that is highly dependent on FiO_2.

CO_2 stores are held in several forms (dissolved, bound to protein, fixed as bicarbonate, etc.) and distributed in compartments that differ in their volumetric capacity and ability to exchange CO_2 rapidly with the blood. Well-perfused organs constitute a small reservoir for CO_2 capable of quick turnover, skeletal muscle is a larger compartment with sluggish exchange, and bone and fat are high-capacity chambers with very slow filling and release. Practically, the existence of large CO_2 reservoirs **2** with different capacities and time constants of filling and emptying means that equilibration to a new steady-state $PaCO_2$ after a step change in ventilation (assuming a constant rate of CO_2 production, $\dot{V}CO_2$) takes longer than generally appreciated—especially for step *reductions* in alveolar ventilation (Fig. 5-3). With such a large capacity and only a modest rate of metabolic CO_2 production, the CO_2 reservoir fills rather slowly, so $PaCO_2$ rises only 6 to 9 mm Hg during the first minute of apnea and 3 to 6 mm Hg each minute thereafter. Depletion of this reservoir can occur at a faster rate.

Measurement of CO_2 excretion is valuable for metabolic assessment, computations of dead space ventilation, and evaluation of hyperpnea. Estimates

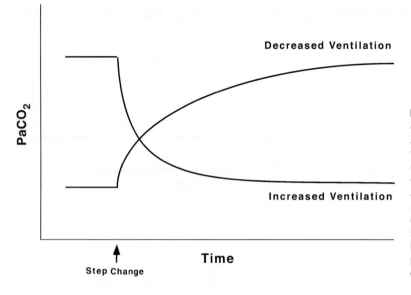

■ **FIGURE 5-3** Effect of step changes in ventilation on $PaCO_2$. After an abrupt change in ventilation, $PaCO_2$ either climbs (step decrease in ventilation) or descends (step increase in ventilation) toward a new plateau. Equilibration is reached more slowly after a step decrease in ventilation because the large storage reservoir for CO_2 can be filled only at the rate of CO_2 production. Elimination of CO_2 can occur more rapidly.

of CO_2 production are representative when the sample is collected carefully in the steady state over adequate time. The rate of CO_2 elimination is a product of minute ventilation ($\dot{V}_E$) and the expired fraction of CO_2 in the expelled gas. If gas collection is timed accurately and the sample is adequately mixed and analyzed, an accurate value for excreted CO_2 can be obtained. However, whether this value faithfully represents metabolic CO_2 production depends on the stability of the patient during the period of gas collection—not only with regard to $\dot{V}O_2$ but also in terms of acid–base fluctuations, perfusion constancy, and ventilation status with respect to metabolic needs. During acute hyperventilation or rapidly developing metabolic acidosis, for example, the rate of CO_2 excretion overestimates the metabolic rate until surplus body stores of CO_2 are washed out or bicarbonate stores reach equilibrium. The opposite obtains during abrupt hypoventilation or transient reduction in CO.

Efficiency of CO_2 Exchange

The volume of CO_2 produced by the body tissues varies with metabolic rate (fever, pain, agitation, sepsis, etc.). In the mechanically ventilated patient, many vagaries of CO_2 flux can be eliminated by controlling ventilation and quieting muscle activity with deep sedation with or without paralysis. $PaCO_2$ must be interpreted in conjunction with the $\dot{V}_E$. For example, the gas exchanging ability of the lung may be unimpaired even though $PaCO_2$ rises when reduced alveolar ventilation is the result of diminished respiratory

drive or marked neuromuscular weakness. As already noted, alveolar and arterial CO_2 concentrations respond quasi-exponentially after step changes in ventilation, with a half-time of approximately 3 min during hyperventilation but a slower half-time (16 min) during hypoventilation. These differing time courses should be taken into account when sampling blood gases after making ventilator adjustments.

Dead space and Dead space Fraction

Dead space
The physiologic dead space (V_D) refers to the "wasted" portion of the tidal breath that fails to participate in CO_2 exchange. A breath can fail to accomplish CO_2 elimination either because fresh (CO_2-free) gas is not brought to the alveoli or because fresh gas fails to contact systemic venous blood. Thus, tidal ventilation is wasted whenever CO_2-laden gas is recycled to the alveoli with the next tidal breath. Alternatively, a portion of the tidal volume is wasted if fresh gas distributes to inadequately perfused alveoli, so CO_2-poor gas is exhausted during exhalation (Fig. 5-4). If this concept is understood, then it becomes clear why V_D cannot be considered accurately as a composite of physical volumes. Nonetheless, wasted ventilation traditionally is characterized as the sum of the "anatomic" (or "series") dead space and the "alveolar" dead space. Because the airways fill with CO_2-containing alveolar gas at the end of the tidal breath, the physical volume of the airways corresponds rather closely to their contribution to

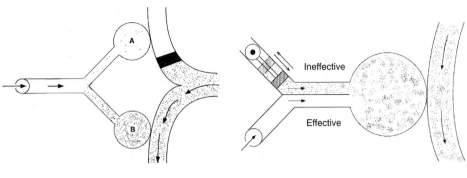

A   **Ventilation Without Perfusion**   B   **Ineffective Ventilation With CO$_2$ Recycling**

■ **FIGURE 5-4** Two definitions of ventilatory dead space. Tidal ventilation is ineffective in eliminating CO$_2$ if fresh gas flows to poorly perfused alveoli that cannot deliver CO$_2$ to the tidal air stream **(A)**. Alternatively, tidal ventilation can be ineffective if the gas flowing to the alveolus during inspiration contains a high concentration of carbon dioxide **(B)**.

wasted ventilation (the "anatomic" dead space)—provided mixed alveolar gas is similar in composition to the gas within a well-perfused alveolus. This is almost true for a quietly breathing normal subject, in whom the alveolar dead space (poorly perfused alveolar volume) is negligible. When the parenchyma is well aerated and well perfused, the anatomic dead space is relatively fixed at approximately 1 mL/lb of body weight. Quite the opposite is true for patients with most lung diseases, in whom alveolar dead space predominates. Here, the lung is composed of well and poorly perfused units, so the *mixed* alveolar gas within the airways at end-exhalation has a CO$_2$ concentration lower than that of pulmonary arterial blood. Although V_D may increase dramatically, the contribution of stale airway gas to V_D is much less important because less amount of airway CO$_2$ is recycled to the alveoli.

For normal subjects, dead space increases with advancing age and body size and is reduced modestly by recumbency, extended breath holding, and decelerating inspiratory flow patterns. External apparatus attached to the airway that remains unflushed by fresh gas (e.g., a facemask) may add to the series dead space, whereas tracheostomy reduces it. The supine position reduces dead space by decreasing the average size of the lung and by increasing the number of well-perfused lung units.

Numerous diseases increase V_D. Destruction of alveolar septae, low output circulatory failure, pulmonary embolism, pulmonary vasoconstriction or vascular compression, and mechanical ventilation with high tidal volumes or PEEP are common mechanisms that often act in combination.

Dead space Fraction

In the setting of parenchymal lung disease, dead space varies in proportion to tidal volume over a remarkably wide range. Series dead space tends to remain fixed but generally constitutes a small percentage of the total physiologic V_D, overwhelmed by the alveolar dead space component. Therefore, except at very small tidal volumes, the *fraction* of wasted ventilation (V_D/V_T) tends to remain relatively constant as the depth of the breath varies. The dead space fraction can be estimated from analyzed specimens of arterial blood and mixed expired ($P_{\bar{E}}CO_2$) gas:

$$(V_D/V_T) = (PaCO_2 - P_{\bar{E}}CO_2)/PaCO_2$$

where $P_{\bar{E}}CO_2$ is the CO$_2$ concentration in mixed expired gas. (This expression is known as the Enghoff-modified Bohr equation.) As already noted, $P_{\bar{E}}CO_2$ can be determined on a breath-by-breath basis if exhaled volume is measured simultaneously. Alternatively, exhaled gas can be collected over a defined period. The PCO$_2$ of gas exiting a mixing chamber attached to the expiratory line provides a continuous "rolling average" value. In collecting the expired gas sample during pressurized ventilator cycles, an adjustment should be made for the volume of any sampled gas stored in the compressible portions of the ventilator circuit (without gaining exposure to the patient).

In healthy persons, the normal V_D/V_T during spontaneous breathing varies approximately from 0.35 to 0.15, depending on the factors noted earlier (position, exercise, age, tidal volume, pulmonary capillary distention, breath holding, etc.). In the setting of critical illness, however, it is not uncommon for V_D/V_T to rise to values that exceed 0.7. Indeed, increased dead space ventilation usually accounts for most of the increase in the $\dot{V}_E$ requirement and CO_2 retention that occur in the terminal phase of acute hypoxemic respiratory failure. In addition to pathologic processes that increase dead space, changes in V_D/V_T occur during periods of hypovolemia or overdistention by high airway pressures. This phenomenon is often apparent when progressive levels of PEEP are applied to support oxygenation. Examination of the airway pressure tracing under conditions of controlled, constant inspiratory flow ventilation may demonstrate concavity or a clear point of upward inflection, indicating overdistention, accelerated dead space formation, and escalating risk of barotrauma. Small reductions in PEEP or tidal volume may then dramatically reduce peak cycling pressure and V_D/V_T.

Monitoring of Exhaled Gas

Capnography analyzes the CO_2 concentration of the expiratory airstream, plotting CO_2 concentration against time or, more usefully, against exhaled volume. Although most capnometers in clinical use currently display PCO_2 as a function of time, much of the attention here will focus on the CO_2 versus volume plot because it provides more information of clinical value. After anatomic dead space has been cleared, the CO_2 tension rises progressively to its maximal value at end-exhalation, a number that reflects the CO_2 tension of mixed alveolar gas. For normal subjects, the transition between phases of the capnogram is sharp, and once achieved, the alveolar plateau rises only gently. Furthermore, when ventilation and perfusion are evenly distributed, as they are in healthy subjects, end-tidal PCO_2 ($P_{ET}CO_2$) closely approximates $PaCO_2$. ($P_{ET}CO_2$ normally underestimates $PaCO_2$ by 1 to 3 mm Hg.) This difference widens when ventilation and perfusion are matched suboptimally, so the alveolar dead space gas admixes with CO_2-rich gas from well-perfused alveoli.

When plotted against a volume axis, as opposed to the more commonly encountered time axis, the capnogram offers data of considerable clinical value. Inspection of such tracings can yield estimates for the "anatomic" (Fowler) dead space, as well as for the end-tidal and mixed expired CO_2 concentrations (Fig. 5-5). Knowing the barometric pressure (P_B), the mixed expired value can be expressed as a percentage of the exhaled volume, which is also

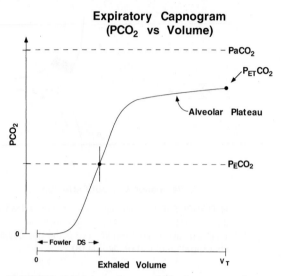

Expiratory Capnogram (PCO₂ vs Volume)

■ **FIGURE 5-5** Information available from an expiratory capnogram plotting PCO_2 concentration against exhaled volume. Under steady-state conditions, mixed expired CO_2 concentration ($P_{\bar{E}}CO_2$), a key component of the physiologic dead space fraction and $\dot{V}CO_2$, is easily discerned. The slope of the alveolar plateau is a measure of ventilation heterogeneity. The Fowler dead space (DS) is a close correlate of anatomic dead space. End-tidal PCO_2 ($P_{ET}CO_2$) reflects the concentration of CO_2 within the alveolar units that are last to empty. Although this value may parallel $PaCO_2$ in normal individuals, it is less reliable in disease.

immediately available from the tracing. If the V_T remains constant, the product of $P_{\bar{E}}CO_2$: P_B ratio and $\dot{V}_E$ is $\dot{V}CO_2$, and the mixed expired CO_2 concentration can be used in the Enghoff-modified Bohr equation to estimate the physiologic dead space fraction.

As with other monitoring techniques, exhaled CO_2 values must be interpreted cautiously. The normal capnogram is composed of an ascending portion, a plateau, a descending portion, and a baseline (Fig. 5-6). In disease, the sharp distinctions between phases of the capnogram, as well as the slopes of each segment, are blurred. Moreover, failure of the airway gas to equilibrate with gas from well-perfused alveoli invalidates $P_{ET}CO_2$ as a reflection of $PaCO_2$, especially as respiratory frequency fluctuates. (The $P_{\bar{E}}CO_2$ per cycle, however, remains valid.) End-tidal PCO_2 gives a low range estimate of $PaCO_2$ in virtually all clinical circumstances, so a high $P_{ET}CO_2$ strongly suggests hypoventilation. Abrupt changes in $P_{ET}CO_2$ may reflect such acute processes as aspiration or pulmonary embolism if the $\dot{V}_E$ and breathing pattern (f, V_T, and $I:E$ ratio) remain unchanged. Although breath-to-breath fluctuations in $P_{ET}CO_2$ can be extreme, the trend of

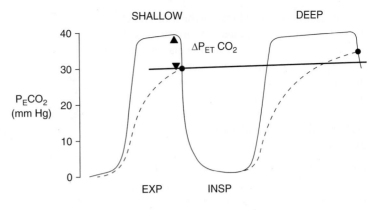

■ **FIGURE 5-6** Expired CO_2 (P_ECO_2) as a function of time. Expired CO_2 tension varies markedly during a breathing cycle in four phases. Wide separation of end-expiratory values of end-tidal CO_2 ($\Delta P_{ET}CO_2$) for a normal subject (*solid line*) and a patient with increased anatomic dead space (*dashed line*) narrows during more complete exhalation.

$P_{ET}CO_2$ over time helps identify underlying changes in CO_2 exchange.

The capnogram also provides an excellent monitor of breathing rhythm. Close examination of the tracing contour and comparison with earlier waveforms may give helpful indications of circuit leaks, patient ventilator dyssynchrony, equipment malfunctions, secretion retention, and changes in underlying pathophysiology. In evaluating the $P_{ET}CO_2$, it is essential to record and examine the entire capnographic tracing, not relying on digital readouts alone. Breathing pattern can be as influential as pathology, especially when gas flow is inhomogeneously distributed, as in airflow obstruction. Failure of the tracing to achieve a true plateau can occur because the sampling technique is inappropriate, exhalation is too brief, or ventilation is inhomogeneously distributed. Thus, the $P_{ET}CO_2$ may fluctuate for a variety of reasons, not all of which imply changes in lung disease. The arterial to end-tidal CO_2 difference is minimized when perfused alveoli are recruited maximally. On this basis, the ($PaCO_2 - P_{ET}CO_2$) difference has been suggested as helpful in identifying "best PEEP" (Fig. 5-5). This technique may have value for patients in whom a clear inflection point observed on the ascending limb of the airway pressure tracing suggests recruitable volume (see following).

■ MONITORING LUNG AND CHEST WALL MECHANICS

General Principles

For cooperative ambulatory patients, respiratory mechanics—those properties of the lung and chest wall that determine the ease of chest expansion—are best measured in the pulmonary function laboratory.

However, because most patients with critical illness cannot cooperate and are often supported by a mechanical ventilator, the clinician must become the analyst of pulmonary function.

Certain properties (e.g., compliance of the chest wall and respiratory system) can be assessed only under passive conditions; others (e.g., maximal inspiratory pressure [MIP]) require active breathing effort. The mechanical properties of the lung—a passive object—can be determined with or without active breathing effort, provided the estimates of pleural pressure as well as airway pressure and flow are available. Although pleural pressure—traditionally estimated by esophageal balloon—is rarely measured, its potential value is high when the pressure applied across the lung is of concern (e.g., in ventilating acute respiratory distress syndrome [ARDS]). Finally, to separate static (e.g., compliance) from dynamic (e.g., flow resistance) variables, points of zero flow within the tidal cycle must be determined exactly; to accomplish this, the clinician may need to impose a well-timed flow stoppage of appropriate length.

Pressure–Volume Relationships

A good understanding of static pressure–volume (PV) relationships is fundamental to the interpretation of chest mechanics. Although this complex topic cannot be addressed thoroughly here, certain key concepts deserve mention. Because the lung is a flexible but passive structure, gas flows to and from the alveoli driven by differences between airway and alveolar pressures—no matter how they are generated. The total pressure gradient expanding the respiratory system is accounted for in two primary ways: (a) in driving gas between the airway opening and the alveolus and (b) in expanding the alveoli against the recoil forces of the lung and chest wall. The pressure required for inspiratory flow dissipates against friction while the elastic pressure that expands the respiratory system is stored temporarily in elastic tissues and then dissipated in driving expiratory flow.

Normal Values for Resistance and Compliance

For clinical purposes, the nonelastic impedance to airflow offered by friction and movement of the lung and chest wall is termed "resistance." The elastic impedance these structures offer in opposing inflation is termed "elastance," and its inverse is the familiar "compliance." For a point of reference, the normal airway resistance of a healthy adult is less than 4 cm $H_2O/L/s$ when breathing spontaneously and rises approximately twofold when orally intubated with a tube of standard size and length (tube diameter is always substantially less than that of the trachea). The elastances of the lungs (E_L) and chest wall (E_{CW}) add in series to comply with that of the respiratory system (E_{RS}): $E_{RS} = E_L + E_{CW}$, and compliances add in parallel (see following). At end-expiration the compliance values for the lung, chest wall, and integrated respiratory system of a spontaneously breathing, healthy adult patient of normal size and weight in the supine position are approximately 200, 150, and 85 mL/cm H_2O, respectively.

Static Properties of the Respiratory System

3 Accurate estimation of respiratory system properties cannot be accomplished in the ventilated patient using airway pressure alone unless the breathing is *passive*. Furthermore, what contributions the lung and chest wall make to the measured compliance requires an estimate of pleural pressure. With these caveats in mind, the PV relationships measured during mechanical ventilation are informative. While increasing the pressure applied across the normal lungs and chest wall increases their volume, the relationship between pressure and volume varies markedly over the vital capacity (VC) range (Fig. 5-7). Over small segments, this relationship can be considered approximately linear over most regions of the PV curve. Therefore, assuming linearity, the elastic properties of the lung, chest wall, and integrated respiratory system can be described by single values for chord elastance ($\Delta P/\Delta V$) or its inverse, chord compliance ($\Delta V/\Delta P$). The tidal compliance measured at the bedside

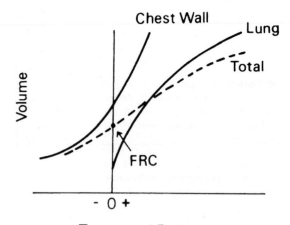

■ FIGURE 5-7 Normal static PV relationships of the lung, chest wall, and total respiratory system. With no pressure applied to the airway opening, the outward recoil pressure of the chest wall at end-expiration counterbalances the inward collapsing pressure of the lung at functional residual capacity (FRC).

(V_t/[Plateau – total PEEP]) is a type of chord compliance. (Chord compliance differs from *tangential* compliance, which is the slope at a single point on the curve.) When tidal recruitment of collapsed lung units occurs over the tidal volume range, calculations of chord compliance may not characterize the elastic properties of the underlying tissue. Examination of the PV relationship indicates that chord compliance differs according to the segment over which it is computed.

Specific Compliance

Because flow and volume are measured in absolute units (L/s and L), the same ΔP will result in a different ΔV for two lungs of identical tissue properties but different capacities (see below). For example, identical pressures drive greatly different volumes into the chest of a patient before and after pneumonectomy. Until very recently, we have had no way to measure lung capacity at the bedside, but the measurement of functional residual capacity (FRC) by gas dilution is now an option on the latest ventilators, allowing the estimation of the *specific* compliance of tissue that is accessible to air.

Respiratory System Compliance and Elastance

The portion of the applied airway pressure that expands the *lung* by a certain volume (ΔV) is the corresponding change in transpulmonary pressure: $P_L = (P_{alv} - P_{pl})$, where P_{alv} = alveolar pressure and

P_{pl} = pleural pressure. The lung elastance (E_L = $\Delta P_L/\Delta V$) is the pressure per unit of inflation volume required to keep the lung expanded under no-flow (static) conditions. In clinical practice, it has been customary to refer to lung compliance, the inverse of elastance ($C_L = 1/E_L = \Delta V/\Delta P_L$). In similar fashion, the distensibility of the relaxed chest wall is characterized by chest wall compliance ($C_w = \Delta V/\Delta P_{pl}$). The slope of the static inspiratory PV relationship for the total respiratory system is C_{RS} ($C_{RS} = \Delta V/\Delta P_{alv}$). In ventilator-derived calculations of compliance, ΔV (normally, the tidal volume) must be measured at the endotracheal tube or expired volume must be adjusted for the volume stored during pressurized inflation in compressible circuit elements. Most modern ventilators do this automatically.

Compliance measurements obtained under passive conditions may have therapeutic and prognostic value for patients with arterial desaturation. In the setting of lung edema (e.g., ARDS), many lung units are collapsed or closed at FRC and reopen at various pressures as the lung distends. At the same time, other lung units distend to the point of overstretching. When PEEP is applied incrementally and the lung is passive, C_L and C_{RS} tend to reach their highest values when the balance of opening and overstretching is most favorable. (Chest wall properties do, however, influence the measurements made.) This zone also tends to be that associated with minimal ventilatory dead space and shunt fraction and often coincides with the zone of maximal oxygen delivery. Because of tidal recruitment, different tidal volumes may be associated with different "optimal PEEP" values. Many experts believe that PEEP is best set after first fully expanding the lung—in other words, on the deflation limb, not the inflation limb of the PV loop. It is a good rule, however, to avoid using values of end-expiratory pressure or tidal volume that depress tidal thoracic compliance—unless objective evidence of significantly improved oxygen *delivery* is available and safe plateau pressure is not exceeded. Generally speaking, lower compliance correlates with a smaller number of aeratable lung units. Followed over time, serial changes in the respiratory PV curve and C_{RS} tend to reflect the nature and course of acute lung injury. Severe disease is implied when compliance falls to less than 25 mL/cm H_2O. Maximal depression of C_{RS} often requires 1 to 2 weeks to develop in the setting of acute lung injury, signifying both fewer functioning lung units and lower specific compliance of those that remain

open. Although C_{RS} provides useful information regarding the difficulty of chest expansion, C_{RS} does not necessarily parallel underlying tissue elastance—both the size of the alveolar compartment and the relative position on the PV curve are important to consider. Ideally, compliance is referenced to a measure of absolute lung volume, such as FRC or total lung capacity (TLC) ("specific" compliance). Furthermore, C_{RS} may differ greatly at the extremes of the VC range, even in the same individual (Fig. 5-8). Thus, most patients with hyperinflated lungs ventilated for acute exacerbations of asthma or chronic obstructive pulmonary disease (COPD) exhibit depressed C_{RS}, despite normal or "supernormal" tissue distensibility; C_{RS} would be a better indicator of tissue elastic properties if measured in a lower volume range. Elastances add in series, so $E_{RS} = E_L + E_{CW}$. Yet, because compliances add in parallel, C_{RS} bears a complex relationship to the individual compliances of the lung (C_L) and chest wall (C_w):

$$C_{RS} = (C_L \times C_w)/(C_w + C_L)$$

The fraction of PEEP transmitted to the pleural space depends on the relative compliances of the lungs and chest wall:

$$\Delta P_{pl} = PEEP \times (C_L/(C_L + C_w))$$

Chest Wall Compliance
The usual assumption that the PV characteristic of the chest wall is normal and remains linear and unchanging throughout its range is often inappropriate for critically ill patients whose chest wall distensibility may be disturbed by abdominal distention,

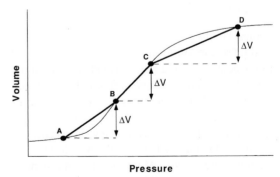

■ **FIGURE 5-8** Computation of tidal (chord) compliance of the respiratory system. An identical tidal volume (ΔV) results in quite different values for compliance (ΔV/Δelastic pressure). In this example, tidal compliance, the inverse of the slope of the chord linking the two volumes over which tidal volume was delivered, is best in the middle third of the inspiratory curve (BC), worst in the top third of the curve (CD), and intermediate in the bottom third (AB).

pleural effusions, ascites, muscular tone, recent surgery, position, binders, braces, and so on (see following). Such changes in C_w are very important to consider in that they dramatically influence P_{PL}. In turn, P_{PL} influences venous return, hemodynamic data (e.g., pulmonary artery occlusion pressure, P_w), and calculations of chest mechanics based on airway pressure. As already noted, an appropriate interpretation of tidal airway pressures depends on a valid assessment of intrapleural pressure. Moreover, specific values for peak airway pressure and C_{RS} have different prognostic significance, depending on whether the lung or chest wall accounts for the stiffness.

Influence of Pleural Effusion

The presence of a large pleural effusion alters the usual interpretation of chest mechanics. Contrary to intuition, the formation of a large pleural effusion often does not substantially reduce the measured compliance of the total respiratory system. With PEEP applied and the chest wall normally flexible, the lung expands into the fluid (rather than directly against the chest wall) during the breath, causing extensive tidal recruitment. In a sense, the fluid "uncouples" the lung from the chest wall. The *apparent* compliance of the total respiratory system—as assessed by our usual tidal compliance—is not reduced but rather tends to improve in the fluid's presence. If the chest wall is unusually stiff, however, the linkage between the lung and the chest wall tightens, and pleural fluid formation impedes lung expansion. Clearly, attempts to identify "best PEEP" in the presence of an effusion are not reliably made by measuring respiratory system compliance.

Clinical Utility
of the Pressure–Volume Curve

In the acutely injured lung, virtually all lung units may sustain initial damage, but not all are equally compromised or mechanically equivalent. In severe cases, perhaps only 20% to 30% of alveoli remain patent, the others being atelectatic or occluded by lung edema, cellular infiltrate, or inflammatory debris. Moreover, the mechanical properties of the lung differ in dependent and nondependent regions. For a supine patient, atelectasis predominates in dorsal sectors, where lung units tend to collapse under the influence of regionally increased pleural pressure and the weight of the overlying lung. This proclivity is greatest at FRC, when transalveolar pressure is

least. In this surfactant-deficient lung, there are tendencies for persisting collapse of dependent alveoli and/or tidal reopening and recollapse of lung units in the middle and dependent zones. The latter process subjects injured tissue to damaging shear forces when high inflation pressures are used. According to current thinking, both persisting collapse of inflamed tissue and the tidal collapse cycle must be avoided. To aid in healing, some knowledgeable investigators believe that the objective is to "open the lung and keep it open" without causing overdistention (see Chapter 24).

Many alveoli—especially those in nondependent zones—remain open and relatively compliant but are subject to overdistention by high peak tidal pressures. These regional differences give rise to an inspiratory PV curve with poor compliance in its initial and terminal segments. Defining the PV relationship may help guide the ventilator settings needed to avoid the damaging effects of both tidal collapse and alveolar overdistention. The PV curve is a composite of information from myriad lung units, and its contours are shaped by the relative numbers of open (recruited) units and the *proportion* of units at various stages of distension (see Chapters 9 and 24). In the setting of ARDS, it appears that recruitment occurs to some degree throughout the total lung capacity range. Therefore, the inflation limb of the PV curve is shaped by two phenomena occurring simultaneously—opening of lung units being recruited and distention or overfilling of those already open. Although not everyone agrees, most investigators of ventilator-induced lung injury currently believe that sufficient end-expiratory alveolar pressure (total PEEP [$PEEP_{TOT}$], see Chapter 9) should be maintained to surpass the lower inflection zone (P_{flex} region) of the inspiratory PV curve when high end-inspiratory (plateau) pressures are in use. Although approximately 12 to 15 cm H_2O generally suffices to approximate P_{flex} in the early stage of ARDS, the PEEP requirement will vary with body size, stage, and severity of lung injury as well as with chest wall compliance. At the same time, peak tidal alveolar pressure should not encroach on the upper *deflection* zone that signals widespread alveolar overdistention. (A few sustained inflations to high static pressure may be necessary to open the lung in the initial stages of ARDS, and periodic "recruiting breaths" may be needed when very small tidal volumes are used.) The relevant opening pressure here may be as low as 25 cm H_2O in some individuals and as high as 60 cm H_2O in others, influenced heavily by the type and duration of lung injury and by chest wall characteristics. It should be noted that PEEP is an *expiratory* pressure and that less pressure is needed to keep lung units open than to open them once they close. (This difference gives rise to hysteresis of the inspiratory–expiratory PV loop.) It follows that setting PEEP is more rationally done by first opening the lung to TLC (opening as many units as possible) and then dropping PEEP from a high value to a lower one that prevents widespread collapse (see Chapters 8 and 24).

Construction of the PV Curve

No simple rules for choosing optimal PEEP apply to all patients because the compliance characteristics of the lung and chest wall differ so radically. Consequently, there is no completely satisfactory alternative to defining the entire PV curve, even though this is not always feasible or safe to undertake. Disconnection of the ventilator may cause a marked drop in mean and end-expiratory transalveolar pressures that can cause hypoxemia, bradycardia, arrhythmia, and/or flooding of the airway with edema fluid. For this reason, many physicians forgo PV curve measurement entirely in their most severely ill patients or elect to use methods whereby the patient remains connected to the ventilator as PEEP and/or tidal volume are varied.

Traditionally, the inspiratory PV curve is constructed by briefly disconnecting the patient from the ventilator and attaching an oxygen-filled, 2 to 3 L "super syringe" to the airway opening. After establishing a uniform inflation "history," airway pressure is followed as serial 100-mL volumes are injected until TLC is reached. Static pressures are recorded 2 to 3 s after injection of each increment. The entire process is completed within 60 to 90 s. The P_{flex} and the upper deflection zones used to guide PEEP and applied pressure or tidal volume selections may be defined carefully by using smaller injection steps in the early and late phases. In recent years, a slow inflation at constant flow (approx. 2 L/min) delivered by the ventilator has been used as a simplified (and even automated) means of obtaining essentially the same information. Unfortunately, reliance on the airway pressure tracing (a synthesis of information from all lung zones) may be misleading, as regional PV relationships of radically different contours may be imbedded within it (Fig. 5-9).

Construction of an *expiratory* PV curve has more theoretical appeal as a means for setting PEEP, as its contours are more directly influenced by the events of expiratory collapse that PEEP is intended to prevent. The construction of such a curve is more difficult and painstaking, however, as it currently requires periodic stoppages of expired flow and measurement of the corresponding alveolar pressure in a series of steps (see Chapters 9 and 24). Assuming that tidal volume has already been selected, tracking tidal compliance

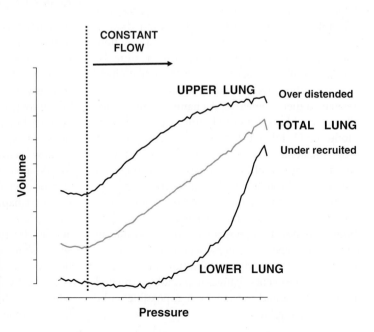

■ **FIGURE 5-9** Regional PV relationships. As the lung fills at a constant rate, the rising total lung pressure bears an apparently linear relationship to volume that actually is a composite of steadily recruiting and overdistending lung units.

during *decrements* of PEEP (proceeding from higher to lower values) has logical appeal for setting PEEP's optimal value. Following this reasoning, the least PEEP associated with preserved tidal compliance and preserved oxygenation is the preferred value.

Calculation of C_{RS} and R_{AW} During Mechanical Ventilation

Inspiratory Resistance and Static Compliance

Although not always elegantly presented or continuously displayed, all ventilators monitor external airway pressure (P_{AW}). When a mechanical ventilator expands the chest of a passive subject, inspiratory P_{AW} furnishes the entire force accomplishing ventilation. Because the PV relationships of the lung and chest wall are approximately linear over the tidal volume range and because the increment in P_{AW} necessary to drive gas flow is nearly unchanging under constant flow conditions, the corresponding P_{AW} waveform resembles a trapezoid, a shape composed of a triangle of elastic pressure and a parallelogram of resistive pressure (Fig. 5-10).

Absolute Lung Volume, Specific Resistance, and Specific Compliance

As already noted, the pressures and flows that determine resistance and compliance are measured in absolute numbers "cm H$_2$O" and "L/s." But a moment's reflection alerts us to the powerful effect that capacity to receive air affects the calculated numbers for compliance and resistance. For example, pressure of 10 cm H$_2$O would drive a huge flow into a healthy elephant, but a tiny flow into a healthy mouse. Moreover, a high value for resistance could reflect the fewer bronchial channels for airflow, rather than hold any information related to their diameters. A change in lung compliance could result not only from a position shift along the PV relationship (e.g., hyperinflation) or from an alteration of tissue elastic properties (e.g., the development of lung fibrosis) but also from a variation in the aeratable capacity of the lung (e.g., pneumonectomy) or the development of consolidation (e.g., pneumonia). Changes in absolute lung volume—now possible with gas dilution built into some ventilators—could tell us more regarding the underlying condition of the lung and about the events changes in pathology (related to recruitment and resistance) than possible without referencing FRC.

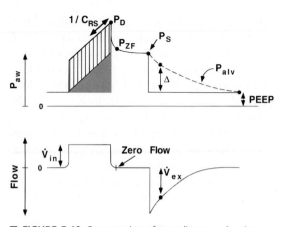

■ **FIGURE 5-10** Computation of compliance and resistance of the respiratory system under passive conditions during constant inspiratory flow ($\dot{V}_{in}$). An end-inspiratory pause is applied to hold the inspired tidal volume before exhalation is begun. Tidal compliance is the quotient of tidal volume and the difference between static plateau pressure (P_S) (equivalent to alveolar pressure, P_{alv}) and PEEP$_{TOT}$. In this example, no AP is present. The difference between peak dynamic pressure (P_D) and plateau pressures, divided by $\dot{V}_{in}$, equals maximum inspiratory resistance. The difference between P_D and the pressure at which flow first becomes zero after the pause is applied (P_{ZF}) reflects the least resistance pressure because it excludes stress relaxation, ventilation redistribution (pendelluft), and viscoelastic pressures. Expiratory resistance requires measurement or calculation of alveolar pressure (referenced to PEEP, Δ) and the corresponding flow it produces ($\dot{V}_{ex}$). Finally, the slope of the airway pressure tracing at the end of inspiration obtained under constant flow conditions reflects elastance of the respiratory system (1/C_{RS}). PEEP, positive end-expiratory pressure.

Role of Dynamics

Although it is customary to characterize the risk for injury to the respiratory system by its static "plateau" pressure after a sustained pause, a growing body of literature indicates that static pressures seriously underestimate the maximal stresses to which some tissues are subjected within the heterogeneous lung and shows that the *rate* at which elastic forces expand should not be ignored. The *pattern* of flow delivery (mean flow velocity and wave form)—not simply the transpulmonary pressure—may be of vital relevance to ventilator-induced lung injury (Chapters 8 and 24). During expansion, some pressure dissipates within the airways, while another fraction of unrecovered (unstored) pressure reshapes the tissues to their static configuration (viscoelastance). Some indication of the latter is offered by the difference between the pressure at which flow first ends after circuit occlusion (zero flow) and the plateau pressure (see Fig. 5-11).

Lung Stretch Depends on Effort and Chest Wall Stiffness

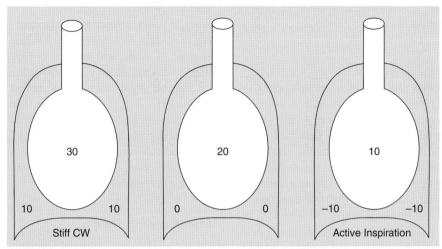

■ **FIGURE 5-11** Importance of chest wall compliance and muscle effort to the "plateau" pressure. The lung's volume and transpulmonary pressure cannot be inferred from knowing the static airway pressure alone. CW, chest wall.

Imaging of Function and Structural Heterogeneity—The Future

To this point in the history of mechanical ventilation, the primary database from which monitored information derives has been limited to global measures of pressure and flow sampled from the airway opening. Yet it is now understood that the diseased lung—whether obstructed or acutely injured—is comprised of heterogeneous subunits whose behaviors and risk susceptibilities vary considerably site to site. Poised to be introduced to the clinical practice are several methodologies designed to monitor regional anatomy and function and thereby help regulate therapy and modify risk. Foremost among these are electrical impedance tomography (EIT), acoustic monitoring, vibration response imaging, and pulmonary ultrasound. Experimental data demonstrate that the distribution and even the nature of lung pathologies can be determined. Surveillance for developing pneumothorax, pleural effusion, consolidation, and tidal recruitment is only one of their potential applications. Although little clinical experience has yet been accumulated, it seems clear from an expanding base of experimental and observational studies that these "real time imaging" methodologies have the potential to elevate respiratory monitoring of the critically ill onto a

new plane of management better aligned with our understanding of underlying pathophysiology and treatment goals.

For most purposes, inspiratory resistance and compliance characteristics of the mechanically ventilated respiratory system are best gauged using translung pressure, which requires esophageal pressure measurement. In clinical practice, these data usually are estimated during volume-cycled, constant flow ventilation using P_{AW} alone. It should be emphasized, however, that calculations of C_{RS} and resistance from P_{AW} can be made only when inflation is *passive*. (During active effort, P_{AW} must be referenced to esophageal pressure to make the relevant calculations.) Both chest wall stiffness and muscular effort may cause the airway pressure to be seriously misleading regarding the lung stess (gauged by the difference between static airway and intrapleural pressures (Fig. 5-11). When gas is prevented from exiting the lung at the end of tidal inspiration, P_{AW} falls quickly to a plateau value. If this end-inspiratory "stop flow," "plateau," or "peak static" (P_S) pressure is referenced to end-expiratory alveolar pressure ($PEEP_{TOT}$), the difference determines the component of end-inspiratory pressure necessary to overcome the elastic forces of inflating the chest with the delivered tidal volume. $PEEP_{TOT}$ is the sum of applied PEEP and ΔP. When tidal volume (adjusted for gas compression) is divided by $(P_S - PEEP_{TOT})$, effective compliance (C_{eff}) can be computed as follows:

$$C_{eff} = V_{Tc}/(P_S - PEEP_{TOT})$$

where V_{Tc} is the corrected V_T.

The maximal pressure achieved just before the end of gas delivery (the peak dynamic pressure, P_D) is the total system pressure required to drive gas to the alveolar level at the selected flow rate and to expand the lungs and chest wall by the full V_T. The difference between P_D and P_S quantifies the gradient driving gas flow ($\dot{V}$) at end-inspiration, a difference that varies with the resistance of the patient and endotracheal tube as well as with the inspiratory gas flow setting. Under these conditions of passive ventilation and constant inspiratory flow, the ratio of $(P_D - P_S)/\dot{V}_{end-insp}$ is the airway resistance (R_{AW}). When corrected for the compression volume of the external circuit, the ratio of delivered volume to $(P_D - PEEP_{TOT})$ reflects the overall difficulty of chest expansion, if V_T and inspiratory flow settings do not change and inflation occurs passively. This index had been termed the "dynamic characteristic" (DC):

$$DC = V_T/(P_D - PEEP_{TOT})$$

Because P_D is influenced both by the frictional and elastic properties of the thorax, it serves as a simple yet valuable indicator of bronchodilator response under passive conditions, again provided that flow rate and V_T remain unchanged. During controlled inflation with constant square wave inspiratory flow and stable airway resistance (R_{AW}), the slope of the inspiratory pressure ramp should reflect C_{RS} (Fig. 5-10). However, estimates of C_{RS} made by this technique (and those by the method described previously) are inappropriately low, unless AP is taken into account. When there is occult PEEP (AP) at the onset of inspiration, the relevant pressure for chest expansion is $(P_S - PEEP_{TOT})$, not $(P_S - PEEP)$.

Stress Index

Noticeable curvature of the inspiratory pressure tracing during passive inflation with constant flow suggests that disproportionate recruitment (concave to the time axis) or disproportionate overdistention (convex to the time axis) is taking place during the tidal cycle. From the standpoint of lung protection, both are undesirable. During constant flow, the relationship between pressure and time can be expressed: $P_{AW} = t^s + (R_{in} flow + PEEP_{TOT})$, where P_{AW} is airway pressure, t is inspiratory time since inflation onset, R_{in} is inspiratory resistance, and s is the shaping coefficient or "stress index." When $s = 1.0$, the contour is linear, and when it is significantly less than or greater than 1, the stress index suggests undesirable tidal recruitment or overdistention, respectively (Fig. 5-12). Modern ventilators can automatically fit a smoothed curve to the inspiratory P_{AW} profile, calculate the stress index, and display "s" as a monitored parameter. Although a quite attractive option, the clinical utility of doing so has not yet been established.

Expiratory Resistance

For the same average flow rate, expiratory resistance routinely exceeds inspiratory resistance, even in the normal airway. This discrepancy can be much larger in the clinical setting, especially when the patient is connected to a mechanical ventilator. This expiratory resistance arises in the endotracheal tube and exhalation valve as well as in the increased expiratory resistance of the native airway. The resistance across the exhalation valve and external tubing can be monitored easily by recording airway pressure and flow in the external airway. Total expiratory resistance, the quotient of expiratory flow and the difference between alveolar and airway opening pressures (or critical closing pressure if expiration is flow limited), is difficult to measure directly. However, it often can be estimated from the knowledge of expiratory flow just before an occlusion of the airway opening and the "stop-flow" pressure (which estimates alveolar pressure). Alternatively, if the time constant of tidal exhalation can be measured under passive conditions, expiratory resistance is the quotient of the time constant and respiratory system compliance.

Expiratory resistance has important consequences, giving rise to AP, neuromuscular reflexes, dyspnea, and differences between mean airway and mean alveolar pressures. Average expiratory flow and expiratory resistance increase as $\dot{V}_E$ rises and the $I:E$ ratio extends, reducing the time available for expiration and boosting average expiratory flow. Except when very mild, the patient must contend with the effects of expiratory resistance by allowing dynamic hyperinflation or by increasing expiratory muscle pressure. For these reasons, certain ventilator manufacturers are now developing techniques to offset the expiratory resistance of the endotracheal tube and circuitry.

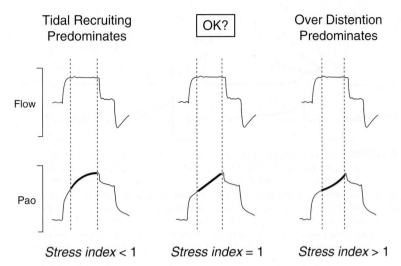

■ FIGURE 5-12 Concept of the "stress index." The slope of the airway pressure during passive inflation with constant flow ("square wave," ACV) may suggest extensive intratidal recruitment (if the curve shaping exponent b [fit to the curve $P_{RS} = at^b + c$] is <1.0, **left**) or extensive overdistention (if >1.0, **right**). When plateau pressure is high, the former suggests that additional PEEP should be considered, while the latter suggests a reducing tidal volume, PEEP, or both are prudent. Even a perfect $b = 1.0$ may hide *regional* problems of either type.

Endotracheal Tube Resistance

The endotracheal tube often contributes greatly to R_{AW}. Depending on the nature, length, diameter, patency, and angulation of the endotracheal tube, the resistive properties of the external airway may dominate computed values for R_{AW}. Marked flow dependence of resistance also may be demonstrated in certain patients, a phenomenon usually attributed to turbulence developing in a narrow or partially occluded tube. If endogenous bronchial resistance is the variable of interest, P_{AW} should be sensed at or beyond the carinal tip of the endotracheal tube. This can be accomplished with an intraluminal catheter or by using a tube specially designed for measuring pressures at this site (e.g., tubes designed for jet ventilation or tracheal gas insufflation). Values for C_{RS} (computed under static conditions) remain valid, whatever the resistances of the endotracheal tube or airway may be.

Auto-PEEP (Intrinsic PEEP) Effects

Definitions of Auto-PEEP, Intrinsic PEEP, and Total PEEP

Considerable confusion has arisen regarding the terms "auto-PEEP" and "intrinsic PEEP." PEEP is the pressure applied to the airway by the clinician. This is also termed "extrinsic PEEP" by some authors. The pressure measured when all airflow is stopped is equivalent to average alveolar pressure and is termed "total PEEP." AP is the difference between $PEEP_{TOT}$ and PEEP (i.e., that component of $PEEP_{TOT}$ attributable to dynamic hyperinflation. The prefix "auto" derives from the Greek term meaning "self."). Different authors use the term *intrinsic PEEP* as a synonym for $PEEP_{TOT}$, and others use it as a synonym for AP. The latter usage allows specific designation of clinician-set (extrinsic) PEEP and dynamic hyperinflation-generated (intrinsic) PEEP without ambiguity. For clarity, we have used the terms PEEP (rather than extrinsic PEEP), AP (rather than intrinsic PEEP), and $PEEP_{TOT}$ throughout this book.

Variants of Auto-PEEP

The need for high levels of ventilation may cause hyperinflation when insufficient time elapses between inflation cycles to reestablish the equilibrium (resting) position of the respiratory system, especially in the presence of increased airway resistance and a lengthy exhalation time constant (Fig. 5-13). Consequently, when a mechanical ventilator powers inflation, alveolar pressure (P_{alv}) remains continuously positive through both phases of the respiratory cycle, and airflow does not cease at end-exhalation.

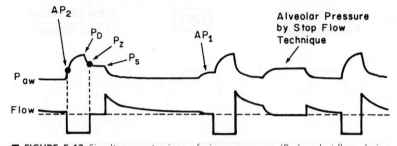

■ **FIGURE 5-13** Simultaneous tracings of airway pressure (P_{AW}) and airflow during controlled volume-cycled ventilation with constant inspiratory flow in a patient with airflow obstruction. P_D, P_Z, and P_S represent end-inspiratory airway pressures during dynamic conditions, at the point of flow cessation, and after complete equilibration among all alveolar and airway pressures, respectively. Alveolar pressure can be estimated by the stop-flow technique in midexpiration or at end-exhalation (AP_1). AP also can be estimated under dynamic conditions as the airway pressure above the set PEEP value that is needed to counterbalance elastic recoil and stop expiratory airflow (AP_2).

5   AP does not necessarily indicate dynamic hyperinflation, unless expiration occurs passively (Fig. 5-14). Even under passive conditions, the extent of dynamic hyperinflation that results from AP is a function of respiratory system compliance. During spontaneous breathing efforts, expiratory muscle activity can raise end-expiratory alveolar pressure, sometimes preventing any hyperinflation at all. AP is also not synonymous with airflow obstruction but, rather, can occur anytime that $\dot{V}_E$ is high enough and/or the combination of frequency and $I{:}E$ ratio leaves insufficient expiratory time—even for normal subjects. Moreover, AP varies markedly from one site to another within the obstructed lung, tending to be greatest in the dependent lung regions. AP can change with variations of body position.

Although deliberate distention of the lungs by dynamic hyperinflation can be used therapeutically for patients with refractory hypoxemia, AP usually occurs inadvertently, often with adverse consequences for hemodynamics, respiratory muscle function, and lung mechanics. Barotrauma is an obvious risk of serious hyperinflation. Unlike restrictive lung disease, obstructive lung disease allows excellent transmission of alveolar pressure to the pleural space. Thus, the hemodynamic consequences of the AP effect may be more severe than those incurred by intentionally applied PEEP of a similar level. Immediately after intubation, CO tends to drop as the AP impedes venous return during passive inflation. With some exceptions, hypotension occurs routinely after intubating a patient with serious airflow obstruction. This

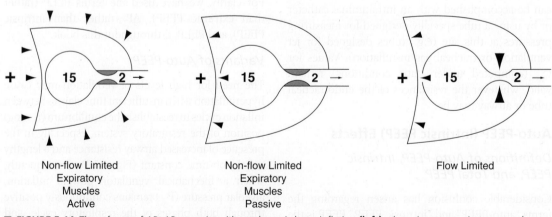

■ **FIGURE 5-14** Three forms of AP. AP can exist without dynamic hyperinflation **(left)** when vigorous expiratory muscle contraction persists to the end of expiration. Under the conditions of passive inflation, however, AP *does* imply dynamic hyperinflation—either without **(middle)** or with **(right)** expiratory flow limitation. The response to exogenous PEEP is influenced greatly by the form of AP encountered.

adverse effect of AP is particularly important to keep in mind during cardiopulmonary resuscitation, when gas trapping secondary to vigorous ventilation further comprosises marginally adequate blood flow

AP also adds to the work of breathing, presenting an increased threshold load to inspiration, impairing the strength of the inspiratory muscles, and depressing the effective triggering sensitivity of the ventilator. For cases in which expiration is flow limited during tidal breathing, the addition of low levels of exogenous PEEP (less than the original AP level) effectively replaces AP and therefore improves subject comfort and the work of breathing, without increasing lung volume or peak cycling pressure. Substitution of PEEP for AP also may improve the distribution of ventilation marginally. At the bedside, $PEEP_{TOT}$ can be quantified by occluding the expiratory port of the ventilator at the end of the period allowed for exhalation between mechanical breaths. As already noted, the AP component is the difference between this measured occlusion pressure and the PEEP value set by the clinician.

Variability of Auto-PEEP

Regional Gas Trapping

AP varies widely throughout a lung composed of individual units with varying time constants. Because pleural pressure follows a gravitational gradient, transpulmonary pressure and alveolar dimensions are least and the tendency for airway closure is greatest in the most dependent regions. Therefore, even if the time constants were otherwise perfectly uniform throughout the lung, there would be a tendency for those units in dependent areas to trap more gas than those located above them. This happens with greater frequency when PEEP is not applied. The gas trapped behind completely closed airways exerts a pressure that cannot be measured at the airway opening. In other words, it is common to have extensive gas trapping without AP that reflects its magnitude.

Vulnerability to Changes in Minute Ventilation

Minute ventilation is a powerful determinant of AP; in fact, in a uniform lung characterized by a single time constant, variations in frequency or tidal volume that do not change the minute ventilation have little effect on the observed AP. On the contrary, relatively small changes in $\dot{V}_E$ can dramatically change the extent of gas trapping in such a single

compartment system. In practice, the diseased lung of an asthmatic patient deflates in a pattern that is better typified as biexponential or multiexponential. For these patients, end-expiratory flows from the slowest compartments are so small that increasing the cycling frequency (and increasing the minute ventilation) may have a negligible effect on gas trapping.

Alterations in Resistance and Compliance

For the same minute ventilation, variations in retained secretions, bronchospasm, apparatus resistance, tissue edema, body position, and muscle tone alter the deflation time constant and the extent of gas trapping encountered at an unchanging $\dot{V}_E$. Partially for this reason, simple maneuvers such as suctioning the airway or changing the patient from the reclining to the upright position can make a dramatic difference in the level of comfort.

Methods for Determining Auto-PEEP

The presence of AP should be suspected whenever **6** detectable flow persists to the very end of tidal expiration (Table 5-1). Such flow often is audible using a stethoscope positioned over the trachea or expiratory valve, and AP (if not dynamic hyperinflation) is certain if wheezing persists to the very end of the expiratory cycle. This flow can be transduced and displayed graphically on the bedside monitor. However, the magnitude of end-expiratory flow does not correlate with the magnitude of AP, whether comparing patients to one another or when observing the same patient over time. End-expiratory flow of a given amount, for example, may result from widespread severe obstruction or from more moderate obstruction confined to a smaller subpopulation of alveoli. Moreover, very high levels of regional hyperinflation and AP can lurk behind airways that have been sealed completely by mucous plugs (with collateral ventilation). Others may open during inspiration but seal before end-expiration is reached, preventing all further discharge of their trapped gas.

TABLE 5-1 CLINICAL METHODS FOR DETERMINING AUTO-PEEP

End-expiratory port occlusion
Pressure needed to initiate inspiratory flow
End-inspiratory plateau pressure difference during volume-cycled ventilation
PEEP substitution
Trapped gas release

Because AP varies on a breath-by-breath basis during spontaneous breathing, it cannot be quantified precisely unless exhalation is passive and the depth and duration of all breaths are equivalent—conditions that only rarely occur when making spontaneous breathing efforts. Once passive conditions are established, an estimate of AP can be determined (or its effects monitored) by a variety of methods. All these methods are approximations, and all are somewhat lower than the highest values existing within the lung. Two methods are based on the principle of counterbalancing AP, either by end-expiratory airway occlusion or by a measured dynamic airway pressure (protoinspiratory counterbalancing, or zero flow method). Alternatively, the AP effect can be characterized by directly measuring the change in end-inspiratory plateau (peak alveolar) pressure with a constant tidal volume and inspiratory time. Finally, the excess (trapped) gas volume that exits during an extended deflation interval reflects the corresponding end-expiratory pressure during tidal breaths. Two of the most important effects of AP—on hemodynamics and work of breathing—are mediated by pleural pressure, which can be assessed directly by measuring esophageal pressure.

End-Expiratory Port Occlusion

For accuracy, occlusion must occur just before the subsequent ventilator-delivered breath and continue for 1.5 to 2.0s (Fig. 2-8). Such timing of occlusion is easiest to achieve during controlled ventilation at modest breathing rates (<20/min) and can be approximated manually or, when the patient is totally passive, automated by modern ventilators that apply a transient expiratory pause. Finally, on older equipment, a three-way inspiratory valve ("Braschi" valve) inserted into the inspiratory limb of the circuit can be turned at any time during expiration to block expiratory backflow through the inspiratory path. When the next tidal breath is delivered, the open limb of the valve diverts the ventilator's inflation volume to atmosphere for one breath as automatic tidal closure of the expiratory valve completes the airway occlusion at exactly the appropriate time.

Pressure Needed to Start Inflation

During passive inflation, inspiratory flow does not begin until the expiratory pressure within the units with the least AP is counterbalanced by an offsetting proximal airway pressure. If flow and airway pressure signals are perfectly synchronous, AP is the airway pressure at the time of zero flow. This estimate for AP is usually less than that given by port occlusion.

End-Inspiratory Plateau Pressure During Volume-Cycled Ventilation

As already noted, alveolar pressures behind occluded airways can be elevated, even if AP measured at the airway opening is low. End-inspiratory plateau pressure is the sum of PEEP, AP, and the quotient of V_T/C_{RS}. Therefore, when tidal volume and PEEP are accounted for and unchanging, plateau pressure reflects the degree of dynamic hyperinflation of all lung units more faithfully than does direct measurement of AP itself, which gives an average of the AP values from only those units that remain in communication with the airway opening. For similar reasons, *changes* in plateau pressure that occur after a prolonged expiration or a variation in a machine setting more reliably index changes in hyperinflation than does direct AP estimation. Assuming passive inflation with a constant tidal volume and applied PEEP, the easiest clinical method at rapid breathing frequencies is to first measure the plateau pressure at the clinically relevant frequency and to then resume the clinical pattern (without the measurement pause) for five or more breaths. Next, the frequency is slowed to less than 5 breaths/min, waiting 15s before reapplying the end-inspiratory pause. The difference in pause pressures estimates the original AP.

PEEP Substitution

When PEEP is added downstream from the site of critical flow limitation, end-expiratory alveolar pressure rises only very modestly until the original level of AP is surpassed, at which point the alveolar and airway pressures rise together. As PEEP is substituted for AP, end-expiratory flow slows or stops completely, and audible flow or wheezing ceases before end-expiration. In flow-controlled, volume-cycled ventilation, plateau pressure changes little until the original level of AP is approximated. In pressure-controlled ventilation, tidal volume may crest at its maximum as PEEP approaches the critical level and AP disappears. Although imprecise and unreliable in (rather unusual) patients with severe airflow obstruction who lack tidal flow limitation, this pragmatic technique lends itself well for both passive and actively breathing patients.

Release of Trapped Gas

A measurement of the *extra* gas released (in excess of the routine tidal volume) in the first exhalation after a sudden and dramatic slowing of ventilatory frequency (to two breaths or less/min) estimates the amount of the total trapped gas (V_{TR}) that can be expelled. If compliance of the respiratory system (C_{RS}) is known, AP can be computed as V_{TR}/C_{RS}.

Flow Limitation

Flow limitation during tidal breathing is a marker of airflow severity and of the collapsibility of the airways. Flow limitation during forceful breathing is what lends reproducibility to the FEV_1 meaurement in the pulmonary function testing laboratory. If a ventilated patient is flow limited during tidal breathing, (s)he cannot respond to a need for more ventilation without suffering further hyperinflation. Flow-limited patients usually show an abrupt L-shaped transition to sharply reduced expiratory flows which then slowly approach the zero-flow baseline in a linear rather than exponential trajectory. Display of flow–volume loops is now an option available on many modern ventilators. One simple way to evaluate flow limitation is to increase pleural pressure selectively during expiration (e.g., by mimicking the action of the expiratory muscles by manually compressing the abdomen firmly and steadily during expiration), and observing whether volume referenced flows improve. Failure to do so may indicate benefit from incrementing external PEEP.

Esophageal Pressure Monitoring

Estimation of intrapleural pressure by an esophageal catheter holds the potential to facilitate clinical decision making. Esophageal pressure measurement enables the calculation of the pressure across the lung during passive or active breathing and permits estimation of the pressure across the chest wall when spontaneous efforts are silenced. Thus, lung and chest wall stresses and compliances can be more accurately estimated than when using plateau pressure alone. The thin esophageal catheter (approx. 2-mm diameter) is relatively comfortable, simple to insert, and poses little risk of esophageal perforation. Appropriate placement is achieved by first inflating the 10-cm-long balloon with approximately 1 mL of air and passing it into the stomach. The catheter is carefully withdrawn 10 cm beyond the position where negative pressure deflections are initially observed during spontaneous inspiratory efforts. The balloon's final position within the lower third of the esophagus is tested by occluding the airway and measuring the simultaneous deflections in P_{AW} and P_{es}. Because no significant change of transpulmonary pressure can occur without a change in lung volume, good balloon position is indicated by nearly identical deflections of esophageal and airway pressures during an occluded spontaneous breath.

As a rule, P_{es} is best measured in an upright position. However, a lateral decubitus position may suffice if the patient must remain recumbent. (The supine position is suboptimal.) Although the absolute value of the average pressure that surrounds the lung cannot be gauged accurately from such a local sampling, fluctuations of average intrathoracic pressure can be estimated acceptably well by an occlusion-tested balloon catheter in any position. Certain commercially available systems are designed to sample esophageal pressure in conjunction with airway pressure and flow, outputting primary and derived mechanics data of clinical interest (e.g., resistance, compliance, and several indices of inspiratory effort during active breathing conditions). Useful graphics of dynamic PV and flow–volume data are also available. Esophageal pressure enables estimation of force generation during all patient-initiated breaths (spontaneous or machine-assisted) and allows partitioning of transthoracic pressure into its lung and chest wall components during passive inflation. The intrapleural pressure provided by the P_{es} tracing also permits calculation of lung compliance and airway resistance during spontaneous breathing. Furthermore, P_{es} aids in interpreting pulmonary artery and wedge pressures under conditions of vigorous hyperpnea or elevated alveolar pressure (PEEP, AP). The P_{es} can be used to compute the work of breathing across the lung and external circuitry or to calculate the product of developed pressure and the duration of inspiratory effort (the pressure–time product). Finally, knowing the transpulmonary lung stress applied by a given plateau pressure may help to prevent ventilator-induced lung injury (Chapters 8 and 24). It has been suggested that fluctuations in central venous pressure can serve similar purposes, but the damped vascular pressure tracing yields a low-range estimate of effort. Such underestimation occurs because venous return tends to rise as intrathoracic pressure falls; conversely, venous return declines when intrathoracic pressure rises.

Transdiaphragmatic pressure (P_{di}), the difference between P_{es} and the balloon catheter-measured gastric pressure, is generated theoretically by a single inspiratory muscle (the diaphragm) and can be used to quantify its effective contractile force. Clinically, the P_{di} is used occasionally in conjunction with phrenic nerve stimulation or voluntary effort to investigate diaphragmatic paralysis.

Abdominal Pressure Measurement

In most patients with acute respiratory failure, increased chest wall stiffness usually occurs because of an increase of intra-abdominal pressure (IAP). In fact, chest wall elastance (the inverse of compliance) relates more or less linearly to IAP, and approximately one fourth of all patients admitted to the ICU have an abnormally high IAP value. Although pressures measured within any flaccid hollow viscus can be used, the bladder pressure has become the de facto standard because of its ease of measurement and established correlation with directly measured values. In healthy subjects, the IAP measured in this way is approximately $0\,cm\,H_2O$ during spontaneous breathing and somewhat higher in mechanically ventilated patients without obvious abdominal pathology (6 to $12\,cm\,H_2O$). Although bladder pressure does not equate to esophageal pressure, it serves two main functions: (a) a high IAP predicts that P_{es} is also high, on occasion prompting direct P_{es} measurement and (b) a very high IAP may result in life-threatening impairment of perfusion to kidney, gut, and other abdominal organs. Values of IAP that rise to exceed $20\,cm\,H_2O$ are a cause for concern regarding the abdominal compartment syndrome (see Chapter 35). It should be noted that while values of abdominal pressure greater than $20\,cm\,H_2O$ are sometimes seen chronically, *without* detectable problems, a rapidly rising IAP in the correct clinical setting and accompanied by a developing anion gap acidosis or otherwise unexplained deterioration of urinary output is a cause for immediate surgical consultation.

Value of Continuously Monitoring P_{AW} and Flow

The Flow Tracing

Most modern ventilators offer the option of displaying both airway pressure and airflow. When used in conjunction with a simultaneously recorded airway pressure, the flow tracing is an invaluable aid in determining a number of parameters of clinical interest. A glance at the flow tracing usually is sufficient to determine the inspiratory mode of the ventilator, and when used in conjunction with airway pressure, it detects patient–ventilator asyn-

chrony. The tracing of flow not only times each breath but also provides crucial data that allow computation of tidal volume, minute ventilation, frequency to tidal volume ratio (rapid shallow breathing index), and breathing pattern variability (see Chapter 10). Flow must be known to compute airway resistance and the work of breathing, as well as to detect (but not quantify) AP without airway occlusion. A smoothly linear, biphasic flow profile, rather than a uniexponential one, may give a clear indication of expiratory flow limitation. A rippling inspiratory flow tracing indicates secretion retention within the central airways. The "zero flow" points of the airway and esophageal pressure tracings define the dynamic mechanical limits of the respiratory cycle, which are required in computations of mouth occlusion pressure ($P_{0.1}$, see following), minimum airway resistance, and AP. The flow tracing also is helpful when adjusting the inspiratory period during time-cycled, pressure-preset forms of ventilation (e.g., pressure-controlled ventilation) to maximize inspiratory tidal volume while avoiding unintended end-inspiratory pauses and/or excessive AP.

The Airway Pressure Tracing

A continuous tracing of P_{AW} provides useful information commonly neglected at the bedside (Fig. 5-15). When the ventilator's display does not automatically provide the tracing, airway pressure can be monitored continuously using transducer and display equipment normally used for measuring pressures in the pulmonary vasculature. A dedicated transducer must be used for this purpose, however, to avoid the risk of air embolism.

Apart from enabling estimation of R_{AW} and C_{RS}, the waveform of inspiratory airway pressure traced during a controlled machine cycle provides graphic evidence of the inflation work performed by the ventilator at the particular combination of tidal volume and flow settings in use. When inflation occurs passively during constant flow, the area under the pressure–time curve is proportionate to the work performed by the machine to inflate the chest, and the pressure measured halfway through inspiration ($\bar{P}$) is the work per liter of ventilation under those conditions. When average flow and tidal volume are matched to spontaneous values, $\bar{P}$ is a good estimate of the pressure needed to ventilate the patient during a conversion to pressure-supported ventilation.

The shape of the airway pressure tracing also should be examined. Using constant inspiratory flow, concavity of the airway pressure ramp under

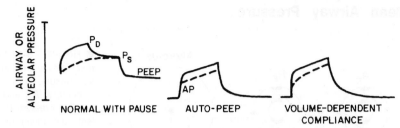

■ FIGURE 5-15 Airway and alveolar pressures during controlled ventilation with constant flow. Airway pressure (*solid line*) and alveolar pressure (*dashed line*) are represented. For the passive subject, the airway pressures measured at end inflation and after a brief inspiratory pause provide the data needed to compute airway resistance: ($[P_D - P_S]$/inspiratory flow rate). Compliance of the respiratory system ($V_T/[P_S -$ Total PEEP]) must take AP into account to avoid underestimation of actual compliance. AP and early volume recruitment are two causes for the normally trapezoidal airway pressure contour to "square off."

passive conditions reflects patient effort during triggered cycles. An upward inflection of the terminal portion of the inspiratory airway pressure tracing (concavity) during passive inflation suggests that the combination of end-expiratory pressure and tidal volume chosen generates pressures that risk overdistention and barotrauma. Conversely, marked convexity of the P_{AW} tracing during constant flow indicates that inflation is becoming easier as the breath proceeds. Such a profile can be seen when volume is alternately recruited and derecruited during the breathing cycle, when AP is present (requiring a range of counterbalancing pressures before units with different AP values are brought "online" for inspiration), or when resistance is highly volume dependent (Fig. 5-15). Cycle-to-cycle variations in the peak dynamic pressure of machine-aided breaths suggest that the durations of inspiratory effort and flow delivery are not well matched or synchronous (Fig. 5-16).

Mean Airway Pressure

Under passive conditions, mean alveolar pressure and its only measurable analog, mean airway pressure (mP_{AW}), relate intimately to the forces that

drive ventilation and hold the lung distended. **7** When the nonelastic pressures dissipated in inspiration and expiration are identical, the airway pressure averaged over the entire ventilatory cycle should be the same everywhere—including the alveolus (Fig. 5-17). This mean pressure is the average pressure that distends the alveolus and passive chest wall and therefore correlates with alveolar size and recruitment as well as with mean intrapleural pressure. Mean alveolar pressure also is the average pressure available to drive expiratory flow, which is indexed by minute ventilation. It follows that mean airway (mean alveolar) pressure, *when measured **without** patient effort*, correlates directly with arterial oxygenation in the setting of pulmonary edema and lung injury, with back pressure to venous return (and consequently with CO and peripheral edema), as well as with minute ventilation.

Mean airway pressure can be raised by increasing $\dot{V}_E$, by raising end-expiratory pressure, or by extending the inspiratory time fraction (see Chapters 9 and 24). To avoid serious and unanticipated problems in the passive patient, mean airway pressure is a crucial variable to monitor when the clinician changes minute ventilation or

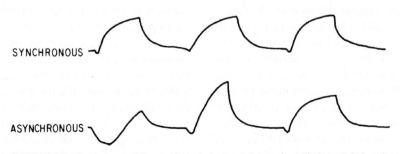

■ FIGURE 5-16 Airway pressure tracings during assist/control ventilation. Variations in contour and peak cycling pressure characterize asynchrony between the respiratory rhythms of the patient and ventilator.

Mean Airway Pressure

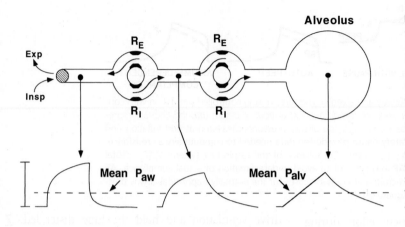

■ **FIGURE 5-17** Relationship of mean airway pressure to mean alveolar pressure. In an airway in which inspiratory (R_{in}) and expiratory (R_{ex}) resistive pressure losses are equivalent, the mean pressure averaged over the entire ventilatory cycle should be equivalent at every point along the path, including airway opening and alveolus. When R_{ex} exceeds R_{in}, mean alveolar pressure exceeds mean airway opening pressure; when R_{in} exceeds R_{ex}, mean airway opening pressure exceeds mean alveolar pressure.

alters the mode of ventilation, breathing pattern, or PEEP setting.

Although the relationship between mP_{AW} and mP_{alv} is a close one, these pressures are not identical. The actual relationship can be expressed mathematically as

$$mP_{alv} = mP_{AW} + V_E (R_{ex} - R_{in})$$

where $R_{ex} - R_{in}$ is the calculated difference between expiratory and inspiratory resistances. For reasons already discussed, this pressure difference generally tends to be positive and may be strikingly so in the setting of severe airflow obstruction with high ventilatory requirements or high frequency or inverse ratio ventilation.

■ MONITORING BREATHING EFFORT

Oxygen Consumption of the Respiratory System

The oxygen consumed by the ventilatory pump ($\dot{V}O_{2R}$) estimates respiratory muscular effort at its most basic level: cellular metabolism. In theory, $\dot{V}O_{2R}$ accounts for all factors that tax the respiratory muscles, in other words, the external workload (W) and the efficiency (e) of the conversion between cellular energy and useful work ($\dot{V}O_{2R} = W/e$). Two patients with different chest configurations, patterns of muscle activation, or degrees of coordination between the muscles of inspiration and expiration may perform identical external work (W) but consume vastly different amounts of O_2 in the process. Because $\dot{V}O_{2R}$ cannot be measured directly, total

body oxygen consumption ($\dot{V}O_2$) is tracked as ventilatory stresses are imposed or relieved, perturbing the respiratory system. Unfortunately, $\dot{V}O_2$ is difficult to measure in unstable patients. Thus, other measures of respiratory muscle effort usually are sought.

Direct Measures of External Mechanical Output

External Work of Breathing

Mechanical work is accomplished when a pressure gradient (P) moves the lung or relaxed chest wall (passive structures) through a volume change. At volumes (V) above relaxed FRC, pressure resulting from a flow ($\dot{V}$) dissipates against frictional and elastic forces in the following way:

$$P = R_{AW} (\dot{V}) + V/C_{RS}$$

Average developed pressure ($\bar{P}$) for the tidal inflation (V_T) can be approximated as follows:

$$\bar{P} = R_{AW} (V_T/t_i) + V_T/2C_{RS} + \text{auto-PEEP}$$

It is numerically equivalent to the work per liter of ventilation. (Work per tidal breath [W_b] can be quantified as the product of $\bar{P}$ and V_T.) Thus, if R_{AW}, C_{RS}, t_i, and V_T are known for the spontaneously breathing subject, the external work rate for inspiration can be computed easily. (Exhalation normally proceeds passively, dissipating elastic energy stored during the inspiratory half cycle.) Such computations also serve to conveniently estimate the pressure support level needed to achieve most ventilatory needs. When the ventilator performs the entire workload for a passive patient, total inflation pressure (P) is simply P_{AW}. (When inflation is achieved with a constant-flow waveform, it is then approximated by the inflation pressure at midcycle.) However, no exertion must occur during inflation and, to be relevant to unsupported natural breathing, V_T and peak flow rate must approximate the spontaneous values. With pressures and volumes expressed in the customary way, a convenient work unit is the joule (or watt–second), approximately $10 \, cm \, H_2O \times 1 \, L$ (equivalent to $1 \, kg\cdot m = 10 \, J$). Total inspiratory mechanical work per minute is the product of P and minute ventilation or of W_b and f, the breathing frequency.

Influence of Auto-PEEP on Work of Breathing

AP imposes a threshold load on inspiration in the sense that the patient must supply a pressure sufficient to counterbalance AP before central airway pressure falls low enough to trigger the ventilator or initiate a pressure-supported breath. The threshold load imposed by AP effectively reduces the triggering sensitivity of the machine to a value equal to the sum of AP and the set trigger sensitivity value. When expiration is flow limited during tidal breathing, low levels of continuous positive airway pressure (CPAP) or PEEP can help restore triggering sensitivity and reduce the work of breathing (see earlier). Moreover, during pressure-supported ventilation, PEEP that counterbalances AP leaves a greater proportion of the inspiratory pressure available to power inflation, often resulting in an increased tidal volume for the same value of pressure support. Although PEEP also tends to improve the distribution of ventilation, additional PEEP should not be used if it causes the peak dynamic cycling pressure to rise significantly.

Work Measurements

Spontaneous Breathing Cycles   An esophageal balloon is required to directly measure work during spontaneous, machine-assisted, or pressure-supported breathing cycles. Fluctuations in P_{es} reflect patient efforts to overcome the impedance of the lung and external circuit. (Clues to the work done against the external apparatus can be gained by examining the P_{AW} tracing.) Inspiratory inflections of the P_{AW} waveform quantify the pressure needed to suck gas through the inspiratory circuitry to the point of pressure measurement. To include the resistance of the endotracheal tube, P_{AW} must be sampled between the tube tip and the carina, a site at which much deeper pressure fluctuations may be seen during inspiration (Fig. 5-18). The resistance of standard endotracheal tubes often exceeds $10 \, cm \, H_2O/L/s$ and is commonly offset during inspiration by pressure support.

Machine-Assisted Breathing Cycles

Volume-Limited Machine Cycles   It is often assumed that patient work becomes negligible during patient-initiated but machine-assisted breathing cycles. Indeed, the ventilator is fully capable of performing the entire work of breathing if the patient were to cease effort immediately after triggering inspiration. However, relaxation does not occur abruptly once the machine cycle begins; instead, patient effort continues in direct proportion to the intensity of respiratory drive. When the ventilation requirement or sense of dyspnea is high (e.g., when the ventilator is poorly adjusted with respect to sensitivity, peak inspiratory flow rate, inspiratory duration, or tidal volume), exertion levels may approach those of unsupported breathing. Interestingly, resistance and compliance do not influence the work of breathing during triggered cycles, provided the

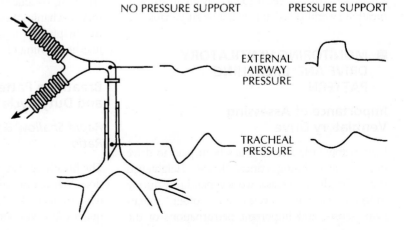

NO PRESSURE SUPPORT   PRESSURE SUPPORT

EXTERNAL AIRWAY PRESSURE

TRACHEAL PRESSURE

■ **FIGURE 5-18** Pressure tracings at the proximal and distal ends of the endotracheal tube during spontaneous breathing. External recordings do not reflect exertion against the endotracheal tube **(left)**. The application of pressure support may overcome endotracheal tube resistance during the inspiratory phase but does nothing to offset the expiratory resistance imposed by the endotracheal tube.

machine fully satisfies the patient's peak inspiratory flow demand (approx. $4 \times V_E$). However, if the patient's flow demand exceeds the delivery rate, the patient works against the resistance of the endotracheal tube and ventilator circuitry as well as against the innate impedance characteristics of the chest. Clues to patient exertion during triggered machine cycles are provided by the airway pressure tracing, as already described. When a P_{AW} tracing is not available, the primary indication of excessive patient effort during a triggered cycle may be the stuttering rise of the manometer needle to its peak value. Peak dynamic pressure itself may not be much different from expected, inasmuch as inspiratory effort slackens near the end of inflation.

Pressure-supported cycles During pressure-supported cycles, inspiratory airway pressure is maintained nearly constant by the machine at the preset level. Therefore, patient effort can be gauged directly only from a P_{es} tracing.

Pressure–Time Product

8 Isometric components of muscle tension that consume oxygen without contributing to volume change fail to register as externally measured work, accounting in large part for the lack of agreement between force generation and W_b. A pressure–time product (PTP = $\bar{P} \times t_i$) parallels effort and $\dot{V}O_{2R}$ more closely than W_b because it includes the isometric component of muscle pressure and is less influenced by the afterload to contraction. When average inspiratory pressure ($\bar{P}$, as computed earlier) is referenced to the maximal isometric pressure that can be generated at FRC (P_{max}) and inspiratory time (t_i) is expressed as a fraction of total cycle length (t_{tot}), a useful effort index is derived:

$$\text{Pressure–time index (PTI)} = \bar{P}/P_{max} \times t_i/t_{tot}$$

Values of PTI that exceed 0.15 identify highly stressful breathing workloads that may not be sustainable.

■ MONITORING VENTILATORY DRIVE AND BREATHING PATTERN

Importance of Assessing Ventilatory Drive

Remarkably little attention has been paid to drive measurement during critical illness. Heightened ventilatory drive increases work expenditure during triggered machine cycles and often signals pain, sepsis, and important perturbations of the

cardiopulmonary system. During machine-assisted breathing cycles, ventilatory drive plays a more important role in determining the energy expenditure of the patient than any indicator of ventilatory mechanics—if the flow delivered by the machine exceeds the patient's flow demand. Derangements in ventilatory drive also furnish clues regarding the ability of the patient to wean from ventilator support. Recent clinical studies demonstrate that patients who fail to wean from mechanical ventilation often have elevated drives to breathe and limited abilities of drive to respond to the increases in ventilatory loads (e.g., increased $PaCO_2$).

Ventilatory Drive Indices

Several methods can be used to index drive. When respiratory mechanics and strength reserves are normal, minute ventilation directly parallels the output of the ventilatory control center. Unfortunately, such preconditions are seldom met in the clinical setting. Minute ventilation can be viewed as the product of mean inspiratory flow rate (the quotient of tidal volume and inspiratory time, V_T/t_i) and the inspiratory time fraction or duty cycle (t_i/t_{tot}):

$$V_e = V_T/t_i \times t_i/t_{tot}$$

Both components yield useful and largely ignored clinical information. Mean inspiratory flow (V_T/t_i) provides another potential index of drive but also depends on the mechanical properties of the ventilatory system. The airway pressure generated against an airway surreptitiously occluded 100 ms after the onset of inspiratory effort (the $P_{0.1}$) is measured before the occlusion is recognized consciously, so the corresponding outflow from the respiratory center is representative of the unimpeded cycles that preceded it. As an isometric measurement, the $P_{0.1}$ is influenced by muscle strength and lung volume but does not depend on respiratory mechanics. Several modern ventilators display this helpful $P_{0.1}$ index, which is obtained by delaying the opening of their expiratory valve.

Breathing Pattern, Frequency, and Duty Cycle

Rapid Shallow Breathing and the f/V_T Ratio

The breathing pattern also offers valuable information. When muscular strength is limited, patients tend to meet $\dot{V}_E$ requirements by increasing frequency (f) without raising V_T. Although smaller breaths require less effort, the cost of rapid, shallow breathing may be increased dead space ventilation and the need for a higher $\dot{V}_E$ to eliminate CO_2. Thus, although work per breath (W_b) is controlled by limiting tidal volume, total work (the product of f and W_b) per minute tends to increase when f exceeds some optimal value. A very high and continuously rising frequency (to rates >30 breaths/min) is generally accepted as a sign of ventilatory muscle decompensation and impending fatigue. It should be noted, however, that some patients increase f to a stable value greater than 35 breaths/min and remain compensated, especially when $\dot{V}_E$ rises proportionally to the rise in breathing frequency.

9   In recent years, considerable attention has focused on the f/V_T ratio, a simply computed bedside index that seems to indicate the ability or inability of mechanically ventilated patients to breathe without mechanical assistance. Discontinuation of ventilator support is likely to prove successful if (f/V_T) does *not* exceed approximately 100 breaths/min/liters within the first minute of a brief trial of fully spontaneous breathing. The f/V_T will tend to rise in anyone as minute ventilation increases, particularly if respiratory system compliance is reduced (see Chapter 10, Weaning). Although hardly infallible, this simple index does have clinical utility.

As the ventilatory muscles fatigue, the duty cycle (t_i/t_{tot}), the fraction of each breathing cycle spent in inspiration, also changes. When there is a breathing stress, the t_i/t_{tot} of spontaneous breathing normally increases approximately from 0.35 to a value of 0.40 to 0.50. ("Inspiratory time" may be fixed by chosen values of inspiratory flow rate and tidal volume during constant flow mechanical ventilation.) At the limits of compensation, the t_i/t_{tot} fails to increase with further stress and may actually decline.

At times of maximal effort, noteworthy alterations may be observed in the pattern of activation and coordination of the ventilatory muscle groups. Although normally passive, expiratory muscles may be called into play whenever the inspiratory muscles face a burden that is stressful in relation to their capability (e.g., during expiratory airflow obstruction, when high levels of PEEP or CPAP are used, when the patient is anxious, when machine-controlled inspiratory duration is excessive, and at high levels of $\dot{V}_E$). Visible use of the accessory muscles, especially the sternocleidomastoid group, may also signal the approach to the limits of ventilatory compensation.

Asynchrony of the Respiratory Muscles

Two indices once believed to always indicate diaphragmatic dysfunction or fatigue—asynchrony between the peak excursions of chest and abdominal compartments and paradoxical inward movement of the abdomen on inspiration—often reflect the normal response of a compensated system to stress. Asynchrony between the excursions of rib cage and abdomen may be a stage in the development of full-blown abdominal paradox. *Respiratory alternans*, another reported pattern of fatigue in which muscles of the chest cage and diaphragm alternate primary responsibility for achieving ventilation, is observed much less commonly than abdominal paradox.

Inductance or Impedance Plethysmography

Inductance (impedance) plethysmography provides a noninvasive means of monitoring f, V_T, t_i/t_{tot}, and respiratory muscle coordination. With this technique, loose elastic bands encircle the chest and abdomen. Changes in compartmental volume create proportional changes in the cross-sectional areas of electrical inductance loops. Fluctuations of compartmental motion can be summed to estimate the overall tidal volume changes. The ratio of maximal compartmental amplitude to tidal volume (the MCA/V_T ratio) correlates with ventilatory distress and provides tangible evidence of mechanical inefficiency. Impedance plethysmography can also be used as an apnea detector in nonintubated patients and may prove helpful in monitoring volume changes during pressure-cycled modes of ventilation (e.g., pressure support, pressure control, and intermittent positive pressure breathing [IPPB]).

■ MONITORING STRENGTH AND MUSCLE RESERVE (ENDURANCE)

The ability of a patient to sustain independent breathing must not be judged on the basis of any absolute value for workload but rather on workload interpreted against the background of muscular strength and endurance.

Strength Measures

The two measures of respiratory muscle strength most commonly used in the clinical setting are the VC and the MIP generated against an occluded airway. Maximal activation of the respiratory musculature requires intense voluntary effort. Therefore, without full patient cooperation, it is questionable that any measure of strength can reflect the full capability for pressure development.

Vital Capacity

In cooperative patients, VC tends to be well preserved relative to MIP for two primary reasons. First, the PV relationship of the thorax is convex to the volume axis, so the small applied pressures achieve relatively large volume changes. Second, whereas many seriously ill patients can generate brief spikes of inspiratory pressure, few can sustain inspiratory effort long enough to achieve the plateau of their volume curve. VC should be generally measured upright rather than supine because certain conditions—diaphragmatic paralysis, for example, may demonstrate a positional reduction of more than 30% (see Chapter 25). Routine measurements of VC involve a single forceful effort from residual volume to TLC (or the converse). However, many weak patients fail to sustain inspiratory effort long enough to achieve their potential maximum. Others simply refuse or cannot fully cooperate with the testing. Thus, for critically ill patients, the VC has proven to be a disappointing and unreliable measure of strength. Cough stimulation may elicit an effort that approximates inspiratory capacity—a useful indicator of breathing reserve. A one-way valve can be used to achieve a "stacked vital capacity," even when patients do not cooperate fully with testing (Fig. 5-19).

Maximal Inspiratory Pressure

The MIP (sometimes erroneously referred to as "maximum inspiratory *force*") is an isometric pressure optimally measured in a totally occluded airway after 20 s or 10 breathing efforts (Fig. 5-19). A one-way valve directed toward expiration can ensure that inspiratory efforts begin from a lung volume low enough to achieve maximal mechanical advantage. The P_{AW} during the MIP maneuver should be measured continuously, either with a needle gauge or (preferably) by a pressure transducer linked to recording apparatus. Ideally, the MIP is sustained for at least 1 s; a transient isometric pressure may bear little relation to true ventilatory muscle strength and endurance. The MIP is perhaps the only involuntary measure of muscle strength that is even moderately reliable. However, it should be kept in mind that the validity of MIP in uncooperative patients depends on the strength of ventilatory drive and that the intensity of a voluntary effort in a fully cooperative patient is likely to exceed that elicited by simple airway occlusion. If sufficient ventilatory drive can be elicited (e.g., by the addition of dead space tubing to the airway), the drive-stimulated involuntary MIP may approximate the voluntary MIP rather closely.

Measures of Endurance

Mechanical Reserve

Two simple indices of ventilatory power reserve— the ratio of $\dot{V}_E$ requirement to maximal voluntary ventilation (MVV) and the V_T/V_C ratio—have long been used to predict the outcome of machine withdrawal. On empirical grounds, it has been suggested that ratios greater than 50% portend weaning failure. Interestingly, laboratory data confirm that only approximately 50% to 60% of the MVV can be sustained longer than 15 min without ventilatory fatigue. During mechanical ventilation, variability of the breathing pattern and involuntary estimates of inspiratory capacity are helpful in gauging the

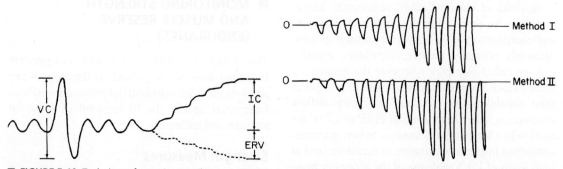

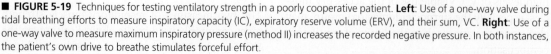

■ **FIGURE 5-19** Techniques for testing ventilatory strength in a poorly cooperative patient. **Left**: Use of a one-way valve during tidal breathing efforts to measure inspiratory capacity (IC), expiratory reserve volume (ERV), and their sum, VC. **Right**: Use of a one-way valve to measure maximum inspiratory pressure (method II) increases the recorded negative pressure. In both instances, the patient's own drive to breathe stimulates forceful effort.

judging reserve and predicting endurance. In the presence of supportive clinical signs and a stable or falling minute ventilation, a rapid shallow breathing index (f/V_T) exceeding 110 suggests an unsustainable breathing workload. This useful indicator has its limitations, however. For example, because relatively rapid shallow breathing patterns may be normal and appropriate for patients with restrictive conditions of lung or chest wall, they may generate f/V_T ratios that are considerably exceed 100, without experiencing respiratory distress or failure.

Electromyography

In the physiology laboratory, an increasing ratio of the integrated diaphragmatic electromyographic (EMG) signal to generated pressure suggests a declining ability of the muscle pump to respond to neural stimulation (i.e., fatigue). Another EMG index of interest characterizes the spectrum of frequencies represented within the diaphragmatic EMG signal. The high frequency to low frequency ratio (H/L) is a good indicator of ventilatory stress and may be a sensitive and specific indicator of developing fatigue. Unfortunately, the diaphragmatic EMG (measured by surface or esophageal electrodes) is not commonly available, and advanced signal conditioning is required to compute the H/L ratio.

Pressure–Time Index

Measured accurately, the MIP can be used in conjunction with $\bar{P}$ to judge endurance and the likelihood of weaning success. In the laboratory setting, a diaphragmatic $\bar{P}/P_{max}$ ratio greater than 40% (with $t_i/t_{tot} = 0.40$) or a PTI (PTI $= \bar{P}/P_{max} \times t_i/t_{tot}$) greater than

0.15 predicts the inability to indefinitely sustain a target workload. No confirmatory data are available yet for the specific clinical setting of the weaning trial.

Sequential Measurements of Drive

A practical indication of declining power reserve may also be provided by a comparison of drive indices (such as the $P_{0.1}$) measured sequentially during the stress period. Patients who fail to increase ventilatory drive in response to increasing $PaCO_2$ are prone to alveolar hypoventilation and weaning failure. In the future, monitoring the response of such indices as $P_{0.1}$ to an imposed stress or to CO_2 loading may provide valuable clinical indications of breathing reserve.

■ SUGGESTED READINGS

Bekos V, Marini JJ. Monitoring the mechanically ventilated patient. *Crit Care Clin.* 2007;23(3):575–611.

Brochard L. Intrinsic (or auto-) positive end-expiratory pressure during spontaneous or assisted ventilation. *Intensive Care Med.* 2002;28(11):1552–1554.

Dooley J, Fegley A. Laboratory monitoring of mechanical ventilation. *Crit Care Clin.* 2007;23:135–148.

Grasso S, Stripoli T, De Michele M, et al. ARDSnet ventilatory protocol and alveolar hyperinflation: Role of positive end-expiratory pressure. *Am J Respir Crit Care Med.* 2007;176(8):761–767.

Lichtenstein DA. Ultrasound in the management of thoracic disease. *Crit Care Med.* 2007;35(Suppl. 5):S250–S261.

Lucangelo U, Bernabe F, Blanch L. Lung mechanics at the bedside: Make it simple. *Curr Opin Crit Care.* 2007;13:64–72.

Marini JJ, Ravenscraft SA. Mean airway pressure: Physiologic determinants and clinical importance—Part 2: Clinical implications. *Crit Care Med.* 1992;20(11):1604–1616.

Owens RL, Stigler WS, Hess DR. Do newer monitors of exhaled gases, mechanics, and esophageal pressure add value? *Clin Chest Med.* 2008;29:297–312.

Putensen C, Wrigge H, Zinserling J. Electrical impedance tomography guided ventilation therapy. *Curr Opin Crit Care.* 2007;13:344–350.

Talmor D, Sarge T, Malhotra A, et al. Mechanical ventilation guided by esophageal pressure in acute lung injury. *N Engl J Med.* 2008;359:2095–2104.

Williams AJ. ABC of oxygen: Assessing and interpreting arterial blood gases and acid–base balance. *Br Med J.* 1998;317(7167):1213–1216.

Airway Intubation

KEY POINTS

1 Noninvasive ventilation may not be appropriate for patients who cannot protect the airway, for those who are obtunded or uncooperative, for those in whom unexpected loss of pressure or enriched oxygen might be immediately hazardous, for those who require high levels of applied pressure, or for those who are hemodynamically unstable. In such cases, endotracheal intubation is the indicated intervention.

2 Orotracheal tube placement is the method of choice during emergencies and most critical care applications. Another option in more elective situations is the nasotracheal route, which requires tubes of generally smaller diameter than tubes used for orotracheal intubation. Although nasotracheal intubation is more comfortable and stable in the conscious or active patient, it is associated with sinusitis, presents higher airway resistance, impedes secretion extraction, and is not recommended for long-term use.

3 Important complications of intubation include a variety of insertion trauma, gastric aspiration, hypoxemia, laryngospasm, esophageal intubation, right main bronchus intubation, cardiac arrhythmias, and hemodynamic impairment.

4 Predictors of difficult intubation include nonvisibility of key oropharyngeal landmarks, poor atlanto-occipital joint mobility, short mentohyoid distance, mentothyroid distance less than 6 cm, mentosternal distance less than 12 cm, and restricted temporomandibular joint excursion. In such cases, the need for special expertise and specialized tools for airway management should be considered before the attempt.

5 Instruments and techniques facilitating the intubation process include fibrobronchoscopy, lighted stylet guidance, specialized laryngoscopes, directed-tip endotracheal tubes, and retrograde wire insertion. Traditional methods to confirm tracheal positioning of the endotracheal tube include stethoscopically audible symmetry of breath sounds, ease of manual insufflation, complete recovery of insufflated tidal volume, loss of voice, expansion of the upper chest, squeeze bulb or syringe recovery of small injected gas volumes, and coughing with expulsion of airway secretions. Currently, CO_2-sensing indicators play an important role for this purpose.

6 Inadvertent extubation is often a life-threatening event that occurs more commonly in orally intubated, lightly sedated patients (who must be carefully restrained). The ability of positive end-expiratory pressure to blow gas freely around a deflated cuff gives some assurance of patency of the larynx above the cuff immediately before a planned extubation.

7 Although its long-term complications can be serious, tracheostomy improves comfort, communication, secretion management, and allows intermittent disconnection of the ventilator. Certain newer variants of conventional tracheostomy (e.g., needle cricothyroidotomy, percutaneous dilatational tracheostomy, and minitracheostomy) do not require an operating room and often prove more convenient or safer to perform in well-selected acutely ill patients.

■ INDICATIONS

Primary indications for endotracheal (ET) intubation include (a) the need for assisted ventilation or the delivery of high levels of inspired oxygen, (b) airway protection against aspiration, (c) clearance of secretions retained in central airways, and (d) relief of upper airway obstruction (Table 6-1).

TABLE 6-1   INDICATIONS FOR ORAL INTUBATION, NASAL INTUBATION, AND TRACHEOSTOMY

ORAL	NASAL	TRACHEOSTOMY
Emergent intubation (cardiopulmonary resuscitation, unconsciousness, or apnea)	Anticipated long-term translaryngeal tube	Inability to insert translaryngeal tube
Nasal or midfacial trauma	Cervical spine ankylosis, arthritis, or trauma	Need for long-term definitive airway
Basilar skull fracture	Oral or mandibular trauma, surgery, or deformity	Obstruction above cricoid cartilage
Epiglottitis	Temporomandibular joint disease	Complications of translaryngeal intubation
Nasal obstruction	Awake intubation	Glottic incompetence
Paranasal disease	Gagging and vomiting	Inability to clear tracheobronchial secretions
Bleeding diathesis	Short (bull) neck	Sleep apnea unresponsive to CPAP
Need for bronchoscopy	Agitation	Facial or laryngeal trauma or structural contraindications to translaryngeal intubation

Need for Assisted Ventilation and Positive End-Expiratory Pressure

1 Intubation of the trachea with a cuffed tube remains the only viable option for simultaneously securing the airway, allowing repeated access to the trachea and providing effective ventilatory support. Recent advances in noninvasive ventilation, however, mandate that the indications for airway intubation must be defined explicitly (see Chapter 7). Tracheal intubation is required when high levels of airway pressure must be applied to ensure satisfactory oxygen exchange or ventilation. Moreover, noninvasive ventilation may not be appropriate or safe for patients who are obtunded or uncooperative, for those in whom even momentary loss of ventilatory pressure or inspired oxygen might be hazardous, for those requiring high levels of applied pressure, and for those who are hemodynamically unstable. When ventilatory support must be continuous and/or extended more than a few days, intubation clearly is a better approach.

Airway Protection

Because protection of the upper airway cannot be ensured without establishing an effective seal, intubation is required for lethargic or comatose patients at high risk for aspiration. Although an inflated cuff prevents massive airway flooding, small quantities of pharyngeal contents are aspirated routinely. Seepage of the infected secretions that pool just above the cuff may help account for the high incidence of pulmonary infections that occur in mechanically ventilated patients. Special tubes that allow continued evacuation of this secretion pool have been reported to reduce the incidence of ventilator-associated pneumonia (see Chapters 8 and 26).

Secretion Clearance

Retained airway secretions predispose to infection, encourage atelectasis, promote hypoxemia, and dramatically increase the breathing workload for patients with neuromuscular weakness and/or underlying airflow obstruction. Translaryngeal intubation and tracheostomy facilitate extraction of these secretions.

Upper Airway Obstruction

Intubation addresses the immediate threat of anatomic or functional obstruction of the upper airway and is often the first step taken before attempting definitive treatment (see Chapter 25).

■ TYPES OF AIRWAYS AND ROUTES OF INTUBATION

Supraglottic Airways

Pharyngeal airways are firm supports placed through the nose or mouth that are intended to bypass the relaxed tongue, thereby splinting open the retropharynx and providing protected access to the hypopharynx (Table 6-2).

TABLE 6-2 INDICATIONS FOR SUPRAGLOTTIC AIRWAYS

ORAL	NASAL
Removal of retropharyngeal secretions	Removal of supraglottic secretions
Maintain patency of oropharyngeal airway	Conscious or unconscious patient
Obtunded patient without gag	Need for repeated cannulation of trachea
Prevention of biting	Limited value in preventing closure of the retropharynx

Oropharyngeal Airways

Oral airways are anatomically contoured plastic devices that displace the tongue from the posterior wall of the pharynx to prevent occlusion. Their primary purpose is to wedge open the hypopharynx and to facilitate secretion extraction during spontaneous breathing or bag-mask ventilation. Well-placed oropharyngeal airways allow unimpeded spontaneous or assisted ventilation and facilitate removal of airway or pharyngeal secretions. Temporary placement of an oropharyngeal airway allows effective delivery of topical anesthetic to the larynx prior to placement of an ET tube. It is not intended to substitute for ET intubation in patients with firm indications for airway protection or who require secure access to the lower airway.

An oral airway can either serve as a "bite block" for an orally intubated patient inclined to jaw clenching. Because they stimulate the retropharynx and promote gagging, oral airways must not be used in alert patients or in those with intact gag reflexes. (Over time, however, some accommodation to this foreign object may develop.) Disturbingly, obtunded patients with depressed gag reflexes are just those who are most inclined to aspirate. These oropharyngeal airways must, therefore, be removed as soon as consciousness returns or evidence for an activated gag reflex appears.

Nasopharyngeal Airways

These firm (but compressible), curved, flanged, and hollow tubes (nasal "trumpets") are available in a variety of diameters and lengths, but none are designed to extend into the glottis. They are inserted through a lubricated, topically anesthetized, and widely patent nasal passage to facilitate extraction of secretions from the hypopharynx or to guide the passage of tracheal suction catheters. For many patients, they are especially useful in the period immediately *after* extubation, when swallowing of oropharyngeal secretions and effective coughing are impaired. Because they induce considerably less pharyngeal stimulation than do oral airways, they can be used for conscious patients and may serve temporarily as an effective conduit for topical anesthetic delivery to the retropharynx and larynx prior to intubation. Nasopharyngeal airways are best transferred to the alternate nasal passage on a daily basis. Continuous use beyond 48 to 72 h is generally inadvisable because of the escalating risk of infective and erosive complications. Although occasionally helpful in keeping the retropharynx open, they do not reliably maintain airway patency and are not an acceptable alternative to ET intubation for high-risk patients.

Laryngeal Mask Airway, King Airway, and Combitube

The laryngeal mask airway (LMA) is a device that is intended to be inserted into the pharynx without direct visualization and yet to allow effective ventilation and isolation of the lungs from the esophagus. Levels of positive pressure ≤20 cm H_2O can be effectively applied. The insertion technique is rather easily mastered and can be implemented without deep anesthesia. Initially, the LMA was intended for out-of-hospital resuscitation, but currently it is used in surgical procedures, noninvasive and invasive radiologic procedures with short or intermediate duration (<2 h). Increasingly, it is an immediate stop-gap measure when ET intubation cannot be immediately established. LMA does not offer protection from aspiration, but new designs (like the Pro-Seal device) can facilitate gastric suctioning and decrease the risk of aspiration. In the intensive care unit (ICU) environment, the LMA may have applications as well; for example, it allows for insertion of a bronchoscope-guided ET tube via an on-board channel while supporting ventilation. An LMA can therefore serve as a useful backup option for intubating—or reintubating—the difficult airway (LMA is included in the American Society of Anesthesia's *Difficult Airway Management Algorithm.*). For emergent placement of a reliable airway, the King airway may represent the easiest and most reliable option. The Combitube, a cuffed, bilumen, perforated tube, performs as a combined esophageal obturator and tracheal conduit. It is usually inserted blindly and affords both ventilation of the lungs and some protection from aspiration, whether or not the lumen ideally intended for the trachea actually rests there. (It usually does not.)

Endotracheal Intubation

Orotracheal Tubes

As a rule, orotracheal (OT) tubes are easier to insert than nasotracheal (NT) tubes, making oral placement the method of choice during emergencies. The larger tube passed by the oral route improves both airway resistance and secretion management and allows passage of a standard caliber fiberoptic bronchoscope (FOB) should the need arise. Variations of OT tubes are available that allow selective main bronchial intubation, allow aspiration of supraglottic secretions (above the cuff), allow direct fiberoptically imaged visualization of the trachea and main carina, provide an intramural lumen for dead space washout by fresh gas injected near the tube tip, and offer a variety of other unusual and occasionally useful functions. However, oral tubes are not without disadvantages, as they are less stable and less comfortable than nasal tubes, and they impair swallowing to a greater extent. Most self-extubations occur in patients who are orally intubated. They often require an additional oral appliance for stabilization and to prevent tube occlusion by biting. During insertion, OT tube placement incurs a higher incidence of retching, vomiting, aspiration, and mainstem bronchus intubation than the nasal approach, and oral tubes seriously compromise oropharyngeal hygiene. Finally, conventional OT intubation should only be attempted very carefully in patients with limited neck mobility (e.g., ankylosing spondylitis, rheumatoid arthritis, cervical spinal trauma, or prior surgery). Devices are now available to facilitate OT intubation and airway management in such difficult cases. These include fiberoptic intubating bronchoscopes, illuminated stylets, and gum elastic bougies (see following).

Nasotracheal Tubes

NT tubes present a comparatively high resistance to airflow because they are relatively long, kink easily, and impose unusually high resistance when lined with thickened secretions. Even when of normal caliber, the nares do not admit tubes as large as those that the oropharynx will accept. NT tubes are often difficult and sometimes painful to insert. Traumatic complications of NT tube insertion include damage to turbinates, polyps, and well-vascularized mucosa. Insertions should never be forced and should not be attempted in patients who do not easily admit a lubricated nasal trumpet on the same side. Severe hemorrhage can result from ill-advised nasal intubation attempts in patients with bleeding predispositions. Coagulopathy, narrow or deformed nasal passages, and nasal polyposis are contraindications. In a significant percentage of patients, purulent nasal discharge or sinusitis may develop after 72 h. Once in place, however, nasal tubes allow better communication, swallowing, mouth hygiene, and anchoring than their oral counterparts. Nasal tubes offer clear advantages for patients with cervical spine disease and for those with a variety of oral, mandibular, and temporomandibular problems. The relative indications for placing OT tubes, NT tubes, and tracheostomies are summarized in Table 6-2.

■ PHYSIOLOGIC RESPONSES TO INTUBATION

During the intubation of a lightly anesthetized normal adult, increases of heart rate and blood pressure are mediated by neural reflexes, catecholamines, and stress hormones. Moreover, bradycardia, cardiac arrhythmias, and arterial hypotension can be provoked. These cardiovascular effects are blunted by sedatives, analgesics, and systemic or topical anesthetics. Conversely, intravenous anesthetics frequently elicit hypotension, especially in patients with hypovolemia. In current ICU practice, a frequent offender is propofol, which should be given at less than customary rates in the elderly, debilitated, and critically ill. Thiopental's myocardial depressive and vasodilating actions are dose dependent and occur routinely in hypovolemic subjects. Ketamine, a drug used commonly for intubations in the operating theater, preserves laryngeal and pharyngeal reflexes, but is not recommended in patients with raised intracranial pressure, except if the patient is hypovolemic and hypotensive. Etomidate is frequently used and is generally safe and effective; however, this drug may interfere with adrenocortical output for days after the dose is given. Laryngoscopy can impressively raise intracranial pressure, and special precautions to minimize this effect are indicated for patients with head trauma or other at-risk condition. Clinically significant laryngospasm and bronchospasm occur infrequently in a well-prepared subject.

By definition, an ET tube cannot exceed the caliber of the larynx, which normally is the site of greatest narrowing within the native airway. Consequently, intubation reduces the dead space of the upper airway by 20 to 60 mL but simultaneously increases the resistance to airflow. Moreover, once inserted, the resistance offered by a bent, kinked, and secretion-lined or clot-obstructed ET tube in situ can be considerably greater than its manufacturing specification. Although certain reports suggest that intubation reduces the resting lung volume and alters the breathing pattern, the available evidence is conflicting and there is no firm consensus on these points.

■ COMPLICATIONS OF AIRWAY INTUBATION

Anatomic Impairment

3 ET tubes bypass the mechanical defenses of the upper airway, contaminate the lower airways, and severely hamper effective coughing. Despite advances in materials and cuff design, all tubes have the potential of inflicting laryngeal and tracheal injury during insertion and none completely protect the lungs against aspiration of liquids. Furthermore, the supraglottic pool of oral secretions that seep past the cuff as well as the biofilm that routinely lines the lumen of the tube serve to repeatedly inoculate the lower airway with potential pathogens.

Insertion Trauma

Inexpert placement of an ET tube may injure delicate labial, laryngeal, nasal, and pharyngeal tissues or cause dental or spinal trauma. Epistaxis occurs in a sizable percentage of patients who are intubated nasotracheally. Mouth trauma, tooth dislodgement, and mandibular dislocation can result from forceful use of the laryngoscope and placement of an OT tube. Most laryngeal injuries that result from intubation with normally inflated tubes having soft, high-volume cuffs are mild and easily healed. The formation of granulation tissue and ulcers by pressure-induced mucosal ischemia, however, can cause major trouble. Such complications may be observed when tight-fitting (oversized) ET tubes and unrelieved excessive cuff pressure are used for long durations. Carinal injury has been reported as consequence of traumatic insertion of

an ET tube. Bilateral vocal cord paralysis and arytenoid cartilage dislocation typically present as postextubation hoarseness and upper airway obstruction. Use of a nasogastric tube in conjunction with oral intubation has been associated with a higher incidence of aspiration, mucosal erythema, and granuloma formation. Rarely, a tracheoesophageal fistula may form generally after prolonged intubation.

Hypoxemia

Patients who require supplemental O_2 often are exposed to room air during intubation, with consequent desaturation of arterial blood. Although this risk is reduced by "preoxygenation," O_2 stored in this way is depleted quickly by deep breathing, especially in patients with seriously impaired gas exchanging function. Therefore, intubation attempts should not be prolonged beyond 30 s before "reoxygenating," especially for patients who continue to breathe actively. Pulse oximetry provides a useful but delayed signal that helps warn of developing hypoxemia during the attempt. Nasal prongs set to deliver 6 to 10 L of oxygen per min can provide supplemental O_2 during oral intubation, as can the use of a laryngoscope adapted for this purpose.

Apneic, Rapid-Sequence, or Ventilation-Assisted Intubation

Depletion of the pulmonary oxygen reservoir can be slowed by maintaining a high FiO_2 within the lung during the attempt at tube placement. This supplementation is effected by first giving a rapidly acting hypnotic agent (e.g., thiopental 3 to 5 mg/kg, propofol 2 mg/kg, or etomidate 0.3 mg/kg intravenously) together with midazolam (amnesic agent, 1 to 5 mg) and an opioid analgesic intravenously. These are followed quickly by an ultra-short-action depolarizing muscle relaxant (customarily, succinylcholine 1 to 2 mg/kg IV) that has onset time less than 60 s. Nondepolarizing muscle relaxants, such as rocuronium (0.6 mg/kg) or vecuronium (0.08 mg/kg), are alternatives with an onset time less than 3 min and are longer acting. This assisted ventilation intubation technique also facilitates cannulation of the larynx, permits control of ventilation, and lessens the hazards of laryngospasm and insertion trauma. Although apneic intubation is often the preferred technique in difficult cases, sedatives and muscle relaxants are not without risk. Relaxed musculature may totally obstruct the upper airway if the intubation attempt is unsuccessful, and barbiturates and propofol may depress cardiac contractility and promote hypotension. The clinician must be certain that manual ventilation by face mask is effective before committing to muscle relaxation, and expert assistance must be immediately at hand. Succinylcholine can induce hyperkalemia or (more rarely) precipitate "malignant hyperthermia," especially in patients with a family history thereof.

In general, the blind NT approach should not be attempted during emergent intubation because of the uncertain time required to secure the airway. Moreover, blind NT intubation is exceedingly difficult if the patient is apneic. Fiberoptic bronchoscopy or direct laryngoscopy may facilitate semiemergent placement of either type of ET tube.

Gastric Aspiration

Stimulation of the oropharynx frequently causes vomiting, especially when the stomach is distended by food or air. In patients with high risk for gastric aspiration, application of gentle cricothyroid pressure (Sellick maneuver) from the start of bag-mask ventilation helps seal the esophagus against air entry and help bring the cords into view, but does not obviate the risk of aspiration. Prior evacuation of the stomach can reduce the aspiration risk; however, gastric decompression should not delay emergent intubation. Patients with high risk for gastric aspiration who will undergo surgery can receive histamine-2 blocker (ranitidine) and/or prokinetic agent as metoclopramide to decrease this risk.

Reflex Glottic Closure and Laryngospasm

Reflex closure of the glottis and true laryngospasm can prevent passage of the ET tube and may severely limit spontaneous ventilation. Prior use of a topical anesthetic (e.g., lidocaine, 4%) or intravenously (1 to 2 mg/kg for 3 to 5 min before intubation) minimizes the risk. In rare individuals, however, lidocaine is irritating and may itself provoke spasm. Rather than attempt forceful intubation (losing valuable time and risking laryngeal trauma), the patient should be ventilated by bag-mask insufflation of oxygen. Spasm usually subsides promptly. However, if adequate ventilation cannot be achieved and the situation becomes urgent, intravenous succinylcholine (1 mg/kg IV) will relax the contracted muscles during ET tube placement. Repeated failure suggests that a bougie, stylet, fiberoptic guide, or other intubation aid is necessary.

Bronchospasm

Tube placement often stimulates irritant receptors, triggering cough and bronchospasm. Such receptors stop firing shortly after tube placement in most cases, unless the tip of the tube continues to touch the carina. In nonemergent cases at higher risk for bronchospasm, prior administration of aerosolized albuterol, ipratropium, or their combination may prove helpful. Infused or aerosolized bronchodilators may relieve bronchospasm but leave the mechanically stimulated coughing reflex unaffected. Although coughing postintubation is often difficult to arrest, an ET bolus of lidocaine (5 mL of a 2% solution) may be effective.

Right Main Bronchus Intubation

In emergent situations, there is a natural tendency to advance the ET tube beyond the carina. The right main bronchus is less sharply angulated from the trachea than is the left main bronchus and will be entered in 90% of low placements. Rarely, this tendency may facilitate intentional isolation of the right and left lungs during management of such problems as massive hemoptysis originating distal to the main carina. The underventilated left lung and right upper lobe may collapse rapidly, especially when previously ventilated with oxygen. Although comparative auscultation is helpful, breath sounds often are surprisingly well transmitted to an underventilated lung.

ET tubes should be advanced a maximum of 2.5 to 5.0 cm beyond the point at which the tube cuff is seen to pass the cords. Use of a lighted stylet facilitates tip localization to the appropriate level. The distance from the frontal incisors to the carina, which is height dependent, is approximately 28 cm in an average man and 24 cm in an average woman. As a general rule, 23 to 24 cm and 21 to 22 cm at the lips, respectively, will approximate the proper tube tip position in adult men and women of average size. A postprocedure chest X-ray is necessary to check the position. A generous distance (at least 3 cm) between tube tip and main carina must be allowed for tube movement due to neck flexion.

■ POINTS OF TECHNIQUE

Intubation of a rapidly deteriorating, critically ill patient can be a dramatic clinical event. In these challenging circumstances, success depends on optimal preparation and experience proportional to the anticipated difficulty of successful insertion. Certain important questions should be addressed before the attempt: (a) Is intubation of the airway likely to be anatomically challenging? If so, who should attempt the intubation? (b) Which is the best approach—oral, nasal, or tracheostomy? (c) Should the attempt be made awake, under sedation, or using rapid sequence (apneic) technique? (d) Is the patient at unusually high risk for aspiration? (e) What is the contingency approach ("backup plan")? (f) Are all necessary materials and personnel at hand to support both the primary and backup plans?

When undertaking the intubation of the airway of a critically ill patient, the physician is obligated to make sure that all appropriate equipment, drugs, personnel, and preparations have been brought to bear whenever possible. Bag-mask ventilation is not invariably effective, and a secondary "backup plan" to secure the airway should be in place for immediate implementation should the first attempts to cannulate the airway fail. In some cases this may mean ensuring the immediate availability of an anesthesiologist, readiness to attempt an alternative mode of intubation (e.g., apneic or rapid sequence), temporary use of a LMA, or performance of needle or surgical cricothyroidotomy. Similar precautions should be taken when a patient with a known or potentially difficult airway is extubated.

The Difficult Airway

In a significant minority of critically ill patients, even a practitioner who is well trained in conventional intubation techniques will experience difficulty with mask ventilation or tracheal intubation. Such problems assume particular importance for the critically ill patient who is hypoxemic, acidotic, or hemodynamically unstable. A plan of action and preparedness for difficult intubation are essential for safe practice. Although prediction of who will present unusual difficulty is not precise, certain

TABLE 6-3 PREDICTORS OF DIFFICULT INTUBATION

Invisibility of faucial pillars, soft palate, uvula
Mentohyoid distance less than three finger breadths
Restricted temporomandibular joint excursion
Restricted excursion of atlanto-occipital joint

TABLE 6-4 TECHNIQUES TO AID DIFFICULT INTUBATION

Forceps-guided insertion
Stylet-guided insertion
Specialized laryngoscopes
Retrograde intubation

"red flag" features are worth noting. Abnormal facial anatomy, inability to open the mouth, pharyngeal and laryngeal abnormalities, and cervical immobility or anomalies account for the vast majority of problems. Very obese patients with short necks and increased circumference often present problems. Other physical features correlate (although quite imperfectly) with the difficulty of intubation (Fig. 6-1). These include the nonvisibility of key oropharyngeal landmarks: faucial pillars, soft palate, and uvula; poor atlanto-occipital joint mobility (<30 degree excursion of the maxillary teeth, neutral to fully extended); short mentohyoid distance **4** (less than three finger breadths); mentothyroid distance less than 6 cm; interincisor distance less than 4.0 cm; sternomental distance less than 12 cm; and restricted temporomandibular joint excursion (maximal oral aperture height less than three finger breadths in the sagittal midline) (Table 6-3). Special caution should be exercised in the presence of a small mouth, large tongue, inability to widely open the mouth, immobile neck, anterior larynx, prior spine surgery, cervical arthritis/arthrosis, and neck masses. Perhaps surprisingly, edentulous patients often present intubation difficulty. Helpful techniques are now available for consideration in such circumstances (Table 6-4).

Aids for Difficult Intubation

The BURP Maneuver

Mandibular advancement alone or combined with Backward, Upward, and Rightward Pressure on the cricoid cartilage (BURP maneuver) may improve the view during direct laryngoscopy (Table 6.5). The BURP is best performed initially by the person attempting to view the cords, with an assistant helping the intubator during the attempt itself.

Airway Exchange (Oxygenating) Catheters

As their name implies, these relatively small diameter tubes act as hollow guides over which to guide a fresh tube after another has been removed

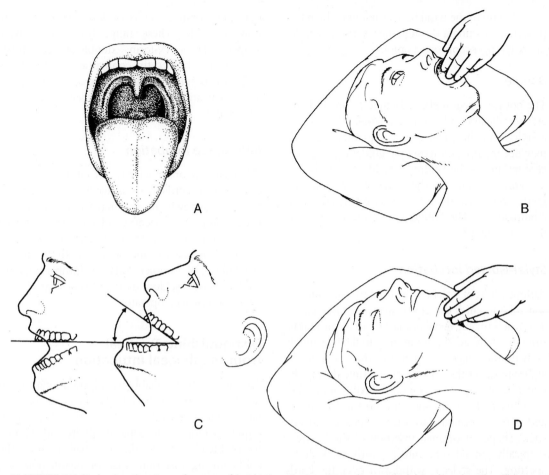

■ **FIGURE 6-1** Evaluating the airway for ease of intubation. **A:** A patient who cannot be intubated easily will have poorly defined oral landmarks (uvula, faucial pillars, and epiglottis) during tongue protrusion. **B:** The mouth aperture should be sufficient to allow entry of three finger breadths on widest opening. **C:** Mobility of the atlanto-occipital joint is ensured by the ability to incline the occlusal surfaces of the maxillary molars by 30 degree or more from the neutral position. **D:** Finally, the chin should allow separation from the hyoid bone by three finger breadths or more. Failure to meet these criteria indicates a potentially difficult oral (and perhaps nasal) intubation.

TABLE 6-5 AIDS AND PRECAUTIONS FOR DIFFICULT INTUBATION

- Optimal positioning
- Availability of:
  - Gum elastic bougies
  - Tracheal tubes of various sizes
  - Tube introducers
  - Varied types and sizes of laryngoscope blade
  - Lighted stylet
  - LMA and cricothyrodotomy kit
- BURP maneuver

<u>5</u> in a high-risk patient, or less frequently, as an introducer during the initial intubation. The fresh gas source helps to "buy time" in patients at a particular risk to rapidly desaturate or suffer adverse consequences of temporary hypoxemia.

Bronchoscope-Guided Airway Management

A FOB may be used to place an oral or nasal tube, position a double lumen or single lumen tube, or assess the feasibility of extubation. Although this procedure may be particularly helpful for patients with difficult airways or poor neck mobility, the field of view is obscured easily by secretions, vomitus, or blood. Bronchoscopic assistance may be particularly useful when an exchange of tubes necessitated by cuff rupture or luminal narrowing can be conducted in semielective time frame.

Forceps-Guided Intubation

When difficulty is encountered in entering the larynx using a nasal approach (or when exchanging an oral for a nasal tube), McGill forceps can be used to grasp the tip of the nasal tube as it enters the retropharynx, directing it through the vocal cords under direct laryngoscopic observation.

Bougie

The bougie (or gum elastic bougie), a small diameter semiflexible tube, serves a similar function as a stylet, but the process is a sequential one and may not require laryngoscopic guidance. The process resembles the Seldinger technique for vascular cannulation in that the bougie acts as a slender guide over which the tube is later gently advanced ("railroaded"). The bougie is inserted in the midline, often blindly.

Stylet-Guided Intubation

Various forms of stylet can be used to configure the soft tube to enter the glottic aperture more easily. These deformable metal or plastic rods span a range from the standard aluminum rods to flexible guides with thumb triggers, which give the operator the ability to direct the tube tip at any time during the insertion attempt. The standard flexible metal stylet is inserted within—not beyond the ET tube—and is often formed into a tip-angulated "hockey stick" shape for optimal insertion of the laryngoscopically guided tube into a poorly seen glottic aperture. The stylet is withdrawn once the cords are passed.

Illuminating Stylets

A battery-operated illuminating stylet ("light wand") has a very bright tip that transilluminates the skin above the thyroid cartilage as it enters the larynx. This "jack-o'-lantern" effect fails to be seen distinctly when the tube enters the esophagus. The light wand accurately guides the ET tube passage in a very high percentage of blind ET intubations (reportedly >95%). This device does not require the sniffing position or laryngoscopy, but requires partially dark room. The light wand has limitations in patients with a very thick neck (e.g., short obese patient) because it is difficult to transilluminate.

Specialized Laryngoscopes

For many years, the primary options for cord visualization were straight and curved blade laryngoscopes, and most clinicians have developed facility with (or preference for) one or the other of them. In response to clinical need, specialized blades that incorporate a variety of desirable features are now available. These range from innovatively shaped blades (V-form, double-angled, tube-shaped, and hinged-tip configurations) to blades that incorporate flexible fiberoscopic bundles to aid visualization or ports for oxygen delivery and suctioning.

Retrograde Intubation

When elective or semielective ET intubation is indicated but the cords defy passage by other methods, a flexible guidewire inserted retrograde through the needle-punctured cricothyroid membrane can be advanced through the mouth to establish the pathway for an introducer and/or tube. With the current availability of simpler aids to intubation, this method is now seldom used and is best performed by an experienced operator.

Distinguishing Tracheal from Esophageal Intubation

Although unquestionably useful, traditional methods for confirming the ET placement of the tube have limited reliability (Table 6-6). These techniques include stethoscopic audibility and symmetry of breath sounds, direct visualization of the cords during insertion, ease of insufflation and recovery of the tidal volume, tidal fogging and clearing of the ET tube, palpation of the ET tube in the larynx, loss of voice, coughing and expulsion of airway secretions, expansion of the upper chest,

---

TABLE 6-6   DISTINGUISHING TRACHEAL FROM ESOPHAGEAL INTUBATION

CONVENTIONAL

Symmetrical breath sounds
Visualization of vocal cords during insertion
Ease of insufflation and recovery of tidal volume
Expiratory fogging of ET tube
Palpation of larynx
Loss of voice
Coughing of airway secretions through tube
Upper chest expansion
Absence of progressive abdominal distention

DEVICES AND AIDS

CO_2 excretion color detector
Capnometry
Tidal gas recovery
Squeeze bulb syringe

and failure of the abdomen to progressively distend during gas delivery.

Pulse oximetry, which is useful in ensuring optimal arterial oxygenation during the procedure for patients with adequate cardiac output, may also help in the evaluation of correct placement. To improve reliability and speed of placement, the phasic detection of CO_2 during expiration by capnography and capnometry can be performed. These devices can be sidestream or mainstream; the latter is more sensitive and more commonly used because it does not require suctioning of gas from the ET connector. For emergent intubations, these devices are not generally available, and a simple color-changing indicator gives an adequate qualitative assessment for most patients. Carbon dioxide detection and measurement by these methods occasionally can be misleading. Little CO_2 is evolved or expelled during shock or circulatory arrest, and conversely, some CO_2 may be liberated initially after esophageal intubation from gas trapped in the gastric pouch. However, this concentration falls rapidly as serial tidal volumes are delivered. Reliability of the detector may be compromised when it is soiled by gastric secretions.

When compressed, a large-capacity squeeze bulb affixed to the ET tube will fail to fill easily if the tube is in the collapsible esophagus. If in good position, however, it recoils effortlessly to its resting volume. Free withdrawal of air via a fitted 50-mL syringe is an equivalent method that is based on the same principle.

Intubation Sequence

Sedation and Neuromuscular Blockade

Rapidly acting benzodiazepines impart amnesia, usually without significantly affecting hemodynamics. Intravenous midazolam, a rapidly acting drug of this class, has a convenient onset (1 to 3 min) and duration (approx. 20 min). Fentanyl or similar narcotic agent often provides effective analgesia. Thiopental or propofol, given as a bolus dose as described previously, has a near immediate onset of action and duration of 7 to 10 min. When required, muscle relaxation can be accomplished with depolarizing (succinylcholine) or nondepolarizing (vecuronium, rocuronium) agents. Etomidate is the ideal induction agent to hold hemodynamic variables unaffected, but it is interesting to note that even a single dose can interfere with determinations of serum cortisol. Ketamine is a good choice in cases with hypovolemia or hypotension.

Oral Intubation

Apart from being well prepared for emergent developments, perhaps the most important thing for the physician to do is to relax and avoid panic. After clearing the airway of secretions and debris, the base of the tongue is displaced from the retropharynx by lifting at the angles of the jaw. For obtunded or comatose patients, an oropharyngeal airway can be inserted to maintain the passage, but such devices may stimulate vomiting in the conscious or agitated subject and in such cases, nasopharyngeal airway may be better. Unless contraindicated, the patient should be positioned with the head (not shoulders) resting on a thin pillow or a doubly folded towel. The optimal "sniffing" position is with the chin lifted, neck flexed, and the head extended (Fig. 6-2). Once positioned, the patient generally can be ventilated by mask without difficulty until the tube is inserted. Bag-mask insufflations should be delivered gently (never forcefully) at a measured rate. During a cardiac arrest in a patient with severe airflow obstruction, special care should be taken to avoid overventilation and iatrogenic "auto positive end-expiratory pressure (PEEP)." If tube placement is not emergent, an alert patient should be lightly sedated and a topical anesthetic used. The antisialagogue glycopyrrolate (0.2 mg IV), given prior to elective intubation, can help preserve a well-visualized field when oral secretions are copious. A cooperative patient can be instructed to pant to concentrate deposition of aerosolized 4% lidocaine on the larynx and upper airway. As a rule, agitated or seriously hypoxemic patients should be sedated and paralyzed quickly (apneic intubation technique). However, this method must be used with special caution for patients who are massively obese and for those with upper airway pathology. In such cases, experienced personnel must be available and the physician should be prepared to undertake cricothyroid puncture in case the airway totally obstructs after paralysis, bag-mask ventilation is unsuccessful, or attempts to intubate repeatedly fail. Even if phasic gas delivery is not undertaken, oxygen insufflated continuously through the needle at 2 to 4 L/min can often maintain acceptable arterial oxygenation (and a degree of ventilation) without hyperinflation until a secure airway is established.

An 8.5-mm (internal diameter) tube for an average male and an 8.0-mm tube for an average female are good sizes to try first. The tube selected should

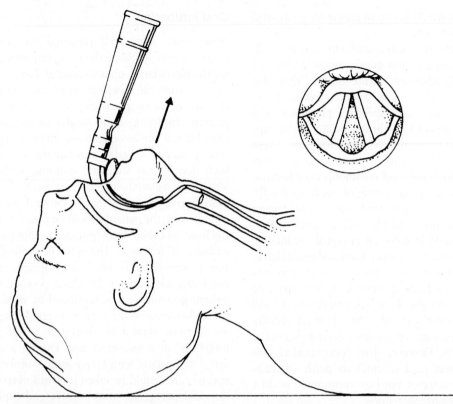

■ **FIGURE 6-2** OT intubation. To align glottis, pharynx, and oral cavity, the neck is flexed and the head is extended. The laryngoscope lifts the tongue and lower jaw away from the posterior pharynx by a motion directed perpendicular to the oroglottic axis.

generally be the largest that will easily pass through the cords.

Curved laryngoscope blades are directed anterior to the epiglottis, with the tip in the vallecula (Fig. 6-2). Straight blades are inserted immediately posterior to the epiglottis and allow a better view of the cords. Both instruments should lift the entire jaw upward to expose the larynx. Neither instrument should use the teeth as a fulcrum for leverage. During intubation, firm cricothyroid pressure (BURP maneuver) helps to bring the cords into view and to seal the esophagus.

When flexible stylets are used to direct the tip of the tube into a glottic opening that cannot be visualized clearly and continuously, care must be taken to ensure that the stylet does not project beyond the tip of the tube. After placement, the cuff should be inflated with the minimum volume that seals without leakage under positive pressure. A variety of useful devices is now available to stabilize an OT tube after placement. A standard ET tube can be anchored effectively by a continuous single band of tape wrapped circumferentially around the neck and secured to the tube (and bite

block, if used) at both ends. The hands must be restrained if there is any possibility for self-extubation. This is especially important after OT intubation in a hypoxemic patient requiring high levels of inspired oxygen or airway pressure. Although a nasogastric or orogastric tube should be used for the orally intubated patient to decompress the stomach when there is gut hypomotility or active air swallowing, its continued use may increase the incidence of aspiration and laryngeal erosion.

Nasotracheal Intubation

Blind NT intubation is not a technique to be performed by the inexperienced caregiver. It should not be used in emergent situations and is especially inappropriate for establishing the airway during apnea. Nasal intubation is especially hazardous in patients with coagulopathy. Because it is usually performed in awake patients, topical anesthesia of the nose, pharynx, and larynx, and sedation are mandatory. A topical vasoconstrictor (typically, phenylephrine) can facilitate tube passage and reduce the risk of mucosal hemorrhage. Before the intubation attempt, a lidocaine-lubricated nasal trumpet should be passed to calibrate the diameter of the passage and deliver topical anesthesia with minimal trauma risk. Selection of an appropriate tube (typically size 6.5 to 7.5), softened with hot water, generous nasal lubrication, and gentle insertion technique are necessary to prevent nasal, laryngeal, or tracheal injury. With the head in an upright orientation, the NT tube should be inserted initially to a level just above the vocal cords. This tube position can be detected by listening to the intensity of expired air flowing through the tube. The tube is then rapidly but gently advanced in synchrony with the next inspiratory effort. Passage through the larynx usually is signaled by a vigorous cough and subsequent inability to speak. Vigilance should be maintained against the development of sinusitis, which complicates approximately one third of placements longer than a few days.

Tube Exchange

Occasionally, a ruptured tube cuff, occlusion of the lumen with secretions or clot, or special care requirements unmet by the tube in place justifies replacement. When ventilation or oxygenation needs are high, the changeout is best conducted under direct vision in an adequately sedated patient, using a conventional laryngoscope or a bronchoscope preloaded with the fresh tube to minimize the risk. Extracting the tube and proceeding as during a fresh intubation is hazardous, particularly in the presence of respiratory failure or laryngeal edema caused by disease or protracted intubation. Using a tube-changing catheter is another option, and here again, laryngoscopy is indicated if airway anatomy is uncertain. A tube changer is a long plastic tube (hollow or solid) that acts as a stent when a fresh ET tube is exchanged for a malfunctioning or less-desirable one along the same insertion path. In an emergency, a tube changer can be fashioned by trimming a standard nasogastric tube.

Extubation

Optimal preparation of the patient is essential before the tube is removed, with special attention to fluid balance, electrolytes, and prevention of cardiac ischemia. Inadvertent extubation can be lethal in acutely ill, agitated patients and must be avoided at all costs. Even planned extubation must not be performed casually. Extubation breaks the seal between the patient's upper and lower airways, potentially allowing purulent secretions pooled above the cuff to enter the lung. Reflex stimulation may also provoke laryngospasm, bronchospasm, or cardiac arrhythmias.

Oxygen should be administered, and the trachea and oropharynx should be cleared of secretions before the cuff is deflated. After a deep inspiration, the tube should be pulled quickly as the patient exhales forcefully from a high lung volume. One simple trick for helping the patient expel those secretions, rather than aspirate them as the tube is extracted, is to raise PEEP to 15 cm H_2O for 3 to 10 breaths before cuff deflation, maintaining the pressure target until removal is complete. This does three useful things: (i) breaks any existing "mucus seal" after cuff deflation; (ii) expands the chest to help with the force of the initial cough; and (iii) generates a mouth-directed flow once the tube cuff is down, favoring expulsion.

Postextubation stridor may occur due to laryngospasm or edema. This usually subsides spontaneously within the first 6 to 24 h if the head is held upright but such patients must be observed carefully to assess the need for urgent reintubation. Although not routinely necessary, inhaled racemic epinephrine, bronchodilators, continuous positive airway pressure (CPAP) and corticosteroids may be helpful after extubation in selected cases—especially those involving small adults or children.

The ability of the patient to inhale and exhale freely around the deflated cuff before extubation gives some assurance that the airway above the cuff is not severely narrowed. This simple test is useful when upper airway obstruction has been the primary indication for intubation. A leak around the partially deflated cuff during ventilation is a sensitive predictor of successful extubation for a patient who meets other criteria for ventilator independence, but the absence of a cuff leak does not reliably predict extubation failure secondary to upper airway obstruction. Noninvasive ventilation, applied with a humidified gas source to minimize secretion inspissation, may provide a useful bridge across the immediate postextubation period. Bi-PAP should be considered not only to ease spontaneous breathing during waking hours, but also to help assure adequate sleep in the first 24–28 hours after extubation. (Functional upper airway obstruction is common after tube removal due to local edema.) In fragile patients with a weak cough, thickened secretions and/or the need for frequent suctioning consideration should be given pre-extubation to inspection of the lower airway for retained secretions. Heliox, a low-density helium–oxygen mixture (70:30, 80:20) reduces resistive pressure losses because of turbulence and may prove useful during the period of maximal edema for selected patients.

Women tend to be predisposed to the long-term complications of intubation. Postextubation stridor may result from vocal cord dysfunction, arytenoid dislocation, laryngospasm, uncleared secretions or blood, or tracheomalacia. If reintubation is needed, a smaller ET tube and a prophylactic epinephrine aerosol directed onto the cords are reasonable measures.

Decannulating the Difficult Airway

Edema, secretions, and local trauma often pose a challenge to reintubation, should that prove necessary. In the case of the airway whose cannulation proved tricky initially, the problem can rapidly advance from difficult to life threatening. In cases with such potential, it is essential to prepare for any contingency *before* the tube is removed. Readiness means having personnel with the required level of experience immediately available and to assure that the aforementioned intubation aids are kept nearby. For this emergent setting, stop-gap stabilizing measures might include an LMA and a large bore needle with attachment tubing for cricothyroid membrane puncture and metered oxygen insufflation. Most importantly, both a strategy and sequence for effectively securing the airway postextubation should be thought through in detail—prior to decannulation.

Postextubation Care

The first 24 to 48h that follow extubation often present a serious challenge to the patient's secretion-clearing mechanisms, as protective reflexes are blunted, laryngeal protection is transiently suboptimal, swallowing is impaired, swelling of periglottic tissues increases airflow resistance, and the patient is characteristically lethargic because of residual drug effects and sleep deprivation. During this time, assiduous secretion hygiene is imperative. To minimize the aspiration risk, the patient should be cared for in the upright position and oral intake must be withheld until proof of effective swallowing is at hand. Noninvasive application of continuous positive airway pressure (CPAP) or Bi-PAP may help ensure upper airway patency and

adequate nocturnal ventilation during this time. Anti-sialagogues, such as glycopyrrolate, may be helpful if oral secretions are excessive and thin. Stridor in the immediate postextubation period may respond to aerosols of racemic epinephrine and relief of bronchospasm, if any. Corticosteroids are often used, but are of uncertain value. When increased upper airway resistance is the primary problem, temporary use of Bi-PAP or heliox may be helpful until the swelling recedes. After 48h, many of the mentioned problems diminish. As noted in Chapter 10, the need for reintubation occurring after a brief period of spontaneous breathing portends a poor prognosis in the setting of critical illness.

■ TRACHEOSTOMY

Benefits and Indications

Tracheostomy improves comfort (potentially allowing the patient to eat, talk, and ambulate), greatly facilitates secretion management, minimizes airway resistance and anatomic dead space, and reduces the risk of laryngeal injury (Table 6-7). However, tracheostomies have the highest associated risk of serious complications (bleeding, stenosis) and the highest incidence of swallowing difficulty and aspiration postextubation. Unless carried out emergently for acute upper airway obstruction, conventional tracheostomy (but not necessarily *percutaneous* tracheostomy) should be performed over an oral or nasal tube in an operating suite. Except when long-term ventilator dependence or need for ongoing secretion management has been established, most experts defer tracheostomy for at least 10 days after intubation.

Variants of Conventional Tracheostomy

Certain variants of tracheostomy recently introduced to clinical practice may be carried out safely at the bedside.

Needle Cricothyroidotomy

In very rare circumstances, life-threatening upper **6** airway obstruction renders all standard methods of airway control invalid or infeasible: pharyngeal airways, bag-mask ventilation, and translaryngeal intubation. Needle cricothyroidotomy can be performed quickly with a 14-gauge or larger needle to provide a temporary conduit for a high-pressure source of oxygen. After the cricothyroid membrane is located, prepared antiseptically, anesthetized, and immobilized, a syringe-mounted needle with

TABLE 6-7   TRANSLARYNGEAL INTUBATION VERSUS TRACHEOSTOMY

	TRANSLARYNGEAL INTUBATION	TRACHEOSTOMY

Advantages	Ease of placement
	Inexpensive
	Fewer severe complications
	No specialized venue
	   needed for insertion
		Comfort
		Ease of mouth care
		Secretion removal
		Stability
		Less airway resistance
		Improved communication
		Ease of swallowing and enteral feeding
		Reduced work of breathing
		Improved mobility
		Ease of reinsertion and ventilator
		   reconnection

Disadvantages	Discomfort Swallowing Secretion clearance Greater work of breathing Impaired speech Upper airway and larynx damage	Expense Severity of complications Swallowing impairment Reduced cough efficiency postdecannulation

external cannula punctures the membrane at a 45 degree angle, and air is aspirated to confirm its position. Once inserted, the outer flexible sheath is advanced as the metallic needle is withdrawn. Attachment of a Y-connector and high-pressure oxygen source at 40 to 60 L/min may then allow manually gated (phasic) insufflations, which usually maintain acceptable oxygenation until a definitive airway can be established.

Percutaneous Dilatational Tracheostomy

An entirely different alternative to conventional tracheostomy has gained considerable popularity as an elective (nonemergent) procedure for establishing long-term airway access, ventilatory support, and secretion clearance at the bedside for those patients who cannot be transported to the operating room (Fig. 6-3). One of two operators uses a bronchoscope to both secure the air channel and to guide the needle puncture of the trachea under direct vision. Using a series of dilators and a modified Seldinger technique, the tube enters the trachea between the cricoid and first tracheal cartilage or between the first and second tracheal cartilages. After dissecting to the anterior tracheal wall, an introducer, sheath, guidewire, and catheter are used to progressively develop and dilate the stoma for acceptance of a standard tracheostomy tube. Bleeding, subcutaneous emphysema, and paratracheal insertion are reported complications.

The incidence of infection is believed to be less than with the open surgical approach.

Minitracheostomy

When secretion retention is the primary concern, a minitracheostomy may be performed to allow suctioning through a small-diameter (4.0-mm) cuffless indwelling cannula that can also serve as an O_2 delivery conduit. Although inadequate for ventilation, transtracheal insufflation via the "minitrach" can be helpful in an emergency, similar to needle cricothyroidotomy, as already described. Candidates for the minitrach should have an intact gag reflex because the airway is not protected. This device does not seriously impede talking, coughing, or eating.

Tracheostomy Tube Displacement

A well-defined track between skin and trachea does not form for 4 to 5 days afterward. Should the tube become displaced during this vulnerable period, the patient is placed at risk for life-threatening consequences. These include dyspnea, tracheal compression with asphyxia, hypoxemia, pneumothorax, pneumomediastinum, and secretion retention. Distortion and swelling of the subcutaneous tissues may prevent easy reentry of the same sized tube through the skin wound. Through this hazardous period, even placing a

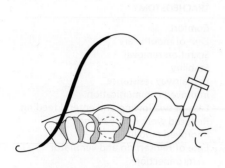

Insertion of guiding catheter

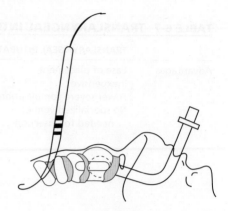

Serial dilation

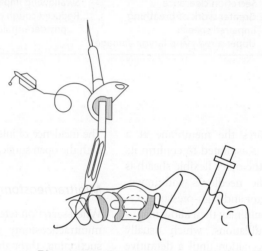

Placement of tracheostomy tube

■ **FIGURE 6-3** Percutaneous dilatational tracheostomy.

tracheostomy tube of smaller size can prove unsuccessful unless traction sutures that identify and spread the tracheal opening are in place. Traditional teaching suggests that oral intubation will be necessary in most of these situations and should be undertaken immediately. Personal experience suggests, however, that an initial attempt to recannulate is prudent, as it is often successful.

■ **SUGGESTED READINGS**

American Society of Anesthesiologists Task Force on Management of the Difficult Airway. Practice guidelines for management of the difficult airway. *Anesthesiology.* 2003;98(5):1269–1277.

Bingham RM, Proctor LT. Airway management. *Pediatr Clin North Am.* 2008;55(4):873–886.

Butler KH, Clyne B. Management of the difficult airway: Alternative airway techniques and adjuncts. *Emerg Med Clin North Am.* 2003;21(2):259–289.

Lavery GG, McCloskey BV. The difficult airway in adult critical care. *Crit Care Med.* 2008;36(7):2163–2173.

Mihai R, Blair E, Kay H, et al. A quantitative review and meta-analysis of performance of non-standard laryngoscopes and rigid fibreoptic intubation aids. *Anaesthesia.* 2008;63(7):745–760.

Rana S, Pendem S, Pogodzinski MS, et al. Tracheostomy in critically ill patients. *Mayo Clin Proc.* 2005;80(12):1632–1638.

Reynolds SF, Heffner J. Airway management of the critically ill patient: Rapid-sequence intubation. *Chest.* 2005;127(4):1397–1412.

Stumper-Groves D, Durbin CG Jr. Tracheostomy in the critically ill: Indications, timing, and techniques. *Curr Opin Crit Care.* 2007;13:90–97.

Walz JM, Zayaruzny M, Heard SO. Airway management in critical illness. *Chest.* 2007;131(2):608–620.

Indications and Options for Mechanical Ventilation

KEY POINTS

1 Prime indications for initiating mechanical ventilation include inadequate alveolar ventilation, inadequate arterial oxygenation, excessive respiratory workload, and acute heart failure with labored breathing.

2 For machine-aided breathing cycles, the physician must determine the minimum frequency of the machine's inspiratory cycle, the pressure or tidal volume to administer, the inspired oxygen fraction, the triggering sensitivity and the levels of certain boundary conditions (e.g., end-expiratory pressure and alarm limits).

3 Positive-pressure inflation can be achieved with machines that control either of the two determinants of ventilating power—pressure or flow—and terminate inspiration according to pressure, flow, volume, or time criteria. Both pressure and flow cannot be fixed simultaneously because once either is set, the other becomes a dependent variable influenced by the interaction of the inflation impedance with the controlled variable.

4 The fundamental difference between pressure-targeted and volume-targeted ventilation is implicit in their names. Strictly pressure-targeted modes regulate pressure at the expense of letting flow and tidal volume vary; volume-targeted modes guarantee flow and/or tidal volume but let airway pressure vary.

5 Standard modes of positive-pressure ventilation include assist/control ventilation, SIMV, and PSV. The first two can be applied using either flow-controlled or pressure-controlled machine cycles.

6 Potentially useful ventilatory options include pressure regulated volume control, automatic tube compensation, airway pressure release ventilation, and Bi-Phasic Airway pressure. Promising newer modes include adaptive support ventilation, proportional assist ventilation, and neurally adjusted ventilatory assist. Each of these innovations is intended to combine desirable features of pressure preset and flow-controlled, volume-targeted ventilation.

7 High frequency ventilation may be useful for those patients who have a bronchopleural fistula, a specialized need for ventilatory support or refractory hypoxemia with high risk for ventilator-induced lung injury. Deep sedation is generally required.

8 Certain adjuncts to mechanical ventilation, including permissive hypercapnia and prone positioning, are now widely applied in clinical practice. The value of other methods, such as inhaled nitric oxide, tracheal gas insufflation, partial liquid ventilation, and extrapulmonary gas exchange, is yet unproved.

9 Noninvasive ventilation seems to be particularly helpful when initiated early in the course of rapidly reversible diseases that respond to modest airway pressures. Good examples are exacerbated COPD and congestive heart failure. It is less often successful for patients whose condition has already deteriorated, for patients who are comatose or noncooperative, and for patients who either cannot be attended closely or are hemodynamically unstable.

■ INDICATIONS FOR MECHANICAL VENTILATION

Although often made concurrently, the decisions to institute mechanical support should be made independently of those made to perform tracheal intubation or to use positive end-expiratory pressure (PEEP) or continuous posture airway pressure (CPAP). This is especially true considering the recently improved noninvasive (nasal and mask) options and interfaces for supporting ventilation. As the ventilator assumes the work of breathing (WOB), important changes occur in

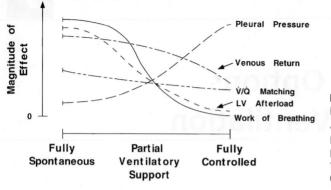

■ **FIGURE 7-1** Important physiologic differences between spontaneous and mechanical ventilation. As the proportion of ventilatory support with positive pressure increases, WOB falls and pleural pressure rises, influencing venous return, left ventricular (LV) afterload, and ventilation/perfusion ($\dot{V}/\dot{Q}$) matching.

pleural pressure, ventilation distribution, and cardiac output (Fig. 7-1). Mechanical assistance may be needed because oxygenation cannot be achieved with an acceptable FiO_2 without manipulating PEEP, mean airway pressure, and pattern of ventilation or because spontaneous ventilation places excessive demands on ventilatory muscles or on a compromised cardiovascular system (Table 7-1).

Inadequate Alveolar Ventilation

Apnea and deteriorating ventilation despite other therapeutic measures are absolute indications for mechanical breathing assistance. Usually in such cases there are signs of respiratory distress or advancing obtundation, and serial blood gas measurements show a falling pH and stable or rising $PaCO_2$. Although few physicians withhold mechanical assistance when the pH trends steadily downward and there are signs of physiologic intolerance, there is less agreement regarding the absolute values of $PaCO_2$ and pH that warrant such intervention; these clearly vary with the specific clinical setting. In fact, after intubation has been accomplished, pH and $PaCO_2$ may be allowed to drift deliberately far outside the normal range to avoid the high ventilating pressures and tidal volumes that tend to induce lung damage. This strategy—permissive hypercapnia—is now considered integral to a lung-protective ventilatory approach for the acute

management of severe asthma and adult acute respiratory distress syndrome (ARDS). Acute hypercapnia has well-known and potentially adverse physiologic consequences. Nonetheless, recent experimental work in varied models of clinical problems—notably, ischemia/reperfusion and ventilator-induced lung injury—clearly indicate that certain forms of cellular injury are actually attenuated by hypercapnia. Whether it is hypercapnia itself or the associated change in hydrogen ion concentration is still a subject of active investigation (ARDS; see Chapter 24).

Blood pH is generally a better indicator than $PaCO_2$ of the need for ventilatory support. Hypercapnia *per se* should not prompt aggressive intervention if pH remains acceptable and the patient remains alert, especially if CO_2 retention occurs slowly. Many patients require ventilatory assistance despite levels of alveolar ventilation that would be appropriate for normal resting metabolism. For example, patients with metabolic acidosis and neuromuscular weakness or airflow obstruction may lower $PaCO_2$ to 40 mm Hg or below but not sufficiently to prevent acidemia. The physiologic consequences of altered pH are still debated and clearly depend on the underlying pathophysiology and comorbidities. However, if not quickly reversible by simpler measures, a sustained pH greater than 7.65 or less than 7.10 is often considered sufficiently dangerous in itself to require control by mechanical ventilation and sedation (with muscle relaxants, if needed). Inside these extremes, the threshold for initiating support varies with the clinical setting. For example, a lethargic patient with asthma who is struggling to breathe can maintain a normal pH until shortly before suffering a respiratory arrest, whereas an alert cooperative patient with chronically blunted respiratory drive may allow pH to fall to 7.25 or lower before recovering uneventfully in response to aggressive

1

TABLE 7-1 INDICATIONS FOR MECHANICAL VENTILATION
Inadequate ventilation to maintain pH
Inadequate oxygenation
Excessive breathing workload
Congestive heart failure
Circulatory shock

bronchodilation, steroids, and oxygen. In less obvious situations, the decision to ventilate should be guided by trends in pH, arterial blood gases, mental status, dyspnea, hemodynamic stability, and response to therapy. The ongoing need for ventilatory assistance must be carefully and repeatedly assessed (see Chapter 10).

■ INADEQUATE OXYGENATION

Arterial oxygenation is the result of complex interactions between systemic oxygen demand, cardiovascular adequacy, and the efficiency of pulmonary oxygen exchange. Improving cardiovascular performance and minimizing O_2 consumption (by reducing fever, agitation, pain, etc.) may dramatically improve the balance between delivery and consumption. Transpulmonary oxygen exchange can be aided by supplementing FiO_2 by using PEEP, by changing the pattern of ventilation to increase mean airway (and consequently, mean alveolar) pressure and average lung size (see Chapter 5), or by prone positioning. In patients with edematous or injured lungs, relief of an excessive breathing workload may improve oxygenation by relaxing the expiratory muscles (improving end-expiratory lung distention) and by allowing the mixed venous O_2 saturation and venous admixture to improve.

Modest fractions of inspired oxygen are administered to nonintubated patients using masks or nasal cannulas. Controlled, low-range O_2 therapy is best delivered to the nonintubated patient by a well-fitting Venturi mask, which automatically adjusts to changes in inspiratory flow demand without change in delivered FiO_2. Without tracheal intubation, delivery of high FiO_2 can only be achieved with a snug nonrebreathing mask that is flushed with high flows of pure O_2. Unfortunately, apart from the risk of O_2 toxicity, masks often become displaced or must be removed intentionally for eating or expectoration. Intubation facilitates the application of PEEP and CPAP needed to avert oxygen toxicity as well as enables extraction of airway secretions.

Although positive airway pressure (noninvasive ventilation [NIV] or CPAP) can be applied to spontaneously breathing, nonintubated patients, these techniques may not be well tolerated for extended periods, especially by confused, poorly cooperative, or hemodynamically unstable patients who require high mask pressures (>15 cm H_2O; see "Noninvasive Ventilation", following). Patients who retain secretions also are poor candidates for these techniques. Moreover, with the airway unprotected, these methods should be used only with extreme caution in patients who are obtunded or comatose. Continuous positive airway pressure is best tolerated at low levels (<10 cm H_2O) for less than 48 h, with sporadic breaks allowed to relieve facial pressure.

Excessive Respiratory Workload

A common reason for mechanical assistance is a lack of ventilatory power or reserve. The respiratory muscles cannot sustain tidal pressures greater than 40% to 50% of their maximal isometric pressure. Respiratory pressure requirements rise with minute ventilation and the impedance to breathing. Patients with hypermetabolism or metabolic acidosis often need ventilatory support to avoid decompensation. Impaired ventilatory drive or muscle strength diminish ventilatory capacity and reserve.

Cardiovascular Support

Although little effort is expended by normal subjects who breathe quietly, the O_2 demands of the respiratory system account for a very high percentage of total body oxygen consumption ($\dot{V}O_2$) during periods of physiologic stress (Fig. 7-2). Experimental animals in circulatory shock who receive mechanical ventilation survive longer than their unassisted counterparts. Moreover, patients with combined cardiorespiratory disease often fail attempts to withdraw ventilatory support for cardiac rather than respiratory reasons. Such observations demonstrate the importance of minimizing the ventilatory O_2 requirement during cardiac insufficiency or ischemia. Doing so helps rebalance myocardial O_2 supply with requirements and/or allows diaphragmatic blood flow to be redirected to other O_2-deprived vital organs. Moreover, reducing ventilatory effort may improve afterload to the left ventricle (see Chapter 1). Therefore, the physician should intervene early to relieve an excessive breathing workload for patients with compromised cardiac function. Although it is possible to use NIV or CPAP alone for mildly to moderately affected patients, fatigue often sets in unless underlying oxygen requirements are reduced substantially, which often requires adequate sedation or higher pressures than can be provided noninvasively.

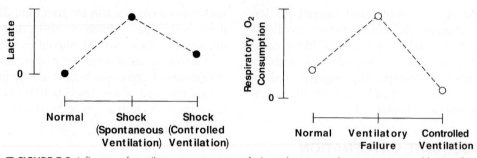

■ **FIGURE 7-2** Influence of ventilatory support on perfusion adequacy and oxygen consumed by ventilatory musculature. The work cost of spontaneous breathing and the increased afterload to LV ejection often contribute significantly to anaerobiosis and lactic acid production during circulatory shock **(left)**. A better balance between oxygen delivery and consumption can be achieved when ventilation is controlled, thereby freeing needed oxygen for other organ systems **(right)**. Conversely, boosting circulatory output in the setting of shock improves oxygen delivery to the fatiguing respiratory muscles, improving their O_2 supply and endurance.

■ OPTIONS IN MECHANICAL VENTILATION

Types of Ventilation

Negative Versus Positive Pressure

To accomplish ventilation, a pressure difference must be developed phasically across the passive lung. This difference can be generated by negative pressure developed by respiratory muscles in the pleural space, by positive pressure applied to the airway opening, or by a combination of both. Although of major historical interest, negative-pressure ventilators are seldom appropriate for the modern acute care setting and will not be discussed further. **2** Whether using negative or positive pressure for machine-aided cycles, the physician must determine the machine's minimum cycling rate, the duration of its inspiratory cycle, the baseline pressure (PEEP), and either the pressure to be applied or the tidal volume to administer, depending on the "mode" selected.

Positive-Pressure Ventilation

3 Positive-pressure inflation can be achieved with machines that control *either* of the two determinants of ventilating power—pressure or flow—and terminate inspiration according to pressure, flow, volume, or time limits. Waveforms for both flow and pressure cannot be controlled *simultaneously*, however, because pressure is developed as a function of flow and the impedance to breathing, which is determined by the uncontrolled parameters of resistance and compliance. Thus, the clinician has the choice of specifying pressure, with tidal volume as a resulting (dependent) variable, or of controlling flow, with pressure as the dependent variable. Whereas older ventilators offered only a single control variable and a single cycling criterion, positive-pressure ventilators of the latest generation enable the physician to select freely among multiple options.

Pressure-Cycled Ventilation

Although pressure-*cycled* (pressure-limited) ventilators generally have been supplanted by more advanced machines that offer multiple modes with different cycling criteria (time or flow), some are still used, especially in economically depressed regions or developing countries. In their simplest form, these low-cost machines allow gas to flow continuously until a set pressure limit is reached. A pressurized gas source is all that is required to operate many of these machines, making them immune to electrical failure. Small size, portability, and low cost make this now obsolete equipment acceptable for low-demand applications in transport and in respiratory therapy, where they can be used for intermittent delivery of aerosols or for deep breathing (intermittent positive pressure breathing [IPPB]).

Pressure-Preset (Pressure-Targeted) Ventilation

Modern ventilators provide pressure-preset or pressure-targeted ventilatory modes (e.g., pressure control or pressure support) as options for full or partial ventilatory assistance. After the breath is initiated, these modes quickly attain a targeted amount of pressure at the airway opening until a

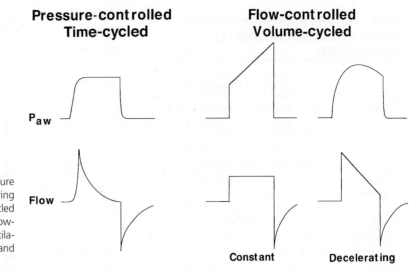

■ **FIGURE 7-3** Airway pressure (P_{aw}) and flow waveforms during pressure-controlled, time-cycled ventilation and during flow-controlled, volume-cycled ventilation delivered with constant and decelerating flow profiles.

specified time (pressure control) or flow (pressure support) cycling criterion is met (Fig. 7-3). Maximal pressure is controlled, but tidal volume is a complex function of applied pressure and its rate of approach to target pressure, available inspiratory time, and the impedance to breathing (compliance, inspiratory and expiratory resistance, and auto-PEEP). High flow capacity, pressure-targeted ventilation compensates well for small air leaks and is therefore quite appropriate for use with leaking or uncuffed endotracheal (ET) tubes, as in neonatal or pediatric patients. Because of its virtually "unlimited" ability to deliver flow and its decelerating flow profile, pressure-targeted ventilation also is an appropriate choice for spontaneously breathing patients with high or varying inspiratory flow demands, which usually peak early in the ventilatory cycle. The decelerating flow profiles of pressure-targeted modes also improve the distribution of ventilation in lungs with heterogeneous mechanical properties (widely varying time constants). Apart from their *potential* to limit the lung's exposure to high airway pressure and risk for barotrauma, pressure-targeted modes also prove helpful for adult patients in whom the airway cannot be completely sealed (e.g., bronchopleural fistula).

Flow-Controlled, Volume-Cycled Ventilation

For many years, flow-controlled, volume-cycled ventilation (assist-control) has been the technique of choice for supporting seriously ill adult patients. Flow can be controlled by selecting a waveform

(e.g., constant or decelerating) and setting a peak flow value or by selecting a flow waveform and setting the combination of tidal volume and inspiratory time. By controlling the tidal volume and "backup" frequency, a lower limit for minute ventilation can be guaranteed. Unfortunately, there are two important trade-offs of controlling flow. First, the pressure required to ventilate with any given PEEP and tidal volume varies widely with the impedance to breathing (Fig. 7-3). Moreover, once the peak and profile are chosen, flow remains inflexible to increased (or decreased) inspiratory flow demands.

Differences between Pressure-Targeted and Volume-Targeted Ventilation

After the decision has been made to initiate mechanical ventilation, the physician must decide to use either pressure-controlled ventilation (PCV) or volume-cycled ventilation. For a well-monitored passively ventilated patient, pressure-targeted and volume-targeted modes can be used with virtually identical benefit and risk. With either method, FiO_2, PEEP, and backup frequency must be selected. If pressure control (sometimes referred to as *pressure assist control*) is used, the targeted inspiratory pressure (above PEEP) and the inspiratory time must be selected (usually with consideration toward the desired tidal volume). Pressure support differs from pressure control in that each pressure-supported breath must be patient initiated (triggered). Furthermore, the off-cycling criterion for pressure support is flow, rather than time, so that cycle length is free to vary with patient effort.

TABLE 7-2 PRESSURE-CONTROLLED VERSUS VOLUME-CONTROLLED VENTILATION

	PRESSURE CONTROL	VOLUME CONTROL
Settings	Pressure target Inspiratory duration Pressure rise rate	Tidal volume target Flow rate Flow wave form
Outcome variables	1°-Tidal volume 2°-Auto-PEEP	1°-Airway pressure 2°-Auto-PEEP
Variables common to both	FiO_2 PEEP Mode Frequency	FiO_2 PEEP Mode Frequency

If volume-cycled ventilation is used, the physician may select (depending on ventilator) either tidal volume and flow delivery pattern (waveform and peak flow) or flow delivery pattern and minimum minute ventilation (with tidal volume the resulting quotient of V_E and backup frequency).

4   The fundamental difference between pressure- and volume-targeted ventilation is implicit in their names; pressure-targeted modes guarantee pressure at the expense of letting tidal volume vary, and volume-targeted modes guarantee flow—and consequently the volume provided to the circuit in the allowed inspiratory time (tidal volume)—at the expense of letting airway pressure float. This distinction governs how they are used in clinical practice (Table 7-2).

Flow and tidal volume are important variables to monitor when pressure targeting, whereas airway pressure is of parallel importance in volume targeting. Gas stored in compressible circuit elements does not contribute to effective alveolar ventilation. For adult patients, such losses (approx. 2 to 4 mL/cm H_2O of peak pressure) usually constitute a modest fraction of the tidal volume. For infants, however, compressible losses may comprise such a high fraction of the V_T that *effective* ventilation varies markedly with peak cycling pressure. Thus, during volume-cycled ventilation, moment-by-moment changes in chest impedance caused by bronchospasm, secretions, and muscular activity can force peak airway pressure and compressible circuit volume to rise and effective tidal volume to fall. Finally, because airway pressure is

controlled, pressure-targeted modes are less likely to cause barotrauma, which is a particularly serious problem for this age group.

Volume-targeted modes deliver a preset volume unless a specified circuit pressure limit is exceeded. Major advantages to volume targeting are the capacity to deliver unvarying tidal volumes (except in the presence of a gas leak), flexibility of flow and volume adjustments, and power to ventilate difficult patients. All ventilators currently used for continuous support in adults offer volume cycling as a primary option. Despite its advantages for acute care, volume cycling also has important disadvantages. Unless the airway is well sealed, volume-cycled modes cannot ventilate effectively and consistently. Furthermore, after the flow rate and profile are set, the inflation time of the machine remains fixed and remains unresponsive to the patient's native cycling rhythm and flow demands. Just as importantly, excessive alveolar pressure may be required to deliver the desired tidal volume. Pressure-targeted modes confer flexibility to flow demand and, when flow cycled, to cycle duration as well.

Standard Modes of Positive Pressure

Controlled Mechanical Ventilation

With the sensitivity adjustment turned off during controlled mechanical ventilation (CMV), the machine provides a fixed number of breaths per minute and remains totally uninfluenced by the patient's efforts to alter frequency. This "lockout" mode demands constant vigilance to make appropriate adjustments for changes in ventilatory requirements and is used only for situations in which pH and/or $PaCO_2$ must be controlled tightly (e.g., some neurologic patients). Most patients require deep sedation to ensure comfort and to ablate breathing efforts. Under these conditions, assist-control ventilation has similar capability and offers additional advantages (less patient–ventilator asynchrony).

Assist-Control Ventilation

During assist-control ventilation (or assisted mechanical ventilation [AMV]), each inspiration triggered by the patient is powered by the ventilator using either volume-cycled or pressure-targeted breaths (Fig. 7-4). When pressure is the targeted variable and inspiratory time is preset, the mode is

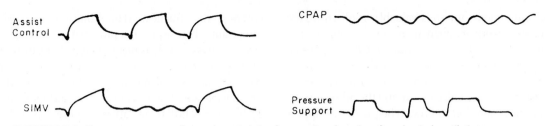

■ **FIGURE 7-4** Airway pressure waveforms characteristic of conventional modes of mechanical ventilation.

known as pressure control or pressure assist control. Sensitivity to inspiratory effort can be adjusted to require a small or large negative pressure deflection below the set level of end-expiratory pressure to initiate the machine's inspiratory phase. Alternatively, modern machines can be flow triggered, initiating a cycle when a flow deficit is sensed in the expiratory limb of the circuit relative to the inspiratory limb during the exhalation period. As a safety mechanism, a "backup rate" is set so that if the patient does not initiate a breath within the number of seconds dictated by that frequency, a machine cycle begins automatically. A backup rate set high enough to cause alkalosis blunts respiratory drive and terminates the patient's efforts to breathe at the "apneic threshold" for $PaCO_2$. In awake, normal subjects, this threshold usually is achieved when $PaCO_2$ is abruptly lowered to 28 to 32 mm Hg; it may be considerably higher during sleep or when sedating drugs are given. Note that unlike CMV or synchronized intermittent mandatory ventilation (SIMV; see following), changes in set machine frequency during AMV have no effect on $\dot{V}_E$ unless this "backup" frequency is set high enough to terminate the patient's own respiratory efforts. Hence, AMV is *not* an appropriate mode for weaning.

Synchronized Intermittent Mandatory Ventilation

During SIMV, the intubated patient is connected to a single circuit that allows both spontaneous breathing and a set number of mechanical cycles timed to coincide with spontaneous effort. Ventilator breaths—volume cycled or pressure controlled—are interspersed to supplement spontaneous ventilation, which is usually pressure supported. Because SIMV can provide a wide range of ventilatory support, it can be used either as a full support mode or as a weaning mode, depending on the mandatory frequency selected.

Pressure-Support Ventilation

Description
Pressure-support ventilation (PSV) is a method with which each breath taken by a spontaneously breathing patient receives a pressure boost. After the breath is initiated, pressure builds rapidly toward an inspiratory pressure target. Airway pressure is then maintained constant at the level set by the clinician until flow decays to satisfy the machine's "off-switch" criterion. At relatively slow respiratory rates, the resulting airway pressure profile resembles a "square" wave. Because PSV is flow cycled (and therefore influenced by pleural pressure), the patient retains control of cycle length and tidal volume. Modern ventilators allow the clinician to modify the aggressiveness with which the pressure target is approached as well as the flow off-switch criterion to span the full spectrum of patient mechanics and requirements. PSV provides the basis for a number of other ventilatory modes, such as SIMV and volume-assured pressure support (VAPS).

Advantages
PSV hybridizes the power of the machine and the patient, providing assistance that ranges from no support at all to fully powered ventilation, depending on the machine's developed pressure relative to patient effort. Because the depth, length, and flow profile of the breath are influenced by the patient, well-adjusted PSV (with well-chosen amplitude, pressure ramp, and off-switch values) tends to be relatively comfortable in comparison with time-cycled modes. Adaptability to the vagaries of patient cycle length and effort can prove especially helpful for patients with erratic breathing patterns that otherwise would be difficult to adapt to a fixed flow profile or set inspiratory time (e.g., COPD, anxiety, Cheyne–Stokes breathing). The transition to spontaneous breathing is eased by the gradual removal of machine support (see Chapter 10). Although PSV has its widest application as a

weaning mode, it also is valuable in offsetting the resistive work required to breathe spontaneously through an ET tube, as during CPAP or SIMV. Another more sophisticated means for doing so, known as automatic tube compensation (ATC), offsets tube resistance by varying the applied pressure in proportion to flow. When used to support ventilation, the pressure-support level should be adjusted to maintain adequate tidal volume at an acceptable frequency (<30 breaths/min). In theory, PSV would provide sufficient power for the entire WOB if set to meet or exceed the average inspiratory pressure required per breath (P_{req}). For a normal subject breathing at a moderate rate, P_{req} is amazingly small, seldom exceeding 7 cm H_2O. For patients who are appropriate for weaning, $\dot{V}_E$ usually approximates 10 L/min or less, and P_{req} commonly does not exceed 10 to 15 cm H_2O. This explains why patients seem to be "weaning smoothly" until some rather low threshold value of PSV is reached at which point further reductions precipitate sudden decompensation.

Problems

PSV requires the ventilatory cycle to be patient-initiated and does not adjust itself to changes in the ease of chest inflation. To draw more help from the machine, the patient often adjusts frequency to reduce effort. PSV is not an ideal mode for patients with unstable ventilatory drive or highly variable thoracic impedance (e.g., bronchospasm, copious secretions, or changing auto-PEEP). Furthermore, because the ability of most ventilator systems to approximate a true square wave of airway pressure deteriorates as ventilatory demands increase, the average inspiratory pressure (and tidal volume) resulting from PSV tends to be frequency sensitive.

Humidifier and Respiratory Circuit

At the start of inspiration, the exhalation valve closes and airway pressure builds. PEEP is applied by causing the exhalation valve to close at a preset pressure level. Older valves imposed substantial expiratory resistance, but modern "active" valves are much more efficient in this regard. Any extra tubing inserted between the ET tube and the Y-connector extends the "anatomic" deadspace with that imposed by the apparatus, impairing ventilation efficiency.

With the upper airway bypassed, pressurized gas must be warmed and humidified before entering the trachea. (Humidification is also important when support is provided by a pressurized facemask [NIV], as many such patients inspire through the mouth, rather than through the nasal passages, and supplemental oxygen is inherently dry.) Disposable low-resistance heat and moisture exchangers (HMEs) or "artificial noses" may be used for patients with modest ventilatory requirements and minimal airway secretions (e.g., in the postoperative setting). By recovering a high percentage of the exhaled water vapor, these units are able to satisfactorily humidify inspired gas for most patients. These devices impose a little deadspace and increase expiratory resistance, especially when saturated with liquid or contaminated by secretions. Consequently, a given unit performs less well when used for extended periods (>24 h) or when provided to patients who cough frequently or whose ventilation power is compromised during spontaneous breathing (unless purposely designed or used with special attachments, disconnection of the ventilator is necessary to suction the airway). With acceptable efficiency, low price, and less maintenance cost, HMEs have become the default humidier choice in many intensive care units.

Another option, the "heated humidifier" ventilator circuits tend to perform better than HMEs when thickened secretions are a problem. These humidifiers maintain a fairly consistent temperature throughout the external circuit, keeping water vapor in its gaseous phase. These are largely successful in keeping condensate from forming before the Y-connector. Because warmed, fully saturated gas cools in unheated connecting tubing, some condensation ("rain-out") should occur in non-heated circuits. Using such equipment, a humidifier maladjustment or malfunction should be suspected if fine water droplets are not evident. The inspired temperature of fully saturated gas should be maintained at approximately 34°C to 37°C. If airway secretions are thick, the temperature should be raised to hydrate them (but not to exceed 37°C). Excessive "rain-out" may result in pooled liquid that can interfere with machine triggering or inadvertently empty into the lung during position changes, thereby injecting a bacterial inoculum or precipitating coughing or bronchospasm. Convincing recent studies indicate that frequent changes, disconnections, or manipulations of the external circuit increase the incidence of ventilator-associated pneumonia. Therefore, it is recommended to follow a circuit maintenance protocol in each intensive care unit.

TABLE 7-3   VENTILATOR SETUP
Mode
Backup frequency
PEEP
FiO_2
Target inspiratory pressure and time (pressure control)
Target tidal volume (volume control)
Inspiratory flow rate and wave shape (volume control)
Alarms
Apnea
Low exhaled tidal volume and/or $\dot{V}_E$
Low inspiratory pressure
Maximum peak airway pressure

Ventilator Setup

Ventilator Options and Settings

Major decisions in ventilator setup (Table 7-3) concern operating mode, FiO_2, tidal volume, guaranteed ventilator frequency, and baseline airway pressure (PEEP). Although minor adjustments can be made safely on the basis of vital signs, physical examination, subjective response, and pulse oximetry, initial choices and major setting adjustments should be verified by checking arterial blood gases drawn within 15 to 30 min of the change.

Mode

The pressure or volume-assist control modes generally are the best choices for full support because they allow the patient to control pH and $PaCO_2$ while the machine powers inflation. Trigger sensitivity should be set at the lowest level that avoids autocycling. It should be recognized, however, that *effective* triggering sensitivity is greatly reduced in the presence of dynamic hyperinflation (auto-PEEP). However, encouraging spontaneous breathing has shown some benefits such as lower requirements for sedation, increased venous return and cardiac output, and improved ventilation/perfusion ratio. For these reasons it seems prudent to promote *comfortable* spontaneous breathing from the onset of ventilatory support if the patient's clinical status permits.

Compared to AMV, SIMV allows lower mean intrathoracic pressure, minimizing impedance to venous return. Currently, SIMV is almost always used with pressure support or ATC for spontaneous (non–time-cycled) breaths. With PSV applied, intermittent mandatory ventilation provides a useful alternative to sedation and control for patients who have difficulty synchronizing rhythmically with the ventilator during AMV or PCV, whose minute ventilation needs vary widely, or who require some mechanical assistance but hyperventilate inappropriately when allowed to trigger the machine on every cycle (e.g., central neurogenic hyperventilation, anxiety). Unless each non-mandated breath is supported with the same pressure used during pressure- or volume-targeted machine cycles, the ventilatory workload of SIMV increases in proportion to the number of spontaneous breaths taken.

CPAP alone may be appropriate for patients who comfortably maintain ventilation but require airway protection and/or improved arterial oxygenation (e.g., mild forms of ARDS). However, a low level of pressure support is usually added to overcome ET tube resistance.

Other Ventilatory Options   Variation of the airway pressure baseline around which spontaneous efforts are made has spawned airway pressure-release ventilation (APRV) and its variants (Bi-Phasic and Bi-Level ventilation). In certain situations, it is desirable either to adjust mid-inspiratory flow in response to changing patient needs or, alternatively, to restrict maximal cycling pressure but ensure delivery of a specified tidal volume. In response, microprocessor capability has given rise to such "combination" modes as pressure-regulated volume control (PRVC) (also branded as autoflow or VC+), volume support (VSV), VAPS, and augmented minute volume (Fig. 7-5). This group of modes is known as dual-control modes, because they allow the clinician to set a volume target as the ventilator delivers pressure-controlled breaths.

Pressure-Regulated Volume Control   This mode satisfies a tidal volume with the least pressure control that accomplishes it within the preset inspiratory time. Pressure is continuously regulated in response to changing inflation impedance to satisfy the tidal volume objective. It should be noted that unlike pressure control, the patient may receive no help at all from the ventilator if a satisfactory tidal volume is attained through patient effort alone.

Volume Support   In VSV, flow-cycled pressure support is adjusted up or down, depending on the tidal volume and minute ventilation that result in comparison with the preset minimums. Minute ventilation is the primary target variable, and a tidal volume minimum is guaranteed. When breathing frequency falls, tidal volume can increase by as much as 50% over the baseline target in an attempt to satisfy the $\dot{V}_E$ minimum. Its advantages are to

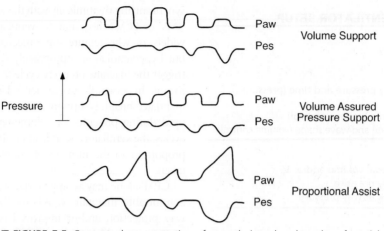

■ **FIGURE 7-5** Conceptual representation of recently introduced modes of partial ventilatory support. In VSV, pressure support is automatically regulated to achieve preset targets for minimum tidal volume and minute ventilation. In VAPS (also known as pressure augmentation), a fixed pressure-support level may be augmented by constant flow at end inspiration, as is necessary to achieve a preselected tidal volume target. Proportional assist ventilation increases the pressure output of the ventilator parallel to the vigor of patient effort, thereby acting as an auxiliary set of ventilatory muscles, the strength of which is regulated by the clinician. P_{aw}, airway pressure; P_{es}, pleural (esophageal) pressure

provide the positive attributes of PSV with assured levels of tidal volume and minute ventilation. Like PRVC, the ventilator's supporting pressure is an inverse function of breathing effort.

Volume-Assured Pressure Support In VAPS, a fixed level of pressure support is supplemented by gas from a backup flow generator if the PSV becomes insufficient to meet a minimum tidal volume objective. Thus, if lung compliance decreases or airway resistance increases, the set tidal volume is delivered by increasing the applied pressure (Fig. 7-5).

Proportional-Assisted Ventilation Proportional-assisted ventilation (PAV) was designed to increase or decrease airway pressure in proportion to patient effort by amplifying airway pressure proportional to inspiratory flow and volume. PAV is designed to adjust the amount of support it provides moment by moment in real time, in accordance with patient need. It was the first mode to allow *intracycle* adjustment to moment by moment patient effort, while starting and stopping with greater precision than ever before possible. PAV does this by sensing flow demand and elastic counter-pressure, assisting ventilation with a uniform proportionally to its perception of patient effort. Resistance and flow guide the pressure component supplied to overcome resistive forces, while elastance and inspired volume guide the pressure supplied to counterbalance elastic forces. Because these may frequently change, resistance and elastance are frequently and automatically estimated in the latest machines. The overall amplitude of pressure assistance (a controllable input) can be varied by the caregiver from negligible to near full support. In effect, PAV acts as a powerful auxiliary muscle whose strength can be adjusted by the caregiver. It requires a backup (apnea) mode and settings in the event that the central drive is suppressed. Early problems with PAV's inherent insensitivity to auto-PEEP, circuit leaks and "runaway" (overassisted) breaths have been addressed, but still present some difficulties. Despite its conceptual attractiveness, few controlled trials convincingly demonstrate PAV's superiority over modern implementations of more traditional options that are set aprropriately.

Neurally Adjusted Ventilatory Assist (NAVA) The ideal of using the patient's own respiratory center nerve traffic to regulate the intensity of machine's output has been brought closer to reality by using the conditioned, integrated electromyographic signal from the phrenic nerve to control machine flow. A purpose-designed esophageal catheter is required to capture the required signal. Whether the respiratory system controller of the diseased patient is a reliable, appropriate, and safe governor for machine output is a question being actively investigated. By side-stepping the need to measure flows and mechanics, NAVA effectively accounts for auto-PEEP and circuit leaks. As a just-introduced option, however, its practical value in daily practice is currently unconfirmed.

Automatic Tube Compensation   ATC compensates for ET tube resistance via closed-loop control of calculated tracheal pressure. In other words, ATC is similar to PSV, but the pressure applied by the ventilator varies as a function of ET tube resistance and flow demand. The proposed advantages of ATC are (a) to overcome the WOB imposed by the artificial airway, (b) to improve patient–ventilator synchrony by varying flow commensurate with demand, and (c) to reduce air trapping by compensating for imposed expiratory resistance. Most of the interest in ATC revolves around eliminating the imposed WOB during inspiration. However, during expiration there is also a flow-dependent pressure drop across the ET tube. ATC may also compensate for that flow resistance by lowering the pressure in the expiratory circuit limb transiently from its PEEP setting, helping reduce effective expiratory resistance and unintentional hyperflation. ATC added to PSV may increase the tidal volume substantially.

Inspired Oxygen Fraction (FiO$_2$)

Initially, FiO$_2$ should be set to err deliberately on the high side, with later adjustment guided by arterial oximetry or blood gases. Immediately after intubation, for example, it is generally prudent to administer pure oxygen until adequate arterial oxygenation has been confirmed. Although adjustments of FiO$_2$ and PEEP are often made using the continuous output from a pulse oximeter, it should be considered that the accuracy of such instruments is frequently suboptimal. It is recommended to use FiO$_2$ less than 0.6, with the objective of decreasing the risk of injury related to biochemically noxious reactive oxygen species.

Tidal Volume

Inspired tidal volume can either be a preset (controlled) parameter or a dependent variable that is taken into account when selecting the controlled pressure during pressure-targeted ventilation. For otherwise healthy individuals, relatively large tidal volumes can be given without generating high pressures and may, in fact, be necessary for adequate

patient comfort. On occasion, tidal volumes higher than 12 mL/kg may be needed to satisfy the demands of a hyperpneic subject with normal ventilatory mechanics. A good starting value for most critically ill patients, however, is 6 to 8 mL/kg of ideal lean body weight (IBW), provided that plateau pressure measured during spontaneous breathing does not rise above 30 cm H$_2$O. (Of course, obese patients do not have larger lungs.) The tidal volume delivered to a patient with a reduced number of available units must be reduced accordingly (e.g., ARDS, pneumonectomy, interstitial fibrosis). Monotonous shallow breaths (<5 mL/kg IBW) encourage microatelectasis unless interrupted periodically by larger inflations or offset by PEEP. If very small tidal volumes and low levels of PEEP are in use, one or more larger breaths (sighs generally 1.5 to 3 times the V_T) may be advisable every 10 to 15 min to avert problems, but this point is controversial. As pressure builds during inspiration, a fraction of the inspired gas is stored in tubing and other compressible elements of the ventilator circuit (internal reservoirs, filters, humidifiers, etc.). Most modern equipment automatically adjusts for the circuit compression losses. Measurements of exhaled volume potentially include compressible volume because tubing contracts during expiratory decompression. Again, most modern ventilators compensate for compressible volume on their readout. Under conditions of controlled ventilation, the discrepancy between set or measured inspiratory tidal volume and exhaled tidal volume can quantitate the severity of a bronchopleural fistula or of the leak past a deflated ET tube cuff.

Frequency

The backup frequency should be chosen in conjunction with V_T or pressure setting to provide minute ventilation ($\dot{V}_E$) adequate to maintain pH and patient comfort. In the assist mode, this "backup" rate should be adjusted to a frequency sufficient to provide 70% to 80% of the patient's usual $\dot{V}_E$, in case of complete failure of the patient to trigger. In the AMV mode, any adjustments in the set frequency—up or down—have no effect on $\dot{V}_E$ or on the level of machine support, so long as the patient triggers each breath.

Other Settings

Flow-controlled, volume-cycled ventilators allow the physician to choose the inspiratory flow rate and to define its contour (square or decelerating).

Inappropriately rapid inspiratory flow rates may worsen the distribution of ventilation in some patients; however, a decelerating flow waveform helps satisfy rapid early inspiratory flow demand. Although peak pressure rises as flow rate increases, the mean airway pressure averaged over the entire ventilatory cycle may remain unchanged or even fall as flow rate increases. The extent to which the ventilator takes up the inspiratory WOB is a function of the margin with which flow delivery exceeds flow demand. It is mandatory that the flow metered by the ventilator meets or exceeds the patient's flow demand throughout inspiration. Otherwise, the ventilator not only fails to reduce the WOB, but also may force the patient to pull against the resistance of the ventilator circuitry, as well as against internal impedance to airflow and chest expansion. This often happens midcycle when flow control is applied with a decelerating waveform.

Comfortably rapid inspiratory flow rates also are desirable to ensure that the machine completes inflation before the patient's own ventilatory rhythm cycles into its exhalation phase. Delayed opening of the exhalation valve causes the patient to "fight" or "pressure limit" the ventilator. When the ventilator pressure limits, the full tidal volume is not delivered but vented to atmosphere. As a rule, the ventilator's *average* inspiratory flow should be approximately 4.0 times the minute ventilation. Peak flow should be set 20% to 30% higher than this average value when the decelerating waveform is used. Peak airway pressure is influenced by inspiratory flow rate and waveform, airway resistance, tidal volume, and total thoracic compliance. During an end-inspiratory pause, the plateau airway pressure reflects the maximum stretching force applied to a typical alveolus and surrounding chest wall. To avoid barotrauma, maximum pressure (alarm and "pop-off" pressure) should be set to no more than 15 to 20 cm H_2O above the peak dynamic cycling pressure observed during a typical breath during constant flow. The pop-off alarm should be set more closely than this (within 10 cm H_2O) if a decelerating flow waveform or pressure control is used because under those conditions, end-inspiratory dynamic and static (plateau) pressures are not as widely separated.

When the patient is passive, the inflation hold setting allows for calculation of respiratory system compliance, estimates maximum alveolar pressure, and when constant flow is in use allows determination of resistance as well. A temporary inflation hold also can be used to check for circuit leaks, as circuit

pressure will continue to decline during the pause interval rather than "plateau" as gas bleeds off.

Pressure control requires selection of the pressure target and either inspiratory time, inspiratory time percentage, or the ratio of inspiratory to expiratory time—the I:E ratio. (In volume-cycled ventilation, the I:E ratio usually is set indirectly by specifying inhaled volume, frequency, and mean inspiratory flow rate.) In general, shorter I:E ratios allow more time for exhalation and reduce mean intrathoracic pressure. To avoid gas trapping, many ventilators provide a visual warning or auditory alarm when the I:E ratio exceeds 1:1 (duty cycle > 0.5). This threshold defines inverse ratio ventilation (IRV).

Newer Modes to Improve Ventilation

The primary purposes of mechanical ventilation are to achieve adequate alveolar ventilation, to relieve an excessive breathing workload, and to improve oxygen exchange. The mainstays of ventilator assistance have been flow-controlled ("volume-controlled") ventilation or AMV, PCV, PSV, and PSV combined with either PCV or AMV–SIMV. Similarly, enrichment of FiO_2 and the addition of end-expiratory pressure (PEEP, CPAP) remain the primary means of supporting oxygenation. Over the years, other interesting techniques have been developed, and a generous handful has now gained traction in clinical practice. These innovations take the form of newer modes of ventilation or of adjuncts to ventilatory support. Several designed for better interfacing with the patient making breathing effort are outlined in the section on "modes" above. Each has a defensible physiologic rationale but little objective supporting data to document clinical benefit. One interesting approach adaptive support ventilation (ASV) uses is conventional ventilation but attempts to modify not only the pressure applied during pressure-controlled SIMV but also the frequency of delivered machine breaths to adapt to changing patient needs. The machine algorithm is guided by the breathing frequency, the depth of the breath, and the estimated WOB. By adjusting backup frequency and magnitude of pressure applied, the breathing pattern is made to lie within a hypothetical ideal "zone"—sufficient ventilation with pressure not too high, frequency not too high, and breathing workload optimized according to the "equation of motion" for the respiratory system (see Chapter 5). In a sense, like PAV and NAVA, this mode is geared to the breathing pattern—not micro managing *within* the breath, but keeping the pattern consistent with *the clinician's* clinical goals under changing conditions of requirement, demand, and mechanics.

High-Frequency Ventilation

7 The collective term "high-frequency ventilation" (HFV) refers to methods of ventilation that intentionally depart from the breathing patterns encountered in spontaneous breathing. Tidal volumes less than or equal to the calculated anatomic deadspace are moved at frequencies ranging from 60 to 3,000 cycles/min. The mechanisms by which these varied forms of HFV establish alveolar ventilation is uncertain and differ among techniques. Peripheral airway pressure is generally higher than measured central airway pressure, and mean alveolar pressures may not differ greatly from—or even exceed—those observed during conventional ventilation of similar effectiveness. Although several variants of HFV (high-frequency positive-pressure ventilation and jet ventilation) are of considerable historical significance, high-frequency oscillation (HFO) has garnered most recent attention for ICU applications.

High-Frequency Oscillation

During HFO, a very small tidal volume (1 to 3 mL/kg) is moved to and fro by a piston membrane at extremely high frequencies (500 to 3,000 cycles/min). Fresh gas is introduced as a continuous flow, and a narrow-gauge venting tube (a "low-pass filter") provides egress for waste gas. Delivered tidal volume is determined by driving pressure and depends on the relative resistances for gas flow through the airway and the bias flow lines. Although the peak alveolar pressure is generally less, *mean* airway pressure is usually set higher than during conventional ventilation to keep the airways patent. Carbon dioxide elimination is a function of stroke (tidal) volume and paradoxically to the inverse of vibration frequency. Unlike jet ventilation, both phases of the ventilatory cycle are controlled actively by the oscillator's piston. Consequently, auto-PEEP less frequently poses a serious problem. Although fresh gas must be provided through the airway, pulsatility of the air column may originate either in the airway or at the lung surface. In experimental animals, mere vibration of the chest wall has successfully established effective gas exchange. Exactly how HFO accomplishes ventilation,

however, continues to be investigated. Although improved gas mixing and facilitated diffusion are undoubtedly important, pulsatility itself does not seem to be a strict requirement for *some* alveolar ventilation to occur. A continuous stream of O_2 introduced just beyond the carina can maintain arterial oxygenation and accomplish significant CO_2 washout in apneic animals, a technique dubbed "apneic diffusion," "continuous flow apneic ventilation," or "tracheal insufflation of oxygen" (TRIO). Although not currently advocated for clinical use, apneic ventilation may have some use as a temporizing measure in emergent settings in which standard ET intubation cannot be accomplished.

Applications of High-Frequency Ventilation

HFV can silence the normal respiratory rhythm and phasic variations of chest volume. This feature has proven advantageous during lithotripsy and in delicate surgical procedures in which gross thoracic motions must be minimized. Because HFV does not require a cuffed ET tube, it has been helpful in bronchoscopy and laryngeal surgery. HFV occasionally is effective in the setting of bronchopleural fistulas that are refractory to closure, in part because of lower peak airway pressures. Fistulas also tend to draw less flow at higher frequencies because the inertance of the fistulous pathway is greater than that of alternative routes. Because high airway cycling pressure may be instrumental in causing airway and parenchymal forms of ventilator-induced lung injury, HFV may have a role in preventing these complications in neonates and perhaps in older children and adults with ARDS as well. If not used in a high PEEP range, "recruiting" maneuvers, in which high pressures are sustained for 0.5 to 2 min, may be needed to avoid atelectasis and to preserve optimal gas exchange. HFO has been reported to compare favorably to conventional therapy in patients with acute lung injury, presumably because its relatively low plateau pressure and relatively high end-expiratory pressure effectively recruit lung tissue, thereby improving oxygenation while applying a "lung-protective" approach. It remains debatable whether any HFV technique holds an advantage over lung-protective approaches using conventional ventilators set to deliver modest tidal volumes and adequate PEEP. With occasional exceptions, HFV appears to offer little advantage with regard to cardiovascular performance, lung water accumulation, or gas exchange at equivalent levels of end-expiratory alveolar pressure. Indeed, some patients with high ventilation requirements or high thoracic impedance cannot be ventilated successfully by HFV. Finally, monitoring alveolar pressure remains a vexing clinical problem during HFV, and currently available machines are quite loud in comparison with conventional alternatives.

Nontraditional Modes to Improve Oxygenation

Pressure-Controlled Inverse Ratio Ventilation

Description and Rationale

To prevent gas trapping, it has long been standard practice to allow at least as much time for exhalation as for inhalation; however, for certain patients with impaired oxygenation, gas exchange may improve when the I:E ratio is extended to values greater than 1:1 (Fig. 7-6). Inversion of the ratio prevents the patient from initiating or expelling a breath during the lengthy inspiratory period. IRV appears to offer no consistent advantage over conventional patterns that achieve similar levels of mean and end-expiratory alveolar pressures and is now seldom used. Occasionally, it may be worth considering when dangerously high plateau pressures would otherwise be required. It is now used only as a technique of last resort in cases of ARDS, even though IRV is most rational and seems to be most effective in the earliest phase, when lung units are most recruitable. At usual frequencies, inverse ratios greater than 2:1 are seldom helpful and may be dangerous. IRV should seldom be used for longer than 48 to 72 h before reassessing its relative advantage over conventional ratio ventilation. IRV is not an appropriate mode of treatment for severely obstructed patients.

When using IRV, a pressure control waveform has the distinct advantage of safety when compared with flow-controlled, volume-cycled methods that leave alveolar pressure unregulated. IRV requires a passive patient, so deep sedation and/or paralysis usually are necessary. With breathing effort silenced, adequate circulating volume is required so as to avoid the hemodynamic consequences of its high mean airway pressure.

Airway Pressure Release and Bi-Phasic Pressure

APRV and Bi-Phasic airway pressure (BIPAP) can be thought of as variants of IRV intended for use by spontaneously breathing patients in acute respiratory failure (Figs. 7-6 and 7-7). In this context, BIPAP should not be confused with Bi-Level, commercially termed "Bi-PAP," a mode designed primarily for NIV and virtually synonymous with pressure support with or without added CPAP. The idea behind APRV is to provide added ventilatory support for a patient who needs high levels of CPAP for oxygenation but who can provide most of the ventilatory power requirement without machine assistance. Both APRV and BIPAP allow ventilatory efforts to occur around an elevated pressure baseline (CPAP or high pressure) over a set time period (time high) but also depressurize the system (partially or completely) to a lower pressure baseline for brief periods (time low) at a frequency set by the physician. After release, fresh

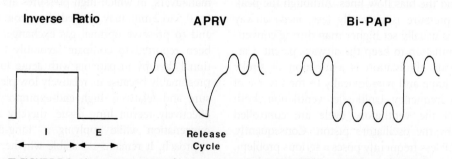

■ FIGURE 7-6 Airway pressure waveforms corresponding to IRV, APRV, and Bi-Phasic airway pressure (BIPAP). In IRV, the airway is pressurized for more than one half of the total cycle length, increasing mean airway pressure. Deep sedation (with or without muscle relaxants) may be necessary to suppress spontaneous breathing efforts. APRV allows the patient to breathe spontaneously around an elevated pressure baseline, which is periodically released and reestablished, thereby aiding spontaneous ventilation. BIPAP extends the release cycle, allowing spontaneous ventilation to occur at each of the two CPAP levels.

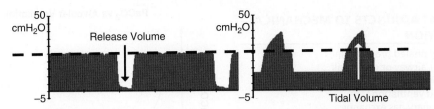

■ **FIGURE 7-7** Machine-aided cycles of APRV and SIMV. APRV emphasizes the maintenance of high lung volume and full recruitment with an open circuit, whereas SIMV achieves similar ventilation assist from the ventilator with lower mean airway pressure. Spontaneous breathing cycles occur in both modes but are not shown (dashed line = maximal alveolar pressure).

gas enters as CPAP rebuilds to its higher value, improving ventilation. With APRV, the original idea was to keep release time very short—about one deflation time constant, re-building to the higher pressure level before lung collapse occurs (deliberate auto-PEEP). PEEP can be added, but this detracts from the driving pressure of release cycles. BIPAP differs from APRV primarily in allowing the option for extended periods of spontaneous breathing at both selected levels of end-expiratory pressure. Typically, APRV has a low time of about 0.8 s—allowing no more than one deflation during the transient circuit decompression, whereas BIPAP allows for an extended low time. Weaning occurs by dropping the high pressure and diminishing the number of release cycles. As commercially implemented, pressure support can be added to the spontaneous breaths that occur on either pressure baseline.

Advantages

These "open circuit" techniques can be viewed as methods to aid in ventilation and/or elevate airway pressure to improve oxygenation. Phasic release cycles function in a manner similar to the machine cycles of SIMV, insofar as they augment ventilation. The difference is that high peak airway pressures generated with a closed expiratory valve are avoided, and spontaneous breathing can occur at any time. As with IRV, sustained higher airway pressure exerts prolonged traction and improves ventilation in slow time constant units. Unlike IRV, however, the patient remains conscious and can adjust alveolar ventilation to the extent that he or she is able to do so, often aided by pressure support. BIPAP can therefore provide the entire range of ventilatory support (ranging from completely controlled ventilation to unsupported breathing), depending on the difference between pressure baselines and the frequency

and duration of the release cycles. For this reason, it serves as the primary platform for ventilatory support in at least one modern ventilator system.

Disadvantages

The efficacy of the pressure-release cycle depends on (a) the duration of release, (b) the mechanical properties of the chest, (c) the level to which airway pressure is allowed to fall, and (d) the cycling frequency between the two pressure baselines. As ventilation support increases, mean airway pressure falls, dissipating some of the oxygen-exchange benefit of the higher CPAP level. More importantly, their value is questionable for patients with significant airflow obstruction or severely reduced lung compliance. In the first instance, the brief release cycles of APRV are relatively ineffectual because of delayed lung decompression. In the second instance, the work of spontaneous breathing may be too great to sustain. Some concern has been raised that like all pressure-targeted modes, excessive transalveolar pressures might be generated during vigorous efforts made on the high pressure baseline. While certainly a potential problem, in practice, observational studies have shown this to be unlikely. Although APRV and BIPAP need more studies to firmly establish their clinical indications, they are used increasingly—especially in the care of patients with acute lung injury and ARDS.

Adjuncts to Mechanical Ventilation

Techniques to Improve Gas Exchange

Recently, there has been increasing interest in developing techniques capable of maintaining or improving pulmonary gas exchange without the need to elevate alveolar and pleural pressures

TABLE 7-4   ADJUNCTS TO MECHANICAL VENTILATION

Nitric oxide/inhaled prostacyclin
Vibration of airway or chest wall
Tracheal gas insufflation
Partial liquid ventilation
Extra-pulmonary gas exchange
Permissive hypercapnia
Prone positioning

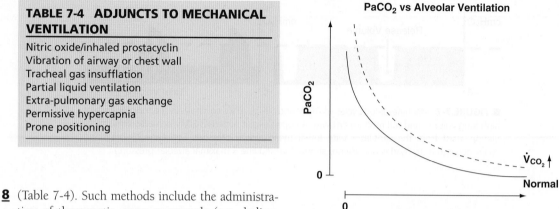

FIGURE 7-8   Relationship of $PaCO_2$ to alveolar ventilation (V_{ALV}). Because this relationship is curvilinear, relatively small changes in V_{ALV} that occur at low levels of ventilation have a dramatic effect on $PaCO_2$. An increase in CO_2 production ($\dot{V}CO_2$) results in a higher $PaCO_2$ for any specified level of ventilation.

8 (Table 7-4). Such methods include the administration of therapeutic gases or aerosols (e.g., heliox, nitric oxide, and inhaled prostacyclin), alterations of body position (prone repositioning), deadspace bypass or washout (intratracheal pulmonary ventilation, tracheal gas insufflation), alteration of the gas exchange medium (partial liquid ventilation), and extrapulmonary gas exchange (extracorporeal membrane oxygenation, extracorporeal CO_2 removal), and intravenacaval gas exchange via gas-permeable catheters (IVOX and Hattler). Some, like the passive arteriovenous and pump-driven venovenous circuits, seem to hold genuine potential to improve the care of patients with life-threatening respiratory failure. Several of these techniques are discussed elsewhere in this volume (see Chapters 24 and 25).

Permissive Hypercapnia

One important "adjunct" to ventilation simply relaxes the ventilation target when the system is severely compromised. Permissive hypercapnia is a ventilatory strategy that assigns higher priority to avoiding injurious pressure than to maintaining normal levels of alveolar ventilation. In the settings of acute lung injury and asthma, high alveolar pressures can injure fragile tissues or compromise hemodynamics. Allowing $PaCO_2$ to rise above baseline values is perhaps the simplest technique for reducing the ventilatory workload, the pressure cost of breathing, and/or the total number of machine cycles needed per minute. As $PaCO_2$ rises, each exhaled breath of a given volume eliminates more CO_2 than it would during normocapnia, thereby improving CO_2 excretion efficiency (Fig. 7-8). With reduced ventilation requirements, smaller tidal volumes can be delivered, lowering the peak and mean inflation pressures and, consequently, the work of spontaneous breathing. Because ventilatory power varies as the second power of $\dot{V}_E$, small reductions in $\dot{V}_E$ can reduce effort and transpulmonary pressure impressively.

Gradual increases in $PaCO_2$ (extending over a few hours) shift *intracellular* pH minimally and are generally well tolerated, even to quite high concentrations of $PaCO_2$. As a rule, patients *without* coexisting β blockade, intracranial pathology, hemodynamic instability, severe pulmonary hypertension, or uncorrected hypoxemia function well at pH values ≥7.15. Indeed, elite athletes typically allow acidosis of this magnitude during maximal exercise. Deep sedation (and occasionally, chemical paralysis) is often required during buildup to the hypercapnic plateau. As clinical status improves, normocapnia is restored gradually. Normalization of pH at a higher level of $PaCO_2$ obligates HCO_3^- retention, which usually blunts ventilatory drive. Although multiple animal experimental studies have shown benefit with the use of permissive hypercapnia, permissive hypercapnia has been reported to be helpful in reducing the mortality of status asthma and ARDS only in single-center retrospective studies. Although still viewed as experimental by some practitioners, lower pH is a natural consequence of a lung-protective ventilation strategy and of itself may actually afford anti-inflammatory lung-protective advantages.

Noninvasive Ventilation

Many patients require only modest pressures to maintain compensated ventilation. With the increasing availability of improved interfaces and efficient valving mechanisms, the option of applying ventilatory support by occlusive mask has become widely exercised—both for chronic nocturnal support and increasingly for acute in-hospital applications. NIV may be used to quickly apply ventilatory assistance without the risk and discomfort of intubation. Infection risk is considerably lower with NIV than in those who are intubated. Such attractive characteristics have numerous applications in emergency centers as well as in-hospital intensive and subacute settings, especially now that much improved, relatively comfortable mask interfaces are available. For example, NIV may sometimes provide a bridge across the treacherous postextubation period in marginally compensated patients recently weaned from ventilatory support. NIV allows communication and, when the mask is temporarily removed, expectoration and eating. There is no major penalty for starting and stopping ventilatory support—indeed, brief intervals off the mask every several hours may help improve tolerance. These methods are often helpful for patients who are not candidates for intubation (e.g., patients with advanced directives not to intubate). For well-selected patients, noninvasive techniques may obviate the need for intubation altogether and help avoid infections and other complications of securing the airway. A few centers report improved mortality rates for patients who are able to accept this treatment. NIV seems to be particularly helpful when implemented at an early stage for noncomatose patients with rapidly reversible diseases (e.g., congestive heart failure, exacerbated chronic airflow obstruction, moderate asthma, transient upper airway obstruction) and for patients for whom intubation is not an acceptable option. The worth of NIV for patients with acute pulmonary edema (especially of the "flash" variety) is now proved, and NIV should be considered strongly in combined cardiorespiratory failure and for those patients with neuromuscular weakness, nocturnal hypoxemia, or hypoventilation.

For marginally compensated patients, noninvasive techniques may prove especially helpful at night, when sleep impairs ventilatory drive or immobilizes the nondiaphragmatic musculature crucial to maintaining adequate ventilation. Indeed, nocturnal nasal ventilation (by nasal mask or other occlusive fitting) seems to be useful over extended periods for selected patients with irreversible neuromuscular disease, sleep apnea, and airflow obstruction. Intermittent rest of fatigued respiratory muscles and, in a minority of cases, improved

lung compliance may result. The precise reason for nocturnal NIV's benefit during waking hours remains undetermined. It has been suggested that nocturnal support may allow the sleep quality needed to preserve adequate ventilatory drive and muscle strength. This is of particular interest in the ICU environment, where sleep architecture is highly abnormal.

Despite its clear value for well-selected patients, NIV has important limitations as well (Table 7-5). NIV helps less consistently in acute parenchymal lung disease (e.g., ARDS), particularly when the ventilatory problem is far advanced, slowly evolving, or unexpected to resolve quickly. Combative or comatose patients; those who cannot be attended or monitored closely; and those with copious secretions, coronary ischemia, or massive obesity are decidedly poor candidates. However, NIV often is successful when applied early enough to cooperative patients by vigilant, well-trained personnel. Gastric distention is unusual at peak mask pressures lower than 20 cm H_2O. Although skin irritation, nasal congestion, sinus discomfort, impeded expectoration, secretion thickening, sleep disruption, and claustrophobia are often troublesome, perhaps the greatest logistical problem continues to be mask leaks, which can develop quickly. These not only compromise ventilation, but also place oxygen or PEEP-dependent patients at risk for hypoxemia and its sequelae. Recent developments in mask technology have dramatically improved the range, quality and comfort of mask interfaces. The need to maintain the patient arousable can limit the application

TABLE 7-5 NONINVASIVE VENTILATION: BENEFITS AND LIMITATIONS

BENEFITS	LIMITATIONS
Easy to implement and remove	Psychic distress
Improves comfort	Slow reversal
Reduces need for sedation	Hypoxemia when removed
Preserves speech/ swallowing	Eye irritation
Preserves cough	Difficult airway hygiene
Avoids tube resistance	No airway protection
Avoids tube complications	Facial discomfort
Upper airway trauma	Gastric distention
"Mini" aspiration	Limited ventilatory capability
Pulmonary infection	
Dilates upper airway	

of sedatives and analgesics. In many hospitals, the burgeoning use of NIV, combined with the need for specialized surveillance, has given rise to nursing units specializing in this modality.

Considering the many factors that potentially may influence the effectiveness of NIV, perhaps it is not surprising that experience and enthusiasm for this technique vary widely across centers. Apart from patient selection, among the most important elements of success with NIV are rigorous training of support personnel, early intervention, and dedicated efforts to coax and encourage the patient to accept NIV in the first few hours of its application. As a rule, attempts to make NIV work should not persist longer than 1 to 2 h without clear evidence for benefit and tolerance.

Devices intended for chronic nocturnal prophylaxis against the upper airway obstruction of sleep apnea are not optimal for use in the acute arena. Many such machines are limited in the concentrations of inspired oxygen they can provide. Modern NIV equipment can provide well-hydrated inspired gas with precisely adjusted FiO_2, minimal CO_2 rebreathing, and good sensitivity to patient cycling rhythm and flow demand. The best units are also appropriately alarmed. Previously, the lack of such features posed serious deficiencies for the application of purpose-designed NIV equipment in ICU applications. Although still imperfect regarding accuracy, the current ability of modern units to monitor delivered tidal volume, minute ventilation, and leak magnitude greatly assist the caregiver in adjusting the applied mask pressures. It should be noted that when deadspace is minimized by reducing the tubing length between the Y-piece and a low-volume mask (similar to that used in bag-mask resuscitation equipment) a modern ICU ventilator can be effectively used in NIV applications, a feature that is especially helpful in the immediate postextubation period.

Generally speaking, NIV is applied with a combination of a modified pressure support and CPAP across a pressure range of 0 to 25 cm H_2O. Higher pressures are very poorly tolerated and require sealing forces, raising the risk for complications. In common parlance, NIV of this type is often referred to as "Bi-PAP," with the inspiratory pressure (sum of pressure support and CPAP) termed "IPAP" and the CPAP level termed "EPAP." The underlying principles of successful application of NIV are identical to those already described for pressure support and CPAP. In the nonintubated patient, CPAP takes

on the added potential role of maintaining upper airway patency—a useful characteristic in the postextubation period, in patients with laryngeal or glottic swelling, and in those with obstructive sleep apnea. As a rule, CPAP levels exceeding 8 to 10 cm H_2O are not well tolerated for extended periods. Because the majority of patients treated in the ICU breathe dry, oxygen-enriched gas with high levels of minute ventilation and are mouth breathers, adequate hydration of the gas stream is essential. This is particularly important to remember when the patient has been recently extubated, has impaired swallowing and/or has a tendency to form and retain mouth and airway secretions.

GENERAL APPROACH TO THE VENTILATED PATIENT

The complex interactions of the patient and ventilator must be approached in a systematic fashion to optimize machine performance, establish synchrony, and minimize hazards (Table 7-6). A number of important questions must be asked in the daily assessment of the ventilated patient.

Patient Status

1. *Are cycling pressures excessive?*
   Have they changed? Are pressures and tidal volumes consistent breath-to-breath? Are any changes attributable to alterations in resistance or compliance? (Or, alternatively, are flow, tidal volume, or PEEP different with unchanging mechanics?)
2. *Are there reversible factors impeding airflow (bronchospasm, secretions) or worsening the compliance of the lung (new infiltrate, atelectasis) or the chest*

TABLE 7-6 BEDSIDE EVALUATION OF THE VENTILATED PATIENT

Mental status
Spontaneous breathing rhythm
Minute ventilation requirement
Muscular strength
Secretion character and volume
Breathing effort and synchrony
pH and gas exchange
Breath sounds (intensity, distribution, symmetry)
Chest radiograph, chest CT, and echocardiogram
Mode of cycling
Cycling pressure (compliance/resistance)
Medications
Complications and practical problems

wall (*agitation, ascites, pleural effusion, abdominal distention*)?

Do secretion volume and character suggest respiratory infection, pulmonary hemorrhage, or ongoing aspiration of oropharyngeal or gastric contents? Is there any sign of unaddressed congestive heart failure, volume overload, volume depletion, or sepsis?

3. *What is the true minute ventilation requirement?*

To determine whether a high $\dot{V}_E$ is related to drive, metabolic requirement, acidosis, or iatrogenic hyperventilation, $\dot{V}_E$ must be interpreted in conjunction with $PaCO_2$, pH, and the physical examination. The variability of $\dot{V}_E$ is an important clue to the contribution of anxiety, agitation, or other reversible drivers of ventilation.

4. *How hard is the patient working to breathe?*

Is the patient making spontaneous breathing efforts? What is the drive to breathe? Are there signs of fatigue—elevated respiratory rate, abdominal paradox, irregular breathing rhythm? What are the pH and $PaCO_2$? During which mode of ventilation, PEEP level, and position were blood gases assessed? The implications of respiratory acidosis, for example, are much different for CMV (underventilation), AMV (reduced drive), or low-level SIMV (reduced drive, inadequate strength).

5. *Is the patient still ventilator-dependent?*

What is the ventilatory requirement and what is driving it (metabolic need, acidosis, agitation, hyperventilation)? Are cycling pressures high or low? Is the patient alert, strong, and able to cough strongly? If the patient is unweanable, is dependency likely to change anytime soon? Should a tracheostomy be scheduled? Can NIV be substituted?

6. *What is the patient's comfort level?*

Is there evidence of agitation or distress? Does any discomfort relate to pain, visceral distention, anxiety, fever, or maladjusted ventilator? Is inadequate or excessive sedation being given? Does discomfort originate in patient–ventilator dyssynchrony?

Ventilator Status

1. Are ventilator connections appropriate? Are the connectors tight? Is the ET tube cuff well sealed and is the circuit tubing unkinked and water-free?

2. Is there a need to raise or lower the overall level of machine support for oxygenation or ventilation? Is there an appropriate $PAO_2:PaO_2$ ratio? Should PEEP be adjusted? Is a change in ventilation mode or cycling frequency indicated to increase or decrease support?

3. Are machine adjustments in mode, flow rate, corrected tidal volume, or PEEP required? Are airway pressures during ventilator cycles uniform and of expected shape, indicating synchrony of patient and ventilator breathing cycles?

■ SUGGESTED READINGS

Branson RD, Johannigman JA. What is the evidence base for the newer ventilation modes? *Respir Care.* 2004;49(7):742–760.

Chatburn RL, Primiano FP Jr. A new system for understanding modes of mechanical ventilation. *Respir Care.* 2001;46(6):604–621.

Kondii E, Xirouchaki N, Georgopoulos D. Modulation and treatment of patient-ventilator dyssynchrony. *Curr Opin Crit Care.* 2007;13:84–89.

MacIntyre NR. Controversies in mechanical ventilation. *Clin Chest Med.* 2008;29(2):225–350.

Marini JJ. Breathing patterns as integrative weaning predictors—variations on a theme. *Crit Care Med.* 2006;34:2241–2243.

Papadakos PJ, Dooley J, eds. Mechanical ventilation. *Crit Care Clin.* 2007;23(2):117–337.

Siau C, Stewart TE. Current role of high-frequency oscillatory ventilation and airway pressure release ventilation in acute lung injury and acute respiratory distress syndrome. *Clin Chest Med.* 2008;29:265–275.

Sinderby C, Beck J. Proportional assist ventilation and neurally adjusted ventilatory assist—better approaches to patient-ventilator synchrony? *Clin Chest Med.* 2008;29:329–342.

Tobin MJ, ed. *Principles and Practice of Mechanical Ventilation.* 2nd Ed. New York: McGraw-Hill; 2006.

Wysocki M, Brunner JX. Closed loop ventilation: An emerging standard of care? *Crit Care Clin.* 2007;23:223–240.

Practical Problems and Complications of Mechanical Ventilation

KEY POINTS

1 Impaired cardiac output is most likely to result from mechanical ventilation when intravascular volume is depleted, vascular reflexes are impaired, and the patient is inflated passively with high mean airway pressures.

2 All forms of alveolar rupture induced by mechanical ventilation—interstitial emphysema, pneumomediastinum, pneumoperitoneum, subcutaneous emphysema, cyst formation, pneumothorax, and systemic gas embolism—have been described in both infants and adults. Certain high- pressure ventilatory patterns are strongly suspected to inflict nonrupture damage, such as diffuse lung injury and bronchopulmonary damage (ventilator induced lung injury).

3 The pathophysiology of tension pneumothorax involves cardiovascular as well as ventilatory compromise. Tension physiology can develop with only a minor portion of the lung collapsed if the lung is infiltrated, the airways are obstructed, or the lung adheres to the chest wall to cause loculations.

4 No single cause is responsible for all barotrauma. High peak airway cycling pressure, necrotizing pneumonia, heterogeneity of lung pathology, copious airway secretions, and duration of positive-pressure ventilation are major predisposing factors. High levels of minute ventilation and cardiac output and very rapid inspiratory flow rates are likely contributors.

5 The thoracostomy tube selected should be of such size and location to adequately drain the pleural air and/or liquid. The lung must be approximated to the parietal pleura whenever possible. Suction may be needed if an air leak is large, if it persists on water seal alone, or if fluid drainage is copious.

6 Failure to limit end-inspiratory plateau pressure and to preserve a crucial minimum level of positive end-expiratory pressure in the early phase of acute respiratory distress syndrome may intensify preexisting alveolar damage, especially when high peak inflation pressures are used. High shearing forces of each tidal cycle may cause small airway damage, capillary stress fracture, and inflammatory changes, as well as overt lung disruption. Later in the disease process, when inflammation has degraded the collagen infrastructure of the lung, minimizing peak pressure helps prevent alveolar rupture, cyst formation, and pneumothorax.

7 Subacute and chronic complications of mechanical ventilation include fluid retention, redistribution of body water, infection, altered ventilatory drive, and respiratory muscle deconditioning.

8 Specific problems encountered after intubation of the critically ill patient include the following: uncontrolled coughing, patient–ventilator asynchrony, excessive work of breathing, and self-extubation. Agitation during mechanical ventilation demands a systematic search through possible causes relating to the patient, the endotracheal tube and circuitry, and the ventilator itself.

■ ACUTE COMPLICATIONS OF MECHANICAL VENTILATION

Cardiovascular Impairment

Patients with an uncompromised heart, normal sympathetic reflexes, and normal or increased intravascular volume tolerate mechanical ventilation well, especially if spontaneous efforts are retained. Venous return is driven across the venous resistance by the difference between the mean systemic vascular pressure upstream (largely determined by intravascular volume and venous tone) and intrathoracic vena caval pressure. For patients who make weak inspiratory efforts, mean intrathoracic pressure rises during ventilation with positive pressure, especially when positive end-expiratory pressure (PEEP) is used or auto-PEEP is generated. This raised intrapleural pressure increases intracavitary right atrial pressure (but reduces the transmural pressure), causing cardiac output to fall unless mean systemic pressure rises sufficiently to compensate (see Chapter 1). Major increases in lung volume may also compress the vena cava and increase resistance in the region of the diaphragm. Initiating ventilatory support is most likely to compromise forward cardiac output in patients with depleted intravascular volume who fail to make breathing efforts. The effect may be quite different in patients with congestive failure in whom relief of the ventilatory burden, in combination with the reduction of left ventricular afterload and reduced transvascular pressures that positive intrathoracic pressure provides, may dramatically improve forward output and reduce pulmonary vascular engorgement. (Conversely, resumption of a high ventilatory workload increases O_2 demands and lowers intrathoracic pressure sufficiently to seriously destabilize the ischemic or failing heart.) Impairment of cardiac output is particularly likely to occur in patients whose mean intrathoracic pressures rise is the highest (e.g., those with chest wall restriction, good lung compliance, and air trapping) and in patients who are volume depleted, β-blocked, or unable to venoconstrict adequately. Profound deterioration may occur in patients developing auto-PEEP immediately after the institution of positive-pressure ventilation. Unlike hemorrhage and other states of volume depletion, compensatory heart rate responses to the lower output and blood pressure associated with positive pressure are often blunted. Usually, adverse reactions are most evident shortly after mechanical ventilation or PEEP is instituted, as slowly adapting compensatory changes in intravascular volume and vessel tone may attenuate these effects over time.

Barotrauma

Pathogenesis of Alveolar Rupture

The varied forms of pulmonary barotrauma—interstitial emphysema, pneumomediastinum, pneumoperitoneum, subcutaneous emphysema, cyst formation, and pneumothorax (PTX)—are among the most troublesome iatrogenic consequences of intensive care. Although PTX may arise from such diverse medical problems as pulmonary infection or infarction, *Pneumocystis* pneumonia, or spontaneous or cough-induced rupture of a pleural bleb, a confined set of etiologies accounts for most PTX in the intensive care unit (ICU): pulmonary and pleural punctures, lung necrosis, and ventilator barotrauma. Projectiles, sharp instruments, and displaced rib fractures cause PTX by direct puncture of the visceral pleura. PTX may also complicate any medical procedure in which a needle enters the thorax, especially thoracentesis, pleural biopsy, transthoracic aspiration of a pulmonary mass, and central line placement. (Therefore, if a subclavian or internal jugular central line must be placed, it is prudent to select the side with an existing chest tube.) If air enters the pleural cavity inadvertently via a needle without inflicting lung injury, the gas will spontaneously reabsorb, often without the need for intervention. Discrete single punctures of the lung are less likely to cause problems than multiple punctures or slashing actions of the bevel of the needle. Disruption of the visceral pleura and necrotizing pulmonary infections may also cause PTX.

With increased awareness of the dangers of high airway pressure, ventilation-associated barotrauma now occurs much less frequently than in previous decades. Direct rupture of the visceral pleura undoubtedly occurs as a consequence of distention by positive pressure in many patients with diseased or injured lungs, but the barotrauma that complicates mechanical ventilation can also develop by a more circuitous path. Rupture of weakened alveolar tissues is particularly likely to affect "nonpartitional" or "marginal" alveoli, which have bases contiguous to relatively immobile structures—vessels, bronchioles, or fibrous septae. During positive-pressure ventilation (or severe blunt chest injury that occurs with the glottis closed), alveolar pressures rise more than interstitial pressures, allowing pressure gradients to develop between marginal alveoli and the contiguous perivascular connective tissues. If rupture occurs, extra-alveolar gas follows a pressure gradient down the path of least resistance, tracking along the perivascular sheaths toward the hilum. The interstitial emphysema produced en route may be detected against the radiopaque background of infiltrated lung as lucent streaks and small cysts that do not correspond to the bronchial anatomy. The gas continues to track centrally, forming a pneumomediastinum that may or may not be evident on routine films (see Chapter 11).

In the absence of preexisting mediastinal pathology, extra-alveolar gas dissects along fascial planes, usually decompressing into the soft tissues of the neck (subcutaneous emphysema) or retroperitoneum (pneumoperitoneum). PTX occurs in a minority of such cases (perhaps 20% to 30%) when soft-tissue gas ruptures into the pleural space via an interrupted or a weakened mediastinal pleural membrane. Interstitial emphysema, pneumomediastinum, and subcutaneous emphysema have little hemodynamic significance and seldom affect gas exchange significantly in adults. Because their presence signals alveolar rupture and the potential for PTX to evolve, these signs are important to detect in the ventilated patient. Pressure gradients usually favor decompression of interstitial gas into the mediastinum. However, when normal bronchovascular channels are blocked, gas accumulates locally or migrates distally to produce subpleural air cysts that compress parenchymal vessels, create dead space, increase the ventilatory requirement, and cause major problems for ventilation–perfusion matching. The development of cystic barotrauma is an ominous finding that usually presages tension PTX a short time afterward.

Bronchopulmonary Injury

Until quite recently, the development of bronchial damage was believed to occur only rarely in adult patients. Autopsy studies of patients ventilated at moderately high pressures for extended periods, however, have demonstrated that small airways unsupported by cartilage can sustain considerable damage at high airway pressures. Airway distortion predisposes to cystic parenchymal damage, disordered gas exchange, and impaired secretion clearance.

Cystic Barotrauma

Widespread cystic barotrauma is most likely to develop in young patients with necrotizing pneumonitis, narrowed airways, and retained secretions. Alveolar rupture and focal gas trapping are key to its pathogenesis. As predicted by the law of Laplace ($P = 2T/R$), the pressure (P) required to maintain a fixed tension (T) in the wall of a spherical structure falls as its radius (R) increases. Therefore, it is not uncommon for a cyst created by positive airway pressure to grow quickly to a large dimension (>10 cm in diameter). Once underway, cystic barotrauma tends to be pernicious and

self-reinforcing. As cysts develop, they compress normal lung tissue, stiffening the lung and increasing the airway pressure needed for effective ventilation. Furthermore, blood flow diverts away from areas of cyst expansion, creating dead space that increases the ventilatory requirement and therefore the mean alveolar pressure. Increased peak and mean airway pressures accentuate the tendency for further lung damage, whereas higher requirements for alveolar ventilation tend to keep the patient dependent on the ventilator. Secretion management, treatment of infection, and most importantly, reduction of airway pressure are fundamental to effective management.

Systemic Gas Embolism

For patients with acute respiratory distress syndrome (ARDS) ventilated with high tidal pressures and maintained with relatively low left ventricular filling pressures (pulmonary arterial "wedge pressures"), peak and mean alveolar pressures may exceed pulmonary venous pressures in certain lung regions. If alveolar rupture opens a communication pathway to the vascular system, this pressure gradient may drive air into systemic circulation. Microbubbles can then cause vasospasm, seizure, stroke, or myocardial infarction (MI). Usually, the MI is inferior, as the buoyant air percolates into the right coronary artery, which lies anteriorly and superiorly in the supine position.

Uncomplicated Pneumothorax

Ordinarily, the visceral and parietal pleural surfaces are approximated during both phases of the respiratory cycle. The negative pressure between them is maintained by the joint tendencies of the chest wall to expand and the lungs to recoil to their natural resting volumes. At equilibrium, these opposing forces create a moderately negative pleural pressure. PTX disrupts the normal relationship of the lung to the chest wall. The lung collapses toward its resting volume. Simultaneously, PTX allows the chest wall to expand toward its unstressed volume, which occurs at approximately 60% of the normal vital capacity. The natural tendency of the chest wall to expand—"the counterspringing effect"—is diminished or lost when thoracic volume increases. The gas that separates them impairs coupling between the lung and chest wall. Outward migration of the chest wall puts the bellows at a mechanical disadvantage. Expansion of the chest wall also shortens the resting length of the inspiratory muscles, placing them on a less advantageous portion of their length–tension relationship. Less obviously, the total force developed by the muscles of the chest wall normally distributes over a larger surface area than that offered by the collapsed lung. Therefore, even if the inspiratory muscles generate the same intrapleural pressure, the total force applied to the lung is reduced in proportion to the degree of lung collapse. As tidal excursions of the unaffected lung increase to maintain ventilation, elastic and flow-resistive work increase. This increase is well tolerated by healthy patients with adequate ventilatory reserve. However, those with significant airflow obstruction, neuromuscular weakness, or parenchymal restriction may experience dyspnea, progressive hypoventilation, and respiratory acidosis.

Tension Pneumothorax

The term *tension PTX* implies sustained positivity of pleural pressure. The intrapleural pressure exceeds atmospheric pressure during expiration and at times during inspiration as well. A tension component can develop when a ball valve mechanism pumps air into the pleural cavity during spontaneous breathing but occurs much more commonly during positive-pressure ventilation. Positive intrapleural pressure expands the ipsilateral chest cage, rendering the muscles less-efficient generators of inspiratory pleural pressure. A shifting mediastinum helps the affected side to accommodate to the increasing pressure but encroaches on and deforms the contralateral hemithorax, compromising lung expansion. (Parenthetically, single-lung transplantation performed in emphysematous subjects can evoke similar "tension" physiology.) Eventually, rising pleural and central venous pressures impede venous return sufficiently to cause hemodynamic deterioration. It should be emphasized that tension can develop without lung collapse or even major volume loss (e.g., when the lung is heavily infiltrated, air trapped, or regionally bound by pleural adhesions). Vigorous inspiratory efforts tend to maintain intrapleural pressure (averaged for both lungs over the entire respiratory cycle) at near-normal levels until the patient fatigues, is sedated, or receives increased machine assistance. Then, abrupt hemodynamic deterioration may occur as mean pleural pressure rises sharply. Such considerations explain why many patients who develop pneumothoraces while mechanically ventilated show a tension component and why ventilated patients with PTX who receive sedating or paralyzing drugs frequently undergo abrupt hemodynamic

deterioration. For the nonintubated patient, muscle fatigue and respiratory arrest may precede the cardiovascular collapse described classically with the tension PTX syndrome.

Risk Factors for Barotrauma

Although the peak airway cycling pressure has been cited frequently as the most important risk factor for ventilator-related barotrauma, it clearly is not the only one (Table 8-1). In fact, magnitude of tidal pressure may be overwhelmed by other cofactors. The correlation between airway pressure or PEEP and barotrauma is not a tight one. A necrotizing parenchymal process, inhomogeneous lung pathology, young age, excessive airway secretions, and duration of positive-pressure ventilation are major predispositions. The process of alveolar rupture is one that seems to require sustained hyperexpansion of fragile alveoli. Therefore, the mean alveolar pressure, averaged over an entire respiratory cycle, may be an important contributing factor. As major determinants of peak and mean alveolar pressures, minute ventilation requirement and high levels of PEEP contribute to the PTX hazard. (PEEP itself without high inflation pressure contributes little to the risk of barotrauma, especially if applied within the range over which lung recruitment is its primary action.) Peak dynamic (P_D) and static (P_S) airway pressures (plateau) seem to contribute most to the multivariate risk equation. Peak dynamic airway pressure can be reduced by improving lung compliance, reducing tidal volume (V_T) or PEEP, lowering airflow resistance, or slowing peak inspiratory flow rate. On first consideration, it might seem that P_S (the pressure that acts in conjunction with thoracic compliance to determine overall lung volume and alveolar stretch) should correlate even more closely with PTX than P_D. However, although P_S does bear a strong relationship to PTX, airway resistance varies greatly among the bronchial channels of a nonhomogeneously affected lung, so that

TABLE 8-1 PREDISPOSITIONS TO BAROTRAUMA

Necrotizing lung pathology
Secretion retention
Young age
Duration of ventilation
High peak cycling pressure
High mean alveolar pressure
High minute ventilation
Nonhomogeneous parenchymal disease

increasing the dynamic pressure within the central airway may encourage regional overdistention and alveolar rupture in channels with open pathways to weakened alveoli. Ball valving may also occur. Therefore, raising the peak flow rate is not risk free. On the other hand, slowing the rate of inspiratory flow prolongs alveolar distention, increasing the mean alveolar pressure. This is true especially for patients with severe airflow obstruction. Improving airway resistance or lung compliance and reducing alveolar pressure by lowering V_T and/or PEEP are preferable methods for lowering P_D.

3 There does not seem to be a sharp threshold value of peak ventilator cycling pressure below which lung rupture fails to occur. As a rule, however, PTX becomes much more likely at peak ventilator cycling pressures greater than 40 cm H_2O. A peak tidal pressure greater than 35 cm H_2O usually achieves or exceeds the alveolar volume corresponding to total lung capacity in a patient with a normal chest wall. Conversely, when the chest wall is stiff, high plateau pressures may be well tolerated. Secretion accumulation, blood clots, or foreign objects can increase the degree of nonhomogeneity or create ball-valve phenomena that increase the barotraumas hazard. The crucial roles of mechanical and structural nonhomogeneity may explain why PTX tends to develop 1 to 3 weeks after diffuse lung injury, a time when some regions are healing while others remain actively inflamed.

Diagnosis of Barotrauma

Clinical Features of Pneumothorax

Early recognition of PTX is of paramount importance for patients ventilated with positive pressure because of their proclivity to develop tension. During episodes of acute clinical deterioration compatible with PTX, the mortality risk rises when physicians delay intervention, awaiting roentgenographic confirmation. Pleuritic chest pain, dyspnea, and anxiety comprise the most common symptoms of uncomplicated PTX. Symptoms indicative of other forms of extra-alveolar air that may precede PTX include transient precordial chest discomfort, neck pain, dysphagia, and abdominal pain. These nonspecific symptoms often are transient. Tension PTX frequently provokes tachypnea, respiratory distress, tachycardia, diaphoresis, cyanosis, or agitation. For patients receiving volume-cycled ventilation, the airway manometer usually (but not always) shows increased peak inspiratory (and peak static or plateau) airway

pressures as PTX develops, especially if tension is present. Compliance of the respiratory system usually falls from previous values. During volume cycling, the ventilator may "pressure limit" or "pop off," resulting in ineffective ventilation. During pressure-controlled ventilation, a decreased tidal volume and/or minute ventilation may be the only clue to increasing ventilatory impedance.

4 Close examination of the affected hemithorax often reveals signs of hyperexpansion with unilateral hyperresonance, tracheal deviation, diminished ventilatory excursion, and reduced breath sounds on the affected side. The examination must be performed carefully, as massive atelectasis can present a similar clinical picture, simulating PTX on the contralateral side. Auscultation and percussion are essential. Massive gas trapping and auto-PEEP is another effective mimic of PTX, especially if hyperinflation or infiltration is distributed asymmetrically. Palpation of the cervical tissues and suprasternal notch is important to detect subcutaneous emphysema or a trachea deviated away from the side of tension. Tension is reflected in elevations of central venous, right atrial, and pulmonary arterial pressures. Such hemodynamic changes generally do not occur during atelectasis.

Radiographic Signs of Barotrauma

Extra-Alveolar Gas

Extra-alveolar air in the lung parenchyma can manifest as interstitial emphysema or as subpleural air cysts. Both are easiest to detect when the parenchyma is densely infiltrated. Sharp black lines that outline the heart, great vessels, trachea, inferior pulmonary ligament, or diaphragm suggest mediastinal emphysema, even when the pleural membrane itself cannot be visualized (Fig. 8-1). The "complete diaphragm" sign indicates that the heart is separated from the diaphragm by a cushion of air. Subcutaneous emphysema, subdiaphragmatic air, and pneumoperitoneum are other manifestations of barotrauma that may precede or coexist with PTX. Subpleural air cysts commonly are often seen in basilar regions.

Pneumothorax

A number of radiographic signs of PTX deserve emphasis (see Chapter 11). A smooth, two-sided visceral pleural line is diagnostic but must be distinguished from a skin fold and other artifacts at the body surface. The magnification feature is often needed if the lung is otherwise normal, especially

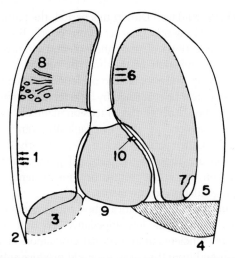

■ **FIGURE 8-1** Radiographic signs of barotrauma: (*1*) visible visceral pleural line, (*2*) deep sulcus sign, (*3*) radiolucency localized to the upper abdomen, (*4*) inverted hemidiaphragm, (*5*) air–fluid level, (*6*) mediastinal shift, (*7*) subpleural air cyst, (*8*) interstitial emphysema, (*9*) complete diaphragm sign, and (*10*) pneumomediastinum.

when digitized films are viewed from a remote monitor. (By providing an air-tissue contrast, infiltrates make the job of PTX detection much easier.) Even when pulmonary infiltrates are extensive, a pleural line may be particularly difficult to detect on a standard supine view if pleural air loculates anteriorly or if ribs or mediastinal vessels obscure the pleural margin. Two useful markers of occult PTX visible on supine films are the "deep sulcus" sign and hyperlucency centered over the ipsilateral abdominal upper quadrant. For bedridden patients, a lateral decubitus view allows air to collect along the upper margin of the hemithorax, facilitating visualization. An expiratory chest radiograph also may prove revealing. (Although the volume of intrapleural air remains constant, it occupies a greater percentage of the available thoracic volume.) PTX under tension can be suspected strongly from a single film when diaphragmatic inversion or extreme mediastinal shift occurs. A sequence of films demonstrating progressive migration of the mediastinal contents into the contralateral hemithorax indicates that the diagnosis was delayed but confirms its validity. Life-threatening tension PTX can exist without complete lung collapse or mediastinal displacement if a portion of the lung adheres to the pleura, if the lung is densely infiltrated, if the airway is obstructed, or if the mediastinum is immobilized by infection, fibrosis, neoplasm, or previous surgery. The mere presence of a chest tube

may *not* prevent tension from developing if the tube is nonfunctional or inadequate to evacuate a large air leak, if the pocket drained is loculated, if the drainage holes are within the major fissure, or if intraparenchymal tension cysts coexist. In fact, by indicating the *presence* of and tendency for tissue rupture, the presence of a chest tube should heighten suspicion for an inapparent PTX on the same side.

Value of the Computed Tomography Scan

The thoracic computed tomography (CT) scan is an invaluable aid in determining whether lucency represents parenchymal or pleural air. In fact, accurate placement of a chest tube into a loculated pocket of gas or fluid may require insertion under direct CT guidance. When doubt exists regarding the effectiveness of the chest tube in draining gas or fluid and/or the exact placement of the tube, CT performed with the tube connected to an appropriate level of suction is currently the "gold standard." Modern CT scanning equipment can acquire a volumetric (helical or spiral) data set very quickly (within seconds). Reconstruction of a two-dimensional image can then be initiated along sagittal and coronal as well as the traditional axial plane. Indeed, highly informative *three*-dimensional reconstruction is now being applied with increasing frequency, imaging that usually leaves little doubt regarding the relevant anatomy.

Management of Pneumothorax and Pleural Effusion

General Principles

Pulmonary barotrauma developing in the setting of acute lung injury is a self-perpetuating, autoamplifying, and potentially lethal process that must be prevented. After extra-alveolar air begins to manifest in its cystic form, impaired gas exchange often forces an increase in minute ventilation requirement and, therefore, in mean airway pressure. In turn, higher mean airway pressure may worsen the tendency for alveolar rupture. Key principles for avoiding barotrauma (Table 8-2) include (a) treat the underlying disease, especially suppurative processes; (b) maintain excellent bronchial hygiene but minimize unnecessary coughing; (c) reduce the minute ventilation requirement by limiting agitation, fever, metabolic acidosis, and bronchospasm; and (d) reduce peak and mean airway pressures by limiting PEEP and tidal volume, by permitting hypercapnia, and by increasing the percentage of

TABLE 8-2 PREVENTING VENTILATOR-RELATED LUNG RUPTURE

Minimize minute ventilation
Limit peak inflation pressure
Use lower V_T
Decrease I:E ratio
Decrease bronchial obstruction
Normalize lung compliance
Improve chest wall compliance
Encourage spontaneous breathing

spontaneous versus machine-aided breaths. During volume-cycled ventilation, reducing tidal volume modestly (e.g., by 100 to 300 mL) may greatly reduce P_D and P_S. Peak flow should be set to the lowest value that satisfies inspiratory demand without incurring additional patient work or auto-PEEP, thus lowering peak dynamic (but not peak static or mean alveolar) pressure. Although several modes of ventilation have been advocated to reduce peak airway pressure (high frequency, pressure supported, and pressure controlled ventilation), their therapeutic efficacy in preventing barotrauma is unproven.

Chest Tube Drainage

Indications for Thoracostomy

Vigilant observation and conservative management are appropriate options in the spontaneously breathing, uncompromised patient with a small PTX. If the patient is breathing spontaneously, simple observation with close radiographic follow-up is often a reasonable strategy for well-compensated patients who experience a small PTX without symptoms after thoracentesis, aspiration needle biopsy, or central line placement. Many such patients will not require more aggressive management. Serial radiographs (or CTs) must demonstrate gradual improvement. (The same is not often true for patients receiving positive pressure ventilation, especially is ventilating pressures are high.) Although spontaneous resolution of PTX is a slow process, an air collection that fails to show convincing improvement over several days may indicate an ongoing leak, with equilibration between the rates of leakage and absorption. After leakage stops, the absorption of intrapleural air occurs at a variable rate (see Chapter 11), averaging approximately (original %)/(1.5%) each day. Even a moderate PTX may take weeks to resolve. (For example, a 15% PTX would be expected to reabsorb completely in

15/1.5 = 10 days.) During this period, the partially collapsed lung may clear secretions poorly. Because large collections of undrained pleural air predisposes to infection of the lung or pleural space, hypoxemia, and proteinaceous pleural fluid collections, it must be evacuated by catheter aspiration or chest tube. The high risk of tension mandates early decompression in the mechanically ventilated patient. Other patients to consider for early intervention are those with ipsilateral pneumonia or secretion retention, ventilatory insufficiency, or high ventilation requirements.

Tube Options   The ideal chest tube system provides a reliable, low-impedance conduit that ensures efficient, unidirectional evacuation of gas and liquid from the chest. It should produce subatmospheric intrapleural pressure and reapproximate the lung to the chest wall. To be in best position for drainage of unloculated air, the tube should be directed superiorly and anteriorly. Small tubes can be introduced anteriorly in the second intercostal space, but for reasons of relative comfort or cosmetics, are often placed laterally. Tubes to be placed in loculated pockets are best inserted by an interventional radiologist. Large tubes are best introduced laterally in the midaxillary line of the sixth-to-seventh interspace and are directed upward, taking care to avoid entry into a fissure. Starting from a lower interspace, the operator should begin far enough posteriorly to avoid subdiaphragmatic placement. When the PTX is distributed evenly (unloculated) and suction is used, the actual position of the tube tip makes little difference. However, if loculations develop, a poorly placed chest tube, especially one not connected to suction, may fail to evacuate the appropriate region. Although large tubes usually are needed to drain substantial collections of fluid, chest tubes placed for simple air drainage are usually 28 French in caliber or smaller. Iatrogenic pneumothoraces without major air leak often can be managed in stable patients with short flexible tubes of very small diameter (usually pigtail catheters). These can be attached to a drainage system (with or without suction) or to a lightweight flutter valve (Heimlich valve) to facilitate ambulation. Such small catheters can be introduced easily but sometimes entail considerable discomfort, especially in young patients. Larger tubes are selected if substantial liquid drainage is also needed. Tube radius is a major determinant of the evacuation capability of the system. However, unless the tube caliber is very small, the leak is very large, or the drainage system is compromised by

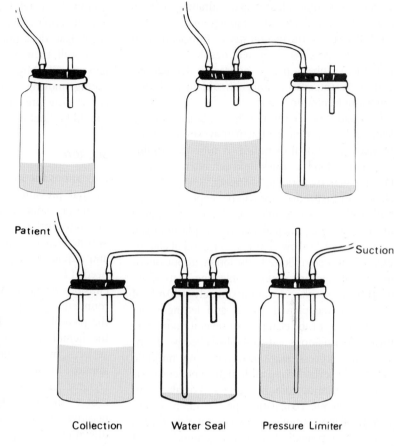

■ **FIGURE 8-2** Elements of a three-chamber drainage system. If a single chamber (here represented as a bottle) were used to collect fluid and to provide the "water seal," compensation must be made for a rising liquid level. Otherwise, there will be increasing back pressure as the tube submerges and foaming will occur as air bubbles through the proteinaceous liquid. Separation of collection and water seal functions in a two-bottle system obviates these problems. The addition of a third "pressure-limiting" bottle enables the application of a safe, constant level of suction from any vacuum source.

fibrin or debris, system resistance usually does not limit the rate of evacuation. (Tube placement and patency are much more important.)

Drainage Apparatus One-way drainage usually is ensured by a water seal (Fig. 8-2). In recent years, lightweight, self-contained, integrated function, disposable plastic units are used almost exclusively. A collection chamber (or "bottle," a label used in deference to the original equipment serving the same function) is inserted in tandem and proximal to the water seal column. The water seal chamber is separated from the collection chamber because accumulated liquid drainage would make air leakage difficult to visualize and, more importantly, would create sufficient back pressure to hinder lung expansion as fluid accumulates. Regulation of the suction pressure applied to the chest tube, a function once done by a water-filled and continuously bubbling "suction regulating" chamber, is now accomplished by a simple noise-free mechanical or needle valve.

Monitoring Tube Function Fluid movements in the water seal tube reflect tidal variations of intrapleural pressure adjacent to the tube. For the spontaneously breathing patient, fluid rises in inspiration and falls during exhalation. The reverse is true during passive inflation with intermittent positive pressure. The direction of tidal fluctuations during triggered machine cycles varies with the vigor of the respiratory effort. Without suction applied, fluctuations of liquid within a dependent loop of drainage tubing or of the water seal ("tidaling") can provide useful clinical information. (Tidal fluctuations are smaller during suction.) An abrupt increase in tidaling magnitude suggests undrained air surrounding the tube, lobar atelectasis, upper airway obstruction, impaired secretion clearance, or hyperpnea. Decreased tidaling can reflect resolution of any of these problems, partial obstruction of drainage, or decreased air leakage through a bronchopleural fistula (BPF). Absent fluctuations may be explained by tube obstruction with fibrin, blood clots, or extrinsic compression. Because of the risks of infection, the chest tube should be removed as soon as it no longer fulfills a useful function. Because 25 to 100 mL of liquid will form each day within the normal pleural space, drainage of this amount is expected through a functioning tube that has full access to the pleural space. (Tubes draining loculated spaces may be patent despite lesser output.) If the tube is patent, noticeable fluctuations within the water seal chamber should occur during moderate respiratory efforts.

A "dead tube" (<50 mL/24 h of drainage, no gas leak, and no respiratory fluctuation) should either be made functional or pulled. A tube that drains empyema, blood, or thick fluid can often be maintained patent by periodic "stripping." Quite often, a clogged or ineffective tube can be reopened at least transiently by sterile injection of an intrapleural fibrinolytic (e.g., alteplase or tissue plasminogen activator, TPA), followed by a brief period of clamping. When a complicated effusion (without ongoing air leak) requires drainage, injecting 25 to 50 mg of 100 mL alteplase in approximately 100 mL of saline into the pleural pocket and letting it act behind a chest tube clamped for several hours may break up loculations and reestablish effective drainage. This process may need repeating multiple times over several days. Although experience has shown that intrapleural bleeding and/or alteration of the systemic coagulation profile rarely occur, TPA instillation is not entirely without risk. A tube that clogs repeatedly presents a genuine risk of infection and probably requires extraction ("pulling"). Another tube or more aggressive surgical approach, such as video-assisted thoracoscopic debridement, should then be considered if the need for draining additional drainage is still apparent. If the water seal level rises (toward the patient) and ceases to fluctuate with respiration after several days of declining drainage, pleural reapposition probably has occurred, and the tube should be removed after radiographic confirmation. The rising level reflects sealing of the air leak and subsequent absorption of the air contained within the chest tube.

Persistent bubbling at the water seal signals an air leak within lung, tubing, or connections. If the leak is within the lung, its magnitude can be quantified during volume-cycled mechanical ventilation by comparing the set inspiratory volume delivered by the machine to the recovered exhaled tidal volume (corrected for the circuit tubing component). (Some drainage systems also provide crude airflow detectors.) If the inspired and expired volumes are nearly equivalent, air leakage is likely to originate external to the lung. Cessation of the air leak when the tube is clamped near the chest wall indicates a BPF or air entry at the incision site. The latter can be excluded by careful approximation of the skin edges and the application of airtight occlusive dressings. If the leak does not stop after clamping near the chest wall, there has been a breach of drainage system integrity. Migratory (transient) clamping of the tubing (moving away from the patient) will then allow more precise localization. Each connection should be carefully inspected.

Suction

Indications for Suction

Natural pressure gradients (fluid siphon effects, expiratory contractions, inspiratory development of positive pressure during mechanical ventilation) are often adequate to empty the pleural space of gas and liquid. However, suction will generally be needed for large air leaks or for drainage of viscous effusions or blood. When the lung is entirely surrounded by gas, pressure applied to one portion of the pleural surface distributes equally throughout the hemithorax. However, when normal pleural surfaces are approximated, the negative pressure applied to one area transmits poorly to other regions. The explanation is that lung tissues adjacent to the tube effectively isolate the pocket of negative pressure. In addition, the tissues may be drawn into the "eyes" of the tube, preventing general transmission of applied negative pressure. When this happens, increasing suction only increases the risk for local tissue injury. For similar reasons, tubes placed inadvertently into a major or minor fissure are surrounded by very pliable lung surfaces and *tend* to drain poorly—but this is not invariably true. Adhesions with loculation also may impede pressure transmission—negative or positive. Massive amounts of fluid or air can collect and tension can develop in sectors remote from a functioning but isolated tube. In this instance, multiple tubes in different locations may be required. Unless the draining fluid is unusually viscid, suction usually can be discontinued (but the water seal maintained) when gas bubbling stops.

Suction Systems

Two types of suction system are used to regulate safe levels of suction pressure. The Emerson suction generator, previously used for decades but now employed with diminishing frequency, links a servomechanism to a fan. A high-capacity, low-impedance, and time-tested system is capable of maintaining essentially constant negative pressure at flow rates up to 40 L/min. If power is interrupted, air escaping from a BPF can vent between the fan blades, preventing tension. If increased gas leakage develops in the system, the servomechanism increases the evacuation rate to maintain constant pressure. It is important to recognize, however, that with older units the pressure is sensed within the apparatus itself, and the manometer will continue to register a substantial level of negative pressure, even if the pump becomes completely disconnected from the patient. If set up as recommended by the manufacturer, the collection and water seal functions are combined. This efficiently protects the motor against damage but causes problems when there is substantial liquid drainage. If suction must be maintained during transport, special battery-operated pumps should be used.

Several commercially available units incorporate a pressure-regulated "three-bottle" (three-chamber) system in a single molded plastic container (Fig. 8-3). A needle valve or a third chamber added in series to fluid collection and water seal columns serves as a pressure governor, modulating excessive wall suction pressures (-80 to $-200\,cm\,H_2O$) to the desired level (typically $<30\,cm\,H_2O$). For unvalved systems of this type, the filling level of the vacuum control column determines and limits the degree of applied suction. Suction is increased until continuous bubbling occurs in the control chamber, indicating that sufficient negative pressure has been applied to the water surface to offset the hydrostatic column. Continuous gentle bubbling in the control chamber must be maintained throughout both phases of the respiratory cycle to ensure the desired level of suction. Increasing the applied vacuum then only serves to increase fluid perturbations in the suction control bottle, leaving the suction applied to the

pleural space unaffected. (The magnitude of bronchopleural air leakage must be gauged from the water seal column.) As opposed to needle valve controllers, these "three-bottle" units are inherently noisy and are slowly disappearing from the clinical scene. When using traditional equipment, three easily remediable problems (Fig. 8-4) commonly cause failure to deliver the desired level of negative pressure: fluid accumulation in the water seal chamber (common with Emerson pump), evaporation from the pressure-limiting tube of a three-bottle system, and the development of a large, fluid-filled dependent loop. Of these, only the latter remains a concern with integrated disposable plastic systems now in widespread use.

Pulling the Tube

Provided that gas leakage ceases and any pleural liquid collection has been effectively drained, the tube can be removed safely 24 to 48 h after suction has been discontinued, provided that no air leakage occurs during coughing and a PTX is not visible radiographically. For patients who have experienced PTX, it is wise to clamp the chest tube for 2 to 4 h prior to the "pre-extraction" X-ray, as very slow leaks may elude brief bedside inspections of the water seal apparatus. Tubes placed to drain pleural effusion *without* PTX can be extracted when no longer functional (see earlier). Even when no gas leak is present and no air collection is suspected, however, some physicians defer extraction of a functional chest tube until a mechanically ventilated patient is extubated. This precaution is controversial, however, and an uncomfortable chest tube may require sedation or analgesia that could delay weaning.

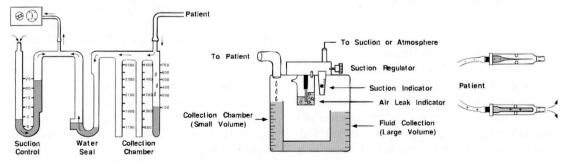

■ **FIGURE 8-3** Pleural drainage apparatus. **Left:** The disposable plastic unit is attached to the chest tube and to a high-capacity suction source to form the equivalent of a three-bottle system. Disconnection from the suction source opens the unit to atmosphere, creating a simple water-sealed two-bottle collection system. **Middle:** Suction regulation can be achieved by a needle valve, reducing the noise associated with the constant bubbling of a suction control water column and obviating the need to replace evaporative water losses from the suction control column. **Right:** The flutter (Heimlich) valve opens only when sufficient positive pressure builds within the chest tube. Such devices are intended primarily for low-volume pleural air leaks without substantial fluid drainage. They enhance mobility for ambulatory patients.

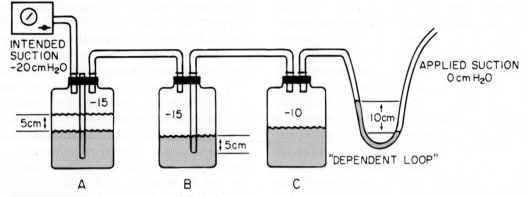

■ **FIGURE 8-4** Factors contributing to failure of applied suction. An intended suction pressure of –20 cm H_2O applied in a three-bottle system can be attenuated by evaporation of water from the pressure limiter bottle **(A)**, by submersion of the water seal tube below the appropriate level of 1 to 2 cm below the water surface **(B)**, and by the presence of liquid in a dependent loop of connecting tubing **(C)**.

Special Problems of Barotrauma

Extensive Subcutaneous Emphysema

A small amount of subcutaneous emphysema frequently is palpable around the chest tube entrance site. However, extensive unilateral emphysema suggests focal accumulation of air under pressure near the thoracostomy wound. Forced exhalation, straining, and coughing tend to drive gas into soft tissues. Extensive subcutaneous emphysema often indicates inadequate evacuation of a large air leak and should prompt careful examination for problems that might decrease system efficiency. In the absence of these, management options include increasing suction pressure, changing to an evacuation system with greater capability, readjusting tube position, or placing a second chest tube to diminish the impedance to pleural emptying. Another potential cause is migration of the most proximal drainage hole from the pleural space and into the soft tissues.

Persistent Bronchopleural Fistula

Nonresolving air leaks occur commonly after rupture of emphysematous blebs, after subtotal pulmonary resection, and during ventilator treatment of ARDS. In the latter setting, the development of a large BPF portends a poor prognosis for survival, largely because BPF is a marker of underlying disease severity—or imprudent ventilator management. Adequate gas exchange usually can be maintained by conventional ventilator adjustments or by one of the following outlined techniques. Interestingly, the effluent from BPF contains considerable CO_2, especially if the lung tissue functions well. Although the "flow-through" ventilation provided by the fistula is less efficient than tidal breathing, the gas that exits the fistula has participated in gas exchange and is not entirely "wasted." For this reason, *effective* tidal volume is greater than that measured from the exhalation line of the ventilator circuit.

Routine Management of a Bronchopleural Fistula

To manage a BPF, the underlying pathology must be reversed, the airway secretions must be cleared, V_E must be minimized, and good nutrition must be ensured (Table 8-3). A large body of clinical data suggests that approximating the visceral and parietal pleura facilitates healing of pleural rents. The initial approach to management may include tube repositioning (preferably with CT guidance), insertion of a second tube, and/or a trial of increased suction in an attempt to appose the pleural surfaces more tightly. However, when the leak remains unsealed, increased suction may simply intensify or perpetuate flow through the fistula. If increasing suction fails, lowering or removing the suction may, in rare instances, promote healing by relieving tension on the margins of the tear. Increased lung collapse may compromise gas exchange, however.

Specialized Techniques

Management of a life-threatening air leak in the mechanically ventilated patient can prove very difficult. Several techniques have been described for

TABLE 8-3 TECHNIQUES FOR MANAGING BPF

GENERAL MEASURES
Reverse underlying pathology
Clear retained airway secretions
Minimize V_E and pressure requirements
Improve nutritional status
Change body position
Reposition chest tubes
Increase suction force if PTX persists
    on radiographs or CT
Trial of decreased suction if high
    suction is ineffective
Chest tube PEEP

SPECIALIZED MEASURES
High-frequency ventilation
Chemical pleurodesis
Endobronchial occlusion
Blood clot
Thrombin/FFP
Tissue glue
Pleural "blood patch"

OPERATIVE CLOSURE
Video-assisted thoracoscopy
Open stapling, resection, or repair

modifying the apparatus, either to prevent flow through the chest tube during inspiration or to maintain a common level of PEEP in the airway and the affected pleural space. None of these has gained widespread support. In some instances, independent lung ventilation has been tried successfully, but this intervention requires heroic supportive efforts. A few studies conducted primarily in children suggest that high-frequency ventilation (HFV) is associated with a lower incidence of barotrauma. Moreover, some reports indicate that HFV can help to close large air leaks by reducing the flow through the low-impedance, high-compliance (leaking) pathway. Whether newly available high-frequency oscillators will prove effective is an interesting but as yet unproven possibility. Surgical intervention may be considered, especially for less critically ill patients with cystic or bullous lung disease. Although long periods (occasionally weeks) of observation and manipulation of the drainage system have traditionally preceded operation, a more aggressive approach is now frequently used because of improved and somewhat less-invasive techniques. Primary suturing or stapling of the injured area often using talc poudrage or pleural abrasion

usually suffice. Closure by video assisted thoracoscopy (VATS) can be attempted in suitably stable, nonhypoxemic patients who can be adequately ventilated during the procedure. In the case of large fistulas, direct tamponade by a pedicle flap, lobectomy, or tissue resection may be needed. Chemical pleurodesis with talc, doxycycline, or tetracycline (where available) has occasionally been used as an alternative to surgical intervention, but this treatment must be considered hazardous and of uncertain merit, especially if the leak is large. Attempts at chemical sclerosis are seldom successful unless performed with meticulous technique. Closure is unlikely to be achieved in the presence of multiple adhesions, large air leaks, or inability to appose the pleural surfaces.

Occasionally successful, transbronchoscopic techniques that occlude the airway with autologous clot, tissue glue, or a mixture of thrombin and fresh frozen plasma may close a persistent BPF and obviate the need for surgery. After identifying a leaking segmental or subsegmental bronchus, occlusion is accomplished by using a balloon-tipped catheter. Then blood (50 mL) or a similar volume of the thrombin/fresh frozen plasma mixture is instilled. Although seldom effective, the results are quickly apparent. Alternatively, pleural instillation of sterile talc (by insufflation or as a slurry), tetracycline, or autologous blood (a blood patch) using a chest tube may seal a very small but persistent leak, but such pleurodesis attempts are generally poorly advised, hazardous, and may complicate a later surgical approach. None can be accomplished safely in the unstable patient, and because such procedures require at least transient clamping of the chest tube, tension physiology may ensue. Interventional bronchoscopy to insert one or more way valves (as is recently done for volume reduction in emphysematous patients) has conceivable merit for a "slow leaker" in an inoperable patient, but there is no published information regarding this highly experimental and unvalidated technique.

Ventilator-Induced Pulmonary Edema, Lung Injury, and Volutrauma

Pathogenesis

Even when alveolar rupture does not occur, excessive tissue stresses are damaging, whether produced by positive or negative pressure. Patients with ARDS seem to be at highest risk for ventilator-induced lung injury (VILI). In experimental animals, the choice of ventilatory pattern dramatically influences the morphology of normal and previously injured tissues, a finding that is not surprising, given that repeated tissue overstretching initiates inflammatory mechanosignaling and that more than 20,000 tidal cycles are undertaken each day.

Effect of Excessive Peak Pressures

6 Ventilatory patterns that apply high transalveolar (static transpulmonary) stretching forces cause or extend tissue edema and damage in experimental animals (Table 8-4). The requisite pressures are often encountered during conventional management of ARDS. Current evidence strongly suggests that static ("plateau") airway pressures greater than 30 cm H_2O commonly produce regional overdistention when the chest wall is normally compliant, especially when end-expiratory pressure is too low to prevent widespread small airway collapse. Judging from the substantial delay to peak incidence of PTX, the lung seems to be able to withstand exposure to somewhat higher distending forces in the earliest phase of ARDS without sustaining radiographically evident barotrauma (see Chapter 24). Later in the course of illness, the strong collagen infrastructure of the lung degrades unevenly, so that similar pressures are more likely to result in overt alveolar disruption (PTX, pneumomediastinum, gas cyst formation). Independent on radiographic evidence for extra-alveolar gas, the lung may sustain edematous injury produced by high tissue strain during inflation.

Randomized, controlled clinical trials of tidal volume and lung protective ventilation strategies aimed at minimizing tissue stresses (limited tidal pressure and high PEEP or high-frequency oscillation) confirm the validity of animal studies of these same variables. A well-conducted, multicenter comparative clinical trial of moderately high (12 mL/kg of ideal body weight) and relatively low tidal volume (6 mL/kg) in patients with ARDS by the NIH-sponsored ARDS network showed a decided mortality advantage for the lower tidal volume limb. Because tidal volumes much higher than this can be applied without injuring healthy lungs (e.g., during exercise), it is logical to assume that it is the *pressures* required to force larger tidal volumes into damaged lungs with reduced aerating capacity that overstretch the individual lung units to mediate the adverse response. Analysis of the data from large clinical trials uncovered that plateau pressure correlates much better than tidal volume with mortality risk, even when adjusted for disease severity. As in Chapter 5, it must be emphasized that the reduced pleural pressure of spontaneous breathing adds to the transalveolar pressure, so that a "plateau" pressure obtained under these conditions may seriously underestimate that recorded under passive conditions. Moreover, while tidal volume is most usefully related to aerating capacity (as indexed by transpulmonary pressure or, ideally measured end-expiratory lung volume), it might also be important for other reasons. The magnitude of tidal volume relates to the *flows* necessary to drive it. Flow itself may have a powerful influence on the expression of injury resulting from any given peak alveolar pressure, as it is a prime determinant of shearing force. Moreover, higher tidal volumes

TABLE 8-4   RISK FACTORS FOR VILI

		HIGH PLATEAU PRESSURE	HIGH TIDAL VOLUME	PEEP	RISK
Normal		No	Yes	No	None
		No	Yes	Yes	Low
		Yes	Yes	Yes	Moderate
ARDS	Early	Yes	Yes	Yes	Moderate
		Yes	Yes	No	High
	Late	Yes	Yes	No	High
		Yes	No	Yes	High
		No	No	No	Moderate

No, not applied; Yes, applied.

are associated with higher expiratory flows that may help disseminate airway biofluids, accentuating injury propagation. (see "Propagation," following). These multiple roles for tidal volume may help explain why very low plateau pressures have been recorded in patients classified as having acute lung injury.

Although there now remains little question that high inflation pressures are damaging, the need to incorporate nontraditionally high levels of PEEP into a lung-protective strategy is likely to depend not only on the number of collapsed units, but also on the driving pressure generated by the difference between end-inspiratory plateau and PEEP. This flow-driving gradient can be thought of as the "lever-arm" for shearing stress at the junctions of closed and open tissues. (Fig. 8-5). Setting exact safety limits for plateau pressures is not an easy task, being complicated by multiple cofactors of

varying importance and by the difficulty of their measurement. (e.g., rate of alveolar pressure development, interstitial pressure, and microvascular pressure gradient). The transalveolar stress that develops in response to building airway pressure is influenced by the relative compliances of the lung and chest wall. Although an imperfect indicator of the interstitial pressure that surrounds the airspace, intrapleural pressure is believed to be a reasonable estimate. Measurement of esophageal pressure (P_{es}), therefore, may be prudent when plateau pressures higher than 30 cm H_2O are contemplated and the chest wall is suspected to be stiffer than normal, as in the setting of abdominal pathology (e.g., ascites, extreme obesity, recent surgery). A bladder pressure measurement is a noninvasive means of estimating intra-abdominal pressure, which, when elevated, may indicate the advisability of measuring esophageal pressure (see Chapter 5).

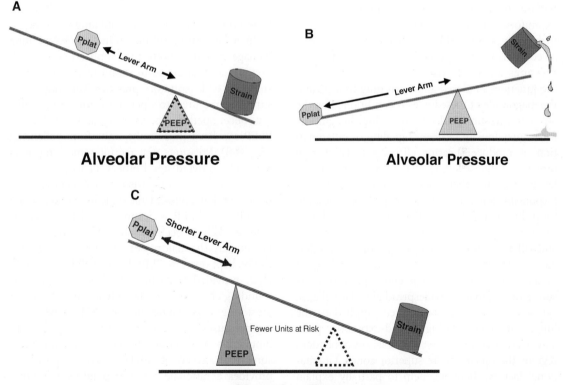

■ **FIGURE 8-5** Conceptual relationship between the elements that cause excessive tissue strain and VILI. Driving pressure for tidal ventilation (the difference between plateau pressure [Pplat] and positive end-expiratory pressure [PEEP]) acts as the lever arm and PEEP acts as the fulcrum. Tissue strain can be kept low by reducing the Pplat or by increasing PEEP when Pplat is high. Thus, although higher PEEP minimizes strain when plateau is high, PEEP does *not* need to be high so long as Pplat does not exceed some threshold value, currently thought to approximate 25 to 30 cm H_2O in patients with normal chest walls. A well-tolerated combination of PEEP and Pplat (moderate Pplat and low to moderate PEEP) **(A)** contrasts with one in which Pplat is raised without adequate PEEP **(B)**. Keeping the same high Pplat while increasing the PEEP again reduces tissue strain to tolerable levels **(C)**.

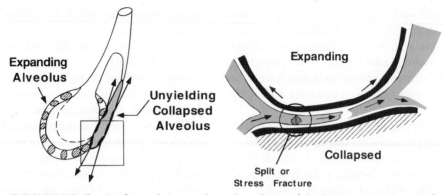

■ **FIGURE 8-6** Shearing forces during mechanical ventilation of the heterogeneous lung. **Left:** The tangential shearing forces at the junction of expanding and collapsed alveolus may far exceed the tensions experienced in the free walls of expanding units, especially at high inflation pressures. **Right:** When junctional tensions rise high enough, the shearing action may exert sufficient force to cause capillary stress fractures and hemorrhagic edema.

Importance of End-Expiratory Lung Volume and PEEP

Failure to preserve a certain minimum end-expiratory transalveolar pressure (i.e., total PEEP) in the early phase of ARDS may intensify pre-existing alveolar damage, especially when high inflation pressures are used. Tissue stress is amplified at the junctions of closed and open lung tissues, and the magnitude of these forces is conditioned by the alveolar pressure. Indeed, these high-magnitude forces may initiate mechanosignaling of inflammation or produce shearing effects associated with repetitive collapse and reinflation of injured alveolar tissues. Together, these phenomena may be responsible for an important component of ventilator-induced lung damage (Fig. 8-6). Extreme forces cause rupture of delicate membranes, hemorrhage, and inflammation; repeated stresses of even moderate amplitude may cause mechanosignaling of inflammation (Fig. 8-7). The end-expiratory pressure required to avert widespread alveolar collapse varies with the hydrostatic forces applied to the lung; consequently, a higher end-expiratory pressure is required to prevent atelectasis in dependent regions than in the more superior zones. Gravitational factors, therefore, help to partially explain the strikingly dependent distribution of radiographic infiltrates shortly after the onset of lung injury, as well as the reversal of these infiltrates and improved arterial oxygenation in the prone position. Experimentally, prone positioning has been shown to even the distribution of ventilation and to avert much of the ventilator-associated lung injury occurring in dependent areas. Applying PEEP sufficient to position the tidal volume above the point of widespread lung unit closure attenuates severe hemorrhagic edema otherwise induced in laboratory animals by high ventilating pressure.

In a laboratory setting, inflicting severe lung damage requires both the application of high pressure and failure to maintain recruitment with sufficient end-expiratory pressure. Very high pressures are required to open refractory lung units, but once opened, considerably lower values of PEEP can keep those same units from collapsing (Fig. 8-8). Pressures that recruit some lung units are likely to overdistend others. (This principle is illustrated in CT comparisons of dependent and nondependent zones.) Unless the lung is kept open by sufficient PEEP, widespread tidal lung recruitment is likely to occur throughout the tidal cycle. Fortunately, the majority of (but not all) lung units can be kept open by PEEP levels well below 20 cm H_2O, provided that the compliance of the surrounding chest wall is relatively normal. Although most lung units of a patient with ARDS have opening pressures of less than 25 cm H_2O, refractory lung units may require sustained opening pressures that exceed 60 cm H_2O. This requirement provides a rationale for incorporating recruiting maneuvers into the ventilation strategy for these patients. In some centers, attempts are made to recruit every possible unstable lung unit—the "open lung" approach. Convincing arguments can be mounted both in favor of and in opposition to this strategy (Table 8-5A and B).

Stress failure of the pulmonary capillaries with resulting extravasation of formed blood elements

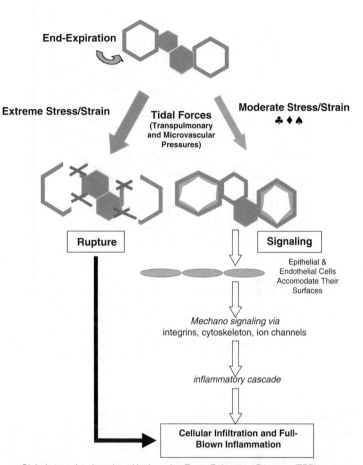

■ FIGURE 8-7 A hypothetical schema of the mechanisms by which ventilatory stress/strain result in inflammation.

♦ Global stress/strain reduced by lowering Trans-Pulmonary Pressure (TPP)
♠ Local stress/strain less if TPP is more homogeneously applied (prone position)
♣ Local stress/strain reduced if PEEP "keeps open"

TABLE 8-5A WHY *SHOULD* WE CONSIDER FULL RECRUITMENT "OPEN LUNG" STRATEGIES?
• Improved gas exchange • Less ventilator associated pneumonia • Reduced VILI hazard • Lower risk of decompartmentalization – Gas – Bacteria – Inflammatory mediators

TABLE 8-5B WHY *SHOULD NOT* WE ATTEMPT TO FULLY "OPEN" THE LUNG?
• Injured lungs may not be recruitable – Recruitability may be limited to *early* phase • ARDS is a heterogeneous disease – Some areas will be overstretched • Open lungs generate "Zone 2" conditions – Dead space – VILI (due to *vascular* stress) • Lung opening has a pressure cost and hazard – Hemodynamic compromise – Heightened tissue strain • Conflicting clinical trials

into the interstitium and alveoli may occur at trans*vascular* pressures that exceed 40 to 90 mm Hg, depending on the animal species. Transcapillary mechanical forces of comparable magnitude may be generated when high tidal airway pressures are applied to diseased, heterogeneous lungs. High *vascular* pressures and blood flows also may be important determinants of lung injury. The breakdown of

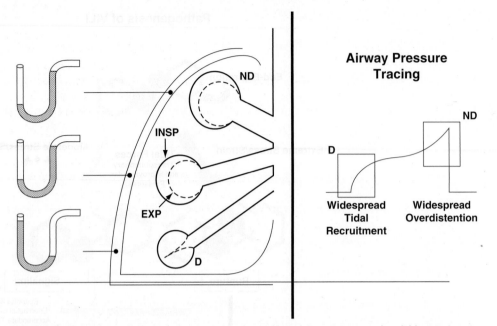

■ FIGURE 8-8 Regional alveolar mechanics during the tidal breath in ARDS. Dependent (*D*) lung units may be surrounded by sufficiently high pressure to collapse at end-expiration and reexpand at some higher pressure achieved during the tidal cycle. Nondependent (*ND*) units that are exposed to low extra-alveolar pressures may overdistend at end-inspiration, risking "overstretch" injury. During controlled ventilation with constant inspiratory flow, the airway pressure tracing may show indirect evidence of these phenomena if it displays segments of rapidly improving and rapidly deteriorating respiratory system compliance.

the alveolar–capillary barrier may create a portal for air, bacteria, and proteinaceous debris to enter the systemic circulation. Vascular pressure appears to be only one of many important cofactors that influence the expression of VILI. Apart from vascular pressure and body position, high inspired fractions of oxygen may contribute by their direct toxic effects or by encouraging absorption collapse. Experimental VILI-associated inflammation may be intensified by fever and attenuated by hypothermia.

Propagation of Lung Injury by Ventilation Pattern and Positioning

The diffuse injury that characterizes ARDS is often considered a process that begins synchronously throughout the lung, mediated by inhaled or blood-borne noxious agents. Relatively little attention has been paid to the possibility that inflammatory lung injury may also begin focally and propagate sequentially via the airway network, proceeding mouthward from distal to proximal. Were this true, modifications of ventilatory pattern and position aimed at geographic containment of

the inflammatory injury process could help prevent its generalization and limit disease severity. If airway propagation of proteinaceous, mediator-laden edema plays an important role in disseminating injury, which would be the key elements of a lung protective ventilation strategy targeted to that specific aspect? (Table 8-6) In the earliest (edematous) stage of lung inflammation, (perhaps the first 48 h)

TABLE 8-6 WHAT MAKES MUCUS AND EDEMA (BIOFLUIDS) MOVE WITHIN THE AIRWAY?

- Bio-fluid volume
  – Antibiotics
  – Steroids
- Biofluid consistency
  – Hydration, mucolytics, β-agents, lubricants
- Exhalation time constant
  – R_x resistance
- Ventilation pattern
  – ↑V_T ↓ Inspiratory flow ↓ PEEP help expel
- Adjuncts to secretion clearance
  – Position, vibration, in-exsufflation

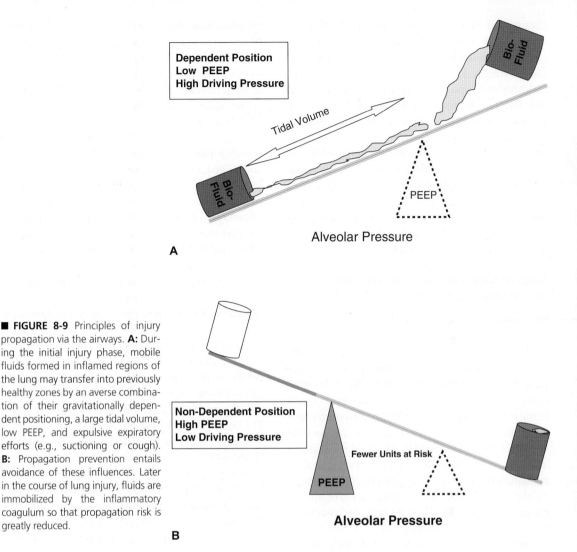

■ **FIGURE 8-9** Principles of injury propagation via the airways. **A:** During the initial injury phase, mobile fluids formed in inflamed regions of the lung may transfer into previously healthy zones by an averse combination of their gravitationally dependent positioning, a large tidal volume, low PEEP, and expulsive expiratory efforts (e.g., suctioning or cough). **B:** Propagation prevention entails avoidance of these influences. Later in the course of lung injury, fluids are immobilized by the inflammatory coagulum so that propagation risk is greatly reduced.

when airway biofluids are mobile, logical steps would include relatively high PEEP to encourage edema to stay at its site of origin or translocate to the interstitial space, to use small tidal volumes to reduce the peak expiratory flows that drive airway fluid mouthward, to minimize minute ventilation (to avoid larger tidal volumes and expulsive expiratory efforts), to avoid fluid excess and edema, to dependently orient the most involved segments or lobes, and to silence vigorous *expiratory* effort (Fig. 8-9A and B). Early intervention would be vital in trying to limit transairway propagation of noxious biofluids during their high mobility phase. Later on, when gelling has occurred, the positioning priority shifts to expulsion of the thickened secretions which otherwise act to plug airways rather than to propagate disease. With fluids relatively immobile or neutralized, PEEP gradually loses its

value in preventing airway flooding. While there is little doubt that certain postural reorientations encourage airway drainage and should be strongly considered when it is safe to do so, it is sobering to think that side-to-side repositioning undertaken from the first hours of care to prevent skin breakdown might actually help to distribute noxious lung fluids more widely into previously unaffected zones before gelling inhibits secretion mobility. Moreover, bacteria contained in situ are neutralized over time by immune defenses and/or antibiotics. After the first few days, clearance of thickened mucus (rather than prevention of spread of mobile liquid) assumes therapeutic primacy.

Propagation avoidance measures do not contradict the basic elements of the "low tidal volume/ open lung" approach to lung protection but, rather, extend their rationale. Such questions as whether altering the ventilatory prescription, position, or their combination could contain (or conversely amplify) an initially focal injury process seem especially attractive to explore.

Injury extension via the airways is certainly *not* the only mechanism at work in ARDS or VILI causation, nor is it important in every case. But when injury is fresh and initially *localized*, the potential for airway propagation reenforces the justification for dependent positioning of the affected zone until secretions are no longer mobile. Furthermore, in the earliest phase of acute lung injury (ALI) and lobar pneumonia it is rational to employ a recruiting strategy and generous PEEP so as to contain highly moblie thin fluids within the minimal number of segments.

Links between VILI and Dysfunction of Systemic Organs

Intriguing laboratory and clinical data have shown that inflammatory mediators originating in the lungs of patients with ARDS may translocate to the periphery when high inflation pressures and reduced levels of PEEP are utilized. Such observations suggest possible links between ARDS, ventilating pattern, and the associated multisystem organ failure that accounts for the deaths of many patients ventilated for this disorder. While dysfunctional initiation of inflammation by circulating signaling mediators is an attractive hypothesis, other experimental data suggest that the upregulation of inflammatory processes in the lung may be associated with net immunosuppressive effects in the periphery, predisposing to infection. Just how lung inflammation incites remote injury is a current research topic of intense interest.

Management

Detailed guidelines are not available regarding the maximum safe peak and mean alveolar pressures that can be applied for extended periods without inducing alveolar damage or retarding lung healing. Clearly, the answer differs among individual patients (Table 8-4). Alveolar stresses undoubtedly vary with PEEP and position and differ from site to site within the damaged lung (Fig. 8-8). The common airway pressure applied to the endotracheal tube (ET) must account for the distensibility and vulnerability of each type of lung unit. Although failure to preserve a certain minimum end-expiratory transalveolar pressure has been shown experimentally to intensify preexisting alveolar damage when endinspiratory alveolar (plateau) pressure is high, this

phenomenon has not yet been convincingly demonstrated in clinical trials. When combined with a small tidal volume, higher PEEP did improve mortality outcome in a Brazilian and a Spanish trial of moderate size. However, the larger ALVEOLI trial of the ARDS network did not show a clear advantage in its higher PEEP limb. (The design of that trial did not allow application of high alveolar pressures to patients of either group.) Similarly, the large Canadian LOVS and French EXPRESS trials demonstrated some intriguing advantages for their higher initial PEEP patients, but no clear mortality advantage overall (see "Suggested Reading" in Chapter 9). Once recruitment has been completed, additional PEEP is probably ineffectual or damaging. Consequently, expert opinion differs regarding whether applying the least PEEP that accomplishes adequate gas exchange or guaranteeing some minimal value of end-expiratory alveolar pressure is the best course to follow during the first few days of the disease process. Initial application of sustained high inflating pressures to recruit unstable lung units continues to be advocated by some knowledgeable investigators, especially when small tidal volumes (<4 to 5 mL/kg) are used or when HFV is employed. PEEP should be withdrawn later in the disease process if no important reduction of PaO_2 occurs upon its reduction.

Allowing $PaCO_2$ to rise to supernormal values (permissive hypercapnia) is an effective strategy for limiting ventilating pressure (see Chapter 24). The full effect of hypercapnia on such important variables as gas exchange, cardiovascular dynamics, and tissue edema is yet to be described in the two settings for which it is most commonly applied—asthma and ARDS. Moreover, there are both relative and absolute contraindications for using this technique (Table 8-7). Elevated FiO_2 and high ventilating pressures often are required to achieve nearcomplete saturation of arterial blood with oxygen. The combinations of O_2 concentration and O_2 exposure duration that produce significant lung damage have not been established firmly for the setting of ARDS and may vary with disease severity

TABLE 8-7 CONTRAINDICATIONS TO PERMISSIVE HYPERCAPNIA

Increased intracranial pressure
Severe cardiovascular dysfunction
Severe pulmonary hypertension
Profound metabolic acidosis

and individual susceptibility. In the absence of definitive data obtained in a clinical context, some knowledgeable practitioners increase lung volume in an attempt to minimize FiO_2, whereas others prefer to use higher inspired fractions of O_2 rather than increase peak, mean, and end-expiratory airway pressures. At FiO_2 levels less than 0.7, limiting P_{aw} to "safe" levels generally takes precedence over limiting FiO_2.

■ SUBACUTE AND CHRONIC COMPLICATIONS

Fluid Retention and Redistribution

7 Extravascular fluid retention tends to develop during positive-pressure ventilation for several reasons: (a) ventilated patients are relatively immobile; (b) as increased intrathoracic pressure limits venous return, stretch receptors located in the atria signal additional antidiuretic hormone (ADH) release to help replenish central vascular volume; and (c) hypotension induced by positive pressure may curtail renal perfusion, redistribute renal blood flow, reduce glomerular filtration, and promote sodium and water retention. PEEP may cause a similar redistribution of intrarenal blood flow by reflex mechanisms. The hypoalbuminemia almost routinely present in the ventilated, critically ill patients is also contributory. As positive-pressure ventilation is discontinued, these fluid shifts reverse and may precipitate cardiac decompensation in patients with poor reserve, as fluid translocates from extravascular sites to the central vessels.

The controversy regarding fluid management in ARDS (liberal vs. restricted) is more than an academic one; published data now exist to indicate that fluid retention correlates with adverse outcomes in several published studies, either because tissue edema is a marker of disease severity or because it relates integrally to organ dysfunction. Whether colloid (e.g., albumin) or crystalloid should be favored as a resuscitation fluid is a controversy that has raged for years and currently seems little closer to resolution. As with most such debates, the answer may vary with the detailed physiology of the individual case.

Fluctuations in pH

The ventilator can powerfully affect acid–base balance. When support is initiated, special care should be exercised not to reverse acidosis too quickly or to cause marked respiratory alkalosis. Metabolic alkalosis tends to develop in mechanically ventilated patients because of intravascular volume contraction, nasogastric suctioning, or use of steroids. If repletion of KCl or intravascular volume fails to correct it, acetazolamide (Diamox) may prove useful in controlling extravascular fluid retention while dumping excess bicarbonate. In the assist/control mode, marked fluctuations in pH and $PaCO_2$ can occur in patients who are alternately agitated and sedated, especially if the ventilator's backup rate is inappropriately low. Mental status and ventilation mode always should be taken into account when interpreting blood gas values.

Infections

Infections of the lung and upper respiratory tract are exceedingly common during mechanical ventilation. Liquid within corrugated ventilator tubing allows bacteria to multiply. Therefore, care should be taken to prevent transfer of the condensate into the trachea during manipulations of the ventilator circuit or changes of patient position. Indeed, such transfers have been suggested to at least partially explain why pneumonia seems to occur more frequently among patients who undergo frequent changes to fresh ventilator circuits. Nasotracheal and nasogastric tubes frequently precipitate sinus infection by blocking their ostia, which prevents drainage. In itself, occult sinusitis is a frequent cause for febrile episodes in intubated patients. Furthermore, blocked sinuses also provide a seeding focus for infections of the lung and bloodstream. Occult sinopulmonary infections often are responsible for the sepsis syndrome in intubated, mechanically ventilated patients, even when the organisms cannot be recovered by conventional culturing techniques.

Ventilator-Associated Pneumonia

Continued intubation of the airway strongly predisposes to hospital-acquired pneumonia, a serious problem associated with high rates of morbidity and mortality. As most patients remain intubated because they require mechanical ventilation, "ventilator-associated pneumonia" (VAP) has received considerable investigative attention. This term is generally reserved for infections that develop by 48 h or more after mechanical ventilation is initiated. It is now certain that patients receiving *non*invasive ventilation by pressurized face mask have an impressively lower incidence of VAP. Although heavy sedation and damaging ventilatory patterns are less likely to be applied during noninvasive ventilation (NIV) because of the inherent pressure limitations of the noninvasive approach. The most intuitive reasons for its relative advantage reside in preservation of clearance mechanisms and prevention of lower airway inoculation.

The oropharynx teems with microbes but in healthy persons the upper airway normally remains sterile below the vocal cords, swept clean by the mucociliary escalator and protected by an effective cough. Bypassing the upper airway with an ET seriously impairs these defenses while facilitating inoculation of the lower airway and lungs with high concentrations of potential pathogens. The rate of developing VAP is strongly influenced by institutional practices such as hand washing and inclining the head of the bed to 30 degrees or more. On average, it approximates 2% to 3% per day, so that the likelihood of developing pneumonia is after the first 10 days of ventilatory support, even when appropriate precautions are taken. Overt pneumonitis, frequently polymicrobial, usually manifests after the first week of hospitalization. Because all new infiltrates are not necessarily pneumonia and because the pathogen may not be obvious, bronchoalveolar lavage (BAL) is quite helpful in establishing the correct diagnosis. Poor dentition, impaired nutritional status, age, immobilization, immune compromise, and the supine position predispose pulmonary infection (Table 8-8). Once under way, pneumonia contributes clearly to the mortality resulting from such underlying conditions as decompensated chronic obstructive pulmonary disease (COPD) and ARDS.

Risk Factors for VAP

Although pneumonia occasionally arises from hematogenous inoculation, most alveolar seeding occurs via the airway. In epidemiologic and experimental studies, the likelihood of developing pneumonia relates to the size of the infective inoculum and the effectiveness of secretion clearance. The ET interferes with the mucociliary escalator and with coughing effectiveness. Colony counts of oral secretions may exceed 10^8/mL, and a rich pool of such fluid often collects above the ET cuff. Aided by gravity, the interstices of the ET cuff may allow continuing seepage of these secretions into the lower airway. Axial movement of the ET may help pump a critical inoculum into the lower airway. ETs that allow aspiration of the supraglottic pool are associated with lower incidence of VAP. Adding to the infection risk, sinus drainage is seriously impaired by extended immobility in the supine position. Moreover, nasal tubes of various kinds impede ipsilateral sinus drainage and increase the reservoir of nosocomial pathogens at risk for aspiration. Frequent breaks, ventilator circuit change, and moisture rain out predispose to lower airway seeding. Nasogastric and orogastric tubes encourage bacterial overgrowth and aspiration, especially in the supine position. While there is general agreement that the head of the intubated patient should be elevated at least 30 degrees, how importantly gastric feedings and antacid therapy contribute to the pneumonia risk is still a matter for debate. An intriguing body of experimental and clinical data suggests not only that high tidal volume and low PEEP ventilatory patterns predispose to the lung damage described earlier but also that lungs injured in this fashion are usually susceptible to pulmonary infections. Moreover, in varied animal models, such patterns cause capillary rupture and allow bacteria, inflammatory products, or mediators to enter the bloodstream.

Diagnosis and Treatment of VAP

Diagnostic techniques and approaches to management of VAP are detailed in Chapter 26. It should be emphasized here, however, that the diagnosis and management strategies for VAP are by no means straightforward. It is known that the bacteriology of the oropharynx and upper airway are different for otherwise healthy individuals recently admitted to the hospital, as compared with debilitated patients, and that colonization patterns shift as hospitalization time lengthens. While fever, purulent sputum, and a new infiltrate certainly *suggest* the development of pneumonia, many commonly encountered conditions are associated with those same features, especially in intubated patients. Although air bronchograms and other features detected by CT scanning are

TABLE 8-8   PREDISPOSITIONS TO VAP
Sinusitis
Poor dentition
Immobilization
Immune compromise
Supine position
Coexisting nasogastric tube
Lengthy period of ventilation
High gastric pH
Condensate within ventilator tubing
Frequent circuit disconnections

highly suggestive, uncertainty often remains and precise bacteriologic diagnosis may be elusive. Sputum cultures are almost invariably positive for several potential pathogens in untreated patients after 2 days in hospital, due to tracheal colonization; moreover, atelectasis and edema can develop confounding the radiographic features. Multiple organisms are frequently recovered from lung tissue of patients with suspected pneumonia. Techniques such as blind catheter lavage (mini-BAL, usually performed by respiratory therapists) and bronchoscope-directed lavage or protected specimen brushing of the suspected region improve the chances of accurate diagnosis. Such data may help modify empirical choices of antibiotic and therefore help prevent emergence of resistance or superinfection with more noxious pathogens, but it is unclear whether such tailoring confers a significant mortality advantage. Antibiotic treatment should begin soon after VAP is suspected, and selection of specific agents is best made considering the underlying medical and physiologic status of the patient, the time elapsed since hospitalization, whether the patient has recently been in a hospital or nursing home, susceptibility patterns of the organisms usually encountered in that specific ICU environment, and prior antibiotic treatment.

Deconditioning

Weakening and discoordination of respiratory muscles may occur as the burden, timing, and breathing pattern are machine controlled for prolonged periods. Substantial work is performed in the effort to trigger the ventilator, especially by breathless patients. As a rule, patients receiving assisted mechanical ventilation expend sufficient effort triggering the ventilator to prevent disuse atrophy, but it is unclear whether original muscle bulk and strength are preserved. The problem of deconditioning seems most serious for those patients who must assume a large workload of breathing when mechanical ventilation is discontinued, for those with preexisting neuromuscular impairment, for those with suppressed ventilatory drive, and for those requiring prolonged sedation or paralysis. Nutritional support, increased spontaneous muscle activity (continuous positive airway pressure [CPAP], intermittent mandatory ventilation [IMV], pressure support), and muscle training may be helpful. It is conceivable (but unproved) that the daily interruptions of sedation and trials of spontaneous breathing that are now advocated could help preserve bulk and strength, even during the acute stage.

■ PATIENT–VENTILATOR INTERACTIONS

Specific "Early Phase" Problems

Poor Coordination Between the Breathing Rhythms of Patient and Ventilator

Initial discomfort may be extreme because of the ET tube, distended hollow viscera, impaired swallowing, pharyngeal or sinus pain, anxiety, disorientation, inability to speak, or discomfort related to recent invasive procedures. Stimulation of bronchial, laryngeal, and carinal irritant receptors triggers bronchospasm and coughing efforts. Furthermore, mechanical ventilators usually are set to deliver higher (and occasionally lower) tidal volumes than the patient would choose spontaneously, whereas inspiratory pattern, flow rate, and cycling frequency differ from those of the presupport period. Hence, shortly after mechanical ventilation begins, attempts to "fight the ventilator" are the rule in alert, awakening, and mildly obtunded patients. Initial mismatching usually abates spontaneously (within minutes) as the settings are adjusted and the patient becomes accustomed to the machine. When deep sedation is not employed, constant attendance by trained medical personnel is often necessary throughout this period, to calm the patient, adjust the settings to the patient's requirements, and ensure that the agitation neither interferes with gas exchange nor has a more serious origin. It is extremely important to secure all tubing connectors and restrain the arms of an intermittently agitated or rousable patient. Ventilator disconnection or self-extubation is a potentially lethal and distressingly common event, especially when nursing resources are stretched too thin. When the patient is connected initially, sensitivity should be adjusted so that the minimal effort avoids autocycling to trigger a ventilator breath. Pressure-targeted modes of ventilation (pressure control and pressure support) adapt automatically to the patient's changing flow needs and are often good choices to avoid dys-synchrony. Pressure control breaths have a set duration, however, so that the I:E ratio varies when frequency changes. When either pressure control ventilation (PCV) or flow-controlled, volume-cycled ventilation is selected and minute ventilation is variable, synchronized intermittent mandatory ventilation (SIMV) may be better tolerated than assist control (see Chapter 7). Pressure (in PCV) or inspiratory flow rate (in assist control ventilation [ACV]) is adjusted to a level commensurate with the vigor and frequency of the patient's efforts. (Peak flows approx. 4 to 5 × V_E usually satisfy flow demands.) Tidal volume may need to be reduced temporarily to achieve an adequate matchup between patient and ventilator frequencies. Although high-level pressure support is generally effective in achieving adequate synchrony and comfort, refractory cases may require temporary disconnection of the circuit and use of a self-inflating anesthesia bag with manual assistance. With the machine properly adjusted, mechanical malfunctioning ruled out, the patient examined, the initial set of blood gases analyzed, and the chest radiograph checked for position of the tube tip and PTX, an opiate, a benzodiazepine, or a propofol may be given to assist smooth linking of endogenous respiratory and ventilator rhythms. Intratracheal lidocaine (2 to 4 mL of 1% to 2% concentration) can briefly arrest coughing spasms and reduce pain. A nasogastric tube helps decompress the gastrointestinal tract and is particularly helpful for patients with gastrointestinal motility impaired by opiates or disease who swallow air around orotracheal tubes.

Special Problems of Patients with High Ventilatory Requirements

Patients with high ventilatory requirements may overtax circuit valving or even the capacity of the ventilator to deliver gas at an adequate rate. Asynchrony markedly elevates the breathing workload, and tachypnea accentuates the importance of resistance within the ET and other circuit elements. Active use of the expiratory musculature may cause hypoxemia by combating the volume recruitment effect of PEEP, altering ventilation–perfusion relationships, and desaturating mixed venous blood. In these circumstances, reducing active effort can improve arterial oxygenation. Although deep sedation and paralysis can be helpful, prolonged immobility encourages regional atelectasis and secretion retention (especially in dependent areas), as well as muscle atrophy. For the paralyzed patient, ventilator disconnections can be rapidly lethal. Under extreme circumstances, adequate ventilation is difficult to achieve, even with paralysis and full machine support. Infused bicarbonate may allow pH to remain

compensated as CO_2 is permitted to stabilize at a higher level. It is not commonly realized that the PEEP and exhalation valves used with older generation ventilators offer substantial airflow resistance, which increases with ventilating frequency and the level of PEEP.

Dys-synchrony

Poor coordination between the patient and the ventilator regarding initiation and termination of breathing cycles, termed dys-synchrony or asynchrony, has been a common problem for traditional modes of ventilation. Whereas time-cycled modes (PCV) are most susceptible to these timing issues because of their fixed inspiratory cycle lengths, pressure support ventilation (PSV) is not immune to them. Newer modes that do not have a fixed trigger for expiration onset (e.g., proportional assist ventilation [PAV]) and/or are geared to phrenic nerve activity (neurally adjusted ventilatory assist [NAVA]) are less susceptible to these cycling conflicts. Dys-synchrony represents more than inconvenience and discomfort, as recent studies demonstrate that duration of mechanical ventilation, sleep quality, and need for tracheostomy are adversely influenced by it. Triggering dys-synchrony can be classified as autotriggering, ineffective triggering, and double triggering (Fig. 8-10).

Autotriggering usually results from a combination of a highly sensitive trigger setting and a circuit problem—condensation, secretions, vigorous cardiac oscillations, or (when flow triggering is used) a gas leak. Fixing sources of circuit "noise," decreasing trigger sensitivity, and/or switching to the pressure triggering option usually correct autotriggering problems.

Ineffective triggering is usually the product of weak inspiratory efforts, a higher than needed pressure support level, or auto-PEEP. Resetting the trigger to greater sensitivity, reducing the level of

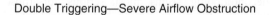

Double Triggering—Severe Airflow Obstruction

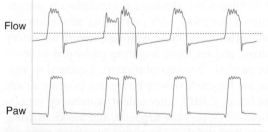

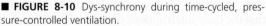

■ **FIGURE 8-10** Dys-synchrony during time-cycled, pressure-controlled ventilation.

pressure applied during PCV or PSV, and reducing auto-PEEP (e.g., by pharmacotherapy or secretion clearance), or counterbalancing auto-PEEP with external PEEP usually resolve the problem.

Double triggering is actually an expiratory off-switch dys-synchrony and results from the patient needing a longer inspiratory time than set. An increase in support (raising the pressure setting or extending the inspiratory time) can be helpful. When it is not, the problem may be that the level of support being given is excessive, mandating a trial of reduced pressure, SIMV rate, or inspiratory flow. Again, clearance of retained secretions is often helpful or sufficient. In this double-triggering situation, therapy is often empirical.

Problems with the expiratory off-switch sometimes arise during PSV. These can be premature termination or delayed termination of the inspiratory period. Convulsive initiation of the breath, as during hiccough, causes flow to fall precipitously and the machine to cycle off. Conversion to a time-cycled, pressure-targeted mode (PCV) is sometimes the answer. In the setting of airflow obstruction, the problem may be the opposite—cycles of excessive length that require active expiratory effort to terminate. When adjustment of the flow off-switch does not succeed in restoring synchrony and setting a time limit is not a machine option, conversion to time-cycled PCV usually is effective.

Specific "Support Phase" Problems

8 Smooth interaction between the patient and machine may be interrupted by malfunctioning of the ventilator system, worsening of cardiopulmonary mechanics, psychic distress, or factors completely unrelated to ventilation. Malfunctions of the ventilator system prevent adequate ventilation or oxygenation and usually present as agitation, worrisome changes in vital signs, or unexplained deterioration in blood gases.

Diagnostic Approach to Agitation During Mechanical Ventilation

When an event develops suddenly during mechanical ventilation, the clinician must efficiently diagnose the problem in an organized fashion. Many latest generation ventilators display helpful and explicit cues to action, such as "circuit disconnect." When the problem is not quickly resolved, the patient should be ventilated manually with pure oxygen until the problem has been diagnosed. The difference between the exhaled versus set tidal volume may provide crucial data. A major difference unexplained by pressure limiting and "pop-off" losses indicates a circuit leak or machine dysfunction. Checking the airway pressure profile and comparing the peak dynamic (P_D) and static (P_S) pressures against previous values also provide essential information. Failure to generate or hold pressure during circuit occlusion usually indicates a system leak. A large disparity between P_D and P_S suggests a resistance problem in the tube or airways (bronchospasm, secretions). It is useful to classify these problems as those that usually elevate peak cycling pressure (pressure limiting) and those that usually do not (Table 8-9). Three components of the system must be checked carefully: the patient, the ET, and the ventilator system.

Patient

The importance of auscultation for signs of PTX, bronchospasm, secretion plugging, and pulmonary edema deserves emphasis. Mucus plugging, accompanied by major airway blockage, is a very frequent cause for sudden high pressures and

TABLE 8-9 SUDDEN CRISES DURING MECHANICAL VENTILATION

PRESSURE LIMITING	NONPRESSURE LIMITING
Central airway obstruction	Cuff deflation/tube withdrawal
Massive atelectasis	Circuit disruption
Tube occlusion	Machine malfunction
Mainstem intubation	PTX without tension
Pain, anxiety, or delirium	Gas trapping (auto-PEEP)
Tension PTX	Hemodynamic crisis
Irritative bronchospasm	Pulmonary embolism
Decreased chest wall compliance	Pulmonary edema
Secretion retention	

hypoxemia. The symmetry of breath sounds and percussion dullness should be determined in one of the first steps of the evaluation. Among the most important distinctions to make is the one between massive atelectasis and tension PTX. A PTX that does not have a tension component may not elevate peak airway pressure (or reduce tidal volume) noticeably. Nonpulmonary causes of discomfort (distention of bladder or intestinal tract, unvarying body position, pain, etc.) are overlooked easily. Pulmonary emboli and cardiac ischemia occur commonly.

Problems occur frequently among patients with combined cardiac and pulmonary disease. Increased VO_2, heart rate, blood pressure, and left ventricular afterload can cause florid congestive failure ("flash" pulmonary edema), ischemia, or other manifestation of circulatory stress within minutes of onset in a patient with coronary insufficiency or myocardial or valvular dysfunction. A quick glance at the cardiac monitor is mandatory. The sudden onset of a tachyarrhythmia, particularly driven by atrial fibrillation and atrial flutter, may be the primary driver of the distress an EKG should be considered very early on if the problem is not otherwise quickly diagnosed and resolved. Quite often, adrenergic bronchodilator therapy is the culprit.

For patients receiving flow-controlled, volume-cycled ventilation (e.g., assist-control or SIMV), the need for increased minute ventilation often causes ventilatory demands to outstrip the ventilator's flow delivery, increasing the work of breathing still further and setting into motion a self-perpetuating cycle of agitation and cardiopulmonary compromise. A boost in ventilatory support and inspiratory flow rate often is required to rectify the situation. Agitated patients often oppose the ventilator, causing dys-synchrony and pressure limiting. In the assist-control mode, dys-synchrony tends to be self-perpetuating, inasmuch as small (pressure-limited) inflations do not allow adequate ventilation and dyspnea continues or increases. A vicious cycle is especially likely to develop in patients with airflow obstruction who hyperinflate, causing auto-PEEP with associated muscle dysfunction and hemodynamic stress. Both the work of breathing and dyspnea escalate markedly as the patient struggles to breathe. Temporarily switching to high-level pressure support (sufficient to achieve an effective tidal volume) often helps relieve dys-synchrony and dyspnea until the situation can be analyzed fully and the underlying cause can be addressed definitively. Disconnecting the ventilator and providing adequate ventilation manually with a resuscitator bag is an alternative strategy that frequently will break the cycle.

It must be stressed that once agitation develops, hypoxemia frequently occurs, increasing both the drive to breathe and dyspnea. Increasing the FiO_2 often reverses hypoxemia and can undo the self-reinforcing process of agitation $\rightarrow$ hypoxemia $\rightarrow$ increased drive $\rightarrow$ agitation $\rightarrow$ hypoxemia. In fact, increasing FiO_2 is a good first option whenever desaturation accompanies agitation. Although agitation often has a trivial origin, it must never be ignored or suppressed with sedatives until possible serious causes are considered. Bradycardia is experienced frequently during temporary machine disconnection for suctioning by patients requiring high levels of PEEP and mean airway pressure. Although hypoxemia occasionally is responsible for these episodes of bradycardia, this phenomenon usually is a reflex effect, which is prevented by pretreatment with systemic atropine, "closed circuit" airway suctioning, or the provision of CPAP during secretion removal.

Endotracheal Tube

Modern ventilators are equipped with audible alarms that sense excessive or inadequate system pressure, failure to exhale a set minimum tidal volume, or disconnection of the patient from the machine. If the cause for distress is not immediately obvious, the caregiver should note the position of the ET in relation to its previous level, listen for cuff leaks during inflation (auscultate over the larynx), and palpate the pilot balloon to sense the pressure in the cuff. ETs often kink, block with secretions, or become constricted by the teeth of a biting patient. After assuring adequate oxygenation, a suction catheter is passed to check patency of the ET and aspirate central airway secretions. Vital signs are checked and auscultation is performed quickly for evidence of PTX, massive atelectasis, or bronchospasm, as the patient is ventilated manually with 100% oxygen. Tubes that are poorly placed or secured may migrate into the larynx or right main bronchus or may rest on the carina, producing cough and bronchospasm.

Ventilator Circuit

The integrity of the ventilator circuit is then inspected quickly, with special attention given to tubing connections and the settings for tidal volume, frequency, trigger sensitivity, and oxygen fraction. Tubing is inspected for accumulated water, which may increase inspiratory resistance or cause inadvertent expiratory retard or PEEP. When heat–moisture exchangers are used, this is less of a problem. Rarely, the swings and vibrations of airway pressure caused by retained secretions or circuit water are great enough to initiate autocycling. If the problem remains obscure, the patient can be reconnected briefly to check delivered versus set minute ventilation. If delivered minute ventilation is too low, all connections should be checked carefully for leaks, especially around the humidifier and the exhalation valve. In a passive patient, the application of an end-inspiratory pause will help detect a circuit leak. If the problem still persists, no cause is detected, and the chest radiograph is negative, judicious doses of morphine or other sedative can be given, as long as gas exchange is well maintained as judged by oximetry or arterial blood gases. Pharmacoparalysis must never be undertaken until an alert patient is adequately sedated.

Other Support Phase Problems

Work of breathing, psychological distress, and depression are prevalent during mechanical ventilation and are discussed at length in Chapter 10.

■ SUGGESTED READINGS

Baumann MH. Top ten list in pleural disease. *Chest.* 2003;124(6): 2352–2355.

Dellinger RP, Levy MM, Carlet JM, et al. Surviving sepsis campaign: International guidelines for management of severe sepsis and septic shock: 2008 section IIA. Mechanical ventilation of sepsis-induced ALI/ARDS. *Crit Care Med.* 2008;36(1):296–326.

Isakow W, Kollef MH. Preventing ventilator-associated pneumonia: An evidence-based approach of modifiable risk factors. *Semin Respir Crit Care Med.* 2006;27(1):5–17.

Kollef MH. Prevention of hospital-associated pneumonia and ventilator-associated pneumonia. *Crit Care Med.* 2004;32(6):1396–1405.

Light RW. Chest tubes. In: *Pleural Diseases.* 5th Ed. Philadelphia, PA: Lippincott Williams & Wilkins; 2007.

Lois M, Noppen M. Bronchopleural fistulas: An overview of the problem with special focus on endoscopic management. *Chest.* 2005;128: 3955–3965.

Marini JJ. Ventilatory management of ARDS. In: Tobin M, ed. *Principles and Practice of Mechanical Ventilation.* 2nd Ed. New York: McGraw-Hill; 2006:625–648.

Marini JJ, Gattinoni L. Ventilatory management of acute respiratory distress syndrome: A consensus of two. *Crit Care Med.* 2004;32(1): 250–255.

Marini JJ, Gattinoni L. Propagation prevention: A complementary mechanism for lung protective ventilation in ARDS. *Crit Care Med.* 2008; 36(12):3252–3258.

Miller LA. Chest wall, lung, and pleural space trauma. *Radiol Clin North Am.* 2006;44(2):213–24.

Woodside KJ, vanSonnenberg E, Chon KS, et al. Pneumothorax in patients with acute respiratory distress syndrome: Pathophysiology, detection, and treatment. *J Intensive Care Med.* 2003;18(1):9–20.

Positive End-Expiratory and Continuous Positive Airway Pressure

KEY POINTS

1 Adding positive end-expiratory pressure (PEEP) can help maintain patency of collapsed lung units or further distend those that are already patent. The former action usually is beneficial, whereas the latter may cause alveolar overdistention. Both effects may occur simultaneously in different lung regions at the same level of PEEP.

2 Positive end-expiratory alveolar pressure or total PEEP is the sum of the PEEP applied intentionally at the airway opening (PEEP or "extrinsic" PEEP) and auto-PEEP ("intrinsic" or "inadvertent" PEEP) that results from dynamic hyperinflation. Expiratory muscle activity may raise the measured value for total PEEP.

3 Transalveolar pressure is the key variable that determines PEEP's effect on lung volume. A patient with a poorly compliant chest wall will require a higher PEEP to achieve adequate lung expansion.

4 Use of PEEP in improving arterial oxygenation, in minimizing ventilator induced lung injury, and perhaps in preventing pneumonia stems primarily from its ability to impede the recollapse of edematous or compressed alveoli recruited by higher pressures experienced during the tidal inspiratory phase or by a sigh or recruitment maneuver. PEEP also improves the distribution of alveolar liquid, translocating edema fluid from the alveolus to the interstitium. When PEEP reduces cardiac output, it also tends to reduce shunt fraction.

5 The volume recruiting effect of PEEP is influenced by the chest wall compliance, the tidal volume, and the activity of the respiratory muscles. Any benefit from PEEP on

oxygen exchange may be offset by expiratory muscle activity and restored by muscle relaxation.

6 A shift to the prone position exerts a selective PEEP-like action in the dorsal regions of the lung and commonly improves oxygenation of patients with lung edema. Proning also has the potential to initiate transfer of secretions, inflammatory edema, and other biofluids to the central airway and to the previously unaffected lung sectors.

7 PEEP tends to decrease both preload and afterload to the left ventricle. Impaired venous return may lower the cardiac output in a passive patient who does not have intact vascular reflexes or adequate circulating blood volume. Conversely, reduced left ventricular afterload resulting from PEEP may benefit the patient in acute congestive heart failure. The hemodynamic effects of auto-PEEP are similar to those of external PEEP.

8 Increased peak and mean alveolar pressures that result from excessive PEEP may produce or extend barotrauma, reduce oxygen delivery, and increase ventilatory dead space. PEEP may either increase or decrease the work of breathing.

9 Good candidates for PEEP have clinically significant hypoxemia that is refractory to inspired oxygen, diffuse acute pulmonary disease, a poorly compliant respiratory system, a tendency for atelectasis, acute cardiogenic edema with increased left ventricular afterload, audible dependent rales during tidal breathing, or severe airflow obstruction with tidal flow limitation. Virtually all intubated patients are candidates for PEEP of 3 to 5 cm H_2O to help offset the lung compressing effects of recumbency.

10 Choosing the optimum level of PEEP is an empirical process determined by the response of multiple gas exchange, mechanics, and hemodynamic variables to a well-monitored PEEP trial. Recruitment maneuvers are integral to the selection process.

11 Auto-PEEP can dramatically increase the work of breathing and provoke patient–ventilator dyssynchrony. In many patients with flow limitation during tidal breathing, these problems can be addressed by adding an appropriate level of PEEP that minimizes end-expiratory airflow without raising the peak alveolar pressure significantly.

Hypoxemia resulting from alveolar collapse or edema often responds to alveolar recruitment and maintenance of lung unit patency with positive **1** end-expiratory airway pressure (PEEP). Adding PEEP helps keep lung units patent but may further distend those that are already open. When PEEP maintains recruited lung volume, it not only improves arterial oxygenation but also may reduce the elastic work of expanding the lung or improve the distribution of ventilation. Conversely, PEEP added to an already "open" lung without compensatory recruitment tends to create dead space and possibly worsen the oxygen exchange. Maintaining end-expiratory lung volume helps prevent ventilator-induced lung injury (VILI) during the initial stages of the acute respiratory distress syndrome (ARDS), reduces alveolar edema, and seems useful in avoiding complications after thoracic and upper abdominal surgery.

This chapter focuses primarily on the use of PEEP in hypoxemic respiratory failure; this objective is quite distinct from that of adding PEEP to reduce the work of breathing and improve

breath triggering (*without* increasing the lung volume) during flow-limiting airflow obstruction. The latter important topic is addressed elsewhere (see Chapter 25).

■ DEFINITIONS

Positive end-expiratory alveolar pressure, or "total **2** PEEP" ($PEEP_T$), is the sum of PEEP applied intentionally at the airway opening (PEEP or "extrinsic" PEEP) and auto ("occult," "inadvertent," or "intrinsic") PEEP ($PEEP_i$). The expressions "assisted ventilation with PEEP" and "continuous positive pressure breathing" are synonymous, referring to mechanically delivered tidal breaths with positive pressure maintained at end-expiration (Fig. 9-1). By convention, when airway pressure is positive at the end of expiration during time limited mechanical ventilation, the acronym is "PEEP." During spontaneous breathing cycles, it is called "continuous positive airway pressure," or "CPAP." In practice, CPAP has come to imply that the patient provides some or all of ventilating power while PEEP suggests that the ventilator is carrying most or all of the breathing workload. The terms are often interchanged, however, as they will be in this chapter—the key principles underlying PEEP and CPAP are identical. When two levels of PEEP are alternated, with spontaneous breaths occurring during each phase, the mode is termed "biphasic positive airway pressure" or "BIPAP." (In this context, the term BIPAP must not be confused with "bi-level," commercially known as BiPAP, which has been applied to a combination of pressure support and CPAP intended for noninvasive ventilation applied via face mask [see Chapter 7].) If the lower level of BIPAP is maintained only transiently (e.g., the span of a single exhalation), the mode is referred to as "airway pressure release." Several of these PEEP variants are discussed elsewhere in this volume (see Chapters 7 and 10). The discussion here will focus on single levels of end-expiratory alveolar pressure.

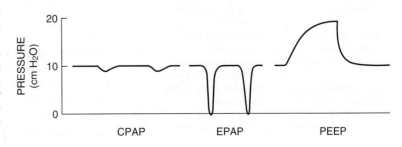

■ **FIGURE 9-1** Three modes of maintaining elevated airway pressure at end-exhalation. CPAP and expiratory positive airway pressure (EPAP) require the patient to supply the energy needed to ventilate. Unlike in CPAP, inspiration only begins in EPAP when airway pressure becomes sub-atmospheric, increasing the inspiratory work.

■ PATHOPHYSIOLOGY

Actions of PEEP in Acute Hypoxemic Respiratory Failure

3 The normal lung requires no PEEP to maintain full recruitment—periodic sighs are sufficient to prevent or reverse the widespread alveolar collapse. When the chest cavity is reduced in size (e.g., after abdominal surgery), the lung is edematous or infiltrated (e.g., pulmonary edema), the alveoli are inherently unstable (surfactant depletion ARDS), and small airways are predisposed to closure during the tidal cycle, particularly in gravitationally dependent regions. Collapsed units open over a spectrum of airway pressures, determined largely by the local pressures that surround them. Even in ARDS, most collapsed units recruit at pressures lower than 25 cm H_2O. Once opened, a lower airspace pressure (PEEP or CPAP) must be sustained to prevent their reclosure. The utility of PEEP in improving arterial oxygenation, in minimizing VILI, and perhaps in preventing pneumonia stems primarily from its ability to impede the recollapse of edematous or compressed alveoli recruited by higher pressures (Table 9-1).

PEEP applied to lung units that are already open increases alveolar dimensions, resting lung volume, and pleural pressure. Distention tends to redirect the blood flow, increase the vena caval resistance to venous return, and create ventilatory dead space, as well as to redistribute alveolar liquid to the interstitial space and favor edema clearance. In a heterogeneous lung with a wide range of unstable alveoli, alveolar opening may occur in different regions throughout inspiration, particularly when PEEP is low and tidal volume (V_T) is

high. When PEEP is added to an unchanging tidal volume, collapsed lung units are opened by the relatively high alveolar pressures (amplified by interdependence) that occur at the end of the inspiratory cycle; PEEP prevents their reclosure **4** during expiration. Oxygenation may benefit by at least two other mechanisms. When PEEP reduces cardiac output, blood flow through shunt regions may also decline, reducing venous admixture. Perhaps more importantly, PEEP improves the distribution of alveolar liquid and translocates fluid from alveolar to interstitial spaces, lowering the diffusion distance for oxygen exchange. In the presence of alveolar edema, PEEP may prevent airway flooding by expanding the alveolar reservoir and encouraging fluid migration into the interstitial space. By inhibiting distribution of proteinaceous and mediator-laden biofluids via the airway network, both actions may play an important role in the prevention of injury propagation, as described in Chapter 8. (Conversely, abrupt removal of PEEP may precipitate translocation of alveolar liquid into the airways, impeding airflow and occasionally generating froth.) Most available data indicate that PEEP redistributes but does not decrease the total lung water; in some instances, lung weight may actually increase because of distention of the interstitial space and raised pulmonary venous and lymphatic pressures.

Interaction of PEEP and Tidal Volume

Recruitment of lung volume is a joint function of PEEP and the opening pressures generated in response to tidal volume. Airways open at higher volumes and trans-structural pressures than those at which they close (see "Recruiting Maneuvers"). Therefore, to achieve the same effect on oxygenation and compliance, higher values of PEEP may be needed when tidal volumes are smaller (Fig. 9-2) (see Chapter 25). Moreover, even if calculated tidal (chord) compliance values are identical, failure to maintain sufficient PEEP may result in tidal opening and closure of dependent lung units, a process that may produce high shearing stresses believed to damage the delicate lung tissues. Some experimental evidence suggests that the *variation* in tidal volume normally observed during health (biologically variable ventilation) serves an important recruiting function. The same minute ventilation achieved after lung injury with monotonous tidal volumes is associated with less-effective

TABLE 9-1 BENEFITS AND PROBLEMS OF POSITIVE END-EXPIRATORY AIRWAY PRESSURE

BENEFITS	PROBLEMS
Improves oxygenation	Predisposes to barotrauma
Reduces work of breathing	Impedes preload and right ventricular ejection
Improves lung compliance	Reduces cerebral perfusion
Aids the left ventricle	Impairs ventilatory pumping efficiency
Splints the chest wall	Increases dead space
Mobilizes distal secretions	Confounds monitoring

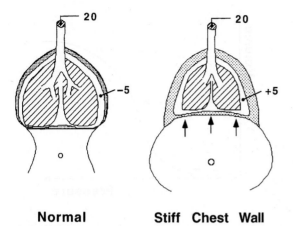

Normal   Stiff Chest Wall

■ **FIGURE 9-2** Effect of chest wall compliance on lung volume. The effect of positive airway pressure (in this case, 20 cm H_2O) on lung volume is influenced by the compliance of the chest wall. In this example, the distending force across the lung is 25 cm H_2O when the chest wall is normal but only 15 cm H_2O when the chest wall is poorly compliant. A patient with a stiff chest wall requires a higher PEEP to achieve the same physiologic effect.

oxygenation than the identical ventilation accomplished with varying tidal volumes. Any benefit is believed to be due (at least in part) to the avalanches of recruitment that occur when the higher inspiratory pressures are transiently applied.

Importance of Chest Wall Compliance

Volume changes resulting from PEEP are shared equally by the lungs and chest wall. Assuming that exhalation occurs passively, the volume recruited by PEEP (ΔV) depends on the compliance of the entire respiratory system, which itself is a function **5** of both lung (C_L) and chest wall (C_W) compliances:

$$\Delta V = PEEP_T \times C_{RS}$$
$$= PEEP_T \times [(C_L C_W)/(C_L + C_W)]$$

As discussed elsewhere (Chapter 5), the pressure distending the lung at end-expiration is ($PEEP_T - P_{PL}$), whereas the pressure that distends the *passive* chest wall is P_{PL} alone. It follows that the volume-expanding and hemodynamic effects of PEEP will vary with the compliance of the chest wall (Fig. 9-3). A very obese patient or one with a recently operated abdomen or rib cage requires relatively more PEEP to keep the lung adequately recruited, and P_{PL} tends to rise disproportionately with each PEEP increment. Local variations in the compliance of the chest wall help explain the heterogeneity of infiltration and lung expansion in the settings of pulmonary edema acute lung injury.

Regional Effects of PEEP

Pressure varies from site to site within the pleural space. In the supine position, a ventral-to-dorsal gravitational gradient causes the pleural pressure that surrounds dependent alveoli to be several centimeters H_2O greater than that in nondependent regions, and this difference increases in the setting of acute lung injury. (This gravitational gradient of pleural pressure is less steep in the prone position.) Because alveolar distention is a function of transalveolar pressure (airspace minus surrounding pressure), regional alveolar dimensions and propensities to collapse differ, despite a common

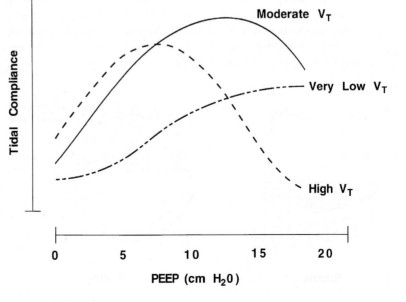

■ **FIGURE 9-3** Interaction of PEEP and tidal volume (V_T) in determining tidal compliance. Assuming that the clinical objective is to maximize tidal compliance, there is no single "best PEEP" value relevant to all tidal volumes. Higher values of PEEP are needed to achieve optimal compliance when small tidal volumes are used. PEEP, positive end-expiratory airway pressure.

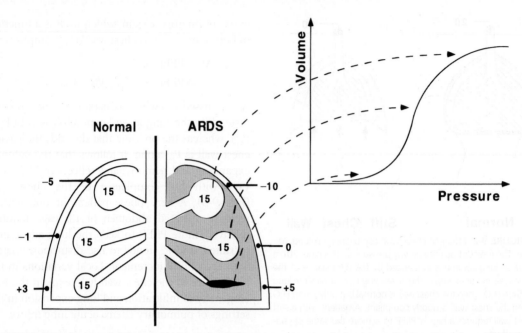

■ FIGURE 9-4 Influence of the gravitational gradient of pressure on regional alveolar mechanics. Dependent alveoli at the base of the lung may remain collapsed at airway pressures that threaten to overdistend those in nondependent regions. Regional mechanics are especially heterogenous in the setting of ARDS. To counterbalance this gradient, higher regional PEEP in dependent areas or modified chest wall compliance in nondependent regions would be needed to improve the uniformity of distention and ventilation. ARDS, acute respiratory distress syndrome.

airway pressure. As progressively higher pressures are applied, individual lung units pop open at some critical opening pressure but collapse abruptly as it is withdrawn. PEEP that is sufficient to hold alveoli in the uppermost regions patent throughout the tidal cycle may be insufficient to prevent the collapse of gravitationally dependent ones (Fig. 9-4). The consequences of this gradient of pleural and transalveolar pressures is likely to explain the marked dependency of computed tomographic (CT) densities evident during the initial stages of acute lung injury, as well as the lower "inflection zone" of improving compliance often observed on the inspiratory pressure–volume curve of the

respiratory system early in the course of ARDS. PEEP tends to narrow the pleural pressure gradient if recruitment occurs or if alveoli in all regions are open. A PEEP value which recruits the most dependent alveoli may be needed to avoid their repeated opening and recollapse during each tidal cycle.

Regional PEEP and the Prone Position

In experimental animals, the gradient of alveolar dimensions and pleural pressure is considerably greater in the supine position than in the prone position. Consequently, the prone position alters the distribution of lung volume corresponding to a

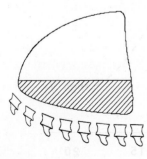

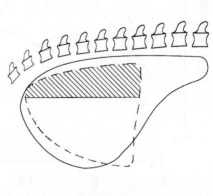

■ FIGURE 9-5 Lung geometry in supine and prone positions. In the supine position, dorsal regions of the lung (crosshatched) are subjected to higher pleural (and lower transpulmonary) pressures than they are in the prone position. These dorsal regions tend to expand dramatically in the prone position, whereas sternal regions are only modestly compressed. The prone position modestly increases the overall resting lung volume (functional residual capacity, FRC) in most patients.

Supine

Prone

given airway pressure, with dorsal regions better expanded (Fig. 9-5). In effect, altering position exerts a differential PEEP-like effect in different lung regions. For the same PEEP, the distribution of tidal ventilation is more homogeneous, and ventilation–perfusion matching and arterial oxygenation tend to improve. Available data suggest that a similar phenomenon also occurs in humans. The effect of prone positioning on overall functional residual capacity (FRC) is debated and is likely to be influenced by any positional changes that occur in chest wall compliance because of the supporting surface. Although the distribution of volume is altered dramatically, FRC increases only modestly or remains unchanged by the turning process.

Active Expiration

If exhalation occurs passively (as it does during quiet, unstressed breathing), PEEP achieves its desired effect—increases in end-expiratory lung volume and in the number of open air channels. However, if the resulting lung expansion proves uncomfortable, spontaneously breathing patients may actively oppose PEEP in attempting to limit the volume increase. Active expiration to a volume lower than the equilibrium position that corresponds to the PEEP applied to the passive patient stores potential energy. In this way, PEEP or CPAP may provide a mechanism by which the dyspneic patient can use the expiratory muscles to share the workload otherwise borne entirely by inspiratory muscles. As the expiratory muscles relax, the outward recoil of the chest wall then provides an inspiratory boost (Fig. 9-6). The expiratory muscles are activated normally during vigorous exercise, hyperpnea, and impeded expiration.

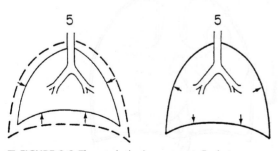

■ **FIGURE 9-6** The work-sharing concept. Expiratory muscles may force the lung below the equilibrium volume appropriate to the applied level of PEEP (in this case, 5 cm H$_2$O). This increases the expiratory work of breathing, reduces FRC, and tends to impair oxygenation. Thoracic compression against PEEP, however, stores the energy for release in early inspiration, thereby sharing the ventilatory workload of the inspiratory muscles.

Opposition to PEEP occurring in a hypoxemic patient may attenuate volume recruitment, especially in the peridiaphragmatic zones. By silencing the expiratory muscles, sedation or paralysis restores the volume recruitment effect of PEEP and can markedly improve oxygenation. In addition, reduced oxygen consumption because of less respiratory effort and agitation undoubtedly contributes as the ventilator assumes the task of powering ventilation.

Time Course of PEEP Effect on Gas Exchange

Although lung recruitment is nearly completed within five to ten breaths, the time course is quite variable; several hours may be required to realize the full effect of a given PEEP increment. On the other hand, desaturation usually occurs quite abruptly upon PEEP withdrawal. Because PEEP's primary benefit relates to the maintenance of lung volume and not to the positive pressure itself, the lung can be expanded by internally positive or externally negative pressure. Therefore, it should cause no concern for lost volume when a patient transiently pulls an inspiratory airway pressure lower than the set PEEP level. To generate a lower airway pressure, pleural pressure must have decreased at least as much as alveolar pressure, so that transpulmonary pressure and end-expiratory lung volume are preserved. (On the other hand, such a decline in pleural pressure may obligate significant ventilatory work.)

PEEP and Mean Airway Pressure

Mean alveolar pressure and its most easily measured analog, mean airway pressure, are discussed at length elsewhere in this text (see Chapters 5 and 24). It is worth noting here, however, that although mean alveolar pressure can be raised in a variety of ways, PEEP has the most predictable effect on oxygenation, combating end-expiratory lung unit collapse as it raises both mean airway and mean alveolar pressures by the amount of the PEEP applied. Just as PEEP$_T$ determines the end-expiratory alveolar dimension, in a passive patient, the mean airway pressure determines the *average* or mean alveolar volume. Most cardiovascular effects of PEEP are mediated by mean alveolar pressure via its effects on mean intrapleural and right atrial pressures. Apart from its effect on mean airway pressure, PEEP$_T$ maintains collapsible alveoli recruited throughout the tidal breath; therefore, it is instrumental in improving oxygen exchange and avoiding VILI. (In fact, it has been argued that raising mean airway pressure while holding PEEP$_T$ constant may not help markedly to improve the arterial oxygen delivery.)

■ ADVERSE EFFECTS OF PEEP

Cardiovascular Impairment

PEEP and Venous Return

At the end of passive exhalation, pressure within the central airway approximates alveolar pressure, provided the expiratory flow has stopped (see "auto-PEEP effect"). Under these quasi-static conditions, an increment of pressure applied to the airway (PEEP) distributes across the lung and chest wall according to the formula:

$$\Delta P_{PL} = PEEP \times [C_L/(C_L + C_W)]$$

where P_{PL} and PEEP refer to pleural and airway pressures and C_L and C_W denote the dynamic compliances of the lung and chest wall, respectively. Normally, the lungs and passive chest wall have similar compliance characteristics in the tidal range near FRC; therefore, approximately one half of the applied PEEP transmits to the pleural space. With abnormally stiff lungs, less is transmitted (typically, one fifth to one third). With compliant lungs and a stiff chest wall (e.g., in a patient with emphysema, obesity, or massive ascites), the pleural pressure increment is a higher fraction of applied PEEP (Fig. 9-2). Because pressures similar to P_{PL} surround the heart and great vessels, PEEP reduces the venous return but tends to raise all intrathoracic vascular pressures. Such pressure changes complicate the interpretation of central venous pressure (CVP) and pulmonary artery occlusion (wedge) pressure.

Depression of cardiac output is seen rarely during the application of modest levels of CPAP to a spontaneously breathing patient. Compared with passive inflation, the magnitude of the CPAP-induced rise of mean intrapleural pressure is routinely small. Moreover, inspiratory descent of the diaphragm (and expiratory effort, if any) boosts intra-abdominal (and therefore upstream) venous pressures relative to their intrathoracic values, improving venous return.

In studies conducted on supine normal animals, it has been shown that high levels of PEEP can compress the inferior vena cava (IVC) at the thoracic inlet, increasing the resistance to venous return (Fig. 9-7). Compression is likely to result, in part, from the lifting effect of PEEP on the heart and seldom occurs in the prone position. Lung expansion lifts the supine heart and depresses the diaphragm, thereby stretching the IVC, which is tethered at the diaphragm, pericardium, and retroperitoneum. Whether caval compression is important when the lungs are stiff (and volume changes are small, as they tend to be in ARDS) is an unanswered question.

PEEP and Ventricular Afterload

Although PEEP may raise pulmonary vascular resistance, this effect is relatively unimportant when the lung has a normal capacity to accept gas. Right ventricular performance remains little affected unless pulmonary capillary reserve is exhausted, the right

7

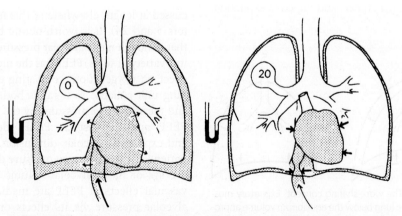

■ **FIGURE 9-7** Effects of PEEP on cardiovascular function. As PEEP holds the lungs distended, increased juxtacardiac pressure tends to compress the heart and great vessels, impeding venous inflow to the thorax while raising intracavitary and intravascular pressures. PEEP may also narrow the inferior vena cava at the inlet to the thorax, thereby increasing the resistance to venous return as well. Alveolar overdistention may significantly afterload the right ventricle.

ventricle is already failing, or peak and mean alveolar pressures rise to quite elevated levels. It is worth noting that only a small fraction of the lung may remain accessible to gas in the later stages of ARDS—typically one third or less of the normal amount. In patients without pleural effusion, the sum of gas, tissue, and liquid in the injured lung is approximately normal and equals the injured volume occupied by the chest wall that surrounds it. In this setting, therefore, the cardiovascular effects of alveolar overdistention, pulmonary hypertension, right ventricular afterload, and left ventricular filling restriction associated with right ventricular dilation may predominate over those caused by the very modest increases of pleural pressure due to PEEP. Even in less-compromised lungs, high levels of PEEP can increase right ventricular (RV) afterload sufficiently to reduce left ventricular compliance by ventricular interdependence.

Left ventricular afterload is decreased by raising intrapleural pressure because the systolic myocardial tension that must be developed to achieve any specified systemic arterial pressure is diminished by the external compression that results from augmented pleural pressure. Although such afterload changes are likely to be of little significance during passive inflation, their importance rises when vigorous inspiratory efforts are made. Applying CPAP to patients with pulmonary edema promotes cardiovascular stability not only by decreasing central vascular volume and improving arterial oxygenation and the work of breathing but also by helping to silence the inspiratory effort, thereby raising intrapleural pressure and reducing afterload. High levels of PEEP have been suggested to cause myocardial dysfunction directly, but such effects, if present at all, are minor.

Compensation for PEEP-induced reductions in cardiac output may be accomplished by increasing heart rate (a compensatory response thought to be blunted by PEEP), raising venous tone, and retaining sufficient intravascular fluid to raise the pressure driving venous return. These counterbalancing effects are maximized within hours to days. Cardiac output usually remains stable when moderate levels of PEEP are used in normovolemic patients with good cardiovascular reflexes and myocardial reserves. Repletion of intravascular volume, guided by the PEEP-adjusted central venous or wedge pressures, should be the primary treatment for depressed cardiac output resulting from PEEP. When adequate intravascular volume is ensured, vasopressors also may be added to improve the driving pressure for venous return.

Barotrauma

Barotrauma during mechanical ventilation is discussed extensively elsewhere in this volume (see Chapter 8). The extent to which PEEP contributes to the tendency for pneumothorax and other forms of extra-alveolar gas accumulation is unclear. When tidal volume remains unchanged, its primary effects may be mediated by increasing peak and mean alveolar pressures. If peak pressure is controlled, PEEP may contribute negligibly to the risk of alveolar rupture. In fact, when high tidal pressures are generated in the early stages of ARDS, PEEP may be instrumental in reducing shear stresses and avoiding ventilator-induced lung edema. It stands to reason that PEEP might accentuate the risk of rupturing alveoli that are weakened by disease if peak pressures are allowed to rise, and once ruptured, a PEEP-induced increase in mean alveolar pressure could promote additional gas leakage. These pressures are reduced effectively by lowering the tidal volume as end-expiratory pressure is raised. A lower tidal volume with increased PEEP often results in hypercapnia, which can be either accepted (permissive hypercapnia) or offset by increasing the ventilator's cycling frequency.

Reduced Oxygen Delivery

Although it usually aids tissue oxygenation, PEEP may adversely affect oxygen delivery via three mechanisms: (a) decreased cardiac output, (b) increased venous admixture, and (c) increased intracardiac or noncapillary shunt. Oxygen delivery declines if the drop in cardiac output caused by PEEP outweighs the rise in arterial oxygen content. Assuming that metabolic demands remain unchanged, additional oxygen will then be stripped from arterial blood, dropping the O_2 saturation of mixed-venous (pulmonary arterial) blood. In turn, reduced mixed-venous O_2 saturation adversely affects arterial O_2 content, unless hypoxic vasoconstriction sufficiently limits admixture. Hence, when the adequacy of tissue oxygen delivery is in question, it is mandatory to follow cardiac output as well as SaO_2 during manipulations of PEEP, supplemented, when feasible, by determinations of central venous or mixed-venous saturation, arterial-venous oxygen content difference $\Delta[(a - v)O_2]$, or other indications of tissue O_2 sufficiency.

PEEP may adversely alter the distribution of pulmonary blood flow, especially in patients with highly regional or asymmetrical lung disease. Positive transpulmonary pressure has its greatest distending effect on compliant alveoli. As PEEP is raised to high levels, resistance to blood flow through compliant lung units increases disproportionately, redirecting the blood flow toward stiffer, more diseased areas. At usual levels of PEEP, any such diversion usually does not outweigh the benefits of alveolar recruitment and hypoxic vasoconstriction. PEEP may reduce PaO_2 by this mechanism in certain patients with highly regionalized disease that produces poorly recruitable (but perfused) lung units (e.g., lobar pneumonia). In a similar fashion, PEEP can increase the shunt flow in a patient with intrapulmonary or intracardiac right-to-left vascular communications. Pulmonary arteriovenous malformations, atrial septal defects, and the pulmonary shunt vessels of cirrhosis may receive a larger percentage of flow as PEEP raises pulmonary vascular resistance and right heart filling pressure.

Impaired Vital Organ Perfusion

Cerebral Perfusion
PEEP increases jugular and intracranial pressures (ICP) by raising CVP. Predictably, these increments are less when the lungs are stiff or heavily infiltrated and transmit less pressure to the pleural space; conversely, the CVP rises more when chest wall compliance is reduced. Lower arterial blood pressure (BP) or raised ICP can reduce cerebral perfusion pressure (CPP): CPP = BP – ICP. However, in the setting of intracranial hypertension, PEEP-related arterial hypotension presents a considerably greater risk for precipitating cerebral dysfunction than does central venous hypertension. (When ICP exceeds CVP, increases in CVP caused by PEEP do not transmit fully to the cerebral veins.) Abrupt application of PEEP can raise ICP and precipitate herniation in patients with intracranial mass lesions or seriously elevated ICP. (If CO_2 clearance is impaired by dead space formation, a rising $PaCO_2$ also can contribute to intracranial hypertension.) Abrupt withdrawal of PEEP can cause a surge in venous return, transiently boosting BP and ICP. Despite its potential dangers, PEEP generally can be used safely if high levels are avoided and if it is applied and withdrawn in small increments.

Hepatic and Renal Perfusion
PEEP-associated reductions of cardiac output, coupled with elevation of CVP, may compromise hepatic perfusion or venous drainage. As with right

heart failure, the resulting passive hepatic congestion can cause mild elevations of bilirubin and hepatic enzymes. PEEP also has been reported to interfere with renal function, even when cardiac output is well preserved. Although a variety of mechanisms (reflex, humoral) have been proposed, none has been generally accepted. If PEEP contributes to excessive intra-abdominal pressure (e.g., after extensive abdominal surgery), prerenal oliguria can result.

Impaired CO_2 Elimination

When alveolar recruitment is marginal or nearly maximized ($PEEP_T$ substantially exceeding P_{flex}), PEEP impairs CO_2 elimination by overdistending patent and well-ventilated lung units, increasing their vascular resistance, and creating high ventilation/perfusion (V/Q) units (Fig. 9-8). Total pulmonary blood flow also may fall if venous return is seriously impeded. Such changes tend to expand the physiologic dead space, increasing the ventilation requirement and encouraging CO_2 retention in patients with marginal ventilatory reserves. Fortunately, these effects usually are modest. Alveolar overdistention may be signaled by a widened difference between arterial and mixed expired or end-expiratory values of PCO_2.

Alterations in the Work of Breathing

Although well-designed ventilator circuits maintain airway pressure nearly constant throughout the spontaneous breathing cycle, many impose substantial airflow resistance, particularly when PEEP is used. PEEP itself may either increase or decrease the work of breathing (W_B). Alveolar recruitment tends to reduce the W_B, but overdistention sometimes proves detrimental on two counts. First, lung compliance may worsen as additional volume is forced into a fully recruited lung, increasing lung tension and elastic workload. Second, chest distention limits the ability of the inspiratory muscles to perform work by placing them on a disadvantageous portion of their length–tension relationship and altering muscle geometry. When the expiratory muscles oppose volume recruitment, the total (inspiratory plus expiratory) W_B tends to increase. As already discussed, however, PEEP may redistribute the ventilation workload by facilitating transfer of inspiratory effort to the expiratory muscles.

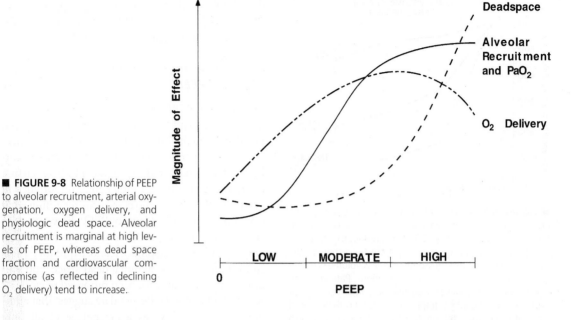

■ **FIGURE 9-8** Relationship of PEEP to alveolar recruitment, arterial oxygenation, oxygen delivery, and physiologic dead space. Alveolar recruitment is marginal at high levels of PEEP, whereas dead space fraction and cardiovascular compromise (as reflected in declining O_2 delivery) tend to increase.

■ CLINICAL USE OF PEEP

Good Candidates for PEEP

9 Based on the foregoing discussion, good candidates for a trial of PEEP are those who have (a) hypoxemia despite an elevated FiO_2, (b) diffuse acute pulmonary disease, (c) a poorly compliant respiratory system, (d) adequate cardiac reserve with normal to increased intravascular volume, (e) a tendency for atelectasis (e.g., after upper abdominal surgery), (f) acute cardiogenic or noncardiogenic pulmonary edema, (g) increased left ventricular afterload, (h) a pressure–volume relationship characterized by a lower inflection zone of rapidly improving compliance, and (i) severe airflow obstruction with flow limitation during tidal breathing, characterized by increased work of breathing and inconsistency in triggering the ventilator-reversible upper airway obstruction, such as that encountered during obstructive sleep apnea, certain variants of asthma, and postextubation laryngeal or glottic edema.

Poor Candidates for PEEP

Although there is a good rationale for using at least 3 to 5 cm H_2O PEEP or CPAP for almost every intubated patient (see the following section), poor candidates for higher levels have (a) unilateral or localized lung disease, (b) normally compliant or emphysematous lungs, (c) subacute or chronic lung or chest wall disease, (d) cardiovascular compromise or hypotension resulting from intravascular volume deficits or right ventricular dysfunction,

(e) severe intracranial disease or hypertension, or (f) pulmonary hyperinflation without tidal flow limitation. Whatever the relative contraindications, a cautious and well-monitored trial of PEEP should not be withheld from apparently poor candidates with refractory hypoxemia.

Physiologic PEEP

Considerable volume loss occurs in moving from the upright to the supine horizontal position in all but severely obstructed patients (Fig. 9-9). (A normal young person loses about 1 L of lung volume in this transition.) Positional volume losses occur disproportionately in juxtadiaphragmatic regions. Because the compliance of the normal respiratory system approximates 80 to 100 mL/cm H_2O, more than 10 cm H_2O PEEP would theoretically be needed to restore the end-expiratory lung volume equivalent to that of the upright position. Other positional changes are also important to consider. Side-to-side turning increases the volume of the upper lung as the shifting abdominal contents alter the regional chest wall compliance. Overall end-expiratory volume is significantly higher in the lateral decubitus position than in the supine position. The prone position helps dramatically for some patients with diffuse lung injury, presumably because it causes a regionally intense PEEP effect in the dorsal and juxtadiaphragmatic regions that most need it and/or because proning increases overall lung volume. PEEP may reduce the work of breathing and, in the earliest stage of ARDS, may also help protect against VILI, lung infection,

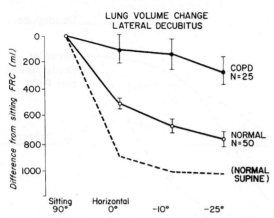

■ **FIGURE 9-9** Influence of lateral decubitus and supine postures on resting lung volume. In a normal subject, a volume loss of approximately 900 mL (equivalent to 5 to 10 cm H_2O PEEP) occurs in the transition from the sitting to the supine horizontal position. Somewhat less volume is lost in assuming the lateral decubitus position. Patients with severe airflow obstruction may lose very little volume but experience positional gas trapping or dramatically increased work of breathing. (Reproduced from Marini JJ, et al. *Am Rev Respir Dis.* 1984;129:101–105, with permission.)

and dissemination of lung bacteria and the products of inflammation to the systemic circulation.

Choosing the Appropriate Level of PEEP

As end-expiratory pressure is raised, the effect is neither smooth nor predictable. Some patients show little response until very high levels (20 to 25 cm H_2O) are reached, at which point oxygen exchange may (or may not) improve remarkably; others respond adequately at 5 cm H_2O or less. As a rule, diffuse infiltrates are most responsive. Highly regionalized diseases, as demonstrated on CT scans, tend to be relatively refractory to PEEP. Because the beneficial effect of PEEP on transpulmonary oxygen transfer parallels recruitment of collapsed lung units, PEEP responsiveness tends to be greatest during the earliest phase of acute lung injury, when edema and atelectasis are most prevalent. Low levels of PEEP may be insufficient to produce or maintain alveolar patency, especially when used in conjunction with modest tidal volumes. As more PEEP is added, peak inflation pressures rise and collapsed alveoli reinflate. As a consequence, venous admixture falls, and improving arterial oxygenation accompanies improving C_{RS}. With a fixed tidal volume or driving pressure, higher values of PEEP boost peak alveolar pressure and may thereby cause end-inspiratory recruitment of units

that PEEP can then keep open. The application of PEEP to the problem of ARDS management is discussed more thoroughly in Chapter 24.

Alternatives for Choosing "Optimal PEEP"

The effects of PEEP on gas exchange may vary with tidal volume, and the maximal response to a given PEEP increment—although generally rapid—may require 1 h or more to establish. As discussed earlier and in Chapter 8, adequate PEEP to ensure recruitment may be of fundamental importance in averting VILI. There is no consensus regarding what constitutes an optimal level of PEEP; however, oxygen saturation, oxygen delivery, venous admixture, lung compliance, inspiratory and expiratory pressure–volume curves, minimal dead space, and volume recruitment all have been proposed to guide its selection (Table 9-2). Recent data suggest that additional "recruitability" as a percentage of all lung units is usually very modest, once 12 to 15 cm H_2O PEEP has been applied. Moreover, because mechanics and gas exchange efficiency are rather tightly linked, the PEEP values selected by these different "optimal PEEP" strategies often—but not invariably—coincide. This is not to say that initial opening of compromised lung units does not require high pressure—it often does. Best results for lung unit recruitment tend to be obtained during the release of a high pressure recruiting maneuver.

A "traditional" method for conducting a PEEP trial is outlined in Table 9-3. It should be understood that, despite its effectiveness in improving O_2 saturation or preventing lung unit collapse, adding PEEP may prove detrimental if it unnecessarily increases tissue stresses, generates significant dead space, or impairs O_2 delivery by reducing cardiac output. Most physicians choose the minimal level of PEEP required to sustain an acceptable arterial oxygen saturation (generally >90%) at a tolerable FiO_2 (generally <0.7). Arterial O_2 saturation alone, however, does not tell the whole

---

TABLE 9-2 OUTCOME VARIABLES FOR "OPTIMAL POSITIVE END-EXPIRATORY AIRWAY PRESSURE"

O_2 saturation (arterial or mixed venous)
O_2 delivery
Minimal venous admixture
Best tidal compliance
Volume recruitment

TABLE 9-3 A "TRADITIONAL" METHOD FOR SELECTING POSITIVE END-EXPIRATORY AIRWAY PRESSURE
Define
Least tolerated PaO_2 or SaO_2 Maximum tolerated FiO_2 Least tolerated cardiac output Maximum tolerated P_{PK} Least tolerated tidal volume
Follow
PaO_2 SaO_2 Cardiac output (if available) Arterial blood pressure Plateau pressure
Sequence in early ARDS

Begin with PEEP approx. 8 cm H_2O
Construct PV curve or increase PEEP in steps
   of 2–3 cm H_2O to tolerance or desired effect
Adjust V_T if peak pressure rises too high
   (volume-cycled ventilation)
Consider raising targeted plateau pressure
Consider adding recruiting breaths if $V_T < 5$ mL/kg

story; the effects of reduced cardiac output can outweigh the benefits of improved arterial O_2 saturation on O_2 delivery. (SvO_2 will fall if O_2 delivery is compromised, even if PaO_2 rises.) A close watch must be kept on peak and mean airway cycling pressures. A marginal boost in PaO_2 or in O_2 delivery may not be worth an increased risk of VILI or lung rupture.

In some centers, an attempt is made to maximize oxygen delivery, even if the airway pressure required is higher than that which achieves 90% saturation. Believing that alveolar inflation reduces the VILI risk and improves the healing of an injured lung, other clinicians attempt to reduce the shunt fraction below an arbitrary limit, as long as adequate cardiac output can be maintained by fluids and vasopressors. An "optimal" PEEP can be selected without the benefit of wedge pressure or SvO_2 measurements by raising PEEP while monitoring "total thoracic compliance." Advocates of this time-honored method believe the level of PEEP, which maximizes (chord) compliance, coincides with the greatest oxygen delivery, lowest alveolar dead space, and maximal alveolar recruitment. Although this is an attractive concept, cardiac output may fall independently of changes in total thoracic compliance, and clinical experience suggests

that this technique is unreliable. (As already noted, chord compliance varies as a joint function of PEEP and tidal volume. Moreover, for some patients, the peak of the compliance curve is not sharp; in others, total thoracic compliance may continue to rise as PEEP is raised to levels that induce hypotension.) Two other methods are variants of this optimal recruitment model. The first compares arterial and end-tidal CO_2 tensions. This difference is minimized at the point of maximal recruitment and widens as overdistention increases dead space. The second variation uses the static airway pressure–volume curve as a guide to identify the point of full lung recruitment. Until recently, the lower inflection "point" of the inflation PV curve was thought to identify the end of recruitment, and, therefore, a slightly higher corresponding pressure identified a suitable PEEP to target. CT imaging has confirmed, however, that this interpretation is misleadingly simplistic. Recruitment of refractory lung units continues until pressures are reached that approach the upper inflection zone. The contours of the *inspiratory* PV curve reflect the simultaneous interplay among lung units that are recruited and overdistended, and the proportions of each vary as airway pressure rises. Factors such as volume-related chest wall compliance changes, gas trapping, and shifts of airway liquids further complicate the analysis. The deflation limb of the PV relationship, that portion of the loop relevant to expiratory events such as relaxation to PEEP, is left-shifted with respect to its inspiratory counterpart. Theoretically, changes in its slope might be more informative. Yet, this curve also reflects the interplay between relaxation of regional overdistention and development of lung unit collapse, and like its inspiratory counterpart, it is influenced by factors unrelated to airway closure.

Selecting PEEP and Tidal Volume in ARDS

Certain principles should guide the approach to PEEP and tidal volume selection in patients with acute lung injury. These include

1. Adjust ventilatory parameters empirically, rather than by formula-driven rules; prioritize patient comfort and safety.
2. Assign the prevention of mechanical trauma precedence over maintenance of normocapnia and avoidance of oxygen toxicity. Both recruitability and VILI risk appear greatest very early on during ventilator support and diminish afterward.

No exact upper limits for acceptable plateau pressure can be specified.

3. During passive inflation, increased chest wall stiffness modifies the implication of plateau pressure for lung stretch, as does active breathing—in the opposite direction. Very high values for FiO_2 risk absorption atelectasis as well as oxygen toxicity. Therefore, FiO_2 be held less than 0.7 whenever possible.

4. Consider the impact of chest wall stiffness (including abdominal contents) on transpulmonary pressure and gas exchange efficiency. In concerning cases, determine the abdominal (bladder) and/or esophageal pressures.

5. Monitor hemodynamics as well as mechanics and gas exchange when regulating ventilatory therapy. A surrogate for measuring hemodynamics directly may be to monitor the central venous oxygen saturation via a sample drawn from the right atrium or pulmonary artery. A value greater than 70% and a difference of 25% or less between arterial and central venous saturations are usually associated with an adequate cardiac index ($>2.5 L/m^2/min$).

6. In severe cases, attempt to minimize ventilatory *demands* and thereby reduce airway pressures, high rates of gas flow, and cardiac output requirements.

7. Incorporate the "challenge" principle—carefully monitored intervention—in revising decisions, both regarding the intensification and the withdrawal of therapeutic measures.

8. Unless otherwise contraindicated, prone positioning should be considered when dangerously high values for ventilatory pressure, PEEP, and FiO_2 are needed to maintain adequate supine arterial oxygen tension.

9. Assess pulmonary interventions in the volume-control mode of ventilation to better track thoracic mechanics and the lung's gas-exchanging efficiency for carbon dioxide. At other times, use pressure-limited forms of ventilation (e.g., pressure control, pressure support, or BIPAP/APRV) for ongoing management. The selections of PEEP and tidal volume for ARDS are discussed in Chapter 24.

Targets for Ventilation and Oxygenation

As a general rule, the desired goal is to use the least PEEP and tidal volume necessary to achieve acceptable gas exchange while minimizing tidal collapse and reopening the unstable lung units. Knowing that moderate hypercapnia is generally well tolerated, therapeutic targeting priorities are directed toward lung protection and maintenance of appropriate hemodynamics and oxygen delivery.

Utility of Recruiting Maneuvers and Auscultation in PEEP/Tidal Volume Selection

All patients should be assessed for severity of disease and for recruitment potential. Recruiting maneuvers help characterize PEEP responsiveness, determine the relative status of intravascular filling and response to altered cardiac loading conditions, and set the PEEP/tidal volume combination. After deficits of intravascular volume have been addressed and hemodynamics have been optimized, recruitment potential is gauged by applying "high-level" pressure control ventilation: PEEP of 15 to 30 cm H_2O, driving pressure of 20 to 30 cm H_2O, and plateau pressure of approximately 50 cm H_2O for 1 to 2 min, as tolerated. Even higher pressures may be appropriate for a patient with a very stiff chest wall—e.g., a burn victim with chest wall edema or eschar. Although sustained inflation with high pressure has been traditionally used, widely employed, and selected for most reported research, it is no more effective and tends to be less well tolerated hemodynamically than a recruiting method based on pressure-controlled ventilation that achieves lower average pressure but similar peak pressure during its inspiratory phase. If oxygenation and lung mechanics do not improve substantially with high-level pressure-controlled ventilation as a recruiting technique, the patient is considered to have low recruiting potential *in that position and at that specific time*. Management goals in the "recruitable" group emphasize the maintenance of high-level end-expiratory pressure, whereas in poorly recruitable patients, PEEP is maintained as low as feasible—generally in the range of 5 to 10 cm H_2O. In both the groups, end-inspiratory plateau pressure is kept less than 30 cm H_2O, except when chest wall compliance is very low.

Patients with an extensive "recruitable" population of lung units respond to increased PEEP and recruiting maneuvers with improved alveolar mechanics and improved gas exchange, reflected both by increased PaO_2 and by better ventilating efficiency, as gauged by a reduced $V_E/PaCO_2$. These salutary changes are accompanied by only marginal effects on hemodynamics, as judged by systemic blood pressure and central venous oxygen saturation. Inspiratory crackles (rales) audible over the dependent zones of the chest during routine tidal cycles suggest that recruitment and derecruitment are occurring with each breath and indicate that recruitment maneuvers followed by higher levels of end-expiratory pressure may be indicated to silence them. Crackles occurring *late* in inspiration are of particular concern, as they may originate in units opening under relatively high pressures. In gauging response to PEEP, it is important to consider CO_2 exchange as well as oxygenation response. With rare exceptions (e.g., when PEEP-impaired cardiac output causes mixed-venous O_2 content to fall), PaO_2 tends to increase when PEEP is applied. However, this oxygenation improvement may be accounted for either by recruitment of lung units or by reduced or redirected blood flow within the injured lung. In the latter circumstance, $PaCO_2$ may also rise. When recruitment is the explanation for O_2 improvement, however, CO_2 exchange is not compromised and may even improve, reflecting increased alveolar ventilation. Similar principles apply during prone positioning.

Initial Preparations Prior to PEEP Selection in ARDS

1. Decide whether to allow inspiratory efforts, using controlled or nearly controlled ventilation to subdue vigorous respiratory efforts for the most severely involved patients during the early stage of support.
2. Establish a ventilation baseline. With the patient gently breathing or passive, a reasonable set of initial ventilatory settings (just after intubation) might be FiO_2 0.8 and PEEP 8 to 10 cm H_2O (depending on the concern regarding hemodynamic tolerance); tidal volume 6 to 8 mL/kg (depending on the inspiratory plateau pressure).
3. Estimate intravascular volume status initially from arterial blood pressure, respiratory variations of pulmonary and systemic arterial pulse pressure, CVP, urinary output, and urinary electrolytes.
4. Confirm adequacy of intravascular volume utilizing echocardiography, results from a volume challenge, and central venous and pulmonary artery catheter data (cardiac index, mixed-venous O_2 saturation, and occlusion pressure), if available.

5. Replete any volume deficits and support the circulation with pressors and inotropes to the extent necessary to safely perform the ventilatory manipulations.
6. Determine the recruitment potential of the patient by using a recruiting maneuver/PEEP trial.

Determining "Best PEEP"

As already noted, no consensus yet exists regarding the best method of conducting a PEEP trial in patients with edematous or injured lungs. Whatever the protocol, however, oxygenation response, ventilatory efficiency, alterations of mechanics, and hemodynamic response should be considered together. During the trial, PEEP level should be the only variable. Position, level of sedation, FiO_2, tidal volume or pressure control level, and all other ventilator settings remain at fixed, safe levels. Given that airways open at pressures higher than those that keep them open, a recruiting maneuver should be considered integral to an adjustment aimed at optimizing the PEEP selection (i.e., recruiting maneuver precedes each PEEP increase). PEEP can either be increased incrementally or decreased decrementally. Step direction should make little difference so long as a recruiting maneuver is integral to setting the step (Fig 9-10). Several PEEP levels should be tried, and the previously mentioned variables that are influenced by recruitment, over-distention, risk of VILI, and hemodynamic response should be monitored. Tidal volume or pressure control level should be adjusted if plateau pressure exceeds 30 cm H_2O in patients with normal chest wall mechanics (Table 9-4).

TABLE 9-4 FINDING THE "BEST PEEP" COMPROMISE

- Minimize effort and ventilation demand
- Choose the V_T or driving pressure to be used in practice (e.g., 6 mL/kg)
- Use least acceptable FiO_2 to keep SaO_2 approx. 92%
- Perform a recruiting maneuver using that V_T with escalating PEEP to 50–60 m H_2O peak pressure (3–5 breaths at each PEEP level)
- Drop PEEP abruptly from its highest value to 20 cm H_2O and then reduce PEEP further in small steps until O_2 sat falls
- Rerecruit and drop PEEP to that value plus one step higher

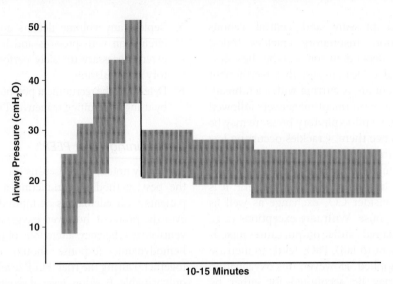

■ **FIGURE 9-10** Stepwise "decremental" selection of best PEEP after a recruiting maneuver. Because PEEP cannot keep open what has never first been opened, an attempt is made to safely recruit the lung (which may require high airway pressures) without hemodynamic compromise. PEEP steps on the down side of the "staircase" are smaller and are made more slowly than those made during the increasing PEEP and recruiting maneuver phases. In this example, recruitment is achieved by using pressure-controlled ventilation and very high PEEP. Best PEEP is found on the deflation limb, monitoring compliance, and oxygenation.

Measurement of esophageal and/or bladder pressure helps to indicate the pressure actually applied across the lung. When using such high levels of PEEP, the need for it should be frequently reassessed and relatively low tidal volumes used. Aggressive efforts must be made to reduce peak and mean cycling pressures as well as oxygen demand and the minute ventilation requirement. Sedation, paralysis, and reducing tidal volume may prove helpful. Prone positioning and inhalation of nitric oxide or aerosolized prostacyclin can sometimes yield dramatic benefits. Once initiated, repeated attempts at cautious PEEP withdrawal and closely regulated fluid management are appropriate.

PEEP Withdrawal

Clinically unstable patients, i.e., those requiring an FiO_2 higher than 0.4 and those with worsening gas exchange, are poor candidates for PEEP withdrawal. However, after the first few days of supporting ARDS, it is important to attempt to withdraw PEEP to the lowest well-tolerated level at an acceptable FiO_2. PEEP should be withdrawn cautiously, with oximetry or arterial blood gas monitoring each step change. A patient who has shown only marginal PEEP response is a possible exception to these guidelines. Abrupt or premature withdrawal of PEEP can cause lung unit collapse with deterioration of gas exchange, which may respond only

slowly to the reinstitution of PEEP if a recruiting maneuver is not performed. Sudden termination of PEEP also can cause cardiovascular overload, increase the work of breathing, result in airway flooding with alveolar fluids, and precipitate dangerous increases in ICP.

"Prophylactic PEEP"

Some physicians administer low levels of PEEP (e.g., 5 cm H_2O) "prophylactically" to all intubated patients. In the past, the practice of applying PEEP to all intubated patients was often defended on the grounds that bypassing the larynx causes FRC to fall. Although FRC may indeed fall post intubation, its physiologic basis remains unclear. The routine application of PEEP to the airway of patients who require intubation after surgery or trauma does, however, rest on firm ground. As noted earlier, lung volume is reduced substantially by recumbency. Moreover, PEEP could offset the additional fall in FRC known to occur in the first few hours to days after thoracic or upper abdominal incisions (a factor contributing to atelectasis and impaired gas exchange). Thus, as long as intubation is required for other reasons and the patient is recumbent, adding a minimum of 5 cm H_2O PEEP seems entirely defensible. At the present time, there is no convincing proof of benefit or danger from this approach. A PEEP of 8 cm H_2O

(generally less than P_{flex}) has not been shown to protect routinely against the development of ARDS, whatever benefit PEEP might confer on O_2 exchange or lung mechanics once ARDS is under way. There is intriguing experimental evidence that PEEP may help in the prevention of propagation of initially localized lung injury (see Chapter 8). PEEP maintenance tends to keep inflammatory biofluids at the periphery of the lung, confined to their sites of origin rather than allowing spread to adjacent sectors (see Chapter 7).

"Auto-PEEP" Effect

Patients who trap air above the relaxed volume of the chest maintain positive pressure in the alveoli and small airways at end-exhalation in excess of the value set at the airway opening. This excess pressure, or auto-PEEP (AP), may create dynamic hyperinflation, which raises intrathoracic pressure and often impedes venous return. As discussed in greater detail in Chapters 5 and 24, AP and dynamic hyperinflation vary with those changes that influence the expiratory time constant (resistance and compliance) or the time available for deflation (minute ventilation and expiratory time fraction). Thus, although classically a problem of patients with severe airflow obstruction, AP can arise in patients with any lung mechanics profile—even ARDS—where tidal gas trapping, primarily in dependent zones, is a product of compressive airway closure, increased airway edema, and high minute ventilation (Fig. 9-11). To reduce AP, it is essential to reduce minute ventilation requirement, improve expiratory flow resistance, and lengthen the percentage of the ventilatory cycle spent in expiration. (When *induction* of AP is the intent, as during Inverse Ratio Ventilation or APRV, just the opposite strategy is followed. See Chapter 7.) Despite many physiological similarities, PEEP and AP are not interchangeable with respect to uniformity. The distribution of AP is often quite heterogeneous, even within the same patient. Many units occluded at end-expiration, for example, are located in dependent regions. Moreover, because overdistention of individual lung units is a direct function of their compliance and fragility, the correlation between AP and the hazard of barotrauma is imperfect, at best.

Unsuspected, this "auto-PEEP" effect can seriously reduce true cardiac filling pressures and confound interpretation of pulmonary artery and wedge pressures, raising them by an amount similar to the pressure transmitted to the pleural space (see Chapters 2 and 5). Because AP must be reversed before inspiratory airflow can begin or the ventilator can be triggered, the ventilatory workload also rises in spontaneously breathing patients. By contributing to total PEEP, AP may have a therapeutic effect in edematous lung disease (e.g., when generated in inverse ratio ventilation). The cardiovascular consequences of AP can be minimized by increasing the rate of fluid or pressor infusion or by increasing the fraction of spontaneous breathing efforts (e.g., by reducing intermittent mandatory ventilation frequency or substituting pressure support). The detection, consequences, and management of AP are discussed in greater detail in Chapters 2, 5, and 25.

PEEP on Auto-PEEP

Although PEEP is the sum of applied PEEP and AP, adding PEEP to existing AP may not raise *total* PEEP proportionately when expiration is flow

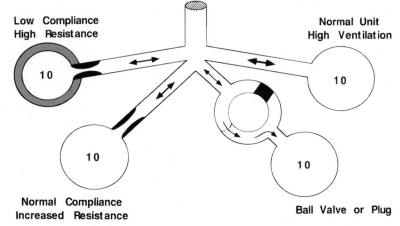

■ **FIGURE 9-11** Mechanisms and implications of AP. AP can be generated in normal lung units because of increased ventilation (**upper right**), one-way or ball valving (as by a secretion plug, **lower right**), or a lengthy expiratory time constant (the product of compliance and resistance, **left**). As illustrated by the two images on the left, the same AP value may or may not be associated with hyperinflation, depending on the mechanism for time constant prolongation.

Low Compliance
High Resistance

Normal Unit
High Ventilation

10

10

10

10

Normal Compliance
Increased Resistance

Ball Valve or Plug

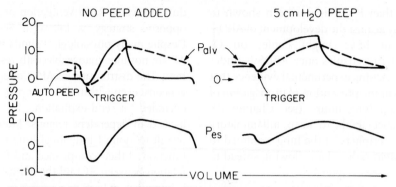

■ **FIGURE 9-12** The effect of PEEP on AP in a patient with expiratory flow limitation during tidal breathing. AP represents a positive end-expiratory alveolar pressure (P_{alv}) that must be overcome by inspiratory effort (reflected by esophageal pressure, P_{es}) before the ventilator can be triggered or spontaneous breathing can begin. PEEP similar to the original AP added downstream from the site of flow limitation does not slow expiratory airflow significantly. As AP is counterbalanced, the inspiratory work of breathing declines. PEEP, positive end-expiratory airway pressure. (Reproduced from Smith TC, Marini JJ. Impact of PEEP on lung mechanics and work of breathing in severe airflow obstruction: The effect of PEEP on auto-PEEP. *J Appl Physiol.* 1988;65(4):1488–1499, with permission.)

limited during tidal breathing (Fig. 9-12 and Chapter 5). Substituting PEEP for AP may help even the distribution of ventilation, improve triggering sensitivity, reduce the work of spontaneous breathing, or increase the tidal volume when pressure support or pressure control is used.

■ **SUGGESTED READINGS**

Acosta P, Santisbon E, Varon J. The use of positive end-expiratory pressure in mechanical ventilation. *Crit Care Clin.* 2007;23:251–261.

Blanch L, Bernabe F, Lucangelo U. Measurement of air trapping, intrinsic positive end-expiratory pressure, and dynamic hyperinflation in mechanically ventilated patients. *Respir Care.* 2005;50(1):110–124.

Brower RG, Lanken PN, MacIntyre NR, et al., for the NHLBI ARDS Clinical Trials Network. Higher vs. lower positive end-expiratory pressures in patients with acute respiratory distress syndrome. *N Engl J Med.* 2004;351:327–336.

Dries DJ, Marini JJ. Optimized positive end-expiratory pressure—an elusive target. *Crit Care Med.* 2002;30(5):1159–1160.

Fan E, Wilcox ME, Brower RG, et al. Recruitment maneuvers for acute lung injury: A systematic review. *Am J Resp Crit Care Med.* 2008; 178(11):1156–1163.

Gattinoni L, Caironi P, Cressoni M, et al. Lung recruitment in patients with the acute respiratory distress syndrome. *N Engl J Med.* 2006; 354(17):1775–1786.

MacIntyre NR. Is there a best way to set positive end-expiratory pressure for mechanical ventilatory support in acute lung injury? *Clin Chest Med.* 2008;29:233–239.

Marini JJ. The "open lung" compromise. *Intensive Care Med.* 2007;33(7): 1114–1116.

Meade MO, Cook DJ, Guyatt GH, et al., for the Lung Open Ventilation Study Investigators. Ventilation strategy using low tidal volumes, recruitment maneuvers, and high positive end-expiratory pressure for acute lung injury and acute respiratory distress syndrome. A randomized controlled trial. *JAMA.* 2008;299(6):637–645.

Mercat A, Richard J-C, Vielle B, et al., for the Expiratory Pressure (Express) Study Group. Positive end-expiratory pressure setting in adults with acute lung injury and acute respiratory distress syndrome: A randomized controlled trial. *JAMA.* 2008;299:646–655.

Sevransky JE, Levy MM, Marini JJ. Mechanical ventilation in sepsis-induced acute lung injury/acute respiratory distress syndrome: An evidence-based review. *Crit Care Med.* 2004;32(Suppl.11):S548–S553.

Soni N, Williams P. Positive pressure ventilation: What is the real cost? *Br J Anaesth.* 2008;101(4):446–457.

Weaning and Discontinuation of Mechanical Ventilation

KEY POINTS

1 A continuing need for ventilator assistance may arise from oxygen desaturation of hemoglobin during spontaneous breathing, cardiovascular instability during machine withdrawal, psychological dependence, or most commonly, imbalance between ventilatory capability and demand.

2 The minute ventilation requirement bears a quadratic relationship to the work of breathing. Three primary factors determine the minute ventilation requirement: the CO_2 production, the efficiency of ventilation, and the central drive to breathe.

3 Ventilatory power is the product of minute ventilation and the mechanical work of breathing per liter of ventilation. For any specific tidal volume and flow rate, the primary determinants of the inspiratory work per liter of ventilation are the resistance and elastance of the respiratory system and auto-positive end-expiratory pressure, a reflection of dynamic hyperinflation.

4 Ventilatory capability is determined by the central drive to breathe and the bulk, strength, and endurance of the ventilatory muscles. The induction of fatigue by excessive effort impairs muscular performance for at least 12 to 24 h afterward. Sleep is essential for optimal neuromuscular performance and for preparing the patient for the weaning attempt.

5 Prediction of success or failure of a weaning trial involves the assessment of oxygen exchange, cardiovascular status, and muscular endurance. Although individual measures of strength, gas exchange, or workload aid in this assessment, "integrative" weaning indices observed during a brief trial of unaided breathing (e.g., rapid shallow breathing index, interpreted in conjunction with the minute ventilation and chest compliance) as well as "integrative"

tests of ventilatory reserve (breathing pattern variability, cough-induced inspiratory capacity) are perhaps the most physiologically sound indicators. Expiratory performance is especially important to evaluate when there is a high secretion load.

6 Persistent failure to wean despite adequate respiratory parameters should prompt consideration of cardiac ischemia, congestive heart failure, psychological dependence or delirium, gas exchange deterioration, lingering effects of sedation, or other nonrespiratory explanation for the failure. A common culprit is net fluid balance that is markedly positive.

7 After the patient has had optimal preparation, the weaning sequence involves estimation of the likelihood of success, a trial of spontaneous ventilation, gradual withdrawal of ventilatory assistance (when indicated), a brief period of observation with minimal pressure support, extubation, and close follow-up after ventilator discontinuance and extubation.

8 Patients experiencing protracted difficulty during removal of ventilatory support should receive adequate ventilator assistance at night to permit sleep. The patient must never be forced to work beyond his or her ability to comfortably sustain it.

9 Reintubation occasionally is necessary in the first few days after extubation. These delayed weaning failures usually arise because of an inability to swallow normally (resulting in oropharyngeal aspiration), glottic swelling, inability to clear thick airway secretions, or congestive heart failure. Appropriate precautions during this period may avert failure. Noninvasive ventilation may provide a useful bridge across this difficult period.

10 Weaning from tracheostomy should be considered when the patient no longer requires frequent airway suctioning, high inspired fractions of O_2, or periodic (nocturnal) connection to the ventilator. Conversion to noninvasive ventilation and/or assisted coughing is possible for many patients previously assigned to permanent tracheostomy.

O nce the underlying reason for initiating ventilator support has been successfully addressed, many patients tolerate abrupt termination of mechanical assistance without needing to gradually adjust to spontaneous breathing. However, evaluating readiness is always a clinical judgment, and in that minority of patients for whom withdrawing machine support proves difficult, a strategy for transferring the respiratory workload to the patient must be developed (Table 10-1). Weaning is the graded removal of ventilator support from patients who cannot tolerate immediate conversion to fully spontaneous breathing. The weaning process often takes place in several stages: weaning from positive-pressure ventilation, weaning from positive end-expiratory pressure (PEEP), weaning from the endotracheal (ET) or tracheostomy tube, and weaning from supplemental oxygen.

■ PHYSIOLOGIC DETERMINANTS OF VENTILATOR DEPENDENCE

1 A continuing need for breathing assistance may arise from O_2 desaturation of hemoglobin during unaided breathing, cardiovascular instability during machine withdrawal, psychological dependence, or from imbalance between ventilatory capability and demand. Often, several of these causes operate simultaneously.

TABLE 10-1   WHO BENEFITS FROM GRADUAL WITHDRAWAL OF MACHINE SUPPORT?

- If workload is disproportionate to capability
  - Muscle reconditioning
  - Reintegration of ventilatory coordination (?)
- If sudden transitions are physiologically or psychologically stressful
  - "Panic" cycles in airflow obstruction
  - Congestive heart failure
    Autotransfusion
    ↑ O_2 consumption
    Diastolic dysfunction
  - Coronary ischemia

Psychological Factors

Prolonged mechanical ventilation is a harrowing experience that may elicit anxiety, depression, or psychosis. Delirium, manifested by inattentiveness, paranoid behavior, and disorientation, occurs very commonly in sleep-deprived and elderly patients receiving medications that interfere with normal mental functioning (e.g., corticosteroids, benzodiazepines). A careful evaluation of mental status often is fruitful, because cooperation and avoidance of panic reactions during the weaning attempt may depend on control of the delirium. Ensuring sleep and the use of appropriate psychotropic agents (e.g., haloperidol or quetiapine) can speed up the process (see Chapter 17).

Arterial Hypoxemia

Mechanical ventilation can improve arterial oxygenation by providing large tidal breaths that oppose atelectasis, sealing the airway to allow delivery of high inspired concentrations of oxygen and PEEP, reducing or offsetting the effects of pulmonary edema, improving the output requirements and loading conditions of a compromised heart, and improving the balance between tissue oxygen delivery and demand. Under a high breathing workload, the respiratory muscles consume a great deal of oxygen. Vigorous expiratory activity reduces end-expiratory lung volume. Stressful breathing may also increase the oxygen demand of other organs by causing agitation or discharge of catecholamines. When cardiac output is compromised, this increased oxygen demand may force greater O_2 extraction. The admixture of the desaturated mixed venous blood that results may then contribute to hypoxemia. Moreover, increased metabolic demands may cause myocardial decompensation, ischemia, or diastolic dysfunction. Mechanical ventilation mitigates these problems by relieving much of the ventilatory workload.

Cardiovascular Instability

Resuming a high ventilatory workload often presents a cardiovascular challenge in the setting of ischemic disease, heart failure, or reduced cardiac reserve. Inappropriately low cardiac output can contribute directly to hypoxemia and weakness of the ventilatory pump. Cardiovascular instability overtly limits the pace of ventilator withdrawal when chest pain, diastolic dysfunction, or arrhythmias develop during the reloading of the respiratory pump. Hypoxemia, abruptly altered cardiac loading conditions, and stress-related release of catecholamines frequently provoke rhythm disturbances in the transition to spontaneous breathing. Resuming spontaneous breathing simultaneously increases both preload and afterload of the left heart, as well as increases anxiety and the respiratory workload. Oxygen consumption (VO_2) and cardiac output can easily double at a time when the heart is least able to provide it. The stress of breathing may trigger coronary ischemia. Careful consideration must be given to optimal preparation of these patients before the weaning attempt.

Oxygen administration, establishing electrolyte and pH balance, antiarrhythmic therapy, afterload reduction, anti-ischemic measures, diuresis, and more gradual conversion to fully spontaneous breathing may be instrumental to the success of machine withdrawal. For patients with coexisting airflow obstruction, assuming a high ventilatory workload can be associated with a fall (rather than a rise) in mean intrapleural pressure. As forceful inspiratory efforts lower intrathoracic pressure, central vascular congestion and effective left ventricular afterload increase (Fig. 10-1). In such circumstances, it is essential to reduce total ventilatory demands by measures that improve lung mechanics and reduce minute ventilation. The use of continuous positive airway pressure (CPAP) or noninvasive ventilatory support may be strikingly effective. Prior pharmacotherapy to improve cardiac performance and/or relieve ischemia before weaning is often helpful.

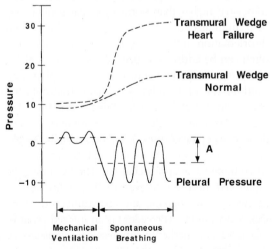

■ **FIGURE 10-1** Influence of spontaneous breathing on left ventricular filling pressure in patients with airflow obstruction. After an abrupt transition to spontaneous breathing, the increased effort results in marked decline of pleural pressure. Transmural wedge pressure increases as mean intrapleural pressure falls (*A*). For patients with left ventricular failure, the increased afterload and oxygen consumption may dramatically elevate transmural wedge pressure, producing pulmonary congestion.

Imbalance of Ventilatory Capability and Demand

To sustain spontaneous ventilation, both ventilatory drive and endurance must be adequate. Impaired ventilatory drive often contributes to CO_2 retention or hypoxemia, especially when excessive sedation or chronic hypercapnia is present. The most common reason for ventilator dependence, however, is the inability to maintain appropriate ventilation without intolerable dyspnea. Ventilatory workload is determined by the product of minute ventilation requirement ($\dot{V}_E$) and the energy expended per liter of gas flow.

Ventilatory Demand: Minute Ventilation Requirement

Reducing the minute ventilation requirement is an important goal because $\dot{V}_E$ bears a quadratic (rather than linear) relationship to the work of breathing. Three primary factors determine the $\dot{V}_E$ requirement: the CO_2 production, the efficiency of ventilation, and the sensitivity of the central drive mechanism (Table 10-2).

CO_2 Production

Fever, shivering, pain, agitation, increased work of breathing, sepsis, and overfeeding are common causes of increased CO_2 production in the intensive care unit (ICU). In the weaning phase, cautious anxiolysis and pain relief can dramatically reduce the ventilatory requirement. Carbon dioxide production is also influenced by underlying nutritional status, as well as by the number and composition of the calories administered. The semistarvation that often precedes critical illness suppresses CO_2 production. Despite the importance

TABLE 10-2 FACTORS AFFECTING VENTILATORY DEMAND		
CO_2 PRODUCTION	↑ V_D/V_T	↑ **DRIVE**
Fever	Lung disease	Neurogenic
Shivering	Hypovolemia	Psychogenic
Pain/agitation	Vascular occlusion	Metabolic acidosis
Trauma/burns	External apparatus	
Sepsis	Excessive PEEP	
Overfeeding		
Work of breathing		

of adequate nutrition, patients should not be overfed. Excess calories may be converted to fat, generating CO_2 as a metabolic by-product unlinked to energy production. Carbohydrate evolves more CO_2 per calorie than fat or protein. However, even though large calorie loads can contribute to ventilatory failure, the importance of calorie composition to ventilator dependence remains to be shown convincingly. Overfeeding also may lead to abdominal distention and discomfort that may adversely impact a patient poised at the boundary of ventilatory failure.

Ventilatory Efficiency

Alveolar ventilation (V_A), the component of ventilation that is effective in eliminating carbon dioxide, is the total minute ventilation adjusted for the fraction of wasted ventilation. Breathing efficiency can be characterized by the following expression:

$$V_A = \dot{V}_E (1 - V_D/V_T)$$

where V_D/V_T is the physiologic dead space fraction (see Chapter 5). Virtually, all the diverse processes that damage the lung or airways of the critically ill patient increase the wasted fraction of ventilation. Certain reversible factors unrelated to underlying lung pathology also can prove to be important. For example, thromboembolic or vasculitic pulmonary arterial occlusion, excessive PEEP, and hypovolemia may reduce perfusion to the ventilated lung, expanding the alveolar dead space. Small tidal volumes are characterized by a high anatomic dead space percentage. By adding "apparatus dead space," disposable heat and moisture exchangers and other devices or tubing interposed between the ET tube and the "Y" of the ventilator circuit may contribute marginally to ventilatory inefficiency.

Central Drive

Although it is unusual for a patient to remain persistently ventilator dependent solely because of a lack of breathing effort, inappropriately depressed or enhanced drive to breathe may limit weaning progress. As a rule, old and debilitated patients are the most susceptible to drive suppression. Suppressed ventilatory drive may be explained by neurologic impairment, hypothyroidism, lingering sedation (very commonly the predominant cause), sleep deprivation, poor nutrition, and metabolic alkalosis (primary or compensatory). Starvation impairs hypoxic and, to a lesser extent, hypercapnic sensitivity. Interestingly, drive is restored rapidly within a few days of reinitiating adequate feeding, perhaps in advance of improved muscle function. The drive to breathe is generally higher, and the breathing pattern is different in the waking state. Minute ventilation occasionally falls markedly during sleep or sedation and accelerates with the return to alertness. (This pattern often applies to the recovering drug overdose victim.) When infused benzodiazepines are given continuously for days to weeks, sufficient drug and drug metabolites may store in brain and fat tissues to suppress consciousness and/or drive for long periods after they are discontinued (occasionally as long as 7 to 10 days). Such unintended effects argue forcefully for the practice of once daily interruption of sedation to assess the need for and rate of their ongoing use. The administration of pharmacologic stimulants such as doxapram or progesterone has been advocated when depressed drive impedes weaning. These drugs, however, usually are not helpful.

Enhanced central drive arising from neurogenic, psychogenic, reflex, or metabolic stimuli augments ventilatory demand and workload. In asthma and acute pulmonary edema, drive-stimulating reflexes arising from the lung or chest wall downregulate after correction of the underlying disorders. Hypoxemia, hypotension, developing sepsis, and acidosis also accentuate ventilatory demands. Correction of metabolic acidosis is one of the most important ways to reduce central drive. It is also important not to force $PaCO_2$ below the patient's usual resting value, as the ensuing bicarbonate diuresis redefines the $\dot{V}_E$ needed to maintain (cerebral pH) homeostasis. In fact, $PaCO_2$ somewhat higher than normal for that patient may help minimize the $\dot{V}_E$ requirement. Anxiety and disorientation influence ventilatory demand and often can be addressed successfully by counseling, co-opting the patient into the weaning plan, and cautious use of anxiolytics or major tranquilizers. Haloperidol (Haldol) is a good first option but often proves inadequate. Quetiapine (Seroquel), risperidone, olanzepine (Zyprexa), and occasionally Depakote may work for delirious or combative patients when more usual approaches fail. The ECG must be monitored, however, to avert the possibility of dangerous QT prolongation and arrhythmia induction. Dexmedetomidine (Precedex) is an infused sedative that does not markedly suppress consciousness or drive to breathe. Given the difficulty of removing the dissociative sedatives (e.g., lorazepam, midazolam) without precipitating delirium, such properties often prove useful in weaning applications. Supplementing the inspired O_2 fraction is often an effective way to reduce drive and interrupt a panic reaction accompanied by worsening hypoxemia.

Ventilatory Demand: Work per Liter of Ventilation

Intrinsic Factors

3 Ventilatory power is the product of $\dot{V}_E$ and mechanical work of breathing per liter of ventilation. The quotient of this mechanical workload and neuromuscular efficiency defines how much energy must be expended in breathing. Once tidal volume and inspiratory time are set, the frictional and elastic properties of the respiratory system determine the pressure generated per breath, as well as the external work output per liter of ventilation. The *average* inspiratory pressure developed by the respiratory system per breath can be approximated by a simple formula:

$$P = R (V_T/t_i) + V_T/2C_{RS}) + \text{auto-PEEP}$$

where R and C_{RS} are the inspiratory resistance and compliance of the respiratory system, V_T is tidal volume, and t_i is the time required for inspiration (see Chapter 5 and Fig. 10-2). Therefore, for the same level of $\dot{V}_E$, more external work must be done if C_{RS} falls or if V_T, auto-PEEP, mean inspiratory flow (V_T/t_i), or R increase. Bronchospasm, retained secretions, and mucosal edema are the primary reversible factors that increase R. Retained secretions greatly amplify the inspiratory workload in patients with already narrowed airways. Lung edema and infiltration, high lung volumes, pleural effusions, abdominal distention, and supine posture reduce C_{RS}. Air trapping and auto-PEEP are highly dynamic phenomena influenced powerfully by minute ventilation and the ease with which gas empties from the lungs (see Chapter 25). Auto-PEEP varies with changes in the breathing impedance (e.g., bronchospasm, secretion retention, minute ventilation, body position, alteration of inspiratory time fraction, and expiratory muscle activity).

These are not the only factors that determine the energy needed by the respiratory muscles, however. For the same tidal volume, the respiratory muscles consume more oxygen (become less effective) when they begin contraction from a mechanically disadvantageous high lung volume or when the pattern of muscle contraction is poorly coordinated. For example, patients with diaphragmatic weakness may allow the abdominal contents to be drawn upward with each inspiratory effort, so that much of the tension developed by the inspiratory muscles of the chest cage fails to translate into the negative pleural pressure that draws air into the lungs.

Extrinsic Factors

The external properties of the ventilator circuit also can play an important role in determining the ventilatory workload. ET tube resistance exceeds the normal resistance of the upper airway. Frictional pressure losses increase rapidly when high flows are driven through small-caliber tubes. Kinks and encrusted secretions may encroach on an otherwise adequate lumen. In some instances, it may be wise to exchange an orotracheal tube for a larger one (e.g., via a tube changer; see Chapter 6) or replace a nasotracheal tube with an orotracheal one. Tracheostomy is worth considering to reduce resistance and to facilitate extraction of airway secretions in particularly difficult patients. In theory, all pressure-support ventilation (PSV) and CPAP should be withdrawn before extubation to test the marginal patient's ventilatory reserve (the "T-piece trial," see following). Even in marginal candidates however, extubation from modest pressure support and CPAP often succeeds, especially when the patient bites the tube or experiences extreme discomfort or a narrow bore tube hinders airflow.

Tracheostomy offers larger tube diameter, shorter axial length, lower resistance and improved secretion clearance. The resistance of other circuit components varies widely and can add significantly to the ventilatory burden. Although the valves of older machines frequently presented problems, they are rarely limiting when using modern equipment.

Ventilatory Capability

The ability to sustain the effort of breathing is determined by respiratory drive, muscle strength and endurance.

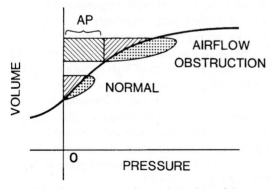

■ **FIGURE 10-2** Pressure–volume relationships of the respiratory system for a normal patient and for one with airflow obstruction. The inspiratory work of breathing is increased in patients with airflow obstruction, due to elevated airflow resistance (*stippled area*), increased elastance at higher lung volume, and auto-PEEP (*AP*).

Central Drive

Although it is unusual for a patient to remain persistently ventilator dependent solely because of a lack of breathing effort, multiple interacting factors can suppress the output of the ventilatory drive center. As a rule, old and debilitated patients are the most susceptible to drive suppression. Sedatives and neurologic impairment generally receive adequate clinical attention. However, other important causes of drive suppression may be potentially reversible. For example, chronic loading of ventilation (as during a severe bout of asthma) can condition the ventilatory center to tolerate hypercapnea. Metabolic alkalosis, hypothyroidism, and sleep deprivation are commonly overlooked causes of impaired ventilatory drive. Because the output of the ventilatory center tends to parallel metabolic rate and caloric intake, nutritional status is important. Starvation impairs hypoxic and, to a lesser extent, hypercapnic sensitivity. Interestingly, drive is restored rapidly within a few days of reinitiating adequate feeding. The drive to breathe is generally higher, and the breathing pattern is different in the waking state. Minute ventilation occasionally falls markedly during sleep or sedation and accelerates impressively with the return to alertness. (A florid example of this pattern is often provided by the recovering drug overdose victim.) The administration of pharmacologic drive stimulants such as doxapram or progesterone has been advocated when depressed drive impedes weaning. These drugs, however, are seldom helpful or used.

Muscular Performance

Strength   Carbon dioxide retention is uncommon if the patient can generate more than 25% of the predicted maximum inspiratory pressure against an occluded airway. The strength of the respiratory muscles is determined by muscle bulk, the intrinsic properties and loading conditions of the contractile fibers, and the chemical environment in which the muscle contracts. Poor nutrition causes muscle wasting and thereby limits maximal respiratory pressures. As overall body weight diminishes, the mass and strength of the diaphragm decrease proportionately. Paralysis that is sustained for more than 24 to 48 h can initiate the process of diaphragm atrophy. Glucocorticoids accelerate the rate of protein catabolism. Optimal concentrations of calcium, magnesium, potassium, phosphate, hydrogen ion, chloride, and carbon dioxide are each important in maximizing muscle performance.

Hypoxemia tends to impair endurance more than muscle strength.

Certain commonly used drugs—particularly aminoglycosides and antiarrhythmics (e.g., calcium channel blockers) contribute to weakness in the setting of myasthenia gravis or other underlying neuromuscular impairment (see Chapter 17). Conversely, aminophylline and β-sympathomimetic drugs may modestly improve contractility and endurance. Intriguing experimental data suggest that the resting potential of the skeletal muscle membrane may remain abnormal for days after sepsis control and perhaps after the crisis period of other critical illnesses as well. Moreover, a "critical illness neuropathy" may help explain the prolonged and impressive muscle weakness observed in many of these patients after the acute phase has passed. The extended suppression of neuromuscular excitation by paralytic agents may result in very profound weakness for lengthy periods after they are discontinued, especially when corticosteroids have been used concomitantly as in status asthmaticus (see Chapter 17).

Contractile Fiber Properties   The contractile force developed by a stimulated muscle fiber relates directly to its resting length at the onset of contraction and inversely to its speed of contraction. Force output is, therefore, compromised when a patient inhales rapidly from high lung volume, as so often occurs in breathless, hyperinflated patients with chronic obstructive pulmonary disease (COPD) or asthma (see Chapter 25).

Endurance   Endurance, the ability of a muscle to sustain effort, is determined by the balance between the supply and demand of muscular energy. Hypoxemia, anemia, and ischemia are especially important to correct, because working muscles require an adequate flow of well-oxygenated blood for optimal performance. Although the respiratory muscles normally can access a large recruitable reserve, even this luxuriant supply may be insufficient under conditions of high stress and a failing cardiac pump. Studies of patients with acute ventilatory failure indicate that spontaneous breathing routinely consumes approximately 25% of the oxygen used by the entire body and even more during flagrant respiratory distress. (The normal percentage of respiratory oxygen consumption at rest is 1% to 2%.)

Over the years, many attempts have been made to gauge endurance by comparing spontaneous breathing cycles with maximal voluntary efforts. For example, the ability to voluntarily double $\dot{V}_E$ or tidal volume has been considered a positive predictive sign. Unfortunately, such voluntary indices require patient cooperation. However, the respiratory pattern gives important clues to ventilatory compensation. The respiratory frequency is the most sensitive but least specific indicator of developing problems. Early in the course of respiratory muscle fatigue, respiratory frequency increases. At the threshold of total exhaustion, frequency may diminish—a harbinger of approaching apnea. The breathing pattern shows variation of tidal volume and I:E ratio when the patient who receives modest support has ample respiratory reserve. In responding to an increased ventilatory workload (e.g., increasing exercise), a well-compensated subject will regularize the breathing pattern and increase both frequency and tidal volume together. Although tidal volume may reach a plateau value while frequency is still rising, tidal volume does not fall during compensated exercise and the ratio of frequency to tidal volume rarely exceeds 50 breaths/min/L, even during vigorous exertion. It has been suggested that a ratio of frequency to tidal volume that exceeds approximately 100 breaths/min/L indicates an unsustainable workload, as the patient fails to generate sufficient pressure to achieve a tidal volume appropriate to the minute ventilation required. The result is inefficient gas exchange and, ultimately, failure to wean from ventilatory support. (There are many exceptions, however, as most patients with restrictive disease naturally start from a higher resting baseline.)

Other components of the respiratory pattern, although harder to quantify, provide equally valuable diagnostic clues. At moderate levels of exertion, pressure in the abdomen rises as the diaphragm contracts, displacing the abdominal contents downward and outward; expiration, which occurs passively at low levels of exertion, often becomes active. Vigorous activity recruits the thoracic musculature, elongating the chest and expanding the rib cage. If diaphragmatic contraction is not proportionately forceful, the abdomen retracts paradoxically during inspiration. When observed in the supine position, this phenomenon, known as paradoxical abdominal motion, indicates a high level of exertion relative to the capability of the diaphragm. Paradoxical abdominal motion may be observed routinely in well-compensated patients with severe airflow obstruction. Some clinicians view the development of this finding as an indicator of established muscle fatigue, but more likely, it should be interpreted as a sign of high workload that may or may not be tolerable. Much less commonly, the ribcage and abdomen alternate primary responsibility for driving inspiration, a pattern known as *respiratory alternans*. Overt respiratory alternans is much less commonly observed than paradoxical abdominal motion and, when present, often has a neuropathologic origin.

Importance of Muscle Rest   To reverse fatigue, **4** the most effective intervention is to rest the muscles. Total rest is not required but a substantial fraction of the imposed workload must be relieved. Assisted mechanical ventilation, optimally adjusted to meet patient demands, usually allows the patient to rest sufficiently. As a rule, the support level can be assumed adequate if the alert patient is made comfortable. How long a skeletal muscle must be rested before it fully recovers from fatigue is not known with certainty. However, physiologic evidence of subnormal performance can be detected in the laboratory setting for at least 12 to 24 h after brief exposure to a fatiguing load. Therefore, a rest period of at least 12 to 24 h seems appropriate after an episode of acute decompensation. Because recovery may be prolonged, labored breathing risks fatigue and must be avoided.

■ PREDICTING INDEPENDENCE FROM VENTILATORY SUPPORT

Many predictive indices based on ventilatory performance have been suggested to accurately fore- **5** cast the outcome of the weaning trial (Table 10-3). However, if the patient is ventilator dependent for reasons unrelated to muscle strength (e.g., hypoxemia, cardiac ischemia, or psychological factors), such indices are of questionable value. Their predictive performance is equally limited after a long period of ventilatory support and for certain patients with permanent neuromuscular deficits. Even when impaired ventilatory power and endurance are responsible, no single index has been universally successful, perhaps because multiple factors cause the patient to remain ventilator dependent. Widely used *panels* of indicators tests are: $\dot{V}_E$, muscle strength, muscle reserve, and respiratory mechanics. Patients who are successfully weaned from mechanical support generally have a $\dot{V}_E$ lower than 10 L/min, a maximally negative inspiratory pressure exceeding $-20 \, cm \, H_2O$, a vital capacity (VC) more than twofold of the spontaneous tidal volume, and an ability to double the baseline $\dot{V}_E$ on command. In practice, the problem with using such a panel of criteria is twofold: only selected components can be measured in uncooperative patients, and there is uncertainty

TABLE 10-3   PREDICTORS OF WEANABILITY[a]

	MEASURED VALUES		CLINICAL OBSERVATIONS	
VENTILATION	STRENGTH	ENDURANCE	NEUROMUSCULAR	OTHER
$V_E \leq 10\text{--}15\,L/min^b$	MIP > –20 cm H_2O	MVV > 2 × V_E	*Absence of:* Scalene or abdominal muscle activity	$FiO_2 \leq 0.470$ < pulse < 120 pH > 7.30 BP > 80 mm Hg
$V_E \leq 175\,mL/kg/min$	$V_T \geq 5\,mL/kg$ VC ≥ 10 mL/kg	VC > 2 × V_T IEQ < 0.15 f < 30/min $f/V_T < 100$ $P_{0.1} < 6$ cm H_2O	Asynchrony Irregular breathing Rapid shallow breathing	

[a]For abbreviations, see text.
[b]Depending on body size.

when only one or two indices lie within the acceptable range. Thus, although these time-honored criteria are reliably predictive when all are satisfied or violated, they are of questionable assistance in difficult cases. While favorable weaning parameters may support a decision to undertake a weaning attempt, poor parameters should not preclude a carefully observed trial of spontaneous breathing or an attempt to wean if clinical judgment otherwise suggests a favorable outcome (Table 10-4).

Noninterventional Measures

Arterial Blood Gases and Pulse Oximetry

Although not reliable predictive indices per se, arterial blood gases and pulse oximetry are invaluable aids in gauging the progress of a weaning trial, especially when trends are followed. Observations

TABLE 10-4   EVALUATION FOR WEANING

AWAKE, OXYGENATED, STABILIZED?

- Power requirement
  - Minute ventilation
  - Work per liter (mean airway pressure)
- Power reserve
  - Cough inspiratory capacity (catheter or saline stimulation)
  - Prior variability of minute ventilation (over 6–8 h)
    (i) Sleep vs. awake
- Breathing test
  - Variation of tidal volume, V_E, I:E ratio
  - Assess f/V_t ratio in relation to:
    (i) Respiratory compliance, chronic neuromuscular background
    (ii) Directional change in minute ventilation

of breathing pattern and muscle activity (see following) as well as expiratory capnometry are also valuable.

Minute Ventilation

Ventilatory requirement and patient capability can be assessed crudely by $\dot{V}_E$ and the maximal inspiratory pressure (P_{max} or MIP) generated against an occluded airway. Although V_E is easy to measure, it should be interpreted with regard for body habitus, metabolic rate, and pH. For example, a 50-kg patient with respiratory acidosis at the time of $\dot{V}_E$ measurement may have a minute ventilation of only 10 L/min and yet be unable to resume spontaneous unaided breathing. Conversely, a patient weighing 100 kg with respiratory alkalosis may wean easily at the same level. As valuable as $\dot{V}_E$ may be, it only partially characterizes ventilatory demand; work per liter of ventilation is equally important in this assessment, as already discussed. Just as importantly, demand always must be related to capability. A low minute ventilation during sleep (as opposed to waking) is a good sign that underlying physiologic demands for ventilation are modest.

Spontaneous Breathing Pattern

Well-compensated patients breathing with pressure support demonstrate considerable variability in tidal volume and I:E ratio. Patients who are well adjusted to the ventilatory workload also choose tidal volumes greater than 4 to 5 mL/kg of lean body weight and breathing frequencies lower than 30/min. Although each breath taken with a shallow tidal volume is less energy costly than a deeper breath, the total energy expenditure necessary to maintain a given $\dot{V}_E$ may be greater, inasmuch as anatomic dead space occupies a larger percentage of each breath during shallow breathing. Therefore, patients with relatively normal chest mechanics who must breathe at frequencies greater than 35/min usually do so because they are too weak or fatigued to inspire to an appropriate depth. Some patients with neurologic disease or severe chronic restrictive disease (e.g., massive obesity, kyphoscoliosis, interstitial fibrosis) assume rapid shallow patterns because of disordered ventilatory control or reflex stimulation and may wean successfully at frequencies exceeding 40/min. The breathing pattern assumed during a brief (5-min) trial of spontaneous breathing under direct observation as well as its *progression* over that interval has proved to be an excellent integrative test of endurance (Fig. 10-3).

It is important to understand that for many patients a rising f/V_T ratio (often referred to as the rapid shallow breathing index, or RSBI) may simply reflect the natural "exercise" response to the increased workload of spontaneous breathing or anxiety. A rising f/V_T in conjunction with an *elevating* minute ventilation means something quite different from the same high f/V_T and a *declining* minute ventilation—compensated exercise response versus evolving ventilatory failure. As always, the appearance of the patient provides essential corroborating information.

Voluntary Measures

Maximal Inspiratory Pressure

Maximal inspiratory pressure (MIP) must be measured carefully to be of value. Although highly negative numbers encourage a weaning attempt, low values may reflect inadequate measurement technique rather than true patient weakness. For poorly cooperative patients, airway occlusion must start from a low lung volume and continue for at least eight to ten efforts before the value is recorded. (A one-way valve that selectively prevents inspiration while allowing unimpeded expiration may be helpful.) The MIP, a good measure of isometric muscle strength, does not yield information regarding endurance. This is better gauged by integrative indices of workload and response (see following).

Vital Capacity and Inspiratory Capacity

Considerably less muscular effort is required to approach the VC or its inspiratory component (IC) than to achieve a valid MIP. Although a one-way valving system can be used effectively to estimate the VC by tidal "breath stacking" without patient cooperation, this involuntary approximation reflects respiratory system mechanics more closely than muscle strength. If a cooperative patient achieves a (single effort) vital or inspiratory capacity twofold greater than the tidal volume, the chances are good that ventilatory reserves are sufficient to allow

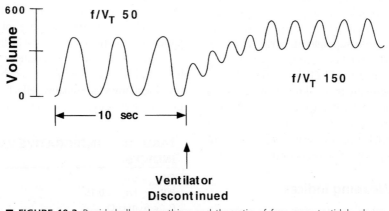

■ **FIGURE 10-3** Rapid shallow breathing and the ratio of frequency to tidal volume (f/V_T) in a patient with airflow obstruction. On ventilator disconnection, a poorly compensated patient with airflow obstruction tends to increase the work of breathing, develop gas trapping (auto-PEEP), and respond by decreasing tidal volume and increasing respiratory frequency. Although many exceptions exist, a patient recovering from acute illness with an f/V_T ratio exceeding 100 breaths/min/L during spontaneous breathing is less likely to be weaned successfully from ventilatory support.

successful resumption of spontaneous breathing. A near inspiratory capacity effort can often be elicited during a vigorous cough provoked by an airway suction catheter or saline instillation. Because modern ventilators have "closed" suction capability and continuously display volumes associated with tidal efforts, a good indication of the patient's IC and VC can be easily assessed.

Cough, Expiratory Pressure, and Maximal Expiratory Flow

Measures aimed at assessing the forcefulness of expiration may be important in gauging the ability to cough and clear secretions and, therefore, the need for continued intubation but have a more limited place in assessing the likelihood of successful weaning from the ventilator (see following).

Other Useful Measures

Nonrespiratory factors (e.g., coronary ischemia) often predominate in the most difficult weaning cases. Observations apart from standard indices of lung mechanics correlate well with an adverse weaning outcome. Very low or high pulse rates, respiratory rates greater than 30/min, forceful abdominal contractions, accessory muscle activity, chaotic breathing patterns, and coma are all negative prognostic factors. When uncertainty exists regarding upper airway patency, the ability of the patient to inspire around the ET tube after cuff deflation is reassuring (but not definitive) evidence that critical structural narrowing (splinted open while intubated) by the tube is not present. Similarly, the ability of moderate ventilating pressure to expel gas around the deflated cuff is encouraging. The oral, retropharyngeal, and supraglottic areas must be suctioned free of secretions prior to conducting either cuff deflation test. A PEEP setting that exceeds 15 cm H_2O helps assure that failure of air leakage is not due to a mucus seal. Passing these tests, although comforting to the clinician, does not ensure that variable (functional) upper airway obstruction will not occur in the postextubation period.

Integrative Weaning Indices

Several clues to the readiness of the patient for ventilator discontinuation are available in the hours preceding the spontaneous breathing trial (Table 10-5). Among the most valuable of these are a minute ventilation that falls during sleep independently of sedation, a nontachycardic sinus

TABLE 10-5 CLUES FOR PREDICTING "WEAN-ABILITY"

- Correlate rapid shallow breathing index (RSBI) with V_E
  - If V_E and RSBI both increase → exercise response
  - If V_E does not rise, high RSBI suggests problems
- Observe variation of breathing patterns
  - V_E before trial
  - Pattern of breathing on low level of PSV
- Observe "cough inspiratory capacity"
  - If $>2 \times V_T$ → good power reserve

rhythm, and a variable breathing pattern characterized by near normal minute ventilation and a wandering I:E ratio. A cough-induced IC that is two to three times the tidal volume is also encouraging. It should be kept in mind that the minute ventilation should be referenced to body size. Any single prognostic indicator is unlikely to prove successful unless it closely reflects the balance of ventilatory capability and demand. Analysis of the breathing pattern during a trial of spontaneous breathing is attractive, in that it allows the brain to integrate the information necessary to relate the workload to work capacity. Among the available options (Table 10-6), the frequency to tidal volume ratio (f/V_T) is perhaps the most useful and readily calculated. A value exceeding 100 breaths/min/L during the first minute of spontaneous breathing indicates extraordinarily rapid (reflected by f) and shallow (reflected by $1/V_T$) breathing. Clearly, patients with restrictive disorders of the lungs or chest wall should adopt a relatively rapid shallow pattern to minimize energy expenditure. Justified concern has been raised over the accuracy of this index for patients with underlying severe airflow obstruction, neuromuscular disorders, or chest wall deformity. It is unclear whether any such index based on respiratory mechanics can reliably reflect cardiac dysfunction or hypoxemia occurring as a consequence of

TABLE 10-6 INTEGRATIVE WEANING INDICES

$\bar{P}/P_{max} < 0.4$

$\bar{P}/P_{max} \times t_i/t_{tot} < 0.15$

$P_{0.1} < 6$ cm H_2O

CO_2-stimulated increase of $P_{0.1} > 4$ cm H_2O

$f/V_T < 100$

$V_T/VC < 0.5$

$\dot{V}_E/MVV < 0.5$

MVV, maximum voluntary ventilation.

spontaneous breathing effort. However, more complex indexes do not seem to offer major advantages over the f/V_T ratio.

■ WEANING TRIAL

Preparations for Withdrawing Ventilatory Support

6 Most patients are easily liberated from mechanical ventilation after the process that initiated the need for this support has improved (Table 10-7). It is now generally recommended that a brief daily trial of spontaneous breathing with low-level support be undertaken in patients whose acute need for ventilation has apparently resolved. If the result is satisfactory, a longer (30- to 120-min) period of unsupported breathing should be observed before an extubation attempt. In such patients, "weaning" in the sense of graded accommodation to unassisted breathing using partial ventilatory support is unnecessary. Patients who fail to tolerate the "minimal support" trial require optimal preparation before another is undertaken (Table 10-8). The inability to discontinue mechanical support often results from failure to correct one or more of the factors that adversely affect strength, capacity for responding to stress, ventilatory requirement, gas exchange, cardiovascular function, or lung mechanics. Significant physiologic problems (infection, renal failure) should not be developing or worsening. The well-prepared patient is in appropriate electrolyte, pH, and fluid balance. Magnesium, potassium, calcium, and phosphate concentrations should be checked especially closely. Infection, arrhythmias, cardiac ischemia, and heart failure must be well controlled.

TABLE 10-7 PREPARATION FOR WEANING

- Encourage sleep; use hypnotics to complement sedation
- Daily wake-up during full support phase of ventilation
- Early conversion to short acting sedatives
  - Propofol
  - Intermittent versed (midazolam)
- Relieve discomfort—skeletal and visceral (bowel, bladder)
  - Opiates relieve pain and improve depth of breathing ($\downarrow f/V_t$)
- Reestablish "baseline" fluid balance
  - Consider albumin and furosemide (drip)
- Address cardiac issues—ischemia, rhythm, CHF
- R_x infection, secretions, pleural effusions, *anemia*

TABLE 10-8 PREPARATIONS FOR WEANING IN DIFFICULT CASES

(i) Consider Depakote, quetiapine (Seroquel), risperidone, olanzepine (Zyprexa), for delerious or combative patients

(ii) Consider antiarrhythmic and ischemia prophylaxis

(iii) Consider lidocaine patch for persistent cough

(iv) Consider trial of methylphenadate (Ritalin) modafenil (Provigil), for patients slow to awaken

(v) Inspect the airway for retained mucus

Airways should be dilated optimally and kept as clear of retained secretions as possible (Fig. 10-4). Adequate sleep and nutritional support are essential. Excessive steroid doses should be avoided.

Patients who are grossly fluid overloaded are often hypoalbuminemic and may not be easy to diurese. Partial repair of the albumin deficit, combined with a furosemide drip (and supplemented by chlorthiazide when necessary) can reduce the excess and greatly improve the chances for independent breathing. Continuous hemofiltration (again in conjunction with albumin, if indicated) is an excellent option to gently but efficiently eliminate tissue water for those whose kidney function is impaired and or in whom diuresis is poorly tolerated or ineffective.

Importance of the Daily "Wake-Up"

Unfortunately, many patients require heavy sedative dosing in the first phase of illness, with unwanted lingering effects. In theory, daily interruption of

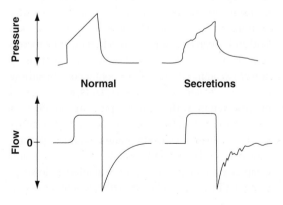

■ **FIGURE 10-4** Flow waveforms generated in a patient with retained central airway secretions. Note the highly irregular flow profile (which ordinarily would be much less apparent during the inspiratory phase of flow-controlled cycles than illustrated here). Such a patient may improve airflow and reduce the work of breathing impressively once the secretions are cleared.

sedative administration (particularly when infused) to the point at which the patient is nearly conscious for a brief period helps ensure that sedative drug accumulation will not delay progress. Conversion to a short-acting agent (e.g., propofol) 12 to 24 h before anticipated disconnection attempt is appropriate. Psychotropic agents such as haloperidol or dexmedetomidine may be needed to combat delirium, avoid panic reactions, and secure cooperation without suppressing consciousness. For patients without organic cause who are very slow to recover consciousness due to lingering drug effects, a trial of an alerting agent such as modafinil (Provigil) may be cautiously administered, especially for whom no clear contraindication exists.

Distention of the abdomen must be relieved. Care should be taken not to ventilate patients with chronic CO_2 retention to an artificially reduced $PaCO_2$ before the spontaneous breathing attempt. If this should happen, the patient may not be able to maintain the lower $PaCO_2$ level during unaided breathing, allowing acute acidosis to develop. Indeed, allowing a higher than usual $PaCO_2$ during the support phase may be appropriate, as already noted. The nursing staff should be advised as soon as the physician has decided that a weaning attempt will be undertaken (preferably the night before). Such warnings can prevent untoward administration of sedatives, nutrients, or procedures that interfere with the trial's success.

Weaning Sequence

7 The steps in removing mechanical support from the stable but ventilator-dependent patient are as follows: (a) estimation of the likelihood of success (physical examination, "parameter" measurement, secretion load and cough assessment); (b) a trial of spontaneous ventilation; (c) gradual withdrawal of ventilatory power (weaning) if the trial of spontaneous breathing is poorly tolerated; (d) for most patients, a brief period of observation with minimal pressure support or CPAP before extubation and/or removal of the ventilator; (e) evaluation of glottic tightness and upper airway patency by the cuff leak test (see earlier and Chapter 6); and (f) close postextubation follow-up, using noninvasive ventilation (NIV), where necessary.

Trial of Spontaneous Breathing

A trial of breathing without inspiratory assistance is a brief but stringent test of the ability to sustain spontaneous ventilation. It is generally undertaken when clinical judgment and a 3- to 5-min observation period of breathing with only minimal levels of pressure support and CPAP suggest the likelihood that the patient can breathe spontaneously without ventilator support. For these patients, a longer test period of breathing with minimal pressure support or CPAP (30 to 120 min, depending on the degree of concern) should be conducted. Passing this minimal support trial justifies an attempt to evaluate for extubation; failing either the brief or extended trial indicates that the causes of respiratory failure have not sufficiently resolved and further support and/or more gradual adaptation are necessary. Should overt fatigue be inadvertently allowed, a new trial should not be conducted before the patient rests for a 24-h period and in the meantime is placed on a comfortable mode of assisted breathing.

Such a trial of spontaneous breathing can be conducted either by the classic T-piece method or simply by allowing the patient to breathe through an efficient ventilator circuit. The latter approach allows tidal volume and frequency to be followed, keeps an apnea alarm in place, prevents infections related to frequent circuit breaks, and avoids time and financial costs associated with circuit manipulation. Using more than 7 cm H_2O of pressure support during the trial does not seem advisable because it may mislead the physician into a false sense of optimism. (Even a low level of pressure support may help a marginally compensated patient.)

Conducting the Trial

One reasonable method for conducting the trial is as follows:

1. Ideally, the initial trials should be undertaken in the morning when the patient is well rested and alert and a full complement of staff is available. This also allows retesting later in the day when the patient's condition may have improved further. If the patient is alert, explain the purpose of the procedure.
2. Place the patient in the sitting or semiupright position for maximal mechanical advantage.
3. Unless PaO_2 is high enough to provide a comfortable margin, increase FiO_2 by at least 10%; desaturation may develop during spontaneous breathing.
4. Suction the airway and oropharynx.
5. Monitor heart rate, blood pressure, tidal volume, respiratory rate, O_2 saturation, and level of comfort before starting and every few minutes

for the first 20 min. Although seldom used, tidal capnometry may be a helpful adjunct, as a steadily rising end-expiratory PCO_2 suggests decompensation. If the outcome is in doubt, arterial blood gases are analyzed.

6. If the patient seems to be doing well, continue. However, if there is any question of tolerance, resume mechanical ventilation immediately. Do *not* let the patient become fatigued or emotionally distressed.

7. Moderate disturbances of vital signs can be seen in successful trials. However, terminate the trial if the patient indicates intolerable dyspnea or if diastolic blood pressure falls or rises by more than 20 mm Hg, pulse rises or falls more than 30/min, respiratory rate increases by more than 10/min over the initial spontaneous value, arterial blood desaturates sharply, mental status deteriorates, or worrisome arrhythmias or signs of coronary ischemia develop. During trials longer than 15 min, periodic suctioning and hyperinflation should be considered.

8 Very prolonged trials of spontaneous breathing are discouraged for patients who have no continuing need for the airway. In general, the duration of the trial should parallel the duration of pretrial mechanical ventilation and vary inversely with the confidence of the physician in the extubation outcome. It should be noted that the first minutes to hours off the ventilator are often the most stressful because tidal volume and functional residual capacity (FRC) may decrease and changes occur in central vascular volume, respiratory work, and pattern of breathing. When the patient has sustained spontaneous ventilation comfortably for 30 min to 2 h, acute deterioration is less likely, and extubation should be considered if no contraindication exists, breathing pattern is stable, and the patient seems to be strong. Preparations for NIV in the immediate postextubation period should be made for the high-risk patient with cardiac insufficiency, massive obesity, or marginal weaning parameters. Special caution is indicated for patients who have undergone a prolonged period of ventilatory support. Patients with potentially unstable respiratory drive should be watched carefully before removing the tube.

An aerosol of racemic epinephrine should be considered for the patient with postextubation stridor. (Although controversial, moderate-dose steroids also may be justified for 48 h afterward.) A nasopharyngeal airway inserted immediately postextubation may help to aspirate secretions from the retropharynx and trachea. For cooperative patients, intermittent positive pressure delivered by mouthpiece or face mask can help maintain open airways, as can the sitting position, CPAP, and bilevel positive airway pressure (commercial Bi-PAP). Although **9** alertness should be maintained, the patient must be kept as comfortable and free from anxiety as feasible. Despite all precautions, it is distressingly common for marginal patients who apparently have been weaned successfully to require reintubation 12 to 48 h after extubation (e.g., due to fatigue, sleep deprivation, aspiration, or upper airway obstruction). Therefore, recently extubated patients must be watched very closely for signs of decompensation and not allowed to eat until adequate swallowing reflexes have been confirmed. Nocturnal support with Bi-PAP should be considered.

■ WEANING STRATEGIES AND METHODS

General Principles

Care must be taken to optimize the physiologic determinants of ventilator dependence ensuring hemodynamic stability (absence of cardiac ischemia, minimal use of pressors), adequate oxygenation (PaO_2/FiO_2 ratio > 200, PEEP < 8 cm H_2O, and an FiO_2 < 0.5), and ability to initiate inspiratory efforts are key to success (Table 10-9). Forcing the patient to work continuously may cause fitful sleep that compromises the weaning effort. The patient must be kept fully informed of the weaning plan, and most patients should be given absolute authority to terminate the trial if he or she experiences intolerable discomfort. Panic reactions must be avoided, especially in patients with COPD who experience a self-reinforcing cycle of dyspnea, hyperinflation, compromised muscle function, and often, pulmonary congestion or chest pain during these episodes. Tracheostomy should be considered after several failed weaning attempts, particularly if rapid recovery of muscle strength is unlikely or impossible. Tracheostomy provides a more stable airway than an ET tube, allows ambulation and oral feeding, improves secretion clearance, and decreases both ventilatory dead space and the work of breathing.

Weaning Priorities

To successfully withdraw ventilatory support, the problems of the patient that dictated the need for machine assistance must be matched to the methods

TABLE 10-9 THERAPEUTIC MEASURES TO ENHANCE WEANING PROGRESS[a]

PROBLEM	HYPOXEMIA	↑ IMPEDANCE	↑ $\dot{V}_E$
	Positioning	Positioning	Sedation
	↓ Secretions	↑ Secretion clearance	↓ Fever
	Bronchodilation	Bronchodilation	↓ Pain
	Diuresis	Diuresis	↓ V_D/V_T
	CPAP	Relieve cardiac ischemia	Correct acidosis
	↑ FiO_2	↓ $\dot{V}_E$	Allow ↑ $PaCO_2$
		↓ Circuit resistance	

PROBLEM	↓ DRIVE	↓ ENDURANCE	PSYCHOLOGICAL FACTORS
	↑ Nutrition	Rest periods	Reassure patient
	↓ Loading	Ensure sleep	Convey plan
	↓ Alkalosis	Optimal positioning	Anxiolytics
	↓ Sedatives	Correct electrolytes	Encourage activity
	↑ Sleep	↑ Calories	Ambulation/physical R_x
	↑ Thyroid	Optimize heart function	Adjust steroid dose
		Steroid replacement	
		Correct anemia	
		Relieve abdominal distention	

↑, increased; ↓, decreased.
[a]Partial listing.

available to address them. Several principles, however, apply to most patients. First, the added external work of breathing must be minimized. Second, adequate lung volume must be maintained to prevent atelectasis, secretion retention, dysfunctional breathing patterns, and inefficient gas exchange. Third, deep tidal inflations should occur periodically to encourage recruitment of marginal lung units.

Methods of Weaning

At the outset, it should be recognized that the need for *any* form of partial ventilatory support in the process of establishing ventilator independence has been seriously questioned. Strong advocates of this doctrine believe that no form of partial assistance is indicated and that a ventilator-dependent patient should be fully supported until their underlying ability to breathe spontaneously has returned. This viewpoint, although understandable, based on the available clinical trial data collected in diverse patient samples, often conflicts with a logical approach to the care of the subset of problematic patients with neuromuscular debility, cardiovascular compromise, and severe airflow obstruction.

Weaning Teams and Weaning Protocols

The complexity of reestablishing independent breathing is reflected by the reported success of weaning protocols that codify the preparations, evaluation, implementation, and pacing of efforts to discontinue ventilatory support. Respiratory therapists who ultimately report to the attending physician can be empowered to make assessments and undertake appropriate changes within the boundaries of agreed protocols. One successful approach is to assign dedicated teams comprised of nurses, therapists, and physicians to the task of consistent protocol-driven evaluation and implementation of weaning for multiple patients under their purview. The demonstrated benefits of weaning teams and weaning protocols appear to contradict the aforementioned "all or none" philosophy of ventilator management, as they infer that the details of the withdrawal process are important to the outcome. Yet, whatever stance is taken regarding partial ventilatory support, simply formalizing and consistently implementing rules governing sedation, daily assessment of spontaneous breathing potential, and ventilator management appear worthwhile in accelerating the "weaning" process.

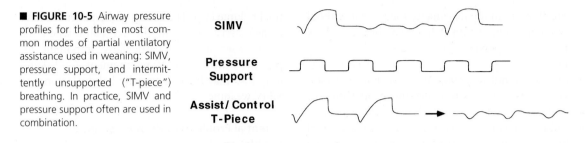

■ **FIGURE 10-5** Airway pressure profiles for the three most common modes of partial ventilatory assistance used in weaning: SIMV, pressure support, and intermittently unsupported ("T-piece") breathing. In practice, SIMV and pressure support often are used in combination.

For patients who fail their daily brief trial of unsupported breathing, three weaning methods have been in widespread use: progressive T-piece trials, intermittent mandatory ventilation (IMV), and PSV (Fig. 10-5). Recent practice has shifted away from gradual withdrawal of the ventilator and toward conducting a spontaneous breathing test once or twice daily, with full support in between failed attempts. Gradual withdrawal of ventilator power does retain a place, however, for the settings already discussed.

Unsupported ("T-piece") Weaning

Using the intermittent spontaneous breathing method (minimal CPAP and pressure support or "T-piece"), the duration of independent breathing is lengthened progressively according to patient tolerance. T-piece weaning provides stress periods punctuated by recovery periods of total rest. Traditionally, the patient is disconnected from the ventilator and is attached to a source of humidified conditioned gas for a brief interval. If well tolerated, these periods of spontaneous ventilation are lengthened progressively. Failure to progress to the next interval mandates reinstitution of continuous ventilator support for 12 to 24 h and a search for correctable problems. If the patient remains comfortable while breathing spontaneously for 30 to 120 min, shows no sign of hemodynamic instability or respiratory decompensation, and maintains acceptable blood gases, spontaneous breathing may continue, punctuated by episodic manual hyperinflation and airway suctioning when needed. The time that a patient must be observed during T-piece breathing before the ventilator is entirely discontinued is a matter of clinical judgment but generally should be governed by the length of time the patient has received mechanical ventilation and the apparent tolerance to spontaneous breathing.

This time-honored approach can be defended, based on current knowledge of fatigue and muscle reconditioning. Furthermore, the T-piece generally provides conditioned gas at negligible resistive work cost. The main disadvantages of using a T-piece are that it requires significant staff time to implement and monitor, involves repeated disconnections and physical manipulation of the circuitry (encouraging infection, see Chapter 8), forgoes respiratory monitoring, and fosters abrupt transitions on and off positive pressure. The latter can prove problematic for patients who must assume a high-impedance workload, for those who are anxiety prone, and for those with ischemic or congestive heart failure.

CPAP as Ventilatory Assistance

It is well known that PEEP and CPAP (>0 cm H_2O) can improve lung compliance for patients with atelectasis and lung edema. Auto-PEEP presents a significant threshold load to ventilation for patients with a critical limitation of expiratory airflow. CPAP helps to counterbalance auto-PEEP and reduce the ventilatory requirement. For weak patients with severe airflow obstruction, the addition of CPAP may cause tidal volume to increase, as pressure support or the natural force of breathing effort becomes more effective. For stronger patients, CPAP may be used as a counterspring against which expiratory muscles can store energy for release during the subsequent inspiration—the "work-sharing" phenomenon.

Partial Ventilatory Support

Synchronized Intermittent Mandatory Ventilation

During synchronized intermittent mandatory ventilation (SIMV), the machine provides a selected number of positive pressure cycles (volume-cycled or pressure-controlled) that support 0% to 100% of the total minute ventilation. A clinician-specified number of machine-supported breaths per minute are interspersed among spontaneous breaths in synchrony with patient effort (see Chapter 7). SIMV provides a method to gradually transfer the work of breathing from the machine to the patient without repeated manipulation of the circuit tubing, thereby reducing the potential for technical error and infection while saving nursing time. Offering a full range of partial ventilatory support is potentially advantageous for patients with congestive heart failure or obstructive lung disease who cannot withstand sudden increments in venous return or the work of breathing and for those who experience anxiety when machine support is withdrawn abruptly. SIMV can provide relatively large breaths at a guaranteed backup rate and, when used expertly, may allow the patient to retrain and strengthen long-rested muscles. Used improperly, however, SIMV can increase the work of breathing, prolong the weaning period unnecessarily, promote chronic "fatigue," or, worse, endanger the patient. SIMV is now used infrequently as a weaning mode.

Pressure-Support Ventilation

In the weaning process, PSV offers an attractive option as an alternative or supplement to SIMV. When inspiratory pressure is set high enough, PSV can provide near-total ventilatory support. At low levels, PSV provides enough of a pressure boost to overcome the inspiratory (but not expiratory) resistance of the ET tube. Each breath is aided by the ventilator to the pressure level set by the physician and is flow-cycled by the patient's ventilatory impedance or expiratory effort. Unlike SIMV delivered without pressure support, PSV lends some flexibility to the amount of power available from the machine. The patient can adapt to decreasing PSV by increasing frequency, thereby taking maximal advantage of machine power. In some instances, it is only when PSV falls below some critical value that the patient must work actively to maintain tidal volume (V_T). The ability of the patient to have greater assistance from the ventilator when the need arises may be particularly important for patients with variable $\dot{V}_E$ requirements, and therefore, PSV may be an especially helpful adjunct to SIMV weaning.

Potential Problems of Pressure-Support Ventilation

Although valuable for overcoming ET tube resistance, in allowing breaths of variable character and in conferring some flexibility in response to changing power requirements, PSV is not the perfect mode for partial ventilatory support, especially in the earlier implementations of this modality. When providing a fixed rate of rise to a set target pressure, PSV does not tailor its output to the changing character of patient effort. Poorly selected pressure targets may elicit discomfort because of a power mismatch or inappropriate tidal volume. When the impedance to inflation is very high, flow may decelerate so quickly that the cycle terminates prematurely. Conversely, for patients with severe airflow obstruction or narrow ET tubes, airway pressurization may need active termination, as inspiratory flow may assume a very slowly decelerating profile (Fig. 10-6). The threshold between tolerance and intolerance to a decrease in PSV is often quite distinct. A difference of only a few cm H_2O per cycle may separate comfort from overt dyspnea. Furthermore, the level of support offered by PSV varies directly with the impedance to chest inflation. Therefore, patients with variable inflation impedance (e.g., those prone to accumulate secretions or who experience bronchospasm during the weaning trial) are less-optimal candidates for its use. The development of auto-PEEP may partially

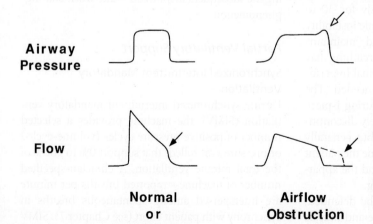

Airway Pressure

Flow

Normal or Restrictive

Airflow Obstruction

■ **FIGURE 10-6** Airway pressure and flow profiles for patients with and without airflow obstruction receiving pressure support. Because inspiratory flow decelerates only slowly when the airway is obstructed, achieving the 25% peak flow off-switch criterion (*solid arrow*) would require an excessive inspiratory time. The patient actively stiffens the chest wall to initiate expiration, as reflected by the end-inspiratory blip in airway pressure (*open arrow*).

or completely nullify the contribution of PSV to the inspired V_T. Interestingly, this curtailment of tidal volume as auto-PEEP develops may give rise to a "feed-forward" process that can cause the ventilatory pattern to show mathematically fractal and even chaotic behavior. These bizarre variability patterns are mathematically determined by the interaction of PSV, the off-switch setting, and the mechanics of the obstructed patient. Theoretically, they have nothing to do with (and may actually disrupt) the patient's own ventilatory control mechanism.

Comparison of SIMV and PSV

At the very onset of the weaning process, SIMV and PSV both support all breathing cycles and provide virtually identical ventilatory assistance for the same tidal volume. Similarly, at the completion of weaning, the patient must eventually breathe without assistance. Unquestionably, however, there are differences in the way that these techniques reload the respiratory muscles as support is withdrawn (Fig. 10-7). The extent of these differences varies from patient to patient. Most patients tend to reload their own ventilatory system later when using pure PSV than when using pure SIMV. In PSV, the machine remains well coupled to the patient's breathing rhythm throughout the power withdrawal process. In SIMV, however, the patient and ventilator seem disconnected in the sense that the patient does not respond to machine cycles by reducing energy output. Such independence becomes overt when SIMV falls below approximately 50% of the assist-control frequency.

Other Ventilatory Modes

Certain modes recently introduced to clinical practice (e.g., proportional assist ventilation [PAV] and neurally adjusted ventilatory assist [NAVA]) have the potential to overcome some of the drawbacks of PSV and SIMV. Both allow patient control over the assisting pressure waveform while allowing the physician to effectively set the strength of the auxiliary muscle they provide. Other approaches such as adaptive support ventilation (ASV) may in theory use respiratory pattern feedback to automatically withdraw pressure assistance. To this point, however, none of these recently introduced modes has seen extensive clinical use (see Chapter 7).

Practical Points in the Weaning Process

General

1. Frequency and tidal volume adapt within seconds to minutes of a change in the breathing workload.

2. The spontaneous breathing pattern during low level PSV or CPAP should be tested once or twice daily for 3 to 15 min (depending on tolerance) in almost *all* patients to detect ventilator independence at the earliest possible time and to avoid unnecessarily protracted weaning schedules.

3. Enough CPAP (3 to 7 cm H_2O) is applied to compensate for positional volume losses and/or auto-PEEP, and enough PSV is used to overcome ET-tube resistance, considering both tube resistance and minute ventilation. Adding some level

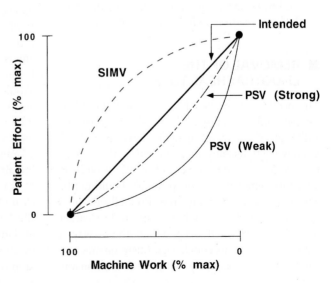

■ **FIGURE 10-7** Rate of reloading of the respiratory musculature during weaning by SIMV and PSV. As breathing frequency is reduced from the assist/control (100%) level, the patient receiving SIMV tends to respond by accepting the ventilatory workload relatively early in the machine withdrawal process. By contrast, relatively strong patients tend to reload the musculature linearly as pressure support is reduced, whereas weak patients tend to defer acceptance of the burden until relatively late in the withdrawal process.

TABLE 10-10 ALTERNATIVE WEANING STRATEGIES

	PRIMARY POWER	
	PSV	SIMV
Timed cycles	0.5–2/min	Assist/control → 0/min
CPAP	3–5 cm H_2O	3–5 cm H_2O
PSV	PSV_{max} 3–7 cm H_2O	3–10 cm H_2O

TABLE 10-11 PERI-EXTUBATION CARE

PRE-EXTUBATION

- Aggressive secretion clearance, respiratory care, and fluid balance
- High PEEP immediately before and during tube extraction
- Consider nasal trumpet *pre*-extubation
- Inspect airway prior to extubation

POST-EXTUBATION

- *Humidified* intermittent and nocturnal Bi-PAP
- Nasal prongs whenever possible

of PSV also lends flexibility to the level of support the patient may draw from, even when SIMV is selected (see previous).

4. The patient must not be allowed to encounter sustained dyspnea and, during weaning efforts extending over days, must be supported adequately at night to allow restful sleep and avoid hypoxemia.

5. With the patient receiving sufficient PSV to seem comfortable with a breathing frequency of less than 20 breaths/min and a tidal volume of approximately 7 to 8 mL/kg (PSV_{max}), pressure support is withdrawn in decrements of 2 to 4 cm H_2O, as tolerated (Table 10-10). If tidal volume or SaO_2 is marginal, one or two deeper SIMV breaths are applied to help avert microatelectasis and triggering of reflex tachypnea.

6. Progression to the next decrement is allowed if the breathing frequency does not exceed 30 to 35 breaths/min and tidal volume remains greater than approximately 3.5 mL/kg for more than 5 to 15 min. If minute ventilation does not fall and the patient appears comfortable, the spontaneous breathing trial may proceed even if the rapid shallow breathing index (f/V_T) > 100.

■ REMOVAL OF THE ENDOTRACHEAL TUBE

The need for continued ET intubation should be assessed independently of the need for ventilation. Although virtually all patients have disordered swallowing transiently after extubation, those likely to have a persisting problem of airway protection after tube removal (e.g., deep coma) should not be extubated. Because airway protection reflexes (pharyngeal gag and laryngeal closure) are lost earlier than cough triggered deep within the airway, a patient who fails to cough vigorously on tracheal suctioning is not likely to protect the airway

effectively when the tube is removed (Table 10-11). For patients with copious airway secretions and ineffective cough, the tube should be retained to facilitate suctioning. VC greater than 20 mL/kg, a cough-induced inspiratory capacity > 2 × V_T, a vigorous expulsive effort on tracheal stimulation (secretions coughed into the external circuit), an MIP more negative than –40 cm H_2O, a measured peak expiratory flow greater than 160 L/min (normal: 360 to 1,000 L/min), and an expiratory pressure generated against an occluded airway greater than 60 cm H_2O predict effective coughing after extubation.

Patients who have had a difficult intubation or who have been reintubated one or more times are at higher risk for glottic swelling and upper airway obstruction after extubation. All such patients should be extubated with appropriate contingency preparations made for immediate reintubation should distress develop precipitously after extubation (see Chapter 6). Assuming that appropriate evaluative tests for ventilation adequacy and glottic patency (deflated cuff "leak" test with high-level PEEP) have already been performed, the extubation procedure itself is straightforward. In preparation, enteral feedings should be stopped, preferably 1 h beforehand, and if a nasogastric tube is in place, it should be connected briefly to suction to evacuate any pools of retained gastric fluid. If the gastric tube is to be removed, ideally it should be pulled *prior* to extubation. Inhaled bronchodilator is given 15 min before extubation in patients with underlying airflow obstruction. A source of supplemental O_2 is readied. The retropharyngeal space should be cleared of supraglottic secretions to the extent possible, and 100% oxygen is delivered in the few minutes immediately prior to tube extraction. It is good practice to elevate PEEP (15 cm H_2O) immediately (approx. five breaths) prior to cuff deflation and to keep higher PEEP throughout the extraction process. (Not only does it help to inflate the lungs and to start the extraction from a relatively high lung volume, but flow from the tube tip propels secretions inaccessible to a suction catheter that remain above the cuff into the mouth for easy expectoration.) With the cuff deflated and PEEP applied, the patient is asked to exhale forcefully as the tube is quickly removed and to cough vigorously immediately afterward. The appropriate concentration of O_2 is administered immediately by face mask or nasal prongs.

In a patient with a tracheostomy, the ability to phonate and expectorate with the tube cuff partially deflated (after oropharyngeal suctioning) is generally considered to be a positive predictive sign. Because compromise of coughing and swallowing in the postextubation period generally parallels the duration of translaryngeal intubation, particular attention should be paid to assiduous tracheobronchial hygiene in these cases. Suctioning, corticosteroids, bronchodilators, Bi-PAP, sitting position, antibiotics, and careful regulation of electrolyte, glucose, and cardiovascular status often make the difference between a patient who bridges the period of difficulty and another who must be reintubated.

■ AVOIDING DELAYED WEANING FAILURES AND REINTUBATION

The need for reintubation carries an adverse prognosis, perhaps partially accounted for by the patient's underlying condition and partially by the hazards of extended intubation/mechanical ventilation. The 24- to 48-h period immediately after ventilator disconnection may be highly dynamic, as the larynx, the upper airway, and the swallowing mechanism may be seriously, but temporarily, dysfunctional. Nonetheless, the patient must readjust to spontaneous breathing and assume responsibility for airway secretion clearance. Stresses arising soon after extubation may result from cardiac ischemia, arrhythmia, pulmonary congestion, atelectasis, secretion retention, oropharyngeal aspiration, or temporary swelling of glottic and subglottic tissues. Appropriate pharmacoprophylaxis, upright positioning, and vigorous attempts to encourage deep breathing, coughing, and mobilization are helpful. In lethargic patients, secretions may pool in the retropharynx and should be aspirated periodically via a nasopharyngeal airway ("trumpet"). Caution should be used when initiating oral feeding after a lengthy intubation. Informal or formal swallowing studies are indicated depending on the clinician's degree of suspicion. Premature resumption of oral intake is hazardous because temporary swallowing dysfunction and impaired glottic defenses are common. Intermittent NIV during this period may help as a bridge across the immediate postextubation period (see following). Anything that can be done to improve sleep quality (including NIV, fewer sleep interruptions, and relatively safe hypnotics, such as zolpidem) is worth implementing to avoid sleep deprivation and eventual exhaustion. The mediation list should be reviewed, and the potential for either mental depression by scheduled narcotics or excessive mental stimulation by high dose steroids and catecholamines minimized. Pulse oximetry, echocardiography, and electrocardiography are helpful monitors during this period as well. Manually or mechanically assisted coughing may be helpful in reaching this threshold in the days that follow extubation.

The Unweanable Patient

The need for continued ventilatory support is often psychological as well as physiological (Table 10-12). A few points are important to keep in mind.

1. The patient must be "co-opted" into the weaning effort and kept fully advised of the treatment plan.
2. Most patients should be given full "veto" power to terminate an overly taxing trial.
3. "Panic" reactions are especially detrimental for patients with airflow obstruction. At such times, these patients generate increased volumes of CO_2 and experience poorly coordinated breathing, hyperinflation, hypoxemia, and extreme dyspnea.
4. A novel sedative and anxiolytic with little respiratory depression (dexmedetomidine) and psychotropic agents may benefit selected patients

TABLE 10-12 AIDS TO WEAN THE UNWEANABLE PATIENT

Co-opt the patient
Confer veto power
Avoid panic reactions
Consider anxiolytics/psychotropics
Rest fully before trial/ensure sleep
Check for "hidden" cardiovascular and endocrine problems
Mobilize and exercise
Respiratory muscle training

who awake into agitated delirium when sedatives are withdrawn.

5. The patient must be fully rested. This can best be ensured by 10 to 12h of full ventilatory support and a good night of sleep before the attempt.

6. Hidden problems such as diastolic dysfunction, coronary insufficiency, endocrinopathy (hypoadrenalism, hypothyroidism), subtle strokes, critical illness polyneuropathy, steroid myopathy, paralytic neuromyopathy, or Parkinson disease may explain protracted ventilator dependence and must be sought aggressively in puzzling cases. Large pleural effusions must be drained, and the stomach must be decompressed.

7. Mobilization aids in general rehabilitation and is often the key to the weaning effort. Prolonged bed rest is attended by multiple adverse physiologic changes related to the changed vector of gravitational forces, including depressed vascular tone, reduced extravascular volume, loss of red cell mass, electrolyte shifts, calcium depletion, aberrations of hormonal balance, and depletion of skeletal muscle mass (see Chapter 18). Prevented from weight bearing, the lower extremities undergo disproportionate atrophy in patients continually at bed rest. Performing arm and leg exercises in bed, and in tracheostomized patients, sitting, standing, and even ambulation aid greatly in the rehabilitation effort. Chronically ventilator-dependent patients demand less nursing attention than other ICU patients. Immobilized and deprived of sensory stimulation, they often become passive, discouraged, or poorly cooperative. Efforts to provide sensory input, to restore the natural diurnal rhythms, normal activities, and social interactions, and to provide physical and occupational therapy may improve mental outlook, strength, and prospects for recovery.

Muscle Training

As soon as the crisis period has passed, it makes good physiologic sense to deliberately stress the ventilatory musculature for brief periods several times daily, encouraging spontaneous breathing (CPAP with low-level PSV). After being fully rested, such "wind sprints" may help strengthen, recoordinate and condition the ventilatory muscles in a fashion similar to athletic training for limb muscles. Many patients with good strength but a tendency to panic do best when extubated directly rather than

being weaned with low levels of machine support. This is particularly true when a highly resistive ET tube is in place (e.g., a small-caliber nasal tube). Although the precise reason for this response is uncertain, expiratory resistance (which may be disproportionately high in the intubated subject) is unchanged by the use of pressure support.

Psychotropics (e.g., respiridone, Seroquel, Zyprexa) are often helpful in such cases. The decision to extubate despite a failed spontaneous breathing trial is encouraged by noting that minute ventilation falls during sleep, rises during the spontaneous breathing trial, and that the breathing pattern is highly variable. Those who cannot be extubated may benefit from tracheostomy, a procedure that lowers airway resistance and apparatus dead space, improves secretion hygiene, and allows mobilization.

For a patient whose primary problem is ventilatory mechanics (and not respiratory drive), it may be worthwhile to allow $PaCO_2$ to rise slowly over several days while maintaining acceptable oxygenation and pH balance. Higher $PaCO_2$ enables each breath to eliminate CO_2 more efficiently. Special attention should be paid to repairing any bicarbonate deficit, which often results from saline administration, diarrhea, or renal tubular dysfunction. Higher bicarbonate levels buffer fluctuations in $PaCO_2$ more effectively and reduce dyspnea.

Noninvasive Ventilation as a Bridge to Ventilator Independence

Over the past decade, the development of appropriate equipment and comfortable interfaces has encouraged the meteoric growth of NIV in a variety of acute applications (see Chapter 7). In the postextubation period, the provision of ventilatory support may maintain upper airway patency and improve sleep quality. Periodic rest may keep the weak patient from the verge of fatigue. COPD patients appear to benefit the most from NIV in the postextubation period. Care must be taken to assure adequate hydration of the inspired airstream, which tends to be dry, increased in quantity, and inhaled through the mouth. If the NIV is unhumidified, secretion thickening in the oropharynx and airway poses a serious risk for retention that may precipitate ventilatory failure and need for reintubation.

Tracheostomy

Timing for tracheostomy must be considered on an individual basis. Some patients in ventilatory failure (e.g., those with slowly reversible or irreversible neurological problems or upper respiratory pathology) should receive early tracheostomy. For patients with acute lung disorders that are expected to reverse, there is no ironclad rule regarding when tracheostomy should be performed. As a guideline, tracheostomy may be appropriate anytime after the first 7 to 10 days. The decision to undertake tracheostomy should consider the pace of improvement; if the patient is progressing sufficiently to be ready for extubation within 3 to 5 days, tracheostomy can be deferred reasonably. Patients who have demonstrated the need to be reintubated without readily correctable cause merit consideration. It should be emphasized, however, that for some patients who are making slow progress—particularly those who do not fight ventilation—ET tubes may be kept in place for longer than 3 weeks without permanent laryngeal or tracheal injury or need for tracheostomy.

Importance of Communication

Intubated patients who require ventilatory support often are frustrated in their attempts to communicate with their families, friends, and caregivers. The psychological value of establishing a reliable means of communication frequently is underestimated. Writing pads and letter, "pick-choice" message boards, and image cards are commonly used for endotracheally intubated patients but are cumbersome at best. For the traceostomized patient, however, better options are available. Effective devices for communication include vibrators placed over the larynx or cheek and for those strong enough to breathe spontaneously, one-way inspiratory valves (Passy-Muir valves). Although specialized tubes that direct a manually gated gas flow through the vocal cords are available, a simpler approach for *any* trached and ventilated patient is to deflate the cuff with 10 cm H_2O of PEEP applied. The ventilator's attempt to maintain pressure will result in flow around the trach tube and across the cords, allowing phonation.

Weaning from Tracheostomy

10 Consideration should be given to removing the tracheostomy tube when the patient no longer requires suctioning for secretion removal, high fractions of inspired oxygen, or periodic reconnection to the ventilator. Replacement of the standard tracheostomy tube with a fenestrated one facilitates talking and allows easier assessment of true cough effectiveness. The predictors of coughing ability were discussed earlier. There are essentially three methods for gradually discontinuing a tracheostomy: use of partial plugs, use of progressively smaller tracheostomy tubes, and use of stomal "buttons." Plugs that progressively occlude a standard-sized tracheostomy orifice (e.g., one-half to three-quarters plugs) can be used to assess the need for continued intubation. (The cuff on the ET tube must be deflated during orifice occlusion.) However, it should be remembered that an occluded tracheostomy tube severely narrows the effective tracheal lumen, thereby increasing the work of breathing and the tendency toward secretion retention. For this reason, many physicians prefer to replace the original tracheostomy with progressively smaller uncuffed (or uninflated) tracheal cannulae, such as silver Jackson tubes. Unfortunately, the stomal orifice rapidly adapts to the smaller-caliber tube as well, so that effective ventilation through the tracheostomy might not be possible if an acute need arose. If the ability to sustain spontaneous ventilation, clear secretions, or protect the airway remains questionable, a well-fitted and snug tracheostomy "button" will maintain the stoma over several days to weeks to allow tube reinsertion, noninvasive nasal or mask ventilation, emergency ventilation, suctioning, and effective administration of inhaled bronchodilators without adding substantially to airway resistance. NIV often aids in providing adequate nocturnal ventilatory assistance, as well as the power necessary to bridge the period of adaptation that follows decannulation.

For certain difficult patients (e.g., those with debilitating weakness, paralysis, or neuromuscular disease), a vigorous program of assisted coughing may be instrumental in achieving airway clearance. This may involve the application of high inflation volumes followed by abdominal thrusts timed to coincide with glottic opening. For patients who cannot maintain glottic closure or for whom abdominal compression is compromised by thoracic cage deformity or extreme obesity, deep spontaneous inspiration and manual abdominal compression may be ineffective; here, a commercially available "insufflation/exsufflation" device (capable of transiently generating 50 cm H_2O of positive and negative pressures when applied to the face mask or ET tube) may be especially useful. A vibratory vest may enhance secretion removal in weakened patients with copious airway secretion who do not respond to other measures (e.g., antibiotics, steroids). For patients with severe obstructive airway disease, however, assisted coughing techniques may be fruitless.

■ **SUGGESTED READINGS**

Butler R, Keenan SP, Inman KJ, et al. Is there a preferred technique for weaning the difficult-to-wean patient? A systematic review of the literature. *Crit Care Med.* 1999;27(11):2331–2336.

Eskandar N, Apostolakos MJ. Weaning from mechanical ventilation. *Crit Care Clin.* 2007;23:263–274.

Girard TD, Ely EW. Protocol-driven ventilator weaning: Reviewing the evidence. *Clin Chest Med.* 2008;29:241–252.

Hess D. Ventilator modes used in weaning. *Chest.* 2001;120 (Suppl. 6):474S–476S.

King C, Moores LK. Controversies in mechanical ventilation: When should a tracheostomy be placed? *Clin Chest Med.* 2008;29: 253–264.

Manthous CA, Schmidt GA, Hall JB. Liberation from mechanical ventilation: A decade of progress. *Chest.* 1998;114(3):886–901.

Marini JJ. Breathing patterns as integrative weaning predictors: Variations on a theme. *Crit Care Med.* 2006;34(8):2241–2243.

Navalesi P. Weaning and noninvasive ventilation: The odd couple. *Am J Respir Crit Care Med.* 2003;168(1):5–6.

Siner JM, Manthous CA. Liberation from mechanical ventilation: What monitoring matters? *Crit Care Clin.* 2007;23(3):613–638.

Wysocki M, Cracco C, Teixeira A, et al. Reduced breathing variability as a predictor of unsuccessful patient separation from mechanical ventilation. *Crit Care Med.* 2006;34(8):2076–2083.

Intensive Care Unit Imaging

Conventional and specialized imaging techniques play key roles in the care of the critically ill. For example, computed tomographic (CT) scanning and magnetic resonance imaging (MRI) are indispensable for neurologic, chest, abdominal, and sinus evaluation. Ultrasound (US) facilitates cardiac, renal, and gallbladder disease diagnosis, and nuclear medicine techniques help to confirm embolic diseases, gastrointestinal (GI) bleeding, and fistulous communications. Availability of high quality US machines has made thoracentesis and

central venous catheter (CVC) placement safer and easier. Interventional radiology assumes an ever-increasing role in performing repairs that once could only be addressed surgically. This list includes embolization of cerebral aneurysms, percutaneous aortic aneurysm grafting, embolization of bowel and spleen bleeding, and pulmonary embolism (PE) disruption. These and other specialized applications are discussed elsewhere in this volume with the specific diseases they help define. This chapter concentrates on studies commonly applied in the critical care setting: the chest X-ray (CXR) and chest CT, and the abdominal plain film.

Huge advances have occurred in ICU radiology in the last decade as digital filming techniques have been perfected, and digital images can now be viewed on almost any computer. This technological revolution has brought a host of advantages:

1. Films are no longer lost or out of chronological order.
2. Delays in availability have decreased.
3. It is possible to manipulate image brightness and contrast and place it side-by-side with previous films.
4. Geographically separated physicians can simultaneously view a study.
5. Physicians no longer need to leave the ICU to view studies.

There are two important disadvantages of the digital revolution. First, the expensive high-resolution monitors necessary to see smallest details are not widely available; hence films are often examined on suboptimal screens. Second, the daily meeting of the intensivist and radiologist that always occurred when X-ray film was used has vanished. These later changes are probably detrimental: they deprive the radiologist of important clinical information, may result in clinicians overlooking subtle but important findings, and eliminate a valuable educational function.

■ CHEST RADIOGRAPHY

Technique

The usefulness of the portable anterior–posterior
1 (AP) CXR is largely determined by positioning
and exposure technique. One simple measure to
improve the ability to interpret CXRs is to reposition overlying devices (e.g., ECG monitoring wires,
ventilator and IV tubing, external pacing pads, and
nasogastric or orogastric tubes) out of the field of
the radiograph. Orientation of the patient with
respect to the radiographic beam is of critical
importance. Kyphotic, lordotic, and rotated projec-
tions have dramatic impact on the apparent
dimensions of intrathoracic structures and detection of pathology. The use of "gravity dependent"
radiopaque markers on the corners of portable
films helps clarify a patient's position. The AP technique blurs and magnifies the anterior mediastinum and great vessels, in some cases by as much as
20%. When radiographs are obtained in supine
patients, cardiovascular structures also appear
enlarged because of augmented venous filling and
reduced lung volume. For example, the azygous
vein distends in the supine normal subject but collapses in the upright position. Conversely, supine
films often render pneumothoraces and pleural
effusions imperceptible. Rotation produces artifactual hemidiaphragm elevation ipsilateral to the
side of rotation. In diffuse infiltrative processes, lateral decubitus positioning accentuates asymmetry—making the dependent lung appear more
affected. Film penetration may emphasize or diminish parenchymal lung markings. Consistency in
exposure technique is critical to allow day-to-day
comparison of radiographs. A properly exposed
CXR should reveal vertebral interspaces in the retrocardiac region. Films on which these interspaces
are not visualized are underpenetrated, exaggerat-
ing parenchymal markings and making visualization of air bronchograms difficult.

Changes in lung volume influence the appearance of parenchymal infiltrates, especially in mechanically ventilated patients and in those receiving
positive end-expiratory pressure (PEEP). Infiltrates
seen on a CXR obtained in full inspiration on the
ventilator usually appear less dense than when
viewed in partial inspiration. Furthermore, roughly
half of all patients will have a "less-infiltrated"
appearing CXR following the application of PEEP.
Unfortunately, there is no predictable relationship
between the level of PEEP applied and its impact on
the appearance of the film. To facilitate comparison,
serial films should be exposed with the patient in
the same position, during the same phase of the
respiratory cycle, and with comparable tidal volume and end-expiratory pressure. CXR appearance
is also influenced by therapeutic interventions and
the development of new medical conditions. Infusions of large volumes of fluids, the development of
oliguria, or superimposed myocardial dysfunction
produces a rapidly deteriorating radiographic picture. Bronchoalveolar lavage may cause the appearance of localized infiltrates due to residual lavage
fluid and atelectasis.

Film Timing

Because of the high likelihood of finding significant
abnormalities (e.g., tube malposition, pneumothorax), it is worthwhile to obtain a CXR on almost all
patients on arrival in the ICU. The frequency with
which radiographs are necessary after admission is
much more controversial. General agreement exists
that CXRs should be obtained promptly after invasive procedures such as endotracheal (ET) intubation,
feeding tube placement, transvenous pacemaker
insertion, thoracentesis, pleural biopsy, and central
vascular catheter placement to ensure proper tube
position and exclude complications. Likewise, a
film should probably be obtained after transbronchial biopsy, although the need for such a study in
the nonintubated patient is debated. In all but
emergency situations, a CXR should follow failed
attempts at catheterization via the subclavian route
before contralateral placement is attempted.

Although many ICUs obtain daily routine or
even more frequent radiographs, regularly scheduled films are not necessary in all patients. Despite
data indicating that a quarter to two thirds of ICU
CXRs demonstrate an abnormality, many of these
findings are chronic or inconsequential and almost
all can be detected by careful examination of the
patient before obtaining the radiograph. Prospective
study indicates that less than 10% of films demonstrate a new significant finding, and only a fraction
of these are not anticipated by clinical examination.
A reasonable compromise position is to obtain daily
"routine" radiographs on mechanically ventilated
patients who have hemodynamic or respiratory
instability (usually 3 to 5 days after admission).
Additional films should be dictated by changes in
the patient's clinical condition and the performance
of procedures. In the stable, mechanically ventilated

patient, especially those with a tracheostomy, films can safely be obtained on a much less frequent basis—perhaps even weekly. Obviously, deterioration should prompt more frequent evaluation.

Placement of Tubes and Catheters

Tracheal Tube Position

Because up to 25% of ET tubes are initially suboptimally positioned, radiographic confirmation of tube location is crucial; positioning the ET tube in the right main bronchus often results in right upper lobe or left lung atelectasis or right sided barotrauma. (Left main intubations are uncommon because the left main bronchus is smaller and angulates sharply from the trachea.) Conversely, if the tube tip lies too high in the trachea (above the level of the clavicles), unintended extubation is likely. When the head is in a neutral position, the tip of the ET tube should rest in the mid-trachea, approximately 5 cm above the carina. In adult patients, the T5-7 vertebral level is a good estimate of carinal position if it cannot be directly visualized. The carina is usually located just inferior to the level of the aortic arch. (Another method to locate the carina uses the intersection of the midline of the trachea with a 45 degree bisecting line which passes through the middle of the aortic knob.) ET tubes move with flexion, extension, and rotation of the neck. Contrary to what might be expected, the tube tip moves caudally when the neck is flexed (i.e., chin down = tip down). Conversely, head rotation away from the midline and neck extension elevates the ET tube tip. Total tip excursion may be as much as 4 to 5 cm.

The normal ET or tracheostomy tube should occupy one half to two thirds of the tracheal width and should not cause bulging of the trachea in the region of the tube cuff. Bulging is associated with an increased risk of subsequent airway stenosis, presumably the result of tracheal wall ischemia from cuff overinflation. Gradual dilation of the trachea may occur during long-term positive pressure ventilation, but every effort should be made to prevent this complication by minimizing ventilator cycling pressure and cuff sealing pressures.

After tracheostomy, a CXR may detect subcutaneous air, pneumothorax, pneumomediastinum, or malposition of the tube. The T3 vertebral level defines the ideal position of the tracheostomy site. (This usually places the tip halfway between the stoma and the carina.) Unlike the orally placed ET tube, the tracheostomy tube does not change position with neck flexion or extension. Lateral radiographs are necessary for evaluation of AP angulation. Sharp anterior angulation of the tracheal tube is associated with the development of tracheoinnominate fistulas, whereas posterior erosion can produce a tracheoesophageal fistula. Massive hemoptysis usually signals the former condition, whereas sudden massive gastric distention with air occurs in the latter.

In patients with previous intubation or tracheostomy, the tracheal air column should be examined for evidence of stenosis. Tracheal narrowing is relatively common and can occur at the level of the tracheal tube tip, at the cuff, or at the tracheostomy tube stoma (most common site). The typical hourglass shaped narrowing can be hard to visualize on a single AP radiograph and stenosis must be substantial (luminal opening <4 mm) to be symptomatic.

Central Venous Catheters

For accurate pressure measurement the tip of the CVC should lie within the thorax, well beyond any venous valves. These are commonly located in the subclavian and jugular veins, approximately 2.5 cm from their junction with the brachiocephalic trunk (at the radiographic level of the anterior first rib). Because CVC catheters in the right atrium or ventricle may cause arrhythmias or perforation, the desirable location for these lines is in the mid-superior vena cava, with the tip directed inferiorly. Radiographically, catheter tips positioned above the superior margin of the right mainstem bronchus are unlikely to rest in the atrium. Catheters should have no sharp bends along their course and should descend lateral and parallel to the spine. Stiff catheters, particularly hemodialysis catheters, inserted from the left subclavian may impinge on the lateral wall of superior vena cava, potentially resulting in vascular perforation. Complications resulting from vascular puncture include air embolism, fluid infusion into the pericardium or pleural space, hemopneumothorax, and pericardial tamponade. Imaging studies reveal that partial thrombosis occurs distressingly often with CVCs and peripherally inserted central catheters (PICC). Postprocedure radiographs reveal complications in up to 15% of CVC placements. On occasion, catheters inserted from the subclavian route can pass across the midline into the contralateral subclavian vein, or even turn cephalad entering the internal jugular veins. Similarly, catheters inserted in the internal jugular veins may track into the subclavian vein of either side. The phenomenon of a subclavian catheter crossing the midline is most common when a triple lumen catheter is threaded through a larger bore placed in the right subclavian vein. Although not evidence based, many clinicians are comfortable leaving CVCs which terminate in the contralateral subclavian in place, provided there are no clinical effects but are much less at ease with CVCs terminating in the internal jugular vein.

As a general rule it is a good idea to obtain a CXR following failed attempts at CVC placement before attempting insertion on the contralateral side. Doing so reduces the already tiny chance of producing bilateral pneumothoraces. Obviously, this safeguard must be abandoned under truly exigent circumstances where venous access must be obtained immediately.

Pulmonary Artery (Swan–Ganz) Catheter

Every insertion-related complication of CVCs, including pneumothorax, pleural entry, and arterial injury, can result from the placement of the pulmonary artery catheter (PAC). Unique complications of PAC placement include knotting or looping and entanglement with other catheters or pacing wires and pulmonary artery rupture and infarction. Knotting or entanglement of PACs with other catheters is frightening to the less experienced practitioner, but can usually be avoided, and need not be dangerous if a few simple steps are followed. Knotting can largely be avoided by proper insertion technique as outlined in Chapter 2. The basic safety measure is to not advance the catheter more than 20 cm before the next chambers pressure tracing is observed. For example, a right ventricular tracing should be seen with less than 20 cm of catheter advancement after obtaining a right atrial pressure tracing, and a pulmonary artery tracing should be obtained before 20 cm of catheter is inserted after obtaining the right ventricular tracing. Doing so prevents the catheter from forming a large loop in the right atrium or ventricle. If the PAC does become knotted or entangled with another device (e.g., pacing wire or vena caval filter), it is essential to resist the temptation to pull on the catheter harder to extract it; doing so only tightens the knot, making eventual extraction more difficult. Almost always knotted catheters can be "untied" under fluoroscopic guidance simply by loosening the knot,

with aid of a stiff internal guidewire. Interventional radiology services are often helpful for disentanglement.

Pulmonary thromboembolism is being recognized with increasing frequency and is now reported in 1% to 10% of PAC placements. The most common radiographic finding is distal catheter tip migration, with or without pulmonary infarction. With an uninflated balloon, the tip of the PAC usually overlies the middle third of a well-centered AP CXR (within 5 cm of the midline). Distal migration is common in the first hours after insertion as the catheter softens and is propelled distally by right ventricular contraction. If pressure tracings suggest continuous wedging, it is important to look for distal migration, as well as a catheter folded on itself across the pulmonic valve or a persistently inflated balloon (appearing as a 1-cm diameter, rounded lucency at the tip of the catheter). Inflation of the balloon of a persistently wedged PAC can result in immediate catastrophic pulmonary artery rupture or delayed formation of a pulmonary artery pseudoaneurysm. Pseudoaneurysms present as indistinct rounded densities on CXR 1 to 3 weeks after PAC placement. The diagnosis is easily confirmed by MRI or contrasted chest CT.

The width of the mediastinal and cardiac shadows should be assessed following placement of PACs and CVCs, because perforation of the free wall of the ventricle may result in pericardial tamponade. Temporary phrenic nerve paralysis due to the lidocaine used in catheter placement rarely precipitates unilateral hemidiaphragm elevation.

Pacing Wires

When transvenous pacing wires are inserted emergently they are often malpositioned in the coronary sinus, right atrium, or pulmonary artery outflow tract. On an AP view of the chest, a properly placed pacing catheter should have a gentle curve with the tip overlying the shadow of the right ventricular apex. However, it is often difficult to assess the position of the pacing wire on a single film. On a lateral view, the tip of the catheter should lie within 4 mm of the epicardial fat stripe and point anteriorly. (Posterior angulation suggests coronary sinus placement.) In patients with permanent pacemakers, leads commonly fracture at the entrance to the pulse generator, a site that should be checked routinely. Pacing wires can also result in cardiac perforation so it is important to examine the CXR for signs of tamponade.

Chest Tubes

The optimal position for a chest tube depends on the reason for its placement. Posterior positioning is ideal for the drainage of free-flowing pleural fluid, whereas anterosuperior placement is preferred for air removal. On an AP chest film, posteriorly placed tubes are closer to the film than those placed anteriorly. This proximity of the chest tube to the film results in a "sharp" or focused appearance of the catheter edge and its radiopaque stripe. Conversely, anteriorly placed chest tubes often have fuzzy or blurred margins. Chest tube location may appear appropriate on a single AP film, even though the tube actually lies within subcutaneous tissues or lung parenchyma. Failure to re-expand the pneumothorax or drain the effusion should be a clue to extrapleural placement. Oblique or lateral films or a chest CT may be necessary to confirm appropriate positioning. On plain film, another clue to the extrapleural location of a chest tube is the inability to visualize both sides of the catheter. Chest tubes are constructed with a "sentinel eye," an interruption of the longitudinal radiopaque stripe that delineates the opening of the chest tube closest to the drainage apparatus. This hole must lie within the pleural space to achieve adequate drainage and ensure that no air enters the tube via the subcutaneous tissue. After removal of the chest tube, fibrinous thickening stimulated by the presence of the tube may produce lines (the tube track), which simulate the visceral pleural boundary, suggesting pneumothorax.

Intra-Aortic Balloon

The intra-aortic balloon (IAB) is an inflatable device placed in the proximal aorta to assist the failing ventricle. Diastolic inflation of the balloon produces a distinct, rounded lucency within the aortic shadow, but in systole the deflated balloon is not visible but the underlying catheter is. Ideal positioning places the catheter tip just distal to the left subclavian artery. Placed too proximally, the IAB may occlude the carotid or left subclavian artery. Placed too distally, the IAB may occlude the lumbar or mesenteric arteries and produce less-effective counterpulsation. Daily radiographic assessment is prudent to detect catheter migration or a change of the aortic contour suggestive of IAB-induced dissection.

Gastric Access Tubes

Whether inserted through the nose (NG) or mouth (OG), it is usually prudent to obtain a CXR to confirm gastric tube position before administration of medication, fluid, or feeding, even when clinical evaluation indicates proper position. Even in intubated patients, a surprising number of tubes intended for the stomach end up in the lung (usually the right mainstem bronchus). Vigorous insertion technique can force the gastric tube through the lung into the pleural space. Inadvertent airway cannulation is most likely to occur when using a small-bore–stylet-stiffened tube, especially when inserted in comatose or deeply sedated patients. When inserted via the esophagus, the side holes of the enteral tube should be fully advanced past the lower esophageal sphincter to minimize reflux. After a percutaneous endoscopic gastric (PEG) tube is placed, an abdominal film should be obtained to search for the most common complications of extragastric placement or peritoneal leakage.

Specific Conditions Diagnosed by Chest Radiography

Atelectasis

Atelectasis is a frequent cause of infiltration on ICU CXRs. The wide spectrum of findings ranges from invisible microatelectasis, through plate, segmental, and lobar atelectasis, to collapse of an entire lung. Differentiating between segmental atelectasis and segmental pneumonia is often difficult, because these conditions often coexist. However, marked volume loss and rapid onset and reversal are more characteristic of acute collapse.

Atelectasis tends to develop in dependent regions and, more commonly, in the left rather than the right lower lobe by a 2:1 margin. Radiographic findings of atelectasis include hemidiaphragm elevation, infiltration or vascular crowding (especially in the retrocardiac area), deviation of hilar vessels, ipsilateral mediastinal shift, and loss of the lateral border of the descending aorta or heart. Each lobe has a characteristic pattern of atelectasis. With right upper lobe collapse, apical density increases as the minor fissure rotates superior-medially producing an easily recognizable curvilinear arch extending to the mediastinum. Because the left lung does not have a middle lobe or minor fissure, upper lobe collapse occurs anteriorly producing a diffuse haziness of the hemithorax and loss of the upper left cardiac border. In both cases the main pulmonary artery shadow moves cephalad. On lateral CXR, right middle lobe atelectasis appears as a prominent wedge with its apex directed toward the hilum, as the minor fissure and major fissure move toward

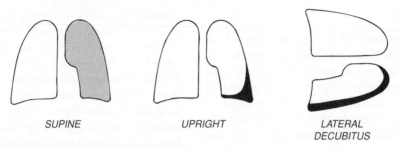

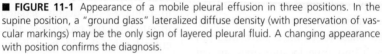

SUPINE   UPRIGHT   LATERAL
                                 DECUBITUS

■ **FIGURE 11-1** Appearance of a mobile pleural effusion in three positions. In the supine position, a "ground glass" lateralized diffuse density (with preservation of vascular markings) may be the only sign of layered pleural fluid. A changing appearance with position confirms the diagnosis.

each other. Unfortunately, on posterior–anterior (PA) CXR findings are typically much more subtle with only obscuration of the right heart border. Partial collapse of either the right or left lower lobe produces a similar pattern of diaphragmatic silhouetting. When lower lobe volume loss is extensive, a triangular posteriomedial density can be seen with its base resting on the diaphragm. Contrary to popular belief, the "silhouette sign" is not always reliable on portable films, particularly in the presence of an enlarged heart or on a film obtained in a lordotic or rotated projection. Air bronchograms extending into an atelectatic area suggest that collapse continues without total occlusion of the central airway and that attempts at airway clearance by bronchoscopy or suctioning are likely to fail.

Pleural Effusion and Hemothorax

Pleural effusions are very common among ICU patients; however, their recognition requires proper patient positioning. On the supine AP CXR, large effusions redistribute—potentially causing a hazy density to overlie the entire hemithorax without loss of vascular definition. Apical pleural capping is another radiographic sign of large collections of pleural fluid in the supine patient. Upright or lateral decubitus radiographs may help confirm the presence of an effusion (Fig. 11-1). If a large collection of pleural fluid obscures the lung parenchyma, a contralateral decubitus film permits visualization of the lung. Pleural fluid is not ordinarily visible until several hundred milliliters have accumulated. On lateral decubitus films, 1 cm of layering fluid indicates a volume that can usually be tapped safely. If there is any question about the quantity or mobility of fluid, bedside US is helpful.

Subpulmonic or loculated fluid may be difficult to recognize. Hemidiaphragm elevation, lateral displacement of the diaphragmatic apex, abrupt transitions from lucency to solid tissue density, and increased distance from the upper diaphragmatic margin to the gastric bubble (on an upright film) are all signs of a subpulmonic effusion (Fig. 11-2). US and chest CT are useful adjuncts in detecting the presence of pleural fluid and in guiding drainage. US has the obvious advantage of portability and real-time imaging for drainage.

Extra-Alveolar Gas/Barotrauma

Extra-alveolar gas can manifest as interstitial emphysema, cyst formation, pneumothorax, pneumomediastinum, pneumoperitoneum, or subcutaneous emphysema (see Chapter 8).

Pulmonary Interstitial Emphysema

Radiographic signs of gas in the pulmonary interstitium include lucent streaks that do not conform to air bronchograms and cysts at the lung periphery, usually at the bases. Interstitial emphysema may also appear as small "target lesions" as air surrounds small peripheral pulmonary arterioles viewed *en face*.

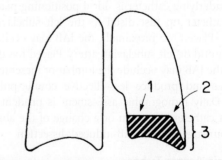

■ **FIGURE 11-2** Radiographic signs of a subpulmonic effusion (*1*) hemidiaphragm elevation with separation of lung from gastric bubble, (*2*) lateralization of the diaphragmatic dome, and (*3*) abrupt transition from lucency to soft tissue density.

These signs, best seen when the parenchyma is densely infiltrated, portend the development of pneumothorax.

Subpleural Air Cysts

Subpleural air cysts, a potential sign of impending pneumothorax in mechanically ventilated patients, are small (3- to 5-cm wide) basilar rounded lucencies. The cysts often appear abruptly and may rapidly increase in size (sometimes to as large as 9 cm). Subpleural air cysts frequently progress to tension pneumothorax in the presence of continued mechanical ventilation. The role of prophylactic tube thoracostomy remains unanswered; however, when subpleural air cysts are noted, the clinician should maintain a high level of vigilance and be prepared to emergently insert chest tubes.

Pneumothorax

Pneumothorax is often difficult to detect on portable CXRs done on ICU patients. Few ICU patients exhibit the typical patterns seen on upright CXRs performed on noncritically ill patients. Proper positioning assumes great importance in detection. On supine films or in patients with pleural adhesions, gas may collect exclusively in the basilar (anterior) regions of the thorax. Thus, gas may outline the minor fissure or may move anteriorly over the heart, mimicking pneumomediastinum or pneumopericardium. Loculated pneumothoraces can be very difficult to detect without CT, and it is surprising how many times a residual localized air collection is found by CT among patients with one or more chest tubes. Radiographic signs of pneumothorax on the supine CXR include a "deep sulcus sign" and lucency over the upper portions of the spleen or liver (see Chapter 8). An upright expiratory CXR is the best film for detecting a pneumothorax. This view confines a fixed amount of intrapleural air within a smaller volume, accentuating the proportion of thoracic volume it occupies and the separation of lung from chest wall.

The visceral pleura provides a specific marker: a radiodense (white) thin stripe of appropriate curvature with lucency visible on both sides and absent lung markings beyond. Skin folds often mimic the pleural edge but can be distinguished by certain features: lucency present only on one margin, poorly defined limits, and extension beyond the confines of the rib cage. Because pneumothorax reduces blood flow to the collapsed lung, its density may be surprisingly normal, even with an extensive gas collection.

Pneumothoraces are often characterized by the percentage of the hemithorax they occupy. This practice is highly imprecise, both because the CXR is only two-dimensional and because apparent percentage changes occur with variations in breathing depth and position. As with pleural fluid, precise estimation of the size of a pneumothorax is neither possible nor necessary. A tension pneumothorax (of any size) and a "large" pneumothorax both require drainage—the former because of its immediate physiologic effects, the latter because it creates a pleural pocket that is unlikely to reabsorb spontaneously over an acceptable time. The reabsorption rate of a pneumothorax has been estimated to be "1% to 2% per day," a crude rule of thumb that emphasizes the slowness of this process. Thus, a 15% pneumothorax would typically take 2 weeks to reabsorb.

Tension Pneumothorax

The diagnosis of tension pneumothorax must be made on clinical grounds if serious morbidity and mortality are to be prevented. Delaying therapy for radiographic confirmation significantly increases mortality. Radiographically, tension pneumothorax often shifts the mediastinum and flattens or inverts the hemidiaphragm ipsilateral to the pneumothorax. Yet, tension is usually difficult to diagnose with confidence on a single film; infiltrated or obstructed lungs fail to collapse completely, and an unyielding mediastinum may not shift noticeably, despite a marked pressure gradient. A comparison of past films with clinical correlation is most often required. When doubt exists and the patient is unstable, tube thoracostomy is indicated.

Pneumothorax occurs in up to 50% of patients receiving mechanical ventilation with peak inflation pressures greater than 60 cm H_2O, and a large fraction of these are under tension. The adoption of lower tidal volume ventilation has decreased the incidence of pneumothorax dramatically. Pneumothorax commonly complicates the course of patients with necrotizing pneumonias, acute respiratory distress syndrome (ARDS), secretion retention, or expanding cavitary or bullous lesions. Tension pneumothorax can be very difficult to distinguish from bullous disease under tension by plain radiograph. Although a chest CT can be revealing, patients in extremis cannot wait for a diagnostic CT scan. In such emergent settings, erring on the side of chest tube insertion is probably the best course of action, even though rupturing a large bullous can create a bronchopleural fistula.

Pneumomediastinum

After gaining access to the mediastinum, gas normally decompresses into adjacent soft tissues. Thus, unless gas trapping occurs, pneumomediastinum rarely produces important physiologic effects in adults. Mediastinal gas may arise from neck injuries, from rupture of the trachea or esophagus, or (most commonly) from alveolar rupture and retrograde dissection of air along bronchovascular bundles. Pneumomediastinum appears radiographically as a lucent band around the heart and great vessels caused by gas within the space separating the parietal pleura from the mediastinal contents. On the heart's inferior border, this lucency can extend across the mediastinum, linking the two sides of the chest with a "complete diaphragm sign." An unnaturally sharp heart border is the first indicator of pneumomediastinum, a sign that must be distinguished from the "kinetic halo" seen at the heart or diaphragm border of an edematous lung. The mediastinal pleura, defined by gas on both sides of a thin radiodense line, can often be detected. On a lateral film, pneumomediastinum usually appears as a thin crescent of gas outlining the ascending aorta. Not uncommonly, extra pleural gas extends from the mediastinum, lifting the parietal pleura off the diaphragm or outlining the inferior pulmonary ligament. Pneumomediastinum is an important harbinger of pneumothorax, which follows in 50% to 70% of mechanically ventilated patients.

Subcutaneous Gas

In the adult, subcutaneous gas, also known as subcutaneous emphysema, usually has important diagnostic but little physiologic significance. Subcutaneous gas produces lucent streaks or bubbles in the soft tissues that typically outline major muscle groups of the chest, neck, and back. However, there is almost no limit to the path the gas may take entering the retroperitoneum, peritoneal cavity, and even the scrotum. During mechanical ventilation, generalized subcutaneous gas usually results from alveolar rupture and medial gas dissection and indicates an increased risk of pneumothorax. Once pneumothorax has occurred, progressive accumulation of gas in the subcutaneous tissue suggests the presence of a bronchopleural fistula or

a malfunctioning chest tube, especially if the gas is bilateral. Small amounts of subcutaneous gas detected shortly after chest tube placement frequently enters via the tube track itself. Subcutaneous gas detected immediately after blunt chest trauma should raise the possibility of tracheobronchial or esophageal disruption (see Chapter 36).

Pulmonary Edema

Without invasive monitoring, distinguishing between normal permeability (fluid overload and congestive heart failure [CHF]) and high-permeability pulmonary edema, ARDS can be difficult. Considerable overlap exists in the radiographic findings of these entities, but certain CXR findings may be helpful in determining the etiology of lung water accumulation. These forms of edema are best distinguished by three features: size of the heart and great vessels, distribution of vascular markings, and the pattern of infiltration (Table 11-1). CHF and volume overload are characterized by a widened vascular pedicle, an even or inverted pattern of vascular markings, and a tendency toward a gravitational distribution of edema ("bat wing" or basilar). Pleural effusions, particularly of substantial size are also more common with CHF than ARDS. The vascular pedicle is measured at the point the superior vena cava crosses the right main bronchus to a perpendicular dropped from the point of takeoff of the left subclavian artery from the aorta. Kerley B lines, due to perilymphatic interstitial fluid, are common in established CHF (usually of several days' to weeks' duration), whereas crisp air bronchograms are unusual. Conversely, the less mobile infiltrates of ARDS are widely scattered, patchy, and often interrupted by distinct air bronchograms. These criteria are better for correctly classifying CHF and volume overload edema and less accurate for identifying ARDS. Widespread application of these criteria to evaluate the etiology of pulmonary edema has shown them to be less successful than originally claimed. Because most of the radiographic deterioration seen in ARDS occurs within the first 5 days of illness, worsening CXR appearance after this time suggests superimposed pneumonia, fluid overload, sepsis, or new CHF.

Although pulmonary edema is usually bilateral and symmetric, it may collect asymmetrically when mediastinal tumor, bronchial cyst, or massive thromboembolism diverts flow preferentially to one lung. The recently transplanted lung is also prone to developing unilateral pulmonary edema. Asymmetry

TABLE 11-1 RADIOGRAPHIC FEATURES OF PULMONARY EDEMA

CHARACTERISTICS	CARDIOGENIC OR VOLUME OVERLOAD EDEMA	HIGH PERMEABILITY EDEMA
Heart size	Enlarged	Normal
Vascular pedicle	Normal/enlarged	Normal/small
Flow distribution	Cephalad	Basal/balanced
Blood volume	Normal/increased	Normal
Septal lines	Common	Absent
Peribronchial cuffing	Very common	Uncommon
Air bronchograms	Uncommon	Very common
Edema distribution	Even/central/gravitational	Patchy/peripheral/nongravitational
Pleural effusion	Very common/moderate-large	Infrequent/small

may also be observed following unilateral aspiration, re-expansion pulmonary edema, or in the presence of extensive bullous disease. Gravity may redistribute edema fluid to dependent lung regions over brief periods—one mechanism for shifting unilateral edema after patient repositioning.

Mediastinal Widening

Mediastinal widening on a well-centered film (particularly following chest trauma or an invasive procedure) provides a clue to aortic disruption. (A rotated or lordotic film may be falsely positive.) Obtaining an upright PA CXR is desirable but is frequently not possible because of injuries or hypotension. Radiographic clues to aortic disruption include a widened superior mediastinum (the most sensitive sign), a blurred aortic knob, rightward deviation of the nasogastric tube or aortic shadow, and tracheal deviation to the right and anteriorly. Inferior displacement of the left main bronchus, left-sided pleural effusion (with or without apical capping), and displacement of intimal calcifications of the aorta provide other signs suggestive of aortic disruption (see Chapter 35). Mediastinal widening with vascular injury is frequently associated with traumatic fractures of the sternum, first two ribs, or clavicle. Widening of the cardiac shadow should prompt careful review of the aortic contour, because blood may dissect from the aorta into the pericardium. If aortic disruption is suspected, angiography probably remains the definitive procedure, although MRI, contrast-enhanced CT scanning, and transthoracic or transesophageal echocardiography may be diagnostic.

Pericardial Effusion

Pericardial effusion is recognized radiographically by enlargement of the cardiac shadow. The classic "water bottle configuration" of the cardiac silhouette, although highly characteristic, is unusual. An epicardial fat pad visible on the lateral CXR should raise the suspicion of a pericardial effusion, as should splaying of the tracheal bifurcation. Echocardiography is the procedure of choice for the detection and evaluation of pericardial effusions, and it simultaneously affords the opportunity to assess heart chamber size, contractile function, and vena caval diameter. When a transthoracic echocardiogram cannot obtain images of adequate quality because of patient weight or chest hyperinflation, transesophageal echocardiogram is usually diagnostic.

Air–Fluid Levels (Lung Abscess vs. Empyema)

Several features help to distinguish whether an air–fluid level lies within the pleural space or within the lung parenchyma. On an AP film, pleural fluid collections generate wide, moderately dense air–fluid levels, whereas intrapulmonary collections are usually smaller, more dense, and rounded. Lung abscesses and liquid-filled bullae tend to project similar diameters on both AP and lateral films. The air–fluid level of pleural fluid collections must abut the chest wall on either AP or lateral film (Fig. 11-3). Fluid collections that cross a fissure line on upright films are located within the pleural space. Lung abscesses generally have thick,

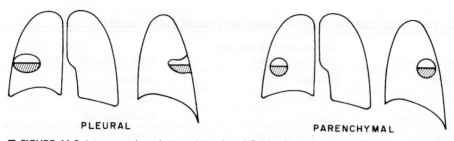

■ **FIGURE 11-3** Intraparenchymal versus intrapleural fluid collections. Fluid collections within the pleural space usually have a greater horizontal than vertical dimension, do not cross fissure lines, and may have sloping attachments to the pleural surface on one or more views. Furthermore, pleural collections typically have different dimensions on AP and lateral views. By contrast, intraparenchymal collections tend to be more spherical, with equal dimensions on AP and lateral views.

shaggy walls with irregular contours, unlike liquid-filled bullae and pleural fluid collections. As the position is altered, pleural fluid collections frequently undergo marked changes in shape or contour. CT scanning reliably differentiates the two conditions.

Postthoracotomy Changes

After pneumonectomy, fluid accumulates in the vacant hemithorax over days to months. Whereas the absolute fluid level is of little significance, changes in the level of fluid are important. A rapid decline in the fluid level should prompt concern for a bronchopleural fistula, a complication that most commonly develops within 8 to 12 days of surgery. If a fistula develops earlier, failure of the bronchial closure should be suspected, prompting consideration of reoperation. On rare occasions, it is necessary that bronchopleural fistulas occurring postthoracotomy are confirmed by instilling a sterile tracer into the pleural space and inspecting the expectorated sputum immediately afterward or, alternatively, by the inhalation of radioactive gas, followed by imaging of the thorax. Bronchopleural fistulas tend to displace the mediastinum to the contralateral side, an unusual occurrence during uneventful postoperative recovery. Small residual air spaces may remain for up to a year following pneumonectomy and do not necessarily imply the presence of a persistent fistula. Very rapid postoperative filling of the hemithorax suggests infection, hemorrhage, or malignant effusion.

Fistulous Tracts

Fistulas between the trachea and innominate artery develop most frequently when a tracheal tube angulates anteriorly and to the right in patients with low tracheostomy stoma, persistent hyperextension of the neck, or asthenic habitus. Because of this association, anteriorly directed tracheal tubes should be repositioned. Fistulas also may form between the trachea and esophagus during prolonged ET intubation. These usually occur at the level of the ET cuff, directly behind the manubrium. Predisposing factors include cuff overdistention, simultaneous presence of a nasogastric tube, and posterior angulation of the tracheal tube tip. The sudden occurrence of massive gastric dilation in a mechanically ventilated patient provides an important clue. A radiographic contrast agent may be introduced into the esophagus after cuff deflation or tube removal in an attempt to confirm the presence of the fistula.

Pulmonary Embolism

Although the plain CXR rarely if ever diagnoses PE, it is quite useful to detect other conditions in the differential diagnosis including CHF, pneumothorax, and aspiration. Despite limited diagnostic utility, large emboli may give rise to suggestive findings: ipsilateral hypovascularity, pulmonary artery enlargement, and (rarely) abrupt vascular cutoff. Local oligemia (the Westermark sign) may be seen early in the course of PE, usually within the first 36 h. "Hampton's hump," a pleural-based triangular density caused by pulmonary infarction, is seldom seen. About 50% of patients with PE have an associated pleural effusion.

For critically ill ICU patients with suspected thromboembolism, it often makes sense to begin the evaluation with US of the limbs. If the US reveals clot in any deep vein, the diagnosis of "thromboembolism" is confirmed, other tests are unnecessary, and anticoagulation is indicated. It has become clear that for ICU patients not only are the legs a potential source of clot, but the neck and arms are as well. Roughly half of all CVCs in place for a week or more are associated with at least a partially occlusive thrombus, and approximately 15% of these patients have concurrent PEs. The initial use of limb US has several advantages including avoidance of contrast exposure and travel from the ICU, as well as lower cost and rapid turnaround time. If the US is negative but the clinical suspicion of PE remains high, ventilation/perfusion (V/Q) scanning or contrasted chest CT may be performed. The rarity of a normal CXR diminishes the value of V/Q scanning in the critically ill. Nonetheless, normal perfusion scans are very helpful and abnormal scans help guide the angiographic search for emboli. If the CXR suggests that the V/Q scan will be uninterruptible, contrasted chest CT represents a reasonable alternative. Although the sensitivity and specificity of chest CT for the diagnosis of PE in the ICU population are unknown, it is probably safe to assume that a filling defect seen in the pulmonary circuit of a technically adequate study represents clot (i.e., high specificity). (Primary tumors of the pulmonary artery, primary lung tumors, cancers metastatic to the mediastinum, nonneoplastic mediastinal adenopathy, hydatid disease, and mediastinal fibrosis can mimic PE.) By contrast, because the sensitivity of CT is variable among institutions, and even in the best centers is as low as 30% for subsegmental clot, a negative CT should not be regarded as definitive data excluding PE. (Sensitivity is optimized by a scanner with many rows of detectors, optimal contrast injection technique and gating, breath-holding by the patient, and experienced interpretation of optimally reconstructed images including three-dimensional views.) Although there is controversy about the importance of subsegmental clots in healthy patients, in critically ill patients with impaired cardiopulmonary reserve, it is probably not wise to overlook such emboli. If the US is negative, V/Q not practical, and CT nondiagnostic but clinical suspicion remains high, angiography is the next step. Frequently, CT and catheter angiography are both contraindicated by renal insufficiency. Angiography can be safely undertaken in most critically ill patients, provided that: (i) care is used in transport, (ii) pulmonary artery pressures are not excessive at the time of contrast administration, and (iii) selective injections guided by perfusion scanning are performed. Septic PE should be considered in patients with multifocal cavitary lesions of varying size. A complete discussion of thromboembolism diagnosis is presented in Chapter 23.

Pneumonitis

Aspiration

Although bacterial infection sometimes supervenes, gastric aspiration initially produces a sterile chemical pneumonitis. When bacterial infection complicates aspiration in the intubated patient, the time from intubation to aspiration can provide valuable clues to the etiologic organism. Events occurring within 4 days of intubation are usually associated with *Staphylococcus*, *Streptococcus*, and *Haemophilus* infections, whereas later episodes are usually due to Gram-negative rods. Massive aspiration, although position and volume dependent, typically appears as bilateral diffuse alveolar and interstitial infiltrates of rapid onset. The extent of the infiltrate does not correlate with outcome and often radiographic improvement is quite rapid. Aspiration in the supine position usually affects the perihilar regions and superior and basilar segments of the lower lobes. Patients who aspirate in a decubitus position often develop unilateral infiltrates. When asymmetrical, the right lung is usually more involved. Significant atelectasis may occur when large pieces of solid food or foreign objects (teeth, dental appliances, pieces of resuscitation equipment) are aspirated.

Pneumonia

Although the CXR is never diagnostic, it may give a clue to the organism producing bacterial pneumonia. Common bacterial pathogens typically produce patchy segmental or lobar involvement. Bulging fissures, although uncommon, suggest *Klebsiella*. A diffuse, patchy, "ground glass" appearance suggests *Legionella*, *Mycoplasma*, or *Pneumocystis*. Small, diffusely scattered nodular densities suggest *Mycobacterium tuberculosis* as the etiological organism. Larger nodular densities are associated with *Cryptococcus*, *Actinomycosis*, or *Nocardia*. *Aspergillus* often gives rise to peripheral wedge-shaped infiltrates caused by vascular invasion and secondary infarction or cavitary formation. Cavitation suggests neoplasm, tuberculosis, fungal infection (e.g., histoplasmosis, cryptococcosis, coccidiomycosis), lung abscess, or septic PE. Pneumonitis that develops in preexisting areas of bullous emphysema often produces air–fluid levels that can be confused with lung abscess or empyema. The thinner contour of the cavity wall, the more rapid pace of development and resolution, and premorbid CXRs demonstrating bullae help to identify this problem.

Nosocomial or ventilator associated pneumonia affects up to 30% of patients with ARDS but is difficult to detect with certainty because focal parenchymal densities may represent edema, atelectasis, and infarction, as well as infection. Hence, radiographic abnormalities must be interpreted in light of the clinical situation. A new unilateral infiltrate in a patient with a previously stable CXR is the best radiographic indicator of a superimposed infection; however, fever, increased sputum production, and progressive hypoxemia are better indicators than the CXR. A focal wedge-shaped infiltrate (especially occurring distal to a PAC tip or in a patient with hemoptysis) is likely to represent pulmonary infarction.

Intra-Abdominal Conditions

The upright CXR can also help diagnose acute intra-abdominal problems. Midline or paraesophageal hiatal hernias usually pose little diagnostic problem. Diaphragmatic disruption may allow abdominal contents to herniate into the chest following abdominal trauma, often displacing a gas-containing viscus into the left chest. Oral contrast aids in the diagnosis, as does CT scan, or injection of a sterile contrast agent into the pleural space. Short of a trip to the CT scanner, the upright CXR also provides the most sensitive method of detecting free air within the abdominal cavity. (A cross-table film of the abdomen taken at least 5 min after decubitus positioning serves a similar purpose.) Intubated patients frequently swallow air, producing gastric dilation. In the appropriate setting, massive gastric dilation can suggest the possibility of esophageal intubation or a tracheoesophageal fistula.

CT and MRI of the Chest

CT scanning and MRI have significant limitations in the critically ill population. Appropriately, concern has been voiced over the risks of moving patients out of the ICU for imaging studies; however, carefully arranged transport can be performed reasonably safely. The range of physiologic changes observed in patients transported to radiology suite is comparable to that of patients who remain in the ICU for a similar time. The most important feature of safe transport is to ensure adequate equipment, and personnel are immediately available to cope with a catastrophic event (accidental extubation or extraction of venous or arterial catheters or chest tubes; or interruption of critical infusions). Patients with bronchopleural fistula and those requiring vasopressors or high inspired oxygen concentrations or PEEP are at particular risk. Although rarely used in practice, interruption of inhaled nitric oxide or nebulized prostacyclin infusions during transport often produces calamitous physiological deterioration. Metallic appliances create artifact on CT scans and may preclude use of MRI because of the powerful magnetic fields involved. Furthermore, both CT and MRI studies are time consuming, and the inability of critically ill patients to remain immobile produces motion artifact on both studies.

CT scanning often requires use of nephrotoxic contrast material. (Enteral contrast used for abdominal scanning does not carry this risk.) Prophylaxis of the patient with marginal renal function is highly variable but should include at least adequate hydration; probably sodium bicarbonate and possibly acetylcysteine. For sometime, MRI was used in place of CT for patients with marginal renal function in an attempt to avoid contrast nephrotoxicity. Unfortunately, the use of some gadolinium-based MRI contrast media may be even more dangerous. Gadolinium has been associated with a progressive often devastating scleroderma-like syndrome known as progressive nephrogenic sclerosis. Many features of this syndrome remain uncertain, therefore, until this condition is better understood it is probably prudent to use gadolinium contrast sparingly, and attempt to avoid it in patients with renal insufficiency.

The financial aspects of imaging should not be overlooked. A chest CT scan typically costs three to four times as much as a portable CXR in addition to the costs of transport which can be substantial. Because patients are placed at higher risk during travel and there are significant financial and manpower costs involved, it is logical to plan ahead bundling studies together when feasible. For example, if an elective head CT is planned tomorrow but an urgent chest CT must be done today, it may make sense to perform both studies today, avoiding the second trip. As a corollary, if an imaging study is likely to yield results that will prompt a radiology-based intervention (e.g., needle or catheter aspiration), it is common sense to confer with the radiologist in advance, to arrange rapid interpretation of the diagnostic study and the intervention in a single trip. Simple preplanning can also avoid wasteful redundant studies. For example, if a chest CT is to be performed today there is little reason to do a "routine" morning CXR.

Despite limitations, the chest CT often provides information not otherwise available. It frequently reveals a small or loculated pneumothorax in patients when previous CXRs are unrevealing. **4** Chest CT also aids discovery of lung abscess or empyema and usually can differentiate between the two conditions. In patients with empyema and persistent, unexplained fever or with a persistent pneumothorax, the chest CT is invaluable to evaluate the location and effectiveness of thoracic drainage tubes. CT scanning has also added greatly to our understanding of the distribution of lung injury in ARDS. The homogeneous-appearing density of the CXR is actually comprised of patchy, dependent consolidation when viewed by CT. The CT has shown that within minutes of repositioning a patient, previously normal-appearing lung regions can become infiltrated. This finding correlates nicely with the clinical observation that positional changes quickly alter oxygenation. CT scanning also demonstrates the severity and distribution of regional barotrauma offering insight into the potential deleterious effects of excessive airway pressure. Normal-appearing lung is seen immediately juxtaposed with densely infiltrated lung. These normal appearing and presumably normally compliant lung units are likely to be overdistended by positive pressure, whereas densely infiltrated lung is likely to remain atelectatic. The physiologic result is shunting of blood past atelectatic alveoli and overdistention of other alveoli, predisposing them to rupture.

In summary, the chest CT represents one of the most useful diagnostics tests available. A short list of indications for chest CT scanning include (i) evaluation of thoracic trauma, (ii) searching for occult or persistent sources of fever (empyema, lung, or mediastinal abscess), (iii) guiding placement of drainage tubes for loculated or persistent pneumothorax or pleural effusions, (iv) detecting mediastinal pathology (especially in the presence of parenchymal infiltrate), and (v) searching for pulmonary emboli.

■ ABDOMINAL RADIOGRAPHY

Screening Film

The plain abdominal X-ray has largely been replaced by the abdominal CT scan. The use of abdominal US **5** and CT scanning is discussed in detail, as it relates to specific disease entities in Chapter 36. Nevertheless, the standard examination of the abdomen consisting of supine kidney–ureter–bladder (KUB) or "flat plate" and upright views can still be useful and does not require a trip outside the ICU. If an upright film cannot be taken, a lateral decubitus view may be substituted. (Cross-table supine radiographs are of little value except to demonstrate calcification in aortic aneurysms.) Systematic review of the KUB may furnish important information, especially after trauma. Fractures of the lower ribs on the left suggest the possibility of a ruptured spleen or lacerated kidney as does medial displacement of the gastric bubble. Breaks in lower ribs on the right suggest the possibility of renal or hepatic damage. Fractures of the lumbar spine, pelvis, and hips may be seen as "incidental" findings on plain abdominal radiographs in trauma patients. A ground glass appearance, displacement of the retroperitoneal fat stripe, or centralization of gas shadows suggests ascites or hemoperitoneum. Free air usually indicates a ruptured viscus, gas-producing infection, barotrauma-induced pneumoperitoneum, or postoperative change. Free air is much more commonly seen as the result of upper GI (stomach or duodenum) perforation rather than from colonic perforation (diverticulitis, appendicitis, colon cancer).

The KUB view is a poor indicator of liver size and should not supplant careful physical examination. The gallbladder is inadequately defined on the KUB view unless it is very distended or calcified. Less than 15% of gallbladder calculi are visible. Gas appearing in the biliary ducts is highly suggestive of infectious cholangitis but can occur following endoscopic retrograde cholangiopancreatography. The ingestion of massive amounts of carbonated beverages, or intake of compounds that can generate gas when mixed with gastric acid (e.g., hydrogen peroxide, sodium bicarbonate), can also cause bile duct gas. Hepatic calcifications, although rare, may be because of healed infection, hemangioma, or metastatic carcinoma. Films taken in different positions may help sort out the location of right upper quadrant calcifications. Calcifications within the kidney or liver maintain a relatively fixed position, whereas stones within the gallbladder are usually mobile. Use of the KUB view in the diagnosis of the "acute abdomen" is discussed in Chapter 36.

Findings Relevant to Specific Organs

Kidneys and Ureters

The visibility of the kidney on the KUB view depends on the amount of perinephric fat and overlying bowel gas. The combination of kidney enlargement and calcification suggests urinary tract obstruction or polycystic kidney disease. If nephrolithiasis is suspected, the renal outlines and course of both ureters should be carefully inspected for calculi (visible in up to 85% of cases). Identifying gas in the renal pelvis is uncommon but is indicative of emphysematous pyelonephritis seen most often in poorly controlled diabetics. Gas-producing infections of the bladder are also seen occasionally.

Pancreas and Retroperitoneum

Asymmetric obliteration of the psoas shadows or retroperitoneal fat lines suggests a retroperitoneal process (most commonly pancreatitis or hemorrhage from a leaking aorta). Similar changes can be seen with spontaneous hemorrhage or traumatic disruption. Although the pancreas is not normally seen on the plain radiograph, calcifications may occur in chronic alcoholic pancreatitis. Localized areas of ileus over the pancreas, such as the "colon cut-off sign" and the "sentinel loop," may also help in the diagnosis of pancreatic inflammation.

Stomach and Bowel

The stomach normally contains some fluid and air, but massive gastric dilation suggests gastric outlet obstruction, gastroparesis, or esophageal intubation. By contrast, the small bowel normally contains little air; gaseous distention indicates ileus or small bowel obstruction. Air–fluid levels of different heights within the same loop of small bowel on an upright film usually indicate mechanical small bowel obstruction and imply residual peristaltic activity. Fluid levels at the same height in a loop of bowel do not necessarily indicate mechanical obstruction. Absence of colonic or rectal gas in patients with small bowel air–fluid levels strongly suggests complete obstruction of the small bowel with distal clearing of gas. Conversely, the presence of gas in the colon (except for small amounts of rectal gas) all but excludes the diagnosis of complete small bowel obstruction. (Incomplete obstruction may be present, however.)

Colonic obstruction due to a sigmoid volvulus may be diagnosed via a KUB view that shows massive sigmoid dilation; the sigmoid forms an inverted "U" whose limbs rise out of the pelvis. Apposition of the medial walls of these bowel segments produces a midline soft tissue density whose inferior extent approximates the site of torsion.

Peritoneal Cavity

On the supine abdominal radiograph, ascites is demonstrated by diffuse haze, indistinctness of the iliopsoas stripes, centralization of small bowel segments, and abnormal separation of bowel loops. Increased pelvic density characterizes ascites on the upright film.

Abnormal gas collections are recognized by their nonanatomic location. Therefore, all gas densities on supine and erect films require explanation. Each must be assigned to an anatomic segment of bowel. Gas may collect under the diaphragm or overlie the liver on erect or lateral decubitus films, respectively. Free air also allows visualization of both sides of the walls of gas-filled bowel. "Bubbly," curvilinear, or triangular gas collections between segments of bowel suggest abdominal abscess. Bowel ischemia may produce a characteristic pattern known as pneumatosis cystoides that represents gas within the bowel wall. Rarely, pneumatosis may rupture to produce free intraperitoneal air, simulating a perforated viscus.

■ SUGGESTED READINGS

Hendriske KA, Gratama WC, ten Hove W, et al. Low value of routine chest-radiographs in a mixed medical-surgical ICU. *Chest.* 2007; 132:823–828.

Krivopal M, Shlobin OA, Schwartzstyein RM. Utility of daily routine portable chest radiographs in mechanically ventilated patients in the medical ICU. *Chest.* 2003;123:1607–1614.

Tagliabue M, Casella TC, Zincone GE, et al. CT and chest radiography in the evaluation of adult respiratory distress syndrome. *Acta Radiol.* 1994;35(3):230–234.

Trotman-Dickenson B. Radiology in the intensive care unit (Part I). *J Intensive Care Med.* 2003;18(4):198–210.

Trotman-Dickenson B. Radiology in the intensive care unit (Part II). *J Intensive Care Med.* 2003;18(5):239–252.

Walser E, Savage C, Zwischenberger JB. Thoracic imaging in the ICU. Interventional radiology. *Chest Surg Clin N Am.* 2002;12(2):209–226.

Acid–Base Disorders

KEY POINTS

1 Viewed in isolation, most ABGs defy unique interpretation for cause or mandate immediate action; each blood gas must be evaluated in light of clinical information and electrolyte status. The technique for obtaining blood gases is critically important for accurate diagnosis.

2 During health, acid–base balance is finely tuned within a narrow range, using complex buffering systems and compensatory responses. Usually, the respiratory system responds quickly to metabolic derangements but ultimately achieves less complete compensation. By contrast, the kidney slowly compensates for respiratory abnormalities but eventually achieves and sustains a near-complete compensatory response.

3 The Stewart and Henderson–Hasselbach approaches to acid–base evaluation use different systems to reach the same point (diagnosis). Using the adjusted anion gap (considering albumin concentration) improves the classic approach to detect hidden acid–base disorders in hospitalized patients. These approaches are of equal validity, differing only in how they approach the understanding of the underlying mechanism.

4 The rules of compensation for primary acid–base disorders in Table 12-1 are important for the accurate evaluation of acid–base disorders. They should be memorized or kept closely at hand.

5 The anion gap provides a valuable tool to determine whether a metabolic acidosis is the result of loss of bicarbonate or the result of titration of bicarbonate with excess hydrogen ion equivalents. It makes good sense to calculate the anion gap whenever evaluating electrolytes and ABGs. The anion gap provides a useful framework for the differential diagnosis of metabolic acidosis. A short list of common conditions usually is

responsible for elevating the anion gap (Table 12-3).

6 Hypoalbuminemia can mask an increased concentration of gap anions by lowering the value of the anion gap.

7 Non–anion gap acidosis often results from administration of large volumes of chloride containing fluids. This occurs frequently in patients with GI loses of bicarbonate.

8 Dilutional acidosis is observed when the patient is infused with high volumes of base-free solutions (e.g., sodium chloride), but the physiological consequences of this type of acidosis are rarely significant at the intracellular level.

9 The management of acid–base disorders requires comprehensive knowledge of the clinical setting. Bicarbonate correction of acidosis is appropriate in extreme cases where acidosis compromises hemodynamic status or when a depleted bicarbonate buffer base must be replenished. THAM, another buffer, has not been associated with the increase of intracellular acidosis and occasionally can be a useful alternative to bicarbonate.

The earliest contemporary definitions of acid and base can be attributed to Arrhenius, who in 1887 defined acid as a hydrogen-ion donor and base as a hydroxyl-ion donor. In 1948, Singer and Hastings proposed the concept of whole blood buffer base (BB) as a quantitative index of the surplus amount of fixed acid or base in the blood. In 1960, Astrup proposed the concept that standard bicarbonate or base excess should be used as an index of the nonrespiratory acid–base status of the blood. Standard bicarbonate is defined as the concentration of bicarbonate in plasma after fully oxygenated whole blood equilibrates with carbon dioxide at PCO_2 of 40 torr. The carbonic acid/bicarbonate system was introduced by Henderson–Hasselbach, whose equation considers the pH to depend on the interactions of these variables. In

1983, the concept of BB was reintroduced by Stewart under the name "strong ion difference" (SID), based on the principles of electroneutrality and mass conservation. Therefore, three related but different methods to analyze acid–base status are currently used: the Henderson–Hasselbach relationship, the base excess, and the SID. To establish an accurate physiologic diagnosis and manage the different disturbances of acid–base balance requires integration of blood gas data with the electrolyte profile and clinical findings.

■ ARTERIAL BLOOD GASES
Obtaining Arterial Blood Gases

Arterial blood gases (ABGs) are valuable only if obtained properly and measured carefully. Patients should have a stable FiO_2 for at least 15 min before sampling to allow the PaO_2 and $PaCO_2$ to equili-

1 brate. Patient position should be noted because PaO_2 may change significantly with varying body position (saturation usually is worse in the supine position). Ventilatory pattern (breath-holding or hyperventilation) also should be noted. Changes in breathing rate or depth may significantly alter the $PaCO_2$ and PaO_2 from the prior condition. Prolonged attempts to obtain an ABG often result in mild hyperventilation as pain and/or anxiety build in the patient.

The patient's body temperature should be recorded. For any given O_2 content, the measured PaO_2 increases as blood is warmed. An increased PaO_2 occurs because of rightward shifts in the oxyhemoglobin dissociation curve and because the solubility of gases decreases in warmer fluids increasing their measurable tensions. Hypothermia shifts the oxyhemoglobin dissociation curve leftward; therefore, as cold blood is warmed to the standard analysis temperature (37°C), O_2 solubility decreases (resulting in a higher measured PaO_2 than exists in vivo). The $PaCO_2$ also will rise as blood is warmed, producing modest declines in the pH.

When sampling or cannulating the radial artery, it is advisable to assess collateral blood flow to the hand, as trauma to that vessel may later result in clotting and/or compromise its patency. The patency of the alternate blood supply, the ulnar artery, is confirmed by the Allen test, first described in 1929. It is performed by elevating the hand, occluding both ulnar and radial arteries, and releasing compression of the ulnar artery. If adequate collateral circulation is present, the hand should flush

pink within 5 to 7 s. It is important to remember that the Allen test has high variability among observers, and its ability to detect inadequate collateral circulation is not high in the hypotensive ICU population. Its performance must be considered, however, prior to placing a radial arterial line. For arterial puncture, the wrist is positioned in mild extension and the skin is cleaned—first with an iodophor or chlorhexidine solution and then wiped with alcohol. Lidocaine (approx. 0.5 mL of 1% solution) may be used to prevent pain in the alert subject. Excessive anesthetic volume may obliterate normal landmarks and arterial pulsations. Commercially prepared ABG syringes are usually used; however, in their absence, a heparin-coated 3-mL syringe tipped with a 21-gauge needle will suffice. The artery is approached from a 45 degree angle, and immediately on vessel entry, pulsatile blood will fill the syringe (aspiration is not necessary in most cases). Blood flow will cease if the needle penetrates the posterior arterial wall, but flow often may be reestablished merely by retracting the needle. After sampling is complete, the needle should be removed and firm pressure should be applied to the puncture site for 5 min (or longer if coagulation disorders exist). The blood and heparin should be mixed by a rolling motion. Prompt analysis is required to obtain accurate results, and icing is needed unless the sample is analyzed immediately.

Pitfalls in Collection, Analysis, and Interpretation
Timing of Analysis

Accuracy depends on prompt analysis. Under most circumstances, the $PaCO_2$ rises approximately 3 to 10 mm Hg/h in uniced specimens, causing a modest fall in pH. The PaO_2 usually remains stable in an iced sample for 1 to 2 h. Samples of body fluids that do not contain sufficient hemoglobin or other protein buffers (e.g., pleural or joint fluid) undergo more rapid pH changes when analysis is delayed.

Pseudohypoxemia

The PaO_2 may dramatically decrease if significant O_2 is consumed in vitro after the blood is sampled—a problem that is most common with marked leukocytosis or thrombocytosis. Leukocyte counts higher than $10^5/mm^3$ or platelet counts higher than $10^6/mm^3$ usually are required to produce significant changes. Addition of cyanide or immediate icing of the blood sample decreases the likelihood of this "pseudohypoxemia." Diffusion of O_2 through the wall of plastic syringes may lead to false reductions in measured PaO_2 (particularly in samples with high O_2 tensions) because plastic syringes are much more permeable than glass to oxygen.

Pseudoacidosis

"Pseudoacidosis" may occur when metabolically active leukocytes generate large quantities of CO_2, causing acidosis to develop in vitro. At room temperature, continued anaerobic glycolysis by red cells and white cells produces organic acids that can induce small reductions in pH and HCO_3^- concentrations.

Air Bubbles

The PO_2 of room air is approximately 150 mm Hg, and the PCO_2 is near 0 mm Hg. Therefore, when large air bubbles are mixed with arterial blood, usually the PaO_2 rises and the $PaCO_2$ falls (if the PaO_2 in the blood exceeds that in the bubble; however, the measured PaO_2 could decline). A small air bubble in a relatively large sample usually has little effect, but when the ratio of bubble to blood volume is large, increases in PaO_2 of up to 30 mm Hg may occur. It is uncommon for bubbles to significantly reduce the $PaCO_2$ unless the baseline CO_2 tension is very high.

Contamination of Arterial Samples with Venous Blood

Normally, the $PaCO_2$ is higher and PaO_2 is lower in venous blood than in arterial blood, as oxygen is extracted and carbon dioxide is added by metabolically active tissues. The degree of oxygen extraction varies greatly among organ systems. The heart is a near complete extractor of oxygen, whereas venous blood from the kidney contains large amounts of venous oxygen and less added CO_2. Furthermore, the degree of O_2 extraction can vary substantially over time for any specific organ. This heterogeneity of venous gas tensions explains why a peripheral venous sample, predominately reflecting skin and muscle oxygen extraction, cannot serve as an accurate indicator of total body oxygen extraction or consumption.

Arterial pH–Tissue pH

It is not always correct to assume that arterial pH reflects the pH at the tissue level. Discordance is a particular problem in patients with severe circulatory failure, in whom pulmonary blood flow is often substantially reduced. In this setting, blood that is delivered to the lungs may be adequately cleared of CO_2, resulting in a relatively normal or even diminished arterial PCO_2. However, the low cardiac output slows the return of CO_2-containing blood from the periphery. As a result, the mixed venous PCO_2, which represents blood that has not yet entered the pulmonary circulation, may be markedly higher than the PCO_2 in arterial blood.

Risks

Risks of arterial puncture are very low for single sticks but increase with frequency of access and when persistent cannulation is used (see Chapter 2). Infection is very rare unless infected tissue is traversed en route to the artery. Arterial thrombosis can usually be avoided by varying sampling sites, using the smallest needle that produces good blood flow and confirming collateral flow before puncture (approx. 3% of hospitalized patients have inadequate collateral circulation). Even when all appropriate precautions are taken, ischemic complications can occur as a result of thrombosis, systemic hypotension, vasopressor use, or an underlying vascular disorder (e.g., Raynaud disease). Nerve trauma usually is because of direct nerve puncture by an inexperienced phlebotomist but also may result from a compressive hematoma if coagulopathy is present or if inadequate pressure is held at the puncture site.

■ BASIC ABG CONCEPTS

Normally, arterial pH, the negative common logarithm of the hydrogen ion (H^+) concentration, varies between 7.35 and 7.45. When breathing room air, normal $PaCO_2$ varies between 35 and 45 mm Hg, and PaO_2 values greater than 80 to 90 mm Hg are considered normal, depending on age. Mixed venous blood gases have a lower pH than arterial gases (normal, approx. 7.30 to 7.35), a lower PaO_2 (normal, approx. 40 to 44 mm Hg), and a slightly increased $PaCO_2$ (normal, approx. 45 mm Hg). Values for $PaCO_2$, PaO_2, and pH are measured directly. By contrast, the reported HCO_3^- concentration usually is not measured but rather is calculated from pH and $PaCO_2$ using a nomogram derived from the Henderson–Hasselbalch equation. In similar fashion, the reported arterial oxygen saturation

(SaO_2) usually is not measured but is calculated from the PaO_2.

Alterations in Oxygenation

Oxygen Tension Versus Saturation

At ambient pressure, oxygen content of blood is determined predominantly by the quantity of O_2 bound to hemoglobin (Hgb), with only a minor contribution from dissolved O_2. The O_2 carried in a volume of blood (mL/dL) is influenced by PaO_2 (mm Hg), Hgb concentration (gm/dL), pH, and the characteristics of the Hgb itself: O_2 content = 1.34 (Hgb)(%Sat) + (0.003)(PaO_2). Normally, the quantity of dissolved oxygen is negligible, but it becomes significant when pure oxygen is administered under hyperbaric conditions. In such circumstances, PaO_2 can exceed 2,000 mm Hg. ABG analysis determines the partial pressure of dissolved O_2 directly but provides only an indirect (and often inaccurate) indicator of O_2 content.

Hypoxemia

Tolerance for hypoxemia depends not only on the extent of desaturation but also on the compensatory mechanisms available and the sensitivity of the patient to hypoxia. If an individual without cardiac limitation or anemia is made hypoxic over a short period of time, no important effect will be noted until PaO_2 falls below 50 to 60 mm Hg. At that level, malaise, light-headedness, mild nausea, vertigo, impaired judgment, and incoordination generally are the first symptoms noted, reflecting the high sensitivity of cerebral tissue to hypoxia. Although minute ventilation increases, little dyspnea usually develops unless the resulting hyperpnea uncovers underlying mechanical lung problems, as in chronic obstructive pulmonary disease (COPD). Confusion resembling alcohol intoxication appears as PaO_2 falls into the range of 35 to 50 mm Hg, especially in older individuals with ischemic cerebrovascular disease (such patients also are prone to heart rhythm disturbances). As PaO_2 falls below 35 mm Hg, renal blood flow decreases, urine output slows, and atropine-refractory bradycardia and conduction system blockade develop. Lactic acidosis also appears at this level, even with normal cardiac function. The patient becomes lethargic or obtunded, and hypoxic drive to breathe is maximal. At a PaO_2 of approximately 25 mm Hg, the normal unadapted individual loses consciousness and minute ventilation begins to fall because of respiratory center depression. This sequence of events occurs at higher O_2 tensions if any of the major compensatory mechanisms for hypoxemia are defective. Even mild decreases in O_2 tension are tolerated poorly by anemic patients with impaired cardiac output or coronary insufficiency. Because the pulmonary vasculature constricts when alveolar O_2 tension falls, hypoxemia may provoke decompensation of the right ventricle in patients with preexisting pulmonary hypertension or cor pulmonale.

Hyperoxia

At normal barometric pressures, venous and tissue O_2 tensions rise very little when pure O_2 is administered to healthy subjects. Hence, nonpulmonary tissues are little affected. However, high concentrations of O_2 eventually replace nitrogen in the lung, even in poorly ventilated regions. Oxygen replacement of nitrogen eventually causes collapse of poorly ventilated units as O_2 is absorbed by venous blood faster than it is replenished. Atelectasis and diminished lung compliance result. More importantly, high O_2 tensions may accelerate the generation of reactive oxygen species and other noxious oxidants, injuring bronchial and parenchymal tissue. Although O_2-induced lung injury certainly occurs in experimental models using healthy animals, the susceptibility of injured lungs to oxygen toxicity is much less certain.

Alterations in Ventilation

Hypercapnia

In addition to its key role in regulation of ventilation, the clinically important effects of CO_2 relate to changes in cerebral blood flow, pH, and adrenergic tone. Hypercapnia dilates cerebral vessels and hypocapnia constricts them—a point of particular importance for patients with raised intracranial pressure. Acute increases in CO_2 depress consciousness, probably a combined result of intraneuronal acidosis, excessive cerebral blood flow, and rising intracranial pressure. Slowly developing hypercapnia is better tolerated, presumably because buffering has time to occur. The adrenergic stimulation that accompanies acute hypercapnia causes cardiac output to rise and helps maintain peripheral vascular resistance. Muscular twitching, asterixis, and seizures can be observed at extreme levels of hypercapnia in patients made susceptible by electrolyte or neural disorders.

As a practical matter, for mechanically ventilated patients, many practitioners permit a modest respiratory acidosis (pH of 7.10 to 7.20) resulting from gradual increases in $PaCO_2$ (<10 mm Hg/h) if the alternative is to markedly elevate airway pressures to achieve normocapnia. The practice of "permissive hypercapnia," a consequence of using lower ventilating pressures and tidal volumes, has become widely accepted. Hypercapnia reduces tissue metabolism, improves surfactant function, and prevents nitration of proteins. Acidosis also decreases sarcoplasmic calcium release, dampens mitochondrial respiration, and reduces the activity of enzymes that produce inflammatory metabolic intermediates. These changes favor adequate cellular functioning, control of inflammatory response, improved cardiac function, and maintenance or reactivation of hypoxic pulmonary vasoconstriction, with resultant improvement ventilation/perfusion matching.

Hypocapnia

The major effects of acute hypocapnia relate to alkalosis and diminished cerebral perfusion. Abrupt lowering of $PaCO_2$ reduces total cerebral blood flow, raises neuronal pH, and reduces available ionized calcium, causing disturbances in cortical and peripheral nerve function. Light-headedness, circumoral and fingertip paresthesias, and muscular tetany can result. Alkalosis caused by sudden reduction of $PaCO_2$ (e.g., shortly after initiating mechanical ventilation) can produce life-threatening seizures or arrhythmias.

Evaluating Hydrogen Ion Concentration

Generation and Excretion of H^+ Ion

Free H^+ ions are present in the body fluids in extremely low concentrations. However, H^+ ions are small and highly reactive, allowing them to bind more strongly than Na^+ or K^+ to negatively charged molecules. As a result, H^+ concentration is critical to the activity of cellular enzymes. Under normal conditions, the H^+ concentration varies little from the normal value of 40 nanoEq/L. The body buffers play an important role in this regulatory process, as they are able to take up or release H^+ ions to prevent large changes in the H^+ concentration. To keep H^+ within physiologic limits, generation and elimination rates must be equal. H^+ ion is generated in two ways:

1. By hydration of CO_2 to form "volatile" acid according to the reaction:

$$CO_2 + H_2O \Rightarrow H_2CO_3 \Rightarrow H^+ + HCO_3^-$$

2. By production of "fixed" acids (primarily sulfates and phosphates) as chemical by-products of metabolism.

The kidneys and lungs play important roles in the maintenance of acid–base balance because they normally adjust the rate of acid excretion to meet homeostatic needs. Each day, approximately 15,000 mmol of CO_2 produced by endogenous metabolism is excreted by the lungs. Similarly, a normal diet generates 50 to 100 mEq of H^+ per day, derived mostly from the metabolism of sulfur-containing amino acids and the subsequent generation of H_2SO_4. These H^+ ions are initially buffered by HCO_3^- and by the cellular and bone buffers to minimize the fall in extracellular pH. Acid–base balance is then restored by urinary H^+ excretion, which regenerates the HCO_3^- lost in the original buffering reaction. If the H^+ concentration is increased, regardless of cause, it can be reduced toward normal by a decrease in the PCO_2 and/or an elevation in the plasma HCO_3^- concentration. Both of these changes occur as alveolar ventilation and urinary excretion of H^+ are enhanced in this setting. Conversely, alveolar ventilation and H^+ secretion diminish when the concentration is reduced. The resultant increase in the PCO_2 and decline in the plasma HCO_3^- concentration raise the H^+ concentration toward normal. If the excretion rate of fixed acid speeds or slows disproportionately in relation to its production rate, or if abnormal metabolic loads of acid or alkali develop, metabolic acidosis or alkalosis occurs. In clinical practice, the concentration of free H^+ ion is tracked by pH = –log [H^+].

Base Excess

The "base excess" is a calculated number that quantitates metabolic abnormality. It hypothetically "corrects" pH to 7.40 by first "adjusting" measured $PaCO_2$ to 40 mm Hg, thus allowing a comparison of the "corrected" HCO_3^- with the known normal value at that pH (24 mEq/L). As a quick rule of thumb, base excess (mEq/L) can be calculated from the observed values for HCO_3^- and pH:

Base excess = HCO_3^- + 10 (pH – 7.40) – 24.

A "negative" base excess means that HCO_3^- stores are depleted. However, the base excess does not indicate whether retention or depletion of HCO_3^- is pathologic or compensatory for long-standing respiratory derangements; that judgment must be made by an analysis of the clinical setting. Likewise, it does not dictate the need for bicarbonate administration. Calculation of base excess is especially helpful when the observed HCO_3^- is nearly normal (24 ± 3 mEq/L). The base excess calculation is unlikely to provide new insights at more extreme HCO_3^- deviations.

Buffer Systems

Carbonic Acid

Chemical and protein buffer systems oppose changes in free H^+. The CO_2/HCO_3^- (carbonic acid) and hemoglobin systems are quantitatively the most important. Clinical attention usually is focused on the carbonic acid system because each of its components is measured readily and because CO_2 and HCO_3^- determinations allow clinical judgments to be made concerning the respiratory or metabolic origin of the problem at hand. To maintain pH at 7.40, the ratio of HCO_3^- to (0.03 × $PaCO_2$) must remain in the 20:1 proportions dictated by the Henderson–Hasselbach equation:

$$pH = 6.1 + \log [HCO_3^-/(0.03 \times PaCO_2)].$$

Noncarbonic (Protein) Buffers

Noncarbonic buffers may be intracellular or extracellular including proteins (albumin, hemoglobin), phosphates, and bone carbonates. On the average, 55% to 60% of an acid load will eventually be buffered by the cells and bone, although higher percentages may occur with severe acidemia when extracellular HCO_3^- stores are markedly reduced. Noncarbonic buffers bind or release H^+ ions, minimizing pH changes while allowing the hydration reaction for CO_2 to continue to run in either direction.

$$CO_2 + H_2O \leftrightarrow [H^+] + HCO_3^-$$
$$\downarrow$$
$$[H^+] + Hgb \leftrightarrow H^+ Hgb$$

For this reason, if $PaCO_2$ changes acutely, there will be a small associated change in HCO_3^- in the same direction (approx. 1 mEq/L per 0.1 pH unit). Such automatic changes in HCO_3^- do not imply a metabolic disturbance, and the "base excess" attributable to this mechanism is zero. Anemic blood fails to buffer fluctuations in H^+ concentration with normal efficiency.

Compensatory Mechanisms

As physiologic stresses on pH balance persist, adjustments in the excretion rate of CO_2 and H^+ counterbalance the effect of these disturbances on pH. In general, renal compensation for a respiratory disturbance is slower (but ultimately more successful) than respiratory compensation for a metabolic disturbance. Thus, although quick to respond initially, the respiratory system will not eliminate sufficient CO_2 to completely offset any but the mildest metabolic acidosis. Furthermore, the respiratory compensatory response is not developed fully until 24 to 48 h after initial activation. The lower limit of sustained compensatory hypocapnia in a healthy adult is approximately 10 to 15 mm Hg. Once that limit is reached, even small additional increments in H^+ ion have exaggerated effects on pH.

Patients with disordered lung mechanics, such as those with COPD or neuromuscular weakness, are highly vulnerable to metabolic acid loads because they lack the normal ability to compensate by hyperventilation. CO_2 retention in response to alkalosis is very limited—only rarely exceeding 60 mm Hg. Moreover, the hypoxemia resulting from hypoventilation helps limit the rise in CO_2 by eventually triggering increased ventilatory effort. Although the kidney cannot respond effectively to abrupt respiratory acidosis or alkalosis, renal compensation may eventually (3 to 7 days) totally counterbalance a respiratory alkalosis of even moderate severity. The kidney also compensates well for chronic respiratory acidosis but cannot compensate completely for a $PaCO_2$ above 65 mm Hg unless another stimulus for HCO_3^- retention (e.g., volume depletion) is present.

Role of Electrolytes in Acid–Base Balance

According to the principle of maintained electroneutrality, the number of positive and negative charges in body fluids must be equal. Accordingly, serum cations (sodium + potassium + calcium + magnesium) must equal anions (chloride + bicarbonate + proteins + sulfate + phosphate + organic acid anions). The main cations are Na^+, K^+, Ca^{2+}, and Mg^{2+}, and the main anions are HCO_3^-, Cl^-, proteins (albumin), and phosphates. The balance among these electrolytes influences acid–base status (see anion gap and Stewart Approach). In fact, evaluation of acid–base status is incomplete without consideration of the clinical setting and the electrolyte profile.

■ ACID–BASE DERANGEMENTS

Terminology of Acid–Base Disorders

The terms *acidemia* and *alkalemia* refer to blood pH. Systemic pH lower than 7.35 defines acidemia. A pH higher than 7.45 defines alkalemia. By contrast, acidosis and alkalosis do not refer to pH but rather to basic pathophysiologic processes or tendencies favoring the development of acidemia or alkalemia. For example, a patient with diabetic ketoacidosis (DKA) (a primary metabolic acidosis) and hypocapnia stimulated by pneumonia (a primary respiratory alkalosis) may exhibit acidemia, alkalemia, or a normal pH depending on the relative changes in $PaCO_2$ and HCO_3^-. Uncomplicated metabolic acidosis is characterized by a decline in HCO_3^-, whereas a primary increase in HCO_3^- denotes metabolic alkalosis. Conversely, respiratory acidosis is defined as a primary increase in $PaCO_2$, whereas respiratory alkalosis occurs when the central feature is a decrease in $PaCO_2$.

Stepwise ABG Analysis

We can use one or both of the following approaches to characterize the acid–base status.

Henderson–Hasselbach Approach

3 Because no set of ABG values has a unique interpretation, concomitant analysis of serum electrolytes and the review of the clinical situation are essential to reach the correct diagnosis in an acid–base disorder. Three specific factors (pH, $PaCO_2$, and the ratio of $PaCO_2$ to HCO_3^-) must be evaluated in a logical stepwise fashion. Interpretation of the pH and $PaCO_2$ rapidly provides a definitive diagnosis in most cases. The remaining disorders can be classified by examining the relationship of the measured $PaCO_2$ to the $PaCO_2$ expected, based on the measured bicarbonate level. Consideration of the anion gap often lends supportive information.

The pH is analyzed first. Values below the normal range indicate acidemia (elevated H^+). A pH value above the normal range (reduced H^+) defines alkalemia. A pH within the normal range has three possible interpretations: (i) no acid–base disorder exists; (ii) two or more acid–base disorders with perfectly offsetting pH effects exist (rare); or (iii) near-complete physiologic compensation has occurred for one or more primary disorders. Deviations of pH from normal usually are quickly acted

on by compensatory mechanisms in an attempt to restore the pH to a normal value. When the primary disorder is respiratory, the kidney attempts to compensate. When metabolic consumption or wasting of BB is the primary problem, the lung attempts to return the pH to normal.

In the acidemic patient, an elevated $PaCO_2$ indicates that some component of respiratory acidosis is present. In such patients, the bicarbonate concentration can be used to decide whether appropriate metabolic compensation is occurring or if a concurrent metabolic disorder is present. If the measured HCO_3^- concentration has increased over baseline by 0.10 to 0.35 unit for each 1-mm Hg change in $PaCO_2$, appropriate metabolic compensation for a respiratory acidosis is taking place. Lesser increases in HCO_3^- are indicative of a complicating metabolic acidosis or suggest that insufficient time has elapsed for the kidney to compensate for the rapidly changing $PaCO_2$. Greater rises in HCO_3^- indicate a superimposed metabolic alkalosis.

Conversely, a reduced $PaCO_2$ in an acidemic patient indicates metabolic acidosis. In the case of a metabolic acidosis, the ultimate diagnosis is reached by comparing the observed $PaCO_2$ to that predicted by directly measuring the serum HCO_3^- content. For any given HCO_3^- value, the expected $PaCO_2 = (1.5 \times HCO_3^-) + (8 \pm 2)$. This equates to roughly a 1.0 to 1.3 mm Hg change in $PaCO_2$ for each mEq change in bicarbonate. Typically, respiratory compensation for a metabolic acidosis is more rapid but less complete than the converse. If the observed $PaCO_2$ equals the expected value, a simple metabolic acidosis with appropriate respiratory compensation is present. If the $PaCO_2$ exceeds the expected value, the patient has both a respiratory and metabolic acidosis. When the observed $PaCO_2$ fails to reach the expected level, the patient has both a metabolic acidosis and respiratory alkalosis.

In the alkalemic patient, a low $PaCO_2$ diagnoses respiratory alkalosis. Determination of whether the disorder is simple or mixed results from examining a concurrently measured HCO_3^- concentration. Reductions in HCO_3^- concentration of 0.2 to 0.5 times the change in $PaCO_2$ will occur slowly to provide the compensation necessary. Failure to lower HCO_3^- by at least 0.2 times the change in $PaCO_2$ suggests a superimposed metabolic alkalosis (or insufficient compensatory time), whereas a HCO_3^- that declines by more than 0.5 times the change in $PaCO_2$ suggests a component of metabolic acidosis (Table 12-1).

4

TABLE 12-1 EXPECTED COMPENSATION FOR ACID–BASE DISORDERS

PRIMARY DISORDER	PRIMARY CHANGE	COMPENSATORY CHANGE	EXPECTED COMPENSATION
Metabolic acidosis	↓ HCO_3^-	↓ $PaCO_2$	$\Delta PaCO_2 = 1.2\ \Delta HCO_3^-$
Metabolic alkalosis	↑ HCO_3^-	↑ $PaCO_2$	$\Delta PaCO_2 = 0.9\ \Delta HCO_3^-$
Respiratory acidosis			
Acute	↑ $PaCO_2$	↑ HCO_3^-	$\Delta HCO_3^- = 0.10\ \Delta PaCO_2$
Chronic			$\Delta HCO_3^- = 0.35\ \Delta PaCO_2$
Respiratory alkalosis			
Acute	↓ $PaCO_2$	↓ HCO_3^-	$\Delta HCO_3^- = 0.2\ \Delta PaCO_2$
Chronic			$\Delta HCO_3^- = 0.5\ \Delta PaCO_2$

The ultimate diagnosis of the alkalotic patient with an elevated $PaCO_2$ is made by comparing the measured $PaCO_2$ value with that expected (calculated), based on the measured serum HCO_3^- concentration. In the presence of a simple compensated metabolic alkalosis, the expected $PaCO_2 = (0.7 \times HCO_3^-) + (20 \pm 1.5)$. A higher observed $PaCO_2$ indicates the presence of a simultaneous respiratory acidosis. A $PaCO_2$ value lower than expected indicates a concomitant respiratory alkalosis.

Stewart Approach (Strong Ion Difference)

In 1983, Peter Stewart published his modern quantitative approach to acid–base chemistry. According to his interpretation, the traditional concepts of the mechanisms behind the changes in acid–base balance are questionable. The main physicochemical principles that must be satisfied are the rule of electroneutrality (mentioned previously) and the principle of mass conservation. Three components in biological fluids are subjected to these principles: (i) water, which is only weakly dissociated into H^+ and OH^-; (ii) strong ions, completely dissociated electrolytes such as Na^+, K^+, Cl^-, and certain molecules or compounds, such as lactate. (Strong ions cannot be created or destroyed to satisfy electroneutrality, but H^+ ions can be generated or consumed by changes in water dissociation to establish this required electroneutrality balance); and (iii) weak acids, incompletely dissociated compounds. Stewart strictly distinguished between dependent and independent variables in accord with these principles. The three dependent variables (bicarbonate, pH, and H^+ concentrations) can only change if the three independent variables allow this change.

These three independent variables are: PCO_2, the total amount of all weak acids ($[A^-]$ called A_{TOT}), and the SID.

A_{TOT} can be calculated from the concentration of the albumin (Alb) and the phosphate concentration (Pi):

$$A_{TOT} = [Alb\ (0.123 \times pH - 0.631)] + [Pi\ (0.309 \times pH - 0.469)]$$

An apparent SID can be calculated using measurable ion concentrations:

$$SID_a = (Na + K + Ca + Mg) - (Cl + lactate)$$

But a simpler formula is

$$SID_a = [Na + K] - [Cl]$$

In healthy humans, the normal SID_a is 40 to 42 mEq/L. Regarding metabolic disturbances of acid base chemistry, changes in pH, H^+, and HCO_3^- are only possible if either SID or A_{TOT} $[A^-]$ changes. If, for example, SID decreases (e.g., in case of hyperchloremia), this increase in "independent" negative charges leads to a decrease in "dependent" negative charges (HCO_3^-) resulting in acidosis (and vice versa). In other words, SID less than 40 mEq/L implies metabolic acidosis. According to Stewart, the decrease in SID during hyperchloremic acidosis results from the increase in serum chloride concentration and is the casual mechanism behind this acidosis. As another example, a decrease in "independent" weak acids $[A^-]$ (e.g., during hypoalbuminemia) leads to an increase in "dependent" HCO_3^-, a subsequent *increase* of SID, and alkalosis. An SID greater than 42 mEq/L indicates metabolic alkalosis. By Stewart's approach, new types of acid–base disturbance, such as "hyperchloremic acidosis" or "hypoalbuminemic alkalosis" (which, of course, can also exist in combination), are identified that had gone unrecognized by the classic acid–base analysis. Consequently, Stewart's analysis complements the understanding of the mechanisms behind the changes in acid–base balance.

Both methods, $HCO_3^-/PaCO_2$ and SID, yield virtually identical results when used to quantify the acid–base status of a given blood sample and clinical condition.

■ SIMPLE ACID–BASE DISORDERS

Metabolic Acidosis

Mechanisms

Metabolic acidosis is the consequence of one of four basic mechanisms: bicarbonate consumption from decreased H^+ excretion, bicarbonate consumption from increased H^+ production, bicarbonate loss, and bicarbonate dilution (Table 12-2).

Bicarbonate Consumption

H^+ normally is excreted renally as titratable acid (phosphates and sulfates) and as ammonia compounds. Renal failure, adrenal insufficiency, distal renal tubular acidosis (RTA), and hypoaldoster-

TABLE 12-2 ETIOLOGY OF METABOLIC ACIDOSIS

INABILITY TO SECRETE THE DIETARY ACID LOAD

A. Diminished NH_4^+ production
   Renal failure
   Hypoaldosteronism (type IV renal tubular acidosis)
B. Diminished H^+ secretion
   Type I (distal) renal tubular acidosis

INCREASED H^+ LOAD OR HCO_3^- LOSS

A. Lactic acidosis
B. Ketoacidosis
C. Ingestions
   Salicylates, methanol or formaldehyde, ethylene glycol, paraldehyde, toluene, ammonium chloride, sulfur, and hyperalimentation fluids
D. Massive rhabdomyolysis
E. Gastrointestinal HCO_3^- loss
   Diarrhea
   Pancreatic, biliary, or intestinal fistulas
   Ureterosigmoidostomy
   Cholestyramine
F. Renal HCO_3^- loss
   Type II (proximal) renal tubular acidosis

DILUTIONAL ACIDOSIS

onism impair this excretion. Patients with renal failure because of a reduced number of functioning nephrons cannot adequately filter and excrete the H^+ load. In distal (type I) RTA, proximal tubular glomerular filtration and HCO_3^- reabsorption are normal but distal tubular H^+ secretion is impaired. Because H^+ excretion in the distal tubule depends on exchange of sodium ions, volume depletion worsens the tendency for acidosis. Through a similar mechanism (reduced tubular sodium delivery), adrenal insufficiency or selective hypoaldosteronism also impairs H^+ excretion. The latter condition may be recognized by the association of metabolic acidosis, hyperkalemia, hyponatremia, and hypercalcemia.

Hydrogen Ion Load and the Anion Gap

An increased H^+ load also may cause metabolic acidosis. In such cases, the disparity between the measured concentrations of serum cations and anions—the anion gap—will widen beyond the normal range. These normally hidden anions are composed of serum proteins (predominantly albumin), phosphate, sulfate, lactate, ketoacids (beta hydroxybutyrate, acetoacetate), and other compounds (e.g., drugs).

The anion gap is based on the principle of electroneutrality mentioned previously. The simplified formula is:

$$AG = (Na^+) - (HCO_3^- + Cl^-)$$

The anion gap has traditionally been simplified and measured as the serum sodium concentration minus the sum of the bicarbonate and chloride concentrations because the potassium concentration is a small quantity that varies only slightly. The normal value for the anion gap ranges from 8 to 12 mmol/L, is dependent of the type of analyzer used, and must be established for each laboratory separately.

The serum anion gap has been proposed to be useful in three clinical settings. The presence or absence of anion gap offers invaluable help in determining the cause of metabolic acidosis. Thus, metabolic acidosis with an increased anion gap is usually attributable to disorders associated with the accumulation of either endogenous organic acids (lactic acidosis, ketoacidosis, mineral acids of renal failure) or exogenous organic acids (methanol, ethylene glycol, salicylate). The magnitude of the increase in the anion gap is important. With an anion gap

TABLE 12-3 ANION GAP AND METABOLIC ACIDOSIS

HIGH ANION GAP

A. Lactic acidosis: D-lactate
B. Ketoacidosis: β-hydroxybutyrate
C. Renal failure: sulfate, phosphate, urate, hippurate
D. Ingestions
   Salicylate: ketones, lactate, salicylate
   Methanol or formaldehyde: formate
   Ethylene glycol: glycolate, oxalate
   Paraldehyde: organic anions
   Sulfur SO_4
E. Massive rhabdomyolysis

NORMAL ANION GAP (HYPERCHLOREMIC ACIDOSIS)

A. Gastrointestinal loss of HCO_3^-
   Diarrhea
B. Renal HCO_3^- loss
   Type II (proximal) renal tubular acidosis
C. Renal dysfunction
   Some cases of renal failure
   Hypoaldosteronism (type IV renal tubular acidosis)
   Type I (distal) renal tubular acidosis
D. Ingestions
   Ammonium chloride
   Hyperalimentation fluids
E. Some cases of ketoacidosis, particularly during treatment with insulin

more than 15 mmol/L, an organic acidosis is nearly always present. However, mild increases in the anion gap may be relatively insensitive for detecting the presence of mild to moderate organic acidosis, such as the lactic acidosis encountered in critically ill patients (Table 12-3).

As a rule, the larger the anion gap, the easier it is to determine the cause of the acidosis. A wide anion gap acidosis usually can be diagnosed rapidly with a clinical history and a limited number of serum tests (i.e., serum creatinine, lactate, and ketone levels). Lactic acidosis generated by anaerobic glycolysis is the most common cause of an elevated anion gap; however, lactic acidosis often is mixed with another form of acidosis. For example, very high serum levels of anionic salicylate molecules may directly elevate the anion gap, but salicylates also raise the anion gap by interfering with carbohydrate metabolism and O_2 utilization, thereby inducing a lactic acidosis. Similarly, DKA produces a mixed anion gap metabolic acidosis by increasing the concentration of unmeasured ketones and by inducing a lactic acidosis, usually from hypoperfusion

(see Chapter 32). Uremia commonly leads to acumulation of titratable acids, producing an anion gap metabolic acidosis.

If the creatine, ketone, and lactate levels are all normal in the setting of a high anion gap, a toxic ingestion becomes the most likely etiology. In such patients, comparing the calculated osmolality to measured serum osmolality proves particularly helpful. An osmolal gap usually indicates some form of alcohol toxicity: ethylene glycol, ethanol, or methanol. Other drugs that can cause an anion gap acidosis include isoniazid, iron, and paraldehyde (see Chapter 33).

The second setting in which the anion gap may be useful is when ascertaining if a *mixed* acid–base disturbance is present through the calculation of the "Delta Ratio" or "Delta/Delta (Δ/Δ)," which is the change in the anion gap divided by the change in the serum bicarbonate. The delta ratio is sometimes used in the assessment of elevated anion gap metabolic acidosis to determine if a mixed acid base disorder is present.

Delta ratio
$$= \Delta \text{Anion gap}/\Delta HCO_3^-$$
$$= (AG_{observed} - AG_{expected})/(HCO_{3normal}^- - HCO_{3expected}^-)$$
$$(\Delta/\Delta) = (AG - 12)/(24 - [HCO_3^-])$$

This calculation is based on the principle that each milliequivalent of acid added to the body should reduce the serum bicarbonate by an equivalent amount. Therefore, when the Delta in the anion gap is larger than the Delta in the serum bicarbonate ($\Delta/\Delta > 1$), this implies an additional source of base (metabolic alkalosis). In other words, if the magnitude of decrease in bicarbonate is less than the magnitude of increase in anion gap, then more base than expected has been added, suggesting an associated alkalotic process.

If all the dissociated acid in the extracellular fluid (ECF) and all the buffering were by bicarbonate, then the increase in the anion gap (AG) should equal the decrease in bicarbonate so the ratio between these two changes (the delta ratio) should equal one. As described previously, however, considerable buffering occurs intracellularly and by bone, not by HCO_3^-. Most of excess anions remain in the ECF because anions cannot easily cross the lipid bilayer of the cell membrane. As a result, the elevation in the anion gap usually exceeds the fall in the plasma $[HCO_3^-]$. In lactic acidosis, for example, the Δ/Δ ratio averages 1.6:1. On the other hand, even though the same principle applies to ketoacidosis, the ratio is usually closer to 1:1 in this disorder because the loss of urinary ketoacid anions (ketones) lowers the anion gap and tends to balance the effect of intracellular buffering. Anion loss in the urine is much less prominent in lactic acidosis because the associated state of marked tissue hypoperfusion usually results in little or no urine output.

A value above 2:1 indicates a lesser fall in $[HCO_3^-]$ than one would expect, given the change in the anion gap. This can be explained by another process that increases the $[HCO_3^-]$, i.e., a concurrent metabolic alkalosis. Another situation to consider when the delta ratio exceeds 2 is a high *preexisting* HCO_3^- level, as would be seen in chronic respiratory acidosis. It should be appreciated that hydrogen buffering in cells and bone takes several hours to complete. Thus, the ratio may be close to 1:1 with very acute lactic acidosis (seizures or exercise to exhaustion) because there has not been time for *nonextracellular* buffering to occur.

When the change in the anion gap is less than that in the serum bicarbonate concentration ($\Delta/\Delta < 1$), this implies an additional source of acid (non–anion gap metabolic acidosis). In other words, more bicarbonate has been consumed than expected and it may be explained by addition of other source of acid, suggesting an associated non–anion gap acidotic process. However, this assumption applies only when the proton and its conjugate base have the same volume of distribution. But as described earlier, more than 50% of the excess H^+ is buffered by the cells, not by the HCO_3^-. By contrast, most of the excess anions remain in the ECF because their distribution is pH dependent. A delta-delta value less than 1:1 indicates a greater fall in $[HCO_3^-]$ than one would expect, given the increase in the anion gap. This can be explained by a mixed metabolic acidosis, i.e., a combined elevated anion gap acidosis and a normal anion gap acidosis, as might occur when lactic acidosis is superimposed on severe diarrhea. In this situation, the additional fall in HCO_3^- is due to further buffering of an acid that does not contribute to the anion gap. (i.e., addition of HCl to the body as a result of diarrhea).

In summary, the Δ/Δ ratio is normally between 1 and 2 in patients with an uncomplicated high anion gap metabolic acidosis. A value below 1:1 suggests a combined *high anion gap acidosis and normal anion gap acidosis*, as might occur when hemoconcentration and lactic acidosis are superimposed on severe diarrhea. On the other hand, a value above 2:1 suggests that the fall in the plasma HCO_3^- concentration is less than expected because of a concurrent metabolic alkalosis.

The third setting in which the anion gap may be useful is in detecting selected disorders that occur when the anion gap is low, rather than high. A low **6** anion gap can occur with a decrease in unmeasured anions, as in hypoalbuminemia. Hypoalbuminemia, a common disturbance in hospitalized patients, can mask an increased concentration of gap anions by lowering the value of the anion gap. For example, in a diabetic patient with hypoalbuminemia significant ketoacidosis can be missed if ketones are not directly measured. The observed anion gap can be adjusted for abnormal albumin concentration, by considering that each g/L decrease in serum albumin causes the observed anion gap to underestimate anion gap by 0.25 mEq/L.

$$Adjusted\ anion\ gap = observed\ anion\ gap + 0.25 \times (normal\ albumin - observed\ albumin)$$

where albumin concentrations are in g/L. (If given in g/dL, the factor is 2.5.)

The low anion gap may be observed if there is an increase in unmeasured cations, as in lithium intoxication, or cases of multiple myeloma in which cationic paraproteins are produced. Rarely, the anion gap may actually be negative, as in severe hyperlipidemia or bromide intoxication. In such rare situations, adjusting for hypoalbuminemia does not correct this error.

Bicarbonate Loss

Bicarbonate loss may produce metabolic acidosis but does not elevate the anion gap because HCO_3^- loss results in compensatory hyperchloremia. Although renal failure usually impairs H^+ excretion, renal failure may also induce direct HCO_3^- loss. In renal failure, the HCO_3^- usually plateaus at 12 to 20 mmol/L, as further H^+ accumulation is blunted by tissue (bone) buffers. Three conditions decrease HCO_3^- disproportionately to reductions in glomerular filtration rate: renal medullary tubular disorders (e.g., proximal RTA), low renin/aldosterone states, and renal failure, in which there is decreased HCO_3^- resorption (due to a constant filtered Na^+ load and an increased filtration fraction through the few remaining nephrons). The mild metabolic acidosis of proximal (type II) RTA usually is an incidental finding resulting from an inability to fully resorb filtered HCO_3^-. In this usually self-limited disease, the impaired reabsorptive capacity for HCO_3^- renders pH correction difficult and produces an alkaline urine. In such patients, exogenous $NaHCO_3$ increases the filtered HCO_3^- load, and raises urinary pH, but seldom affects serum pH. In addition to metabolic acidosis and alkaline urine, ancillary features characteristic of proximal RTA are as follows: decreased serum urate, HCO_3^-, and potassium, aminoaciduria, and glycosuria.

7 The gastrointestinal (GI) tract frequently provides a route for HCO_3^- loss in patients with chronic diarrhea. Diarrhea related to human immunodeficiency virus (HIV) or laxative abuse is relatively common. In such patients, urinary pH can be a helpful diagnostic test—a normal kidney will increase acid excretion (and reclaim HCO_3^-), resulting in a urine pH lower than 5.0. Cholestyramine also may cause metabolic acidosis by exchanging HCO_3^- for Cl^-. Because the ileum and colon have ion pumps that exchange HCO_3^- and for Cl^-, hyperchloremic (nongap) acidosis frequently develops in patients with ureterosigmoidostomy.

Dilutional Acidosis

This type of acidosis is observed mainly when a high volume of saline solution has been given. The simplest explanation for dilutional acidosis from a physicochemical point of view is that admixture of **8** large volumes of a solution less alkaline than blood, such as saline (which contains no bicarbonate), will result in less alkalinity (i.e., more acidity of the solution). Because most body metabolism is performed intracellularly and there is no practical method to obtain intracellular samples, we sample the blood and often presume that it reflects intracellular acid–base kinetics. However, the acidosis resulting from normal saline infusion does not reflect an intracellular metabolic derangement. For the same degree of acidemia, a dilutional acidosis might be expected to be less worrisome than a metabolic acidosis caused by an intracellular metabolic derangement for at least two reasons. First, there is no underlying metabolic derangement associated with simple dilutional acidosis. Second, for the same degree of acidemia, the initial pH change in the dilutional acidosis occurs extracellularly, and a lesser or delayed pH change occurs intracellularly. Conversely, in the metabolically deranged patient, the initial pH change occurs intracellularly and a lesser or delayed change occurs extracellularly.

Urine Anion Gap

Calculation of the urine anion gap may be helpful diagnostically in some cases with a normal anion gap metabolic acidosis. The major measured cations and anions in the urine are Na^+, K^+, and Cl^-; thus, the urine anion gap is

$$\text{Urine anion gap} = ([Na^+] + [K^+]) - [Cl^-]$$
$$\text{Urine anion gap} = \text{Unmeasured anions} - \text{Unmeasured cations}.$$

In normal subjects excreting between 20 and 40 mEq of NH_4^+ per liter (NH_4^+ being the major unmeasured urinary cation), the urinary anion gap (UAG) generally has a positive value or is near zero. In metabolic acidosis, however, the excretion of NH_4^+ (and of Cl^- to maintain electroneutrality) should increase markedly if renal acidification is intact, resulting in a UAG value that varies from -20 to more than -50 mEq/L; the negative value in this setting occurs because in keeping with the principle of electroneutrality, the Cl^- now exceeds that of Na^+ plus K^+. In comparison, the acidemia in renal failure and Types I and IV RTA are primarily due to impaired H^+ and NH_4^+ excretion, and the UAG typically retains its normal positive value.

There are two conditions in which the urine anion gap cannot be used. The first is a high anion gap acidosis, such as ketoacidosis, where the excretion of unmeasured ketoacid anions in the urine will counteract the effect of NH_4^+. The second is volume depletion with avid Na^+ retention (urine sodium <25 mEq/L). The associated decrease in distal Na^+ delivery impairs distal acidification, and the associated increase in Cl^- reabsorption prevents the excretion of NH_4Cl. This represents a reversible form of type I RTA, despite the development of a negative anion gap.

Signs and Symptoms

Unlike those with respiratory acidosis, patients with metabolic acidosis usually have an increased depth and rate of respiration unless ventilatory drive is depressed. If the acidosis is severe, lethargy or coma may occur. Neurologic changes are less prominent with metabolic than with respiratory acidosis, perhaps because the hypercapnia and hypoxemia of respiratory acidosis exert independent effects and because intracerebral pH may be considerably lower, due to easier movement of CO_2 across the blood–brain barrier. Moderate metabolic acidosis may decrease blood pressure, depress heart function, alter the effects of catecholamines on the cardiovascular system, and impair smooth muscle function, leading to such complications as gastroparesis, emesis, and regurgitation of gastric contents.

Compensation

There are several compensatory mechanisms for metabolic acidosis. Initially, extracellular buffers (predominantly HCO_3^-) blunt the falling pH. Rapidly thereafter, the metabolic acidosis stimulates both the central and peripheral chemoreceptors controlling respiration, increasing alveolar ventilation to reduce $PaCO_2$, and raising the extracellular pH toward normal. The increase in ventilation begins within 1 to 2 h and reaches its maximum level at 12 to 24 h. Hyperpnea is characterized more by an increase in tidal volume than by an increase in respiratory rate and may, if the acidemia is severe, reach values exceeding 30 L/min. This degree of hyperventilation (called Kussmaul's respiration) is usually apparent on physical examination and should alert the physician to a possible underlying metabolic acidosis. The $PaCO_2$ declines at a rate of approximately 1.2 mm Hg/mEq/L reduction in serum HCO_3^- but rarely falls below 10 mm Hg. The $PaCO_2$ expected in response to an established metabolic acidosis may be predicted from the following equation: expected $PaCO_2 = 1.5 \times$ measured $HCO_3^- + 8$ (±2).

As a simple rule of thumb for *chronic* metabolic acidosis, the expected $PaCO_2$ approximates the last two digits of the pH value (e.g., the expected $PaCO_2$ for a pH of 7.25 is 25). Although respiratory compensation is relatively prompt (fully developed within 24 to 48 h), it is rarely complete. If the $PaCO_2$ is above that expected for a given HCO_3^-, either the time for compensation has been too short or respiratory acidosis is present. If the $PaCO_2$ is less than expected, concomitant respiratory alkalosis is present. Buffering of H^+ by intracellular protein and fixed buffers in bone (calcium salts) represents a third major mechanism for blunting the decrease in pH. Finally, the kidneys may enhance H^+ excretion, but this function requires the active excretion of H^+ in combination with phosphate (titratable acidity) and ammonium. Such losses of H^+ are limited approximately to 50 to 100 mEq/day, a rate that approximates the normal pace of mineral acid production. In general, 10 to 40 mEq of H^+ is excreted each day as titrable acidity and 30 to 60 mEq as ammonium.

$$H^+ + HPO_4^{2-} \leftrightarrow H_2PO_4^-$$
$$H^+ + NH_3 \leftrightarrow NH_4^+$$

These processes are essential for maintenance of acid–base balance because the rate of excretion of free H^+ ions is extremely low. The kidneys respond to an increased H^+ load by augmenting production and subsequent excretion of NH_4^+. The net effect is that NH_4^+ excretion can exceed 250 mEq/day with severe acidemia. By contrast, there generally is only a limited ability to enhance titratable acidity because phosphate excretion remains relatively constant. One exception occurs in ketoacidosis, where excreted ketone anions can act as urinary buffers, increasing titrable acid excretion by up to 50 mEq/day.

Treatment

If pH disturbances are severe, therapeutic measures **9** may be necessary to alter the PCO_2 or bicarbonate content directly. However, the treatment of acid–base disorders usually should be directed at the underlying cause. Mistakenly, the lack of definitive evidence proving efficacy of bicarbonate therapy in some forms of metabolic acidosis has been interpreted to imply that base therapy is futile in all situations. Potential indications for direct treatment of metabolic acidosis are (i) pH less than 7.10, (ii) overt physiologic compromise attributable to acidosis, and (iii) excessive work of breathing required to maintain an acceptable pH (>7.20). Exogenous HCO_3^- may need to be repleted when the "buffer base" has been depleted by chronic respiratory alkalosis, GI or renal losses of HCO_3^-, and resolved metabolic acidosis.

If bicarbonate therapy is used, calculation of the HCO_3^- dose assumes a distribution into half of total body water. Total body water (in L) is approximately 0.6 times the lean body weight (in kg). The following expression

$$HCO_3^- \text{ deficit} = (0.5 \times \text{total body water}) \times (24 - [HCO_3^-])$$

approximates the HCO_3^- deficit in mEq. Larger bicarbonate doses may be required to repair profound reductions in serum bicarbonate levels, as the apparent volume of distribution for bicarbonate then increases. Because $NaHCO_3$ has potentially adverse effects and because the effectiveness of a given dose is not entirely predictable, it is customary to replace one half the calculated HCO_3^- deficit over several hours while following the pH response closely. $NaHCO_3$ partially equilibrates in total body water within 15 min of administration; however, cellular equilibration requires approximately 2 h to complete.

NaHCO$_3$ administration presents several potential problems. In large doses, hypertonic hypernatremia and fluid overload may occur (an ampule of NaHCO$_3$ contains nearly as much Na$^+$ as 0.5 L of normal saline). Bolus injection of NaHCO$_3$ may elicit a biphasic ventilatory response. Immediately after administration, peripheral pH rises and the drive to breathe falls. However, soon thereafter, rising CO$_2$ (due to both metabolic load and buffered H$^+$ ion) diffuses across the blood–brain barrier to reduce intracerebral pH and stimulate breathing ("paradoxical central nervous system [CNS] acidosis"). Rapid bolus injection of NaHCO$_3$ is potentially dangerous—it may cause a rapid leftward shift of the oxyhemoglobin dissociation curve, alter cerebral hemodynamics, or induce life-threatening hypokalemia. A pH greater than 7.10 usually is sufficient to maintain near-normal vascular tone and myocardial contractility and can almost always be obtained using small doses of NaHCO$_3$. Furthermore, some types of acidosis (e.g., proximal RTA) are very difficult to correct with exogenous bicarbonate. In organic acidosis (DKA or lactic acidosis), NaHCO$_3$ therapy eventually may lead to an alkalosis as the organic acids (ketones, lactate) are recycled to HCO$_3^-$ by the liver. There is no loss of potential bicarbonate in these disorders; therefore, bicarbonate therapy is rarely necessary.

Dichloroacetate (DCA) is a compound that stimulates pyruvate dehydrogenase activity, thereby minimizing lactate production by allowing pyruvate to be oxidized to CO$_2$ and H$_2$O. Although there is evidence of benefit in experimental models of lactic acidosis, a controlled trial in humans showed that DCA produced a minor increase in the plasma bicarbonate concentration and arterial pH, but no improvement in systemic hemodynamics or mortality. Tromethamine (THAM) is an inert amino alcohol that buffers acids and CO$_2$ by virtue of its amine moiety. THAM is excreted in the urine at a slightly higher rate than creatinine clearance in conjunction with either chloride or bicarbonate. Thus, THAM supplements the buffering capacity of blood without generating carbon dioxide but is less effective in patients with renal failure. Published clinical experience with THAM is limited, but the drug has been used in treating severe acidemia because of sepsis, hypercapnia, DKA, RTA, and drug intoxication.

Metabolic Alkalosis

Metabolic alkalosis, a pH higher than 7.45 with a normal or elevated PaCO$_2$, usually is generated and maintained by two distinct pathophysiologic mechanisms. Metabolic alkalosis always occurs because of the gain of HCO$_3^-$, loss of H$^+$ ions, or loss of body fluid rich in chloride compared to its plasma concentration. In the first situation, exogenous base may accumulate when excess bicarbonate, citrate, lactate, or acetate is administered. The second mechanism for establishing metabolic alkalosis occurs when H$^+$ is lost. Loss most commonly occurs in gastric juice from nasogastric (NG) suctioning or vomiting, but this occurs less commonly with the widespread use of H$_2$ blockers and proton pump inhibitors. Rarely, H$^+$ excretion may result from a renal disorder in which losses may be mediated by excess mineralocorticoids, increased distal tubule Na$^+$ delivery, or excessive filtration of nonreabsorbable anions (e.g., calcium, penicillin). Interestingly, renal mechanisms almost never generate metabolic alkalosis but are almost always responsible for its perpetuation. The normal kidney rapidly excretes alkaline urine in response to a HCO$_3^-$ load, provided that serum Cl$^-$, K$^+$, and Mg^{3+} are normal and perfusion is adequate. However, hypokalemia, hypomagnesemia, and hypochloremia all inhibit the excretion of excess HCO$_3^-$.

Diagnostic Criteria

Metabolic alkalosis is characterized by an elevated pH, elevated HCO$_3^-$, and often a compensatory increase in PaCO$_2$ if the disorder is chronic. The anion gap may increase because of the increased "charge equivalency" of albumin and stimulation of organic anion synthesis.

Signs and Symptoms

Patients with metabolic alkalosis may be asymptomatic or complain of symptoms related either to volume depletion (weakness, muscle cramps, postural dizziness) or to hypokalemia (polyuria, polydipsia, muscle weakness). Complaints directly related to alkalemia, however, are uncommon. Metabolic alkalosis impairs neural transmission and muscular contraction, especially when accompanied by hypokalemia and hypophosphatemia—two commonly coexisting abnormalities. Indeed, metabolic alkalosis mimics hypocalcemia in its symptomatology. Changes in mental status and thirst because of volume depletion occur commonly.

Precipitants of Metabolic Alkalosis

NG suctioning or vomiting can deplete circulatory volume as well as H^+, Mg^{3+}, and Cl^- concentrations. In replacing these H^+ losses, HCO_3^- is generated and retained. Volume depletion causes hyperaldosteronism (HCO_3^- retention, K^+ loss). Aldosterone also promotes maximal Na^+ resorption, leading to high rates of tubular Na^+ for H^+ exchange, which further worsens the alkalosis.

Relief of long-standing respiratory acidosis (e.g., with institution of mechanical ventilation) results in a rapidly evolving metabolic alkalosis because of the HCO_3^- previously retained in compensation. For unknown reasons, chronic respiratory acidosis promotes urinary Cl^- wasting, which further helps to perpetuate alkalosis. Mineralocorticoid excess (primary or secondary) is commonly accompanied by K^+ loss and impaired renal tubular HCO_3^- excretion. When loop diuretics are given to volume-depleted patients, increased amounts of Na^+ are presented to the distal renal tubule and the resulting intensified exchange of Na^+ for H^+ perpetuates metabolic alkalosis. If Na^+ is administered along with a nonresorbable anion (e.g., penicillin) to volume-depleted patients, the Na^+ will be reabsorbed in the renal tubule and H^+ will be secreted to maintain electroneutrality.

The weak aldosterone-like properties of glucocorticoids may cause metabolic alkalosis in Cushing syndrome or with exogenous administration of corticosteroids. Excess HCO_3^- retention may occur after therapeutic administration, but if circulating volume and K^+ are normal, the kidney has a remarkable ability to excrete excess HCO_3^-. Iatrogenic metabolic alkalosis often complicates therapy of acidosis because of DKA, or lactate because HCO_3^- is regenerated in the recovery period.

The contraction of diuretic use accounts for perhaps the most commonly encountered cause of metabolic alkalosis. Contraction alkalosis is a state in which losses of intravascular volume, K^+, and Cl^- act in conjunction with hyperaldosteronism to deplete ECF while HCO_3^- remains nearly constant. The reactive increase of aldosterone favors reabsorption of Na^+ and excretion of urinary H^+. Although this problem is most commonly seen with loop or thiazide-type diuretics, it can also occur with vomiting (high gastric loss of Cl^-).

Maintenance of Alkalosis

Metabolic alkalosis can be maintained by the same four mechanisms responsible for its development: Cl^- deficiency, mineralocorticoid excess, and depletion of circulating volume or K^+. However, in a given patient, metabolic alkalosis often is maintained by a different mechanism from the one that established it. For example, NG removal of Cl^- and H^+ may generate a metabolic alkalosis, but it is associated depletion of intravascular volume and Cl^- that maintain it, even after NG suctioning is discontinued. Cl^- and volume must be administered for reversal. Given a choice, the body chooses to maintain adequate circulating volume status at the expense of Cl^- and pH homeostasis.

Compensation for Metabolic Alkalosis

In metabolic alkalosis, the $PaCO_2$ normally rises approximately 0.6 mm Hg/mmol increase in HCO_3^-. (Lower $PaCO_2$ values indicate a superimposed respiratory alkalosis.) When breathing room air, it is rare to see a compensatory increase in $PaCO_2$ that exceeds 60 mm Hg, at least in part because at this level of hypercarbia, the PaO_2 falls to approximately 60 mm Hg and hypoxemia begins to drive respiration.

Diagnosis

As already indicated, the clinical history, the medication profile, serum chemistry, and intravascular volume status are keys to the differential diagnosis. The laboratory evaluation should be directed at differentiating chloride-responsive from chloride-resistant alkalosis (see following). A chloride-responsive alkalosis usually can be identified by measuring urine electrolytes. Such measurements are useful, provided that they are not obtained within 24 h of diuretic administration, because most diuretics result in Cl^- and K^+ losses. Urinary Cl^- concentrations lower than 20 mEq/L characterize a chloride-responsive condition, suggesting volume depletion or posthypercapnic alkalosis as potential mechanism. If the urine Cl^- concentration exceeds 20 mEq/L, mineralocorticoid excess, diuretic use, and severe hypokalemia or hypomagnesemia are common causes. Marked disparity between urinary Cl^- and Na^+ concentrations strongly suggests mineralocorticoid excess.

Treatment

Metabolic alkalosis often is considered in two general categories—"salt" (NaCl) responsive or salt unresponsive (Table 12-4). NaCl frequently reverses volume contraction and secondary

TABLE 12-4 CLASSIFICATION OF METABOLIC ALKALOSIS BASED ON CHLORIDE RESPONSIVENESS

CHLORIDE RESPONSIVE	CHLORIDE RESISTANT
Volume depletion	Hyperaldosteronism
Vomiting/diarrhea	Exogenous steroids
Nasogastric suction	Cushing syndrome
Diuretics	Alkali ingestion
Posthypercapnia	
Chronic medications (e.g., penicillin)	

hyperaldosteronism. The "chloride dose" required to correct a chloride-responsive alkalosis can be approximated as the desired change in chloride concentration times 25% of body weight in kilogram. NaCl also provides Cl^- ions for reabsorption, with Na^+ obviating the need for H^+ secretion. (The effectiveness of NaCl replacement may be determined by measuring urinary pH—if Na^+ replacement is sufficient, urinary pH will rise above 7.0.) Chloride, the only absorbable anion, is the critical component in NaCl administration. For example, administration of other sodium salts (e.g., sodium sulfate) will not improve metabolic alkalosis even though Na^+ is provided and the volume is corrected. Because K^+ depletion contributes to maintenance of metabolic alkalosis by preventing adequate HCO_3^- excretion, potassium chloride replacement is the preferred therapy, but quantities of potassium that can be safely given limit the rate and volume of administration.

Patients with the edematous states associated with heart failure, cirrhosis, or nephrotic syndrome often develop metabolic alkalosis following diuretic therapy, but the administration of saline is not indicated because it will increase the degree of edema. Preferred corrective therapy consists of withholding diuretics if possible, using acetazolamide, HCl, or dialysis. Acetazolamide is a carbonic anhydrase inhibitor that increases the renal excretion of sodium bicarbonate. The dose is 125 to 500 mg orally or intravenously, given with a maximum total of 1,000 mg daily.

Chloride-resistant alkaloses (adrenal disorders, corticosteroid administration, excess alkali ingestion or administration) usually occur due to mineralocorticoid excess. Therefore, in most such disorders, hypokalemia (sometimes severe) is a predictable feature. Therapy of mineralocorticoid excess may be directed at removal of the hormonal source

(tumor control, withdrawal of steroids) or blockade of mineralocorticoid effect (spironolactone). K^+-sparing diuretics or the combination of Na^+ restriction and K^+ supplementation also is effective. Caution is mandated in patients who are oliguric. Rarely, metabolic alkalosis is sufficiently protracted or severe to warrant the administration of intravenous HCl. This therapy should be reserved for patients with normal volume status and potassium concentrations and refractory severe symptomatic alkalosis. HCl may be infused as a 0.1- to 0.2-M solution, but must be given directly into a central venous catheter at a rate not exceeding 0.2 mEq/kg/h. In a similar manner as calculating bicarbonate deficit, the appropriate HCl dose may be approximated from the product of the desired change in HCO_3^-, assuming distribution in 50% of the total lean body water. Ammonium chloride may be used instead of HCl but should not be administered to patients with renal or hepatic failure.

Respiratory Acidosis

Although CO_2 is not an acid, it combines with H_2O as it is added to the bloodstream, resulting in the formation of H_2CO_3. The ensuing elevation in the H^+ concentration is then minimized because most of the excess H^+ ions combine with extracellular buffers, including hemoglobin (Hgb) in red cells.

$$H_2CO_3 + Hgb^- \leftrightarrow HHgb + HCO_3^-$$

The HCO_3^- generated by this reaction leaves the erythrocyte and enters the ECF in exchange for extracellular Cl^-. The net effect is that metabolic CO_2 is primarily carried in the bloodstream as HCO_3^- with little change in the extracellular pH. These processes are reversed in the alveoli. As HHgb is oxygenated, H^+ is released. These H^+ ions combine with HCO_3^- to form H_2CO_3 and then CO_2, which is excreted. The respiratory acidosis can be acute or chronic (Table 12-5).

Acute Respiratory Acidosis

From an acid–base perspective, the body is not well adapted to handle an acute elevation in CO_2 concentration. Little extracellular buffering occurs, because HCO_3 cannot buffer H_2CO_3 and the renal response takes time to develop. Consequently, the cellular buffers, particularly hemoglobin and proteins, constitute the primary modulators of acidosis related to acute hypercapnia.

$$H_2CO_3 + Buf^- \leftrightarrow HBuf + HCO_3^-$$

TABLE 12-5 ETIOLOGY OF ACUTE AND CHRONIC RESPIRATORY ACIDOSIS

INHIBITION OF THE MEDULLARY RESPIRATORY CENTER

A. Acute
1. Drugs: opiates, anesthetics, sedatives
2. Oxygen in chronic hypercapnia
3. Cardiac arrest
4. Central sleep apnea
B. Chronic
1. Extreme obesity (Pickwickian syndrome)
2. Central nervous system disease (rare)
3. Metabolic alkalosis

DISORDERS OF THE RESPIRATORY MUSCLES AND CHEST WALL

A. Acute
1. Muscle weakness: myasthenia gravis, periodic paralysis, Guillain–Barré syndrome, severe hypokalemia, or hypophosphatemia
B. Chronic
1. Muscle weakness: spinal cord injury, poliomyelitis, amyotrophic lateral sclerosis, multiple sclerosis, myxedema
2. Kyphoscoliosis
3. Extreme obesity

UPPER AIRWAY OBSTRUCTION

A. Acute
1. Aspiration
2. Obstructive sleep apnea
3. Laryngospasm

DISORDERS AFFECTING GAS EXCHANGE ACROSS THE PULMONARY CAPILLARY

A. Acute
1. Exacerbation of underlying lung disease
2. Adult respiratory distress syndrome
3. Acute cardiogenic pulmonary edema
4. Severe asthma or pneumonia
5. Pneumothorax–hemothorax
B. Chronic
1. COPD: bronchitis, emphysema
2. Extreme obesity

MECHANICAL VENTILATION (Permissive Hypercapnia)

As a result of these buffering reactions, there is an increase in the plasma HCO_3^- concentration, averaging 1 mEq/L for every 10 mm Hg rise in the PCO_2.

The common causes of acute respiratory acidosis include acute exacerbation of such underlying lung diseases as severe asthma or pneumonia, pulmonary edema, and suppression of the respiratory center following a cardiac arrest, a drug overdose, or the administration of oxygen to a patient with chronic hypercapnia.

Chronic Respiratory Acidosis

The persistent elevation in the $PaCO_2$ stimulates renal H^+ excretion, resulting in the addition of HCO_3^- to the ECF. The net effect is that, after 3 to 5 days, a new steady state is attained in which there is roughly a 3.5 mEq/L increase in the plasma HCO_3^- concentration for every 10 mm Hg increment in the $PaCO_2$. The efficiency of the renal compensation has allowed some patients to tolerate $PaCO_2$ values as an ongoing bases as high as 90 to 110 mm Hg, without a fall in the arterial pH to less than 7.25 and without symptoms as long as adequate oxygenation is maintained. Chronic respiratory acidosis is a relatively common clinical disturbance that is most often because of chronic obstructive lung disease (bronchitis and emphysema) in smokers.

Symptoms

Severe acute respiratory acidosis can produce a variety of neurologic abnormalities. The initial symptoms include headache, blurred vision, restlessness, and anxiety, which can progress to tremors, asterixis, delirium, and somnolence (called CO_2 narcosis). The cerebrospinal fluid pressure is often elevated, and papilledema may be seen. Arrhythmias and peripheral vasodilatation can produce hypotension if the systemic pH falls below 7.10. Chronic respiratory acidosis is also associated with cor pulmonale and peripheral edema. The cardiac output and glomerular filtration rate are usually normal in this disorder.

Diagnosis

The presence of an acid pH and hypercapnia associated with a ventilatory disorder is diagnostic of respiratory acidosis. However, identifying the underlying acid–base disorder is more complicated than in metabolic acidosis or alkalosis, and the clinical context is essential. Compensated chronic respiratory acidosis is recognized by clinical history of pulmonary pathology, elevated CO_2, and a blood pH that is maintained at a nearly normal level. Uncompensated chronic respiratory acidosis is recognized by the clinical history of pulmonary pathology, elevated CO_2, and acidotic blood pH.

Treatment

Patients with acute respiratory acidosis are at risk of both hypercapnia and hypoxemia. Although the PO_2 can usually be raised by the administration of supplemental oxygen, reversal of the hypercapnia requires an increase in effective alveolar ventilation. This can be achieved by control of the underlying disease (as with bronchodilators and corticosteroids in asthma) or by mechanical ventilation delivered via either a tight-fitting mask or an endotracheal tube. The role of an alkalinizing agent in this setting is controversial and usually considered primarily when the hemodynamic status of the patient is compromised. THAM has been used in this setting, and the results have been satisfactory. Under some conditions, bicarbonate can increase intracellular acidosis.

The primary goals of therapy in patients with chronic respiratory acidosis are to maintain adequate oxygenation and, if possible, to improve effective alveolar ventilation per se. Because of the effectiveness of the renal compensation, it is usually not necessary to treat pH, even in patients with severe hypercapnia. The appropriate treatment varies with the underlying disease.

Respiratory Alkalosis

Inciting Mechanisms

Respiratory alkalosis—primary or compensatory—is defined by hypocapnia, a finding that implies alveolar hyperventilation. Central neurologic disorders, agitation, pain, inappropriate mechanical ventilation, hypoxemia, and restrictive diseases that reduce respiratory system compliance all may produce primary respiratory alkalosis.

Symptoms

Acute respiratory alkalosis usually is manifest by tachypnea; however, when chronic, this disorder may be associated with large tidal volume breaths at near-normal respiratory rates. The symptoms of acute respiratory alkalosis, "the hyperventilation syndrome," vary only in intensity from those of any alkalosis—most notably impaired neuromuscular function (e.g., paresthesias, tetany, tremor). A constellation of symptoms has been described with respiratory alkalosis, including chest pain, circumoral paresthesias, carpopedal spasm, anxiety, and light-headedness.

Compensatory Mechanisms

Protracted respiratory alkalosis induces renal HCO_3^- wasting to offset hypocapnia. When the stimulus for hyperventilation is removed, hyperpnea tends to continue, driven by CNS acidosis until intracerebral HCO_3^- and pH are fully corrected.

■ MIXED ACID–BASE DISORDERS

Renal and respiratory compensation returns the pH toward, but rarely to, normal. Thus, a normal pH in the presence of changes in the $PaCO_2$ and plasma HCO_3^- concentration immediately suggests a mixed disorder. Complex (mixed) acid–base disorders occur most frequently when lung and renal diseases coexist, when compensatory mechanisms are rendered inoperative, or when mechanical ventilation is used. The presence of a complex or mixed acid–base disorder is discovered by applying the rules of expected compensation given earlier and in Chapter 5.

One particular condition, the "triple acid–base disorder," deserves special mention. It should be recognized that the term "triple acid–base disorder" has no unique interpretation. It could refer to three simultaneous metabolic acidoses or alkaloses or any combination of metabolic processes. However, because respiratory acidosis and respiratory alkalosis cannot coexist, the so-called triple acid–base disorder is the result of two metabolic derangements and a single ventilation abnormality.

■ SUGGESTED READINGS

Carreira F, Anderson RJ. Assessing metabolic acidosis in the intensive care unit: Does the method make a difference? *Crit Care Med.* 2004;32(5):1227–1228.

Corey HE. Stewart and beyond: New models of acid-base balance. *Kidney Int.* 2003;64(3):777–787.

Kaplan LJ, Kellum JA. Comparison of acid-base models for prediction of hospital mortality after trauma. *Shock.* 2008;29(6):662–666.

Kellum JA. Disorders of acid-base balance. *Crit Care Med.* 2007;35: 2630–2636.

Kraut JA, Madias NE. Approach to patients with acid-base disorders. *Respir Care.* 2001;46(4):392–403.

Moe OW, Fuster D. Clinical acid–base pathophysiology: Disorders of plasma anion gap. *Best Pract Res Clin Endocrinol Metab.* 2003; 17(4):559–574.

Peixoto AJ. Critical issues in nephrology. *Clin Chest Med.* 2003;24: 561–581.

Rose BD, Post T. *Clinical Physiology of Acid–Base and Electrolyte Disorders,* 5th Ed. New York: McGraw-Hill; 2001.

Story DA, Morimatsu H, Bellomo R. Strong ions, weak acids and base excess: A simplified Fencl–Stewart approach to clinical acid–base disorders. *Br J Anaesth.* 2004;92:54–60.

Fluid and Electrolyte Disorders

KEY POINTS

1 The diagnosis of the etiology of hyponatremia relies on serum osmolality and an accurate assessment of fluid status of the patient. In most cases, the etiology can be determined by history and physical examination. For cases in which the diagnosis is uncertain after examination, serum and urine osmolality measurements are useful.

2 Severe hyponatremia (serum Na$^+$ < 120 mEq/L) defines an urgent clinical situation in which levels of the ion should be raised to 120 mEq/L or above. Correction should be approximately 1 to 2 mEq/L/h in patients with severe neurologic symptoms (stupor, coma, seizures, etc.), then slower once the life-threatening symptoms are reversed. Water restriction or isotonic saline or hypertonic saline is an appropriate treatment for hypervolemic or hypovolemic or symptomatic isovolemic hyponatremia, if present, respectively.

3 Hypernatremia usually is the result of restricted access to free water or absence of the sensation of thirst. Rarely, central diabetes insipidus, a fatal condition unless recognized and treated with antidiuretic hormone, is the etiology. Diabetes insipidus can be recognized by noting large volumes of dilute urine in a patient with hyperosmolar serum.

4 Because little of the body's K$^+$ is in the extracellular compartment, significant hypokalemia signals total body depletion of K$^+$, usually more than 200 mEq. Because of the importance of K$^+$ in maintaining normal neural and muscular function, prompt correction of the deficit is prudent. When possible, oral replacement avoids the rapid swings of IV dosing. When IV replacement is used, dosing should probably be limited to 40 mEq/h.

5 Significant hyperkalemia usually is the result of renal insufficiency. Hyperkalemia sufficient to induce electrocardiographic changes should be treated aggressively with volume expanders, loop diuretics, insulin, glucose, bicarbonate (in the presence of acidosis), and Ca^{2+}. K$^+$ removal using dialysis or binding resins is indicated.

6 Both Ca^{2+} and Mg depend on their ionized forms for biologic action; therefore, total serum concentrations do not accurately reflect bioactivity. Total Ca^{2+} and Mg levels, and possibly the ionized forms of each, should be measured when unexplained neuromuscular disorders occur in the ICU.

■ DISORDERS OF SODIUM AND OSMOLALITY

Despite great variability in sodium (Na$^+$) and water intake, circulating intravascular volume, serum Na$^+$ concentration, and osmolality normally remain quite stable. As a consequence of dehydration and/or hypovolemia, there are increases in serum osmolality, which trigger thirst, and antidiuretic hormone (ADH) secretion. Although they often coexist, it is essential to recognize that dehydration (loss of water) is different from hypovolemia (inadequate circulating volume). ADH secretion increases dramatically as osmolality rises above 285 mOsm/L or extracellular volume declines by 10% to 15%. ADH then acts on the medullary collecting duct of the kidney to stimulate water reabsorption. The renin–angiotensin–aldosterone system restores the circulating volume in response to its contraction. The combined effects of ADH and the renin system balance the retention of Na$^+$ and water. When plasma osmolality declines, ADH release is inhibited, and excess water is lost in an attempt to return osmolality toward normal. Hence, usually the serum Na$^+$ concentration has little to do with the amount of Na$^+$ in the body, but much to do with the amount of water.

Hyponatremia

Disorders of fluid and Na$^+$ balance occur daily in the intensive care unit (ICU) because patients have multiple organ system failures, are usually denied self-regulation of water balance, and are administered medications that disturb fluid and electrolyte status. Hyponatremia, defined as a serum Na^+ concentration less than 134 mEq/L, is one of the most common electrolyte disorders and implies excess water in the body. The manifestations of hyponatremia range from the subtle to the neurologically profound but generally are proportional to the magnitude of the hyponatremia and the speed with which it develops. Symptoms span the spectrum from muscle cramps, nausea, vomiting, and anorexia to confusion, lethargy, coma, and seizures.

1 In combination with a thorough history, medication review, and physical examination, the serum osmolality, glucose, creatinine, and albumin provide essential data for determining the etiology of hyponatremia. Because Na^+ is the predominant osmotically active extracellular action, serum osmolality is normally determined largely by the relative proportions of water and Na^+. Measurements of serum osmolality help to separate hyponatremic disorders into three distinct categories summarized in Table 13-1. Apart from disturbances in sodium/water balance, marked elevations of glucose or exogenous substances (alcohols and complex carbohydrates) can elevate serum osmolality. Conversely, reductions in osmolality virtually always are reflected in the Na^+ concentration as illustrated by the equation commonly used to calculate serum osmolality:

Osmolality = $2[Na^+]$ + glucose/18 + BUN/2.8 + [serum ethanol]/4.6 + ("unmeasured" osmoles)

Categories of Hyponatremia

Hypertonic Hyponatremia

Hypertonic hyponatremia results from the infusion or spontaneous generation of (nonsodium) osmotically active substances. Hyperglycemia and therapeutic administration of hypertonic glucose, mannitol, or glycine can cause hypertonicity while depressing Na^+ levels. (Although urea also increases osmolality, it fails to affect serum Na^+ concentration because it freely traverses cell membranes, dissipating any potential osmotic gradient.) Extracellular hypertonicity draws water from cells in an attempt to reduce the osmotic gradient. This effect not only partially corrects the hyperosmolality but also lowers the Na^+ concentration and causes cellular dehydration. The cause of hypertonic hyponatremia usually can be diagnosed by measuring serum glucose and reviewing a list of the patient's drugs. When hyperglycemia is the etiology, Na^+ levels decline approximately 1.6 mEq/L per 100 mg/dL rise in serum glucose. Thus, hyperglycemia has a negligible effect on Na^+ levels in concentrations less than 200 to 300 mg/dL.

Hypotonic Hyponatremias

Hypotonic hyponatremia is the most common form of hyponatremia and can be subclassified into three categories based upon the estimation of the patient's volume status. Hypotonic hyponatremia almost never develops unless the patient has unrestricted access to water or receives a hypotonic fluid.

Hypovolemic Hypotonic Hyponatremia Hypovolemic hyponatremia with low serum osmolality results from replacing losses of salt-containing plasma with hypotonic fluid. Volume depletion is a potent stimulus for ADH release. Intake of hypotonic fluid, when combined with the decreased free water clearance that results from ADH release, causes hyponatremia. Physical examination reveals signs of volume depletion. Thirst and postural hypotension are more objective and reliable signs than are skin turgor, sunken orbits, or mucous membrane dryness.

TABLE 13-1 HYPONATREMIA: DIAGNOSTIC CATEGORIES AND CAUSES

HYPERTONIC HYPONATREMIA	HYPOTONIC HYPONATREMIA			ISOTONIC HYPONATREMIA
	HYPOVOLEMIC	ISOVOLEMIC	HYPERVOLEMIC	
Osmotic agents	Hemorrhage	Inappropriate ADH	Heart failure	Hyperproteinemia
Glucose	Vomiting	Polydipsia	Cirrhosis	Hyperlipidemia
Mannitol	Diarrhea	Hypothyroidism	Nephrosis	Isotonic infusions of
Starch	Sweating	Hypocortisolism	Chronic renal failure	Mannitol
			Hypoproteinemia	Glycine
	Diuretics (thiazide, loop, and osmotic) Third-space loss Salt-wasting nephropathy			Starch

Hypovolemic hypotonic hyponatremia may result from renal or nonrenal causes. Bleeding, diarrhea, vomiting, and profuse sweating are common nonrenal mechanisms of circulating volume loss and are usually apparent clinically. Third-space losses (e.g., pancreatitis or gut sequestration) may be less obvious. Renal causes of volume depletion and hyponatremia include diuretic use (particularly thiazide diuretics), osmotic diuresis from ketones, glucose, or mannitol and the less common conditions of mineralocorticoid deficiency, and salt wasting nephropathy.

For patients with well-functioning kidneys and normal levels of mineralocorticoid hormones, small volumes of hypertonic urine with a very low Na$^+$ concentration reflect intense conservation of Na$^+$ and water. If the cause of the syndrome is not clear from the history and physical examination, measuring urine Na$^+$ and osmolality and serum cortisol and aldosterone may be diagnostically helpful. If urine Na$^+$ concentration is high and urine osmolality normal, renal salt wasting is the probable etiology. With mineralocorticoid insufficiency, the urine Na$^+$ concentration is high and the urine osmolality is elevated. Because hypovolemia reduces renal blood flow, thereby slowing tubular flow, urea may "back-diffuse" into the bloodstream, so the BUN/creatinine ratio rises. Similarly uric acid levels tend to rise.

Isovolemic Hypotonic Hyponatremia Isovolemic hypotonic hyponatremia is a misnomer; almost always a clinically undetectable, slight excess of total body fluid (3 to 4 L) exists. Inappropriate secretion of antidiuretic hormone (SIADH) and water intoxication are the two most frequent causes. Most cases of water intoxication occur in patients with impaired ability to clear free water or ADH excess. For example, water intoxication occurs with increased frequency when renal disease (decreased clearance) complicates schizophrenia (increased ADH and increased water intake). Another common clinical setting is the postoperative patient given hypotonic IV fluid or tap water enemas (increased ADH and increased water intake). Diuretics can also cause isovolemic hyponatremia in a patient with unlimited water access, as natriuresis impairs free water clearance and sensitizes to ADH. Since hypothyroidism and hypocortisolism are relatively common causes of isovolemic hypotonic hyponatremia, thyroid and adrenal function must be tested. Ecstasy (MDMA) use should be suspected in otherwise healthy young patients presenting with isovolemic hypotonic hyponatremia. Users know ecstasy causes water loss by increasing body temperature and activity and sometimes obsessively drink water to prevent dehydration.

Inappropriate ADH syndrome (SIADH) is a diagnosis of exclusion, which requires near normal volume status, normal cardiac and renal function, and a normal hormonal environment (exclusive of ADH). Because the requisite conditions are often not met, SIADH is overdiagnosed. SIADH-induced volume expansion increases cardiac output and glomerular filtration rate (GFR), eventually depleting the stores of total body Na$^+$. (Because a constant fraction of filtered Na$^+$ is reabsorbed, there is obligatory renal loss of Na$^+$.) Serum values of Na$^+$, creatinine, and uric acid are all subnormal because of the expanded circulating volume and increased GFR. SIADH is most frequently associated with malignant tumors, particularly of the lung; however, central nervous system (CNS) or pulmonary infections, drugs (Table 13-2), and trauma also may be causative. SIADH is characterized by inappropriately concentrated urine where urine osmolality typically exceeds that of plasma. Urine Na$^+$ concentrations are more than 20 mEq/L, and the urine cannot be diluted appropriately in response to water loading. (When water-challenged, patients with most other types of hyponatremia completely suppress ADH release to excrete maximally diluted urine of <100 mOsm/L.)

Cerebral salt-wasting syndrome is an uncommon problem described in patients with intracranial

TABLE 13-2 CAUSES OF INAPPROPRIATE ADH SYNDROME

NEUROLOGIC DISORDERS	CANCERS	PULMONARY DISORDERS	DRUGS
Trauma	Lung carcinoma	Tuberculosis	Narcotics
Stroke	Pancreatic carcinoma	Pneumonia	Chlorpropamide
Infections			Tolbutamide
			Cyclophosphamide
			Vincristine
			Carbamazepine

pathology, particularly subarachnoid hemorrhage. There is a high urine Na^+ concentration thought to arise from the release of a brain natriuretic peptide-like substance. As with SIADH, the urine has a high Na^+ concentration and a low uric acid level. Once there is reversal of hyponatremia, the uric acid remains low in cerebral salt-wasting but corrects in SIADH.

The treatment of isovolemic hypotonic hyponatremia depends on the cause. If tumor related, appropriate antineoplastic therapy can be helpful. Replacement of thyroid hormone or cortisol reverses the defect in hypothyroidism or adrenal insufficiency. In SIADH, treatment restricts free water. Vaprisol, a vasopressin receptor 2 blocker, acts in the renal collecting duct to accentuate free water loss. Unfortunately, the drug is quite expensive and has only transient effects.

Hypervolemic Hypotonic Hyponatremia Edema is the hallmark of hypervolemic hypotonic hyponatremia, a syndrome in which water is retained in excess of Na^+. Because approximately 60% of total body water is intracellular, a 12- to 15-L excess of total body water must be present before sufficient interstitial fluid accumulates to cause detectable edema (unless hypoalbuminemia or vascular permeability is increased). Despite increases in both total body water and Na^+, effective intravascular volume usually is modestly decreased.

The basic problem in this condition is that the kidney cannot excrete Na^+ and water at a rate sufficient to keep pace with intake. Reduced Na^+ and water clearance can be the result of intrinsic renal disease or conditions that decrease effective renal perfusion (congestive heart failure, cirrhosis, malnutrition, and nephrotic syndrome). Renal causes include almost any form of acute or chronic renal failure.

If the cause is extrarenal, there is intense conservation of Na^+ and water with very low urinary Na^+ concentrations (<10 mEq/L), low urine volumes, and high urine osmolality. Urine electrolytes and osmolality are more variable (and less helpful) in kidney disorders. Because diuretics impair the ability to conserve Na^+ and water, at least 24 h must elapse between the last dose of diuretic and determinations of urinary electrolytes and osmolality.

Isotonic Hyponatremia

Hyponatremia with normal serum osmolality occurs when large volumes of isotonic, non–salt-containing solutions (glucose, hydroxyethyl starch, mannitol, glycine, etc.) are retained in the extracellular space. This volume expansion does not cause a transcellular shift of water. One of the most common settings for the syndrome is following transurethral prostatectomy. Massive absorption of bladder irrigants containing 5% mannitol can cause isotonic hyponatremia. However, if the irrigant used is 1.5% glycine or 3.3% sorbitol, hypotonic hyponatremia may ensue. Such patients can develop severe symptomatic hyponatremia. It is unclear if the clinical impact is the result of the Na^+ and water imbalance or the solutes of the irrigants themselves. Isotonic hyponatremia can also occur in severe paraproteinemia (usually protein concentrations higher than 12 to 15 g/dL) or hypertriglyceridemia. In this condition, a large proportion of the water composing the liquid portion of blood and the corresponding Na^+ is displaced by fat leading to an artifact in the laboratory measurement.

Treatment of Hyponatremia

Regardless of etiology, hyponatremia primarily affects the CNS. As the Na^+ concentration drops below 125 mEq/L, changes in cognition and motor function occur commonly. Confusion and seizures often occur at serum values less than 120 mEq/L, particularly if the decline occurs acutely. The severity of the complications increases rapidly with a declining Na^+ concentration; half of all patients with severe hyponatremia ($Na^+ < 105$ mEq/L) die.

While clearly there are risks from hyponatremia, there are also risks of treating it. Even though there are no definitive studies of the topic, it is generally agreed that the speed of correction should be in proportion to the chronicity of the problem. Unfortunately, the clinician oftentimes does not know the duration of hyponatremia. Practically speaking, most symptomatic hyponatremic patients should have the Na^+ corrected to an initial level of 120 to 130 mEq/L over a 12- to 24-h period, at an hourly rate not to exceed 1 to 2 mEq/L. (Without little supporting data, some experts sanction rapid normalization of hyponatremia, even when severe, if <1 to 2 days duration.) Slower correction (i.e., 0.5 mEq/L/h) is prudent in patients with chronic hyponatremia. Rapid correction of long-standing hyponatremia is associated with serious neurologic sequelae—central pontine myelinolysis (CPM). CPM is a CNS demyelinating syndrome characterized by weakness, dysarthria, dysphagia, coma, and potentially death. Risk factors include not only the rate of hyponatremia correction but also severity of the hyponatremia, advanced age, preexisting liver or CNS disorders, diuretic use, and alcoholism.

The treatment of hyponatremia depends on its cause and severity. In hypervolemic hyponatremia, restrictions of salt and fluid are the mainstays of therapy. However, diuretics or dialysis may be required when renal function is impaired. In most patients with hypovolemic hyponatremia, isotonic saline should be used to restore circulating volume. In isovolemic hyponatremia, free water restriction and treatment of the underlying disorder are preferred. In less-acute cases of SIADH, hyponatremia may respond to demeclocycline (600 to 1,200 mg/day). Rarely vaprisol (40 mg IV over 24 h) may be useful.

Most patients with severe and symptomatic hyponatremia (stupor, coma, seizures, etc.) require hypertonic saline and/or diuretics to achieve safe serum Na$^+$ with adequate speed. (Remember that 0.9% saline is significantly "hypertonic" for severely hyponatremic patients.) Relatively small increases in serum Na$^+$ on the order of 5% should decrease cerebral edema. One should slow correction once life-threatening manifestations have improved, typically to approximately 0.5 mEq/L/h. One way to calculate the amount of Na$^+$ to be given using 3% saline follows. Multiply the desired change in serum Na$^+$ times the estimated total body water to get the number of mEq of Na$^+$ to be administered. Divide that amount by the concentration of Na$^+$ in the fluid to be infused (513 mEq/L for 3% saline) to obtain the total volume to be administered. Then divide the total volume by the time over which the correction is desired to yield the infusion rate.

Example: A 60-kg woman with normal preoperative electrolytes develops seizures postoperatively while receiving hypotonic fluid. The serum Na$^+$ is 116 mEq.

Calculation to raise the serum Na$^+$ to 120 mEq over 4 h is as follows:

- Na$^+$ required (mEq) = $(120 - 116) \times (0.5 \times 60 \text{ kg})$ = 4×30 (120 mEq)
- Volume of 3% saline (mL) = 120 mEq / 513 mEq/L = (233 mL)
- Infusion rate = 233 mL/desired infusion time (4 h) = 58 mL/h

Hypernatremia

Etiology and Pathophysiology

Hypernatremia, defined as a serum Na$^+$ level more than 145 mEq/L, occurs when more water than Na$^+$ is lost from the body or when highly concentrated Na$^+$ solutions are administered or ingested. Hypernatremia is rare in patients with intact ADH

secretion, a sensitive thirst mechanism, and access to free water. Hence, it is primarily a disease of patients who are unable to obtain and drink fresh water (e.g., infants, elderly, bedridden, and critically ill), particularly those simultaneously sustaining increased water losses (e.g., diuretics, sweating). Hypernatremia implies hyperosmolarity, the major mechanism of toxicity.

Similar to hyponatremia, the problem can logically be thought of in three categories: high, normal, or low extracellular volume. Hypervolemic hypernatremia occurs from ingestion or infusion of hypertonic Na$^+$ containing solutions. For example, "normal" saline (0.9% NaCl) is modestly hypertonic (Na$^+$ 154 mEq/L, 308 mOsm/L) and without adequate free water, it tends to raise the serum Na$^+$ concentration while expanding extracellular volume. Hypernatremia is much more common when osmolarity is intentionally increased by hypertonic (3%) saline (Na$^+$ 513 mEq/L, 1,026 mOsm/L) or unintentionally by sodium bicarbonate (NaHCO$_3$) with a Na$^+$ of 595 mEq/L and 1,190 mOsm/L. Even though data on effectiveness are limited, 3% saline is now a widely used therapy for intracranial hypertension from cerebral edema. In this setting, serum hypertonicity attracts water from cerebrospinal fluid and brain cells thereby facilitating cerebral blood flow. For effect, serum Na$^+$ is typically maintained in the 145 to 155 mEq/L range (roughly 300 to 320 mOsm/L). Hypertonic saline is now also being used for field resuscitation of hemorrhagic shock because the fluid is low in cost, does not require refrigeration or cross-matching, and produces substantial intravascular volume expansion for the amount of fluid that must be transported. Hypernatremia can be an unintended consequence of NaHCO$_3$ if large volumes are administered to treat metabolic acidosis or cyclic antidepressant overdose. For patients with impaired Na$^+$ clearance, the Na$^+$–K$^+$ ion exchange resin, Kayexalate, can raise serum Na$^+$ by transferring significant salt loads across the bowel wall. Na$^+$ accumulations from primary hyperaldosteronism or salt or sea water ingestion are rare causes of hypernatremia.

Extracellular volume is normal, at least initially in a number of hypernatremic conditions. For example, both central and nephrogenic diabetes insipidus (DI) produce hypernatremia by preventing appropriate water reabsorption by the distal convoluted tubules and collecting ducts of the kidney. In central DI, ADH secretion is inadequate and in nephrogenic DI, the kidney does not respond normally to the secreted ADH. Hypernatremia with

TABLE 13-3 URINARY OSMOLALITY IN HYPERNATREMIA

URINE OSMOLARITY (mOsm)	DIFFERENTIAL DIAGNOSIS	THERAPY
>800	Dehydration Hypodipsia Sodium intoxication	Free water replacement
300–800	Osmotic diuretics Partial or mild DI	Free water replacement Trial of ADH
<300	Central or nephrogenic DI	Free water replacement and ADH therapy

near normal extracellular volume can also result from insensible (skin and lung) water losses of burns, tachypnea, or hyperthermia (high fever, heatstroke, neuroleptic malignant syndrome, malignant hyperthermia, etc.). Note that a high minute ventilation does not cause dehydration in mechanically ventilated patients because fully humidified gas is used.

Hypernatremia can also result from conditions that cause low extracellular volume such as vomiting, diarrhea, and osmotic diuretics such as glucose, mannitol, or glycerol. In each case, the tonicity of the fluid lost must be less than that of serum for hypernatremia to develop.

Diagnosis

Regardless of cause, the common symptoms of hypernatremia are thirst, nausea, vomiting, agitation, stupor, and coma. Unfortunately, all these symptoms are nonspecific, hence their cause often goes unrecognized. The history and physical examination typically lead to the correct diagnosis. It is usually obvious when $NaHCO_3$, 3% NaCl, or osmotic diuretics have been administered. The impressive urine output of the volume-replete patient with full-blown DI (up to 1 to 2 L/h) is also almost always noted. It is important to note that the diagnosis of DI may be missed if free water losses have progressed to the point that profound intravascular volume depletion has occurred. Caution must be exercised in the diagnosis of DI; in the unstable, volume-depleted patient in the ICU, the often recommended "water deprivation test" may prove harmful. A better strategy is to replace the circulating volume and empirically give a trial of ADH. When hemodynamically stable, additional endocrine testing, including a water deprivation test, may be safely performed. Although hypernatremia usually does not present a diagnostic challenge, the

urinary osmolarity can be particularly helpful if the etiology is unclear (Table 13-3).

Treatment

Treatment of hypernatremia consists of the replacement of water (either given enterally or as D_5W or a hypotonic NaCl solution), with frequent evaluation of electrolytes and osmolality. The speed of correction should depend on the chronicity of the problem and the severity of neurologic symptoms, but as a general rule, correction at a rate of 0.5 to 2 mEq/L each hour is an appropriate target. Expert recommendations also suggest that correction rates not exceed 12 mEq/L in a day or 18 mEq/L over two days. Like hyponatremia, very rapid correction, especially of longstanding hypernatremia, can precipitate CPM or cerebral edema. The latter condition results from rapid swelling of neurons which have accumulated "idiogenic osmoles" in an attempt to match the tonicity of serum during hypernatremia. If endogenous ADH is deficient or ineffective, it may be replaced with desmopressin (DDAVP), an ADH analog (see Chapter 32). In the less common cases of hypernatremia resulting from Na^+ gain, such as after the $NaHCO_3$ administration (cardiac arrest), the use of loop diuretics addition to Na^+ poor fluid may be necessary.

Unnecessarily precise calculations of "water deficit" are often performed in hypernatremia. It is important to recognize that the use of the conventional water deficit formula—Water deficit = (0.6 × weight) × (1 − [140/serum sodium concentration])—has limitations. It may underestimate the free water need in cases of hypotonic fluid losses (e.g., vomiting) and does not take into account the ongoing insensible losses. Because Na^+ concentrations less than 155 mEq/L rarely concern clinicians, by the time the decision is made to treat hypernatremia in the average sized adult, water deficits average 4 to 6 L. If the goal is to correct the deficit over 1 to 2 days, IV infusion of D_5W at 200 mL/h is usually effective unless the initial Na^+ concentration is much higher or ongoing water losses are substantial.

■ POTASSIUM DISORDERS

Hypokalemia

Ninety-five percent of total body potassium (K^+) is intracellular, but the K^+ concentration in the small extracellular compartment critically influences the neuromuscular and cardiac function. Humans consume an average of 100 mEq of K^+ daily of which normally 90 mEq is excreted by the kidney and almost all the rest leaves the body through the gastrointestinal (GI) tract. Because normal *obligatory* K^+ losses are only 5 to 10 mEq/day, and because the intracellular storage pool of K^+ is very large, hypokalemia is uncommon unless losses or impaired intake occurs for a substantial period of time. As a corollary, once hypokalemia (K^+ < 3.5 mEq/L) is manifest, the average deficit is large—250 to 300 mEq (5% to 10% of the total body stores). Similarly, because repleting intracellular K^+ requires the ions to traverse the small intravascular compartment, even modest K^+ doses may induce hyperkalemia if given rapidly. Systemic pH significantly influences extracellular K^+ concentrations. In patients with acidosis, hydrogen ions move into cells raising extracellular K^+. Therefore, hypokalemia during acidosis suggests an even larger total-body deficit.

Etiology

Hypokalemia may result from decreased intake, increased losses, or redistribution of K^+. Measurement of urinary K^+ and chloride (Cl^-) concentrations and pH is very helpful in determining the etiology of hypokalemia (Table 13-4). If urinary K^+ levels are less than 20 mEq/L, either decreased intake or excessive GI losses are to blame. (The normally functioning kidney can reduce K^+ excretion to <10 mEq/day, a level almost always less than intake.) Furthermore, although the K^+ content of stool may reach 60 mEq/L, with the exception of cholera-like illnesses, cathartic abuse, and villous adenomas, GI losses are rarely severe enough to produce symptomatic hypokalemia. Likewise, losses of K^+ directly from gastric fluid are minimal. Thus, vomiting induces hypokalemia—not through direct losses, but by promoting renal K^+ wasting as a result of volume depletion and hypochloremic metabolic alkalosis.

If the urinary K^+ concentration is high (>20 mEq/L), measurement of arterial pH and urinary Cl^- helps determine the diagnosis. High urinary K^+ with acidosis usually is caused by renal tubular acidosis or diabetic ketoacidosis. If high urinary K^+ losses are accompanied by alkalosis, urinary Cl^- becomes key to diagnosis. A low value (<10 mEq/L) is indicative of diuretic use, vomiting, or nasogastric suction, all of which are usually clinically evident. Diuretic use constitutes the most common cause of hypokalemia. Diuretics increase distal tubular flow, promoting the exchange of Na^+ for K^+, induce secondary hyperaldosteronism, and

TABLE 13-4   URINE ELECTROLYTES IN HYPOKALEMIA

	IF URINARY POTASSIUM > 20 mEq/L		
		ALKALEMIA	
NORMAL ACID–BASE STATUS	ACIDEMIA	URINE Cl^- < 10 mEq/L	URINE Cl^- > 10 mEq/L

Drug or electrolyte disorder likely
  Amphotericin B
  Penicillin
  Aminoglycosides
  Platinum compounds
  Hypomagnesemia
	Diabetic ketoacidosis
	Renal tubular acidosis
		Diuretics
		Vomiting
		Gastric suction
			Mineralocorticoid excess

IF URINARY POTASSIUM < 20 mEq/L			

Extrarenal mechanism is etiologic
  Decreased dietary intake
  Diarrhea			

encourage alkalosis, resulting in a shift of K⁺ from the extracellular to the intracellular compartment. A high urinary K⁺ accompanied by an elevated urinary Cl⁻ concentration (>10 mEq/L) and alkalosis usually is due to mineralocorticoid excess (e.g., primary hyperaldosteronism, Cushing syndrome, cirrhosis, or intravascular volume depletion). Magnesium is a cofactor for the enzyme Na⁺–K⁺ ATPase, which may be a partial explanation for high renal K⁺ losses observed in patients with hypomagnesemia.

A number of events which facilitate K⁺ entry into cells may cause hypokalemia without loss of K⁺ from the body. For example, high insulin levels, whether exogenous or induced by continuous parenteral or enteral alimentation, increase cellular uptake. Metabolic alkalosis also causes K⁺ to enter cells in exchange for H⁺. (On average, K⁺ levels decline 0.1 to 0.4 mEq/L for each 0.1-unit increase in pH.) In turn, hypokalemia increases renal HCO_3^- absorption, perpetuating the alkalosis. In addition, administration of β-adrenergic agonists facilitates transport of K⁺ from blood into cells but plasma K⁺ rarely declines by more than 0.5 mEq/L.

Pathophysiology

Hypokalemia increases the resting membrane potentials of neural and muscular tissues, reducing excitability. Hypokalemia impairs muscle contractility and, when severe (K⁺ < 2.5 mEq/L), may cause profound, even life-threatening muscle weakness. The severity of the muscular effects of a given K⁺ level depends on pH, calcium, and the rapidity with which hypokalemia developed. The muscles of the lower extremities usually are the first to be affected, followed by those of the trunk and the respiratory system. Even moderate degrees of hypokalemia may impair smooth muscle function, producing ileus, or intestinal pseudo-obstruction. Severe hypokalemia

also impairs the vascular smooth muscle response to catecholamines and angiotensin, influencing blood pressure stability. Severe hypokalemia can cause cell membrane damage, resulting in rhabdomyolysis. Although focal neurologic findings rarely result from hypokalemia, lethargy and confusion can occur in severe K⁺ depletion. Virtually any arrhythmia may surface during hypokalemia, especially in the presence of digitalis. Mild hypokalemia delays ventricular repolarization and is manifested by ST segment depression, diminished or inverted T waves, heightened U waves, and a prolonged QU interval. When hypokalemia is severe (K⁺ < 2.5 mEq/L), P wave amplitude, PR interval, and QRS duration increase (Fig. 13-1).

Treatment

Total body deficits of K⁺ usually exceed 200 mEq in patients with hypokalemia. Hence, it should not be surprising that the common practice of administering a small KCl replacement dose (i.e., 20 to 40 mEq) almost always is inadequate for correction. However, because the intracellular space must be accessed via the small intravascular compartment, K⁺ therapy (especially intravenous replacement) must be cautiously and closely monitored to avoid potentially harmful hyperkalemia. Because of the limited capacity to excrete K⁺, special care must be exercised when replacing K⁺ in patients with renal disease or diabetes and in those receiving drugs that block renin, angiotensin, or prostaglandin activity. Angiotensin-converting enzyme (ACE) inhibitors, angiotensin receptor blockers (ARBs), potassium-sparing diuretics (e.g., spironolactone), and nonsteroidal anti-inflammatory drugs (NSAIDs) are all examples of such medications. Almost every condition which causes hypokalemia also causes magnesium wasting. Hypomagnesemia aggravates the physiologic effects of hypokalemia and renders

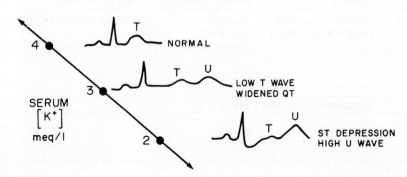

■ **FIGURE 13-1** ECG manifestations of hypokalemia.

deficit correction difficult. Therefore, it makes some sense to empirically administer magnesium to severely hypokalemic patients. Possibly the most vexing situation occurs when hypokalemia and acidosis coexist. Correction of acidosis aggravates the hypokalemia and often requires very aggressive K⁺ administration. In this uncommon situation, consideration should be given to the use of $KHCO_3$ for replacement rather than the more common KCl. Alternatively, hemodialysis using a bath containing HCO_3 and a higher K⁺ concentration is an effective treatment strategy.

As a general rule, K⁺ should not be infused more quickly than 40 mEq/h, and only in urgent circumstances. In fact many pharmacies now limit dispensed quantities of IV KCl to 40 mEq. Infusion into a peripheral vein is often painful; it occasionally induces chemical phlebitis, and if extravasated into soft tissue, it can cause necrosis. Rapid infusion of K⁺ into a central venous catheter terminating in or near the heart can result in arrhythmias. It is best to administer intravenous K⁺ diluted in non–glucose-containing solutions. (When glucose is coinfused, insulin release is stimulated, causing rapid incorporation of K⁺ into cells which can potentially aggravate hypokalemia.) When possible, K⁺ deficits should be replaced with enteral preparations. One note of caution: If KCl solutions are repeatedly placed directly into the small bowel via feeding tube, irritation and even ulceration may develop.

Hyperkalemia

It is difficult for healthy subjects to develop hyperkalemia because even minimally functional kidneys efficiently excrete excess K⁺. Furthermore, when renal clearance decreases, the colon may increase excretion. Cellular buffering (particularly by muscle and liver) acutely blunts the impact of a K⁺ load while the kidneys eliminate the excess. Insulin deficiency inhibits cellular buffering, whereas excretion requires functioning kidneys. Therefore, K⁺ handling is greatly impaired in patients with diabetes and renal insufficiency. K⁺-sparing diuretics (e.g., spironolactone), ACE inhibitors, ARBs, and, less commonly, nonsteroidal anti-inflammatory agents can induce hyperkalemia, especially in patients with baseline reductions in GFR or intrinsic renal disease.

Diagnosis

Pseudohyperkalemia may occur if venous blood is analyzed after prolonged tourniquet application or if the blood is hemolyzed. Serum K⁺ values are normally 0.5 mEq/L higher than the plasma values because K⁺ is released from platelets during clotting. However, marked hemolysis, severe leukocytosis (>100,000/mm³), or thrombocytosis (>10⁶/mm³) also may raise the K⁺ of the clotted specimen to extraordinary levels. The diagnosis of clot-related "pseudohyperkalemia" is confirmed by detecting a disparity between simultaneous determinations of plasma and serum K⁺. Hemolysis can usually be confirmed by simple visual inspection of the sample.

Mechanisms

Three basic mechanisms contribute to hyperkalemia: (i) increased K⁺ intake, (ii) redistribution of K⁺ from the intracellular to the extracellular compartment, and (iii) decreased K⁺ excretion.

Even with the wide distribution of K⁺ supplements, hyperkalemia from excessive intake alone is uncommon. (However, the simultaneous intake of KCl with a K⁺-sparing diuretic and an ACE inhibitor often results in hyperkalemia.) Likewise, iatrogenic K⁺ overloading often is seen in hospitalized patients with limited excretory power. Ringer's lactate contains 4 mEq/L of K⁺ and therefore should be administered carefully to patients with renal insufficiency. Potassium penicillin G contains 1.6 mEq of K⁺ for each 10⁶ units of penicillin, constituting a significant K⁺ load in patients receiving high penicillin doses. Packed red cells, stored for long periods, may deliver more than 7 mEq/unit. Renal transplant recipients receive significant intraoperative K⁺ loads when donor kidneys perfused with Collins' solution (140 mEq/L) are implanted.

Acidosis is the most common cause of redistributive hyperkalemia. Changes in serum K⁺ are more sensitive to changes in the bicarbonate concentration than to pH itself. Therefore, respiratory acidosis has relatively little effect on K⁺, whereas metabolic acidosis exerts a potent effect. Insulin stimulates intracellular transport of K⁺ from plasma, thus when its deficiency leads to the development of ketoacidosis, two mechanisms are operative to redistribute K⁺ from cells to plasma. Digitalis toxicity poisons the cellular Na⁺/K⁺ pump and may produce severe refractory hyperkalemia. β-adrenergic blockers also can increase the serum K⁺ by blocking adrenergic-receptor–mediated cellular uptake of K⁺. Hyperkalemia may follow the breakdown of red blood cells from hemolytic transfusion reactions or from large hematomas.

Any injury that produces extensive tissue necrosis, but particularly rhabdomyolysis, crush injuries, burns, and tumor lysis, can cause hyperkalemia. Finally, succinylcholine (a depolarizing neuromuscular blocker) predictably produces a small rise in plasma K^+ (approx. 0.5 mEq/L) but may precipitate striking hyperkalemia in patients with burns, tetanus, or other neuromuscular diseases. These effects are minimized by pretreatment with a subparalyzing dose of a nondepolarizing neuromuscular blocker.

Even though 80% to 90% of normal GFR must be lost before the kidney noticeably fails to excrete K^+, renal insufficiency remains the most common cause of hyperkalemia. Among patients with renal insufficiency, concomitant drug therapy often is a complicating factor (Table 13-5). Acidosis induced by renal failure further impairs the ability of the kidney to excrete K^+ and promotes the shift of K^+ from cellular stores into the circulation. In renal failure of abrupt onset, serum K^+ tends to rise faster than the BUN or creatinine, especially when exogenous K^+ is given; low tubular flow rates immediately prevent exchange of Na^+ for K^+, whereas creatinine and BUN require time to accumulate to noteworthy concentrations. However, even when complete renal shutdown occurs, the serum K^+ concentration seldom rises more than 0.5 mEq/L/day in response to the usual loads. (When normal K^+ intake is exceeded or excessive release occurs from the damaged cells, this rate may be surpassed.)

Aldosterone is required to maintain circulating volume and to enable tubular secretion of K^+. Therefore, primary adrenal insufficiency should be strongly considered in patients with hyperkalemia and prominent fluid deficits. Though even with primary adrenal failure, hyperkalemia usually is not significant in the absence of another confounding factor (e.g., increased K^+ intake or low GFR). Drugs that interfere with the formation or action of aldosterone (e.g., potassium-sparing diuretics, heparin, and ACE inhibitors and ARBs) also may produce overt hyperkalemia, especially as GFR declines.

Signs and Symptoms

Hyponatremia, hypocalcemia, hypermagnesemia, and acidosis potentiate the neuromuscular effects of hyperkalemia. Therefore, levels of Na^+, calcium, and magnesium should be evaluated and corrected concurrently. Functional impairment of skeletal muscle rarely occurs at K^+ levels less than 7.0 mEq/L. Hyperkalemia usually spares the respiratory muscles, cranial nerves, and deep tendon reflexes but commonly causes weakness of the proximal lower extremities. The most devastating effect of hyperkalemia is cardiac arrhythmias; however, the myocardial-impairing and vasodilatory effects of severe hyperkalemia may precipitate refractory hypotension.

An electrocardiogram (ECG) should be obtained for every patient with a K^+ more than 5.5 mEq/L (Fig. 13-2). Narrowing and peaking of T waves and QT interval shortening are typically seen with levels of 5.5 to 7 mEq/L. Lengthening of the PR interval and widening of the QRS complex (because of delayed depolarization) are often seen when concentrations reach 6.5 to 8.5 mEq/L. Atrial activity usually is lost shortly before the characteristic sine wave hybrid of ventricular tachycardia/fibrillation appears at levels greater than 8 mEq/L.

Treatment

The aggressiveness with which hyperkalemia is treated should parallel the severity of the clinical manifestations of the disorder—largely the ECG manifestations. When an elevated K^+ develops in a patient with risk factors for hyperkalemia (e.g., renal insufficiency, tumor lysis) and significant clinical or ECG manifestations are present, immediate treatment is indicated. In situations which **5** are less obvious or urgent, the diagnosis should be confirmed before initiating therapy due to the potential risk of inducing hypokalemia if the initial high K^+ value is spurious. (A repeat K^+ and leukocyte and platelet counts and an ECG should be obtained.) If the ECG is normal, treatment can usually await a repeat confirmatory K^+ determination. If the ECG is diagnostically abnormal, muscle weakness is present, or a reliable K^+ determination is more than 7 mEq/L, immediate action is indicated. Continuous ECG monitoring should be initiated, followed by treatment on five fronts as

TABLE 13-5 DRUGS ASSOCIATED WITH DECREASED RENAL POTASSIUM EXCRETION

ACE inhibitors
ARBs
Cyclosporine
Heparin
NSAIDs
Potassium-sparing diuretics

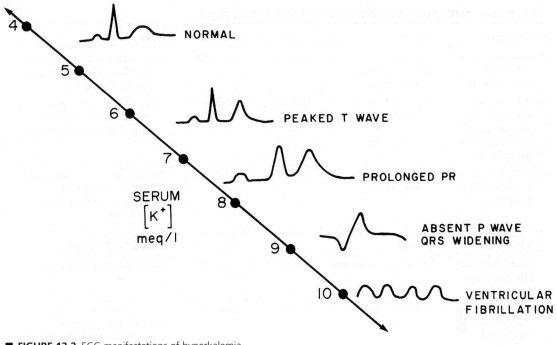

■ **FIGURE 13-2** ECG manifestations of hyperkalemia.

outlined in Table 13-6: (i) stop all K+ administration, (ii) expand intravascular volume, (iii) begin removing K+ from the body, (iv) administer drugs to shift K+ into the cellular compartment, and (v) stabilize neuromuscular and cardiac function with calcium.

While it may seem obvious, surprisingly often K+ therapy is not discontinued. It is important to consider all sources including standing orders for oral and IV supplementation and enteral and parenteral feedings. In patients who have intravascular volume depletion and those who are volume replete but can tolerate fluid administration, rapid infusion of isotonic saline can increase GFR promoting K+ excretion and will dilute the plasma K+ concentration. After achieving adequate intravascular volume, a loop diuretic can enhance excretion in patients making urine. Ion exchange resins lower K+ levels by trading Na+ for K+ across the bowel wall. (More Na+ is gained than K+ is lost, and electroneutrality is maintained by additional losses of magnesium and calcium.) Resultant Na+ gain may produce volume overload in oliguric or anuric patients. A typical 50-mg dose of resin decreases K+ levels by 0.5 to 1 mEq/L. When given orally, ion exchange resins require a vehicle to prevent constipation (usually 20% sorbitol solution). Dialysis is usually required for effective K+ removal from patients with renal insufficiency, severe hyperkalemia, or high K+ loads that result from multiple trauma or tumor lysis. Hemodialysis may extract 40 mEq/h or more, whereas peritoneal dialysis removes only 5 to 10 mEq/h.

Shifting K+ from blood into cells using insulin, *β*-2 adrenergic agonists, or $NaHCO_3$ rapidly lowers the serum concentration, but it is short-lived. A 10-unit intravenous bolus of regular insulin usually is sufficient to produce at least transient reduction in K+ levels. Patients with normal blood sugar levels should receive glucose (25 to 50 gm) concurrently to prevent hypoglycemia. Insulin produces a reduction in serum K+ of 1 to 3 mEq/L within minutes, and it may last several hours. Nebulized *β*-2 adrenergic agonists have been shown to act synergistically with insulin to decrease K+ levels, but high doses or prolonged therapy is usually required. $NaHCO_3$ causes an exchange of H+ for K+ across cell membranes in patients with intracellular acidosis but its effectiveness in nonacidemic patients is questioned.

When the K+ concentration exceeds 8 mEq/L or there is demonstrable lengthening of the PR interval or widening of the QRS complex, calcium treatment is indicated. Calcium (1 to 2 g of IV $CaCl_2$) rapidly stabilizes cardiac conduction and though it acts within minutes, its effect usually persists less than 2 h. Calcium salts should be administered with caution to patients receiving digitalis preparations.

TABLE 13-6 THERAPEUTIC OPTIONS FOR HYPERKALEMIA

TREATMENT	ACTION	ONSET	DURATION	NOTES
Intravenous saline (0.9% NaCl, 200–300 mL/h)	Diluent Enhances renal excretion	Minutes	Hours to days	Risks hypervolemia, hypernatremia, hypocalcemia, and hypomagnesemia
Insulin (10 U regular), add one to two ampules D50W for normoglycemic patients	Enhances cellular uptake	Minutes	Several hours	Risks hyperglycemia and hypoglycemia. Requires careful glucose monitoring
NaHCO$_3$ (one to two ampules over 5–10 min)	Enhances cellular uptake	Minutes	Several hours	Risks hypervolemia, alkalosis, and hypernatremia Probably only effective in acidemia
Nebulized β agonist (albuterol)	Enhances cellular uptake	Minutes	Minutes to hours	Modest effect Risks tachyarrhythmias
Calcium gluconate (10–20 mL over 5 min)	Membrane stabilizer	Minutes	Minutes to hours	May induce hypercalcemia
Diuretics (furosemide 40–160 mg)	Enhances renal excretion	Minutes	Several hours	Ineffective in renal failure Risks volume depletion Loop plus thiazide diuretic synergistic
Dialysis	Direct removal	Minutes	Hours to days	Hemodialysis most effective Risks all complications of dialysis
Potassium-binding resins (Kayexalate 50 g p.o. or rectally)	Enhances GI excretion	Hours	Hours to days	Risks hypernatremia, volume overload Delayed effect Add sorbitol for catharsis

■ CALCIUM DISORDERS

Normally each day approximately 1,200 mg of calcium (Ca^{2+}) is ingested, but only one third of that total is absorbed; renal excretion varies to balance serum levels between 8.5 and 10.5 mg/dL. Vitamin D serves to increase the gut absorption and renal tubular reabsorption of Ca^{2+}. Parathyroid hormone (PTH) also exerts significant influence over serum Ca^{2+} balance by increasing the release of Ca^{2+} from bone and promoting reabsorption of Ca^{2+} in the kidneys' distal tubule.

Hypercalcemia

Etiology

Although there is some mechanistic overlap, the long list of possible causes of hypercalcemia (Table 13-7) can be thought of as having three basic mechanisms: increased gut absorption, decreased renal excretion, or redistribution of Ca^{2+} from bone to serum. Relatively few disorders are responsible for most cases of hypercalcemia and the list can be rapidly culled by taking a careful history and obtaining a few basic laboratory tests. Neoplasia and primary hyperparathyroidism together account for 80% to 90% of cases, with all other causes comprising the remainder. Furthermore, the hypercalcemia associated with hyperparathyroidism is usually mild and only uncommonly causes significant intravascular volume depletion. Thus, most cases of significant hypercalcemia are the result of malignancy. Interestingly, when neoplasia is the cause, 50% of patients have no evidence of bony metastases.

Signs and Symptoms

The signs and symptoms of hypercalcemia are nonspecific but most commonly result from the two major pathophysiologic derangements—dehydration

TABLE 13-7   CAUSES OF HYPERCALCEMIA

INCREASED GUT ABSORPTION	DECREASED RENAL EXCRETION	ENHANCED BONE RELEASE
Vitamin D or A intoxication	Thiazide diuretics	Nonbone malignancy
Milk–alkali syndrome	Adrenal insufficiency	Multiple myeloma
Sarcoidosis	Intravascular volume depletion	Immobilization
Hyperparathyroidism (via increased Vitamin D levels)		Hyperparathyroidism
		Hyperthyroidism
		Paget disease

and depressed neuromuscular function. Hypercalcemia induces an osmotic diuresis, but if fluid intake is unrestricted, severe Ca^{2+} elevations are unlikely. Unfortunately, the decreased gut motility of hypercalcemia often produces nausea, vomiting, abdominal pain, and constipation, negating this mode of compensation. The most common manifestations of hypercalcemia are neuromuscular disturbances (lethargy, weakness, fatigue, delirium, and coma). **6** Symptoms correlate poorly with Ca^{2+} concentrations, but severe manifestations are rare unless levels exceed 14 mg/dL. The ECG reflects the altered cellular electrical potential when it demonstrates a truncated QT or increased PR interval. Rarely, complete heart block occurs. Ca^{2+} salts form and are deposited in the tissue when a critical calcium-phosphate product (usually >60) is reached. In the kidney, renal stones and renal insufficiency may result from these complexes; skin deposits may induce pruritus. Muscle and other soft tissue also may be affected by this "metastatic" calcification. Pancreatitis or peptic ulcer diseases are rare presentations. Hypercalcemia may produce hypertension by increasing the peripheral vascular resistance, an effect that is usually offset by significant volume depletion.

Laboratory Evaluation

Ca^{2+} is predominately an extracellular cation, and because as much as one half of the total serum Ca^{2+} is bound to proteins (predominately albumin), Ca^{2+} levels must be evaluated in light of the serum protein level. For example, hyperproteinemic states such as myeloma can raise the total serum Ca^{2+} levels. Vulnerable to dietary influences, the serum PO_4^{3-} level is a highly labile measurement but, normally, an inverse relationship exists between the serum PO_4^{3-} and Ca^{2+}. When this usual relationship is violated and both serum Ca^{2+} and PO_4^{3-} levels are elevated, vitamin D–related disorders and thyrotoxicosis are likely causes. PO_4^{3-} levels are usually low in primary hyperparathyroidism and malignancy. Urinary Ca^{2+} usually is very high in hypercalcemic disorders that are not dependent on parathyroid hormone (PTH) activity (i.e., sarcoid or vitamin D intoxication). Vitamin D levels are useful in confirming suspected toxicity but are not diagnostic in any other form of hypercalcemia. Although frequently assayed, PTH levels are not helpful diagnostically unless markedly elevated in a patient with severe hypercalcemia and normal renal function. Even mild renal insufficiency severely limits the use of certain PTH assays because it decreases the clearance of the commonly assayed carboxy-PTH fragment. For this reason, midmolecule or amino-terminal assays are superior.

Treatment

Among the various causes of symptomatic hypercalcemia, malignancy is the most common; therefore, effective therapy usually requires treatment of the primary tumor. As with hyperkalemia, the simplest and most rapid method to begin reducing Ca^{2+} is to expand the circulating volume with isotonic saline. Although the absolute magnitude of this intervention is usually small (reductions of 1 to 3 mg/dL), such corrections often are critical in reducing the symptoms. After volume expansion, loop diuretics, like furosemide, are rapidly effective in lowering the Ca^{2+} concentration if good urine flow is established. By blocking Ca^{2+} reabsorption in the kidney, furosemide can reduce the serum levels as much as 4 to 5 mg/dL each day. A reasonable goal for saline and diuretic therapy is to establish and maintain a urine output of 200 mL/h. Corticosteroids are relatively ineffective at lowering serum

Ca^{2+} unless the cause is adrenal insufficiency, vitamin D intoxication, sarcoidosis, or a corticosteroid responsive malignancy. (Corticosteroids are also an adjunctive treatment for hyperthyroidism.) In situations where they might be expected to have effect, corticosteroids work within hours. Phosphate binds Ca^{2+} in the gut, rendering it insoluble and decreasing its absorption. Diarrhea sometimes limits the dose.

Calcitonin decreases renal tubular Ca^{2+} reabsorption, inhibits osteoclast function, and promotes the incorporation of Ca^{2+} into bone but is expensive and subject to tachyphylaxis. In symptomatic patients with severe hypercalcemia, doses of 2 to 8 units given every 6 to 12 h (IV or subcutaneously) can produce prompt (4 to 6 h) but modest (1 to 2 mg/dL) reductions in serum Ca^{2+} levels. (Calcitonin's effectiveness is augmented by glucocorticoids.) Biphosphonates are more potent than calcitonin but require days before effects are seen. Biphosphonates decrease Ca^{2+} release by inhibiting the osteoclast function. They are the preferred agents for hypercalcemia of malignancy. The currently used agents are etidronate (7.5 mg/kg/day in 250 mL of NS over 4 h, given for 3 days). Only one dose of pamidronate (60 to 90 mg infusion over 2 to 4 h) maintains lower Ca^{2+} levels for 2 to 3 weeks. A single dose of zoledronic acid (4 to 8 mg IV over 15 min) is the most potent and convenient of the three, lowering the Ca^{2+} levels for up to a month. Gallium also decreases bone resorption but must be given by continuous infusion and can be nephrotoxic. In the truly emergent setting, serum Ca^{2+} levels of the hypercalcemic patient can be reduced rapidly by hemodialysis.

Hypocalcemia

Mild hypocalcemia occurs commonly but rarely is symptomatic. Overt hypocalcemia is less common than symptomatic hypercalcemia but is just as life threatening. The urgency of evaluation and treatment depends on the severity of symptoms.

Clinical Manifestations

Hypocalcemia usually is asymptomatic if ionized Ca^{2+} remains normal despite low total Ca^{2+} levels or if hypocalcemia develops slowly. Alkalosis, however, lowers the fraction of ionized Ca^{2+}, aggravating the symptoms. The threshold at which symptoms develop in hypocalcemia is highly variable; most symptoms are due to neuromuscular irritability. The most common complaints are paresthesia, cramps, or tetany. Dyspnea or stridor may occur if ventilatory or upper airway muscles are affected. Although usually a consequence of hypocalcemia, tetany also may develop in acute respiratory alkalosis and acute hyperkalemia. Rare but more specific signs of neuromuscular irritability, including carpopedal spasm (Trousseau's sign) or facial muscle hyperreflexia (Chvostek's sign), may be elicited in patients with hypocalcemia. Other potential CNS effects include seizures, papilledema, hallucinations, confusion, and depression. In humans, the relationship between hypocalcemia and impaired circulatory system performance is speculative, but in experimental models, hypocalcemia may compromise perfusion by lowering the systemic vascular resistance and decreasing the cardiac contractility. The QT prolongation seen with hypocalcemia may result in a variety of arrhythmias (most significantly, *torsades de pointes*).

Causes

There are four mechanisms of hypocalcemia: (i) decreases in serum protein concentration, (ii) binding and sequestration of Ca^{2+}, (iii) inability to mobilize bone Ca^{2+}, and (iv) decreased Ca^{2+} intake or absorption. Because most Ca^{2+} is bound to the serum proteins, reductions in protein concentration result in hypocalcemia. A reduction in albumin of 1 gm/dL reduces the serum Ca^{2+} level by approximately 0.8 mg/dL. Ca^{2+} may be removed from the circulation by binding to other drugs or chemicals such as phosphate, chelating agents (e.g., ethylenediaminetetraacetic acid [EDTA]), or the citrate anticoagulant used to prevent the clotting of dialysis circuits or transfused blood. Ca^{2+} may also bind inflamed intra-abdominal fat in pancreatitis. Hyperphosphatemia induces hypocalcemia in patients with renal failure or in those who are otherwise unable to excrete PO_4^{3-} normally. Reductions in Ca^{2+} intake or impaired absorption resulting from reduced activity of vitamin D also may induce hypocalcemia. Anticonvulsants and glucocorticoids impair Ca^{2+} absorption (probably by inhibiting vitamin D action). Although renal failure decreases vitamin D production, symptomatic hypocalcemia usually is prevented by the development of secondary hyperparathyroidism. PTH deficiency and resistance to PTH are rare causes of hypocalcemia, except in patients undergoing thyroid or parathyroid surgery. For such patients, life-threatening hypocalcemia may develop within hours of surgery.

TABLE 13-8 CAUSES OF HYPOCALCEMIA

Alkalosis
Anticonvulsant use
Citrate
Dialysis anticoagulation
Massive transfusion
Fat embolism syndrome
Foscarnet
Gadolinium (pseudohypocalcemia)
Hypoparathyroidism
Hypoalbuminemia
Hypomagnesemia
Hyperphosphatemia
Burns
Renal failure
Rhabdomyolysis
Tumor lysis syndrome
Renal failure—chronic
Pancreatitis
Severe sepsis
Vitamin D deficiency

Therefore, monitoring postoperative Ca^{2+} assumes added importance after surgical procedures in the neck, which have the potential to injure the parathyroid glands. Very rarely, protracted, severe hypotension may result in parathyroid infarction and subsequent hypocalcemia. Magnesium (Mg) levels should be obtained in hypocalcemic patients because Mg is necessary for both PTH secretion and action. Hypocalcemia secondary to hypomagnesemia is particularly common in alcoholics and in malnourished patients and those receiving diuretics. Some Gadolinium-based contrast agents interfere with the laboratory assays of Ca^{2+} causing spurious hypocalcemia. The causes of hypocalcemia are outlined in Table 13-8.

Treatment

The first step in the treatment of hypocalcemia is to ensure airway patency and adequate ventilation and perfusion. Serum levels of K^+, Mg, vitamin D, and PTH should be obtained. Alkalosis should be corrected to raise the ionized Ca^{2+} fraction. In non-emergent settings, hyperphosphatemia should first be corrected with PO_4^{3-} binders and a low PO_4^{3-} diet, preferably before administering Ca^{2+}. Ca^{2+} administration in the setting of profound hyperphosphatemia is unlikely to correct the defect because calcium phosphate salts will rapidly deposit in tissues. Ca^{2+} replacement is always empiric because deficits are impossible to calculate accurately.

Therefore, correction must be guided by serial determinations of serum Ca^{2+}. Symptomatic patients should be given intravenous Ca^{2+}, preferably via a large central vein because of the tendency of Ca^{2+} solutions to induce chemical phlebitis or tissue necrosis when given in peripheral veins. Intramuscular injection should be avoided. Slow infusion of 10 to 20 mL of 10% calcium gluconate is the preferred method of supplementation. Concomitant vitamin D deficiency should be treated. Therapy with the costly, 1,25-OH vitamin D analog may be required if renal and liver functions are compromised, but for patients with preserved hepatic and renal functions, nonhydroxylated vitamin D preparations suffice. Because thiazides increase the renal tubular Ca^{2+} reabsorption, they are useful adjuncts to increase serum Ca^{2+}.

■ PHOSPHATE DISORDERS

Phosphate (PO_4^{3-}) and Ca^{2+} coexist in the body in a complex inverse relationship. As PO_4^{3-} levels rise, serum Ca^{2+} concentrations decline and vice versa. The bulk of both ions is located in bone; hence, the treatment of hypocalcemia is often an intervention directed at lowering PO_4^{3-} concentrations.

Hyperphosphatemia

Because of the huge excess capacity of the normal kidney to excrete PO_4^{3-}, it is difficult to become hyperphosphatemic (>5 mg/dL) from increased intake alone. Vitamin D intoxication can cause hyperphosphatemia by enhancing GI absorption of PO_4^{3-} and increasing tubular reabsorption of PO_4^{3-} in the kidney, especially if intake is high. Deficiency of parathyroid hormone impairs renal PO_4^{3-} excretion, but it is alone a rare explanation for hyperphosphatemia. In the ICU, high levels of PO_4^{3-} usually reflect impaired excretion (i.e., renal insufficiency with GFR < 25 mL/min) with or without increased cellular release of PO_4^{3-} (e.g., rhabdomyolysis, hemolysis, tumor lysis, etc.). Symptoms, however, are few, apart from those of hypocalcemia induced by excess PO_4^{3-}. In treating hyperphosphatemia, attention should first be directed to the primary cause of PO_4^{3-} elevation. Obviously, it also makes sense to minimize PO_4^{3-} intake. Acutely, sevelamer (two to four capsules tid), calcium acetate (two tablets tid) or carbonate (1 gm tid), lanthanum carbonate (500 mg tid), and aluminum hydroxide (four tablets tid) all effectively bind PO_4^{3-}. In cases where hyperphosphatemia is causing severe hypocalcemia, dialysis may be required.

Hypophosphatemia

As the major intracellular anion, PO_4^{3-} plays an important role in lipid, protein, and sugar metabolism. Serum values imperfectly reflect the depletion of intracellular PO_4^{3-} stores responsible for clinical symptomatology. Although PO_4^{3-} is easily depleted from skeletal muscle and erythrocytes, levels tend to be well preserved in most other tissues, such as cardiac muscle. Hypophosphatemia results from impaired intake, increased GI or renal losses, or uptake by cells. Hence, malnutrition and alcoholism are major risk factors. Low levels of vitamin D tend to decrease PO_4^{3-} absorption and increase renal losses. Likewise, hyperparathyroidism increases renal excretion of PO_4^{3-}. GI losses (starvation, antacids and sucralfate binding, malabsorption, nasogastric suctioning, emesis, diarrhea, etc.) are common contributing factors. Renal losses from tubular dysfunction or more commonly from diuretics (loop, thiazides, and osmotic) are also prevalent. Extracellular to intracellular transfer of PO_4^{3-} occurs during anabolism, with insulin administration, during correction of metabolic acidosis, and in the acute phase of respiratory alkalosis. In the ICU, hypophosphatemia is commonly observed in alcoholics, during refeeding of the malnourished, during recovery from diabetic ketoacidosis, and during hyperventilation. In many such patients, hypophosphatemia is transient and does not reflect pathological PO_4^{3-} depletion.

As a rule, serum PO_4^{3-} must fall below 1.0 mg/dL before overt symptoms develop. Dysfunction of the cellular elements of the blood, muscle weakness, GI upset, neural dysfunction, and (rarely) tissue breakdown are the major clinical consequences. Depletion of 2,3-diphosphoglyceric acid (2,3-DPG) diminishes the ability of erythrocytes to unload oxygen to the tissues. Skeletal muscle dysfunction can rarely produce ventilatory failure or prolonged weaning. A sensorimotor neuropathy is occasionally observed 4 to 7 days after PO_4^{3-}-poor nutrition is started. Very rarely, severe PO_4^{3-} depletion can produce hemolysis, rhabdomyolysis, or congestive cardiomyopathy, especially when generous feeding is abruptly initiated in severely malnourished patients (the "refeeding syndrome").

Oral supplementation usually will suffice when the serum PO_4^{3-} is modestly reduced (>1.0 mg/dL). Because enteral absorption is incomplete, typically 2.5 to 3.5 gm of PO_4^{3-} supplementation is needed each day to achieve desired effects. Caution is advised because each 250 mg of PO_4^{3-} is accompanied by approximately 13 to 14 mEq of Na^+ or K^+ depending upon the product. Concurrent hypomagnesemia must be corrected for optimal effect. Oral PO_4^{3-} supplementation should continue for 5 to 10 days after reestablishing a normal serum level. Urgent correction should be reserved for situations in which clinical symptoms accompany serum PO_4^{3-} levels less than 1.0 mg/dL. As with K^+, PO_4^{3-} must traverse the small intravascular compartment to reach its intracellular target, so repletion must proceed cautiously. A daily IV infusion of 10 mg/kg of sodium or potassium phosphate will replete levels but doses should not exceed 2.5 mg/kg over 6 h so as to avoid raising the calcium-phosphate product to dangerous levels (>60 mg/dL). (Each milliliter of intravenous PO_4^{3-} repleting compounds provides 93 mg of PO_4^{3-} and approximately 4 mEq of K^+ or Na^+, respectively.)

■ MAGNESIUM DISORDERS

Of the roughly 25 gm of magnesium (Mg) present in the human body, more than 95% is intracellular (most in bone and muscle). Thus, similar to K^+, large Mg deficits exist before hypomagnesemia becomes evident and administration of Mg transiently increases the levels in the relatively small intravascular space even though intracellular deficits may persist. In contrast to K^+, Mg in blood is protein bound, hence hypoalbuminemia can reduce serum levels even when total body stores are adequate. To further complicate matters, the kidney is exquisitely effective in excreting Mg when plasma levels rise above normal. To highlight this fact, each day the average human ingests approximately 30 mEq of Mg, of which only 10 mEq is absorbed, and promptly, the kidney excretes 9.5 mEq and the gut loses the balance. Despite the high frequency of abnormal serum Mg values, clinical manifestations of hypermagnesemia or hypomagnesemia are uncommon, and the value of measuring Mg on a regular basis is uncertain.

Hypermagnesemia

Under normal circumstances, the gut and kidney work in concert to tightly regulate serum Mg levels. When deficient, gut absorption of Mg increases and renal excretion decreases. When a larger enteral Mg load is presented, the gut absorbs a smaller fraction and the kidney excretes a greater proportion. Therefore, hypermagnesemia is uncommon unless very large intravenous doses of $MgSO_4$ are infused for pre-eclampsia or Mg salts are given to patients with renal insufficiency. (For patients with severe renal insufficiency or ileus, gut absorption of Mg-containing cathartics may overload the excretory capacity.) Hypermagnesemia also has occurred after absorption of kidney stone "dissolving" drugs (e.g., Renacidin) that contain high concentrations of magnesium carbonate.

Clinically, hypermagnesemia presents as hyporeflexia and hypotension when levels exceed 4 mEq/dL, somnolence develops at levels greater than 7 mEq/dL, and heart block and paralysis present at levels greater than 10 mg/dL. Hypermagnesemia prolongs the PR interval on ECG, impairs conduction, and may produce heart block. Initially, calcium gluconate (1 to 2 g intravenously) should be administered to counter the neuromuscular effects. If renal function is preserved, administration of isotonic saline and loop diuretics can facilitate Mg excretion. (Emergent dialysis is usually necessary because hypermagnesemia is rarely seen in the absence of severe renal insufficiency.)

Hypomagnesemia

Hypomagnesemia is one of the most common electrolyte abnormalities in hospitalized patients, but its clinical importance often is unclear. Its common causes are presented in Table 13-9. Hypomagnesemia can result from inadequate intake, increased GI or renal losses, or movement into cells. (Excessive renal or GI losses are most common.) Because Mg is predominately absorbed in the small bowel, inflammatory bowel disease, chronic diarrhea, and malabsorption are common precipitants. Hypomagnesemia, from poor intake and increased renal and gut loss, is particularly common and important in alcoholics because Mg is a required cofactor for the action of thiamine. Although several types of renal disease may produce Mg wasting, it most commonly results from the use of diuretics (thiazides, loop, and osmotic). The osmotic diuresis produced by the glycosuria of diabetes is a common precipitant. "Forced saline diuresis" also may waste Mg during cancer chemotherapy or treatment of hypercalcemia or rhabdomyolysis. Aminoglycosides, cyclosporine, foscarnet, pentamidine, amphotericin, platinum, and alcohol all cause renal Mg loss. Perhaps more importantly, by encouraging K^+ egress from cells and Ca^{2+} release from bone, over the long run, hypomagnesemia may induce hypokalemia and hypocalcemia. Mg deficiency should be considered in patients with hypokalemia, hypocalcemia, and hypophosphatemia, especially if encountered together. There are also numerous less common conditions in which transport of Mg from plasma into the cells producing hypomagnesemia (e.g., refeeding syndrome, tumor growth, rhabdomyolysis, and pancreatitis) takes place.

Like hypocalcemia, hypomagnesemia causes neuromuscular irritability manifest as muscle cramps, increased reflexes, tremor, Trousseau's and Chvostek's signs, cranial nerve abnormalities, and even seizures. (Neuromuscular or cardiac effects rarely occur until serum levels are <1.0 mg/dL.) Hypomagnesemia predisposes to almost all types of arrhythmias (including *torsades de pointes* and those of digitalis toxicity); however, large clinical studies have been unable to confirm beneficial antiarrhythmic and survival effects of Mg in patients suffering from myocardial ischemia. The ECG effects of hypomagnesemia are nonspecific and rarely diagnostic.

Plasma levels imperfectly reflect total body Mg stores and correlate even less well with ionized Mg levels. Mg is inexpensive, and for patients with normal renal function, it is safe, even in large doses. For asymptomatic hypomagnesemic patients, oral MgO or $MgCl_2$ compounds usually are effective at raising the Mg level, but sometimes produce such severe diarrhea that hypomagnesemia actually worsens. If the oral route is chosen, 0.5 mEq/kg represents a good starting dose. In mildly symptomatic hypomagnesemia, 6 to 8 gm of $MgSO_4$ can be given IV each day. In life-threatening hypomagnesemic crises, $MgSO_4$ (1 to 2 gm) is given IV over 2 to 3 min, followed by 2 to 4 gm every 15 to 30 min until cardiac or neuromuscular abnormalities abate. In life-threatening cases, daily replacement of 6 to

TABLE 13-9 CAUSES OF HYPOMAGNESEMIA

Alcoholism
Diabetes
Diarrhea
Inflammatory bowel disease
Malnutrition, starvation
Medications
Aminoglycosides
Amphotericin
Cisplatinin
Cyclosporine
Digitalis
Diuretics (loop, thiazides, and osmotic)
Foscarnet
Pentamidine

8 gm of $MgSO_4$ is usually required to replete body stores. (It is prudent to measure serum levels once or twice daily to assure hypermagnesemia does not result.) Rapid intravenous Mg infusions can produce hypotension and therefore should be avoided except in emergent circumstances.

■ SUGGESTED READINGS

Adrogue HJ, Madias NE. Hypernatremia. *N Engl J Med.* 2000;342: 1493–1499.

Adrogue HJ, Madias NE. Hyponatremia. *N Engl J Med.* 2000;342: 1581–1589.

Ariyan CE, Sosa JA. Assessment and management of patients with abnormal calcium. *Crit Care Med.* 2004;32(Suppl. 4):S146–S154.

Bhardwaj A, Ulatowski JA. Hypertonic saline solutions in brain injury. *Curr Opin Crit Care.* 2004;10:126–131.

Charron T, Bernard F, Skrobik Y. Intravenous phosphate in the intensive care unit: More aggressive repletion regimens for moderate and severe hypophosphatemia. *Intensive Care Med.* 2003;29(8): 1273–1278.

Gaasbeek A, Meinders AE. Hypophosphatemia: An update on its etiology and treatment. *Am J Med.* 2005;118(10):1094–1101.

Gennari FJ. Disorders of potassium homeostasis: Hypokalemia and hyperkalemia. *Crit Care Clin.* 2002;18(2):273–288, vi.

Milionis HJ, Liamis GL, Elisaf MS. The hyponatremic patient: A systematic approach to laboratory diagnosis. *CMAJ.* 2002;166(8):1056–1062.

Moe SM. Disorders of calcium, phosphorus, and magnesium. *Am J Kidney Dis.* 2005;45(1):213–218.

Murase T, Sugimura Y, Takefuji S, et al. Mechanisms and therapy of osmotic demyelination. *Am J Med.* 2006;119(7 Suppl. 1):S69–S73.

Palmer BF. Hyponatremia in neurosurgical patients: Syndrome of inappropriate antidiuretic hormone versus cerebral salt wasting. *Nephrol Dial Transplant.* 2000;125:262–268.

Palmer BF. Managing hyperkalemia caused by inhibitors of the renin-angiotensin-aldosterone system. *N Engl J Med.* 2004;351:585–592.

Stewart AF. Clinical practice: Hypercalcemia associated with cancer. *N Engl J Med.* 2005;352(4):373–379.

Verbalis JG, Goldsmith SR, Greenberg A, et al. Hyponatremia treatment guidelines 2007: Expert panel recommendations. *Am J Med.* 2007;120(11 Suppl. 1):S1–S21.

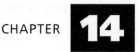

Blood Conservation and Transfusion

KEY POINTS

1 In hemodynamically stable, nonbleeding patients, reasonable target levels for hemoglobin are 7 to 9 gm/dL and greater than 20,000/mm³ for platelets. Higher levels may be appropriate in patients actively bleeding or those at particularly high risk from anemia or hemorrhage.

2 Many transfusions can be avoided if careful thought is given to blood conservation measures, including reevaluating transfusion triggers, limiting laboratory determinations to only those necessary, minimizing the volume of blood for each test, and thoughtfully using erythropoeisis stimulating agents.

3 Use of blood components effectively targets specific patient deficiencies and is a much more efficient use of the limited blood supply than use of whole blood.

4 Transfusion of leukocyte blood that has been stored less than 2 weeks is associated with better clinical outcomes including fewer organ failures; shorter time in the ICU and on the ventilator; and lower rates of death.

5 Massive transfusion of the actively bleeding patient should be guided by frequent measurements of hemoglobin, coagulation parameters, and platelet counts. Supplemental fresh frozen plasma and platelets are usually required after 5 to 10 units of packed red blood cells have been transfused.

■ INDICATIONS FOR BLOOD PRODUCTS

No blood is as good as your own. Setting aside concerns of transfusion-related infection and immune reactions, transfused blood is substantially less robust than native blood in its primary function of carrying O_2 to tissues and leaving it there. In addition, receiving another's blood is associated with numerous risks outlined below, some of which are only partially understood. Therefore, unless absolutely necessary, it is not a good idea to receive allogeneic transfusion or perhaps even one's own blood if it has been stored for more than several weeks. Despite the risks and limitations of transfusion, there are three situations in which blood product can be useful and even lifesaving: (i) to increase O_2-carrying capacity, (ii) to reverse deficiencies of clotting factors, and (iii) to correct thrombocytopenia.

Tissue oxygen delivery (DO_2) is the product of cardiac output, hemoglobin (Hgb) concentration and its saturation, plus the normally trivial contribution of O_2 dissolved in plasma. DO_2 remains adequate even in the face of profound anemia (Hgb of 3 to 4 gm/dL) if arterial saturation is normal and reductions in Hgb are offset by proportional increases in cardiac output or O_2 extraction. Unfortunately, these compensatory mechanisms are often impaired in critically ill patients and saturation is rarely normal without supplemental O_2. For these reasons, Hgb concentration has traditionally been maintained greater than 10 gm/dL, a value that corresponds to a hematocrit (Hct) $\geq$ 30%. By contrast, experimental evidence suggests that for most hemodynamically stable patients, substantially lower Hgb concentrations (approx. 7 gm/dL) are not only tolerated, but are also associated with better outcomes. **1** Similarly, the lower acceptable limit for Hgb can be relaxed in patients with long-standing anemia and in those whose tissues and cardiac performance accommodate to chronically reduced O_2 delivery (e.g., chronic renal failure). Conversely, traditional Hgb goals may be more important in patients with coronary or carotid ischemia, refractory hypoxemia, or limited cardiac reserve. Increasing Hgb however, does not always increase DO_2; as the Hct rises above 40%, increases in viscosity eventually reduce overall DO_2 (Fig. 14-1). In addition, depletion of 2,3-DPG (diphosphoglyceric acid) in stored blood results in a leftward shift in the oxyhemoglobin dissociation curve resulting in less tissue O_2 delivery

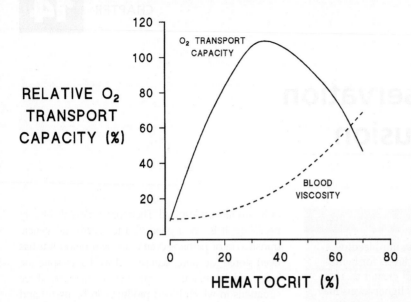

■ **FIGURE 14-1** Relationship between hematocrit, oxygen transport capacity, and serum viscosity. At low hematocrit values, oxygen transport capacity (*solid line*) is impaired because of anemia. Oxygen transport increases with a rising hematocrit reaching a maximum value when hematocrit nears 35% to 40%. Transport capacity declines after this peak because of nonlinear increases in blood viscosity (*broken line*).

than that of an identical concentration of native Hgb. Numerous other changes in stored red blood cells (RBCs), outlined below, further limit DO_2.

Administration of blood products solely to increase circulating volume is probably only rational in the setting of acute bleeding where there is concomitant anemia and coagulopathy (e.g., massive hemorrhage in trauma or bleeding in the patient with hepatic failure or disseminated intravascular coagulation [DIC]). However, even in hemorrhagic shock it makes sense to replace deficits with a combination of packed red blood cells (PRBCs) and crystalloid, unless massive losses necessitate supplemental plasma and platelet transfusion. In most settings, intravascular volume depletion can be corrected as quickly, with less risk and cost, using crystalloid solutions or non-blood-colloid.

There are clear indications for treatment with clotting factors, where no other option will suffice. These situations include (i) bleeding from congenital or acquired isolated factor deficiencies; (ii) hemorrhage due to multiple factor deficiencies from warfarin toxicity, hepatic failure, or consumptive or dilutional coagulopathy; and (iii) correction of severe thrombocytopenia resulting in hemorrhage.

■ ANEMIA

Approximately one third of patients are anemic at the time of intensive care unit (ICU) admission, and nearly half develop anemia by the third day in ICU. Greater than 85% of all patients with an ICU stay exceeding a week receive a blood component; and of the transfused group almost half receive more than 5 units of blood products. The incidence of anemia is understandable because patients enter the ICU with chronic diseases and while their RBC production is blunted by functional iron deficiency and by decreased erythropoietin production and sensitivity. Critically ill patients are also subjected to intense phlebotomy typically losing 40 to 70 mL of blood daily, a value that outstrips production capacity.

■ BLOOD PRODUCT CONSERVATION

Because of stricter rules for donation, blood supplies are decreasing while demands are increasing. The good news is that donor selection and enhanced blood testing have made blood supply safer now than ever with regard to traditional transfusion risks (e.g., viral hepatitis, human immunodeficiency virus [HIV]). Unfortunately, emerging data suggest transfusions may be associated with heretofore under or unappreciated hazards (e.g., immune modulation). Furthermore, blood products are very expensive in many locations: a unit of PRBCs now costs approximately $1,000. Because blood is increasingly scarce, expensive, and has potential dangers, it makes sense to limit the need for its use.

Perhaps half of all RBC transfusions could be averted if the volume and frequency of blood drawing were minimized, thresholds for transfusion were sensibly reduced, and erythropoiesis stimulating agents (ESAs) thoughtfully administered. Simple first steps to RBC conservation are the prohibition of "standing orders" for blood tests, reduced use of indwelling catheters, and whenever possible, use of alternative monitoring methods to minimize phlebotomy. Routine morning evaluations of chemistry and hematology panels and arterial blood gasses are unnecessary and wasteful for most patients. Blood test orders should be driven by clinical indication, not habit, or the solar cycle. Because they make obtaining samples easy, central venous and arterial catheters encourage sampling more frequently than is clinically necessary. Techniques such as bedside testing of blood glucose and the use of pulse oximetry and capnography to determine arterial O_2 and CO_2 tensions, respectively, can decrease bloodletting. ICU-based, small-volume, multichannel chemistry-blood gas analyzers can further reduce the quantity of blood used for monitoring as long as clinicians do not increase the frequency of testing because results are easy to obtain. Use of "cell savers" in trauma victims and in patients undergoing bloody surgical procedures is also prudent. Highly automated systems now collect shed blood from operative sites, mix it with an anticoagulant, wash the collected mixture, concentrate the RBCs, and then reinfuse them through a filter. For patients undergoing some elective operations, autologous transfusion is another technique to avoid donated cells.

ESAs like erythropoietin and darbepoetin comprise another element of an RBC conservation strategy. When administered just once a week, 40,000 U of recombinant human erythropoietin (rhEPO) has been shown to reduce the volume of RBCs transfused. Perhaps more important, about 10% of patients have avoided RBC transfusion altogether. Use of rhEPO requires the clinician to plan ahead; on average, a dose given today stimulates manufacture of the equivalent of roughly 1 unit of RBCs by next week. The lag time to produce results and the cost of rhEPO (about $300 weekly) have been barriers to use. One rational strategy for ESA use is (i) begin weekly ESA injections at the time of admission for all anemic, critically ill patients who are thought to be salvageable and likely to have at least a 7-day hospital stay (e.g., severe sepsis, ARDS); (ii) at the time of admission, withhold ESA treatment from moribund patients, nonanemic patients, and those anticipated to have short ICU stays (e.g., asthma or COPD exacerbation, drug overdose, diabetic ketoacidosis); and (iii) reassess the therapeutic plan at 4- to 7-day intervals. For example, it is reasonable to begin therapy for an anemic COPD

patient initially thought likely to have a short stay but who develops nosocomial pneumonia and progressive anemia, or a patient initially believed to be moribund who rallies. Conversely, it is sensible to discontinue ESAs from a patient dying with inexorable multiple organ failure. When using ESAs, the target should not be a normal or supranormal Hgb, doing so is associated with a higher risk of complications including thromboses.

The use of fresh frozen plasma (FFP) and platelets can also be sharply curtailed by knowing a few simple facts and making several safe, easy changes in practice. The first is recognizing that bleeding, either spontaneous or following procedures or surgery, is uncommon with platelet counts greater than 20,000/mm³ and exceedingly rare with platelet counts greater than 50,000/mm³. Hence, unless the patient is bleeding or platelet function is known to be abnormal, withholding platelet transfusions until counts are less than 20,000/mm³ (certainly <50,000/mm³) can dramatically reduce the number of platelets transfused without compromise of safety. (There is some data to suggest that patients with consumptive coagulopathy may have a higher bleeding risk than patients with equivalent platelet counts without consumption.) Although not evidence based, some experts recommend maintaining periprocedural platelet counts greater than 50,000/mm³ for patients undergoing surgery or invasive procedures, especially if bleeding would pose a high risk. The administration of platelets to thrombocytopenic patients with thrombotic thrombocytopenic purpura (TTP) or heparin-induced thrombocytopenia (HIT) is not only wasteful, but it may also be harmful by producing thrombotic complications.

FFP is often administered to nonbleeding patients in an attempt to normalize a prolonged prothrombin time (PT) or activated partial thromboplastin time (aPTT), based upon the assumption that correcting the laboratory value is possible and doing so will decrease the risk of bleeding. This practice is perhaps most common in patients presenting with excessive warfarin effect or hepatic failure, but is also done for patients with DIC, vitamin K deficiency, or dilutional coagulopathy. Several observations suggest this practice should be limited if not abandoned; only a minority of patients given FFP have in vitro clotting studies corrected and the correction typically lasts only 2 to 4 h. Perhaps more fundamental is the fact that there is a poor correlation between modest PT and aPTT prolongations and risk of bleeding. Therefore, it makes sense to withhold FFP from nonhemorrhaging patients with PT and aPTT prolongations less than three times normal. When vitamin K deficiency, warfarin effect, or hepatic dysfunction are etiologic, administration of vitamin K can often correct in vitro clotting abnormalities in less than a day, at much lower cost and risk. (An exception to this guideline occurs in patients with INRs > 10 to 20 from warfarin, in whom the risk of spontaneous bleeding is quite high and prompt correction with FFP may warrant the additional risks and costs of transfusion.) A nonevidence based and especially wasteful practice is the formulaic administration of platelets or FFP to patients, after a fixed number of red cells have been transfused.

Emerging data suggest that reducing or better yet avoiding transfusion altogether can shorten the length of stay, and reduce organ failure rates, and mortality. Attention to blood conservation during a protracted ICU stay reduces cost, risk of transfusion complications, and workload for nurses and laboratory personnel.

■ SOURCES OF BLOOD LOSS

Because Hgb and clotting function measurements are sensitive to error and artifact, each time a physician is confronted with an abnormal value, the validity of the result should be questioned. Failure to do so will result in unnecessary diagnostic tests and transfusions. One should be particularly skeptical when abnormalities develop suddenly and are large in magnitude, especially if they do not match the patient's clinical appearance. In stable patients with no "visible" blood loss, an acute decline in Hct of nine points or more (the equivalent of 3 units of RBCs) should make the laboratory result suspect. Similarly, sudden apparent "pancytopenia" with proportional decreases in white cells, red cells, and platelets is likely to indicate that the sample was obtained from a catheter and was diluted by infusate.

When convinced that abnormal laboratory data are accurate, it is important to carefully consider the cause of the abnormality. Simply stated, where did the blood clotting factors or platelets go? With few exceptions, it is difficult to rapidly lose substantial red cell mass without external evidence of blood loss. In the ICU, the most common sources of visible blood loss are the gastrointestinal tract or surgical and traumatic wounds. Because blood is an emetic and cathartic, rarely will large quantities of blood be "concealed" in the gut for long. When a

true acute drop in Hct is not accompanied by obvious bleeding, retroperitoneal, rectus muscle, or thigh (soft tissue) bleeding, alveolar hemorrhage, and hemolysis should be suspected. Retroperitoneal bleeding may be spontaneous in patients with thrombocytopenia or soluble factor deficiencies or warfarin excess, but more commonly therapeutic anticoagulation and trauma (including femoral artery or vein cannulation or vena caval filters placement) are the causes. Soft tissues of the thigh can clandestinely harbor large amounts of blood following femoral vessel puncture. Alveolar hemorrhage is most common in immunocompromised thrombocytopenic patients, occurring less often with Goodpasture disease, Wegener's granulomatosis, or systemic lupus. Hemolysis may occur spontaneously, but in the ICU is more commonly drug or transfusion induced.

When production of platelets is diminished but consumption is not excessive, platelet counts usually decline slowly over 3 to 5 days. Therefore, sudden (<1 day) decreases in platelet counts are usually indicative of a consumptive process, often, for example, DIC or drug- (e.g., heparin) associated thrombocytopenia.

Similar to the situation with platelets, when production of soluble clotting factors is curtailed but consumption is not excessive, changes in the PT and aPTT times occur over several days. Rapid development of a coagulopathy is most likely related to accelerated factor consumption of sepsis-induced DIC or resulting from dilution of clotting factors by massive transfusion or resuscitation. The problems of thrombocytopenia and abnormal clotting studies are discussed at length in Chapter 30.

■ THE COMPONENT SYSTEM

Most patients receiving transfusions do not require all the components available in whole blood (Table 14-1). Component therapy "stretches" the blood supply by allowing prolonged storage of stable constituents and by permitting several patients to receive the specific components they need from a single donation. For example, RBCs are routinely stored 5 to 6 weeks and after freezing, can be stored up to 10 years. FFP can be stored for months and purified clotting factors can be stored for years. The time limited component of blood is the platelet fraction, which lasts only days. By limiting administered volume, component therapy also reduces the risk of fluid overload,

TABLE 14-1 WHOLE BLOOD COMPONENTS

Erythrocytes
Fresh frozen plasma
Platelets
Factor VIII concentrate
Factor IX concentrate
Cryoprecipitate
Plasma protein fraction
Albumin
Leukocytes
Immunoglobulin
Antithrombin III

the amount of transfused anticoagulant, and the risk of infection.

Consequences of Blood Storage

4 In the 1970s and 1980s, some physicians insisted their patients receive fresh whole blood because they believed better outcomes were achieved compared to use of component therapy. Advocates of the practice were often ridiculed because it seemed incredulous that giving whole blood could be any different than "remixing" just the needed components. Despite their advocacy, whole blood transfusion largely ended as the product became scarce; and with the rise of the AIDS epidemic, more dangerous. Two decades later, it is apparent that fresh whole blood may well have produced better outcomes, but we now know that important part of the equation was that the blood was *fresh*, not that it was whole. So what are the important differences between fresh and stored blood? Numerous abnormalities, collectively known as the "storage lesion," have been identified in RBCs stored for two or more weeks. RBC rigidity, aggregation, and vessel wall adhesiveness are increased due to nitric oxide depletion and altered membrane lipid content. RBCs that lyse during storage release free Hgb which neutralizes endothelial bound nitric oxide causing vasoconstriction. Together, these changes impair capillary transit of RBCs. In addition, reductions in adenosine triphosphate (ATP) and 2,3-DPG inhibit tissue O_2 release by shifting the oxyhemoglobin dissociation curve leftward. The 2,3-DPG depletion persists for 1 to 2 days after transfusion. Because of metabolism of glucose in the storage media and spontaneous lysis of RBCs, the plasma portion of stored blood also contains higher levels of lactate, ammonia, potassium, and iron than fresh

blood. Finally, inflammatory cytokines and microvesicles of shed RBC cell membranes increase in stored blood.

Red Blood Cell Components

Whole Blood

Whole blood can be used for emergent restoration of circulating volume and O_2-carrying capacity, but unless fresh, it is a poor source of clotting factors and platelets. (Platelets are nonfunctional within 24 h; within 48 h, essentially all factor VIII is depleted; and within a week, factors V and VII levels are negligible.) Furthermore, transfusion of whole blood may produce circulatory overload in the euvolemic patient who requires only RBCs (e.g., sickle cell disease, chemotherapy-induced anemia, myelodysplasia). A 500 mL "unit" of whole blood contains approximately 60 mEq of Na^+ and has an average Hct of 35% to 40%. Whole blood is also more likely to contain microaggregates of leukocytes and platelets which may be detrimental. The only remaining indication for whole blood is in support of massively bleeding patients. Even then, whole blood must usually be supplemented by transfusions of platelets and/or plasma.

Packed Red Blood Cells

Removing the plasma from whole blood leaves a 200- to 300-mL unit of PRBCs having a Hct of 65% to 75%. PRBCs are used to restore O_2-carrying capacity. A unit of transfused PRBCs should raise the Hct of an adult patient by approximately 3%. (Continued bleeding or excessive volume expansion blunts the expected increase.) PRBCs contain few platelets, clotting factors, or leukocytes and are not particularly effective as volume expanders when used alone. PRBCs can be infused as rapidly as whole blood when viscosity is reduced by adding approximately 75 mL of normal saline per unit.

PRBCs offer several advantages over whole blood: (i) less volume expansion for a given increase in O_2-carrying capacity (each unit of PRBCs contains only 8 to 20 mEq of Na^+, a particularly helpful feature in patients with heart or kidney failure); (ii) PRBCs contain less anticoagulant, reducing the potential risk of citrate toxicity; and (iii) lower plasma volume, reducing the risk of allergy, anaphylaxis, viral hepatitis, and immunologic reactions from transfused antibodies. There are several disadvantages of using stored PRBCs: (i) there is a significant decrement in posttransfusion viability of the cells; (ii) stored RBCs release K^+ into the surrounding plasma as they age with concentrations often reaching 90 mEq/L; and (iii) plasma ammonia concentrations rise.

Specialized RBC Components

Five processing methods are employed to improve the safety or longevity of RBCs (Table 14-2). Leukocyte-poor RBC transfusions are used in patients who have experienced white cell or leukoagglutinin reactions; and for seronegative patients at-risk for cytomegalovirus (CMV) (CMV lives in white blood cells [WBCs]). Leukoreduction can be achieved by filtering, repeated washing, or freezing collected blood. Each method destroys some platelets while reducing the WBCs and plasma by approximately 75% to 90%. Because of the loss of RBCs in processing, a unit of leukocyte-poor RBCs contains less Hgb than a unit of PRBCs. Even leukocyte-poor RBCs contain small numbers of viable WBCs; therefore, blood products transfused into immunosuppressed patients must be irradiated to prevent graft versus host disease (GVHD). Even though it is probably a good idea to leukoreduce all RBCs, it is not done universally because the costs of doing so are prohibitive. Freezing or washing RBCs has additional advantages over filtration: the former two processes also minimize reactions caused by allergy to transfused proteins and those resulting from presence of anti-IgA or IgE antibodies.

White Blood Cell Transfusions

Because of the risk, expense, and limited benefit of WBC transfusions, they are rarely used. WBC transfusions are indicated only for neutropenic patients with overwhelming infections failing conventional antimicrobial therapy. WBC transfusions are fraught with problems: Febrile and allergic reactions are nearly universal, and because WBCs have a circulating half-life of only 6 h, frequent transfusion is required. WBCs must also be ABO-compatible. Historically, hepatitis was commonly transmitted by WBC infusions, and CMV infection remains a risk. In patients with bone marrow depression, WBC transfusion also carries a nearly certain risk of GVHD. WBCs often aggregate, a tendency that precludes the use of transfusion filters and frequently leads to acute lung injury.

Platelet Components

Random Donor Platelets

The risk of hemorrhage rises as functional platelet concentrations decline, but thrombocytopenia must be marked before the risk of bleeding increases significantly. The risks of bleeding are amplified at any given platelet concentration by concomitant abnormalities in platelet function, soluble clotting factor levels, and vascular integrity. Commonly used platelet counts to guide the need for transfusion are illustrated in Table 14-3. Platelet concentrations greater

TABLE 14-2 RBC PROCESSING METHODS AND RATIONALE

PROCESSING TECHNIQUE	METHOD	PURPOSE	LIMITATIONS
Freezing	Glycerol preservation	Long-term storage of strategic blood supply and for rare blood types	Thawing and washing process are time consuming Reduces but does not eliminate leukocytes
Irradiation	2,500 Gy exposure	Kill lymphocytes to prevent graft vs. host disease in immunocompromised recipients	Time consuming Added expense Does not reduce infection or allergy risk.
Leukoreduction	Filtration	Reduction in WBC numbers to lower risk of febrile reactions, CMV, and alloimmunization	Does not prevent graft versus host disease
Volume reduction	Plasma removal by centrifugation	Reduce infused volume while preserving oxygen carrying capacity	Does not remove WBCs. Less effective than washing to prevent allergic reactions
Washing	Saline washing/ centrifugation	Removal of plasma proteins and electrolytes to deter allergic reactions and hyperkalemia	

TABLE 14-3   PLATELET TRANSFUSION GUIDELINES FOR NONBLEEDING PATIENTS

PLATELET COUNT (no./mm³)	SPONTANEOUS BLEEDING RISK	PLATELET TRANSFUSION GIVEN?
<5,000	High	Almost always
5,000–20,000	Moderate to high	Usually given to raise counts >20,000
20,000–50,000	Low	Occasionally given if platelets dysfunctional, soluble factors abnormal, or invasive intervention planned.
50,000–100,000	Low	Transfuse only if actively bleeding, or critical site invasive procedure planned
>100,000	Low	Should be very rare

than 50,000/mm³ are rarely associated with significant bleeding, even in trauma or surgical patients, and are more than sufficient to provide hemostasis in patients undergoing invasive procedures. Platelet counts less than 20,000/mm³ are associated with an increased risk of spontaneous hemorrhage (especially if counts fall below 5,000/mm³). Therefore, "prophylactic" transfusions are sometimes performed for counts in the 10,000 to 20,000/mm³ range, often undertaken with platelet counts of 5,000 to 10,000/mm³, and are almost always given when counts fall below 5,000/mm³. Practice is highly variable for nonbleeding patients when counts are in the 20,000 to 50,000/ mm³ range. Even though the practice is not evidence based, patients with ongoing hemorrhage and those planned to undergo invasive procedures in critical locations (e.g., intracranial surgery) are often given platelet transfusions even when the levels are above 50,000/mm³. Regardless of number, platelet transfusions are also performed for therapy of platelet dysfunction because of uremia, liver disease, and nonsteroidal anti-inflammatory drugs in bleeding patients.

Most platelets are collected by centrifuging whole blood. A unit of pooled random donor platelets (RDPs) contains 40 to 70 mL of platelet concentrate and large numbers of WBCs that may be removed by filtration (leukoreduction). For each 5 to 6 units of transfused RPDs, patients receive roughly the equivalent of 1 unit of plasma. The usefulness of RDPs is limited by many factors: (i) repeatedly transfused patients develop alloantibodies to common platelet surface antigens and may eventually require human leukocyte antigen (HLA)-matched platelets to prevent rapid immune destruction of the transfused platelets; (ii) platelet infusions often produce

minor allergic reactions including chills, fever, and rash; (iii) WBCs contained in platelet transfusions may produce GVHD in the immunocompromised patient; and (iv) platelet transfusions are unlikely to be helpful and may be harmful in the "immune thrombocytopenias" (idiopathic thrombocytopenic purpura [ITP], TTP, or HIT) because of rapid platelet destruction. In such cases, plasmapheresis, corticosteroids, and intravenous immunoglobulin (IVIG) preparations may extend the circulating half-life of transfused platelets.

Platelets may be administered as rapidly as they will infuse (5 to 10 min/unit). The normal life span of circulating platelets is 3 to 4 days; therefore, platelet transfusions are usually needed every 2 to 3 days if production is reduced without accelerated destruction. There is some evidence that giving a larger dose less frequently results in fewer total transfusions than giving smaller doses more frequently. Each unit increases the count by 5,000 to 10,000 platelets/mm³ unless destruction is ongoing. When assessed 1 h after transfusion, an increment of less than 2,000/mm³/unit confirms platelet destruction. Platelets are usually administered as "five-packs" or "six-packs," which raise the platelet count by approximately 25,000 to 50,000 platelets/mm³. A blunted increment is common in patients with burns, splenic sequestration, fever, severe sepsis, infection, and/or platelet antibodies. Because young (large) platelets have enhanced hemostatic function, the presence of many large platelets may indicate a lower risk of bleeding at any given count.

ABO-compatible platelets minimize formation of antiplatelet antibodies and survive longer in the circulation. Because of the very small volume of plasma present in transfused platelets, incompatibility between donor plasma and recipient RBCs is usually insignificant. However, if multiple units of platelets and incompatible plasma are transfused, a positive Coombs test or overt hemolysis may occur. The small number of RBCs transfused in platelet concentrates makes RBC cross-matching unnecessary. (However, 10% of massively transfused patients will develop ABO sensitization.) Platelets do not contain Rh antigens and therefore, Rh sensitization is not a problem. Although platelets should be administered through a filter to prevent aggregation, filtration lengthens infusion time and decreases the number of viable platelets transfused.

Platelets are the least stable blood component requiring special handling and limiting shelf life to just 5 days. To maintain functionality for even this length of time, platelets must be stored in plasma, constantly gently agitated (to maximize oxygenation) and maintained near room temperature. Unfortunately, this requirement dramatically increases the risk of bacterial proliferation in contaminated units. Current estimates suggest somewhere between 1 in 500 and 1 in 5,000 units of platelets are contaminated with bacteria. (Diphtheroids, coagulase-negative staphylococci, and other skin flora are the most common pathogens.)

Single-Donor Platelets

In patients refractory to RDPs, single donors may be pheresed as often as two or three times weekly to provide large numbers of platelets for transfusion. Administration of these pheresed concentrates (typically, approx. 300 mL) commonly produces a rise of 30,000 to 60,000 platelets/mm^3, roughly the increment seen with six random donor units. Single-donor pheresed platelets often at least transiently raise platelet counts even if not HLA-matched. In patients failing to respond to RDP or single-donor pheresed platelets, HLA-matched pheresed platelets usually will boost platelet counts. The effective survival of HLA-matched platelets can be nearly normal if used in patients alloimmunized to platelet antigens by random donors, but if accelerated destruction is caused by non-HLA antigen mechanisms (e.g., DIC), HLA-matched platelets will not offer a substantial advantage over RDPs. A less cumbersome alternative to HLA matching is to cross match potential donor platelets with recipient serum. Regardless of the matching method, single-donor platelets have the advantage of reducing transfusion-related infection risk.

Clotting Factor Concentrates and Plasma Products

Fresh Frozen Plasma

Each 180 to 300 mL unit of FFP contains fibrinogen; clotting factors II, V, VII, VIII, IX, X, XI, XIII; and von Willebrand factor. Factors V and VIII and fibrinogen are present in the highest functional concentrations. FFP also contains donor antibodies and a substantial number of WBCs (even if the blood is leukoreduced at the time of collection). FFP is indicated to treat bleeding due to deficiency of multiple clotting factors, including (i) dilutional coagulopathy in the massively transfused patient, (ii) excessive anticoagulation with warfarin, and (iii) bleeding associated with hepatic synthetic failure.

FFP dosing is commonly guided by the degree of PT or partial thromboplastin time (PTT) prolongation. In practice, PTs less than 18 s, INRs less than 1.5, and aPTTs less than 55 s are usually not treated unless patients are actively bleeding. The practice of treating an elevated PT or aPTT less than three times normal in a nonbleeding patient is commonplace but not evidence based. In cases where hemorrhage is ongoing, the endpoint of FFP administration is usually "normalization" of the PT and PTT. In most cases, factor levels of 25% to 30% of normal are sufficient to achieve hemostasis. Because humans have about 40 mL/kg of circulating plasma, a minimum of 10 to 15 mL/kg of FFP (2 to 4 units) is necessary to restore hemostasis in patients with profound deficiencies. Hence, if the decision is made to give FFP, it makes sense to administer at least 2 units, then reassess in vitro clotting times. Congenital or acquired coagulation factor deficiencies, including those of factors VIII and IX and von Willebrand factor, are better treated with specific concentrates of superior efficiency and safety. FFP should not be used primarily for intravascular volume expansion or as a source of albumin because less costly, equally effective alternatives exist.

FFP use has risks and several disadvantages: (i) each milliliter of transfused plasma contains only 1 unit of each clotting factor; therefore, relatively large volumes are needed to correct deficiencies compared to factor concentrates; (ii) the risk of allergic (anaphylactoid) reactions is high because of plasma proteins and residual platelets and leukocytes; (iii) because FFP and other clotting factor concentrates have been common sources of viral infection in the past, they have been the targets of efforts to reduce viral contamination. Treatment with solvents and detergents has been shown to destroy enveloped viruses (i.e., HIV, CMV, Epstein–Barr virus, hepatitis B and C) but unfortunately, nonenveloped viruses (i.e., parvovirus, hepatitis A) are resistant to such treatments. The detergent process modestly reduces clotting factor concentrations (von Willebrand factor levels are affected most) and is expensive. Because RBCs and platelets are not routinely detergent treated, controversy exists as to the wisdom of using detergent-treated FFP in patients concurrently receiving nontreated blood products; and (iv) FFP must be ABO compatible with the recipient's RBCs.

Cryoprecipitate

Cryoprecipitate forms when plasma separated from fresh whole blood is rapidly frozen and then allowed to rewarm. This small-volume (10 to 15 mL) extract contains most of the factor VIII (about 100 units), fibrinogen (200 mg), fibronectin, factor XIII, and 40% to 60% of the von Willebrand factor present in the original unit of plasma. Cryoprecipitate may be used to treat (i) hypofibrinogenemic states (e.g., thrombolytic therapy, congenital deficiency, and dilutional or consumptive coagulopathy); (ii) factor XIII deficiency; (iii) von Willebrand disease; and (iv) hemophilia A (factor VIII deficiency). In hypofibrinogenemic states, 1 bag of cryoprecipitate/5 to 10 kg of body weight is a usual dose. When used for von Willebrand disease, 1 bag/10 kg is usually adequate. Because infection risk is now eliminated by using pasteurized or recombinant factor VIII, both these products are favored over cryoprecipitate for the treatment of hemophilia A. A role for cryoprecipitate may remain in the treatment of von Willebrand disease.

Hemophilia Factor Replacement

Because of the complexity of treatment, intensivists should seek help from coagulation specialists when treating hemophilia A or B and von Willebrand disease. Although FFP can be used to replace factor VIII or IX, it is an inefficient way to do so requiring large-volume infusions. The more concentrated cryoprecipitate reduces the required volume somewhat but is still suboptimal because of the risk of infection. Factor VIII concentrates solve this problem for patients with hemophilia A by pooling plasma of many donors (frequently hundreds) and then purifying the clotting protein using one of a variety of methods. Another, albeit more costly, option is the use of one of several recombinant human factor VIII products. For clotting factor replacement in patients with hemophilia B, monoclonal antibody purification of pooled plasma or recombinant factor IX is optimal, although the so-called prothrombin complex concentrates rich in factor IX are still widely used.

In the bleeding hemophiliac, either factor VIII or IX activity is negligible and should be increased to greater than 50% of normal levels to arrest hemorrhage. (Levels of 80% to 100% should be targeted for life-threatening bleeding and patients destined for the operating room.) The initial dose of clotting factor may be calculated by replacing 1 unit of factor VIII or IX per milliliter of calculated plasma volume per percent of desired factor activity. Because plasma volume is approximately 40 mL/kg, the simple calculation is given by the equation: dose (units) = $40 \times$ (wt in kg) $\times$ (% factor activity desired). Because of a larger volume of distribution, higher doses of factor IX may be required.

Because administered factor VIII has a half-life of only 8 to 12 h, close monitoring of clinical signs of bleeding and specific factor levels are necessary. The half-life of factor IX is longer (approx. 16 h). Historically, factor VIII and IX concentrates carried a high risk of viral infection; however, careful donor selection and the institution of pasteurization, monoclonal antibody purification, microfiltration, detergent treatment, and serologic testing have all but eliminated the risk of viral hepatitis and HIV.

Antithrombin Supplements

Antithrombin (AT) concentrate is available for treatment of congenital AT deficiency and represents a preferable alternative to use of large volumes of FFP. AT treatment of acquired deficiency states (e.g., sepsis) has been ineffective.

Intravenous Immunoglobulin

IVIG, a pooled immunoglobulin fraction from multiple donors, is useful in three basic situations: (i) replacement therapy of humoral immune deficiency states such as congenital agammaglobulinemia, common variable immunodeficiency, and chronic lymphocytic leukemia; (ii) control of selected infections such as neonatal group B streptococcal disease, disseminated CMV infection in transplant recipients, and *Pseudomonas* infections in burn victims; and (iii) treatment of ITP, TTP, and refractory thrombocytopenia because of repeated platelet transfusions. IVIG is not without risk;

patients with immunoglobulin A deficiency may develop anaphylactic reactions from preformed anti-IgA antibodies, and antibody aggregates in IVIG may cause other allergic reactions. IVIG preparations may also transmit infections such as non-A, non-B hepatitis; however, the risk of HIV is very low.

Recombinant Human Factor VIIa (rhVIIa)

rhVIIa was developed as a treatment for hemorrhaging patients with hemophilia who had high titers of antibodies to either factor VIII or IX. It is also useful for treatment of inherited factor VII deficiency and may help in cases of antiplatelet antibodies causing refractory thrombocytopenia by initiating thrombin activation on the surface of platelets. The use quickly expanded well beyond these indications to include exsanguination from trauma, coagulopathy of liver failure, warfarin toxicity, and intracranial hemorrhage. Controlled clinical trials have now shown no survival benefit and little difference in amounts of transfused blood among trauma patients treated with rhVIIa compared to those given placebo. Likewise, formal study of rhVIIa in intracranial hemorrhage shows that the volume of bleeding is reduced but clinical outcomes are not improved. In nonhemophilia-related bleeding, clinicians should be dissuaded from the use of rhVIIa because of uncertainty about optimal dosing, lack of efficacy, extremely high cost, and anecdotal reports of clinical thromboses. If use of rhVIIa is considered, the expertise of a coagulation specialist should be sought.

■ PROBLEMS ASSOCIATED WITH MASSIVE TRANSFUSION

Exsanguination and Cross-Matching

A formal cross-matching procedure requires 45 to 60 min. Therefore, when the patient's condition does not allow completion of a formal cross-match, O-negative (universal donor) or type-specific (ABO- and Rh-compatible) blood may be given. The small amount of plasma in O-negative blood often contains antibodies to the recipient's RBCs and can provoke delayed transfusion reactions. ABO determination alone usually takes less than 10 min. Therefore, type-specific blood is preferred except in cases in which transfusion must occur even more urgently.

Massive Transfusion

The rate at which blood products can be administered is proportional to the driving pressure for delivery and the fourth power of the IV catheter radius and is inversely proportional to the length of the IV catheter and viscosity of the fluid to be infused. Hence, using multiple, (usually peripheral), short, large-bore IV catheters will usually be more efficient than smaller, longer, centrally placed catheters, except when large-bore introducer sheaths are already in place. Obviously, flow rates can be augmented by increasing the driving pressure through use of pressure bags. Fluid viscosity is rarely a limiting factor except when transfusing cold PRBCs. Viscosity can be dramatically reduced by warming the blood or by adding 100 to 200 mL of sterile isotonic saline to the PRBCs before infusion.

Massive transfusion is variably defined as the administration of greater than 10 units of blood (or 50% of the patient's blood volume) in less than 24 h. Problems resulting from massive transfusion include (i) dilutional thrombocytopenia and coagulopathy, (ii) hypokalemic alkalosis as HCO_3^- is generated from transfused citrate, (iii) hypocalcemia, (iv) hypothermia, and (v) hyperkalemia.

In previously healthy persons, dilutional clotting disorders begin to emerge when one blood volume equivalent (5 to 10 units of blood) has been replaced. Clotting factor levels then commonly drop below 30% of normal, and platelet counts fall below 100,000/mm³. Hence, after 5 units of blood have been transfused, platelet counts, PT, and an aPTT should be monitored.

RBCs are collected in an acidic environment (pH 7.1) using sodium citrate and citric acid as preservatives. As blood ages the pH drops further because of the cellular production of pyruvate and lactate. Surprisingly, when transfused, this "acidic" solution does not cause acidosis in the absence of profound shock. To the contrary, when infused, each unit of blood yields 23 mEq of bicarbonate from the hepatic metabolism of citrate. If impaired kidney function limits bicarbonate excretion, metabolic alkalosis results. Similarly, in the presence of renal insufficiency, the K⁺ challenge of PRBCs (up to 90 mEq/L) can induce hyperkalemia. If alkalosis occurs, serum K⁺ and ionized Ca^{2+} concentrations both may decline, but symptomatic hypokalemia is uncommon because of the K⁺ in transfused PRBCs. Even during massive transfusion, the incidence of citrate-induced hypocalcemia is very low. (Typically, more than 10 to 20 units of PRBCs must be infused

5

each hour to provide a citrate load sufficient to depress Ca^{2+} levels.) Although replacement is rarely necessary, it is prudent to monitor calcium levels. If symptomatic hypocalcemia develops, administration of 10 to 20 mL of 10% calcium gluconate, or 5 mL of 10% $CaCl_2$, for each unit of PRBCs usually suffices.

Systemic hypothermia has numerous adverse effects (see Chapter 28), but fortunately hypothermia is rarely seen outside the setting of massive transfusion. Perhaps the most important effect of hypothermia is inhibition of clotting enzyme activity. In the profoundly hypothermic patient, this can translate into a significant functional coagulopathy despite normal levels of clotting proteins. Blood warming is a reasonable practice with (i) massive transfusion, (ii) transfusion rates exceeding 50 mL/min, or (iii) cold agglutinin disease. Blood may hemolyze if heated above 38°C.

■ COMPLICATIONS OF TRANSFUSION

Receiving blood products is now safer than it has ever been in the history of transfusion medicine; nevertheless, there are still numerous risks, the approximate frequencies of which are presented in Table 14-4. Conceptually, most complications can be thought of as either immunologic or infectious.

Immunologic Complications

Febrile, Nonhemolytic Transfusion Reactions

Febrile, nonhemolytic transfusion reactions are the most common transfusion-related adverse event. Febrile reactions are an immunologic response by the recipient to surface antigens on WBCs, or less commonly inflammatory cytokines in donor blood. Between 15% and 20% of RBC recipients develop fever during transfusion, but only a fraction of these cases are of sufficient magnitude that they are reported as a transfusion reaction. In the severe cases, flushing, fever, and chills are prominent within 60 min of starting the RBC infusion. In patients with previous febrile reactions, the use of leukocyte-poor RBCs and HLA-matched components reduce the risk.

Allergic/Anaphylactoid Reactions

Allergic reactions, ranging from mild urticaria to frank IgE-mediated anaphylaxis, occur with about 3% of RBC transfusions. Because such reactions are more common among IgA deficient recipients, it has long been thought that the mechanism was preformed IgG recipient antibodies directed against IgA in donor blood. Data now suggest that recipient antibodies to haptoglobin also may be involved. Stopping the transfusion and administering antihistamines are usually sufficient to abort the reaction. Full-blown anaphylaxis should be treated with intravenous epinephrine and volume expansion. Inhaled β-adrenergic agonists may moderate bronchospasm. Despite widespread use of corticosteroids, they are not effective. To avert future episodes, blood products from IgA deficient donors or washed RBCs or platelets are usually selected.

Immediate Hemolytic Reactions

Hemolytic reactions can be immediate or delayed. If immediate, they are usually because of major ABO incompatibility, the most common cause of which is misidentification of the patient sample or transfusion of properly matched blood into the wrong patient. As a result, stringent rules have been instituted in most hospitals requiring two licensed health care providers to check the blood product against patient identification to avoid this mistake. As a corollary when notified by the blood bank that they have received an improperly labeled sample, repeat collection is indicated. Fortunately, these mistakes are rare (1/10,000 to 1/100,000 transfusions) with fatalities even less common ($1/10^6$ transfusions). Although HIV and viral hepatitis are often cited by clinicians as the most concerning risks of transfusion, simple administrative or clerical error resulting in transfusion of blood into the wrong patient may be 10 to 100 times greater. Any process that causes lysis of the donor cells ex vivo (e.g., overheating, freezing, administration through a small bore needle, or mixing RBCs with hypotonic fluid) can mimic an immunologic hemolytic reaction when those cells are infused.

Most severe reactions occur rapidly as the first 50 to 100 mL of blood is infused. For this reason, frequent vital signs should be taken in the initial period of transfusion. Major reactions are potentially fatal because they produce intravascular hemolysis, coagulopathy, shock, renal failure, and pulmonary dysfunction. New-onset anxiety, dyspnea, fever, back or infusion site pain, and diffuse bleeding are all clues to transfusion reaction. (Such signs and symptoms may be difficult to recognize in the unconscious, critically ill patient.) Primary treatment of a major reaction is to stop the

TABLE 14-4 FREQUENCY OF TRANSFUSION-RELATED RISKS

CONDITION	APPROXIMATE RISK PER RBC UNIT TRANSFUSED
Immune Mediated Conditions	
Minor allergy/urticaria	1/75
Febrile reactions	1/300
Alloimmunization	1/400
Transfusion-related lung injury	1/5,000
Delayed hemolysis	1/6,000
Immediate hemolysis	1/20,000
Fatal immediate hemolysis	1/1,000,000
Anaphylaxis	1/30,000
Immunomodulation	Unknown
Graft vs. host disease	Unknown
Infectious Complications	
Hepatitis B	1/2,000,000
HTLV 1 and 2	1/600,000
Hepatitis C	1/1,000,000 to 1/2,000,000
HIV	1/2,000,000 to 1/3,000,000
Malaria	1/4,000,000
RBC bacterial contamination	1/5,000,000

transfusion. Using sterile technique, donor blood and blood tubing should be returned to the blood bank. Clotted and anticoagulated samples of the recipient's blood and a urine sample should also be sent to the blood bank with notification of a suspected transfusion reaction. Fluids and vasopressors should be administered as required to maintain perfusion. Intravenous $NaHCO_3$ may be given to prevent precipitation of Hgb in the renal tubules and subsequent acute kidney injury. Loop and osmotic diuretics may also be useful to preserve urine flow and avert renal failure.

Alloimmunization and Delayed Hemolytic Reactions

Alloimmunization is common, occurring roughly once for each 100 transfused units, fortunately, delayed hemolytic reactions are much less common occurring in only 1/6,000 RBC transfusions. Low-titer alloantibodies (often undetectable by Coombs test) can cause delayed hemolysis in previously transfused or multiparous patients, as the transfused RBCs recall an amnestic response that produces IgG antibodies directed against donor cells. Over the next 10 to 14 days, antibody levels rise, the direct Coombs test becomes positive and transfused RBCs lyse resulting in a sudden (but often asymptomatic) drop in the Hct. Concomitantly, serum haptoglobin levels fall and lactate dehydrogenase levels increase. Although usually benign, a falling Hct and rising bilirubin, especially in a postoperative patient, may raise concerns of hepatic failure or occult bleeding.

Transfusion Associated Lung Injury

Transfusion associated lung injury (TRALI) is a relatively common (1/1,200 to 1/5,000 transfusions) syndrome of acute lung injury which promptly (within 1 to 6 h) follows transfusion of RBCs or more commonly plasma. Typical manifestations are cough, dyspnea, and hypoxemia; one third of patients exhibit either hypotension or hypertension. The chest radiograph is typical of noncardiogenic pulmonary edema. Although the mechanism remains debated, the observation that risk of the syndrome is highest with donations from multiparous women suggests that the cause could be donor alloantibodies to recipient leukocytes or plasma proteins. For this reason, some countries have adopted a policy of only transfusing FFP from men. The incidence of TRALI appears to be higher in older recipients and among heavy alcohol drinkers. Treatment is supportive, similar to other forms of ALI, and the syndrome typically resolves more rapidly that acute lung injury of other causes.

Graft versus Host Disease

GVHD occurs when donor T lymphocytes colonize the recipient, subsequently attacking the new host as foreign. GVHD was long thought to only occur in immunocompromised patients (e.g., following marrow ablative chemotherapy or radiation therapy), but it is now clear that normal hosts are also at risk. Manifestations range from subclinical microchimerism to minor skin and gut disease to death. Because freshly collected blood contains higher numbers of viable lymphocytes, it poses a higher risk of GVHD; the risk is lowered by leukoreduction but can only be eliminated by irradiation of the donor blood to kill lymphocytes.

Transfusion-Related Immune Modulation

It has long been known that receiving preoperative allogeneic blood transfusions improved the survival of transplanted organs. Although hotly debated, more recent observations suggest that patients receiving perioperative RBC transfusions are more prone to infections and recurrence of resected tumors, a process called transfusion-related immune modulation (TRIM).

Infectious Complications

Bacterial Infections

Bacterial infections transmitted through transfused blood are most frequently due to breaches in sterile technique at the time of the transfusion and prolonged infusion time. When a contaminated blood component is to blame, platelets are the most likely source. (If contaminated when obtained from the donor, bacterial growth can proceed unabated because platelets must be stored at room temperature, without preservative.) It should be noted that *Listeria monocytogenes* is capable of growing at the usual storage temperature of RBCs and may cause transfusion-related bacteremia.

Viral Infections

Because of the large number of donors required for preparation, the risk of viral infection has been highest with pooled blood products (e.g., factor VIII concentrate and activated factor complexes). Better selection of donors and biochemical and serologic testing have reduced the prevalence of these infections in the donor pool. Processing of blood including filtration and treatment with solvents and detergents has dramatically reduced the risk of acquiring enveloped viruses (i.e., HIV, CMV, Epstein–Barr virus, hepatitis B and C) but unfortunately, nonenveloped viruses (i.e., parvovirus, hepatitis A) are still a problem because they resist treatments designed to inactivate them. Other infections potentially transmitted via blood include malaria, syphilis, brucellosis, and toxoplasmosis.

Depending on the region of the country, screening tests for HIV have lowered the risk of transfusion acquired AIDS infection to between 1/50,000 and 1/500,000 for each unit of transfused blood component.

Miscellaneous Complications

RBCs, WBCs, platelets, and cryoprecipitate should all be administered through standard blood filters to prevent transfusing aggregates of these components. All filters reduce the maximal infusion rate and should be changed after every 2 to 4 units because of filter plugging.

Hyperkalemia may occur in massively transfused patients, given that PRBCs are stored for long periods of time (especially patients with renal dysfunction). Potassium concentration in the transfused plasma may rise as high as 90 mEq/L in PRBCs stored more than 3 weeks. Hyperkalemia may be prevented by using fresh blood or by using RBC products containing little plasma, such as washed or PRBCs.

Citrate-induced hypocalcemia has been touted as a problem in the massively transfused patient but is a rare event. Prophylactic administration of calcium is not recommended, but if the patient exhibits signs of hypocalcemia, determination of ionized calcium is warranted. Because sodium citrate is used to anticoagulate most blood components, alkalemia may develop as the liver converts citrate to bicarbonate. Patients with normal liver function are able to metabolize massive amounts of citrate (that contained in up to 20 units of PRBCs per hour). Therefore, metabolic alkalosis of citrate infusion is usually clinically insignificant and self-correcting.

■ BLOOD SUBSTITUTES

Extracted, purified, and stabilized Hgb and genetically engineered Hgb solutions continue to be investigated as blood substitutes but are not ready for clinical use. In the past, Hgb solutions have carried substantial risk of renal tubular damage. Limited application of O_2-carrying perfluorochemical solutions in coronary reperfusion has shown promise in experimental settings, but there is no evidence supporting their safe and effective systemic use.

■ SUGGESTED READINGS

Corwin HL, Surgenor SD, Gettinger A, et al. Transfusion practice in the critically ill. *Crit Care Med*. 2003;31(Suppl. 12):S668–S671.

Gajic O, Dzik WH, Toy P, et al. Fresh frozen plasma and platelet transfusion for nonbleeding patients in the intensive care unit: Benefit or harm? *Crit Care Med*. 2006;34:S170–S173.

Hebert PC, Wells G, Blajchman MA, et al. A multicenter, randomized, controlled clinical trial of transfusion requirements in critical care. Transfusion requirements in critical care investigators, Canadian Critical Care Trials Group. *N Engl J Med*. 1999;340(6):409–417.

Key NS, Negrier C. Coagulation factor concentrates: Past, present, and future. *Lancet*. 2007;370:439–448.

Klein HG, Spahn DR, Carson JL. Red blood cell transfusion clinical practice. *Lancet*. 2007;370:415–426.

Koch CG, Li L, Sessler DI, et al. Duration of red-cell storage and complications after cardiac surgery. *N Engl J Med*. 2008;358:1229–1239.

O'Shaughnessy DF, Atterbury C, Bolton Maggs P, et al. Guidelines for the use of fresh-frozen plasma, cryoprecipitate and cryosupernatant. *Br J Haematol*. 2004;126(1):11–28.

Shorr AF, Jackson WL, Kelly KM, et al. Transfusion practice and blood stream infections in critically ill patients. *Chest*. 2005;127(5):1722–1728.

Slichter SJ. Evidence based platelet transfusion guidelines. *Hematology*. 2007;2007:172–178.

Stroncek DF, Rebulla P. Platelet transfusions. *Lancet*. 2007;370:427–438.

Tinmouth A, Fergusson D, Yee IC, et al. Clinical consequences of red cell storage in the critically ill. *Transfusion*. 2006;46:2014–2027.

Walsh TS, Garrioch M, Maciver C, et al. Red cell requirements for intensive care units adhering to evidence-based transfusion guidelines. *Transfusion*. 2004;44:1405.

Weiskopf RB, Viele MK, Feiner J, et al. Human cardiovascular and metabolic response to acute, severe isovolemic anemia. *JAMA*. 1998;279:217.

Pharmacotherapy

KEY POINTS

1 It is essential to review the medication list of every patient daily, preferably with a pharmacist specializing in critical care.

2 In choosing a cost-effective course of therapy, consider not only the cost of the drug, but also the costs associated with administration and monitoring of its effect and reduced costs for other resources.

3 Avoiding continuous infusions, ultra-short-acting compounds, and frequent intermittent dosing are the best methods of reducing drug costs.

4 The volume of distribution and half-life of most medications are increased in the critically ill.

5 Drugs should generally be selected for use based on their putative duration of action and method of clearance.

6 The multiple organ dysfunction present in most patients in the ICU dramatically alters the pharmacokinetics of most drugs. Experience with any drug's actions in healthy patients is difficult to translate to the ICU population.

◼ QUALITY IMPROVEMENT AND COST-CONTROL

The intensive care unit (ICU) is one of the hospitals' highest consumers of pharmacy services and uses some of the most expensive (e.g., rasburicase, 4-methylpyrazole, drotrecogin alfa activated) and potentially dangerous (e.g., tissue plasminogen activator, radiographic contrast) drugs. Critically ill patients often receive ten or more medications each day, and the potential for dosing errors, drug interactions, and adverse events is high.

In addition, medication charges can account for 20% of a patient's ICU bill. While it can be argued that almost any cost for a truly "life-saving" drug is justified, there are not many drugs that live up to that description. Obviously, therapies known to be inferior should not be chosen just because they are less expensive but careful deliberation reveals that equally effective, less-expensive alternatives often exist. Undoubtedly, medications represent an area for cost savings but drug costs are often unreasonably targeted. This happens partly because the pharmacy is one of the few departments of the hospital that has any idea of acquisition costs, how much is used, and how much they are reimbursed. Yet, there are practical limitations to what can be accomplished. Consider the most extreme case where all medications were eliminated; even if such a practice did not worsen outcomes, such a radical change could only reduce costs by approximately 20%.

Role of the Pharmacist

Numerous studies indicate that making a pharmacist part of the ICU team helps identify numerous potential opportunities for care improvement and cost saving. Cynically, some physicians believe that pharmacy involvement is intended only to cut costs but careful study reveals otherwise. While approximately 40% of pharmacist-suggested changes reduce costs; 40% are cost neutral; and 10% of suggestions actually increase costs. Regardless of the effect on cost, ample data indicate that when a pharmacist experienced in the care of ICU patients is included in rounds, pharmacotherapy is simplified, important overlooked treatments are initiated, and drug-related adverse events decline. Unfortunately, sometimes shortsighted hospitals are reluctant to provide pharmacist support even though the cost of the small amount of time needed each day is quickly recouped.

Quality Improvement Strategies

Perhaps the most important step in improving pharmacotherapy is a thorough daily examination of all prescribed medications. Regular review of the **1** medication list routinely reveals redundant, unnecessary, or competing drugs and commonly exposes a drug or drug interaction responsible for a major problem (e.g., renal failure, thrombocytopenia, delirium). The incidence of adverse events is magnified by allowing multiple consulting physicians to write medication orders. Numerous ways in which medication practices can be improved are discussed below.

Using Guidelines and Protocols

A fundamental step in improving medication safety is to establish guidelines and protocols for drugs that are frequently overlooked, are difficult or dangerous to use, or are of high cost. Written or electronic tools to prevent prophylactic therapies from being overlooked (or overused) are wise. For example, patients at high risk for developing gastric ulceration should receive prophylaxis, but it is clearly not necessary that every patient in the ICU receives gastrointestinal (GI) bleeding prophylaxis. Hence, guidelines to help physicians decide who are appropriate candidates, will match risk to treatment. Because of the costs, ease of therapy, and effectiveness, histamine blockers or proton pump inhibitors represent good therapeutic options when indicated (see Chapter 39). Another case in point is deep venous thrombosis (DVT) prophylaxis. Without prevention, DVT is so frequent in the critically ill that it makes sense to use preventative therapy in almost all patients but it can be overlooked. Unfractionated heparin (UFH) and low-molecular-weight heparin (LMWH) are generally safe and so inexpensive that they should be the agents of choice unless contraindications to anticoagulation are compelling (e.g., active hemorrhage, recent high-risk trauma or surgery, potential neuraxial bleeding, significant thrombocytopenia). For patients unable to receive anticoagulants, a combination of graded compression stockings and intermittent pneumatic devices is a less satisfactory nonpharmacological alternative. From an economic standpoint, the annual costs of prophylaxis for an entire ICU may be dwarfed by the price to treat just one case of thromboembolism or massive GI bleeding. The importance of DVT prophylaxis has been magnified, now that funding and regulatory agencies are holding hospitals responsible for un-prevented thromboembolism. A related example is implementation of a *treatment* protocol for UFH dosing. Without such guidance, therapeutic failure is commonplace and complications frequent (see Chapter 23).

To prevent excessive or inadequate treatment, it is also an excellent idea to develop guidelines for dosing mediations to objective endpoints. Using a validated pain scale to guide opioid dosing can achieve better analgesia with fewer side effects. Use of sedation dosing tools (e.g., Richmond Agitation Sedation Scale [RASS]) with mandated drug interruptions has been shown to reduce total doses of administered drugs and shorten the length of mechanical ventilation and ICU stay while lowering costs (see Chapter 17). Although the best target value for glucose can be debated, validated glucose control protocols are also very sensible to minimize risks of hypoglycemia while improving glycemic control. For some medications that are used infrequently, providing a checklist or protocol to maximize the chance a patient can benefit from and safely receive the drug makes sense. Examples include drotrecogin alfa activated for severe sepsis, tissue plasminogen activator for ischemic stroke, and nitric oxide for hypoxemic respiratory failure.

Restricted Prescribing

For the most complicated or dangerous drugs, it even makes sense to restrict prescribing to physicians with special training or qualifications. Cancer chemotherapy is a prime example. Another case in point is infectious disease consultation for decisions regarding use of side effect prone or expensive antimicrobial therapies (e.g., ganciclovir, liposomal amphotericin B, voriconazole). Another instance would be restricting prescribing of tissue plasminogen activator and glycoprotein IIb/IIIa inhibitors to qualified cardiologists. A final example would be to restrict drotrecogin alfa activated prescribing to critical care physicians experienced in treating severe sepsis. However, it is a very bad idea to design impediments to timely use of therapies merely for cost control. Doing so *might* reduce acquisition costs for that drug but are not likely to save any money as outcomes worsen and stays lengthen.

Eliminating Duplicative Treatment

Another step toward optimizing medication use is to eliminate duplicative or overlapping therapies. It is common to see patients' prescribed suboptimal doses of two or more narcotics and a similar number of benzodiazepines for pain and sedation, respectively. It is also reasonably common to see a patient with asthma or chronic obstructive lung disease to have inhaled corticosteroids wastefully coadministered on top of high dose of oral or parenteral corticosteroids. Antibiotic therapy is frequently duplicated. Examples include concomitant use of a third generation cephalosporin and extended spectrum penicillin; two simultaneous quinolones; coadministration of clindamycin and metronidazole; or perhaps simultaneous treatment with oral vancomycin and metronidazole. In each case, a much better strategy is to reduce the number of drugs and dose each to optimal effect. Parsimony reduces costs and risks of adverse effects and drug interactions. In addition, if something does go wrong, it is much easier to identify the culprit when there are fewer medicines.

Double Dipping

It is always a good idea to ask if one drug can be used to accomplish two purposes. For example, in a patient with suspected pneumonia and a possible urinary tract infection, is there one antibiotic, or combination, that will effectively treat both? Another example of this principle would be selecting a benzodiazepine or propofol for sedation over another drug class in a patient who has had a seizure. Choosing the benzodiazepine or propofol provides a "free" anticonvulsant. Likewise, choosing a nonsteroidal anti-inflammatory drug like ibuprofen to control fever also provides free nonnarcotic analgesia that is much more effective than acetaminophen.

Making Safer and Less Costly Choices

In most cases, more than one drug alternative exists, and often there are differences in safety between choices. When two drugs are equally effective, choosing the safer alternative makes sense. A prime example is using fluconazole or voriconazole in place of amphotericin B to reduce the risk of kidney injury. Another situation would be use of a fluroquinolone in place of an aminoglycoside–ampicillin regimen for a hospitalized patient with urinary tract infection, to avoid renal injury. Sometimes, the safer alternative is more expensive but now and then not. For each patient, the clinician must decide if the safety advantages between two equally effective options justify cost differences.

When two courses of therapy are equally safe and effective, cost should be considered. For example, *Escherichia coli* bacteriuria could be treated with generic enteral amoxicillin for pennies or with a proprietary intravenous (IV) extended spectrum penicillin for hundreds of dollars. Generic equivalents are almost always less expensive, and the good business practice of competitive bidding further

reduces costs. Sometimes, the choice is between two expensive therapies, as is the case with nitric oxide and nebulized prostacyclin. Neither compound has proven outcome benefits but both lower pulmonary artery pressure and may at least temporarily improve oxygenation in life-threatening hypoxemia. A protocol detailing who might receive these treatments and substitution of inhaled prostacyclin for nitric oxide can save a hospital hundreds of thousands of dollars annually with no decrement in quality.

Establishing an automatic substitution program in which the least expensive therapeutically equivalent compound is substituted for a brand name medication also saves money. Excellent areas in which to realize these savings are with antibiotics (e.g., quinolones, advanced-generation cephalosporins), gastric acid–modifying drugs (histamine blockers and proton pump inhibitors), and sedatives (e.g., brands of propofol). The process of therapeutic substitution requires a proactive pharmacy committee and consensus, though not universal agreement, of local experts that the substitutions are reasonably "equivalent." Reducing the number of like medications stocked by the pharmacy can also produce benefits. Pharmacy size is reduced, fewer personnel are necessary to track and manage inventory, and waste is reduced as fewer expired drugs are discarded. In the case of restriction or substitution, however, a multidisciplinary pharmacy committee must remain open to well-reasoned arguments for formulary additions or exceptions and a mechanism must exist for waiver of formulary rules under emergency circumstances.

Modifying Frequency and Route of Administration

There are numerous other ways to cut costs while maintaining or improving safety and efficacy. Surprisingly, the cost of a course of therapy often depends more on the route and frequency of administration than it does on the drug acquisition cost. Because patient *charges* for preparation of a dose of any IV medication average $20 to $40, it is apparent that charges for a drug purchased for $1/dose that must be given six times daily will exceed those for a drug that costs $100/dose given but once daily. In most cases, a very cost-effective measure is to minimize the number of times a day a drug is given, even if that requires using a more expensive drug. Prime examples are the substitution of once daily tiotropium for chronic obstructive pulmonary disease treatment instead of four times daily ipratropium; use of ceftriaxone or cefepime once daily instead of cefotaxime thrice daily; and once daily LMWH instead of UFH every 8 h. Reducing the number of scheduled administrations each day has also been shown to be associated with fewer missed doses.

The route of therapy can have profound impact on costs. In general, the cost of an equivalent dose of an oral medicine is one tenth to one hundredth that of the same drug given intravenously. This vast discrepancy exists because IV preparations are usually more expensive to purchase, some drug is wasted, and there are substantial labor costs associated with stocking, retrieving, mixing, transporting, and administering an IV preparation. Essentially, all patients eating or tolerating tube feeding can receive enteral medications. In fact, many medications (including benzodiazepines, gastric acid-suppressing drugs, narcotics, and some antibiotics) have equal bioavailability when given orally and intravenously. Hence, almost any time an IV preparation can be changed to an oral route, substantial savings can be achieved. Fluconazole, quinolone antibiotics, and parenteral nutrition are great examples.

Continuous infusion is the most costly method of administration, because a dedicated line, infusion pump, and specialized cassettes and tubing, all of which are expensive, are required. Also, each infusion site increases the risk of infection, and the mere presence of an IV catheter in a patient with fever is likely to prompt an expensive evaluation and empiric antibiotic therapy. Furthermore, if a central venous catheter must be inserted for access, the danger of infection persists and the risks of arterial puncture and pneumothorax are incurred. Sometimes, even switching from continuous infusion to intermittent IV dosing is cost effective. A constant infusion of a short-acting agent usually requires a dedicated line and a pump for precise control. By contrast, intermittent dosing of a longer acting agent can free up an IV line for administration of other required medications and in the process may avoid inserting another catheter. Examples of this principle would be substitution of intermittent IV or even enteral metoprolol for continuous esmolol and intermittent IV lorazepam for continuous infusion midazolam.

The belief that giving medications by continuous infusion automatically confers accurate control over drug effects is fallacious even when the practice achieves precise regulation of plasma drug levels. Exact titration of a plasma drug level is rarely necessary or achievable, and drug levels often do not correlate with effects. Critically ill patients commonly have such altered pharmacodynamics that "short-acting drugs" have prolonged actions. Accumulation of medications given by continuous infusion is frequent enough to be considered routine (lidocaine, fentanyl, theophylline, and midazolam are prime examples). In addition, continuous infusion may obscure signs that the drug is no longer necessary. A prime example is the continuous infusion of a sedative or neuromuscular blocker in which recognition of the ability to do without sedation or paralysis is delayed by the therapy itself.

Drug Monitoring Costs

A "hidden" cost of drug use is monitoring drug levels or indices of organ toxicity (e.g., creatinine, liver function tests). Although aminoglycosides and vancomycin are inexpensive to purchase and are typically dosed infrequently, their cost can be enormous: patients have peak and trough serum levels tested on multiple occasions (at about $100/determination) along with frequent creatinine determinations, not to mention the costs associated with renal failure if it develops. (Moreover, it is far from clear that knowing the blood levels of these compounds improves efficacy, and perhaps not even safety.) Another example is the use of warfarin versus LMWH for DVT prophylaxis. At 1 cent/tablet, compared to about $15/injection, warfarin seems to be the clear choice. However, the costs of prothrombin and hemoglobin determinations typically performed on patients treated with warfarin, but not done in patients treated with LMWH rapidly outstrip the savings for the drug itself. The same situation exists for UFH versus LMWH where multiple venapunctures and the costs of activated partial thromboplastin time (aPTT) determinations are avoided by using LMWH.

Avoiding Competing Therapies

It makes no sense to provide one drug that negates or counteracts the effect of another, yet it happens frequently. Common examples of this problem include simultaneous use of a histamine blocker or proton pump inhibitor and sucralfate (sucralfate requires gastric acid for mucosal binding), or coadministration of oral fluroquinolones and aluminum-magnesium containing antacids (antacids chelate quinolones). Another situation which leads to antagonistic therapy is forgetting to stop certain chronic outpatient medications. One example would be continuing a regimen of outpatient antihypertensive drugs for a patient in vasopressor dependent septic shock.

Optimizing Dosing

One of the most important areas for safety improvement, which also often reduces drug costs, is careful attention to dosing as organ function changes. Whole books have been written on the dose adjustment of drugs cleared by the kidney, but one basic principle is clearly important. Bedside calculation of creatinine clearance using the Cockcroft–Gault equation, which typically serves as the basis for dose adjustments, is not valid until renal function plateaus. The practical implication is that calculated creatinine clearance lags behind actual declines in renal function, usually by 1 to 3 days. Hence, a defensible strategy for adjusting renally cleared drugs is to assume a glomerular filtration rate (GFR) of zero as soon as patients develop significant oliguria (urine output < 0.5 mL/kg/h). Once the creatinine stabilizes then recalculate the GFR. Just as there are times when doses must be reduced, occasionally drug requirements go up. For instance, a higher dose of renally cleared medications may be needed in situations where GFR is increased (e.g., pregnancy and fully resuscitated major burns).

Contrary to conventional wisdom, organ failure is not always bad news for pharmacotherapy. For example, the treatment of a methicillin resistant staphylococcal infection can be simpler and more economical in a patient with established renal failure where postdialysis vancomycin dosing reduces the frequency of administration. Another instance would be intentionally selecting a neuromuscular blocking agent that is cleared by an organ that is failing (liver or kidney) when long-term therapeutic paralysis is required.

Stopping Ineffective/Unnecessary Treatments

Another method to improve safety while reducing costs is to simply discontinue medications which were never or are no longer beneficial. "Renal dose" dopamine is a prime example; the drug increases the heart rate and mandates a dedicated IV catheter without benefit. One more unneeded treatment is the use of dilute UFH to prevent clotting of IV catheters. It is clear this process is rarely necessary (saline works as well), increases costs, and can lead to heparin-induced thrombocytopenia. An additional example is administration of repeated doses of serotonin (5-HT) antagonists for nausea and vomiting. Even though 5-HT antagonists are effective when single doses are given to prevent chemotherapy-induced nausea and vomiting, there is little data to suggest efficacy for most causes of vomiting seen in the ICU. In addition, there is essentially no data to suggest that 5-HT drugs treat established nausea and vomiting or that multiple doses offer benefit over a single dose.

Sometimes, medications which might have been clearly indicated when started are not appropriately stopped. The most frequent examples come from the use of antibiotics. Perhaps the most common situation results from initiation of broad spectrum antibiotic therapy that is not trimmed appropriately as culture data return and the patient improves. Failure to stop empiric vancomycin in the face of negative cultures is a regular occurrence. Another almost daily event is the continuation of an antibiotic for days or sometimes even weeks longer than it could reasonably be expected to be needed to treat a proven infection. The arbitrariness of the duration of antibiotic therapy is spotlighted by the common practice of treating for calendar period (e.g., a week) instead of a physiologic or biochemical endpoint.

Oftentimes medication review reveals continuation of outpatient medications of questionable or no value during the time a patient is critically ill: alpha blockers given to men with an indwelling urinary catheter, oral hypoglycemic agents for patients receiving insulin. The value of continuing outpatient osteoporosis drugs and antidepressants is also arguable. In almost every case, these treatments serve only to increase the risk of adverse events.

Sometimes, out of habit or absentmindedness, a treatment is prescribed that not only makes no sense but may also be harmful. One example is prescribing acetaminophen for a patient admitted with fulminant hepatic failure due to acetaminophen overdose. Another is continuing an outpatient treatment, like potassium, in a patient who develops renal failure. Obviously, mistakenly prescribing any drug to which the patient is known to be allergic falls into this category.

Shortening of ICU or Hospital Stay

Sometimes, the choice of a more expensive drug may result in net cost savings by reducing the use of other resources. One example would be the use of intermittent injections of a LMWH instead of a continuous infusion of UFH. The former choice can result in substantial institutional savings by permitting early discharge. This principle may even extend to expensive drugs such as drotrecogin alfa activated, where timely administration to patients with severe sepsis has been reported to reduce mortality and shorten the duration of mechanical ventilation and ICU stay.

■ PHARMACOKINETICS

Patients in the ICU are often given ten or more medications simultaneously. As the number of medications, severity of illness, and patient age increase, so does the risk of an adverse drug reaction. Although many physicians have little enthusiasm for studying pharmacokinetics (the science of drug absorption, distribution, and clearance) or pharmacodynamics (the practical application of pharmacokinetics to the patient), understanding these concepts is essential to provide quality care. The critical care physician must develop a healthy respect for medications with narrow therapeutic margins and serious side effects. Intensivists must also learn how drug absorption, distribution, and clearance differ between critically ill and ambulatory patients. Ignorance of such differences predisposes patients to side effects, drug interactions, and the potential for ineffective therapy. Four major concepts are key to understanding drug dosing: bioavailability, volume of distribution (V_d), clearance, and half-life ($t_{1/2}$).

Bioavailability

When a drug is given intravenously, the entire dose is almost always available to body tissues. Exceptions include coadministration of two incompatible medications resulting in an inactive precipitate (e.g., heparin with an aminoglycoside or dopamine with amphotericin B). All other routes of administration reduce bioavailability (i.e., the fraction of unmetabolized drug reaching the circulation, compared to the total dose given). For enterally administered drugs, impaired absorption and hepatic metabolism are the most important determinants of bioavailability. The severely ill patient often has reduced peristalsis and gut blood flow, which both alter absorption. Furthermore, many enterally administered drugs have reduced bioavailability because splanchnic blood flows first through the liver (possibly the major drug clearing organ) en route to the systemic circulation. Drugs highly subject to first-pass clearance include morphine, verapamil, propranolol, and furosemide; others, such

as theophylline and phenytoin, have insignificant first-pass metabolism. Administration of some medications like fentanyl transcutaneously avoids the hepatic first-pass effect, allowing much lower analgesic doses to be effective. Severe liver damage commonly increases available concentrations of orally administered medications because of hepatocellular dysfunction and portal-to-systemic shunts (particularly in cirrhosis).

Dose, concentration, route of administration, solubility, rate of dissolution, absorptive area, GI motility, and drug–drug interactions all influence bioavailability. Problems of altered bioavailability abound in the ICU. For example, some drugs (e.g., ketoconazole, tetracycline, sucralfate) require an acidic gastric environment for absorption of effect. Hence, concurrent use of gastric acid reducing drugs like antacids, histamine blockers, and proton pump inhibitors significantly reduces bioavailability. By contrast, the same acid-suppressing medications increase the absorption of other drugs like the hypoglycemic agent glyburide. The formation of inactivated drug complexes is also very common among patients receiving medications (e.g., antacids) containing divalent or trivalent cations (calcium, magnesium, aluminum, iron). In addition to antacids, activated charcoal and bile acid binders may also complex with drugs inhibiting their absorption. Although the drugs whose absorption is limited by these agents are too long to list, warfarin, theophylline, digoxin, n-acetylcysteine, isoniazid, tetracycline, valproate, barbiturates, carbamazepine, and phenytoin are all subject to this effect. Similarly, an inhibitory effect of sucralfate on quinolone absorption is well known.

Alterations in GI motility have unpredictable effects on drug absorption. For example, the increased motility induced by metoclopramide and erythromycin increases the absorption of acetaminophen and lithium, but decreases the absorption of cimetidine and digoxin. Circulation to the site of drug deposition (intramuscular [IM] or subcutaneous injections) or to the gut mucosa (enteral route) also affects absorption and bioavailability—a key consideration in states of hypoperfusion. For example, absorption of subcutaneous insulin or heparin may be impaired in shock or in patients with anasarca. After absorption, bioavailability can actually be increased by certain drug interactions. For most drugs, the free or non–protein-bound form of the drug is the active moiety. Therefore, coadministration of any two avidly protein-bound drugs can result in higher free concentrations of one or both compounds as they compete for serum protein binding. Examples of drugs that when given together raise each other's active concentration include warfarin, diazepam, phenytoin, valproate, tolbutamide, and salicylates.

Another issue of bioavailability relates to the use of "pro-drugs" that require metabolism for activity. The best example of this issue may be use of fosphenytoin instead of phenytoin. The misinformed practitioner may believe that because the fosphenytoin can be administered more rapidly, it acts more rapidly. That is not the case: after infusion, 30 to 60 min is required for the metabolic conversion of inactive fosphenytoin to the active compound, a period of time almost identical to the time it takes to safely infuse the older active drug, phenytoin. This is not to discount potential advantages of fosphenytoin in certain settings (i.e., IM dosing capability and a reduced incidence of chemical phlebitis).

Volume of Distribution

Drugs distribute unevenly among the intracellular and extracellular compartments, in accordance with serum protein binding, cardiac output, pH, vascular permeability, and tissue solubility. The volume of distribution (V_d) relates the total amount of drug in the body to its plasma concentration. Knowledge of V_d is most useful in determining loading doses of drugs, particularly those that distribute in multiple compartments (like lidocaine). Distribution effects may account for such phenomena as ultra-rapid buildup and termination of drug effects and prolongation of drug action with repeated dosing (e.g., fentanyl). The critically ill patient often has an abnormally large volume of distribution for hydrophilic drugs (e.g., aminoglycosides) because of the accumulation of large amounts of extracellular water. On the other hand, drugs like digitalis and procainamide, which are highly tissue bound, are less subject to changes in the volume of distribution as a result of edema formation. Drugs with a large V_d can require a massive loading dose of medication to initially become saturated. Later in the course, this same reservoir of drug must be metabolized or excreted to fully terminate a drug's effect. This alteration can explain why it can be difficult to achieve a drug effect at first, but that same effect can be prolonged in duration. Perhaps the most common examples occur with the sedatives midazolam and propofol when they persist days after their discontinuation.

Clearance

In simplest terms, clearance reflects the rate at which a drug is eliminated from the circulation. Drug clearance may occur through chemical conversion and subsequent excretion of metabolites or through excretion of unchanged drug. It is plain that important genetic differences exist among patients in the ability to metabolize drugs. Although other tissues may participate, the liver is the central site of most drug metabolism. Hepatic metabolites are secreted into bile and then either directly eliminated in the stool or, alternatively, reabsorbed across the gut wall, assimilated into the bloodstream, and eliminated by the kidney. In addition to inherent genetic variability, the administration of one hepatically degraded drug can impact bioavailability or clearance of another by inducing metabolizing enzymes (The P450 cytochrome system is best characterized). The most common examples involve drugs that when taken chronically rev up hepatic metabolism (e.g., barbiturates, cyclosporine, phenytoin, rifampin, ethanol), thereby accelerating the clearance of other hepatically metabolized drugs (e.g., oral contraceptives, warfarin, ketoconazole, theophylline, glucocorticoids). Use of medications that induce hepatic metabolism can also increase formation of toxic metabolites (e.g., ethanol and acetaminophen). By contrast, patients treated acutely with cimetidine, ciprofloxacin, diltiazem, erythromycin, ketoconazole, metronidazole, and propranolol may demonstrate decreased metabolism (higher drug levels) of theophylline, warfarin, cyclosporine, barbiturates, and midazolam as two drugs compete for the same metabolic pathways. On occasion, drug-induced, enhanced bioavailability or reduced clearance can be used to great therapeutic advantage. For example, administration of even low doses of some calcium channel antagonists to patients receiving cyclosporine can elevate cyclosporine levels (and reduce drug costs) dramatically.

Half-Life

After administration, most drugs exhibit a two-phase concentration profile corresponding to initial distribution and then elimination. The serum half-life ($t_{1/2}$) is the time required for drug concentration to fall by 50% without further supplementation. The $t_{1/2}$ incorporates distribution and clearance effects to give a useful index for predicting the time required to achieve steady-state concentration and determine dosing interval. With repeated intermittent dosing, most drugs accumulate and wash out exponentially to their final

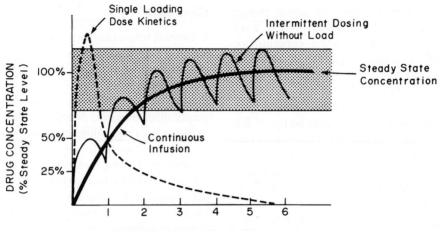

■ **FIGURE 15-1** Dosing and elimination kinetics. After a single dose, drug concentration falls exponentially to undetectable levels over approximately five half-lives (*dashed line*). During continuous infusion or intermittent administration of smaller maintenance doses (without load), a steady-state concentration is not achieved until five half-lives have elapsed (*solid line*). The therapeutic range can be achieved and maintained quickly by combining a large initial loading dose with a maintenance schedule of either type.

concentrations (first-order kinetics). Usually, five half-lives are required before drugs administered in constant dosage achieve a steady-state concentration—a delay that may compromise treatment. Therapeutic drug levels may be achieved more rapidly by the use of loading doses, but loading doses will not shorten the time to reach the steady state. Drug level monitoring before five half-lives have elapsed will underestimate the eventual steady-state peak and trough concentrations (Fig. 15-1). Unfortunately, the half-life of drugs is determined in relatively healthy individuals and rarely accurately reflects the kinetics of a compound in the critically ill. Commonly, long-term dosing and dysfunction of several organ systems leads to a prolonged half-life. In fact, the practitioner should be suspect of any claim of a "short half-life" for any drug repeatedly administered to ICU patients. Examples include the "expanding" half-life seen with chronic midazolam, propofol, or fentanyl infusions. Furthermore, the plasma half-life may not accurately portray the duration of biological effect: If a drug is highly tissue bound, effects can be observed even when plasma drug levels approach zero. This principle is exemplified by lorazepam where avid gamma amino butyric acid (GABA) receptor binding provides anticonvulsant activity longer than drug is detectable in the circulation. The previous comments notwithstanding, as a general rule in the ICU the half-life of a chosen drug should parallel the desired duration of effect.

■ **PHARMACOKINETICS IN DISEASE**

To a greater or lesser extent, dysfunction of every major organ system alters the distribution, metabolism, and clearance of medications. Specific organ system failures and their impact on drug metabolism are discussed following.

Circulatory Failure

In circulatory failure, blood flow is diverted from the skin, splanchnic bed, and muscle to maintain cerebral and cardiac perfusions. Thus, depressed cardiac output impairs drug absorption from subcutaneous, IM, and GI sites. Reports that plasma activity of LMWHs are reduced by shock with vasopressor use serves as a relevant example. Although IV dosing averts the problem of absorption, the smaller V_d observed in shock often results in high blood levels immediately after injection. (For example, usual doses of lidocaine commonly cause central nervous system [CNS] toxicity after bolus injection.) Even in the absence of overt liver or kidney failure, circulatory failure compromises the clearance of many drugs by diminishing glomerular filtration and hepatic metabolism. Reduced clearance increases the steady-state drug level for any given dosage and prolongs the time necessary to reach equilibrium. These two facts help explain why circulatory failure frequently results in the delayed expression of toxicity of drugs like lidocaine, quinidine, and theophylline.

Hepatic Failure

As the primary organ of drug metabolism and serum protein formation, the liver plays a key role in pharmacokinetics. Hepatic failure depresses the synthesis of albumin and other serum proteins, causing the total serum levels of highly protein-bound drugs to fall. On the other hand, serum concentrations of free drug may be normal or increased. (Phenytoin is a classic example.) Reduced liver blood flow impairs hepatic drug clearance. Specifically, portosystemic shunts (as in cirrhosis) decrease "first-pass" metabolism, thereby increasing bio-availability of orally administered drugs. Unstable patients with vacillating hepatic blood flow or parenchymal function can be difficult to manage with medications subject to extensive first-pass metabolism (e.g., diltiazem, morphine, nifedipine, propranolol). To avoid the vagaries of fluctuating liver function, it is often useful to use renally metabolized and excreted drugs in patients with impaired hepatic function. (For example, oxacillin is a logical substitute for nafcillin and pancuronium, a reasonable replacement for vecuronium.)

Biliary obstruction impairs the ability of the liver to concentrate drugs (particularly antibiotics) in the bile. Even drugs that normally enter the bile (e.g., ampicillin) fail to do so in the setting of complete biliary obstruction. Drug therapy may also cause artifactual elevations in liver-related laboratory tests. For example, tetracycline and IV lipid preparations may elevate reported values of serum bilirubin, and hydroxyethyl starch may spuriously elevate serum amylase. Metronidazole and para-amino salicylic acid cause artifactual elevations in aspartate aminotransferase (AST).

Renal Failure

For many, perhaps most drugs (e.g., aminoglycosides, acyclovir, quinolones, cyclosporine) dosages must be modified to prevent accumulation of the parent drug or its metabolites. Often a nonrenally excreted compound may be successfully substituted for one dependent on the kidney for removal (e.g., voriconazole for amphotericin B). Renal failure is frequently accompanied by a reduced albumin concentration and diminished protein binding. As in hepatic failure, these changes may lower total serum drug concentrations while raising free drug levels. The clearance of most renally excreted drugs is proportional to the GFR, which in turn parallels creatinine clearance. At steady state, drug dose (as a percentage of normal) can be calculated by estimating creatinine clearance (see Chapter 29). The Cockcroft–Gault equation is commonly used for this purpose. It is critical to recognize that this equation is only valid at steady state. Early in the course of kidney injury when the creatine is just beginning to rise, calculated creatine clearance dramatically overestimates actual GFR. Hence, when severe oliguria or anuria develops, it is probably best to calculate drug doses based upon a GFR of zero until creatinine plateaus. Although reduced GFR is the usual concern, some conditions increase GFR and hasten drug elimination. For example, during pregnancy increases in GFR outstrip weight gains. Similarly, the GFR is often supranormal in fully resuscitated young burn patients. Cefoxitin, trimethoprim-sulfa, and flucytosine can produce misleading elevations of creatinine by competing with creatinine for renal tubular excretion.

Lung Disease

Although lung disease rarely affects drug metabolism (one exception may be prostacyclin infusion), cor pulmonale, positive pressure ventilation, and positive end-expiratory pressure may reduce cardiac output and hepatic and renal blood flow, thereby predisposing to drug toxicity.

Burns

Beginning immediately after the injury, burn patients translocate fluid from the intravascular to the extravascular space, changing V_d and reducing renal and hepatic blood flows. However, after successful resuscitation, the GFR and metabolic rate accelerate and the concentrations of serum albumin and protein-bound drugs decline. Consequently, larger doses of many drugs (e.g., cimetidine, vancomycin, aminoglycosides) are needed to achieve therapeutic levels.

Acid–Base Disorders

Acid–base status plays a significant role in the absorption, distribution, and elimination of drugs. Ionized drugs traverse cell membranes poorly. Systemic acidosis inhibits the ionization of weak acids (e.g., salicylates, phenobarbital), thereby promoting their translocation to target tissues. For similar reasons, weak bases (e.g., amphetamines, quinidine) enter cells more readily under alkalemic conditions. These same acid–base properties can be used to alter drug distribution within the body and bolster drug excretion. Urinary alkalinization traps weak acids in the urine, increasing the renal excretion of salicylates and phenobarbital, whereas acidosis promotes excretion of amphetamines, quinidine, and phencyclidine (PCP). pH also impacts the binding of certain drugs to serum proteins. Therefore, manipulation of acid–base status can rapidly influence drug activity by altering distribution—a principle useful during crisis intervention. (A good example is the use of bicarbonate to facilitate transfer of tricyclic antidepressants from cardiac tissue to plasma in the treatment of overdosage.) An important clinical situation with regard to pH occurs in patients with salicylate toxicity. When spontaneously breathing, such patients often have massive increases in minute ventilation to offset the effects of metabolic acidosis. However, if sedation or intubation results in a lower minute ventilation than that selected by the spontaneously breathing patient, pH plummets and causes intracellular salicylate levels to skyrocket.

■ GOALS OF DRUG ADMINISTRATION

The aim of drug therapy is to rapidly achieve and maintain effective, nontoxic tissue drug concentrations. In critically ill patients, these goals are met by combining appropriate loading and maintenance regimens. During intermittent dosing, drug levels may demonstrate peaks and troughs that potentially expose patients to toxicity and subtherapeutic levels (Fig. 15-1). In an attempt to avoid these fluctuations, many drugs used in the ICU are infused at a constant rate. Unfortunately, even constant infusions do not guarantee constant drug levels. Highly lipid-soluble drugs, drugs with long half-lives, and those with a large V_d may accumulate for long periods of time before toxic side effects emerge. Deterioration of renal or hepatic function may impair drug excretion. The addition of new drugs to an established regimen may also alter metabolism, compete for protein binding, or alter absorption.

■ ROUTES OF ADMINISTRATION

Inhalation (Aerosols)

Endobronchial administration normally achieves high local drug concentrations without adverse systemic effects. β-Agonist and anticholinergic

bronchodilators, inhaled corticosteroids, and pentamidine serve as examples. However, certain inhaled solutions reaching the pulmonary parenchyma both act locally and can be rapidly absorbed across the massive surface area of the capillary bed (e.g., prostacyclin, isoproterenol, and lidocaine). Inhaled nitric oxide, a vasodilating gas, both acts locally on pulmonary vessels but is then inactivated as it enters the bloodstream.

Intratracheal Instillation

The intratracheal route may be used to produce therapeutic drug levels rapidly in settings where IV access is limited or denied (e.g., cardiopulmonary resuscitation). Drugs given via the intratracheal route must be delivered in at least 10 mL of liquid to permit the majority of the dose to access the alveolar compartment where absorption occurs. The intratracheal route has been demonstrated effective for emergent use of lidocaine, epinephrine, naloxone, and atropine (Table 15-1). Interestingly, intratracheal administration may prolong the duration of action of certain drugs (e.g., lidocaine, atropine). It is unwise to mix drugs when dosing via the intratracheal route. Furthermore, some commonly used drugs should not be given intratracheally (i.e., norepinephrine and calcium chloride) because they may cause pulmonary necrosis. Since sodium bicarbonate depletes functional surfactant, massive atelectasis may result from intratracheal use.

Intravenous Injection

IV injection is the most reliable route of drug administration and avoids problems of bioavailability and delays associated with absorption. Unfortunately, IV injections can result in potentially detrimental high peak drug concentrations, especially when a drug is infused rapidly through a central venous catheter. Good examples of this phenomenon are the cardiac toxicity of phenytoin or potassium sometimes seen with rapid IV

TABLE 15-1 INTRATRACHEAL DRUGS	
DRUG	DOSE (mg)
Lidocaine	50–100
Atropine	1–2
Naloxone	2–5
Epinephrine	1 (1:10,000 dilution)

infusions of these medications. IV injection also allows the administration of drugs that otherwise would be too caustic, unstable, or poorly absorbed to dose via other routes. At steady state, uninterrupted, continuous IV infusion sustains drug levels, limits peaks and troughs, and avoids the associated problems of subtherapeutic levels and toxicity. It should be noted, however, that impaired drug clearance, especially that resulting from deteriorating renal function, might cause important changes in drug concentrations—even at an unchanging rate of infusion.

Constant IV infusion is the most costly method of drug administration and is often not necessary. Costs come from two sources: not only are IV drugs typically the most expensive formulations, but substantial costs are also incurred in securing and maintaining IV access. Often overlooked, the incremental costs of inserting an IV line are huge if that insertion results in hemothorax, pneumothorax, or catheter-related sepsis. These complications become particularly tragic if similar therapeutic effect could have been achieved by using a different method of administration, or if the drug was not truly necessary. Many medications achieve similar blood concentration when given by the enteral or IV route. When enteral absorptive function is intact, oral doses of fluconazole, clindamycin, tetracycline, metronidazole, doxycycline, trimethoprim-sulfa, and fluoroquinolones produce comparable blood levels as after IV dosing.

Intramuscular Injections

Because uptake of drug from muscle into the intravascular compartment is a gradual process, the duration of action of an IM injection is usually longer than that of an equivalent IV bolus. Under normal circumstances, aqueous solutions are more promptly absorbed than oily or viscous preparations. Drug absorption may be erratic if local perfusion is impaired, as during shock or cardiopulmonary arrest. IM injections cause pain, fever, and routinely raise the serum creatinine phosphokinase, thereby interfering with the diagnosis of myocardial infarction and rhabdomyolysis. Some compounds (e.g., phenytoin) are sufficiently caustic that IM injections can cause extensive tissue necrosis. Others which are very safe when given subcutaneously (e.g., heparins) in the muscle can cause significant hematoma formation. IM injection of any drug in a patient receiving therapeutic anticoagulation can have the same result.

Subcutaneous Injections

Subcutaneous injections (particularly of insulin, epinephrine, or heparins) may be appropriate if the drug is nonirritating and administered in a small volume (approx. 1 mL). Rates of absorption vary widely, depending on the drug and local blood flow. For example, subcutaneous epinephrine is absorbed with sufficient speed to be a mainstay of therapy in anaphylactoid reactions. Conversely, insulin should probably not be given subcutaneously to the hypotensive diabetic. Delayed absorption of some drugs (e.g., UFH) may be useful to allow prolonged low-level drug effects (i.e., DVT prophylaxis).

Intra-arterial Injections

Direct injection into peripheral arteries delivers massive concentrations of drug to a local region and may produce serious complications (tissue ischemia and necrosis), particularly if vasoactive drugs are infused. Consequently, the only common use of intra-arterial therapy is the deliberate, selective, and closely metered administration of vasoconstrictors by catheterization of mesenteric vessels in the treatment of GI bleeding or vasodilators in mesenteric ischemia. Rarely, selective infusions of antineoplastic agents into visceral arteries may be performed.

Intrathecal Therapy

Intrathecal therapy is rarely used, except when high CNS concentrations of drugs that cross the blood–brain barrier poorly must be obtained. Refractory CNS infection (i.e., fungal meningitis, Gram-negative meningitis, or abscess) constitutes one such indication. Intraventricular or spinal access to the cerebrospinal fluid may be appropriate, depending on the organism and clinical condition of the patient. Rarely, intrathecal antineoplastic drugs may be used for leukemic meningitis.

Intraperitoneal Therapy

Intraperitoneal antibiotics are often used to treat peritonitis in patients undergoing peritoneal dialysis. (Gram-positive coverage is usually provided by a cephalosporin or vancomycin, and Gram-negative coverage using an aminoglycoside.) IV loading doses are given initially and then serum levels are sustained by absorption of drug given via the intraperitoneal route. Because intraperitoneal concentrations of drug equilibrate with those in the serum, the concentration of drug in the dialysate should equal that desired in the serum. For example, if a serum level of 7 mg/dL is desired, the dialysate concentration of drug should be kept at 7 mg/dL. Because peritoneal dialysis is now uncommon and advantages over IV dosing are uncertain, the practice of intraperitoneal dosing is a dying art.

Transcutaneous Administration

Cutaneous drug absorption depends on skin permeability, temperature, blood flow, moisture content, and the presence of dermatologic disorders. The highest penetration of transcutaneously administered drugs is for lipid-soluble preparations applied to moist skin under an occlusive dressing. At the present time, nitroglycerin, clonidine, fentanyl, nicotine, estrogen, and scopolamine are the only systemic drugs commonly administered transcutaneously in the ICU. Diffusion of drug through the skin often requires a significant period of time, delaying the onset of action. Because the skin and subcutaneous tissue act as a reservoir, removal of medications (e.g., fentanyl patches, nitroglycerin paste) does not immediately terminate the action of the drug.

High concentrations of topical corticosteroids applied over large areas may occasionally result in significant systemic absorption. Chronic use of long-acting (fluorinated) topical corticosteroids can suppress the pituitary–adrenal axis, particularly if applied to inflamed skin under occlusive dressings. Certain topical antibiotics used in burn therapy may also produce metabolic acidosis (i.e., mafenide) or salt-wasting (i.e., sodium nitrate) (see Chapter 41).

Intraocular Drugs

Even eye drops may be absorbed systemically in significant concentrations if given frequently, in high doses, or if there is significant corneal inflammation or trauma. Corticosteroids and β-blockers both have the potential for producing systemic effects when administered intraocularly. (Thus, intraocular β-blockers are viewed by many physicians as contraindicated in asthma or congestive heart failure.)

Enteral Administration

Bioavailability of enterally administered drugs can be limited by gastric acid digestion, poor absorption, and first-pass metabolism by the liver. Effective enteral therapy requires gut motility, mucosal perfusion, and epithelial integrity. Patients with ileus, gut hypoperfusion, or atrophic or injured epithelium are poor candidates for enteral therapy because absorption will be limited. Drugs given in aqueous solutions are more rapidly absorbed than those given in oily solutions, and nonionized drugs are more readily absorbed than ionized drugs. A few poorly absorbed drugs (e.g., vancomycin, polymyxin) are intentionally given enterally to act only in the gut. Drugs destroyed by an acidic pH may be partially protected by enteric coating. Conversely, other drugs require acid for activation or absorption (e.g., sucralfate, ketoconazole, and iron), a point that deserves consideration in patients receiving acid suppressive therapy. It is important to note that many "sustained release" drug formulations (e.g., proton pump inhibitors, clarithromycin) cannot be reliably administered through an enteral tube either because they plug the lumen or because the delayed-release properties of the drug are destroyed by crushing the medication (e.g., extended-release diltiazem, theophylline, or procainamide). Although not often considered, significant volume overload may result from giving such fluid intensive oral preparations as sodium–potassium exchange resin (e.g., kayexalate) or bowel preparations (e.g., saline or polyethylene glycol).

Sublingual Administration

Because only minute quantities of drug are absorbed across intact oral epithelium, an effective sublingual drug must be potent and lipid soluble. Nitroglycerin, nicotine, and fentanyl are the few drugs that fit this description. If swallowed and absorbed enterally, nitroglycerin is rapidly eliminated by first-pass liver metabolism. However, because drugs absorbed from the sublingual space drain directly to the superior vena cava, such first-pass clearance is bypassed, increasing bioavailability.

Rectal Administration

Rectal administration of certain drugs can occasionally be useful in children, combative patients, and patients with problematic venous access or refractory vomiting and/or ileus. Hepatic first-pass metabolism is less extensive with rectally administered drugs than with orally administered drugs, but it is still significant. Unfortunately, rectal administration sometimes results in erratic and incomplete absorption and therefore is less desirable than either oral or parenteral dosing. Rectal dosing is best confined to sedatives (e.g., diazepam), antiemetics (e.g., phenergran), antipyretics (e.g., acetaminophen), laxatives, and theophylline compounds.

Intravesicular Administration

In the past, amphotericin bladder lavage was commonly used when yeast was found in the urine, but it is cumbersome and of limited usefulness. Systemic antifungal therapy (i.e., fluconazole, voriconazole, caspofungin, or some form of amphotericin) should be used if evidence of hyphal forms, or clumps, of fungus, urine, or histologic evidence of bladder wall invasion suggests invasive cystitis with *Candida* or *Aspergillus*. Yeast in the urine of an asymptomatic patient rarely requires treatment (particularly in patients with indwelling urinary catheters), and when treatment is necessary, oral imidazoles are highly effective. Intravesicular therapy may result in hyponatremia if aqueous solutions are used, and fluid overload may result from isotonic saline. Bladder lavage with glycine-containing solutions is often used to control bleeding after urinary tract surgery.

■ SUGGESTED READINGS

Kucukarslan SN, Peters M, Mlynarek M, et al. Pharmacists on rounding teams reduce preventable adverse drug events in hospital general medicine units. *Arch Intern Med.* 2003;163(17):2014–2018.

MacLaren R, Bond CA, Martin SJ, et al. Clinical and economic outcomes of involving pharmacists in the direct care of critically ill patients with infections. *Crit Care Med.* 2008;36(12):3184–3189.

Nielson C. Pharmacologic considerations in critical care of the elderly. *Clin Geriatr Med.* 1994;10(1):71–89.

Reynolds JR. Pharmacokinetic considerations in critical care. *Crit Care Nurs Clin North Am.* 1993;5(2):227–235.

Romac DR, Albertson TE. Drug interactions in the intensive care unit. *Clin Chest Med.* 1999;20(2):385–399, ix.

Vargas E, Terleira A, Hernando F, et al. Effect of adverse drug reactions on length of stay in surgical intensive care units. *Crit Care Med.* 2003;31(3):694–698.

Nutritional Assessment and Support

1 For patients with preexisting nutritional deficiencies, profound hypermetabolic states, or prolonged ICU stays, nutritional support is probably important. By contrast, for patients with normal nutritional status and brief ICU stays, nutrition is much less critical.

2 Detailed nutritional assessments and metabolic cart studies are expensive and offer little benefit for most ICU patients.

3 Enteral feeding delivered to the stomach using a small-bore nasal or oral tube is preferred over total parenteral nutrition in essentially all circumstances where the gut is functioning.

4 Both enteral and parenteral nutrition are associated with significant complications: aspiration with the former and metabolic and septic complications with the latter.

5 If intravenous nutritional support is required, central total parenteral nutrition delivered through a freshly placed dedicated catheter is the best option. The total parenteral nutrition prescription should be customized to meet patient requirements and limitations based on underlying organ failures.

Perhaps even more so than ventilator or hemodynamic management, critical care nutrition is controversial. Discussions are polarizing with strong opinions held about when, what, how, and how much support should be provided. Unfortunately, the controversies are yet to be resolved by large, randomized, controlled clinical trials, so much of current practice defaults to habit and belief. However, four basic facts are rarely disputed: malnutrition is associated with poor outcomes, starvation for weeks to months is fatal, several days without food is well tolerated by previously healthy

humans, and enteral or parenteral nutrition support is far different than eating a regular diet.

■ WHY FEED CRITICALLY ILL PATIENTS?

In the intensive care unit (ICU), pressing concerns of hemodynamic and respiratory instability often divert attention away from nutrition. Yet, by impairing immunity, prolonging ventilator weaning, and delaying wound healing, malnutrition could prove decisive in the fragile patient with a long stay. However, most patients stay only a few days in the ICU, which raises the question of how important it is to begin support rapidly or to achieve full caloric goals. Despite the inherent appeal of providing nutrition, there is surprisingly little credible evidence that nutritional support improves important clinical outcomes among the critically ill, and there are significant complications associated with "feeding," especially after long periods of starvation. Even though a convincing survival benefit has not been demonstrated for either enteral or parenteral support, studies demonstrating improvement in surrogate markers of nutritional status (e.g., serum protein concentrations or lymphocyte counts) and length of stay or infectious complications and the visceral appeal of "feeding" have promoted an entire industry.

■ WHY WITHHOLD NUTRITION SUPPORT?

Historically, many physicians and nurses have assumed the gastrointestinal (GI) tract is so dysfunctional that enteral nutrition in the critically ill patient was not feasible. Given this belief only two options existed: begin *parenteral* nutrition or withhold all support. Thus, many patients were not given nutrition because of the risks, costs, and complexity of the parenteral route. However, the realization has come over time that there are advantages of enteral nutrition over parenteral nutrition and that enteral feeding is much more practical than once believed. Furthermore, it is likely that some catabolic patients, especially those with severe sepsis, ineffectively utilize nutrients in any form. Even if nutritional substrate could be fully used by the tissues of seriously ill patients, the high likelihood of survival and brief stay of most ICU patients raises serious doubt about the ability of any form of nutritional support to improve survival or shorten length of stay (or at least to demonstrate such benefit in a clinical trial). Despite widespread advocacy for early and full feeding, studies of current practice indicate most critical care physicians are content to delay the institution of nutritional support for days. Expert consensus statements suggest that even a week of delay is acceptable. In addition, several small studies suggest that early full enteral nutrition may be associated with worse outcomes; perhaps due to enhanced inflammation. Once a decision has been made to provide supplemental nutrition, three basic questions need to be answered: (i) What route of feeding will be used? (ii) How many calories and how much protein will be delivered? and (iii) Are there any special considerations related to the patient's underlying diseases?

■ SELECTING CANDIDATES FOR NUTRITION SUPPORT

Most previously healthy patients readily tolerate calorie deprivation for a week or more before supplementation is necessary. Although benefit is **1** unproven, candidates likely to benefit from nutritional supplementation include (i) those unable to eat for long periods because of endotracheal intubation or GI tract interruption; (ii) patients with high caloric requirements (e.g., burns, severe sepsis, major surgery, or trauma); (iii) patients who sustain high protein losses (e.g., corticosteroid or tetracycline usage, nephrotic syndrome, or draining fistulas); and (iv) patients already malnourished at the time of ICU admission.

Complex nutritional assessment scales have been developed that incorporate anthropomorphic measurements and laboratory studies. Whereas such **2** precise indices of nutritional status may occasionally be helpful, simple clinical evaluation—a history of weight loss, dietary habits, and knowledge of underlying disease—provides a good working

assessment. Of the widely available clinical measures of nutritional status, clinical history, absolute lymphocyte count, cholesterol, and serum protein levels at the time of admission are perhaps the most useful data.

Malnutrition is almost certain in patients losing 5% of their body weight in the past month or more than 10% in the 6 months preceding admission. Absolute lymphocyte counts less than 1,200 cells/mm^3 and less than 800/mm^3 signify moderate and severe malnutrition, respectively. It is widely believed that because albumin normally has a long half-life (approx. 18 days), weeks of nutritional deficiency is needed to produce hypoalbuminemia. This is not true in the ICU population because vascular permeability for albumin is often dramatically increased; the liver ceases to produce albumin during severe illness; and extracellular water is often dramatically expanded. The net effect of these processes is to cause hypoalbuminemia within hours to days. Even faster declines may occur during intense catabolic stress. Transferrin and thyroid-binding globulin (TBG) prealbumin may be more sensitive acute indicators of response to nutritional depletion or therapy because they have shorter half-lives. In the absence of hypothyroidism, severe liver disease, or nephrotic syndrome and profound depressions of serum cholesterol reliably indicate calorie deprivation. Fever, severe sepsis, steroids, tumors, and immunosuppressant drugs reduce the value of the antigenic skin test response to the point of making it not clinically useful.

■ NUTRITIONAL REQUIREMENTS

Energy/Calories

Formulas for calculating calorie requirements (basal energy expenditure [BEE]) are often complicated, as exemplified by the Harris–Benedict equation:

$$BEE \text{ (men)} = 66 + (13.7 \times wt) + (5 \times ht) - (6.8 \times age)$$

$$BEE \text{ (women)} = 655 + (9.6 \times wt) + (1.8 \times ht) - (4.7 \times age)$$

Weight (wt) and height (ht) are expressed in kilograms and centimeters, respectively, and BEE is kcal/day.

Despite their complexity and seeming precision, the Harris–Benedict formulas still require upward adjustment for additional stress. For example, a well-nourished, minimally active patient should receive 1.25 times the BEE, whereas a severely anabolic patient may expend up to 1.75 times the

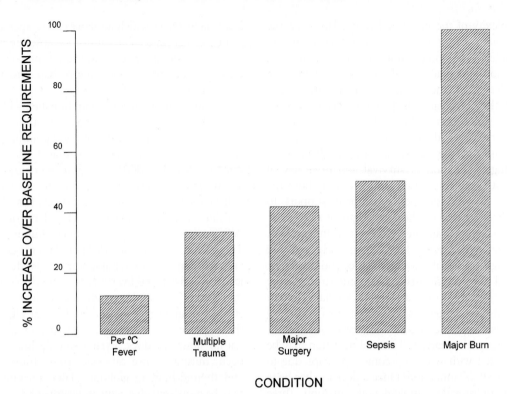

■ **FIGURE 16-1** Caloric requirements in stress.

BEE. Although detailed calculations may occasionally prove helpful, adequate caloric requirements can usually be estimated by simple assessment of the patient's general condition and lean body weight. Rather than calculating the Harris–Benedict equations, simply providing 25 to 35 kcal/kg/day will be close to the mark for most patients. In the severely stressed patient, two to three times that number of calories may be required (Fig. 16-1).

Bedside indirect calorimetry (metabolic cart study) provides a direct measure of caloric expenditure during the period the test is performed (usually 15 to 20 min). Resting energy expenditure (REE) is determined using the Weir equation (see following) by measuring oxygen consumption (VO_2), carbon dioxide production (VCO_2), and minute ventilation (V_e). Accuracy of REE determinations are highly dependent on proper setup and calibration of the measuring device and are less reliable in patients receiving greater than 50% oxygen. Furthermore, calorimetry disrupts the patient care routine, is expensive, and is not universally available. Calorimetry is not necessary for most patients. REE measurements might be helpful in difficult-to-wean patients who may be overfed and in obese or edematous patients in whom current

body weight may not provide an accurate estimation of caloric requirements.

$$\text{Daily REE} = [(VO_2)\,(3.94) + (VCO_2)\,(1.11)] \times 1{,}440$$

(VO_2 and VCO_2 are in L/min, and REE is in kcal/day.)

About 80% of all calories should be supplied by nonprotein sources. Typically, glucose provides one half to three quarters of this (2 to 4 gm/kg/day), with the remainder provided as lipid. The exact proportions of glucose and lipid are not of crucial importance. However, at least 100 to 150 nonprotein kcal/gm of nitrogen (approx. 20 cal/gm protein) must be provided to avoid using amino acids as an energy source. Some glucose is required for protein-sparing effects and to supply those tissues with an obligate requirement for glucose (e.g., brain). However, when given in excess of 7 mg/kg/min, glucose is largely converted to fat, leading to potential complications of overfeeding (volume overload, hyperglycemia, increased CO_2 production, and fatty liver).

Protein

Normal adults require 0.5 to 1.0 gm/kg/day of protein; however, the average ICU patient may need up to 1.5 to 2.0 gm/kg/day (Fig. 16-2). The

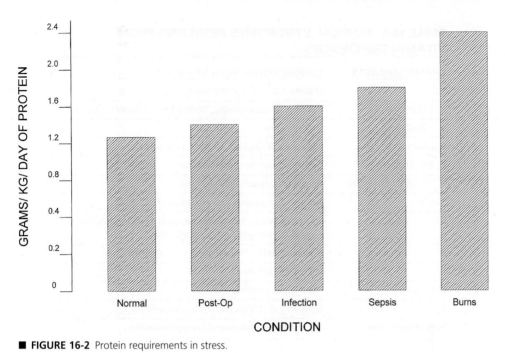

■ **FIGURE 16-2** Protein requirements in stress.

corresponding amount of nitrogen supplied may be calculated by dividing grams of protein by 6.25 (about 0.15 gm of N_2/kg/day). Nutritional supplements provide amino acids capable of being reassembled intracellularly to form structural proteins and enzymes. Providing greater quantities of amino acids than required is not likely to be beneficial. (Excess amino acids cannot be stored; therefore overfeeding requires the oxidation and excretion of these compounds as urinary nitrogen wastes.) For most patients, anabolism or protein-sparing effects are not enhanced by administration of protein in amounts above 1.5 gm/kg/day. In addition to the normal routes of catabolism, important protein losses may also occur through the urine (in nephrotic syndrome), surgical drains, or chest tubes (especially chylothorax). The adequacy of protein delivery can be assessed using a urinary nitrogen balance study (detailed following); however, in practice, such studies are laborious and expensive and hence, are uncommonly performed.

The classical distinction between "essential" and "nonessential" amino acids is artificial. Histidine, isoleucine, leucine, lysine, methionine, phenylalanine, threonine, tryptophan, and valine have been considered to be essential, but for critically ill patients all amino acids are probably "conditionally essential." (Glutamine, alanine, and aspartate are the only nonessential amino acids, but now some data even suggests benefits of supplementing glutamine.)

Lipids

Some lipid intake is required to prevent the occurrence (over several weeks) of essential (linoleic) fatty acid deficiency. Minimal daily linoleic acid requirements are estimated to be between 3 and 20 gm, an amount easily supplied by providing as little as 5% of calories in the form of lipid. Usual lipid doses are in the range of 0.5 to 2.0 gm/kg/day. (In most patients, the limits of lipid metabolism are approximately 4 gm/kg/day.) Lipids also provide a rich source of calories in a small volume. This fact is supported by the observation that sedation using propofol with its lipid vehicle supplies 1 to 2 kcal/mL of drug infused. The lower respiratory quotient observed from the oxidation of fats as compared to carbohydrates indicates that fats generate a lower CO_2 burden for any given caloric intake. Effective lipid metabolism requires a functioning liver; therefore, lipids may not represent the best caloric choice for patients with hepatic dysfunction.

Vitamins and Trace Elements

Vitamins and trace elements serve as antioxidants and play key roles as intracellular cofactors for enzymatic and energy generating reactions. More

TABLE 16-1   CLINICAL SYNDROMES RESULTING FROM VITAMIN DEFICIENCIES

VITAMIN DEFICIENCY	CLINICAL SYNDROME/SYMPTOMS
A	Decreased vision, dermatitis
B_1 (thiamine)	Peripheral neuropathy, Wernicke–Korsakoff syndrome
B_2 (riboflavin)	Glossitis, cheilosis, pruritus
B_3 (niacin)	Pellagra (dermatitis, diarrhea, dementia)
B_6 (pyridoxine)	Calcium oxalate urinary stones
B_{12} (cyanocobalamin)	Pernicious, macrocytic anemia
Biotin	Alopecia, myalgias, paresthesias, dermatitis
C	Scurvy (anemia, hemorrhage, gum swelling, muscle weakness), poor wound healing
D	Osteomalacia
E	Hemolytic anemia
Folic acid	Macrocytic anemia
K	Bleeding diathesis (warfarin-like effect)
Pantothenic acid	Paresthesias, abdominal cramping/pain

than a dozen different vitamins and trace minerals have been identified as essential for normal physiologic function. It is well recognized that levels of these substances are often abnormal in the plasma of critically ill patients.

In general, fat-soluble vitamins (K, E, D, A) are less prone to acute changes induced by critical illness by virtue of their relatively large storage pool in most patients. Fat-soluble vitamin levels can be reduced in patients suffering from prolonged starvation or malabsorption and in patients treated with broad-spectrum antibiotics, warfarin compounds, or bile-sequestering drugs. By contrast, the water-soluble vitamins (C, folate, and other B complex vitamins) are prone to rapid declines when patients are subjected to dietary deprivation. (Vitamin B_{12} is an exception to this rule.) Table 16-1 provides a list of clinical conditions associated with specific vitamin deficiencies.

Individual deficiencies of the trace minerals, copper, zinc, selenium, chromium, manganese, and molybdenum, have all been associated with specific syndromes. A full discussion of these syndromes is well beyond the scope of this text. Suffice it to say that significant clinical deficiencies of these elements are rare given even meager nutritional support. Luckily, all commercially available tube feeding products and now essentially all parenteral nutrition solutions contain at least the daily minimum requirements of vitamins and trace minerals, making clinical deficiencies uncommon.

■ THE ADVERSE EFFECTS OF MALNUTRITION

Malnutrition depresses the immune system by reducing immunoglobulin levels and by decreasing T cell function. Deficiencies of glutathione and other antioxidant compounds (vitamin E, β-carotene) may be associated with impaired resistance to the oxidative stress of sepsis, cancer chemotherapy, or high levels of inspired oxygen. Low colloid osmotic pressure caused by hypoalbuminemia predisposes to pulmonary and peripheral edema at a lower-than-normal hydrostatic pressure. Poor nutrition may impair wound healing and increase rates of infection in burns, trauma, and postoperative states. Starvation impairs ventilatory capacity by decreasing drive and diaphragm bulk. Severe nutritional deficiencies may be fatal, even in otherwise healthy patients. (Even under optimal conditions, otherwise healthy adults succumb to subacute losses greater than 40% of lean body mass.) When patients with prolonged starvation are refed, hypophosphatemia may cause muscle weakness.

■ INDICES OF ADEQUATE SUPPORT

The same indices used to detect malnutrition may also be used to determine the effectiveness of nutritional supplementation. Because albumin is slowly repleted, it is not a very useful index of acute improvement or deterioration in nutritional status. With much shorter half-lives, prealbumin and transferrin may be more helpful. Note that iron deficiency can increase transferrin levels independent of nutritional status. Weight gain is not a dependable sign; edema may produce rapid weight increases without improvement in nutritional status, and the average critically ill patient gains approximately 1 L of fluid each day.

Nitrogen balance is possibly the best indicator of nutritional homeostasis. Because nonurinary (skin and stool) losses of nitrogen are usually small (approx. 2 gm/day), the 24-h urine collection effectively quantitates nitrogen losses. Urine urea nitrogen (UUN) accounts for 80% of total urinary N_2 losses, and acute illness promotes urinary excretion of nitrogen as a result of catabolism. Hence, unless excessive nonurinary nitrogen losses occur (e.g., through fistulas or open surgical wounds), the balance between nitrogen intake and loss can be approximated using this formula:

$$N_2 \text{ balance} = (\text{Protein intake}/6.25) - ([UUN + 20\%] + \text{nonurinary losses})$$

■ ROUTES OF NUTRITIONAL SUPPLEMENTATION

Enteral Therapy

3 The numerous advantages of enteral feeding almost always make it preferable to the parenteral route (Table 16-2). Enteral feeding is less expensive, deters GI ulceration, promotes immune function, and preserves small bowel mucosal integrity and function better than intravenous nutrition. Because enteral feeding stimulates insulin secretion, hyperglycemia is less likely than during total parenteral nutrition (TPN). Enteral feeding stimulated release of cholecystokinin and gastrin preserves normal emptying of the gallbladder and pancreatic secretions. Enteral feeding also provides iron and trace elements more effectively than TPN. Although the importance of any individual component found in enteral feedings is uncertain, nucleic acids, medium- and short-chain amino acids, fiber, glutamine, and intact proteins are not present in TPN solutions.

The GI tract is often not used for nutrition in favor of TPN because of concerns that the gut is immotile. Because gastric peristalsis is often lost while small bowel function is preserved, air may not move into the small bowel to generate the characteristic gurgling bowel sounds in critically ill

TABLE 16-2 **ADVANTAGES OF ENTERAL NUTRITION**
Maintains gut mucosal structure
Decreases bacteria and toxin translocation
Promotes enteric hormone secretion
Eliminates need for central catheter Reduced risk of sepsis and line related complications
Buffers gastric acid
Less likely to induce hyperglycemia
Provides unique and complex nutrients not available by TPN Glutamine Dietary fiber Medium- and short-chain fatty acids
Dramatically reduces cost

patients. Likewise, patients receiving continuous gastric suction or neuromuscular blocking drugs do not swallow air or fluid necessary to produce bowel sounds. Therefore, neither mild abdominal distention nor reduced bowel sounds should deter a trial of enteral feeding. In fact, it is often only after feeding is begun that bowel sounds return.

When the upper GI tract must be bypassed, soft small bore (6 to 8 French) feeding tubes passed through the nose or larger tubes passed through the mouth are both acceptable conduits. Inserting feeding tubes through the mouth minimizes the risk of nosocomial sinusitis. (For patients who are already orally intubated, passage of a feeding tube through the mouth does not add risk or increase discomfort.) In most patients with ileus, peristalsis of the small bowel returns before gastric and colonic motility; therefore, it may be advantageous to deliver nutrients directly to the small bowel. Surprising to some, the vast majority of ICU patients tolerate gastric food delivery quite well; only vomiting or a persistently elevated gastric residual volume mandates interruption of feeding. When reduced gastric motility becomes problematic, advancing the feeding tube into the distal duodenum or use of prokinetic agents may improve tolerance. Pancreatitis may be one condition where postpyloric feeding is useful but recent data suggest that even gastric feeding is feasible. Unfortunately, achieving and maintaining a postpyloric tube position is often easier said than done. In some patients short-term use of metoclopramide or erythromycin can facilitate migration of the tube past the duodenum.

Before starting gastric feeding using a freshly placed tube, it is important to ensure proper placement by radiograph. Neither the aspiration of what appears to be stomach contents nor characteristic gurgling with air insufflation guarantees satisfactory positioning. Feeding tubes malpositioned in the airway may produce similar sounds. (Clinical hints to intratracheal placement of a feeding tube include persistent coughing in an alert patient or in mechanically ventilated patients, a reduction in exhaled tidal volume as gas insufflated by the ventilator is vented through the feeding tube.) Recently, it has been demonstrated that connecting the gastric tube to an end-tidal CO_2 monitor can be used to detect errant intratracheal placement. Initiating feeding before confirming the tube is in the GI tract invites disaster. By contrast, it is not necessary to reconfirm tube location with a radiograph before beginning feeding if the gastric tube has been in place for days being used for gastric suctioning or administration of medications. In patients requiring long-term enteral support, endoscopic placement of a percutaneous gastrostomy (PEG) tube or surgical placement of a jejunostomy feeding catheter may be advantageous for tube stability.

Continuous feedings are preferable to bolus feedings because they constantly buffer gastric acid, reduce aspiration risk, produce less bloating, and generate smaller residual volumes. Gastric residuals may be checked to ensure that the stomach is not overfilling but contrary to widespread belief over a broad range, there is no clear relationship between the risk of regurgitation and aspiration and residual volume. As a general rule, "normal" gastric residuals approximate one to two times the hourly infusion rate of continuous tube feeding and are usually less than 200 mL. Large (>300 mL) gastric residuals present before initiation of feeding should urge caution, but not prohibit, a trial of enteral feeding. A measured gastric residual that increases hourly by exactly the volume of feeding infused suggests that eventual failure is likely but surprisingly, many patients will not empty the stomach until residual volumes reach 200 to 400 mL. A safe and reasonable approach is to liberalize the traditional gastric residual volume tolerated to 300 to 400 mL and then only interrupt the feedings if two consecutive residuals reach this threshold. This practice is supported by the observation that even when feeding is continued, nearly 80% of patients with an elevated gastric residual will have a lower residual volume when rechecked just 2 h later. Regurgitation is a clear sign of intolerance that should prompt temporary interruption of enteral feeding. Even when delivered to the duodenum, tube feeding stimulates additional gastric secretion (sometimes up to 3 to 4 L/day). In patients with depressed gastric motility, metoclopramide or erythromycin may help normal gastric egress of food. Recently, methylnaltrexone has shown promise in restoring opiod-induced gut hypomotility.

Selection of Formula

Numerous products are available to supplement oral diets and enteral feedings. A calorie boost can be provided by complex carbohydrates (Polycose 2 kcal/mL) or oils (MCT oil, Microlipid 4.5 kcal/mL). Certain protein supplements may be particularly helpful for patients on liquid or fat-restriction diets (Citrotein, ProMod provide 5 gm protein/scoop). Puddings made from complete formulas are ideal for fluid-restricted patients.

Nutritionally balanced feedings may be obtained either in polymeric form in which protein, fat, and carbohydrates are all present as complex molecules, or as elemental diets, wherein amino acids provide nitrogen and oligosaccharides serve as the carbohydrate source. Polymeric feedings are inexpensive, widely available, and almost always suffice. The most commonly used formulations (Isocal, Isosource, Ensure, Ultracal, Osmolite, and Precision LR) can provide adequate protein, fat, and between 1 and 2 kcal/mL. The higher fat content of polymeric feedings enhances palatability if taken orally. The potential for diarrhea from polymeric feedings, generally, is low because they have no lactose, a low residual, and an osmolarity close to that of serum. However, the higher calorie preparations (e.g., TwoCal, Novosource 2.0, Deliver 2.0), have higher osmolarity and hence, a greater risk for diarrhea. Certain formulations containing fiber (e.g., Enrich, Ultracal, Jevity, Fibersource, and Complete B) may help to regularize bowel evacuation. Essentially, all commercially available feedings are gluten free. Characteristics of commonly available enteral formulas are provided in Table 16-3.

Elemental diets consisting of oligosaccharides as the carbohydrate source and amino acids as the nitrogen source (Vivonex, Vital-HN, and Travasorb) contain virtually no fat, have no lactose, and have little residual material. Therefore, they require minimal digestion, making them ideal for patients with short bowel syndrome, inflammatory bowel disease, and pancreatic insufficiency. Their low viscosity also renders them useful for

TABLE 16-3   CATEGORIES OF ENTERAL NUTRITION PRODUCTS

FORMULA TYPE/ CHARACTERISTICS	PATIENT USES	EXAMPLES
Polymeric, nutritionally complete tube feeding, 1 kcal/mL	General purpose, normal digestion	Osmolite, Isocal
Polymeric, nutritionally complete concentrated tube feeding, 2 kcal/mL	Normal digestion, fluid restricted	Magnacal, Isocal-HCN
Polymeric, nutritionally complete oral supplement, 1–1.5 kcal/mL	Oral supplement	Sustacal, Ensure Plus
Elemental, nutritionally complete tube feeding, 1 kcal/mL	Malabsorption (short bowel, pancreatic insufficiency)	Vivonex TEN, Vital-HN
Fiber containing, nutritionally complete tube feeding, 1 kcal/mL	Diarrhea or constipation	Enrich, Ultracal, Jevity
Peptide based, nutritionally complete tube feeding, 1–1.2 kcal/kg	Hypoalbuminemia with malabsorption	Reabilan, Peptamen

TABLE 16-4   DISEASE-SPECIFIC NUTRITIONAL SUPPLEMENTS

DISEASE CONDITION	SOLUTION CHARACTERISTICS	EXAMPLES
Acute renal failure (without dialysis)	Low protein and electrolyte 2 kcal/mL	Amin-Aid, Suplena
Acute renal failure (with dialysis)	Moderate protein and electrolytes 2 kcal/mL	Nepro, Novasource-renal
Hepatic failure (with encephalopathy)	Increased branched-chain amino acids Low aromatic amino acids, 1.1 kcal/mL	Hepatic-Aid, Travasorb-hepatic
Respiratory failure (with CO_2 retention)	Increased fat, decreased carbohydrate 1.5 kcal/mL	Pulmocare, NutriVent
Diabetes (glucose intolerance)	Increased fat, decreased carbohydrate 1 kcal/mL	Glucerna, Nutren
Immunocompromised (trauma, burns, AIDS?)	Enhanced arginine, omega-3 fatty acids nucleotides, beta carotene, 1–1.3 kcal/mL	Impact, Immun-Aid, Perative
Physiological stress states (burns, trauma, sepsis)	Increased branched-chain amino acids, high protein, or both, 1–1.2 kcal/mL	Stresstein, TraumaCal
Long-term NPO, stress	Enhanced glutamine	AlitraQ, Reconvan
Acute lung injury	Enhanced omega-3 fatty acids	Oxepa

catheter-needle jejunostomy feeding. Unfortunately, such preparations are expensive, and their high osmolarity predisposes to diarrhea, despite their low residual. Essential fatty acids must also be supplemented. Although specific advantages of individual products have not been convincingly demonstrated in specific disease states, Table 16-4 provides a listing of enteral supplements that may have niche indications.

When initiating higher calorie, hypertonic (550 to 850 mOsm) tube feedings, infusion is usually begun at 25 to 50 mL/h. At this rate, discomfort, bloating, and diarrhea are seldom encountered. If diarrhea occurs, reduction in the rate of infusion rather than further dilution is the preferred remedy. However, prolonged reduced infusion rate delays full calorie and protein supplementation. Isotonic formulas are best started full strength, but at a rate one quarter to one half of the projected target (typically 25 to 50 mL/h). Although definitive data are lacking, it is reasonable to advance feeding to target infusion rates over no more than a 1- to 2-day period, as tolerated.

Tube Types

Gastrostomy tubes offer the advantages of stable position and large caliber. The large-bore gastrostomy tube allows administration of pulverized medications, an advantage over jejunostomy or nasogastric (NG) tubes, which frequently obstruct. Although gastrostomy tubes enter the stomach directly through the abdominal wall, they do not prevent regurgitation and aspiration. Endoscopic placement of PEG tubes, the "PEG" tube, has recently gained popularity, avoiding expense and scheduling delays inherent in open surgery. Percutaneous placement is far from risk free, and malpositioning at the time of insertion and displacement can prove fatal by causing peritonitis. Jejunostomy feeding requires direct surgical placement of a small-bore catheter. Jejunostomy prevents regurgitation and may later be withdrawn (without reoperation) to leave a self-closing fistula. An interesting innovation in tube design is the jejunostomy–gastrostomy or J–G tube, which has ports in both structures allowing jejunal infusion of nutrition and gastric suctioning simultaneously.

Problems and Complications of Enteral Nutrition

Feeding by infusion rather than bolus and elevating the head of the bed to at least 30 degree from horizontal may reduce aspiration, the most important and life-threatening complication of enteral alimentation. Whether protection against aspiration is provided by a postpyloric tube position or smaller gastric residuals is uncertain.

The most common problem encountered in the use of enteral nutrition is putative "intolerance." Often "intolerance" equates to reluctance to initiate a trial of tube feeding in a patient with mild abdominal distention or minimal bowel sounds. On other occasions, intolerance represents excessive concern over an arbitrary "gastric residual volume" or mild abdominal distention. Sometimes, tube feedings are interrupted for gastric residuals as low as 100 mL (seven tablespoons). In general, more liberal limits should be allowed for gastric residuals (300 to 400 mL) with greater emphasis placed on the trend in residual rather than any absolute value. It is safe and reasonable to require two consecutive elevated residual volumes before interrupting feeding. A residual that increases every hour by exactly the amount of feeding infused suggests that eventual regurgitation is likely.

Diarrhea occurs in 30% to 40% of ICU patients and is given as a common reason to interrupt tube feedings. Most cases of diarrhea in enterally fed patients are not because of tube feeding but rather concurrent use of other medications, hypoalbuminemia, or enteral infection (Table 16-5). In cases where another cause of diarrhea cannot be determined, reductions in feeding volume, solution osmolarity, and carbohydrate content can sometimes reduce the frequency of diarrhea. The addition of pectin or other bulking agents to the feeding solution may be a useful countermeasure. Diarrhea in patients receiving tube feedings may result from bacterial overgrowth if feeding is contaminated in the process of preparation; therefore, the formula should not dwell at ambient temperature for greater than a few hours. It is also good practice to rinse feeding infusion bags and administration tubing on a regular basis and to use good hand washing practices in the preparation and administration of tube feedings. The problem of bacterial overgrowth has been counteracted by some manufactures who now supply formulae in ready-to-infuse containers.

Gastric tubes often become obstructed and require unclogging or replacement. Using a metal stylet for this purpose risks GI tract perforation and should be avoided. One trick to unclog an obstruction is to instill a cold carbonated beverage into the tube using a syringe. As the solution warms, CO_2 comes out of solution raising pressure in the tube, which then expels the blockage.

TABLE 16-5 CAUSES OF DIARRHEA IN ICU PATIENTS

MEDICATIONS
Antibiotics
Antacids (especially those containing magnesium)
Histamine blockers
Peristalsis-promoting drugs (metoclopramide, erythromycin)
Cholinergic agents (physostigmine)
Sorbitol-containing oral medicines (KCl, digitalis, and theophylline elixirs)
Quinidine
α-methyl dopa

COLONIC INFECTIONS
Clostridium difficile
Enteric pathogens (*Salmonella, Shigella, Campylobacter*)

HYPOALBUMINEMIA

COLONIC IMPACTION (Overflow diarrhea)

Obstruction may be avoided if pill fragments are not administered and if the lumen is flushed with water several times daily. Placement of small-bore feeding tubes using a metallic stylet must be done cautiously to avoid esophageal perforation or translaryngeal introduction of the catheter into the lung or pleural space.

The pH-neutralizing effect of enteral feedings encourages overgrowth of pathogenic bacteria, predisposing to GI and pulmonary infections. Paradoxically, fiber-containing tube feedings may occasionally cause fecal impaction because of colonic hypomotility and the indigestible nature of fiber. The correct diagnosis is often missed because patients often demonstrate "overflow" diarrhea and have impaction in the transverse or ascending colon (beyond the reach of the rectal exam). Cathartics are usually effective after the diagnosis is confirmed by abdominal radiograph.

Even with the best of intentions, patients rarely receive the daily intended amount of enteral feeding. The most common practice which undermines full feeding is interruption of formula infusion in response to an artificially low gastric residual volume. The common practices of interrupting feeding to bath or transport patients contribute. Finally, the frequent practice of interrupting feeding for 12 h before planned extubation or endoscopic evaluation is completely irrational; each time it is done, patients lose half a day of nutritional support.

Parenteral Feeding

There are no demonstrated benefits of intravenous nutrition over enteral nutrition if the latter can be accomplished. The costs of intravenous nutrition (TPN) and its attendant laboratory monitoring often reach hundreds of dollars each day. TPN solutions may be delivered into peripheral or central veins, with each route having specific advantages and disadvantages.

Peripheral TPN

Peripheral TPN alone is an expensive way to supplement patients with minimal requirements; however, it is not acceptable for catabolic patients requiring protracted support. Similar protein solutions are used in both central and peripheral TPN mixtures. However, to avoid osmolality-related phlebitis, the glucose concentration of peripheral TPN is lower than that of centrally administered TPN. Consequently, fewer calories are available in a given infused volume. If lipid is not used as a major calorie source, up to 7 L/day of peripheral TPN may be needed to fully satisfy calorie and protein requirements. Even when approximately 60% of calories are derived from intravenous lipid, 3 to 3.5 L of fluid is still needed to deliver 2,100 cal (3 L of glucose plus amino acids and 500 mL of 20% lipid solution). Consequently, underfeeding is common when peripheral TPN is used.

The corrosive nature of the TPN solution presents a major problem for peripheral administration. Venous inflammation results from the high (glucose) osmolarity and potassium content of TPN solutions. Used alone, glucose and amino acid mixtures are highly irritating. Up to 50% of patients receiving 600 mOsm (standard) TPN solutions in a peripheral vein develop phlebitis within 2 days. Therefore, peripheral intravenous sites should be changed at least every other day. However, the concurrent infusion of lipid through a Y connector reduces the risk of chemical phlebitis. Because of numerous practical problems of peripheral TPN, it is rarely used.

Central TPN

Central administration of TPN incurs all the risks of large-vessel cannulation. Catheter tip position must be checked before starting feeding to prevent inadvertent infusion of fluids into the pericardium or pleural space. To minimize the infection risk, it is **5** best to insert a fresh dedicated central venous pressure (CVP) line to initiate therapy. A balance exists between the risk of repeated catheter insertions and the risk of infection if catheter sites are not changed on a regular schedule. For multiuse catheters (those inserted or used for fluids other than TPN), catheter changes at approximately 7-day intervals probably best balances these two competing risks. Although controversial, a 10- to 14-day interval between catheter changes is probably acceptable in cleanly inserted single purpose catheters. When a skin-tunneled catheter is placed exclusively for TPN, it is not clear that the catheter ever needs changing unless it malfunctions or becomes infected. To minimize the risk of infection, feeding catheters should not be used for phlebotomy, medication delivery, or non-TPN solutions unless absolutely necessary. Although controversy surrounds the optimal management of the patient with a TPN catheter who develops fever without an obvious source, the safest course of action is usually removal of the catheter (culturing the catheter tip and blood) with reinsertion at a new clean site. The decision to remove the catheter is made easier if severe sepsis rather than just fever is the problem. Changing catheters over a guidewire makes little sense unless no other alternate site exists for a clean insertion. If the catheter being removed is colonized, the wire effectively transfers the organisms to the freshly inserted catheter.

After a central catheter is properly positioned, a highly concentrated (usually 1,000 to 2,000 mOsm/L) solution composed of 5% to 10% amino acids (approx. 400 mOsm/L) mixed with 40% to 50% glucose (approx. 2,400 mOsm/L) is administered. An 8.5% to 10% amino acid solution is usually mixed with an equal volume of D50 or D75 glucose to yield a solution containing 150 to 200 kcal/gm N_2. The specific vitamins and trace metals added to standard TPN solutions vary on a hospital-to-hospital basis. To prevent bacterial growth in TPN solutions, individual bottles should not hang longer than 24 h.

Normal electrolyte composition of TPN solution includes sodium (40 to 50 mEq/L), potassium (30 to 45 mEq/L), chloride (40 to 220 mEq/L), phosphate (14 to 30 mEq/L), magnesium (5 to 20 mEq/L), and calcium (5 to 20 mEq/L), plus an anion (usually acetate) needed to electrically balance the solution.

Soybean (Intralipid) or safflower (Liposyn) oil mixtures provide extra calories and prevent essential fatty acid deficiency. Iso-osmolar lipid solutions normally provide all essential fatty acids (linoleic, linolenic, and oleic acid). As little as 500 mL of 10% lipid solution given weekly will prevent essential fatty acid deficiency. Lipid solutions also serve as a concentrated source of calories, providing 1.1 kcal/mL for 10% solutions. No more than 60% of total daily calories should be provided as fat. Rapidly administered large-volume lipid infusions may produce pulmonary dysfunction or thrombocytopenia. Adding low concentrations of unfractionated heparin to lipid solutions (up to 1,000 U/L) may accelerate triglyceride clearance by activating lipoprotein lipase. It should be noted that the vehicle used to solubilize the sedative agent, propofol, provides substantial lipid supplementation (1 to 2 kcal/mL).

Monitoring TPN

Careful monitoring is required to prevent complications and to ensure that TPN accomplishes its goal. Daily weights should be obtained to monitor fluid status. (Weight gains in excess of 1 lb/day are likely to result from accumulating fluid.) Frequent sampling of glucose during the initiation of TPN therapy is necessary to avoid hyperglycemia and hyperosmolarity. Gross examination of the serum for lipemia 3 to 6 h after fat infusion or ingestion may confirm hyperlipidemia induced by lipid supplements. Electrolytes (including magnesium, calcium, phosphorus), liver function tests (LFTs), creatinine, protein, and albumin should be monitored at least twice weekly. Each week a 24-h determination of urine urea can be done to assess nitrogen balance.

Complications of TPN

Complications of parenteral nutrition are reduced by an experienced team versed in all aspects of TPN, including the local care of infusion catheters. Insertion of a central TPN catheter carries all of the potential complications of central venous catheter insertion (e.g., pneumothorax and arterial cannulation). Fortunately, complications related to catheter insertion occur at a very low (less than 5%) rate in most series. Catheter-related sepsis occurs in less than 3% of patients when proper precautions are taken.

Metabolic complications are more likely to occur in starved and severely malnourished patients and those with diabetes or impaired hepatic or renal function. Sudden refeeding, especially with concentrated carbohydrate loads, can rarely trigger a severe, sometimes fatal refeeding syndrome. Dextrose challenge stimulates excessive insulin secretion that in turn decreases distal renal tubular excretion of sodium and water. Hyperinsulinemia also promotes the intracellular migration of phosphate, potassium, and magnesium, occasionally resulting in profound disturbances of muscular function and cardiac conduction.

Hyperosmolarity is common when glucose is infused at rates greater than 0.5 mg/kg/h, particularly in dehydrated patients. Certain free fatty acids (linoleic, linolenic, and arachidonic acid) are considered essential because the body cannot synthesize them. Essential fatty acid requirements are met easily by 500 mL lipid emulsion (10%) given once or twice weekly. Deficiency of essential fatty acids may also be avoided by giving 15 to 30 mL of corn oil orally each week. Vitamin deficiencies are common during TPN use. Many hospitals do not include vitamin K, vitamin B_{12}, or folic acid in TPN solutions. Vitamin B_{12} injections are not required more than monthly, and weekly injections are usually adequate to prevent vitamin K deficiency. Folate requirements do not exceed 1 mg/day, except in patients undergoing dialysis. During prolonged use, deficiencies of trace elements (including zinc, iron, cobalt, iodine, copper, selenium, and chromium) may produce skin disorders, immunologic defects, and other metabolic problems.

Bone pain and increased alkaline phosphatase may occur with the chronic use of TPN, but the mechanism is unknown. (Both are usually associated with normal vitamin D levels and decreased serum phosphorus.) Hypophosphatemia occurs in about one third of patients started on TPN and is particularly likely when markedly elevated serum glucose levels induce an osmotic diuresis. Hypophosphatemia shifts the oxyhemoglobin dissociation curve leftward and decreases glycolysis but does not produce obvious weakness until levels fall below 1 mg/dL. Hemolysis, impaired phagocytosis, and rhabdomyolysis may all be seen with severe phosphate depletion. Hypomagnesemia may present as refractory hypocalcemia, hypokalemia, or both. Hypomagnesemia is particularly common in patients with pancreatitis and underlying alcoholism. Mild increases in serum glucose (to <250 mg/dL) are desirable because they produce protein-sparing effects. More profound hyperglycemia, however, causes hyperosmolality (seizures and coma), osmotic diuresis, and depressed immune function. However, problematic hyperglycemia occurs commonly in infants, diabetics, cirrhotics, the elderly, and patients receiving corticosteroids. To avoid hyperglycemia, glucose infusions should be limited to 5 gm/kg/day. If this proves ineffective, insulin should be added to TPN if the serum glucose remains greater than 200 mg/dL for more than 1 day. It is best to add insulin directly to the TPN bottle to match insulin dosing to the rate of TPN infusion. (Hypoglycemia is particularly common when insulin is continued, as TPN is tapered or discontinued.) To prevent hypoglycemia as TPN is stopped, the infusion rate may first be slowly tapered to approximately 1 L/day. D10W can then be substituted for an additional 24 h. (The need for tapering TPN, however, is debated.)

Acalculous cholecystitis and cholelithiasis are seen with increased frequency in patients receiving TPN, probably secondary to diminished gallbladder secretion and emptying. The incidence of symptomatic gallbladder disease may reach one in four patients receiving TPN for more than 12 weeks.

It is especially high in patients with impaired small bowel absorption (e.g., Crohn disease).

Lipid administration encourages cholestasis by inhibiting hepatic bilirubin excretion. Restricting lipid intake to less than 2 gm/kg/day and keeping a 200:1 ratio of calories to protein may help prevent this problem. Rapid infusion of amino acids (particularly histidine, alanine, and glycine) may cause hyperchloremic acidosis. The addition of acetate to TPN solution can prevent these changes. Amino acid infusions also promote gastric and pancreatic secretions and stimulate ventilatory drive.

Mild selective increases in LFTs are almost universal in patients receiving TPN for greater than 10 days. About half of all patients experience a 50% rise in alkaline phosphatase and serum aspartate aminotransferase (AST). Serum alanine aminotransferase (ALT) is less commonly affected. Fatty infiltration is the presumed cause. High insulin levels produced by continuous glucose infusion may inhibit lipolysis and favor triglyceride synthesis. Decreases in the glucose infusion rate usually correct the problem. LFT abnormalities may be decreased or prevented by giving less than 60% of nonprotein calories as glucose. Patients who remain normoglycemic rarely develop hepatic function test abnormalities. Even when TPN solutions are continued, LFT abnormalities usually revert to normal in 3 weeks.

■ DISEASE SPECIFIC CONSIDERATIONS

Chronic Obstructive Lung Disease

Malnutrition is common in chronic obstructive pulmonary disease patients because they have reduced intake and increased caloric expenditure. Such patients may devote massive energy expenditure to power ventilation when respiratory failure supervenes. Even after the institution of mechanical ventilation, caloric requirements remain elevated by an average of 10%. Rarely, respiratory failure may be precipitated or prolonged by overfeeding or disproportionate carbohydrate intake. Overfeeding causes excessive CO_2 production, further stressing a limited excretory capacity for CO_2. Overfeeding is particularly likely to result in hypercapnia when carbohydrates are the predominant energy source because oxidation of sugars generates 30% more CO_2 than that produced by burning the amount of fat necessary to supply an equal number of calories. To avoid the problem of carbohydrate overfeeding, carbohydrates should be limited to no more than 50% of the total caloric load and should be administered no faster than 4 mg/kg/min. Several commercially available enteral feeding products rich in fat are designed to avoid the problem of excessive CO_2 generation. Rarely when nutritional support is reinstituted after a prolonged absence, profound hypophosphatemia, hypokalemia, and hypomagnesemia (refeeding syndrome) may occur resulting in glucose intolerance, impaired respiratory muscle function, and depressed myocardial contractility.

Acute Lung Injury

Acute lung injury (ALI) is an inflammatory disorder with high oxidant stress. Because survivors typically require more than a week of ventilation, they are often provided nutritional support. ALI victims have been found to have reduced plasma levels of specific omega-3 (n−3) fatty acids (i.e., eicosapentaenoic acid and docosahexaenoic acid) and proportionally higher levels of the omega-6 (n−6) arachidonic acid. This observation may be important since arachidonate metabolism yields highly inflammatory dienoic prostaglandins and series 4 leukotrienes, whereas n−3 fatty acid metabolism produces less-inflammatory trienoic prostaglandins and series 5 leukotrienes. In addition, n−3 fatty acid supplementation has been associated with lower levels of inflammatory cytokines in plasma and lung lavage. Three small studies of humans with ALI now suggest that supplementation with n−3 fatty acids and antioxidants can reduce inflammation and may improve clinical outcomes. Currently, a large randomized blinded trial to confirm or refute these findings is underway.

Renal Failure

Studies reveal that generally acute renal failure by itself has little impact on resting rates of energy expenditure. The major problems renal failure poses are the inability to normally excrete fluid, potassium, phosphorus, and nitrogenous wastes. Therefore, it makes sense to provide whatever calories and protein are needed in the smallest volume possible using a product poor in potassium and phosphorus. If renal replacement therapy has not been started, limiting protein intake to avoid uremic complications may make sense but a better strategy is to provide the high quality protein needed and the dialytic support to remove the generated wastes. If enteral support is chosen, there are numerous commercially available concentrated products high in calories but low in potassium and phosphorus to meet patient needs.

Regardless of route of support, goals in acute renal failure are to provide 2,000 to 3,000 cal and 0.6 to 1.5 gm/kg of protein with high biologic value daily. If TPN is used, reaching this goal often requires administration of sufficient fluid, sodium, and protein to necessitate earlier institution of maintenance dialysis than might be necessary in the starved state. Concentrated glucose concentrations are used to minimize administered volume, but this often creates another problem—glucose intolerance. A beneficial effect of parenteral nutrition on outcome in acute renal failure is uncertain. Use of essential amino acids and histidine as protein sources may stimulate hepatic protein synthesis and anabolism more effectively than standard TPN formulations. The recycling of nitrogen into nonessential amino acid synthesis can theoretically decrease urea production, hence reducing the need for dialysis. Some amino acids like glutamine may be conditionally essential in patients with severe catabolism. Solutions low in sodium and potassium are used unless volume depletion or sodium wasting is a problem.

In chronic renal failure, an appropriate goal is to provide 0.5 to 1.0 gm/kg/day of high-grade protein; intake should seldom be restricted to less than 20 gm/day. Because losses can be massive in the nephrotic syndrome, protein intake should not be limited in this group. Patients with end-stage renal disease should be dialyzed at a rate sufficient to allow nearly normal protein ingestion. Vitamin depletion is a potential problem of patients with renal failure because almost all low-protein diets are vitamin deficient, and water-soluble vitamins are lost during dialysis.

Hepatic Failure

The nutritional prescription must be radically altered in hepatic failure. Because fat metabolism is impaired (long-chain triglycerides are metabolized by the liver), hyperlipidemia may result when a large fraction of nonprotein calories are provided as lipid. Carbohydrate intolerance is also common, and high carbohydrate loads may lead to fatty liver. Heightened aldosterone secretion and depressed free water clearance require low sodium and low volume when TPN is used. Large protein loads may precipitate encephalopathy, particularly when aromatic amino acids (e.g., phenylalanine, tyrosine, and tryptophan) are the major nitrogen source. Although controversial, the substitution of intravenous branched-chain amino acids for their aromatic counterparts may reduce the frequency of hepatic encephalopathy but offers no benefit to patients with liver disease lacking encephalopathy. Therefore, efficacy and cost considerations dictate use of branched-chain amino acid preparations only in the setting of encephalopathy.

Cancer

TPN improves the weight and nutritional parameters of many patients with cancer. However, a survival benefit remains questionable. The catabolic mediators (e.g., tumor necrosis factor) released in response to many neoplasms often blunt the anabolic effects of TPN. Protein gain is not as rapid in cancer patients as in other TPN candidates but fat gain is similar. TPN may improve the tolerance to chemotherapy in some patients; one study of TPN in patients undergoing bone marrow transplantation suggests that both short- and long-term outcomes are improved.

Burns

Burned patients have extremely high caloric requirements and protein losses during the hyperacute phase of care. Protein losses can reach levels ten times normal. Enteral nutrition is the preferred route for supplementation. Preliminary data support inclusion of three specific nutrients for burn victims: glutamine, arginine and omega-3 fatty acids. Of these compounds, glutamine appears to be the most promising. By preserving mucosal barrier function and diminishing infectious complications, glutamine has contributed to improved clinical outcomes.

■ SUGGESTED READINGS

A.S.P.E.N. Board of Directors and the Clinical Guidelines Task Force. Guidelines for the use of parenteral and enteral nutrition in adult and pediatric patients. *JPEN J Parenter Enteral Nutr.* 2002;26(Suppl. 1): 1–138SA.

Drakulovic MB, Torres A, Bauer TT, et al. Supine body position as a risk factor for nosocomial pneumonia in mechanically ventilated patients: A randomized trial. *Lancet.* 1999;354:1851–1858.

Gramlich L, Kichian K, Pinilla J, et al. Does enteral nutrition compared to parenteral nutrition result in better outcomes in critically ill adult patients? A systematic review of the literature. *Nutrition.* 2004;20:843–848.

Heyland DK, Dhaliwal R, Drover JW, et al. Canadian clinical practice guidelines for nutrition support in mechanically ventilated, critically ill adult patients. *JPEN J Parenter Enteral Nutr.* 2003;27:355–373.

Heyland DK, Novak F, Drover JW, et al. Should immunonutrition become routine in critically ill patients? A systematic review of the evidence. *JAMA.* 2001;286:944–953.

Krishnan JA, Parce PB, Martinez A, et al. Caloric intake in medical ICU patients: Consistency of care with guidelines and relationship to clinical outcomes. *Chest.* 2003;124:297–305.

McClave SA, DeMeo MT, DeLegge MH, et al. North American summit on aspiration in the critically ill patient: Consensus statement. *JPEN J Parenter Enteral Nutr.* 2002;26:S80–S85.

Rice TW, Swope T, Bozeman S, et al. Variation in enteral nutrition delivery in mechanically ventilated patients. *Nutrition.* 2005;21(7):786–792.

Analgesia, Sedation, and Therapeutic Paralysis

KEY POINTS

1 Sedatives should be administered to achieve specific target levels of an objective sedation scale and for most patients, should be interrupted at least once daily as part of a planned spontaneous awakening trial.

2 Agitation is often a manifestation of discomfort or physiologic distress that can be resolved without the use of pharmacologic agents. Ventilator adjustments, repositioning, relief of GI and bladder distention, and reassurance are essential nonpharmacologic methods of agitation control.

3 When pharmacotherapy is deemed necessary, drug selection should be based on desired effect, duration of action, and costs, taking into account the organ dysfunction of each patient. In general, intermittent dosing of longer-acting compounds is the preferred strategy to smooth peak and trough effects, prevent oversedation, and reduce costs.

4 Pharmacodynamics in the ICU often differ greatly from those of less ill patients. Most drugs have longer durations of action and larger volumes of distribution when given to ICU patients than to less ill patients.

5 A narcotic (morphine or fentanyl) with a benzodiazepine (lorazepam) offers a safe, effective, economical analgesic–sedative combination for most ICU patients.

6 Propofol is a good choice for short-term sedation (hours) and for sedating patients with neurological conditions requiring frequent reassessment.

7 Haloperidol or droperidol represents an excellent choice for treatment of the extremely agitated or delirious patient not experiencing pain.

8 Neuromuscular blockers should be used sparingly because of numerous risks, which include awake paralysis, hemodynamic instability, prolonged muscle weakness, and obscuration of intercurrent illnesses. When necessary for long-term paralysis, pancuronium or vecuronium are safe, economical choices for most patients.

■ GOALS OF THERAPY

The relief of pain and anxiety is often overlooked while efforts focus on life-threatening crises. A growing awareness of the stress imposed by the intensive care unit (ICU) and the increasing popularity of some modes of mechanical ventilation that are intolerable without sedation have highlighted the need for effective pharmacotherapy. In the ICU, the overall goal is to use just enough of an optimally chosen sedative or analgesic for the shortest possible time. Doing so avoids immediate deleterious cardiopulmonary effects and may minimize late neuropsychological and muscular effects. Nonparalyzed patients should be comfortable but sufficiently awake to communicate their needs and cooperate in their care. By contrast, sedation to unconsciousness is mandated during paralysis in all but the most exceptional circumstances. Reluctance to provide analgesia or sedation to nonintubated patients is understandable but has its own liabilities: it can result in unrelieved pain and anxiety, causing splinting, atelectasis, and increased O_2 consumption; it discourages activity; it promotes venous thrombosis and deconditioning; and it adversely affects immune function.

■ MONITORING TREATMENT

It has become clear that poorly regulated or monitored sedation exacts a high price by increasing sedative costs, predisposing patients to delirium, prolonging ventilator time, and even increasing mortality. In the short term, excessive sedation causes respiratory depression, hypotension, and gastrointestinal (GI) hypomotility and masks the presence of intercurrent illnesses. Long-term, excessive sedation results in cognitive impairment and neuromuscular weakness.

There are several effective strategies to minimize the adverse effects of sedatives and analgesics. One measure is to begin therapy using intermittent doses instead of a continuous infusion. (Propofol is the obvious exception.) If intermittent doses of analgesics or sedatives are being given more frequently than every 2 to 3 h, it then makes sense to start a continuous infusion. Continuous infusions should only be used when needed by the patient, not for the convenience of the staff because continuous infusions have been associated with higher total medication doses and longer times on mechanical ventilation. Another strategy to avoid excessive sedation or analgesia is to use a well-validated **1** assessment scale. For sedation one such measure is the Richmond Agitation Sedation Scale (RASS) where targets selected by a physician are achieved by nurses giving carefully considered doses of sedatives. The RASS is the best current tool because it encompasses the full range of patient actions from completely unresponsive to wildly agitated, has mutually exclusive categories, is easily learned and highly reproducible. Incorporating a review of the current RASS and the target RASS into rounds each day aligns physician and nurse goals and holds each accountable to a realistic objective and practice to achieve it. In some ICUs, bispectral index (BIS) monitoring has been implemented in an attempt to prevent inadequate sedation of paralyzed patients. (Obviously, such patients cannot have RASS assessments.) Although unlikely to be harmful, the usefulness of BIS monitoring is uncertain; recent reports suggest awareness is possible despite BIS scores that would suggest otherwise. It has also been recognized that artifact can increase the BIS score, falsely suggesting awareness and perhaps prompting unnecessary sedative administration. Hence, BIS monitoring should not replace clinical (e.g., pulse, blood pressure) monitoring.

In addition to use of an objective sedation scale, daily sedation-free periods, (spontaneous awakening trials) facilitate recognition of the time when less or no sedative is needed. In several clinical trials scheduled sedation interruption results in fewer days of ventilation, fewer days in the ICU and hospital, and fewer neurological evaluations. A recent study of spontaneous awakening suggests that mortality may even be reduced by the practice. Some physicians are reluctant to interrupt sedation

TABLE 17-1 CORRECTABLE FACTORS CAUSING AGITATION

Endotracheal tube malposition or obstruction
Hypoxemia
Pneumothorax
Ventilator malfunction
Stomach, bowel, or bladder distension
Pain
Impaired communication
Sleep deprivation

for fears of patient self-harm (e.g., extubation) or psychological damage. Although studies of these end points are limited, current data suggest that sedation interruption does not increase neuropsychological nor physiological risks.

■ CORRECTABLE FACTORS CAUSING AGITATION

Initially, agitation should not be regarded as a "sedative deficiency" but rather as a potential sign of unrelieved pain or physiologic or psychological distress. Hence, before sedating or certainly paralyzing agitated patients, especially those being **2** mechanically ventilated, it is critical that common correctable problems be excluded (Table 17-1). Difficulty interfacing with the ventilator shortly after intubation is often improved by suctioning and varying ventilatory mode, tidal volume, flow rate, and trigger sensitivity (see Chapters 7 and 8 on mechanical ventilation). Often, nonpharmacologic actions such as reorientation, reassurance, repositioning, and relaxation therapy suffice.

■ CHOOSING PHARMACOLOGIC AGENTS

The choice of an analgesic, sedative, or paralytic, its dosage, and route of administration should be based on the desired duration of effect, pharmacologic properties of the drug, and individual patient factors. The most common errors in *initial* sedative analgesic selection are insufficient doses given **3** too infrequently and use of short-acting agents when long-term sedation is desired. Whereas use of short-acting agents offers the theoretical advantage of sedation titration, in most cases rapid reversal is unnecessary. Furthermore, undersedation is common with short-acting drugs, and prolonged infusions of short-acting drugs often result in drug accumulation and prolonged effects. In addition, use of short-acting drugs for long-term sedation is often costly (sometimes hundreds or thousands of dollars per day). The most common

4 error during *ongoing* sedation is failure to minimize sedative dosing and intermittently interrupt therapy; problems typically the result of not regularly reassessing patients using an objective sedation scale.

Analgesics

Opioids

Opioids are potent, predictable, and reversible analgesics but are poor amnestic agents. When analgesic doses of opioids are used alone, few hemodynamic

5 or respiratory effects are observed; however, when large "anesthetic-range" doses (often ten times the analgesic dose) are used or when narcotics are combined with neuromuscular blockers or other sedatives, the risk of cardiopulmonary instability is magnified. Opioid complications are minimized by (i) ensuring intravascular volume is adequate, (ii) using the lowest effective dose, and (iii) slow administration. The histamine-releasing (vasodilating) potential of opioids is minimal unless rapid, large intravenous doses are given (meperidine and morphine are the most common offenders). Although rarely necessary, histamine effects can be attenuated by pretreatment with H_1 and H_2 blockers. A feature common to all narcotics is blunting of the hypercapnic and hypoxic respiratory drives. Although often considered a liability, lessening respiratory drive often benefits mechanically ventilated patients by reducing their sense of dyspnea and minute ventilation requirement and can therefore decrease the tendency for breath stacking. Blunting of respiratory drive can also provide great comfort for dyspneic patients at the end of life.

Unfortunately, opioids and their breakdown products accumulate in patients with hepatic and/or renal failure, especially in those receiving prolonged treatment. Hepatic biotransformation typically precedes renal excretion of drugs and their metabolites. Initially, the synthetic, highly lipid-soluble opioids (e.g., fentanyl, sufentanil, alfentanil) have their actions terminated by redistribution, not metabolism. With chronic use, however, patients become "saturated" with the drug, requiring metabolism for termination of effect. Another synthetic opioid, remifentanil, has its effects terminated within minutes by rapid plasma esterase metabolism. Opioids, especially in high doses, may complicate attempts at

enteral feeding by reducing GI motility and inciting nausea. Although still preliminary, recent reports suggest subcutaneous administration of the μ receptor antagonist methylnaltrexone may attenuate this effect. Rarely, biliary spasm may be precipitated by opiate use, but for the patient with biliary colic the analgesic benefits far outweigh the theoretical risks. Regional and epidural blocks, patient-controlled analgesia, multimodal analgesia using nonopioid analgesics (e.g., ibuprofen), and addition of anxiolytic agents which potentiate analgesics (e.g., benzodiazepines) are significant advances in pain control, providing superior pain relief with a lower total narcotic dose and lower risk of oversedation. Reluctance to use narcotics for long-term pain relief for fear of dependence or addiction is unfounded; addiction is rare among patients with real pain who lack a history of substance dependence. However, there is a growing appreciation that withdrawal does occur in long-term recipients of high doses of opioids who have their therapy abruptly discontinued. Withdrawal syndromes in the ICU may masquerade as infection because they manifest as fever, tachycardia, tachypnea, and confusion.

Morphine is an inexpensive drug with a rapid onset of action and a 1- to 3-h half-life. Intermittent intravenous (IV) doses of 2 to 10 mg or 1 to 3 mg/h (0.03 to 0.15 mL/kg/h) by constant infusion usually are adequate for relief of moderate to severe pain in the average adult. Administration rates less than 10 mg/min minimize the risk of hypotension. Although morphine is an excellent analgesic, high doses or the addition of a benzodiazepine are usually required to produce unconsciousness. Morphine's action is prolonged by both renal and hepatic failure because a fraction of each morphine dose is directly excreted unchanged by the kidney, but most is metabolized hepatically before renal excretion. One advantage of morphine over synthetic opioids, especially in the oliguric patient, is its high water solubility, permitting analgesia to be administered in a minimum volume. Hydromorphone, is an even more potent (approx. 10-fold) semisynthetic opiod derived from morphine. Its half-life of 2 to 3 h provides a similar or slightly longer analgesic effect than morphine. However, because the half-life of hydromorphone can increase 20-fold in patients with renal failure, extreme caution must be exercised in this population.

Fentanyl is a potent, highly lipid-soluble, synthetic opioid possessing a very rapid onset and brief duration of action—at least with initial use. With repeated injections or when given by continuous infusion, large stores of drug may accumulate in lipophilic tissues that then must be metabolized to terminate the drug's action. Because of this accumulation, fentanyl's effective half-life after days of use may exceed that of morphine. Initial analgesic doses of 0.5 to 10 µg/kg IV may be titrated upward as necessary. Because fentanyl cannot be prepared in highly concentrated aqueous solutions, it is one of the few medications that can present a "volume" challenge. With chronic use, it is common to req uire several hundred milliliter of fluid each day to administer the analgesic dose. Fentanyl's perceived chief advantage is its minimal hemodynamic effect for a given level of analgesia. Very rarely, fentanyl causes seizures or a bizarre syndrome of chest wall rigidity (most common when large IV doses are given rapidly to elderly patients). Thoracic rigidity may be so severe that intubation, neuromuscular paralysis, and mechanical ventilation are necessary. Transdermal patches bypass the substantial first-pass hepatic clearance seen with IV dosing, offering a useful alternative method of administration. Unfortunately, the skin slows diffusion, resulting in a long lag time between patch application and effective analgesia, and removal of the patch fails to rapidly terminate the drug's effect because the skin serves as a "reservoir." For patients with modest analgesic requirements and good perfusion, the patch delivery system is especially worth considering. Unfortunately, a very high incidence of nausea has been reported with transdermal dosing. As an aside, patients presenting with a clinical syndrome of opioid overdose should be carefully examined to make sure they do not have one or more fentanyl patches affixed.

Alfentanil is a short-acting, lipid-soluble, synthetic opioid that is more potent than morphine but less so than fentanyl. Consciousness returns rapidly after high doses, making this drug useful for brief but painful procedures. Absence of active metabolites results in minimal drug accumulation unless hepatic failure is present. Sufentanil is perhaps 1,000 times as potent as morphine but, except for a potentially smaller volume requirement, does not offer any significant advantages over fentanyl. Remifentanil, a very potent, short-acting, synthetic opioid, is metabolized by plasma esterases, thus its metabolism is not altered by hepatic or renal failure. Alfentanil, sufentanil, and remifentanil are expensive options without unique therapeutic effect.

Meperidine should be avoided. It is a poor pain reliever; offers no substantial advantage over other opioids, and its myocardial depressant effect and vagolytic and histamine-releasing tendencies often cause tachycardia and hypotension. The perceived superiority of meperidine for patients with ureteral or biliary colic is unfounded. Meperidine's major metabolite, normeperidine, is active, accumulates in renal failure, and causes seizures when present in high concentrations.

Reversing Opioid Effects

In the event of opioid overdose, the antagonist naloxone promptly reverses excessive sedation. Intravenous doses of 0.4 to 2 mg are usually sufficient, at least transiently, although doses as high as 10 mg are occasionally required. Naloxone given in repeated smaller doses or by slow intravenous infusion can undo the respiratory depressant effects of narcotics without reversing the analgesia. Low-dose naloxone is particularly useful for chronic opioid users who unintentionally develop excessive sedation. Naloxone's duration of action is not as long as many commonly used opioids, necessitating close observation and sometimes-repeated administration to prevent recurrence of sedation.

Nonsteroidal Anti-inflammatory Agents

Nonsteroidal anti-inflammatory agents (NSAIDs) are often avoided in the ICU because of their antiplatelet activity and reputation to cause bleeding and renal insufficiency. The frequency and severity of these adverse events are overestimated, and unfortunately drugs with more serious side effects are often chosen as alternatives. Oddly, NSAIDs are often blamed when renal insufficiency develops in patients with multiple potential causes of kidney injury (e.g., low cardiac output, hypotension, contrast exposure, high-dose vasoconstrictors, angiotensin converting enzyme [ACE] inhibitors). Whereas the cyclooxygenase and platelet-inhibiting activities make NSAIDs less than ideal choices for patients with impaired renal function, coagulopathy or active bleeding, antiplatelet activity may be advantageous for patients with ischemia. These potent, inexpensive compounds (e.g., aspirin, ibuprofen, and COX-2 inhibitors) often suffice for pain relief and act synergistically with narcotics. (In studies of postoperative pain, opioid doses may be reduced by 1/4 to 1/3). No credible data support enhanced GI safety of selective COX-2 inhibitors in the ICU population. The major drawback is that most NSAIDs can only be given via the GI tract. (Ibuprofen is well absorbed from the rectum, and a liquid formulation can be used in patients unable to tolerate gastric administration.) Currently, only ibuprofen and ketorolac are offered in parenteral form.

Sedatives

Benzodiazepines

Benzodiazepines are sedative, anxiolytic amnestics with a wide therapeutic margin. Because pain and anxiety are synergistic and often indistinguishable, benzodiazepines can reduce analgesic needs even though they have no intrinsic analgesic properties. Benzodiazepines also induce amnesia and provide anticonvulsant and muscle-relaxant properties. Although not as potent as barbiturates or propofol for the purpose, benzodiazepines reduce cerebral O_2 consumption, intracranial pressure, and cerebral blood flow. Although they may induce unconsciousness, this state is not normal slumber. Sleep fragmentation occurs without the full range and depth of normal sleep stages. When sleep is the primary objective, a hypnotic (e.g., zolpidem or triazolam) are better choices than benzodiazepines intended for sedation (e.g., midazolam, lorazepam, or diazepam). Benzodiazepines are associated with the development of delirium in the critically ill and paradoxically, can excite patients by disinhibiting normal social behavioral control. Similarly, amnestic and dissociative effects may linger after consciousness returns, resulting in an agitated, confused state that prompts additional doses of the very medication that precipitated it—a potentially vicious cycle. Droperidol and its parent drug, haloperidol, are effective agents to break this cycle.

Unless used in large doses or combined with narcotics, propofol, or neuromuscular blockers, benzodiazepines have few cardiovascular effects. Mild tachycardia and minimal reductions in blood pressure are most commonly observed in elderly or dehydrated patients, patients using β-blockers, and patients with underlying cardiac disease. Benzodiazepines cause mild dose-dependent respiratory depression but rarely cause apnea. (Apnea is most common after rapid administration of large IV doses to chronically ill patients or elderly patients or patients receiving concomitant narcotics.) The highly lipid-soluble benzodiazepines (e.g., midazolam, diazepam) accumulate in fat after repeated or prolonged use, resulting in delayed recovery. The avid protein binding of benzodiazepines leads to frequent interactions with other protein-bound drugs and exposes hypoproteinemic patients to high concentrations of free (active) drug. Most benzodiazepines require hepatic metabolism and/or excretion; therefore, liver disease can prolong the action of these drugs (lorazepam and oxazepam are least subject to this effect). Conversely, patients with induced liver enzymes (e.g., alcoholics, barbiturate users) may require enormous doses for effect. Currently, all the commonly used benzodiazepines are inexpensive and comparably priced based on hourly use. The properties of the three most frequently used parenteral benzodiazepines are contrasted in Table 17-2.

Diazepam is a long-acting sedative-amnestic-anxiolytic agent available in oral or parenteral forms. Unpredictable absorption from muscle usually limits use to the IV route. Unfortunately, phlebitis is common after IV injection in peripheral veins (Midazolam shares this liability to a lesser degree.) Diazepam's high lipid solubility, active metabolites, and large volume of distribution result in a rapid onset and prolonged action. Doses of 2 to 10 mg (0.04 to 0.2 mg/kg IV) given every 5 to 10 min are reasonable to initiate therapy. Because diazepam contains the preservative propylene glycol, use of high doses for long periods of time can cause hyperosmolarity and metabolic acidosis.

Because of its lesser lipid solubility, smaller volume of distribution and high gamma amino butyric acid (GABA) receptor affinity, lorazepam has a slower onset and longer duration of action than midazolam or diazepam. Prolonged action generally is a desirable characteristic for an ICU sedative because of the common need for long-term sedation. Because glucuronidation, rather

TABLE 17-2 COMPARISON OF THE PROPERTIES OF PARENTERAL BENZODIAZEPINES

COMPOUND	DURATION OF ACTION	HEPATIC METABOLISM REQUIRED?	METABOLITES ACTIVE?	RELATIVE HOURLY COST
Diazepam	Long	Yes	Yes	$
Lorazepam	Long	No	No	$
Midazolam	Variable	Yes	Yes	$

than oxidation, is the mechanism of metabolism, lorazepam is the benzodiazepine least subject to prolongation of effect with changing hepatic function. Minimal cardiovascular effects and excellent amnestic properties make lorazepam a good choice for performing "awake" endotracheal intubation and as a premedicant for procedures. Lorazepam is also the preferred benzodiazepine for termination of status epilepticus because of its prompt but prolonged duration of action. Initial IV doses of 1.0 to 2.0 mg (0.03 to 0.04 mg/kg) may be repeated every few minutes until the desired degree of sedation is achieved. Predictable absorption with oral dosing permits an easy transition from intravenous to oral therapy not possible with midazolam. Like diazepam, lorazepam contains propylene glycol and can cause hyperosmolarity and metabolic acidosis when used in high doses over days.

Midazolam is a potent, (initially) short-acting benzodiazepine. High lipid solubility and the ability to cross the blood–brain barrier produce a rapid onset of action (2 to 3 min). A steep dose–response curve dictates that, initially, low doses and close observation are indicated to avoid excessive sedation. Starting doses of 0.5 to 1.0 mg (0.01 to 0.1 mg/kg) given intravenously at 5- to 15-min intervals are customary. Whereas isolated doses of midazolam are eliminated rapidly by hepatic extraction and metabolism, the effective half-life of midazolam is prolonged after extended IV infusion as the drug accumulates in fat. After days of use, accumulation can produce an effective duration of action exceeding that of diazepam or lorazepam. Prolonged effects are also partially explained by formation of active midazolam metabolites. When combined with local anesthetics, midazolam is a good agent to provide sedation and anxiolysis during brief procedures.

Chlordiazepoxide is limited to the oral route and is historically used for prevention of delirium tremens. Despite its popularity, chlordiazepoxide has no unique properties distinguishing it from the other available benzodiazepines.

Benzodiazepine Antagonism

Flumazenil is an expensive competitive receptor antagonist capable of reversing the respiratory and central depressant effects of benzodiazepines in most patients. Chronic or high-dose benzodiazepine use lowers the success rate. Flumazenil has no beneficial effect on ethanol, barbiturate, narcotic, or tricyclic antidepressant-induced central nervous system depression. Because flumazenil is cleared rapidly by the liver, its duration of action is substantially shorter than that of most of the compounds it antagonizes. As occurs with naloxone opioid use, up to 10% of patients given flumazenil relapse into a sedated state, making close observation essential. Doses of 0.2 mg at 1-min intervals (up to 1 mg total) are customary. Although flumazenil may confirm a diagnosis of benzodiazepine overdose, it rarely alters patient management significantly and thus, is seldom needed in the ICU. Flumazenil should be used cautiously because it may precipitate withdrawal (agitation, vomiting, and seizures), especially among chronic benzodiazepine users. For patients with suspected combined (benzodiazepine and tricyclic antidepressants) drug overdose, flumazenil can precipitate seizures, presumably as a result of unmasking tricyclic effects.

Propofol

Propofol is a mixture of an alkyl-phenol sedative in an egg and soybean oil emulsion. Initial doses of 1 to 2 mg/kg IV result in profound, easily titrated sedation (but not analgesia) that may be maintained using similar hourly doses. With short-term use, propofol has a rapid onset and offset of action, thus it is particularly useful for patients who require brief (<24 h) sedation and for patients requiring repeated neurological assessment. Similar to other highly lipid-soluble agents, long-term administration can lead to saturation of fatty tissue and prolonged recovery times. Because propofol is hepatically conjugated to inactive metabolites, which are renally excreted, it is a good choice for patients with multiple organ failure. Despite these advantages, propofol has significant limitations. Potent cardiovascular depression causes hypotension in up to one third of patients, especially when loading doses are used. Because of its fat content, the vehicle provides 1.1 cal/mL and can cause hypertriglyceridemia and even hyperlipidemic pancreatitis. For unclear reasons, a small minority of patients develop a potentially lethal syndrome of metabolic acidosis and acute renal failure called the propofol infusion syndrome (see Chapter 33). The vehicle may cause allergic reactions, and users should not be surprised by the green-tinged urine produced by excretion of the phenol metabolites. Previous problems with bacterial contamination have largely been overcome by addition of compounds to inhibit microbial growth. Regardless, sterile precautions must be used when infusing propofol, and the duration of infusion of an individual vial should be limited to a few hours. Even though generic forms are now available, costs can still reach hundreds of dollars daily. Thus, propofol should be reserved for short-term use and for patients with neurological conditions who require frequent awakening.

Dexmedetomidine

Dexmedetomidine is a centrally acting α_2 agonist that produces sedation but not analgesia. The drug has gained popularity in the postoperative setting because it has relatively little effect on respiratory drive or alertness, has a short onset and offset of action, and is easily titrated. Patients given dexmedetomidine in the postoperative setting receive less propofol and benzodiazepines, but the clinical significance of this observation is unclear since patients do not report an improved surgical experience. It allows sedation to be maintained while patients are extubated, after which the drug is tapered as tolerated. Dexmedetomidine has many of the desirable properties as propofol. Unfortunately, it also shares many of propofol's liabilities: loading doses cause bradycardia and hypotension in many patients and the drug can induce apnea. In addition, dexmedetomidine costs can reach $400 a day. Because it does not have sufficiently unique properties, a favorable risk benefit ratio, or a cost advantage, dexmedetomidine cannot be recommended for routine long-term sedation at this time.

Etomidate

Etomidate is an imidazole sedative-hypnotic lacking analgesic properties. Because etomidate rarely causes hypotension and has a rapid onset (seconds) and a brief duration of action (5 min), it is a popular choice for conscious sedation for brief procedures and for intubation. A dose of 0.3 mg/kg is customary and a wide therapeutic margin exists. Even though the sedative effect of etomidate lasts only minutes, the imidazole structure of the compound is capable of inhibiting adrenal glucocorticoid synthesis for a day. The clinical importance of this biochemical observation is unclear after a single dose, but long-term etomidate administration has been associated with higher mortality rates. Since etomidate is often chosen as the sedative because a patient has tenuous cardiovascular function, a cause and effect relationship with mortality is speculative. One practical implication of the glucocorticoid suppressing effect is that adrenal function (ACTH) testing after etomidate use will routinely conclude the patient to have at least "relative" adrenal insufficiency. This finding is likely to prompt exogenous, almost certainly unnecessary, glucocorticoid administration by the physician unfamiliar with this phenomenon. Given the undeniable advantages of etomidate for short-term use and the uncertainties of long-term safety, etomidate use should probably be restricted to one or two doses in any given patient.

Barbiturates

The most lipid-soluble barbiturates (e.g., thiopental, thiamylal, and methohexital) have a rapid onset of action because the luxuriously perfused lipophilic brain becomes saturated rapidly with drug after dosing. By achieving high brain concentrations, barbiturates depress the reticular activating system. Occurring almost as rapidly as the onset of action, redistribution terminates drug effects. Less lipid-soluble barbiturates (e.g., phenobarbital) have a slower onset of action and longer recovery time. The nearly immediate onset of action of ultra-short-acting barbiturates makes them useful for "rapid sequence intubation" of carefully selected patients. Barbiturates have a limited role in the ICU because of their narrow therapeutic margin and propensity to cause hypoventilation, cardiac depression, and vasodilation and because in most settings safer alternatives exist. Hypotension is common in patients with underlying cardiovascular disease, the elderly, and volume-depleted patients. Barbiturates do not produce muscle relaxation or analgesia; rather, they may enhance the perception of pain. Tolerance and physiologic dependence occur rapidly, and withdrawal symptoms occur frequently. Because most barbiturates are highly protein bound and alter hepatic metabolism of other compounds, drug interactions are common. Diseases that reduce the serum protein concentration (e.g., severe sepsis, nephrotic syndrome, malnutrition, and cirrhosis) potentiate barbiturate effects by increasing the free fraction of drug in plasma. After hepatic metabolism, barbiturates are renally excreted; therefore, liver or kidney dysfunction potentiates these agents as metabolites. Reduced intracranial pressure and cerebral O_2 consumption account for the neuroprotective effects of barbiturates; however, fluid and vasopressor therapy is almost always required to maintain the blood pressure. In the ICU, barbiturate use should probably be limited to: (i) second- or third-line anticonvulsant therapy, (ii) induction of coma for cerebral preservation, and (iii) rapid-sequence induction/intubation.

Neuroleptics/Antipsychotics

Haloperidol/Droperidol

Haloperidol, a butyrophenone, has become popular for control of severely agitated patients in the ICU, particularly when agitated delirium is prominent. **7** Initial IV doses of 1 to 2 mg commonly are doubled every 15 to 30 min until behavioral control is obtained. (Some clinicians begin with larger doses 5 to 10 mg, when agitation is violent.) Afterward, a recurring dose of 2 to 5 mg every 6 to 8 h is often sufficient to render a calm, awake patient. For severely agitated patients the combination of a benzodiazepine and haloperidol is superior to either agent alone. Haloperidol has a large volume of distribution and half-life approaching a day in patients with normal hepatic function. The cost of parenteral haloperidol has skyrocketed such that it now often costs hundreds of dollars per day to achieve adequate sedation. Both haloperidol and droperidol lower the seizure threshold and very rarely precipitate *torsades de pointes,* neuroleptic malignant syndrome, transient extrapyramidal reactions, and potentially permanent tarditive dyskinesia. Surprisingly, extrapyramidal effects of intravenous haloperidol appear to be less common than with oral use. Recently, use of the haloperidol derivative, droperidol, has increased because the drug has nearly identical actions and toxicities as haloperidol but can be given at a tiny fraction of the cost. (Perhaps, hypotension is more common with droperidol.) When using droperidol, initial intravenous doses of 2.5 mg are common.

Olanzapine

Olanzapine is an atypical antipsychotic that has also been used to treat agitated delirium in the ICU. Few data exist on use of this drug among critically ill patients but one small trial suggests comparable effect to haloperidol. Although olanzapine can cause tarditive dyskinesia and neuroleptic malignant syndrome, QT prolongation and cardiac arrhythmias are rarely reported.

Phenothiazines

Phenothiazines (e.g., Phenergan) are sedative antiemetics that may be used to potentiate the analgesic and sedative effects of opioids. With the exception of their antiemetic effects, the combination of phenothiazines and narcotics offers no substantial advantage over the more commonly used benzodiazepine–narcotic combination. Phenothiazines have the potential disadvantage of inducing dystonic (extrapyramidal) reactions in a small minority of patients.

Neuromuscular Blocking Agents

Mechanism of Action

Normally, electrical impulses reach the neuromuscular junction, causing calcium-mediated release of acetylcholine into the junctional cleft. Acetylcholine binding to nicotinic muscle receptors then causes a sodium–potassium flux (depolarization). Through a combination of acetylcholine reuptake and local degradation by "true or specific" acetylcholinesterase, muscle repolarization occurs and the opportunity for subsequent contraction is restored. A second nonspecific plasma enzyme, pseudocholinesterase, metabolizes acetylcholine and acetylcholine-like molecules. Depolarizing neuromuscular blockers stereochemically resemble acetylcholine and mimic its action at the neuromuscular junction resulting in Na^+–K^+ flux across the muscle. Depolarizing blockers are not metabolized in the neuromuscular junction by acetylcholinesterase; therefore, persistent depolarization occurs until the neuromuscular blocker diffuses out of the synaptic cleft, where it is metabolized by plasma or pseudocholinesterase. Nondepolarizing blockers act by passively occupying acetylcholine binding sites or sodium–potassium ion channels, thereby competitively blocking acetylcholine's depolarizing action.

Indications

With the exception of endotracheal intubation, paralytic agents rarely are needed in the ICU when adequate sedation is used; yet, carefully selected patients can benefit. Unless absolutely necessary to preserve life, awake paralysis is never an acceptable alternative to sedation. Experience with these inherently dangerous agents should come from carefully supervised use and cannot be learned safely by only reading about them. Because of the potential for numerous complications, paralytic agents should be used in the lowest possible doses, for the shortest possible time, and only after sedation alone has proved inadequate.

TABLE 17-3 POTENTIAL INDICATIONS FOR PARALYSIS

Endotracheal intubation
Muscle relaxation during surgery
Facilitation of mechanical ventilation refractory to deep sedation
Reduction of oxygen consumption
Injury prevention (e.g., electroconvulsive therapy)
Termination of tetanus/convulsive activity
Prevention of intracranial hypertension

Commonly accepted indications for paralytic drug use are given in Table 17-3. Facilitation of endotracheal intubation is the most common indication, but extreme caution is indicated; as a rule, the hazards of paralysis for intubation parallel the perceived need for muscle relaxation. For example, use of paralytics in morbidly obese patients or those with spinal instability can precipitate complete upper airway obstruction. Ideally, expert backup and provisions to secure the airway endoscopically and surgically should be available when using paralytic drugs.

Diseases in which muscular contraction is itself harmful (e.g., tetanus and hemodynamic instability resulting from status epilepticus) may benefit from neuromuscular blockade. It is important to remember that although paralytics terminate the muscular convulsive activity, they do *nothing* to terminate chaotic cerebral electrical activity damaging the brain. Because paralytics obscure clinical assessment of seizure (convulsive) activity, it is best if continuous electroencephalographic monitoring is provided when seizing patients are paralyzed.

High levels of positive end-expiratory pressure (PEEP) and modes of ventilation with prolonged inspiratory times (e.g., extended ratio or airway pressure release ventilation) are sometimes actively opposed by patients. The practices of lower tidal volume ventilation or "permissive hypercapnia" also drive ventilation. In these settings, sedation alone is almost always sufficient to provide comfort, aid ventilation, and lower peak airway pressures. Neuromuscular blockers, however, are rarely necessary to facilitate ventilation, especially when respiratory drive is very high (e.g., severe metabolic acidosis). Paralysis also can reduce oxygen consumption in patients with

marginal oxygenation, but there is little evidence that paralysis is superior to deep sedation in this situation. When sedation is optimally managed, use of neuromuscular blockade to facilitate mechanical ventilation is a rarity.

Cautions

Neuromuscular blockade has many dangers: ranking behind loss of the airway, the most frightening is the potential for awake paralysis. Insufficient sedation is difficult to recognize: hypertension, **8** tachycardia, diaphoresis, and lacrimation are the only possible physiologic manifestations. Hopes that BIS monitoring would eliminate awareness during paralysis have not been realized. Paralyzed patients are helpless—unrecognized extubation, ventilator malfunction, or vascular catheter disconnection can be fatal. Paralysis also predisposes patients to developing decubitus ulcers, nerve compression syndromes, corneal erosions, deep venous thrombosis, and muscle atrophy. By preventing patient communication and concealing physical signs (e.g., abdominal rigidity, rigors), paralysis obscures the diagnosis of intercurrent conditions (e.g., intra-abdominal disasters, myocardial ischemia, hypoglycemia, seizures, and stroke). Essentially, all data on paralytic drugs come from their short-term use in the operating room; therefore, actions, interactions, and side effects for critically ill patients in the ICU after long-term administration are less certain. For example, it took substantial time before reports emerged regarding prolonged muscle weakness after use of corticosteroid-derived neuromuscular blockers.

The terms *critical illness polyneuropathy or myoneuropathy* have been coined to describe the residual weakness observed in some ICU patients. Profound, prolonged weakness can develop as a result of critical illness itself; however, this syndrome is probably more common following continuous long-term use of neuromuscular blockers, especially when corticosteroids are administered concomitantly. Some cases of myopathy or neuromyopathy are associated with elevation of creatine phosphokinase (CPK) or aldolase levels; however, normal levels of these compounds do not preclude the syndrome. The particular neuromuscular blocker, the total paralytic dose, the duration of therapy, the presence of renal failure, and the quantity and duration of corticosteroids all may be risk factors for development of this syndrome. Unfortunately, there is no credible data to indicate that selecting one agent over another or monitoring the depth of neuromuscular blockade decreases the risk. Avoidance of corticosteroids is likely beneficial.

The potency and duration of paralytic agents are affected by the duration of therapy and by the presence of concomitant medications and medical conditions. Burns and use of methylxanthines, phenytoin, lithium, corticosteroids, and carbamazepine all reduce the effectiveness of paralytics (Table 17-4). Edematous states produce more complex problems: by increasing the volume of distribution, edema makes initial paralysis more difficult to achieve; however, the large reservoir of drug that accumulates in edema fluid may prolong recovery. Tachyphylaxis is often seen with long-term use.

Respiratory acidosis and metabolic alkalosis, hypokalemia, hyponatremia, hypocalcemia, hyper-magnesemia, and hypothermia all potentiate neuromuscular blockade. Patients with "denervation hypersensitivity" caused by diseases such as myasthenia gravis and Guillain–Barré syndrome are particularly sensitive to depolarizing paralytic agents. β-blockers, calcium channel blockers, cyclosporine, aminoglycosides, tetracycline, clindamycin, and the antiarrhythmics procainamide and quinidine also potentiate neuromuscular blockade.

Specific Blockers

Depolarizing Neuromuscular Blockers

Succinylcholine is the drug of choice for many intubations because it has a very rapid onset of action (seconds) and a brief duration (<10 min). Because it is degraded rapidly by plasma cholinesterase, most of an administered dose never reaches the neuromuscular junction (see also Chapter 6). Succinylcholine causes fasciculations (depolarizations) in skeletal muscle but does not affect smooth muscle action. Despite its brief duration of action, succinylcholine is not without side effects. Most adult patients develop a sympathomimetic response; however, hypotension may occur, especially when succinylcholine is combined with propofol or barbiturates. Succinylcholine is not suited for repeated injection or constant infusion because when given in this manner, it causes vagal stimulation and bradycardia. If more than one dose of succinylcholine is required, atropine should be given before the second dose.

Depolarization causes muscle contraction and hence, potassium release from muscles. Plasma potassium increases of 0.5 to 1 mEq/L are common; but among patients with peritonitis, burns, multiple trauma, or rhabdomyolysis, hyperkalemia may be severe. Patients with increased numbers of acetylcholine receptors because of denervation hypersensitivity are especially prone to hyperkalemia. Vomiting caused by abdominal muscle contraction and postparalysis muscle pain commonly result from succinylcholine use but may be attenuated by pretreating with a subparalyzing dose (10% to 15% of the usual dose) of a nondepolarizing blocker. Succinylcholine raises intraocular pressure and should be avoided in patients with glaucoma or ocular injuries.

Nondepolarizing Neuromuscular Blockers

Nondepolarizing neuromuscular blockers act by preventing the action of acetylcholine at its receptor. Nondepolarizing blockers may be grouped conveniently by several basic properties: duration

---

TABLE 17-4 CONDITIONS INFLUENCING THE INTENSITY OF NEUROMUSCULAR BLOCKADE

CONDITIONS THAT POTENTIATE BLOCKADE

Acidosis
Hypocalcemia
Hypokalemia
Hypermagnesemia
Hyponatremia
Hypothermia
Neuromuscular diseases
Myasthenia gravis, Guillain–Barré, Amyotrophic
  lateral sclerosis, Polio
Drug interactions
Aminoglycosides
β-blockers
Calcium channel blockers
Clindamycin
Cyclosporine
Procainamide
Quinidine
Tetracycline

CONDITIONS THAT INHIBIT BLOCKADE

Alkalosis
Burns
Prolonged paralytic use
Tissue edema
Drug interactions
Azathioprine
Carbamazepine
Corticosteroids
Lithium
Methylxanthines
Phenytoin

of action, route of metabolism and excretion, propensity to release histamine, and the tendency to cause vagal blockade (Table 17-5). Many of these compounds (e.g., pancuronium, vecuronium, rocuronium, pipecuronium) chemically resemble corticosteroids. Each of the nondepolarizing blockers has a slower onset of action than succinylcholine but produces paralysis longer than succinylcholine. The duration of action ranges from 20 min for mivacurium to often more than an hour for pipecuronium, pancuronium, doxacurium, metocurine, and tubocurarine.

Pancuronium is the longest acting of the nondepolarizing agents but falls short of being the perfect paralytic drug for the ICU because it requires renal excretion like tubocurarine, metocurine, doxacurium, and pipecuronium. Pancuronium also undergoes substantial (approx. 20%) hepatic metabolism yielding active metabolites and complicating its use in hepatic failure. Pancuronium also has modest histamine-releasing properties and vagolytic effects that may cause tachycardia and hypotension.

Vecuronium is used widely because of its intermediate duration of action and paucity of cardiovascular effects. Because vecuronium is cleared in large part (approx. 80%) by hepatic metabolism and biliary excretion, it is a less than ideal choice for patients with liver disease. Although not cleared directly by the kidney, vecuronium has active metabolites that are cleared renally. Hence, reports of prolonged paralysis after vecuronium administration in patients with renal insufficiency are not surprising. Paralysis using vecuronium, pancuronium, and atracurium and cisatracurium are now all of comparable hourly cost.

Atracurium, cisatracurium, and mivacurium have theoretical advantages for patients with hepatic or renal failure because these drugs undergo extensive plasma degradation. Mivacurium is broken down by pseudocholinesterase, whereas atracurium undergoes esterase degradation and spontaneous breakdown at physiologic pH and temperature called "Hoffman elimination." Because of its metabolism, atracurium is probably least affected by the presence of renal failure, but is altered by hypothermia and acidosis. Atracurium's metabolism yields laudanosine, a renally cleared excitatory amine that may precipitate seizures. Breakdown of atracurium is delayed by hypothermia and acidosis, but unlike most other neuromuscular blockers, its termination is not impaired by advanced age. Cisatracurium may result in lesser laudanosine generation.

General Recommendations: Intubation

The rapidity of onset and brief duration of action make succinylcholine the drug of choice for most ICU intubations, unless neuromuscular diseases, burns, or electrolyte disorders dictate otherwise. Mivacurium's nondepolarizing properties, short duration of action, and plasma metabolism make it a second-line choice for patients with contraindications to succinylcholine. Rocuronium is an acceptable alternative.

Long-acting, nondepolarizing neuromuscular blockers may be used as well. The onset of paralysis is hastened by administration of low doses or subparalytic "priming doses" given several minutes before the paralytic dose. Vecuronium and mivacurium represent good alternate choices for rapid-sequence intubation because both drugs exhibit a priming effect and have an intermediate duration of action and even large doses have minimal side effects. Although atracurium and vecuronium can be used for intubation, their long duration of action can be problematic if the airway cannot be cannulated.

Long-Term Paralysis

For patients with reasonable hemodynamic reserves and near-normal hepatic and renal function, paralysis for longer than 1 h can be accomplished safely and economically with pancuronium. Patients with tenuous hemodynamic status may be less likely to experience adverse cardiovascular effects if paralyzed with vecuronium, atracurium, or cisatracurium. Hepatic failure would be an additional consideration favoring atracurium or cisatracurium. Renal failure favors using vecuronium. Doxacurium, pipecuronium, and vecuronium do not offer any substantial advantage over pancuronium with respect to cost, duration of action, or side effect or elimination profiles. Tubocurarine and metocurine do not have a niche in the ICU because they require intact renal function for clearance and are potent histamine releasers. Despite the limitations of pancuronium, it can be used safely even for patients with advanced hepatic and renal insufficiency if care is taken to avoid massive overdose through close clinical monitoring.

Complications of Paralysis

Pseudocholinesterase Deficiency

Pseudocholinesterase is the plasma enzyme that metabolizes acetylcholine, succinylcholine, and mivacurium. Genetic or acquired reductions in this

TABLE 17-5 PROPERTIES OF NEUROMUSCULAR BLOCKERS

DRUG	INITIAL DOSE (mg/kg)	ONSET (min)	DURATION	HISTAMINE RELEASE	VAGAL BLOCKADE	METABOLISM	EXCRETION
Atracurium	0.4–0.6	2–3	Intermediate	+	0	Mostly nonenzymatic	Renal metabolite excretion
Cisatracurium	0.15–0.2	3–6	Intermediate	< atracurium	0	Mostly nonenzymatic	Renal metabolite excretion
Doxacurium	0.025–0.08	3–5	Long	0	0	Minimal	Renal
Mivacurium	0.15	2–3	Short	In large doses	0	Extensive in plasma	Minimal
Pancuronium	0.06–0.1	1–3	Long	0 to +	+	Moderate	Renal >> hepatic
Pipecuronium	0.07–0.85	1–3	Long	0	0	Moderate	Renal
Rocuronium	0.6	1–2	Intermediate	0	0	Moderate	Hepatic
Suyccinylcholine	1.0–1.5	1–2	Short	0	0	Extensive in plasma	Minimal
Vecuronium	0.08–0.10	1–3	Intermediate	0	0	Moderate	Hepatic >> renal

315

enzyme increase the duration of paralysis when using these drugs. Up to 5% of patients are heterozygous for plasma cholinesterase, resulting in prolongation of paralysis by several minutes. Approximately, 1 in 3,000 persons has a homozygous pseudocholinesterase deficiency, extending the duration of the paralysis to 6 to 8 h. Because the goal of therapy in the ICU, unlike the operating room, is usually to produce paralysis that lasts for hours, prolonged paralysis usually is of little consequence. There is no certain clue to pseudocholinesterase deficiency short of a clear history of prior prolonged paralysis; however, cholinesterase levels tend to decrease in patients with liver disease, renal failure, advanced age, pregnancy, marked anemia, and organophosphate toxicity.

Malignant Hyperthermia

Malignant hyperthermia is a calcium channel-mediated genetic disorder that is rarely precipitated by use of neuromuscular blockers, but when it occurs it is usually in combination with an inhalational anesthetic (see Chapter 28). Clinical features include the rapid development of muscular rigidity, high fever, and enormous increases in metabolic rate resulting in metabolic acidosis with massive CO_2 production and O_2 consumption. Untreated, lethal cardiac ischemia and ventricular arrhythmias are common. Treatment consists of removing the offending agent(s) and administering intravenous dantrolene.

Assessment of Neuromuscular Blockade

Approximately, 50% receptor blockade is required to cause some muscle weakness, with 95% percent blockade needed for complete muscular relaxation. Interestingly, the diaphragm is one of the muscles most resistant to paralytic drugs, requiring 90% or more of receptors to be blocked to develop paralysis. It can be difficult to clinically assess the degree of neuromuscular blockade in the ICU, but as a practical bedside test, the ability to sustain a head lift for several seconds indicates reversal of paralysis and is more reliable than tests of negative inspiratory force, vital capacity, tongue protrusion, or grip strength. Simply observing that the patient is overbreathing the rate set on the ventilator indicates that paralysis is not complete.

A peripheral nerve stimulator (PNS) provides the objective index of the intensity of neuromuscular blockade but is rarely used in ICU practice.

This fact is probably because there is little or no data to suggest improved outcomes with PNS compared to clinical evaluation. If employed, the goal of PNS use is to prevent complete obliteration of a "train of four" electrical stimulus. If patients are able to produce one to three muscular contractions per four electrical stimuli, paralytic overdose is presumed to have not occurred. Unfortunately, appropriate monitoring sites can be difficult to find and maintain, and it is possible to have complete obliteration of "train of four" stimulus, even with intact diaphragm function. The practical implication of this observation is that patients may still exhibit ventilator dyssynchrony despite profound peripheral skeletal muscle blockade or the desired obliteration of diaphragm function may require excessive peripheral blockade.

A more commonly used monitoring strategy is to allow the patient to move before subsequent doses of a paralytic agent are given. This practice has several practical advantages: (i) it does not require special equipment or training or induce patient discomfort; (ii) it allows early discovery of patients who are inadequately sedated; (iii) it permits assessment that may discover new intercurrent conditions; and (iv) it often reveals that continued paralysis is not necessary, thereby reducing duration of paralysis and expense. Regardless of the method of minute-to-minute monitoring, it is prudent to interrupt the administration of neuromuscular blockade at least once each day to prevent inadvertent overdose.

Reversal of Neuromuscular Blockade

The reversing agents (e.g., neostigmine, pyridostigmine, and edrophonium) act by raising acetylcholine levels in the neuromuscular junction and therefore, will not reverse blockade of succinylcholine or the profound (ion channel) blockade due to nondepolarizing blockers. Reversal of paralysis is rarely necessary in the ICU, and use of these agents risks muscarinic stimulation (bradycardia, bronchorrhea, and salivation). Muscarinic effects may be countered by pretreatment with the anticholinergic atropine or glycopyrrolate.

■ SUGGESTED READINGS

Avidan MS, Zhang L, Burnside BA, et al. Anaesthesia awareness and the bispectral index. *N Engl J Med.* 2008;358:1097–1108.
Ely EW, Truman B, Shintani A, et al. Monitoring sedation status over time in ICU patients: Reliability and validity of the Richmond Agitation-Sedation Scale (RASS). *JAMA.* 2003;289(22):2983–2991.

Girard TD, Kress JP, Fuchs BD, et al., Efficacy and safety of a paired sedation and ventilator weaning protocol for mechanically ventilated patients in intensive care (Awakening and Breathing Controlled trial): A randomised controlled trial. *Lancet.* 2008;371: 126–134.

Kress JP, Hall JB. Sedation in the mechanically ventilated patient. *Crit Care Med.* 2006;34(10):2541–2546.

Kress JP, Pohlman AS, O'Connor MF, et al. Daily interruption of sedative infusions in critically ill patients undergoing mechanical ventilation. *N Engl J Med.* 2000;342(20):1471–1477.

Ostermann ME, Keenan SP, Seiferling RA, et al. Sedation in the intensive care unit: A systematic review. *JAMA.* 2000;284(4):441–442.

Pun BT, Gordon SM, Peterson JF, et al. Large-scale implementation of sedation and delirium monitoring in the intensive care unit: A report from two medical centers. *Crit Care Med.* 2005;33(6): 1199–1205.

Riker RR, Fraser GL. Adverse events associated with sedatives, analgesics, and other drugs that provide patient comfort in the intensive care unit. *Pharmacotherapy.* 2005;25(5 Pt 2):8S–18S.

Shapiro BA, Warren J, Egol AB, et al. Practice parameters for intravenous analgesia and sedation for adult patients in the intensive care unit: An executive summary. Society of Critical Care Medicine. *Crit Care Med.* 1995;23(9):1596–1600.

General Supportive Care

KEY POINTS

1 Failure to systematically review the available database relevant to prior history, events immediately preceding presentation, vital organ performance, and therapy prescribed before and during hospitalization often leads to misinterpretation, inappropriate care plans, or ineffective communications among caregivers that translate into adverse outcomes or protracted hospital stays.

2 Although the ICU practitioner must intercede quickly and decisively when action is needed to avert disaster, in most circumstances, the clinician's prime objective should not be to reestablish "normal physiology" as quickly as possible but rather to encourage smooth resolution or adaptation to the pathophysiologic insult.

3 In the presence of uncertainty, conducting a closely observed "therapeutic minitrial" is a key element in the successful management of fragile or unstable patients. After the initial evaluation has been completed and a course of action has been decided, the patient and physician are often well served by implementing the proposed change under close observation for a brief interval, before formalizing the ongoing orders.

4 Uncertainty regarding the needed dose of medication (e.g., diuretics) often can be addressed, valuable time can be saved, and prescription errors can be avoided by verbalizing therapeutic intent and boundaries to the nurse and writing goal-oriented orders when possible to do so.

5 Concerned family members may seek or be offered information from multiple caregivers with differing perspectives, knowledge, and attitudes. One or two physicians must be identified as the primary contact(s) and one responsible family member identified as the conduit for important medical interchanges. To maintain confidence, the family must understand the logic of the management plan. Each ICU needs to establish and enforce a policy for family–caregiver communications that encourages trust, inspires confidence, meets the emotional needs of the family, and facilitates rather than impedes optimal care delivery.

6 Although certain consequences of protracted bed rest are well known to most practitioners, many subtle repercussions are either unknown or ignored. Physiologic adaptations to gravity affect nearly all organ systems, and release from gravitational stress may set in motion changes that delay recovery. Unrelieved recumbency has particularly adverse implications for the respiratory, cardiovascular, and neuromuscular systems.

7 Bedridden patients must be repositioned every 2 h unless there is an important contraindication to do so. Motion about the gravitational plane (Fowler's, reverse Trendelenburg, sitting positions) helps preserve vascular reflexes and reduces the tendency for peridiaphragmatic (basilar) atelectasis. The lateral decubitus and prone positions effectively stretch and drain the nondependent lung. Modern low air-cushioned beds can be programmed to effectively rotate the patient around the craniocaudal axis in an attempt to ensure such benefits and preserve skin integrity.

8 Anxiety and pain occur almost universally in the ICU setting. The skillful team blends the use of anxiolytics with psychotropics, analgesics, physical measures, environmental modifications, and concerted attempts to establish two-way communication. Attempts to encourage "normal" sleep–wake, lighting, and activity cycles may include "batching" of the routine monitoring observations and patient manipulations as well as the systematic use of hypnotics, analgesics, and anxiolytics where appropriate. Early intervention and the synergistic use of psychotropics help alleviate pain and disorientation.

9 Aggressive respiratory therapy is essential to the care of patients with impaired lung expansion, retained secretions, and bronchospasm. These techniques, which include repositioning, deep breathing, coughing, inhalation of a bronchodilator, and chest physiotherapy, must be targeted to the specific problem at hand and used only as long as clearly indicated—either as a prophylactic measure or as a treatment of demonstrated benefit.

10 Oxygen supplementation can be accomplished by nasal prongs and catheters, closed or open face masks, or a sealed airway (endotracheal tube). The selection is influenced by the range and precision of the FiO_2 required, patient tolerance, and the empirical response. The need for external humidification and the efficiency of humidifier required are determined by the flow of oxygen delivered relative to the total minute ventilation and the need to bypass the upper airway. Because disposable hygroscopic (heat-moisture exchanging) units may clog, impose dead space, and exhibit declining efficiency at high levels of ventilation, they may be unsuitable for severely ill patients and for those who have a high secretion burden or a marginal ventilatory reserve.

Certain aspects of management are common to critical care, independently of the precipitating cause for admission. These background details of day-to-day nursing and respiratory care help determine the eventual success or failure of specific management approaches leveled at the primary problems. This chapter reviews the basic elements of evaluation and therapy that apply to most patients in an intensive care unit (ICU) environment.

■ BEDSIDE EVALUATION OF THE CRITICALLY ILL PATIENT

Therapeutic Perspective

The term *intensive* care implies the potential for rapid changes in clinical status. Therefore, the patient must be monitored carefully, and the lines of communication among caregivers must be kept open. To care for the most critically ill, a knowledgeable and responsive physician must be continuously accessible and committed to reevaluating the patient as often and as long as required. The complexity of many critical illnesses demands that the physician evaluate each case with a strong background in physiology, intervene thoughtfully but promptly when indicated, and reassess frequently. There must be a short "feedback loop" linking intervention, result, and midcourse correction. In a field in which many key disorders are poorly defined (acute respiratory distress syndrome [ARDS], sepsis, etc.), it is often impossible to apply with confidence the results of population-based clinical trials to the individual patient. Decision support tools such as computer-aided displays of patient data, handheld digital databases for drugs and diseases (e.g., PDAs loaded with medical text information), and immediate access to the entire electronically encoded medical record make impressive contributions to the goal of correct and timely intensive care. Remote access, however, cannot take the place of frequent bedside visits and effective verbal communications regarding goals, problems, and progress.

Except under exceptional circumstances, vital communications concerning a complex database are too severely strained by long-distance discussions for complicated decision making. In recent years, however, advances in telecommunications have facilitated economical and timely transfer of massive data files (e.g., as required for radiographic imaging and streamed video), thereby improving the capacity for decision making at a distance. Although not yet equivalent for bedside evaluation, such techniques are rapidly improving and clearly offer the future possibility for care delivery of a uniform standard "24/7" or for a single specialty-trained physician to be involved simultaneously in the care of multiple patients at different sites.

Although isolated measurements are unquestionably important, *trends* in the data stream are often of equal or greater value. For many variables, the trending interval ideally should include the prehospital period. Answers to such questions as "What is the patient's chronic blood pressure, weight, cardiac rhythm, blood chemistries, medication listing, or $PaCO_2$?" may determine the appropriate management goals.

The ICU practitioner must intercede quickly and decisively when action is clearly necessary. In most circumstances, however, the clinician's prime

2 objective should *not* be to reestablish "normal physiology" as quickly as possible, but rather to encourage smooth resolution or adaptation to the pathophysiologic insult. A working diagnosis and updated plan of action must be clearly formulated and communicated. Because the clinician cannot always foresee the consequences, it is important to question the data quality and to consider alternative explanations before intervening—what really is known for certain and what must be better established?

Elements of the Bedside Evaluation

To be maximally effective, the intensivist must quickly probe, organize, prioritize, and integrate an extensive body of information flowing from verbal and written communications, monitored data, laboratory output, and imaging studies (Table 18-1). Using the available database and his/her own observations at the time of evaluation, the physician formulates a listing of current problems, ranks their urgency and relative priority, and thoughtfully devises a plan of action. When things become hectic and/or risk is high for errors of omission or commission, 5 or 10 min spent away from the bedside

TABLE 18-1 ELEMENTS OF THE BEDSIDE EVALUATION

Verbal communication
   Caregivers
   Patient
   Family
   Referring physician or institution

Written communication
   Chart record
   Nursing notes
   Current orders
   Medication/therapy lists
   Data board

Laboratory record

Imaging studies

Physical examination
   Vital signs
   Systems review
   Directed examination

Monitored information
   Ventilator
   Hemodynamics
   Electrocardiogram
   Other apparatus

in a quiet setting to analyze the database, identify the major problems and possibilities, and decide on the management approach nearly always is time well invested.

Caution is indicated whenever making management decisions without diagnostic certainty. Conducting a closely observed "therapeutic minitrial" is a key element in the successful management of fragile or unstable patients, especially when the physician is uncertain regarding the outcome of a planned intervention. After the evaluation has been completed and a course of action has been decided, the patient and physician are often well served by implementing the proposed change under direct observation for a brief interval, before formalizing the order. This approach is particularly helpful when making ventilator adjustments, position changes, or alterations in the infusion rates of fluids or rapidly acting drugs, the effects of which can be monitored directly (see "Volume Challenge" in Chapter 2). **3**

Accessing the Decisional Database

Skillful ICU practitioners not only integrate a vast array of data pertaining to the individual under treatment but also bring to bear the most appropriate therapy. Many decisions need to be made very quickly, and securing the needed information has the potential to consume enormous time. Faced with uncertainty and many competing priorities, the temptation is strong to forgo making a decision, to rely on memory, or to trust the verbal counsel of readily available colleagues. Potential for error and, consequently, the opportunity to improve care are high. The dramatic development of computer and communications technology has enabled partial closure of the information gap. Over a few short years, most physicians have been made aware of or now make active use of computerized medical records, remote digital access to laboratory data, and imaging studies from unit-based workstations or personal computers. Impressive displays of trended information as well as raw and processed data can be configured to the user's specific needs. A somewhat smaller but growing proportion of physicians now use the powerful search engines of public or private electronic libraries to rapidly identify and retrieve relevant articles from the medical literature. The first steps toward this goal of timely information access have already been taken—not only by bedside computers, but also by hand-carried computers and PDAs of ever-increasing power. These units not only package vital references, drug information, and periodically updated digests of evidence-based practice (e.g., Up-to-Date) but also allow wireless access to the Internet and to the hospital's own local network (intranet) for timely retrieval of patient-specific data. Without question, the potential benefits and consequences of this extraordinary leap into the information age have only begun to develop.

Verbal Communications

As most experienced practitioners realize, the ICU tends to function best with a team approach in which caregivers of varied descriptions (physicians, nurses, therapists, etc.) are professionally acquainted, mutually respected, and equally committed. All must be apprised of the current therapeutic objectives. The day-to-day routines and the expectations for the unit must be well understood, ideally with an awareness of the work schedules and priorities of all involved. Despite the unquestioned value of "hard data," overreliance on "the numbers" to guide decision making fosters an immature and dangerous style of practice. Drawing from moment-by-moment observations made over extended periods, a well-trained nurse or therapist is often the caregiver with the best insight regarding the relation of events and medications to evolving problems, tolerance of current therapy, and the probable effects of intended interventions (weaning from mechanical ventilation, mobilization, transport, reaction to medication, mental status, airway secretions, etc.). The clinician must seek their active involvement and advice in the planning process. For the team to operate with maximum effectiveness, the nurse, respiratory therapist, and unit pharmacologist (if available) should make formal rounds with the physician to share observations and advice as well as to be kept abreast of the doctor's current thinking and care plan. The specific objectives of therapy and conditions or developments for which the doctor desires to be contacted should be communicated explicitly. Enormous benefit accrues from well-thought-out protocols and goal-directed orders that account for patient response. Uncertainty regarding the appropriateness and dosage of certain medications often can be addressed, valuable time can be saved, and prescription errors can be avoided by communicating the intent of treatment. The latter strategy lends flexibility and allows timely dosage adjustment (e.g., for fluids and/or diuretics). A very common error is to write an order,

to assume that it was carried out, and then to fail to **4** follow up on the result of its execution. Setting clear goals for the nurse or the therapist, allowing for "online" modification of dosing in accordance with those goals, and automatic notification when the goals cannot be met tighten the linkage between patient and caregivers. ("Adjust the furosemide drip to maintain output > input by at least 1 L per shift" is more likely to succeed than "Give 40 mg furosemide IV TID.") Goal-directed order writing extends many of the same advantages offered by formalized care protocols (e.g., for heparin adjustment or insulin delivery) to a much broader and less-constrained therapeutic context.

Family Communications

It is difficult to overestimate the importance of **5** direct, unambiguous communication with the family. The ICU environment holds undeniable potential for miscommunication as the concerned family member may seek or receive information and advice from many caregivers with differing perspectives, knowledge, and attitudes. Generally speaking, trust in the fast-paced, high-tech unit and in the care team that makes potentially life-saving or life-threatening decisions has eroded somewhat over the years. Respect and engagement are the two watchwords. Families usually wish to know the "real story" and to understand the perceptions and approach—primary and contingency plans—of the attending physician. If care is obviously futile or should be withdrawn, a frank discussion is in order, especially if the family has initiated the conversation. But if the outcome is uncertain and there are logical steps to be taken to reverse the crisis, the family needs to know this as well. They also must perceive the physician's positive attitude toward resolution of the illness, whenever this is possible to realistically convey. Telling the family that there is little hope when the situation is ambiguous is likely to alienate the family, as often they perceive that the team is not genuinely trying or has already given up.

The tone and content of communication should not always be serious—humor does wonders to bridge the gap between caregiver and the vulnerable recipients of care. One or two physicians must be identified as the primary contact(s). Clearly, the family must be allowed to visit the patient as soon as appropriate after admission or in an unanticipated emergency. Continual presence of at least one family member at the bedside may be culturally mandated. In fact, there is a strong trend to design or modify ICUs so that the family can remain close to the patient at all times, encouraged to directly observe many aspects of care that were previously "out of bounds"—even cardiopulmonary resuscitation. Some recently published data support this newer practice. Even though some caregivers with the best intentions maintain unrestricted access to the patient, many believe it wisest to restrict routine visiting hours to two or three predictably "quiet periods" in the work day (e.g., late morning, late afternoon, early evening), especially in high-acuity ICUs. The approach should be individualized. Continual contact often threatens to confuse and emotionally exhaust the worried family, seldom benefits the comatose or sedated patient, encourages interchange of microbial pathogens, and interferes with caregiving. Whatever the local policy, it is wise to set aside a time in the day when the physician reliably communicates progress and plans and receives vital feedback from family members. Some well-functioning units reserve a specific hour each day (e.g., 1:00 to 2:00 PM) during which the intensivist can be scheduled (by the unit clerk) to discuss progress and plans with the patient's relatives. To reduce the emotional strain on both family and staff in an inherently unstable environment, it is important to emphasize that monotonic improvement (albeit desirable) seldom occurs, that minor setbacks and complications are to be anticipated, and that it is often most appropriate to view the general trend over days to weeks—not minutes to hours. Clearly defining the likely diagnoses and plausible alternatives, the team's approach, the strategy for action, and contingency plans helps instill confidence and trust.

Communications and Records

In addition to discussions with other caregivers, the physician must review the chart record, nursing notes, orders, medication and therapy lists, bedside data board, ventilator sheet, and laboratory record. Increasingly, all such information is incorporated into an electronic medical record (EMR) and the caregivers are given direct responsibility for detailed documentation and for entering orders that are not transcribed but are immediately entered. This new emphasis on electronic documentation—in many cases designed as much as a billing instrument than a communication tool—has given rise to templated notes laden with "cut and paste" entries and unnecessary replication of laboratory data. The need to communicate and document through the computer

has taken its toll on effective communication among caregivers and discourages the physician from returning to the bedside. Just how the benefits and detriments of the electronic medical record (EMR) play out in the ICU has yet to be fully experienced.

The need to carefully review the current listing of medications with the patient's ongoing and resolved problems clearly in mind cannot be overemphasized. To prevent delays and errors, it is a good idea to enter intended orders at the time of the bedside visit. The nursing record often provides an overlooked and valuable source of information. Puzzling entries with the potential to influence decision making should be clarified by direct verbal communication. Calculations required to synthesize the clinical picture and formulate revisions to the care plan (e.g., anion gap, systemic vascular resistance, respiratory compliance, airway resistance) should be automated or made quickly available at the bedside. Specific attention should be directed to the patient's weight, net fluid balance, intake, urinary and fecal output (Ins and Outs), diet, and drugs (those scheduled and those given as needed). Sedatives, antibiotics, vasoactive agents, and diuretics tend to be of special interest. The volume and description of expectorated or suctioned airway secretions and gastric aspirates should be noted.

Laboratory Data

The most recently obtained values for arterial blood gases, hemoglobin concentration, leukocyte and platelet counts, serum glucose, blood urea nitrogen (BUN), creatinine, electrolytes, and urinalysis must be reviewed in every patient for whom they are available. Serial tests for liver or cardiac enzymes, leukocyte differential, coagulation profile, drug levels, renal function tests, and so on may be of unusual interest in specific patients. As already noted, trends in such data often are more meaningful than individual test results.

Physical Examination and Monitoring

The contribution of the physical examination has become devalued as our technical abilities to image noninvasively, to monitor cardiorespiratory function, and to use laboratory data have improved. However, certain key bits of information that are impossible to gather quickly by other means should be assessed by physical examination one or more times daily in virtually every patient with cardiorespiratory instability or compromise.

Although the directed physical examination is the practical standard, outstanding clinicians are sufficiently disciplined to quickly but systematically assess certain aspects of the physical examination each day, not only to detect areas of concern but also to develop the background against which to gauge any future changes.

Vital Signs

Review of the vital signs record is a frequent starting point in the bedside evaluation. What are often overlooked, however, are the degree of variability and telling relationships among individual parameters. For example, heart rate may not parallel the height of fever or may be inappropriately slow for the clinical setting of congestive failure, as suggested by a disjunction between elevations of heart rate and respiratory rate. Extreme respiratory variation evident on an arterial or pulse oximetry tracing suggests relative hypovolemia and/or the paradox associated with severe airflow obstruction, severe left heart failure, or pericardial disease. Vital signs may change markedly with sleep or level of alertness. In the ventilated patient who makes spontaneous efforts, minute ventilation should be considered a vital sign. Wide variations of minute ventilation, especially when they occur abruptly, suggest that agitation may be responsible for the higher values. (This variability becomes an important consideration when prescribing sedatives and analgesics and when evaluating the ventilation requirements of a weaning candidate.)

Mental Status and Neuromuscular System

The categories of the Glasgow Coma Scale serve as a reminder of the gross characteristics to be screened and followed: best verbal, motor, and eye opening (and pupillary) responses. Muscle tone and strength, facial appearance, eye movements, pupillary size and reactivity, peripheral reflexes, and asymmetry should be noted. Signs of fear, anxiety, depression, and delirium should be elicited actively by attempting to engage the patient in meaningful conversation as well as light banter. (A well-timed sense of humor tests high-level integrative mental capacity, builds trust, reduces anxiety, and serves to narrow the communication gulf that separates patient and physician.) It is important to question the nursing staff regarding how well the patient has been sleeping, especially if delirium is suspected, dyspnea is questioned, or weaning is contemplated.

Cardiovascular System

Sequential cardiovascular examinations can reveal a new gallop, murmur, rhythm disturbance, paradoxical pulse, neck vein distention, basilar rales, dryness of the mucous membranes, diaphoresis, edema, impaired capillary refill, and other signs that provide clues to underlying pathophysiology. This knowledge should be interpreted in conjunction with an examination of electrocardiographic and arterial pressure tracings, echocardiographic and radiographic information, and data from a pulmonary artery catheter, when available. Serial examinations are especially important in the setting of myocardial infarction, acute endocarditis, or other potentially life-threatening, rapidly changeable conditions.

Respiratory System

Consecutive physical examinations of the respiratory system should focus on the quality, intensity, and symmetry of breath sounds; the presence or absence of regional percussion dullness; the breathing pattern; the audibility and distribution of wheezes, rales, rubs, rhonchi, and bronchial breath sounds; and the vigor and effectiveness of breathing efforts. Pulse oximetry can be extremely helpful when adjusting inspired oxygen fraction (FiO_2), positive end-expiratory pressure (PEEP), position, or ventilator settings. Mechanically ventilated patients require a careful review of the record documenting minute ventilation, oxygen, pressure requirements (peak, plateau, mean, and end-expiratory), gas exchange efficiency, patient–ventilator synchrony, integrity of the breathing circuit, and machine mode and settings (as detailed in Chapter 5).

Renal and Electrolyte Status

Although urine output and composition often should be followed closely, not every patient in the ICU requires an indwelling bladder catheter. However, because the urinary output of the healthy kidney tends to parallel intravascular fluid volume and serves as a useful indicator of vital organ perfusion, patients with questionable cardiovascular status often benefit from continuous urometry. The clinician should allow a trend to evolve over 1 to 3 h before making radical interventions based primarily on urinary output because oliguria may be transient or may respond only slowly to corrective action. Moreover, it is prudent to keep in mind the recent changes in therapy, cardiovascular status, sleep–wake cycles, and serum electrolytes in making the interpretation. The color, pH, specific gravity, glucose and electrolyte concentrations, results of tests for leukocyte esterase, erythrocytes, hemoglobin, and a review of sediment characteristics and pending urine cultures aid in assessing fluid status as well as in determining the etiology and severity of many common disorders. BUN and creatinine should be compared with previous values. This data should be considered in conjunction with the daily and cumulative I&O record, the daily weight trend, and the listing of medications in assessing the fluid balance. Weight should be compared with those of previous hospital days and the admission value as well as with weights recorded previously in clinical or prior admissions. Arterial blood gases and serum electrolytes should be reviewed, and anion gap and serum osmolality should be estimated.

Gastrointestinal/Nutritional Status

Daily assessments should include a review of nutritional intake. The volume and character of gastric aspirates and stool output also must be tracked. To evaluate gut motility, the physical examination of the abdomen always should include auscultation. The persistent absence of stool or gas output despite enteral intake may suggest obstipation or bowel obstruction, especially when the abdomen becomes noticeably distended. When confronting a quiet abdomen, it is important to palpate deeply and to attempt to elicit signs of peritoneal inflammation. Ascites, excessive bowel gas, gastric distention, and gut edema may explain a visibly distending abdomen. A "tight belly" may explain high ventilator cycling pressures or, if extreme, a dwindling urinary output. In such cases, bladder pressure should be transduced and measured (see Chapter 5).

Apparatus

Extensive use of equipment and devices characterizes the care delivered to critically ill patients. Intravascular lines and pumps should be inspected quickly, and their sites of entry should be examined for evidence of phlebitis, local cellulitis, or purulence. The dressings that cover suspicious points of catheter insertion must be taken down, and the wound beneath must be examined carefully, preferably at the time of routine dressing changes. When specialized life-support equipment is used (e.g., balloon pump), the key variables relevant to its operation and the level of support must be noted. Enteral catheters and endotracheal tube anchoring devices should be inspected and the ventilator circuit examined for collected water. The essential data provided by the bedside cardiac monitor and the ventilator display are reviewed with each visit to the bedside.

Imaging Data

Radiographs, computed tomograms (CT), and ultrasonic images have become integral to the evaluation of the critically ill patient. Rounds should incorporate a review of such data, which often redirect thinking or confirm diagnoses made by other means.

■ THERAPEUTIC SUPPORTIVE CARE

Intensive life support has no evolutionary precedent. Before modern civilization, our primate ancestors were at constant risk of predatory attack and disease. Survival required foraging and continuous vigilance; our predecessors seldom remained off their feet or motionless for longer than a few hours at a time. Most conditions that now prompt admission to the ICU would previously have resulted in a quick demise. Deprived of food and water and unable to take shelter from the elements and natural enemies, the sick individual became vulnerable to many of the traumatic, infectious, and environmental problems that now are easily manageable. A philosopher or anthropologist could argue effectively that evolutionary pressures encourage elimination (rather than survival) of those weak enough to fall prey to catastrophic disease or severe trauma. Because the recumbent position is central to the extended life support but is inherently unnatural, a working knowledge of the physiology of sustained bed rest and immobility is fundamental to understanding the rationale and consequences of ICU confinement.

Physiology of Bed Rest

Noncardiorespiratory Effects of Recumbency

Certain consequences of protracted bed rest are well known to most practitioners, whereas other, subtler repercussions are either unknown or ignored. Physiologic adaptations to gravity affect nearly all organ systems, and release from gravitational stress may set in motion changes that impede recovery.

Neuromuscular

While under the influence of gravity, contracting skeletal muscles compress the veins and lymphatics, counteracting the gravitational forces that would otherwise cause the body fluids to pool in the legs and lower abdomen. Contraction of muscles used in maintaining the upright posture and locomotion preserves muscle bulk and strength. Symmetry of upper as well as lower extremities should be noted and tracked. Lack of movement, hypoalbuminemia, and the persistently upright torso encourage edema to form in the hands and the lower arms. *Asymmetry* of the edema that forms suggests an upper extremity thrombosis—which occur quite commonly in patients with ipsilateral PICC and subclavian or internal jugular catheters. Moreover, muscular traction and gravitational stresses help the bones retain calcium. It is not known what level of fiber tension or duration of contraction is necessary to sustain these benefits. It is clear, however, that release of the skeletal muscles from their diurnal activity for longer than 24 to 48 h initiates metabolic processes that eventually culminate in tissue atrophy and impressive physiologic changes.

Aerospace science and experiments in healthy volunteers have yielded impressive data on the effects of bed rest in healthy individuals (Table 18-2). Skeletal muscles quickly lose tone when not supporting the body's weight. After only 72 h, the loss of myofibrillar protein is under way—even in a well-nourished, physiologically unstressed subject. The greatest protein losses occur in the muscle groups that normally bear the greatest postural burden—legs and dorsal trunk. The rates at which

bulk and strength diminish are believed to be functions of the length at which the muscle fiber is immobilized as well as the completeness of relaxation. As indicated by the devastating weakness that results from extended pharmacologic paralysis, neural excitation may be a crucial factor in preserving muscle function. Intense stimulation may not be required to dramatically slow the pace of sarcomere depletion, and although active movement is clearly better than passive manipulation of resting muscle, physical therapy of the immobilized patient aids significantly in preventing contractures.

As any sleepless physician understands, periodic rest in the recumbent position is essential for optimal cerebral functioning. Even during sleep, however, the healthy adult turns or makes a significant positional adjustment multiple times per hour. As noted following, there may be important physiologic advantages to such frequent repositioning. Most adults do not prefer to initiate sleep in the supine horizontal position that is used routinely in the ICU. Many individuals express great difficulty in falling asleep in this position or awaken quickly if they inadvertently shift into it. In fact, all nonarboreal four-footed mammals—including the primates—ambulate prone, with vulnerable vital structures protected by proximity to the ground. Most animals sleep in that position as well.

With the development of modern intensive care and the need to cannulate blood vessels and access the various orifices of the respiratory, gastrointestinal, and urinary systems, the recumbent critically ill patient was kept oriented in the supine position for extended periods, often immobilized by sedation or paralyzed pharmacologically by muscle relaxants. Periodic turning is known to be important in the avoidance of pressure trauma (decubitus ulcers, see following), which is most likely to develop over the points of high contact pressure—especially when the patient is cared for on a firm traditional bed. (Perhaps such vulnerability helps explain the need for frequent movement during sleep.)

Endocrine and Metabolic

Release of many hormones normally is timed to a diurnal cycle. For example, cortisol and epinephrine normally vary in a circadian fashion, with trough levels occurring in the early morning hours. Cholinergic (vagal) tone also increases at night. The unnatural activity, lighting, and noise within many ICU environments disrupt these cycles. Moreover, bed rest itself alters certain biorhythms; cycles for

---

TABLE 18-2 PHYSIOLOGIC EFFECTS OF BED REST

Noncardiorespiratory effects
  Reduced muscle bulk and strength
  Altered biorhythms
  Decreased glucose tolerance
  Endocrine dysfunction
  Fluid shifts and diuresis
  Calcium, potassium, and sodium depletion
  Immunologic impairment
  Nasal congestion/impaired sinus drainage
  Reduced gastrointestinal motility/esophageal
    reflux

Cardiovascular effects
  Pulmonary vascular congestion
  Impaired vasomotor tone and reflexes
  Increased preload and stroke volume
  Altered autonomic activity

Respiratory effects
  Reduced functional residual capacity
  Altered distribution of lung volume
  Altered airway drainage

insulin and growth hormone (and consequently glucose) often demonstrate multimodal patterns, time-shifted peaks, and other perturbations in normal healthy subjects, even when feeding schedules remain unchanged. The activity of the pancreas gradually declines, and glucose intolerance may develop after as little as 3 days of enforced bed rest. These changes usually reverse within 1 week of resuming normal activity. Thyroid hormones tend to rise as bed rest continues beyond a few weeks, whereas androgen levels fall. Oxygen consumption declines significantly during recumbency.

Fluid and Electrolyte Shifts

Recumbency shifts about 10% of the total blood volume (approx. 500 mL) cephalad, away from the legs. Almost 80% of the shifted volume migrates to the thorax; the remainder translocates to the head and neck. The nasal mucosa swells, and the patient may experience nasal congestion. Diuresis begins on the first day of recumbency for the normal subject, who loses approximately 600 mL of extracellular fluid by the second day (more if edema was present initially). Bed rest initiates losses of sodium and potassium but reduces the amplitudes of the diurnal excretory cycles for water, sodium, potassium, and chloride. Weight bearing seems to be an important stimulus to osteoblastic activity, and during prolonged bed rest, approximately 0.5% of total body calcium stores are leached per month from the bones and muscles. Rarely, impaired renal excretion of the increased calcium load results in hypercalcemia.

Gastrointestinal Changes

Well-known gastrointestinal responses to inactivity include anorexia and constipation. Recumbency impairs the efficiency of swallowing and may precipitate esophageal reflux in those with lax esophageal sphincter function. The gut may lose all but a vestige of its natural motility if food is not provided, gastric secretion is pharmacologically suppressed, and air swallowing is inhibited—even if opiates are not prescribed (see Chapter 17).

Immunologic Defenses

Bed rest impairs the body's resistance to infection, even when no catheters enter the vascular, urinary, respiratory, or gastrointestinal compartments. The normal rate of catabolizing immunoglobulin G doubles, and neutrophilic phagocytosis slows. The mucosal colonization rate for certain pathogens, such as the staphylococcus, may increase. An adverse gravitational bias results in stasis, secretion pooling, and bacterial overgrowth within the maxillofacial sinuses and tracheobronchial tree—further predisposing patients to infection.

Blood Components and Coagulation

It generally is understood that patients on protracted bed rest are vulnerable to thrombosis—largely because of venostasis and unrelieved compression of the leg veins. Subtle changes also occur in the coagulation profile; procoagulant synthesis and fibrinolytic activity increase, and the thromboplastin time shortens. Independent of any coexisting disease process, the red blood cell mass tends to decline during the first several weeks of inactivity, primarily because of a decrease in erythropoiesis.

Cardiovascular Effects of Recumbency

Vasomotor changes in arterial resistance both maintain blood pressure relatively constant and regulate the distribution of blood flow. In the active and fully conscious normal individual, fluctuations in regional tissue blood flows occur naturally and spontaneously. In the immobile supine patient, these fluctuations gradually disappear over the first hour of recumbency. Alert subjects may then experience sufficient discomfort to impel a change in position.

Many significant cardiovascular changes occur in the normal individual during the transition to the supine position (see Table 18-2). In the conscious subject, heart rate declines as stroke volume increases. Cerebral, renal, and hepatic blood flows increase, whereas blood pressure and systemic and pulmonary vascular resistances tend to decline. Sympathetic tone decreases, and parasympathetic tone increases. The renin–angiotensin axis downregulates, promoting diuresis. The baroreceptive reflexes that are instrumental in adapting to the upright position are blunted after sustained bed rest; therefore, chronic orthostatic stress seems necessary, both for the preservation of an adequate blood volume as well as for maintaining adaptive cardiovascular reflexes.

The Trendelenburg (head down) position offers no significant hemodynamic benefit over that provided by the supine position, and despite its widespread use, it has no confirmed place in the management of shock (other than for central line placement). The gravitational bias of the Trendelenburg position increases intracranial arterial and venous pressures equally and, therefore, leaves cerebral perfusion unimpaired in normal individuals. However, elevated intracranial pressures may compromise cerebral perfusion in the patient with preexisting head injury. Head inversion also increases the tendency for esophageal reflux. These drawbacks do not mean that the Trendelenburg position cannot be useful when used briefly for specific purposes; airways drain more effectively, and distention of neck veins facilitates the insertion of central venous catheters while helping to avoid air embolism.

In the lateral and prone positions, gravitational effects on hydrostatic pressure are of less importance, but venous obstruction occasionally may pose significant problems. Extreme flexion of the trunk in infants, obese adults, and advanced pregnancy may not only result in hypoxemia but also may impede venous return. For a woman in the advanced stages of pregnancy, lying in the supine position may compress the vena cava, causing hypotension that is relieved by lying on the left side. Increased abdominal pressure leading to inferior vena cava obstruction also has been associated with the prone position, especially when there is exaggerated knee–chest positioning or an unusually noncompliant abdominal support.

Respiratory System

7 Conversion from the upright to the supine position is accompanied by important changes in ventilation, perfusion, secretion clearance, muscle function, gas trapping, and tendency for and distribution of lung collapse. In normal subjects, reclining decreases functional residual capacity (FRC), primarily because of the upward pressure of the abdominal contents on the diaphragm and to a lesser extent to declining lung compliance. The functional residual volume declines by approximately 30% (or 800 mL) in shifting from the sitting to the horizontal supine position and by about half as much in the sitting to lateral decubitus transition. Head-down tilting causes only a marginal additional volume loss. The magnitude of these reductions is somewhat less in older than in younger patients. Conversion from the supine to the prone position is accompanied by an increase of resting lung volume of approximately 15%, with most of this change occurring in dorsal regions. Patients with airflow obstruction generally lose much less volume in supine recumbency (Fig. 18-1) (see Chapter 25).

Position also influences pulmonary hemodynamics. Hydrostatic pressures and blood flows tend to distribute preferentially to the dorsal regions in the supine position. Recumbency redistributes lung

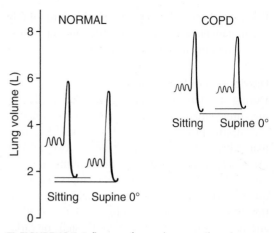

■ **FIGURE 18-1** Influence of recumbency on the spirograms of the normal subject and the patient with chronic obstructive pulmonary disease (COPD). Note that the positional changes in FRC are not matched by corresponding changes of residual volume in either instance. Patients with COPD may lose very little volume in the transition to the supine position—in part due to gas trapping.

volume because it alters the geometry of the thorax. The heart tends to compress the left lower lobe bronchi and is supported partially by the lung tissue beneath. This anatomy helps account for the tendency for atelectasis to develop so commonly in the left lower lobe in postoperative and bedridden patients—especially those with cardiovascular disease. The pleural pressure adjacent to the diaphragm is considerably less negative than at the apex. The vertical gradient of transpulmonary pressure (alveolar minus pleural pressure) is approximately 0.25 cm H_2O per cm of vertical height for normal subjects in the erect position and approximately 0.17 cm H_2O per cm for normal subjects in recumbency; therefore, alveolar volumes are greatest in the nondependent regions. For patients with edematous lungs, an intensified gravitational gradient of pleural pressure accentuates dorsal atelectasis and consolidation.

Available data indicate that the gradient of pleural pressure is considerably less in the prone than in the supine position, perhaps in part because of the shifting weight of the heart and mediastinal contents. The prone position also favors airway drainage. The lateral decubitus position causes the upper lung to assume a resting volume nearly as large as it has in the sitting position and to undergo better drainage, whereas the lower lung tends to pool mucus and is compressed to a size similar to or less than it has in the supine position. *Total* resting lung volume is considerably greater in the lateral decubitus than in the supine horizontal orientation.

Positional losses of lung volume are considerably less in patients with airflow obstruction, in part due to gas trapping in dependent regions.

Distribution of Ventilation

During spontaneous breathing, ventilation distributes preferentially to the dependent lung zones in the supine, prone, and lateral positions. The normal subject also takes "sigh" breaths two to four times deeper than the average tidal volume approximately 8 to 10 times/h. Postural changes occur frequently. Microatelectasis and arterial O_2 desaturation tend to develop if breathing remains shallow and uninterrupted by these periodic sighs or variations of position. In contrast to spontaneous breathing, the nondependent regions receive the most ventilation when the patient is inflated passively by a mechanical ventilator. Dependent regions not only have the least end-expiratory (resting) lung volume but also receive less ventilation, further promoting atelectasis in those areas.

Positional Dyspnea

Certain positions may relieve or exacerbate dyspnea. Orthopnea, although most emblematic of congestive heart failure, also characterizes severe airflow obstruction, pregnancy, extreme obesity, pericardial tamponade, and diaphragmatic weakness. Conversely, patients with quadriplegia or extreme orthostatic hypotension and those who experience abdominal or back pain accentuated by the upright position may not tolerate sitting without breathlessness.

Immobility: Preventative and Therapeutic Measures

Against the physiologic background just described, it is clear that prolonged immobility must be avoided. In profoundly weak or pharmacologically immobilized patients, range-of-motion exercises and high-top tennis shoes or foot boards may help prevent foot drop. As a rule, bedridden patients must be repositioned every 2 h unless there is an important contraindication (e.g., hemodynamic instability or spinal injury). Inclining the upper torso above the horizontal plane (Fowler's, reverse Trendelenburg, sitting position) helps preserve the vascular reflexes, limits the risks of esophageal reflux and aspiration, and reduces the tendency for peridiaphragmatic (basilar) atelectasis. The lateral decubitus and prone positions effectively stretch and drain the uppermost lung regions. Certain

automated beds can effectively rotate the patient about the craniocaudal axis in an attempt to ensure such benefits and preserve skin integrity (see "Specialty Beds," following).

■ SKIN BREAKDOWN AND PRESSURE ULCERS

Etiology

When local surface pressures exceed capillary pressure, the resulting ischemia can produce necrosis of the integument. Breakdown of the skin over pressure points is a common and costly problem for critically ill patients. Pressure ulcers tend to prolong hospitalization and increase morbidity. The toll that skin breakdown takes is not easily measured. But it has been estimated that each year more than one million patients receiving treatment in an ICU are affected with pressure sores at enormous financial costs. Although decubitus ulcers develop frequently in elderly and/or diabetic patients, any patient with one or more of the major risk factors (high local pressure, increased shear force, friction, reduced capillary perfusion, anemia, malnutrition, tissue edema, or prolonged moisture exposure) can develop a pressure ulcer. Because mechanically ventilated patients often are sedated or paralyzed, malnourished, edematous, hypotensive, or confined to bed for lengthy periods, they are especially vulnerable.

Pressure ulcers are most likely to develop over bony prominences where compressive forces may exceed the normal capillary filling pressure of approximately 25 to 30 mm Hg for an extended period, thereby promoting ischemic injury. Relieving local pressure is especially important for patients in the prone position, when the nose, chin, shoulders, knees, and hips are the contact points rather than the broad surface of the back and upper legs. Pressure ulcers also can develop without high compression when the skin is subjected repeatedly to friction or shear or becomes macerated because of prolonged exposure to urine or feces.

Prevention and Treatment

Varied measures can be used to interrupt and reverse the progression toward ulceration (Table 18-3). Frequent repositioning and mobilization relieve local pressure and forestall skin breakdown. Massage of reddened skin and areas of bony prominence improves local circulation. Prevention of decubitus ulcers is one reason to avoid deep sedation or

TABLE 18-3 PREVENTION OF CUTANEOUS PRESSURE SORES

Avoidance of high local pressure

Avoidance of:
  Malnutrition
  Edema
  Maceration
  Ischemia

Mobilization
Topical coverings
Specialty mattresses and beds

paralysis whenever possible. As already noted, adjustments of position occur frequently during sleep. Motionless patients should be repositioned no less frequently than every 2 h, unless such manipulation disrupts wounds, impairs oxygenation, or promotes homodynamic instability. When frequent repositioning is not possible, careful padding of bony prominences can help prevent injury. Many air-cushioned specialty beds limit and vary the gravitational forces applied to specific high-risk areas, decreasing the likelihood of skin breakdown (see following).

Preventing the development of pressure ulcers is much easier than treating the established lesions. Once established, however, more than 100 topical products can be brought to bear. These are organized into several categories: wet gauze, ulcer-covering films (e.g., Tegaderm), foams (e.g., Lyofoam), hydrocolloids (e.g., DuoDERM), hydrogels (e.g., Carrington), and alginates (e.g., Sorbsan). Each product group claims superiority in specific settings and, because of the complexity of this topic, it is best to consult a wound care specialist for significant problems. (Depending on the institution, this service may be offered by burn, wound, or plastic surgery professionals.) In the healing process, the importance of optimizing nutritional status, of avoiding extended moisture exposure (especially that due to incontinence), and of early mobilization cannot be overemphasized.

For patients whose decubitus ulcers fail to heal despite such measures, infection of soft tissue or underlying bone is often responsible. To optimize healing, devitalized tissue should be debrided and appropriate antibiotics administered. Although the site of ulceration may influence the spectrum of flora recovered, infected wounds often contain a mixture of Gram-positive cocci and Gram-negative

rods and anaerobes, making blanket antibiotic recommendations difficult. In non–life-threatening infections, cefazolin used in combination with gentamicin or ofloxacin may suffice. However, in most cases of serious infection, an extended-spectrum penicillin and an aminoglycoside or quinolone—with or without metronidazole—are necessary for complete coverage. Vancomycin usually is indicated when methicillin-resistant *Staphylococci* are recovered.

For the comatose or immobilized patient, prevention of pressure sores emphasizes frequent turning, early mobilization, and avoidance of deep sedation or paralysis. Although automated "specialty beds" (see following) have largely supplanted their need, prophylactic use of thick or quilted foam (egg carton) or air-flotation mattresses should be considered for high-risk patients where these are not in use; they are effective preventative devices when used for short periods in patients exhibiting some spontaneous movement. Adjunctive measures include maintenance of an adequate tissue perfusion pressure (avoidance of hypotension), prevention of malnutrition, and elimination of tissue edema. When pressure sores develop, consultation with a wound care specialist for appropriate topical treatment can help prevent the devastating complications of cellulitis and systemic sepsis.

Specialty Beds

Air-fluidized, inflatable segment, low-air-loss beds have gained great popularity in ICU practice, not only for their skin-sparing benefits but also for their ability to vary the distribution of pressure, to vary the body angle on a programmable schedule, to administer vibropercussion, to provide precise automated weights, and to facilitate cleanup, body positioning, and patient transfer. They most effectively prevent decubitus ulcers. Although extremely expensive, the latest generation of these instruments sufficiently extends capability to provide quality ICU care to make them the de facto equipment standard.

Beds with segmented air cushion capability can help in a variety of settings in which skin breakdown is well established or imminent. Soft beds of this type are particularly helpful for patients who must be positioned prone for extended periods, as they both cushion the contact points and facilitate the "flipping" process. Massively obese patients can benefit from "chair convertible beds," which allow easy transitions between the supine and upright postures.

Isolation Precautions

In a busy ICU, transfer of communicable pathogens is facilitated by the variety and multiplicity of the interactions that occur between patient, family, and caregivers. Certain principles of infection prevention in the individual patient are detailed in Chapter 26. Frequently, patients will require special attention to avoid transmitting infections to themselves or to others. To protect staff and fellow patients, the need for isolation should be reconsidered frequently, and ICU nursing staff should be notified immediately of isolation plans. Visitors as well as staff must adhere to hygienic guidelines.

Several levels of protection are used in most ICUs (Table 18-4). *Universal Precautions* require the use of gloves with any direct patient contact, including handling of body fluids. They generally are recommended as the basal level of care for all patients in the ICU, but in reality, these standards are sometimes violated. Hand washing and use of antiseptic foams (foam in–foam out) between patient contacts are mandatory when gloves are not used because they are among the most effective simple measures for avoiding spread of communicable pathogens. When used properly, antimicrobial gels, foams, and lotions may be as effective as hand washing and have recently gained popularity as their convenience fosters compliance with prophylaxis guidelines. Using gloves does not entirely eliminate the need for hand washing as the warm, moist environment of the tight-fitting glove can serve as an effective incubator for small inocula of pathogens trapped beneath the fingernails, under the rings, and between the fingers. Relatively large innocula can then be transferred via fomites, coworkers, visitors, or subsequent ungloved contact with patients. It should be pointed out to poorly compliant staff that hand washing, gloves, and cidal gels help to protect the caregiver from viral contamination, presumably reducing their own likelihood of colds and other transmissible diseases spread by skin contact. Any caregiver with a cold should wear a face mask.

Strict isolation demands the donning of gowns, gloves, and masks whenever entering a patient's room and the removal of these items before exiting.

Respiratory isolation is observed in cases in which there is potential for airborne transmission of a dangerous, communicable pathogen. Well-fitting masks that meet a rigorous filtration standard high efficiency particulate air (HEPA) are mandated or recommended in most hospitals for pathogens such as tuberculosis. Isolation rooms for respiratory pathogens are designed for one-way (outside room to inside room) airflow to prevent the dissemination of airborne pathogens to corridors and public areas.

Contact isolation requires the practitioner to take appropriate precautions (gloves, mask, and/or gown) when dealing with the affected area. Hand washing or gel usage should follow glove removal.

Reverse isolation is used for immunocompromised patients or at any time the clinician may transfer a communicable pathogen to the patient.

Ambient Environment

Modern ICUs recognize the need for critically ill patients to be cared for in a pleasant, temperature-controlled environment that encourages a normal sleep–wake cycle. Many units are required to provide visual access to the outdoors and appropriately ventilated and temperature-conditioned rooms. However, equipment and external temperatures during peak summer hours may cause even well-designed rooms to overheat. Such simple measures as drawing the shades during times of sunlight exposure and use of fans to improve air circulation can moderate any resulting discomfort.

Noise levels should be reduced whenever possible; gentle music provided via headphones or a bedside radio may comfort the conscious patient. It comes as no surprise that sleep quality is seriously compromised in the ICU. Sedative-induced unrousability does not equal quality rest. Sleep architecture is fragmented, and even though total sleep time may be normal, sleep depth and phase content are not. The vast majority of ICU survivors relate sleep disruption as a serious problem—with as yet undetermined physiologic consequences. Earplugs should be considered for use during sleeping hours in unusually noisy (e.g., multipatient) rooms. In many instances, the volume of certain alarms can be muted safely at the bedside or "remoted" to the nursing station. Attempts to encourage a normal

TABLE 18-4   CATEGORIES OF PROTECTION AND ISOLATION

Universal precautions

Isolation
  Strict
  Respiratory
  Contact
  Reverse

sleep–wake lighting and activity cycle may include "batching" of routine monitoring observations and patient manipulations as well as the systematic use of hypnotics, analgesics, and anxiolytics when appropriate. The importance of adequate high-quality natural sleep cannot be overrated. Providing adequate sleep markedly diminishes the incidence of disorientation and delirium. Hypnotics that preserve normal sleep architecture (such as zolpidem) are probably underutilized in the high-stress ICU environment.

Comfort Measures

8 Anxiety and pain occur almost universally in the ICU setting. The skillful team blends the use of anxiolytics with psychotropics, analgesics, physical measures, and concerted attempts to communicate. Vigilance to prevent or treat bladder and bowel distention, muscular skeletal discomfort, and pain arising from medication infusions (e.g., potassium, amphotericin, diazepam, bicarbonate, and erythromycin) are essential. Slowing the rate of administration, coadministration with a more swiftly flowing diluent, local use of lidocaine, hydrocortisone (e.g., for traditional amphotericin, 1 mg per mg of drug), or heparin (0.5 to 1.0 U/mL), and administration via a central vein are helpful strategies to minimize local pain. For certain medications (e.g., nonlipophilic or nonliposomal amphotericin), premedication with an antipyretic and antihistamine (e.g., diphenhydramine) can blunt the chills and fever that predictably accompany their administration.

Although benzodiazepines, propofol, and opiates are used universally to reduce ongoing discomfort, psychotropics such as haloperidol and olanzapine have been recognized as valuable adjuncts for some (see Chapter 10). Anxiety and pain reinforce each other; early intervention can pay high dividends in aborting a spiraling pain—anxiety cycle (see Chapter 17). Such simple measures as variation of body position, back rubs, and heating pads may make an important difference. It has been shown that directing a stream of air over the face (using a fan) may reduce the sense of dyspnea, even in an intubated, mechanically ventilated patient.

Gastrointestinal Care

Impairment of gastrointestinal motility occurs frequently in critically ill patients, even in the absence of primary gastrointestinal disease. Prolonged abstinence from oral intake, dehydration, nasogastric suctioning, bed rest, opiates, and sedatives slow the gastrointestinal motility, especially in elderly patients. Simultaneously, air swallowing and/or fixed-rate enteral feedings encourage abdominal distention that might impair diaphragmatic excursion. On the other hand, mucosal atrophy, edema of the bowel wall, antibiotics, and alterations of the native gut flora encourage malabsorption and diarrhea. Strategies to cope with these disturbances emphasize mobilization and the institution of oral intake as soon as feasible. Enteral feedings given at well-tolerated rates generally are preferred to parenteral nutrition. Bedside commodes are preferred to bedpans by many patients who otherwise would voluntarily retain and tend to obstipate. Appropriate hydration, stool softeners, bulk-forming agents, gentle enemas, laxatives, motility stimulants (e.g., metoclopramide, erythromycin, low-dose enteral physostigmine), and manual disimpaction are helpful options for problematic patients.

Copious diarrhea is a difficult management problem that carries the potential for nutritional depletion, electrolyte disturbances, and skin maceration (see Chapter 16). Tests for detecting *Clostridium difficile* should be ordered, whether or not the patient has received antibiotics recently. Ointments and coverings serve as an effective barrier when skin breakdown is imminent. Although occasionally useful, fecal bags seldom work well, usually leak, and may be difficult to remove without spillage or tissue trauma. When diarrhea is profuse and thin, rectal tubes may be inserted for brief periods. To avoid serious complications because of erosion of the rectal mucosa, the tube should be removed periodically. Generally speaking, balloon inflation is inadvisable.

Bladder Care

Although invaluable for collecting and monitoring urinary output, Foley catheters should not be viewed as innocuous or inserted merely as a convenience. Intermittently catheterizing the bladder via a straight catheter and using an external collection apparatus are useful options when they are feasible to use and continuous urometry is not required. In the face of oliguria, a dysfunctional or clogged Foley catheter should be irrigated and/or replaced.

Dressing and Wound Care

Dressings around central lines and arterial catheters should be changed every other day unless required earlier. Transparent plastic windows in the specialized dressing placed over the catheter allow the skin puncture site to be monitored. These routine procedures usually are undertaken in the morning in conjunction with other hygienic maneuvers. Dressings should not be allowed to remain soaked in wound drainage (blood, serum, pus). Communication with the nursing staff will enable the interested physician to examine the wound at the time that it is scheduled for exposure, obviating unnecessary dressing changes.

Transportation Issues

Transportation of the critically ill patient to a site outside the ICU tends to be a complicated and somewhat hazardous process that requires coordination among multiple caregivers. Patients requiring studies outside the ICU (most commonly for imaging studies and interventional radiology) must be well monitored, and all vital life-support systems must remain functional in transit. Emergency drugs and supplies should accompany the patient. Available transport monitors allow display of all important variables tracked at the bedside. As a rule, at least one ICU nurse is needed to observe the patient, to monitor cardiorespiratory function, and to intervene rapidly if difficulty arises. Two or more additional persons generally are required to maintain appropriate ventilation and move the bed, pumps, and ancillary equipment. Consequently, the nursing staff must know as early as possible about the need for and the time of the intended transport.

Because of the considerable risk and resource commitment, it is wise to consolidate studies and interventions that take place outside the ICU whenever feasible to do so. For example, a CT scan performed in search of an abscess or loculated effusion should serve simultaneously to guide catheter insertion by a radiologist or physician who is standing by for that purpose. Sequential imaging procedures should take place during the same session, whenever possible; it is not unreasonable to conduct CT scans in a predetermined exploratory sequence during the same transport episode when the patient is critically ill and several diagnostic possibilities are at hand. To judge the wisdom of proceeding to the next step, the physician must be available to make the appropriate decision to proceed with, extend, or abort the planned studies.

Unstable patients are not good candidates for transport, especially when extended elevator and hallway exposure is required. Stable patients can be manually ventilated with the help of oximetry and cardiovascular monitoring. A "minitrial" of manual ventilation adequacy should be conducted at the bedside for several minutes before the actual move is attempted. Those more seriously ill may require a specialized transport ventilator capable of maintaining the required ventilatory pattern.

With modern drainage systems, thoracostomy (chest) tubes present little difficulty in transport if no suction is required to keep the lung adequately inflated. If a mobile suction system is not available for patients who are suction dependent (e.g., those with large bronchopleural fistulae), a water seal should be attempted at the bedside for a duration similar to that projected for the transport before its execution during the "minitrial" of transport ventilation—manual or automated. Prior arrangements should be made to reestablish suction drainage at the remote site.

Communication

The experience of receiving intensive care is simultaneously isolating, frightening, and disorienting; perhaps never before has the patient felt as powerless, vulnerable, or dependent on others. Almost invariably, it is life disrupting and anxiety provoking for family and close relations as well. Establishing trust with the caregivers is vital to alleviating worry and achieving compliance with indicated measures. Seriousness, honesty, and respect must be conveyed whenever addressing medical issues. A clear plan and contingency arrangements must be communicated to reinforce the perception that the clinician is truly the patient's advocate and that the situation—however difficult—will be appropriately addressed. When not discussing serious medical matters, the opportunity should be taken to break down the artificial "white coat" barrier that keeps the patient and family feeling in subordinate. Good-natured light banter and humor—the great "leveler" of interpersonal relations—help enormously. Intubated patients cannot verbally express needs, sensations, or emotions. Familiar photographs, a clock plainly visible to the patient, and a readable calendar help maintain proper orientation. Although no strategy works effectively for all patients, caregivers should remain sensitive to the possibility of hearing or sight impairment. The fact that the patient normally wears a hearing aid or uses glasses may be forgotten in the highly charged, technology-driven setting of the ICU. Alert patients may be able to express basic needs or pose questions via note writing, lip-reading or letter boards, or graphic charts. Close friends and family members may interpret gestures more effectively than the medical staff, especially if the patient has been chronically disabled. For patients with tracheostomies who require ventilator support, cuff deflation allows vocalization if PEEP of about 10 cm H_2O is applied to provide adequate leakage airflow across the vocal cords. Patients with adequate strength who are not ventilator dependent and breathe spontaneously can speak through a one-way (Passy-Muir) valve attached to the cuff-deflated tracheostomy tube. For patients who are fully alert and sufficiently strong, written messages offer an effective, albeit tedious, method of interaction.

Gastrointestinal Ulcer Prophylaxis

Before the availability of selective histamine receptor antagonists, proton pump inhibitors of gastric acid production, early enteral nutrition and sucralfate, gastrointestinal bleeding that resulted from stress ulceration presented an annoying and occasionally a life-threatening problem. Fortunately, these complications currently are encountered much less frequently. Patients receiving effective enteral feeding seldom experience erosive stress ulcers and may not require special measures to prevent them. Whether acid inhibition encourages the overgrowth of bacteria within the stomach and thereby predisposes patients to aspiration pneumonia remains an unsettled and contested issue.

Leg-clotting Prophylaxis

Trauma, recent surgery, sepsis, dehydration, immobility, venostasis, procoagulants, clotting factor aberrations, and a variety of other predisposing factors accentuate the tendency to form lower-extremity clots. Prophylactic interventions—both mechanical and pharmacologic—to prevent venous thrombosis in the lower extremities are indicated in most patients placed on bed rest in the ICU setting. Support stockings are used for otherwise mobile patients. High-risk patients are usually given subcutaneous heparin or low-molecular-weight heparin unless there is an overriding contraindication (e.g., ongoing blood loss, heparin-induced thrombocytopenia [HIT], or coexisting risk of bleeding complication) (see Chapter 23). Compressive "pneumo boots" and "foot pumps" are more effective than support stockings and do not present the risks of anticoagulants. They may, however, be uncomfortably warm or may result in skin breakdown in poorly nourished, edematous patients

with circulatory insufficiency. Patients with known lower-extremity clot and a contraindication to unfractionated heparin and its low-molecular-weight derivatives may be offered a *removable* intra–vena caval filter if a nonheparin-based anticoagulant (e.g., lepirudin or argatroban) is not advisable.

Respiratory Care

Few hospital services are as valuable to patient care as respiratory therapy (RT). However, RT is often ordered indiscriminately at substantial discomfort, morbidity, and financial cost. Respiratory care services are now under pressure to become optimally cost effective as hospitals face the constraints imposed by prospective payment and managed care. Therapist-driven protocols for ventilator management and other RT services streamline and generally improve care delivery. Because the physician usually determines the treatment type and intensity when protocols are not used, understanding the indications and contraindications for RT procedures is vital to appropriate patient management (Table 18-5).

Procedures

Assisted Coughing

Encouraging the reluctant patient to cough productively is among the most effective services a therapist provides. Cooperative patients with cuffless or fenestrated tracheostomy tubes can be taught to cough effectively by momentarily occluding the tube orifice as a forceful effort is made against a closed glottis. Pressure can then build to a level sufficient to expel secretions through the pharynx on glottic release. Many patients can be assisted by applying a pillow to splint the painful areas of the abdomen or chest. Exhalation pressure can be increased in patients with quadriplegia by abdominal compression coordinated with the patient's spontaneous efforts. Mechanical devices are available to

TABLE 18-5 **RESPIRATORY CARE SERVICES**
Assisted coughing
Deep breathing
Incentive spirometry
CPAP/Bi-PAP/IPPB
Chest percussion and postural drainage
Airway suctioning and hygiene
Bronchodilator administration
Oxygen therapy

encourage effective coughing by pressurizing and depressurizing the air column.

Deep Breathing

Healthy individuals spontaneously take breaths that are two to three times greater than the average tidal depth multiple times per hour. Sighs to volumes approaching total lung capacity (TLC) occur less often but are by no means unusual. Animated, uninterrupted speech also requires deep breathing. Many influences, including sedatives, coma, and thoracoabdominal surgery, abolish this pattern, encouraging atelectasis and secretion retention. Although the main purpose of deep breathing (hyperinflation) is to restore prophylactic lung stretching, stimulation of a productive cough is an additional benefit for some patients. Useful deep breathing starts from FRC, ends at TLC, and sustains inflation at a high lung volume for several seconds. Maneuvers that encourage exhalation rather than inhalation actually may be counterproductive.

Appropriate positioning is perhaps the most effective means of sustaining a higher lung volume in the nonintubated patient. In moving from the supine to the upright posture, a normal lung may experience a 500- to 1000-mL increase in volume, a change equivalent to 5 to 10 cm H_2O PEEP. Changing the position of patients with unilateral disease may notably affect both gas exchange and secretion clearance. Turning is especially important for patients immobilized by trauma, sedation, or paralysis.

Incentive Spirometry, IPPB, CPAP, and Biphasic Airway Pressure

Several methods are used to encourage sustained deep breathing in nonintubated patients. An incentive spirometer is a device that gives a visual indication of whether the inhalation effort approaches the targeted volume. The frequency of deep breathing also may be tabulated. Despite their potential utility, only the highly motivated patient can cooperate fully in their use, and lung volume falls to near baseline immediately after the exercise.

Recently, traditional pressure-cycled intermittent positive pressure breathing (IPPB) has yielded to noninvasive ventilation (e.g., biphasic or bi-level positive airway pressure [Bi-PAP]) and continuous positive airway pressure (CPAP; see Chapter 7). Intermittent use of CPAP or Bi-PAP applied by a tight-fitting mask often succeeds in improving gas exchange. Its primary advantages are that little patient cooperation or personnel time is required and that the increment in lung volume is sustained, improving efficacy. Unfortunately, many patients most in need of CPAP and Bi-PAP cannot tolerate their sustained application.

Bronchodilator Administration

A nebulizer used with a mouthpiece or simple face mask can be used to deposit a small amount of drug on the airways if no other method is feasible. Metered-dose canisters do not deliver the intended dose unless the patient coordinates the puff with the breathing cycle or a spacing chamber attachment is used. The latter is essential for marginally cooperative or maladroit-hospitalized patients and may be comparable in efficacy to the compressor-driven method when a sufficient number of puffs are given through a spacing inhalation chamber. If the patient is mechanically ventilated, medication delivery is accomplished through the inspiratory limb of the circuit. This can be accomplished either with a traditional "wet" nebulizer or by insufflation of multiple puffs from a metered-dose unit. For patients with severe airflow obstruction, continuous nebulization is sometimes used rather than episodic administration of the same total dose over the same interval. The data supporting this practice, however, are unconvincing.

Chest Percussion and Postural Drainage

The objectives of chest percussion and postural drainage (chest physiotherapy [CPT]) are to dislodge the secretions from peripheral airways to help reverse atelectasis and to aid in the clearance of sputum retained in the central airways. Vibration or hand percussion of the involved region is performed for 5 to 15 min, optimally with the involved segment(s) in the position of best gravitational drainage and with the postural drainage position maintained for an additional 5 to 15 min afterward. (As already noted, some specialty beds can provide automated vibropercussion of variable frequency and amplitude, and this availability has all but supplanted the manual chest percussion.) For well-selected patients with diffuse airway disease and copious secretions (e.g., cystic fibrosis or bronchiectasis), a vibrating inflatable vest powered by a compressor may be effective as an aid in secretion clearance. Bronchodilator administration should precede CPT, and deep breathing and coughing should be encouraged before, during, and after the 10 to 15 min of optimal positioning.

These resource-intensive and intrusive methods are best reserved for patients with unusually copious secretions who can safely undergo them and empirically demonstrate unequivocal benefit.

Patients are most likely to improve after treatment are those who retain secretions because of impaired clearance mechanics (e.g., airflow obstruction, neuromuscular weakness, or postoperative pain). Although CPT may benefit patients with acute lobar atelectasis, patients with a vigorous cough experience little benefit. CPT may be helpful for patients with pneumonia who are unable to clear secretions pooled in the central airways. CPT is appropriate in the ICU setting, provided hypotension, cardiac arrhythmias or ischemia, thoracic incisions, tubes, position limitation, rib fractures, or other mechanical impediments do not contraindicate its use.

Many patients experience dyspnea during CPT, presumably because of increased venous return, positional hypoxemia, increased work of breathing, or decreased muscular efficiency in head-dependent positions. Available data warrant prophylactic oxygen supplementation and oximetric monitoring during and shortly after treatment.

Airway Suctioning

Nasotracheal suctioning serves two purposes: (a) to stimulate the coughing efforts that bring distal secretions to more proximal airways and (b) to aspirate secretions retained in the central bronchi. Traumatic and uncomfortable, the airway must be suctioned sparingly, especially in patients with heart disease; associated vagal stimulation and hypoxemia can be arrhythmogenic. Inherently traumatic, hazardous, and less effective than a productive cough, tracheal suctioning should be performed only when a sputum specimen must be obtained or when ventilation or oxygenation is compromised by secretions retained in the central airways. A blindly placed suction catheter usually reaches the lower trachea or right main bronchus and recovers sputum from the more distal airways only if cough propels the sputum forward. Soft nasal "trumpets" facilitate retropharyngeal clearance and act as guiding channels to the glottic aperture (see Chapter 6). Shaped catheters favor cannulation of the left main bronchus. For mechanically ventilated patients, closed systems allow the simultaneous provision of PEEP.

Proper technique emphasizes hygienic but not rigidly sterile precautions. "Preoxygenation" is first accomplished by several deep inflations of pure oxygen. After the trachea is entered, the catheter is advanced 4 to 5 in. and then is withdrawn as intermittent suction is applied and released for no longer than 5 s. Several "hyperinflations" of oxygen are given before resuming the usual ventilatory pattern.

TABLE 18-6 METHODS OF OXYGEN ADMINISTRATION

Nasal cannulae and catheters

Masks
  Open
  Closed
    Simple
    Partial rebreather
    Nonrebreather
    Venturi
  Tracheostomy dome

Sealed airway (endotracheal tube or tracheostomy)/ragged right

Methods of Oxygen Administration

Most patients admitted to the ICU will require supplementation of inspired oxygen. To apply this vital treatment most effectively, the clinician must be aware of the advantages, drawbacks, and limitations of each available technique (Table 18-6).

Nasal Cannulae (Prongs) and Nasal Catheters

Nasal prongs are perhaps the best choice for most applications requiring moderate oxygen supplementation. Continuous flow fills the nasopharynx and oropharynx with oxygen. These reservoirs empty into the lungs during each tidal breath, even when breathing occurs through a widely open mouth. One of the two prongs can be taped flat (or cut off and the hole sealed) without a notable change in FiO_2, allowing effective supplementation to continue despite the presence of an occlusive nasogastric tube, nasotracheal suction catheter, or bronchoscope in the other nostril. Nasal prongs allow an uninterrupted flow of oxygen while eating or expectorating and during procedures involving the oropharynx (such as suctioning and orotracheal intubation). Prongs taped in place reliably deliver oxygen to patients who tend to remove their face masks.

Rates of nasal oxygen administration vary from 0.5 to 8 L/min, depending on the clinical situation, duration of application, patency of the nasal canals, and size of the patient. At a fixed oxygen flow rate, the FiO_2 achieved depends on minute ventilation. Therefore, a "low-flow" rate of 2 L/min may correspond to a low or moderately high FiO_2, depending on whether it is diluted with a large or small quantity of ambient air. For an average patient, 0.40 approximates the upper limit of FiO_2 achievable by this method.

The jet of oxygen dries the nasal mucosa, encourages surface bleeding, and may invoke pain in the paranasal sinuses at high flow rates. Oxygen must be humidified if given faster than 4 L/min with two prongs or 2 L/min with one prong. A non–petroleum-based lubricating jelly applied to each nostril is a useful prophylactic measure against local irritation.

A nasal catheter is a single-perforated plastic tube advanced behind the soft palate. Somewhat more secure than nasal prongs, catheters deliver similar concentrations of oxygen. They are less popular than prongs because of greater irritation to nasal tissues, because location must be checked frequently, and because the catheter must be alternated between the nostrils every 8 h.

Oxygen-conserving devices that inject gas only during inspiration have been introduced successfully to outpatient practice. Whether similar units will prove cost effective in the hospital setting has not yet been determined.

Face masks

Face masks can provide higher oxygen concentrations than are available with open tents and nasal devices but are inherently uncomfortable and less stable than other methods that deliver similar inspired fractions of oxygen (Fig. 18-2). Masks must be removed when eating and expectorating, allowing the oxygen concentration to fall during these activities. Unrestrained patients often dislodge them when agitated, dyspneic, or sleeping.

There are five common types of face masks: simple, partial rebreathing, nonrebreathing, open tent, and Venturi. Simple masks have an oxygen inlet at the base and 1.5-cm-diameter holes at the sides to allow unimpeded exhalation. Because the peak inspiratory flow rate usually exceeds the set inflow rate of oxygen, room air is entrained around the mask and through the side holes. Therefore, the FiO_2 actually delivered depends not only on the oxygen flow rate but also on the patient's tidal volume and inspiratory flow pattern. In an "average" patient, the oxygen percentage delivered by a simple mask varies from approximately 35% at 6 L/min to 55% at 10 L/min. The addition of short lengths of circuit tubing to each hole of the mask creates the appearance of "tusks," which act as T-piece oxygen reservoirs. At low flow rates, CO_2 can collect in the mask, effectively adding dead space and increasing the work of breathing. Venturi masks provide a concentration of oxygen no higher than that specified. Oxygen is directed into a jet that entrains room air to flood the facial area with a gas mixture of fixed oxygen concentration. If the patient's peak inspiratory flow rate does not exceed the combined flow of the oxygen–air mixture, the FiO_2 will be the nominal value, provided the mask fits snugly. Venturi masks are available to deliver selected oxygen

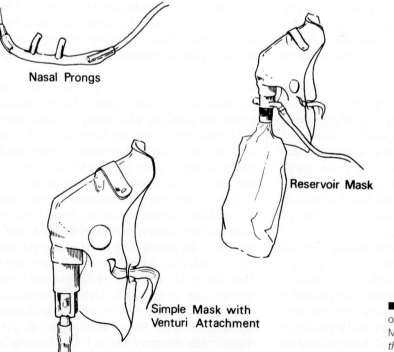

Nasal Prongs

Reservoir Mask

Simple Mask with Venturi Attachment

■ **FIGURE 18-2** Three types of oxygen delivery devices. (From Marini JJ. *Respiratory Medicine for the House Officer.* Baltimore, MD: Williams & Wilkins; 1987:95.)

percentages varying from 24% to 50% and have all but replaced simple masks in routine ICU practice. Some masks allow rapid switching of the delivered concentration by adjustment of a collar selector, which changes the entrainment ratio.

The structure of the partial rebreather (reservoir) mask is virtually identical to the simple mask, but oxygen flows continuously into a collapsible reservoir bag attached to the base. If the mask is well sealed, the patient inspires from the bag when demand exceeds the constant line supply. Peak efforts draw less air from the room and a higher FiO_2 is achieved. The reservoir must be kept well filled; if the bag is allowed to collapse, the partial rebreather converts to a simple mask. Although these masks may make more efficient use of oxygen, the highest FiO_2 usually achievable with this device is approximately 0.65.

Nonrebreather masks are identical to partial rebreather masks, except for two sets of one-way valves. One valve set is placed between the reservoir and the breathing chamber so that exhaled gas must exit through the side ports or around the mask. The second valve set seals one or both side ports during inspiration in such a fashion that nearly all inhaled gas is drawn directly from the oxygen reservoir. With a tightly fitting mask, inspired oxygen concentrations exceeding 80% can be delivered. Oxygen inflow must be high enough to prevent collapse of the reservoir bag. If collapse occurs, oxygen delivery rate would be insufficient to meet ventilation requirements, causing the patient to struggle against the one-way valves to entrain additional room air. Masks without a safety release mechanism could conceivably allow a weak or restrained patient to suffocate. Therefore, patients on nonrebreather masks should remain under direct observation.

Open-face troughs can deliver either oxygen or mist and can serve a useful purpose for patients who will not tolerate tight-fitting masks or nasal cannulae. They allow the patient to communicate and expectorate easily but impede eating. The FiO_2 varies widely with the set flow rate, tent position, and minute ventilation. Inspired oxygen fractions cannot be boosted above approximately 0.6 because of entrainment of ambient air. With all the methods of oxygen delivery discussed thus far, FiO_2 can vary depending on the patient's breathing pattern. In certain clinical situations, such as decompensated chronic obstructive pulmonary disease (COPD) with CO_2 retention, more precise control of FiO_2 may be desired.

Endotracheal Tubes

Any inspired fraction of oxygen can be delivered when a cuffed endotracheal tube prevents access to room air. If the patient is not connected to a ventilator circuit, humidified gas is administered either by a T-piece adapter or a tracheostomy tent. If no "tail" (wide-bore tubing) is attached to the T-piece adapter, the concentration of oxygen delivered will be less than that in the afferent tubing because of dilution by room air during inspiration. A length of tubing attached downstream from the endotracheal tube orifice provides an inspiratory reservoir to counteract this effect without adding dead space. The length needed depends on the source flow rate and the patient's peak flow demand.

A tracheostomy mask is a small, open-domed hood that creates a tentlike area over the tracheostomy orifice. Some room air entrainment occurs, tending to reduce both humidity and FiO_2. The latter usually can be overcome by increasing the FiO_2. The tracheostomy mask is less unwieldy than a T piece and does not produce traction on the tracheostomy tube.

Humidification

During spontaneous normal breathing, humidification is accomplished by the well-vascularized mucosa of the nasal and oral passages. At normal rates of breathing, the nose is an efficient air conditioner, filtering out particles greater than $10\,\mu$m in size and completing the warming and humidifying process before gas enters the larynx. The mouth is somewhat less effective, especially at high minute ventilation. If humidification is not completed in the upper airway, water must be drawn from the tracheobronchial mucosa, causing desiccation, impaired mucociliary clearance, and thickened sputum.

Unlike ambient air (which is, on average, 50% saturated), medical gases contain no water vapor, so the entire amount must be supplied. Unhumidified gas rapidly dries the nasal and oral mucosae, especially when oxygen is being administered. If the upper airway is bypassed, as by endotracheal intubation, drying of the sensitive lower tract occurs, with the attendant risk of infection and ventilatory impairment. The object of external humidification is to provide gas containing acceptable amounts of water vapor to the respiratory tract. Gas introduced at the tracheal level must be fully prewarmed and saturated. If the upper tract is not bypassed, humidity and temperature similar to those of ambient air suffice.

Without the upper airway bypassed, low flow rates of oxygen (e.g., up to 3L by nasal prongs) admix with sufficient ambient air to preclude the need for humidification, unless the ambient environment is exceptionally dry. External humidification is required with higher flow rates by prongs and with masks that deliver moderate to high oxygen concentrations. Humidification is required in most patients receiving mask Bi-PAP as well, especially as many breathe at elevated levels of minute ventilation, with high concentrations of dry oxyygen through an open mouth. For intubated patients, humidification can be accomplished either by disposable heat and moisture exchangers (see following) or by units that fully saturate the inspired airstream as they warm it to near body temperature (32°C to 37°C) (see Chapter 7). Heated wire circuits often are used to maintain a nearly uniform temperature within the inspiratory tubing and thereby prevent airstream cooling and excessive "rain-out" of the supersaturated water vapor.

In recent years, disposable hygroscopic filters placed in the common limb of the ventilator circuit have supplanted sophisticated mechanical humidifiers for many less-demanding applications. These "artificial noses" are designed to recover much of the exhaled moisture that otherwise would be lost to the atmosphere, releasing it to the inspirate. Such units economically serve the needs of patients without severe illness who have adequate breathing reserve and modest ventilation requirements. However, because they clog easily, impose dead space, increase airway resistance, and exhibit declining efficiency at high levels of ventilation, hygroscopic filters are less well suited to some severely ill patients and those who have a high secretion burden or marginal ventilatory reserve.

■ SUGGESTED READINGS

Azoulay E, Pochard F. Communication with family members of patients dying in the intensive care unit. *Curr Opin Crit Care.* 2003;9(6): 545–550.

Baudouin SV, Evans TW. Nutritional support in critical care. *Clin Chest Med.* 2003;24:633–645.

Crowther MA, Cook DJ. Thromboprophylaxis in medical-surgical critically ill patients. *Curr Opin Crit Care.* 2008;14:520–533.

Kane-Gill S, Weber RJ. Principles and practices of medication safety in the ICU. *Crit Care Clin.* 2006;22:273–290.

Kollef MA. Pneumonia in the hospital setting. *Clin Chest Med.* 2005; 26:1–158.

Martin SJ, Dasta JF. Pharmacotherapy. *Crit Care Clin.* 2006;22(2): 187–374.

Ozsancak A, D'Ambrosio C, Garpestad E, et al. Sleep and mechanical ventilation. *Crit Care Clin.* 2008;24:517–531.

Pavy-Le Traon A, Heer M, Narici MV, et al. From space to Earth: Advances in human physiology from 20 years of bed rest studies (1986–2006). *Eur J Appl Physiol.* 2007;101(2):143–194.

Quintiliani R. Pharmacokinetics and pharmacodynamics for critical care clinicians. *Crit Care Clin.* 2008;24:335–348.

Topp R, Ditmyer M, King K, et al. The effect of bed rest and potential of prehabilitation on patients in the intensive care unit. *AACN Clin Issues.* 2002;13(2):263–276.

Weinhouse GL. Effects on sleep of commonly used ICU medications. *Crit Care Clin.* 2008;24:477–491.

Quality Improvement and Cost Control

KEY POINTS

1 Quality, cost-efficient care requires dedicated, open-minded, and well-trained ICU leaders who are provided with accurate performance data and the power to establish unit policy.

2 Critical care is best delivered by on-site, critical-care-trained physicians, using well-reasoned, standardized care plans, in units in which all patients are treated primarily by intensivists.

3 The entire ICU staff must work as a team toward well-defined, patient-directed goals. Daily multidisciplinary rounds are an essential feature of quality care and team building.

4 Patient charges for critical care services bear little relationship to actual costs because of high inflexible "overhead," inherent excess capacity of the ICU, use of expensive and rarely needed services, and arbitrary price fixing by hospitals and payers.

5 Nursing labor costs comprise the bulk of ICU spending; therefore, profound reductions in costs will almost certainly be associated with fewer or less well trained nursing staff.

6 Wise use of diagnostic laboratory, radiology, and pharmacy services can reduce costs. Protocols or pathways for using these services must be crafted individually to meet the needs of each ICU and patient population.

resource utilization *and* costs while improving efficiency. Typically such savings are achieved by (a) reducing length of stay, (b) preventing complications and readmissions, (c) limiting ineffective or excessive care, (d) reducing staff turnover, and (e) reducing family complaints and litigation.

■ BUILDING QUALITY

ICU Leadership

Quality care begins by hiring respected, competent, and experienced critical care trained physician and nurse leaders who are devoted to providing first-rate care. While ICUs essentially always have a designated nursing leader, surprisingly less than half of ICUs have a dedicated medical director. Almost as bad as not having a director is having one who is a "figurehead" uninvolved in the daily workings of the unit. The director must be easily reached and should play a central role in smoothing the admission, discharge, and transfer processes; in establishing standard policies, procedures, and protocols; and in assembling a competent, effective, and efficient staff. Although it is a tall task, it is helpful if the leaders serve on hospital committees that have a large impact on ICU practice, such as the pharmacy, resuscitation, and laboratory services groups. To improve quality and control costs, ICU leaders **1** must be provided with accurate performance data, remain open to new solutions, and have the authority to change practice by establishing policy. Ideally, the medical and nursing directors of all ICUs in a hospital meet regularly and work together to implement the best practices.

The Available Intensivist

Despite the trend to having all medical care delivered by a primary care provider, critical care is not just internal medicine, pediatrics, or general surgery **2**

Running an ICU requires managing three inextricably linked factors: quality of care, efficiency, and cost control. While increasing resource utilization usually does not lead to improved quality, inefficiency almost always hurts quality. Along the same lines, in most cases, improving quality reduces plus a few procedures. The ICU poses a wide range of potentially lethal problems and uses sophisticated technology to which the primary care provider typically has limited exposure. Because of the rapid pace of illness and events in the ICU, decisions must be made quickly, often using incomplete information. The non-ICU practitioner typically has little experience with inevitable diagnostic uncertainty in this setting.

Ideally, physicians working in ICUs should be critical care trained and readily available, yet less than 5% of ICUs have a senior physician present around the clock, and less than one third of all ICUs have even continuous "resident" level coverage. More striking is the fact that fewer than 20% of hospitals have a critical care trained physician on-site continuously even during daylight hours. This situation is unfortunate because numerous studies indicate that establishing a "closed unit," where patients are cared for by a critical care physician, reduces the length of stay, mortality, *and* costs. There are several potential reasons for improved outcomes with intensivist staffing. ICU physicians are more likely to be on-site without the distraction of a busy clinic or operating room schedule. The advantages of dedicated intensivists are eroded when physicians are not physically present, for example, when they provide care in geographically widely separated units. Benefit may also result from the fact that intensivists have a body of experience which allows them to anticipate and preempt serious problems before they become fatal or costly. For example, to an intensivist at the bedside, subtle increases in airway pressure and modest declines in saturation and blood pressure are likely to signal an early pneumothorax that can be successfully treated long before it results in serious injury. An off-site physician is less likely to appreciate and promptly act upon these very same findings. The presence of a dedicated intensivist also increases consistency of care and compliance with recommended practices. Examples abound: when no standards exist, deep venous thrombosis prophylaxis, fluid resuscitation for septic shock, glucose control, nutrition, and normal tidal volume ventilation are inconsistent in method and application. When a different method is used for every patient, it is likely that the therapy will be overlooked for some patients and suboptimal in others. Despite fierce arguments for physician autonomy and "customization" of care, there, usually, is a best way to *begin* treating the typical patient and reducing unnecessary variation contributes to improved quality. Furthermore, knowing which treatments have succeeded or failed in a given patient leads to more efficient and less costly care. In an era in which patient turnover is rapid, and staff changes are frequent, well-crafted policies, protocols, and checklists are essential to maintain consistent care. Variability in care can be magnified in teaching hospitals where trainee duty hours are now tightly constrained, necessitating frequent handoffs. Another potential advantage of the on-site critical care physician is that he or she is less likely to summon multiple consultants. Care is inefficient, costly, and potentially dangerous when a physician, especially one off-site, "practices" using multiple consultants. In this model, each consultant responds at a pace dictated by his or her schedule, and the communication between the consultants, the primary physician, and the family is often suboptimal. The intensivist is the best person to adjudicate and coordinate the consultant recommendations and to communicate with the family and with the physicians who will provide care after ICU discharge. Without effective coordination, it is possible for numerous, often redundant, diagnostic tests to be ordered as subspecialists attempt to justify their involvement by searching for evermore obscure conditions. An even worse situation occurs when the therapeutic goals of consultants are at odds or when one consultant is oblivious to the thoughts of another.

Perhaps no one is better attuned to the potential for and limitations of the ICU than the intensivist, the person who is most qualified to identify patients who cannot benefit from ICU care because they either are not sufficiently ill or are unsalvageable. Patients at low risk of death or complications tie-up needed beds and are more likely to experience an adverse event as a result of ICU admission than they are to experience benefit. Hence, "low risk admissions" should be avoided. Likewise, moribund patients are not well served by ICU admission, where they occupy beds that could be used for salvageable patients, may suffer isolation from family and friends, are exposed to nosocomial hazards, and pay a high financial price. Even with all the difficulty in determining what "futile" care is, reasonable limits can be developed on a case-by-case basis. The intensivist is the best person to help the patient and family develop these boundaries by having honest, open, and recurring discussions of expectations. Regular, preferably daily, consultation with the patient and family is important to maintain common goals. Such consultations often require 30 to 60 min/patient each day, a time requirement that few physicians with responsibilities outside the ICU can manage. Beginning routine family discussions early in the ICU stay makes later meetings when weighty decisions must be made much less daunting. This plan of communication has other benefits: patient and family satisfaction is enhanced by communication with fewer physicians delivering a consistent message.

The role of the "hospitalist" in the care of the critically ill patient remains to be defined. Although one would expect that a hospitalist providing around-the-clock care would be superior to no in-house physician, the training, experience, and scope of responsibilities of the hospitalists are heterogeneous and results unknown. For example, many hospitalists are internists with no formal critical care training who have chosen to limit their practice to inpatient medicine. It is also not clear if a physician providing coverage for many patients throughout the hospital provides the same level of care as a physician dedicated to the ICU.

Similarly, the role of the "tele-physician" remains uncertain, and the implementation of a telemedicine program is quite expensive. In practice settings lacking any organized critical care presence, the addition of telemedicine oversight could be imagined to produce significant improvements in outcome. However, in settings where critical care physicians are already present during the day, improved outcomes have not been demonstrated. Interestingly, it is not clear if the benefits of telemedicine come from the oversight function of the service or from establishing the standardized methods of dealing with common issues.

Undoubtedly, an experienced on-site critical care trained physician is the best person to care for critically ill patients with the input of necessary consultants. Unfortunately this ideal model is currently impractical because even in large tertiary care centers, there are rarely sufficient numbers of critical care physicians to provide in-house, 24-h-a-day coverage.

Critical Care Nurses

Critical care nurses are the patient's lifeline and family's salvation. Today's nurses are being asked to do more highly technical, labor-intensive tasks with a greater level of independence than ever before. In this environment, making sure that nurses are not overburdened is as important as making sure that they are well educated and current in their training. Given the intensity of ICU activity, anytime a nurse is asked to care for more than two (sometimes more than one) critically ill patient(s), it is likely that less than ideal care is being delivered. When task saturation occurs, it is common for nurses to keep performing essential patient-centered work but care of the family and documentation suffer. Although a heretical idea to some, lapses in documentation are usually unimportant, unless a critical event or adverse occurrence is inadequately described, leading to its repetition. Nonetheless, it is best to avoid any inconsistency in care or documentation by providing adequate staffing. To this end, bedside nurses, ICU leaders, and administrators must work together to ensure that the process of care is efficient. New programs and initiatives should be thoroughly vetted before implementation to make sure that additional work or documentation requirements do not detract from care of the patient or family. Common examples of process of care changes that can impose substantial burdens are institution of intensive glucose control, early mobilization programs, and continuous renal replacement therapy. Sometimes seemingly trivial requirements can impose significant work; for example, simply documenting that mouth care and repositioning have been done every few hours can be time intensive, especially if the system for documentation is inefficient.

ICU nurses are not interchangeable cogs in a large critical care machine. They develop specialized skills to serve the most common problems they see and become familiar with the policies, procedures, and layout of the unit in which they most often work. Simply not knowing where supplies or equipment are stored in an unfamiliar unit results in inefficiency and, in some cases, even danger. In addition, the teamwork and camaraderie that develops among nurses who work consistently together provide physical and emotional support to complete the difficult tasks they are called upon to do. For these reasons, the use of temporary nurses or rotating nurses between ICUs of different disciplines should be discouraged.

Nursing excellence requires much more than a caring attitude, technical knowledge, and careful documentation; experience brings priceless insight, intuition, or judgment. Every savvy critical care physician knows the folly of not promptly responding to an experienced nurse who says "I'm not sure what's wrong, but the patient just doesn't look right." Not only can one not buy experience, but it is also very expensive to retrain or orient a nurse to a new ICU; some have estimated costs at tens of thousands of dollars. Hence, it makes sense to do everything reasonably possible to retain quality nurses. While nurses certainly care about salary, benefits, and work hours, satisfaction at work is a much more important factor for staff stability. There are numerous ways to improve nurse's job satisfaction. The first and probably the most important factor to enhance satisfaction is to treat nurses as the indispensible elements of a team providing care. Just like the copilot of an aircraft, nurses provide critical information and accomplish crucial tasks for successful mission completion. Airlines long ago recognized that an intimidating, unapproachable captain was a dangerous and divisive employee; the same is true of a dictatorial ICU physician who disregards a nurse's ideas or observations. Although it is clear that one person (the attending physician) must make the key decisions, there is no room for paternalism, patronization, or dismission. For satisfaction, but more importantly for patient safety, everyone caring for patients should understand the plans for care and must feel free to speak up when a course of action appears to be not working. Another method to promote staff satisfaction is to develop an environment where learning and teaching are valued and inquiry is welcomed. Conducting formal clinical trials or quality control projects helps establish an environment where questions are welcomed and a culture of discovery flourishes. Conducting regular educational programs designed to answer the questions that arise during patient care is also valuable and vastly superior to an arbitrary or irrelevant schedule of topics. By having all members of the health care team present at educational sessions, the knowledge of the group is boosted, the stature of the presenter is enhanced, and, as a result, care improves.

Pharmacists, Nutritionists, and Physical and Occupational Therapists

The ICU pharmacist is pivotal for optimal patient outcomes and cost control. The role of pharmacists and methods to optimize pharmacotherapy are covered in detail in Table 19-1 and Chapter 15. Similarly, the ICU dietitian or nutritionist provides valuable guidance for nutritional requirements and is essential to help navigate the dizzying variety and the number of products available. While clearly an oversimplification, merely having someone on rounds each day to prompt the team to begin enteral feeding and to discourage irrational interruptions in support is valuable. Attention to immediate life-threatening concerns often lowers the perceived importance

TABLE 19-1 PHARMACY QUALITY IMPROVMENT STRATEGIES
Elimination of unnecessary and duplicative medications
Dose adjustment optimization
Avoidance of drug interactions
Substitution of less-toxic regimens of equal efficacy
Substitution of less-costly regimens of equal efficacy
Converting parenteral medications to an oral route as soon as feasible
Reducing the frequency of administration
Avoiding drugs that require monitoring
Preferential use of enteral nutrition

of problems that can affect the long-term quality of life. Perhaps no better example exists than lack of attention to physical therapy or occupational therapy needs. Saving the life of a young severe sepsis patient is profoundly rewarding until it is realized that the patient is left with the potentially avoidable problems of foot drop and wrist contractures which prevent return to employment and recreation. In addition, it has recently been recognized that early mobilization of some critically ill patients may even accelerate ventilator weaning and ICU discharge. Therefore, it is important to involve physical and occupational therapists as soon as feasible during the ICU stay.

Processes and Practices

Team Communication

An automobile journey would prove long, expensive, and potentially dangerous if there were no clear destination, defined route, or even a map and numerous people took turns driving. In the same way, successfully negotiating the path through the ICU becomes perilous and expensive if the "driver" does not understand the route or destination. It is also impossible to plan an efficient route without knowing all the relevant trip information. For most of the day, bedside nurses "drive," and if the plan and priorities are not clear, a wandering route is likely. For the ICU patient, confusion is manifest as redundant or irrelevant diagnostic testing, inappropriate therapeutic interventions, missed critical opportunities, and miscommunication.

The most practical solution to such problems is to have a senior physician lead the ICU team to execute a carefully developed plan. To accomplish this goal, it is essential to have at least daily multidisciplinary bedside rounds where participation (not just attendance) of key team members is required. This group should include the physician, nurse, pharmacist, dietician, and respiratory therapist. Attendance of consultant physicians is desirable but often not feasible. When circumstances suggest that they would be beneficial, occupational/physical therapists, social workers, case managers, palliative care specialists, and clergy should be included. Each day, the success or failure to achieve goals set the previous day should be evaluated. New problems and organ system function should be reviewed. Diagnostic information gained since the previous day and its implications should be discussed. The need for all medications, tubes, and catheters should be questioned. Changes in therapy should be agreed upon (not just what to do, but in what order to do it, with contingency plans for unexpected events). The information to be communicated to the patient, family, and referring physicians should be discussed, and plans for transfer or discharge should be finalized. Following these steps all but guarantees that members of the team move efficiently in the same direction. This cooperative process offers the physician in charge the most current and accurate information upon which to make decisions, and as a major benefit, the staff becomes more cohesive, knowledgeable, happy, and respectful of one another.

In most hospitals, nursing and respiratory therapy personnel change shifts two or three times daily while physicians typically trade responsibilities less often. Personnel changes have advantages and disadvantages. While a new caregiver provides a rested body and mind, the oncoming provider lacks key information and recent experience with the patient. The process of "handing off" a patient may occur much more frequently though than just once or twice daily as personnel may differ during transport of patients to or from the CT scanner, operating room, recovery room, or general care floor. It is important that transfers be done in an orderly and systematic way to prevent miscommunication. The oncoming staff must be made aware of the patient's history, life support technology, medications, recent events and problems, and future plans. This review is often accomplished at two levels as bedside nurses exchange information and review medications, indwelling lines, and pertinent examination features. Separately, charge nurses review critical elements of illness and care to plan which nurses might need help or which patients are likely to require higher or lower levels of staffing. In the handoff process, respiratory therapists likewise review ventilator settings, treatment requirements, and recent problems and plans for weaning. For physicians, the process of care transfer often involves making formal beside rounds together daily in teaching institutions. In nonteaching hospitals, a face-to-face or telephone exchange of information is often conducted.

Family Visitation and Communication

There is no blanket approach to family communication, rather it is best to learn about the patient, family, and their preferences for receiving information and making decisions and then attempt to meet their goals. For example, do they want to attend rounds, have a face-to-face meeting daily, or talk by phone at a specified time? Including families in daily rounds is not an unreasonable option but can be time consuming and has met with mixed results. If done, it takes special physician talent to translate medical issues to lay-language and answer questions accurately but efficiently while avoiding the appearance of haste. Some family desires cannot be met; no physician can meet or even call multiple family members at a set time each day. For large, especially large involved families, it is a very good idea to have them appoint a spokesperson with whom communication will occur if the entire clan is not in attendance. This practice is obviously not to withhold information from others who wish to be present for such discussions but rather to prevent physicians and nurses from being inundated by sometimes dozens of calls or visits each day requesting the same information. Furthermore, even when the exact same words are spoken to different family members, their interpretations are often dissimilar. As typically happens, after several family members compare what *they* "heard," yet more calls are placed to the doctor or nurse to reconcile seemingly discordant communications. Even when the message provided is consistent, the perception of the family is often one of inconsistency leading to dissatisfaction. In addition to scheduled discussions, families should be notified in a reasonable time frame of major changes in status including procedural complications, significant clinical deterioration *or* improvement, and certainly if the patient is being transferred from the unit. Because the time shortly after admission is particularly stressful, it is important not to let families languish without information during the period of initial evaluation and stabilization. Even a brief visit from the patient's nurse, the charge nurse, a doctor, or even a receptionist can be soothing. Keeping families updated on the progress of procedures and surgery is very comforting, especially if a procedure takes longer than planned or does not start when scheduled. Providing families a phone number that can be called at all times to obtain information should be a standard practice. It is important to respect the patient's right of confidentiality; hence, it is essential to find out if there are family members or friends who should not receive information—a practice that is facilitated by issuing passwords to persons authorized to receive information.

The policies surrounding visitation are highly variable, but more than two thirds of hospitals have some restrictions regarding the number of visitors and hours for visitation. While some of these policies may simply be tradition, a sound case can be made for some periods of each day being visitor free (or limited). For example, space limitations in many ICUs practically limit the number of visitors at one time. Restricting visiting times can also be justified to guard the privacy of the patient being visited and other patients as they undergo physician examinations, bathing, and procedures. The presence of visitors can also hinder some important but routine duties such as handoffs, teaching rounds, and housekeeping functions.

Some family members have a driving need for physical proximity to the patient, wanting to stay at the hospital, sleep in the patient's room, and even help provide nursing care. Just as many family members care as deeply but cannot stand the sights, sounds, and smells of the ICU. For others, despite the strong desire to be present, their wishes cannot be fulfilled because of work or family obligations or simply geographic remoteness, and for them, a great guilt can result. Having families stay with patients for extended periods has good and bad aspects. Visitors can be very helpful in the care of patients or can be dangerous disruptions. Because of their familiarity with the patient, vigilant visitors can alert the staff to subtle findings which may presage a true physiologic crisis. A helpful visitor can also provide valuable information such as a patient's usual medications, allergies, and previous illnesses and therapeutic misadventures. In theory, visitors could even prevent problems like drug dosing errors, taking the wrong patient for a procedure, or performing an operation at the wrong site. Helpful visitors can offer the patient comfort and familiarity and sometimes can even be a care extender. When visitors participate in the care of the patient, valuable knowledge can be transferred that may be needed for a successful transition home

(e.g., tracheostomy care) and they also get a realistic sense of how hard staff work and how many things must be done to care for a critically ill patient. Having a family member present can also enhance communication with other relatives who are not at the hospital.

On the other hand, a hyper-vigilant visitor can be a profound disruption if he or she obsesses over each beep or buzzer resulting from a cough on the ventilator, the completion of a medication infusion, or artifactual heart rate alarm. Similarly, if visitors prevent patient rest, or cause frustration by repeatedly asking the same question of a patient with delirium or impaired communication, they can impair care. The continuous presence of visitors in the ICU can also present significant challenges to patient confidentiality and privacy. Special care should be taken to prevent visitors from overhearing conversations or seeing things from other patients that should remain confidential. Visitors also present important infection control issues, especially for patients in contact isolation because of transmissible infections. Visitors' failure to comply with isolation procedures can contaminate themselves and other visitors in the waiting area. Finally, the continuous presence of the same family member or visitor also presents a real problem of exhaustion and sleep deprivation for the visitor since facilities for rest and nourishment are rarely adequate.

Critical illness is frightening, and each family member has a different desire for knowledge and a different way of coping with the stress. For some, acquisition of information is comforting. These family members relish participating in rounds, search the internet, read informational pamphlets, ask probing questions about the diseases and procedures, and may even investigate the training and qualifications of the physicians and nurses. They often want to be present during procedures or sometimes even during cardiopulmonary resuscitation. Such family members appreciate the discussions of the risks and benefits of various possible courses of action. However, for just as many family members, the very same information is terrifying, incomprehensible, or overwhelming. For them, hearing the problems of even minor transient instability and the seemingly infinite number of laboratory and radiographic abnormalities is disconcerting. Similarly, team discussions of the likely next events or complications produce a sense of dread. All they want to know are answers to simple questions like are the lungs getting better? Family members also have vastly different responses to the inherent uncertainty of much of medicine, especially critical care. Learning that there may be disagreement about the best path to take or that some questions just cannot be answered can erode confidence in providers and sometimes even produces anger. "How could there not be an answer?"

Prognostication is difficult, yet it is one of the most desired features of family–physician communication. For some families, precision is important, insisting on specific "percentages," but for others, questions are much more general: Do you think she will make it? Predicting outcomes is hard because except at the extremes of illness, survivability is uncertain. Because survival data are derived from populations not individuals, it makes little sense to communicate prognosis with precision. No person has 55% mortality—survival is dichotomous. For this reason, without being evasive, many clinicians use nonnumerical phrases like "hardly ever," "very unlikely," "more likely than not," and "almost certainly" when describing outcomes. Another reasonable approach is to emphasize that outcome predictions come from populations using phrases like "Of 100 patients with a condition similar to your mother 85 will survive." The obvious problem is that there are not 100 patients sufficiently similar to anyone's mother to make such a comparison meaningful. Along similar lines, it is a folly to provide families precise timelines for improvement, deterioration, or even death; doing so is doomed to failure. For example, any precise time is *probably* going to be wrong, and when wrong confidence in the providers is undermined not just for the patient at hand but also for future health care encounters. All experienced providers have heard something along the lines of: "Five years ago the doctors told me my brother would not live through the night but lived almost a week, so why should I believe you now?" Again the best course of action is to be as honest as possible in providing estimates of outcomes and timing while avoiding false precision.

It is important to explore cultural and religious issues with the family. In some cultures, life support is viewed as interference with the natural order, for others not providing full support is akin to suicide. For some patients, a successful outcome is defined as a well-functioning mind regardless of the state of the body; for others, physical limitations define failure. Some cultures find it incomprehensible that the patient is provided all the information regarding his or her condition, especially if the diagnosis is a terminal one like metastatic cancer. In other cultures, some diagnoses (e.g., severe sepsis) imply personal or moral failure and are therefore poorly accepted. For some patients, avoidance of transfusion and transplant are paramount, whereas others have specific prohibitions against use of recombinant or animal-derived medications. The only way to cope with the wide variety of beliefs and preferences is to talk openly with patients and families exploring these issues. A spiritual leader or clergyman of the patient's faith can be very useful to help the providers understand the patient's beliefs.

Consent

Before performing nonemergent procedures or surgery, seeking informed consent from patients or ascent from families is a common but far-from-uniform practice. Which risks are discussed and who carries out the discussion are highly variable. In addition, the procedures by which consent is sought vary by location with some hospitals seeking consent for transfusion, others for HIV testing, and some only for mechanical or surgical interventions. By contrast, formal consent or ascent discussions using a detailed approved consent form are almost always required for the conduct of prospective human research. Regardless of this, in both settings, the risks, benefits, and alternatives to the proposed intervention should be discussed and questions answered. It is best to think of consent as a process rather than an event where continuing discussions occur sometimes over hours or perhaps even days until the risks and benefits are clear. There is general agreement that consent is not required to perform immediately necessary life-saving procedures (i.e., chest tube placement for tension pneumothorax). Despite the expectation to seek consent, there is a huge variability in the depth of information families seek during discussions, and little is known about what is actually understood. In fact, it is likely that no matter how well the discussion is conducted, there will be some knowledge deficit on the part of the patient or the family. In addition, there is legitimate debate about the value or need to seek reconsent for a third or fourth central line during a long ICU stay. Accordingly, some ICUs have instituted the concept of "preconsent" where families are provided information regarding all commonly performed procedures at or near the time of admission and provide a single consent or assent for care. While this practice makes sense in many ways, some practical issues can be envisioned. First, the sheer volume of information presented all at once might be overwhelming. Second, since the risks and benefits of any given procedure change somewhat over time, a discussion closer to the time of a given procedure might provide a more accurate assessment of the risk-benefit ratio. Moreover, a patient's or a family's acceptance of a given procedure may change over time as the patient improves or deteriorates, even if the risks and benefits have not changed. And finally, who knows what the legal interpretation of a single consent is.

Medical Errors and Adverse Events

Errors and complications occur in all phases of medical care and it is probably unrealistic to think that all such events can be avoided. Short of elimination, the most important things are having a program to try to continuously reduce errors and having a plan about what to do when errors are discovered. If errors are concealed only to be repeated, patients continue to be put at risk and the system does not improve. As dangerous are accusatory investigational practices which cultivate a culture of fear and cover-up. Clearly, patients and families should be made aware of errors as soon as they are known and a reasonable amount of information can be provided regarding the cause and the effect on the patient. A good example would be informing the patient and/or family about a pneumothorax following central catheter insertion and laying out the plan to deal with the complication. In most cases, the potential for this adverse event should have already been discussed with the family or patient during the consent process—another reason for taking the consent process seriously. In other cases, it is clear that an error has occurred, perhaps administration of a medication to the wrong patient, but the reason for the error is not immediately apparent; here inquiry is needed. Fortunately, in most such cases, there is no physical harm to the patient but clearly even minor errors undermine the confidence in care givers. An essential step to building quality is promoting an environment where factual error reporting is encouraged. For some employees to feel comfortable with the process, there must be a mechanism for anonymous reporting. The next step is an objective dispassionate investigation to determine why the error occurred. Sometimes the cause is clear; in other cases, even extensive investigation cannot determine how an adverse event occurred. Some errors are so preventable that they

should probably never happen: wrong patient or wrong-site surgery. Regardless, the goal should be zero errors and whenever possible *systems* should be put in place to prevent or minimize errors so that one does not have to rely on the flawless performance of people.

Rapid Response, Transport, and Airway Teams

For many patients transferring to the ICU from a general care floor, looking back on the 12 to 24 h before admission is terrifyingly instructive, often like watching an accident occur in slow motion. Frequently modest patient complaints and marginally abnormal vital signs are responded to in a leisurely series of escalating treatments, often ordered by telephone without physician examination. Occasionally, there are substantial delays between when physicians are called and when they respond. If there is an in-person examination, it is often conducted by a doctor unfamiliar with the patient. Commonly, the magnitude of physiologic abnormalities increases as does treatment intensity. Many times, nurses know the prescribed treatment is not working or the problem is more serious than the consideration it is being given. The most assertive and experienced nurses demand more aggressive action, but unseasoned or more timid nurses simply execute orders provided. The sense of the patient's downhill trajectory is often lost as personnel change shifts. Eventually, a crisis is manifest and the patient suffers a cardiac or respiratory arrest or is rushed to the ICU *in extremis*. One way to lessen this all-too-common scenario is by developing independent in-house teams to respond to deteriorating patients that can be activated by anyone who perceives an impending crisis. These responders known variously as medical emergency teams (MET) or rapid response teams (RRT) have garnered wide endorsement. The composition of the responding teams varies widely but often includes an ICU charge nurse, a respiratory therapist, and a physician. The physician's background is highly variable and he or she may be an emergency medicine doctor, an intensivist, or a hospitalist. While most activations end with transport of a critically ill patient to the ICU, surprisingly as many as 10% of MET/RRT calls end with a decision not to move the patient but rather establish comfort care with a "do not attempt resuscitation" designation. Another significant proportion of patients have a different or a more aggressive therapeutic approach initiated but are not moved to the ICU. In some cases, the call is a "false alarm."

Some studies report dramatic (approx. 50%) reductions in unexpected cardiac arrest rates following implementation of such teams, and for patients transferred to the ICU, shorter stays with better outcomes are the rule. In many cases, cost savings have been also demonstrated, probably because delaying transfer until a patient experiences a cardiopulmonary arrest on the floor is bad medicine and ends up costing *more* to treat multiple postarrest complications. Interestingly, in some studies, benefits of MET/RRT teams have not been observed. The reason for heterogeneous findings is not certain; however, an explanation may stem from the pattern of use of such services. Amazingly, in many hospitals, well-trained, easily accessible MET/RRT groups exist but they are called late or not at all. Reasons for suboptimal use are speculative but could include inadequate staff education about the program, inability of the staff to recognize early signs of critical illness, established patterns of care, or fear of retaliation from the primary care team for usurping their authority. As a result, some hospitals are now experimenting with mandatory MET/RRT calls when patients reach certain physiologic or treatment thresholds.

Admission and Discharge Practices

To ensure that adequate resources are available to treat salvageable critically ill patients while costs are minimized, admission and discharge criteria must be implemented. These criteria should curtail the number of "unnecessary" admissions and minimize the safe length of stay. Admissions only for "observation," in which no specific ICU intervention occurs, are probably most wasteful. Despite being at very low risk, patients who are admitted for observation still consume substantial resources and block access to the ICU for more seriously ill patients. This group, although fully deserving of close observation, should not occupy beds better used for those requiring intensive treatment. Furthermore, it is intuitive that such low-risk patients cannot experience an incremental benefit in outcome from ICU care because their prognosis is excellent to begin with. Stable postoperative patients and patients with diabetic ketoacidosis, hemodynamically stable gastrointestinal bleeding, and inconsequential drug ingestion comprise most of this group. The propriety of ICU admission for moribund patients or patients who choose not to receive life-support technology because of personal, family, or physician preference is also questionable. For such patients, palliative care or hospice services are much more appropriate; clearly, not all deaths must occur in an ICU. Research is now attempting to identify the patients likely to return to the ICU because they are liable to redevelop instability or are simply too much work for the staff of a regular hospital floor. Moreover, there obviously are times when patients not requiring the "technology" of the ICU are appropriately admitted for intensive nursing care or pain control.

Triage

There never seems to be enough beds in the ICU to meet peak demand, and a policy of "first-come first-served" rarely provides an equitable solution for limited resources. Because each physician views (and should view) his or her own patient to be the most deserving of an ICU bed, someone must prioritize the need and adjudicate disputes. Thus, when the ICU is at 100% occupancy, it is important to have a triage officer to judge the severity of illness of both current ICU occupants and potential admissions. The triage function is best performed by an experienced critical care physician because although nurses usually have more than sufficient medical knowledge, they rarely have the political clout necessary to enforce a contentious decision. Triage problems are minimized when only a small number of trained critical care physicians admit patients to the ICU (a "closed unit") and maximized when physicians with little ICU training or experience control the process. When triage is absent, the most powerful, belligerent, or persistent physician's patient usually gets the bed—not necessarily the patient who needs it most. In some hospitals, the emergency department physician determines the destination of each emergency admission, but obviously this practice is flawed because that physician cannot know the condition of all other patients in the ICU. Furthermore, possibly the worst-case scenario occurs when a patient at another hospital is directly admitted "sight unseen" by any physician.

Prophylaxis Practices

Roughly a dozen practices are reasonably proven to be safe, cost-effective preventative therapies (Table 19-2). Since few people can reliably remember all these interventions, it makes sense to construct a "checklist" or standardized order set to

TABLE 19-2 PROPHYLAXIS PRACTICES

Venous thromboembolism prevention
Gastrointestinal bleeding prophylaxis
Turning-repositioning decubitus ulcer prophylaxis
Pain control protocol
Targeted sedation protocol
Anemia prevention and transfusion protocol
Elevation of the head of the bed
Oral hygiene
Immunization—influenza, pneumococcal vaccine
Hand washing
Standardized enteral feeding protocol
Preprocedural "timeouts"

prevent inadvertent omissions and to ensure appropriate application.

Treatment Protocols

Many physicians oppose the concept of using treatment protocols largely based upon three objections: (a) patients are too variable to have a set plan, (b) results of clinical trials do not translate to individual patients because of the study's inclusion and exclusion criteria, and (c) use of a plan or a protocol usurps the value of the expert clinician. Often this debate is polarized with claims that treatment plans are always evil or good, but the truth certainly lies between these extreme positions. Protocols have immense value when the treatment plan is complex, especially if elements are time sensitive and there are steps which are likely to be overlooked or misapplied. Examples include initial evaluation of the trauma patient and early management of acute coronary syndrome, ischemic stroke, or septic shock. Protocols with a narrower focus are also helpful to empower nonphysicians to expedite the agreed-upon best practices (e.g., ventilator tapering, spontaneous breathing trials [SBTs], scale targeted sedation, enteral feeding management). Even though it is hard for physicians to acknowledge the fact, many are not expert in all aspects of critical illness and for them having guidance on how to start treatment can be valuable. On the other hand, application of protocols to patients who should not receive them makes no sense and in some cases might be dangerous (e.g., permissive hypercapnia in the setting of intracranial hypertension). In addition, it is incumbent upon the physician ordering protocol-based treatment to know the exceptions to the protocol and when to reassess the plan. Deviation from protocol-based treatment is essential when the patient does not fit the protocol criteria or the plan fails. Regardless, if protocols are used, they should be carefully constructed and thoughtfully implemented. Whenever possible, performance data should be gathered to evaluate the success of such efforts.

Medical Records and Order Systems

Computerized medical records, order systems, and digital radiographs have improved care in many ways. Multiple persons can now simultaneously review the same record, even from remote locations. The "chart" or "films" are never lost, and changes to the medical record have clear date and time stamping. Legibility and clarity of orders and notes are dramatically improved and there is accountability if ordered treatments are not delivered in a timely fashion. In addition, the ready availability of diagnostic test results and decision support tools, especially with regard to medication ordering, are clear advantages. However, electronic systems have produced some problems. Perhaps the worst results from nurse documentation systems which use only standardized phrases or terms selected from a menu to document actions. Such charts are difficult to read and, in some cases, almost impossible to understand when the charting involves a string of digits which refer to standardized "footnotes." Similarly, in an effort to standardize charting, the ability to enter free text descriptions is tacitly, if not overtly, discouraged. Sometimes computerized nursing documentation is difficult to access and as a result less often read than in the past when the nurses' notes were prominently displayed on a flow sheet at the bedside. In some electronic systems, the location of certain pieces of information is not intuitive, making it difficult for non-nurses to find information. As a result, understanding what really happened during a physiologic crisis becomes difficult if face-to-face communication with the nurse cannot occur. For physicians, there is a parallel problem. Instead of using handwritten-free text to describe the patient's problems and the thinking behind the decision making, the physician's electronic note has devolved into little more than a list of "standardized diagnoses" for billing purposes. Both of these developments make it difficult to know what really happened to a patient, even when just a few days have passed.

Tragically, in some cases, care of the chart has subsumed care of the patient and the computer terminal now holds a near-magnetic pull drawing nurses and doctors away from the patient. This is especially acute in hospitals where administrative electronic monitoring of documentation now occurs, putting unnecessary pressure on providers for "timely" documentation. In such settings, nurses, respiratory therapists, and other personnel are placed on a treadmill where reaching documentation landmarks becomes a surrogate for caring for the patient.

■ FACTORS INFLUENCING CRITICAL CARE COSTS

To many, "intensive care" equals "expensive care." Unarguably, ICU care is costly; a patient's life savings can be spent in hours, with costs now averaging thousands of dollars per day. First day costs often approach $7,000 to $10,000 and then plateau at $3,000 to $5,000. The 5% to 10% of US hospital beds used for critical care generate nearly one third of all hospital charges; astonishingly, critical care expenses approach 1% to 2% of the US gross national product, with the vast majority of that money spent in the last few days or weeks of a patients life. Even more impressive is that one clinical situation, the chronically ventilated patient, is responsible for half of all the money spent. With the global trend toward more care delivered in the outpatient setting, over time hospitals are devoting a higher proportion of beds to critically ill patients.

Critical care is expensive for a variety of reasons, some influenced by patients and their families, some determined by physicians, and some as a result of the sheer volume and complexity of treatments provided. An aging population brings many chronic problems to the hospital with each acute illness, making ICU admission ever more likely. It is not just the elderly patients who are incurring ICU costs, however; the increasing frequency of trauma and prevalence of immunocompromised states (e.g., HIV infection, transplants, and cancer therapy) account for the increasing demand for ICU care. Expanding numbers of middle-aged patients suffering the effects of lifelong smoking, alcohol, inactivity, and obesity represent a large segment of the coronary care unit and medical ICU populations. Against the backdrop of increasing severity of illness and costs, the population has shown little restraint in its desire for critical care. The public perceives that miracles occur regularly in the ICU, and it seems that everyone wants his or her miracle when the need arises. This perception is not without some basis in fact: most large ICUs have mortality rates well under 20% despite a gravely ill patient group. In addition, in the last 10 years, dramatic progress has occurred in treating critically ill patients with severe sepsis and acute lung injury. Undoubtedly, a more realistic view of critical care by the public would help allocate the limited resources most effectively, but there is little evidence that the public perception is changing. Likewise, physicians not trained in critical care frequently have unrealistic perceptions of the capabilities of the ICU.

Physicians and nurses also contribute to the high costs of critical care. Some of these costs are the result of well-intentioned desires to provide the best care; others are the result of inflexibility, intransigence, ignorance, and the practice of "defensive medicine." Unfortunately, some members of the medical profession share the view, along with much of the rest of the society, that more is better. More diagnostic tests, more monitoring, more medicines, and longer stays all have been (consciously or unconsciously) equated with quality care. Furthermore, historically physicians have been rewarded financially for increasing the resource use. Times are changing; we now recognize that more is often *not* better. For example, more blood sampling eventually causes anemia, requiring transfusion with its attendant risks and costs. "Unnecessary" tests will yield some false-positive results, which then prompt more, increasingly expensive, and potentially dangerous tests. More imaging studies expose patients to more radiation and radiographic contrast, often require travel from the ICU, and all such studies are expensive. Administration of radiographic contrast presents a special risk to patients with volume depletion, diabetes, or underlying renal insufficiency. More medications increase the risk of an adverse drug reaction often prompting additional diagnostic or therapeutic intervention. There are many examples, but in particular, imprudent use of antibiotics increases the risk of an antibiotic-resistant infection, not only for the treated patient, but also for the subsequent patients admitted to the ICU.

Another factor leading to increased cost of care is physicians' shortsightedness to exploit inexpensive or even free preventative measures to prevent catastrophic consequences. Examples include failure to use maximal barrier precautions when inserting vascular catheters, omission of deep venous thrombosis or gastrointestinal bleeding prophylaxis, and failure to elevate the head of the bed of mechanically ventilated patients. Finally, mortality, resource utilization, and costs may increase when physicians fail to adopt proven treatment strategies, such as lower tidal volume ventilation for acute lung injury.

By focusing only on providing critical care, the medical profession generally has ignored its costs. Many practitioners have no idea what tests and treatments cost, and even when aware of costs, some believe that no amount is too much to spend, provided there is even the smallest chance of recovery. Although charges vary widely by region and hospital, Table 19-3 presents a realistic picture of the potentially staggering bill that can accrue on the first day in the ICU. Moreover, this illustration does not include charges for emergency services, surgery, transfusion, transportation, or physicians' professional fees.

The ICU, like the emergency department, must be constantly prepared to accept a nearly unlimited number of admissions at any time and must be prepared to provide a full range of services for these admissions. Most US ICUs operate at approximately 85% capacity to satisfy this requirement for flexibility. In business terms, this excess capacity and its accompanying technology are "wasted." Moreover, a perverse competition occurs as the hospital with the greatest range of services and amenities entices doctors to hospitalize patients in that facility, promoting geographic duplication of services. Regionalization of ICU care represents one potential solution to the problem of excess capacity, but without strong financial incentives, it is not likely to occur.

Tests and interventions are performed at a greater rate in the ICU than anywhere else in the hospital. Selecting which of these events are appropriate and reducing the rate at which unneeded interventions occur reduce cost. Thus, much of the discussion that follows focuses on methods of reducing needless resource use and eliminating waste. Unfortunately, rapid deployment of new operations, devices, and drugs, many of which have not been demonstrated to be sufficiently useful to justify their cost, inflate the price of care. It should be the role of the intensivist to be certain that new technology passes muster for safety, efficacy, and cost-effectiveness in well-designed clinical studies before being embraced. To fully grasp the cost-control strategies, it is important to be able to distinguish costs from charges and to know the sources of ICU expenditures.

TABLE 19-3 ITEMIZED TYPICAL ICU FIRST-DAY CHARGES[a]

ITEM	CHARGE (IN $)
Room	2,500
"Routine" admission laboratories	750
Blood, sputum, and urine cultures	250
Electrocardiogram	100
Portable chest X-ray	150
Urinary drainage system	50
Mechanical ventilator	1,000
Noninvasive monitors (oximeter, blood pressure cuff)	100
Intravenous pump, tubing, and fluids	225
One intravenous antibiotic	150
Pulmonary artery monitoring catheter, tubing, and fluids	900
Simple sedative, analgesic regimen	200
Total	~6,500

[a]Exclusive of physician fees.

■ DIFFERENCES BETWEEN COST AND CHARGE

Charges are easy to measure and are undoubtedly important. They are what patients and insurance companies pay and, at the hospital level, are the major determinant of the success or failure of attempting to secure contractual relationships to care for groups of patients. Charges do not track **4** costs for several reasons. First, the cost of providing care for a specific diagnosis has multiple components, many of which, like utility or capital equipment costs, cannot be itemized but must be passed along to patients. Hence, arbitrary charges are set that vastly exceed true "cost." Second, a large fraction of patients do not pay all or any of their bills, and these losses are recovered from private paying or insured patients. Third, some treatment options are so costly or used so rarely that no patient could bear the true cost. Therefore, charges are distributed, or "shifted," to other patients who do not receive the service to ensure that the treatment remains available. For example, helicopter/air ambulance service is so expensive that users of the service cannot bear costs by themselves. This cost shifting is manifest as inflated charges for more commonly used therapies (e.g., "the $5 aspirin"). Moreover, certain high-volume services may be targeted as high revenue generators. Finally, over time, insurers and hospitals have come to agreement on "reasonable and customary charges" for services that do not even remotely reflect the cost.

Patient charges for a service, especially drug treatment, can differ greatly from the hospital's acquisition cost for that drug because of the introduction of labor costs. For example, penicillin is a very inexpensive antibiotic to purchase; the cost for a day's supply of the intravenous form is probably less than $10. Why, then, is the daily patient charge likely to exceed $100? How could this drug be more expensive per day than an antibiotic costing 50 times as much per dose? The answers lie in the dosing schedule and costs for preparation. The less-expensive compound may require more frequent administration and laboratory monitoring. In the end, the patient is charged much more for this "less-expensive" drug because of the labor costs associated with repeatedly measuring, mixing, transporting, infusing, and monitoring the drug. The bottom line is that in today's environment, costs do not equate with charges, and many hidden charges (e.g., drug toxicity and interactions and monitoring of levels) exist in prescribing a course of drug therapy; therefore, the cost of the entire therapeutic package must be considered.

■ **WHERE THE MONEY GOES**

Potential cost control targets come from examining the pattern of ICU spending (Fig. 19-1). Well more than half of expenditures go to labor costs (the largest portion of which is nursing salaries and benefits). About 10% to 15% of expenditures pay physicians; a similar amount is divided among other support personnel. It would be easy to say that fewer or less well trained nurses (or physicians) are the answer, but generally you get what you pay for. Lower pay usually means less experience, and quality care is not delivered with fewer nurses or physicians or a less-qualified staff. In fact, perhaps the single most influential organizational factor for outcome is the nurse-to-patient staffing ratio. The use of physician assistants or nurse practitioners to provide critical care, especially after hours care, is in its infancy. It remains to be seen if outcomes will be better or worse and if sufficient numbers of practitioners can

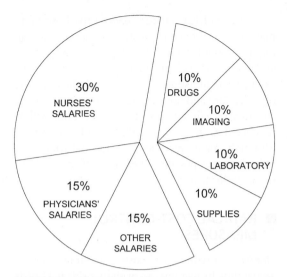

■ **FIGURE 19-1** Typical distribution of intensive care unit spending. The majority (approx. 60%) of expenses are labor costs—in large part those necessary for constant bedside nursing. Costs for drugs, imaging procedures, laboratory studies, and supplies vary by individual patients, but each category averages about 10% of total expenses. This figure highlights the difficulty associated with significant cost reduction—substantial saving usually requires reducing personnel and risks lowering the quality of care.

be trained and enticed into providing night and weekend coverage.

As highly skilled and paid nurses are replaced with less-expensive "care extenders," quality of certain essential ICU features may deteriorate. This process may have an unforeseen effect on professionalism, morale, and other difficult-to-quantify factors that reduce the efficacy and efficiency of care delivery. Furthermore, forcing highly trained healthcare professionals to undertake tasks for which they have little interest (e.g., supply restocking and cleaning), suboptimal training (e.g., phlebotomy), or inadequate experience (e.g., renal replacement therapy) is demoralizing and accelerates turnover. These problems can offset any potential cost saving, and over time, staff retraining becomes necessary. "Cross-training" ICU employees to perform a variety of tasks (e.g., food service, transport, phlebotomy, bathing, inventory, maintenance, and housekeeping) can reduce the total number of employees, but the reduction of lower paying jobs results in little net cost savings. In addition, there can be adverse consequences. For example, shoddy phlebotomy technique resulting in contaminated blood cultures ends up being very costly. For the near future, major reductions in the single largest area of expenditure, labor costs, seem unlikely.

Portions of ICU charges pass to the hospital to maintain the physical plant, durable equipment, required infrastructure (radiology, laboratory, etc.), and administrative staff and to provide a profit. The extensive administrative structure of managed care organizations and hospitals raises concerns that *real* cost savings will not happen; instead, funds will be redirected from patient care to administration. Although many methods of hospital-wide cost reductions are possible, they are well beyond the scope of this text.

RADICAL COST-CONTROL MEASURES

One way to reduce ICU costs is to limit resource availability. In many parts of the world, ICU beds constitute a tiny fraction of the total number of hospital beds compared to the United States. Limited availability means de facto "rationing" a distasteful term for many. Undoubtedly, it would be reasonable to reduce or even eliminate ICU beds at many small hospitals in favor of transfer of critically ill patients to more specialized facilities, much like what is done with trauma victims, or critically ill neonates. Doing so could eliminate the substantial capital and labor costs of having an ICU in the referring hospital and could improve the quality by getting sick patients to expert care. In addition, such a system could avoid any chance of biased referrals where tertiary care facilities are sent the critically ill uninsured patient but the insured patient remains at the original hospital. It is clear that patients who are transferred to tertiary facilities after a period of critical illness at a referring hospital have substantially worse outcomes and cost more to care for.

Sadly, many existing cost-control measures have been arbitrary and externally imposed, rather than being thoughtfully, internally fashioned. Regardless of the source of the spending restraint, quality will suffer if cost becomes the major determinant of care. The most effective way to reduce overall hospital costs is to reduce the length of stay; the same is true for the ICU. The most obvious, radical, and possibly effective cost-control strategies (rationing admission, limiting the duration of support, or prohibition of certain therapies) are not now, and may never be, palatable to the public or to conservative physicians. Ideally, improved therapeutics shorten the ICU stay, resulting in a salutary effect on cost without such policies. Dramatic therapeutic advances have occurred in sedation practice, glucose control, mechanical ventilation for acute lung injury, and treatment of severe sepsis. However, in large part, we are left with less-grand cost-control strategies: making optimal use of available beds, minimizing labor costs, improving efficiency of care delivery, and reducing equipment, imaging, laboratory, and drug expenditures.

SPECIFIC COST-CONTROL SUGGESTIONS

Imaging Costs

Imaging studies account for 10% to 20% of an ICU patient's hospital charges. In addition, use of radiographic contrast media can cause catastrophic and expensive complications (e.g., acute kidney injury, nephrogenic fibrosing dermopathy). Furthermore, many of today's imaging studies require costly transport to the radiology department, during which time any number of complications can occur. Thus, reducing the number of radiological studies can trim costs in at least three ways. Strategies to sensibly limit the procedures include (a) eliminating low-yield portable studies (e.g., abdominal flat plate, sinus studies, bone films); (b) for stable patients, reducing the frequency of "routine" studies, especially the daily portable chest X-ray (CXR); (c) when two options of comparable quality and cost exist, using the one that can be performed in the ICU to avoid transport costs and risks; (d) optimizing scheduling to minimize the number of trips to the radiology department; (e) using the absolutely necessary visits to the radiology department as an opportunity to substitute higher quality images for less-optimal portable studies; (f) when a series of procedures are done in rapid succession, wait until all are completed and then obtain just one radiograph to evaluate placement and look for compilations; (g) putting in place measures to avoid or minimize radiographic contrast exposure, especially in patients at highest risk for injury; and (h) when a diagnostic study is performed in the radiology department, it should be interpreted immediately so that additional views, complementary studies, or therapeutic intervention can be performed without a second trip. (This mandates the ready availability of a physician decision maker.)

Even though some studies are ordered by custom, they are of low yield or only partially informative. One example is the abdominal flat plate—even though it may rarely find free air, or intra-abdominal calcifications sensitivity is very low and even if positive, almost certainly a more detailed study will be required before definitive intervention. For this reason, if viscous perforation or obstructive uropathy is suspected, it probably makes most sense to proceed directly to an abdominal CT scan or ultrasound, respectively.

Overall, the portable CXR is the most common and costly radiographic procedure for most ICU patients. As discussed in Chapter 11, the CXR provides vital information but has many limitations. Unless imaging guidelines are established, most ICU patients undergo one to two portable CXRs each day at a charge of several hundred dollars. Although the CXR usually is abnormal in ICU occupants, in stable patients, abnormalities are often insignificant or equally evident through other less-costly means (i.e., physical examination). When hemodynamic status and respiratory status are stable, typically 2 to 3 days after admission, the practice of ordering "routine" daily CXRs should be reconsidered. A justification commonly given for daily films is the necessity to evaluate endotracheal tube and vascular catheter position. However, because the CXR captures much less than 1 s of each day, that argument rings hollow and obviously loses validity for patients with a much more stable nasotracheal or tracheostomy tube in place. Paradoxically, the very act of obtaining the CXR may displace tubes as the patient is repositioned (see Chapter 6). Forgoing "routine" daily CXRs for stable patients (even those on mechanical ventilators) is safe and can reduce imaging costs by up to one third. Obviously, a significant change in cardiopulmonary status should prompt consideration of a CXR, as should insertion or manipulation of tubes or catheters. Practically, even when "routine" films are not obtained, patients are likely to have at least one CXR each day because of changing physiology or insertion of monitoring devices. Additional savings can be had by performing only one CXR after a series of procedures (e.g., thoracentesis, central catheter insertion) instead of a film between each intervention. Obviously, imaging should not be delayed if a life-threatening complication from the initial procedure is suspected.

Other potential cost savings can be realized when patients must leave the ICU for an imaging study. Substantial expense and risk are associated with transporting patients from the ICU—one report suggests costs of $300 to $500 for transport alone. Regardless of the true cost, it makes sense to travel as little as necessary. When a diagnostic study can be performed in the ICU with comparable quality to that performed in the radiology department, opting for the portable examination avoids transport cost, risk, and inconvenience. One example would be the search for gallstones or biliary obstruction, in which both portable ultrasound and department-based CT scan are viable options but the portable study offers substantial cost advantage. Another example of when ICU imaging could avert a trip to the radiology department is with regard to thromboembolism diagnosis. A patient with a suspected pulmonary embolism could have the diagnosis of *thromboembolism* confirmed by portable ultrasound of the legs instead of traveling for a chest CT or VQ scan. In the vast majority of cases, the treatment will be identical for the diagnosis of deep venous thrombosis and pulmonary embolism and such a strategy avoids contrast and ionizing radiation exposure.

Arranging several studies to be performed in the radiology department during the same visit is also cost effective. For example, if plans exist to perform an elective chest CT today and head CT tomorrow, it is reasonable to consider rescheduling to accomplish both in a single trip. Finally, it makes sense to anticipate the need for therapeutic intervention when ordering diagnostic studies. For example, a patient with pancreatitis experiencing high fever and clinical deterioration is likely to have an area of the pancreatic bed that will need to be aspirated or drained. Thus, it makes great sense to plan the aspiration at the time of initial imaging and then abort the intervention if not necessary.

Supplies

Equipment savings can be substantial if stocking is well planned. Almost all disposable equipment (e.g., sutures, dressings, sterile trays, intravenous and suction catheters) has an expiration date. None of these items are inexpensive, and careful inventory will often reveal that much is discarded because it "expired" without ever being used. The justification for continued stocking of seldom-used items is often "we needed it once." Do not do away with immediately essential equipment, but reconsider all materials stocked. Limit the variety and quantity of supplies to a safe level that minimizes waste. For example, many different sizes and types of tracheal suction catheters or pulmonary artery monitoring catheters are not necessary. Likewise, it is not necessary to have immediately available every type and size of suture and needle. Take stock of what is used regularly and what is rarely used but must be available immediately. Stock only those items, and stock them in reasonable quantities.

A considerable amount of time can be saved and complications avoided if sets of commonly used supplies are packaged together. One example is placing all needed materials for central venous catheter insertion in a single container. Packaging in this way not only saves time but also encourages best insertion practice by ensuring that the appropriate disinfectant, gowns, gloves, caps, drapes, etc. are all present.

Respiratory Therapy

Some types of respiratory care equipment are ineffective or obsolete and should be eliminated. For example "room humidifiers" do not augment the water content of tracheal gas and provide little, if any, benefit for patients with sinus disease. They do, however, generate a substantial patient charge and, more importantly, present a source of nosocomial infection. By contrast, it may be cost effective to add other equipment. For example, in selected patients (i.e., few secretions and minute ventilation <10 L), use of heat-moisture exchangers in the ventilator circuit can provide significant benefits. Avoidance of the heated circuit may decrease nosocomial pneumonia rates and avoids the frequent problem of obstructed ventilator tubing by water "rainout."

Another simple, effective cost-control measure involves the process of weaning and extubation. For most patients, "weaning" is not complex or prolonged. Because many physicians do not consider withdrawal of mechanical ventilation until certain targets are met for FiO_2 and positive end-expiratory pressure (PEEP), it makes sense to empower the respiratory therapist to automatically reduce the levels of support using predetermined unit-based guidelines. Doing so can reduce the time required for a patient to "qualify" for an SBT. The vast majority of patients who are not paralyzed or in shock and who are receiving ≤10 cm H_2O of PEEP and an FiO_2 ≤0.5 can safely undergo an SBT conducted by nurses or respiratory therapists using an established protocol. When spontaneous breathing is tolerated for 30 to 120 min (under observation), the physician can be consulted for a decision to extubate. Making the process of testing automatic avoids inherent delays in physicians "ordering" an SBT, or, even worse, overlooking the possibility altogether.

Other simple measures can safely decrease costs of the weaning process. One is to avoid "T-piece" weaning. Charges for the equipment and labor for setup are often substantial; instead, use the continuous positive airway pressure (CPAP) mode of the ventilator. When necessary, CPAP can be combined with a low level of pressure support to overcome intrinsic resistance of the ventilator circuit. For most patients, no significant increase in work of ventilation is realized in breathing through well-adjusted ventilator circuitry, and the machine provides the advantage of an "apnea alarm." Another example is to immediately place patients on nasal cannula oxygen rather than some variety of mask or face tent. In common practice, the mask is discarded within minutes or hours in favor of a nasal cannula anyway. Going directly to the cannula avoids the cost of the equipment and the therapist's time. Obviously, patients extubated from high FiO_2 and those with conditions that would impede nasal oxygen flow are poor candidates for such a strategy. Finally, once the patient is extubated, remove the ventilator from the room if safe to do so. When not connected to the patient, the ventilator offers little more than expensive psychological comfort. Many hospitals charge ventilator fees in 12-h blocks, and if the ventilator is still in the room, the patient will be charged for unneeded equipment.

In many cases, additional savings can be realized through the use of metered dose inhalers (MDIs) instead of old-style updraft nebulizers. For most spontaneously breathing patients, MDIs are capable of providing equal bronchodilating effect, although on occasion, the number of puffs must be increased. Use of MDIs is particularly advantageous for the ventilated patient where the bias flow of an in-line nebulizer can create triggering problems and all but obscures the evaluation of minute ventilation. Dramatic charge reductions can also be realized by substitution of long-acting inhaled drugs for short-acting medications. For example, hundreds of dollars a day in charges can be avoided by using once daily tiotropium and patient-administered short-acting beta agonist compared to repeated nebulized doses of an ipatropium-albuterol product. Finally, the common practice of routinely providing most or all mechanically ventilated patients with inhaled bronchodilators should be reconsidered. Obviously if bronchospasm is present on exam such treatment makes sense, but the mere use of mechanical support does not justify universal application of bronchodilator therapy.

■ LABORATORY STUDIES

Legitimate concern over physiologic and chemical abnormalities is a major factor driving laboratory use. Unfortunately, the range and frequency of laboratory use are determined in large part by habit and a physician's comfort and experience in the care of critically ill patients. For example, less-experienced physicians often order chemistry and hematology profiles and blood gases daily. In addition, standing orders for blood, sputum, and urine cultures are often written to evaluate temperature elevations. Frankly, there is little justification for such rigid practices; more flexibility and thought are required. Although laboratory use should be customized for each patient, reasonable guidelines for the frequency of laboratory monitoring for the "average" patient can be proposed (Table 19-4). In addition, there are numerous studies demonstrating that development of testing guidelines decreases laboratory use without compromising outcomes.

Another unappreciated problem is that of improper sampling. In some hospitals, up to 25% of samples delivered to the clinical laboratory are improperly collected or labeled. The majority of these "preanalytical" errors are under-filled tubes, blood collected in the wrong tube, or mislabeled or inadequately labeled samples. In many cases, this results in the sample being discarded. The impact in terms of wasted time and blood is enormous, and it logically follows that at some point, wasted blood will be replaced by transfusion. The problem of mislabeled samples is particularly keen if the sample is unique or difficult to obtain (e.g., spinal or bronchoalveolar lavage fluid). Clearly, measures such as point-of-care testing and dedicated phlebotomy teams should be implemented to prevent this wasteful practice.

TABLE 19-4 ONE SCHEME FOR ICU LABORATORY MONITORING

All Patients on Admission
  12-lead electrocardiogram
  Portable chest radiograph
  Urinalysis
  Hemoglobin, platelet count, and white cell
    count with differential
  Automated chemistry profile
    Electrolytes Na^+, K^+, Cl^-, HCO_3^-
    Liver function tests: serum aspartate amino
      transferase, serum alanine amino
      transferase, bilirubin, alkaline phosphatase
    Renal function tests: creatinine, blood urea
      nitrogen
    Nutritional indices: cholesterol, total protein,
      albumin
    Glucose
  Prothrombin time

Individualized Studies
  Arterial blood gas
  Partial thromboplastin time
  Magnesium
  Calcium
  Creatinine phosphokinase
  Brain naturetic peptide
  Troponin
  Blood, urine, sputum cultures

Daily Assessment for Patients with Hemodynamic or Respiratory Instability
  Portable chest radiograph
  Electrolytes
  Creatinine, blood urea nitrogen
  Glucose
  White blood cell count, hemoglobin

After Stabilization (tests to be done once or twice weekly)
  Electrolytes and renal function tests
  Hemoglobin, platelet count
  Portable chest radiograph
  Automated profile of nutritional status and liver
    function
  Arterial blood gas

Indications for Cultures
  New-onset fever or hypothermia
  Reculture approximately every 3 days for
    persistently febrile patients
  New, unexplained hemodynamic or respiratory
    deterioration

Microbiology Laboratory

Fever evaluations are most fruitful when performed for new-onset fever in the absence of antibiotic therapy. A temperature threshold for obtaining cultures of less than 96°F or more than 101.4°F is rational in the absence of other alarming indicators. For patients with continuous or near continuous fever, it is reasonable to repeat cultures every 3 days, an interval sufficient for full evaluation of previously obtained cultures and for empiric antibiotics to work. An obvious exception includes patients with suspected endocarditis or septic thrombophlebitis in whom bacteremia may be continuous and patients who have dramatic physiologic deteriorations associated with worsening of fever. Up to one half of all "positive" blood cultures grow organisms ultimately deemed to be "contaminants." These false-positive cultures prove costly (>$10,000/episode), as they prompt additional diagnostic studies (more cultures and imaging studies) and antibiotic therapy as well as prolong hospital stay. Meticulous technique for obtaining blood cultures, perhaps even using dedicated phlebotomists, will minimize the problem of contamination.

Chemistry Laboratory

Evaluation of electrolytes is often prudent several times a day during a period of instability, especially early in the hospitalization. During this time, provision or removal of large amounts of fluid often leads to dramatic changes in sodium, chloride, and potassium concentrations. Likewise, acid–base disorders alter the bicarbonate and potassium levels in these unstable patients. However, after 2 to 3 days in the ICU, daily chemistry evaluations are needed in only the occasional patient. Granted, patients with acute renal failure, especially those receiving renal replacement therapy, and patients with severe hypokalemia or hyperkalemia warrant more frequent monitoring. Although very reasonable on admission, extensive automated blood chemistry profiles are rarely needed more than once weekly. If specific components of the profile are necessary (e.g., liver function tests, albumin), it is often more cost effective to order the individual components. When automated chemistry profiles are used to track nutritional status, evaluation at more than weekly intervals is probably wasteful; the slow pace at which nutritional parameters change rarely makes more frequent monitoring necessary.

It is also wasteful to repeatedly monitor the values without instituting reasonable corrective action. A good example is potassium replacement in patients with severe hypokalemia. When potassium values fall below 3 mEq/dL, administering 20 or 40 mEq of potassium and rechecking the value are near useless—the ion deficit is close to ten times as great.

Perhaps two of the most overused chemistry tests are those for calcium and magnesium. As largely intracellular cations, both are highly susceptible to variations in plasma protein concentration and acid–base status changes. In addition, changes in plasma values have little biological effect over broad ranges. Unless obtained to evaluate a specific clinical problem (e.g., refractory arrhythmia, neuromuscular weakness, or irritability), neither test is likely to be helpful. Because the therapeutic margin of magnesium is broad unless a patient has

significant renal insufficiency, a very reasonable strategy is to simply administer magnesium in situations where depletion is likely and potentially related to clinical findings. Magnesium depletion is common in the same clinical situations in which hypokalemia is observed (diuretic use, alcoholism, etc.) (Table 19-4).

Hematology Laboratory

Like chemistry measurements, with some notable exceptions, daily or more frequent monitoring of hemoglobin, platelet count, and white blood cell count is probably not necessary after the initial period of instability. Patients undergoing therapeutic anticoagulation are prone to declines in hematocrit and possibly the thrombocytopenic effects of heparin suggesting that monitoring should be more frequent. Thus, once-daily monitoring of each parameter is not unreasonable. Similarly, patients with active hemorrhage (especially trauma victims, patients with active gastrointestinal bleeding, and others receiving transfusion) probably should be monitored on at least a daily basis. But even for these patients, there is potential for cost reduction: white blood cell, particularly differential, counts are not necessary for patients in whom the purpose is to track hemorrhage. Furthermore, differential counts are seldom helpful after admission, except for patients with neutropenia from sepsis or chemotherapy.

Coagulation Laboratory

Tests of coagulation frequently are abused at great expense. At the time of admission, it is very reasonable to assay the prothrombin time (PT). Measuring the activated partial thromboplastin time (aPTT) is unlikely to yield useful information unless heparin therapy or hereditary coagulopathy (e.g., hemophilia, von Willebrands) is suspected. The combination of normal PT and aPTT all but excludes hereditary coagulopathy, consumptive coagulopathy, and profound nutritional deficiency. After admission, the PT is subject to change by consumption, dilution, or decreased production of vitamin-K-dependent clotting factors. Hence, disseminated intravascular coagulation (DIC), dilutional coagulopathy, progressive liver disease, or warfarin anticoagulation would be a clear indication for monitoring the PT over time. The PT will not respond quickly to warfarin therapy and is essentially useless as a measure of heparin effect. Hence, it is wasteful to obtain repeated PT determinations from patients receiving heparin alone. The aPTT is increased by dilution, consumption, heparin therapy, or congenital coagulopathy. Therefore, it is reasonable to obtain aPTT measurements for patients being treated for DIC or dilutional coagulopathy, and it is essential for patients being treated with continuous infusion unfractionated heparin therapy. There is no indication for repeated aPTT determinations in patients being treated with low-molecular-weight heparin or those receiving warfarin alone.

Another coagulation test that is vastly overused in the hospitalized patient population is the d-dimer test. Although a low result from an ultrasensitive d-dimer test is very useful in the outpatient setting to truncate the evaluation of venous thromboembolism, among inpatients, testing is usually wasteful. Essentially every condition which provokes ICU admission (e.g., surgery, trauma, severe sepsis, hepatic failure, DIC, etc.) also raises the d-dimer, negating its usefulness for exclusion of thromboembolism.

Blood Gases

Before wide application of pulse oximetry and realization that the arterial CO_2 concentration rarely needs to be normalized, arterial blood gases (ABGs) were recommended after every ventilator change and were performed routinely on a daily basis for ventilated patients. Even daily ABGs are not necessary in the absence of a change in clinical status or noteworthy ventilator parameter change. Furthermore, changes in administered oxygen concentrations do not routinely require ABGs when saturation is monitored. In several centers, the application of simple clinical guidelines as to when ABGs should be obtained has been associated with dramatic declines in use without detectable harm. Obviously, ABGs prove most useful in the initial period of hemodynamic and ventilatory instability or when metabolic acid–base disorders are suspected (see Chapter 5). There have been numerous advances in capnography technology but it still has limited value among patients with advanced lung disease in whom end-tidal CO_2 rarely equilibrates with arterial CO_2. Despite its limitations, capnography is useful for confirmation of proper endotracheal tube placement and as an early warning to airway loss during the transport of patients. When clinically indicated, ABGs are still necessary for evaluation of arterial CO_2 content in patients with severe lung disease.

■ SUMMARY

Dedicated and experienced leadership; a team approach to care; a defined procedure for admission, discharge, and transfer; restriction of attending privileges; and comprehensive guidelines for the use of drugs, imaging studies, and laboratory tests can produce substantial cost savings while simultaneously improving the quality of care. Clear, frequent communication among health care providers and with patients and families is essential for good outcomes. In the end, the best hope for cost containment and quality care lies in the education of caring physicians and nurses so they can choose wisely from the ever-expanding set of diagnostic and therapeutic alternatives.

■ SUGGESTED READINGS

Burns SM, Ervin S, Fisher C, et al. Implementation of an institutional program to improve clinical and financial outcomes of mechanically ventilated patients: One-year outcomes and lessons learned. *Crit Care Med.* 2003;31(12):2752–2763.

Curtis JC, Cook DJ, Wall RJ, et al. Intensive care unit quality improvement: A how to guide for the interdisciplinary team. *Crit Care Med.* 2006;34:211–218.

Dasta JF, McLaughlin TP, Moody SH, et al. Daily cost of an intensive care unit day: The contribution of mechanical ventilation. *Crit Care Med.* 2005;33(6):1266–1271.

Devita MA, Bellomo R, Hillman K, et al. Findings of the first consensus conference on medical emergency teams. *Crit Care Med.* 2006;34: 2463–2478.

Gajic O, Afessa B, Hanson AC, et al. Effect of 24 hour mandatory versus on-demand critical care specialist presence on quality care and family and provider satisfaction in the intensive care unit of a teaching hospital. *Crit Care Med.* 2008;36:36–44.

Halm MA. Daily goals worksheet and other checklists: Are our critical care units safer? *Am J Crit Care.* 2008;17:577–580.

Holcomb B, Wheeler AP, Ely EW. New ways to reduce unnecessary variation and improve outcomes in the intensive care unit. *Cur Open Crit Care.* 2001;7(4):304–311.

Sebat F, Johnson D, Mustafa AA, et al. A multidisciplinary community hospital program for early and rapid resuscitation of shock in nontrauma patients. *Chest.* 2005;127(5):1729–1743.

Truog RD, Campbell ML, Curtis JR, et al. Recommendation for end of life care in the intensive care unit: A consensus statement by the American academy of critical care medicine. *Crit Care Med.* 2008;36: 953–963.

Walter K, Siegler M, Hall JB. How decisions are made to admit patients to medical intensive care units (MICUs): A survey of MCIU directors at academic medical centers across the united states. *Crit Care Med.* 2008;36:414–420.

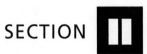
Medical and Surgical Crises

Cardiopulmonary Arrest

By necessity, most recommendations for treating cardiopulmonary arrest are not derived from high quality randomized human studies but rather come from retrospective series, animal experiments, and expert opinion. Treatment recommendations traditionally have been intricate and most applicable to patients who sustained cardiac death, especially outside the hospital. Since the focus of this book is on the hospitalized critically ill patient, some of the discussion that follows will naturally differ from widely disseminated generic recommendations. Outside the hospital, and in the coronary care unit and cardiac catheterization lab, most arrests are due to ventricular tachycardia (VT) and ventricular fibrillation (VF) in patients with ischemic heart disease. As a corollary, because VT or VF is so likely to be the cause of death in cardiovascular ICU, such patients should almost always be treated immediately with unsynchronized cardioversion. This fact underscores the utility of installing automated external defibrillators (AEDs) in public places. By contrast, a respiratory event (aspiration, excessive sedation, pulmonary embolism, airway obstruction) is much more likely to occur in a hospitalized patient. It follows that arrests on a general ward or noncardiac ICU are more likely to respond to a nonarrhythmia directed intervention, often one involving the lungs.

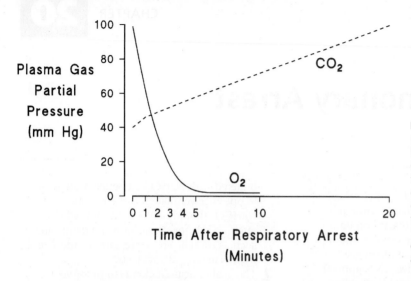

■ **FIGURE 20-1** Change in arterial partial pressure of oxygen and carbon dioxide after respiratory arrest (normal lungs). Oxygen concentrations fall precipitously to dangerously low levels within minutes. By contrast, the rise in carbon dioxide tensions is much slower, requiring 15 to 20 min to reach levels sufficient to produce life-threatening acidosis.

■ PRIMARY PULMONARY EVENTS (RESPIRATORY AND PULMOCARDIAC ARREST)

Patients found unresponsive without respirations but with an effective pulse have suffered a respiratory arrest. Failure to rapidly restore oxygenation results in hypoxemia and progressive acidosis that culminate in reduced contractility, hypotension, and eventual circulatory collapse. Although the etiology of many respiratory arrests remains uncertain even after thorough investigation, the cause often can be traced to respiratory center depression (e.g., sedation, coma, stroke, high intracranial pressure) or to failure of the respiratory muscle pump (e.g., excessive workload, impaired mechanical efficiency, small or large airway obstruction, or muscle weakness). Tachypnea usually is the first response to stress, but as overloading continues, the respiratory rhythm disorganizes, slows, and eventually ceases. Initially, mild hypoxemia enhances the peripheral chemical drive to breathe and stimulates heart rate. Profound hypoxemia, however, depresses neural function and produces bradycardia refractory to sympathetic and parasympatholytic influences. At this point, cardiovascular function usually is severely disordered, because cardiac and vascular smooth muscle function poorly under conditions of hypoxia and acidosis and cardiac output falls as heart rate declines. The observation that nearly one half of hospitalized arrest victims exhibit an initial bradycardic rhythm, underscores the role of respiratory causes of circulatory arrest.

In hospitalized, especially critically ill patients, the partial pressure of arterial oxygen (PaO_2) plummets shortly after ventilation ceases because limited

O_2 stores are rapidly consumed. Reserves are diminished by diseases which reduce baseline saturation (e.g., chronic obstructive pulmonary disease [COPD], pulmonary embolism), lower functional residual capacity (e.g., morbid obesity, pregnancy), or both (e.g., pulmonary fibrosis, congestive heart failure). Ambulatory patients who suffer sudden cardiac arrest have substantially greater O_2 reserves because they typically do not have diseases causing significant desaturation or thoracic restriction. For this reason, attention to oxygenation is much more important in the hospitalized arrest victim, whereas establishing artificial circulation and prompt rhythm correction are priorities for the "cardiac" death patient. Unlike O_2, CO_2 has a huge storage pool and an efficient buffering system. Therefore, $PaCO_2$ initially builds rather slowly, at a rate of 6 to 9 mm Hg in the first apneic minute and 3 to 6 mm Hg/min thereafter (Fig. 20-1). However, as the apneic patient develops metabolic acidosis from tissue hypoxia, H^+ combines with HCO_3^- to dramatically increase the rate of CO_2 production. The net effect of these events is that life-threatening hypoxemia occurs long before significant respiratory acidosis.

■ PRIMARY CARDIOVASCULAR EVENTS (CARDIOPULMONARY ARREST)

The heart may abruptly fail to produce an effective output because of an arrhythmia or suddenly impaired pump function resulting from diminished preload, excessive afterload, or decreased contractility. The normal heart compensates for changes in heart rate over a wide range through the Starling mechanism. Thus, cardiac output usually is maintained by compensatory chamber dilation and increased stroke volume despite significant slowing of rate. Children and adults with dilated or stiff hearts lose this reserve and are highly sensitive to bradycardia.

Decreases in left ventricular preload sufficient to cause cardiovascular collapse usually are the result of venodilation, hemorrhage, pericardial tamponade, or tension pneumothorax. In contrast to the left ventricle, which is constantly adapting to a widely changing afterload, the right ventricle is not adept at adjusting quickly to increased impedance. Therefore, abrupt increases in right ventricular afterload (e.g., air or thromboembolism) are much more likely to cause catastrophic cardiovascular collapse. Acute dysfunction of the cardiac muscle fiber can result from tissue hypoxia, severe sepsis, acidosis, electrolyte disturbance (e.g., hypokalemia), or drug intoxication (e.g., β-blockers). Regardless of the precipitating event, patients with narrowed coronary arteries are particularly susceptible to the adverse effects of a reduced perfusion pressure.

Neural tissue is disproportionately sensitive to reduced blood flow. Circulatory arrest always produces unconsciousness within seconds, and respiratory rhythm ceases rapidly thereafter. Thus, ongoing respiratory efforts indicate very recent collapse or the continuation of effective blood flow below the palpable pulse threshold. (In a person of normal body habitus, a systolic pressure of approximately 80, 70, or 60 mm Hg must be present for a pulse to be detected at radial, femoral, or carotid sites, respectively.)

■ CARDIOPULMONARY RESUSCITATION

Cardiopulmonary resuscitation (CPR) was conceived as a temporary circulatory support procedure for otherwise healthy patients suffering sudden cardiac death. In most cases, coronary ischemia or primary arrhythmia was the inciting event. Since its inception however, CPR use has been expanded to nearly all types of patients who **1** suffer an arrest. Understandably, with wider application, its success rate has declined. Currently, less than one half of all patients undergoing CPR will be resuscitated initially, and well less than one half of these initial survivors live to hospital discharge. Even more discouraging, at least one half of the discharged patients suffer neurological damage

severe enough to prohibit independent living. Despite the success portrayed on television, as few as 5% of all CPR recipients enjoy even a near-normal postarrest life. In addition, pharmacoeconomic analyses suggest that in hospital, resuscitation may be the least cost effective treatment delivered with any regularity. The likelihood of successful CPR (discharge without neurological damage) depends on the population to whom the procedure is applied and the time until circulation is restored. **2** Brief periods of promptly instituted CPR are highly successful when applied to patients with sudden cardiac death, but when CPR is used as a "last rite" for progressive multiple organ failure, the likelihood of benefit approaches zero.

Principles of Resuscitation

This chapter emphasizes general principles of resuscitation which are enduring, intentionally omitting details that are not evidence based or are likely to change. Current expert recommendations for resuscitation are much simpler than those in the past and stress the importance of effective circulatory support and prompt shock of VT and VF de-emphasizing respiratory support. While that advice makes sense for most out of hospital events, in the hospital the resuscitation team must quickly **3** consider the specific circumstances of each arrest to determine the best course of action (Table 20-1). For example, a mechanically ventilated patient found in VF will not be saved by a formulaic approach to arrhythmia treatment if it is not recognized that the cause of the event is a tension pneumothorax or airway obstruction. Because survival declines exponentially with time after arrest (Fig. 20-2), most successfully resuscitated patients

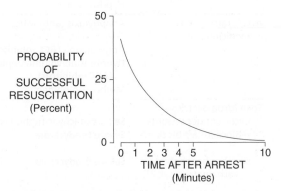

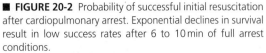

■ **FIGURE 20-2** Probability of successful initial resuscitation after cardiopulmonary arrest. Exponential declines in survival result in low success rates after 6 to 10 min of full arrest conditions.

4 **TABLE 20-1 COMMON CLINICAL SCENARIOS OF CARDIOPULMONARY ARREST**

SETTING	LIKELY ETIOLOGY	APPROPRIATE INTERVENTION
Early during mechanical ventilation	Misplaced ET tube	Confirm proper location by visualization and auscultation, CO_2 detector
	Tension pneumothorax	Physical examination, chest tube placement
	Hypovolemia	Fluid bolus
	Auto-PEEP	Reduce V_t, increase expiratory time, bronchodilator, suction airway
	Hypoxemia	Check ET placement, oximeter saturation, administer 100% O_2
During chronic mechanical ventilation	ET tube displacement	Confirm proper ET placement by auscultation and chest radiograph
	Hypoxemia	Confirm oxygenation with oximeter or ABG, increase FiO_2
	Tension pneumothorax	Physical examination, chest tube placement
	Auto-PEEP	Reduce V_t, increase expiratory time, bronchodilator
	Mucus plugging	Suction airway
Post-central line placement/attempt	Tension pneumothorax	Physical examination, chest tube placement
	Tachyarrhythmia	Withdraw intracardiac wires or catheters, try cardioversion/ antiarrhythmic
	Bradycardia/heart block	Withdraw intracardiac wires or catheters, try chronotropic drugs, temporary pacing
During dialysis or plasmapheresis	Hypovolemia	Fluid therapy
	Transfusion reaction	Stop transfusion; treat anaphylaxis
	IgA deficiency: allergic reaction	Stop transfusion, treat anaphylaxis
	Hyperkalemia	Check K^+, treat empirically if ECG suggests hyperkalemia
During transport	Displaced ET tube	Early identification using end-tidal CO_2
	Interruption of vasoactive drugs	Restart IV access
Acute head injury	Increased intracranial pressure (especially with bradycardia)	Lower intracranial pressure (ICP): hyperventilation, mannitol, 3% NaCl
	Diabetes insipidus: hypovolemia (especially with tachycardia)	Administer fluid
Pancreatitis	Hypovolemia	Fluid administration
	Hypocalcemia	Calcium supplementation
After starting a new medicine	Anaphylaxis (antibiotics)	Stop drug, administer fluid, epinephrine, corticosteroids
	Angioedema (ACE inhibitors)	
	Hypotension/volume depletion (ACE inhibitors)	Volume expansion
	Methemoglobinemia	Methylene blue
Toxin/drug overdose		
Cyclic antidepressants	Seizures/tachyarrhythmias	Sodium bicarbonate
β-Blocker/Ca^{2+} blocker	Severe bradycardia	Chronotropes, pacing, glucagon, insulin + glucose
Organophosphates carbamates	Severe bradycardia	Decontamination, atropine, pralidoxime

(continued)

TABLE 20-1 COMMON CLINICAL SCENARIOS OF CARDIOPULMONARY ARREST (*Continued*)

SETTING	LIKELY ETIOLOGY	APPROPRIATE INTERVENTION
MAO inhibitor	Hypertension	Drug removal
CO, cyanide	Hypoxia	Oxygen, sodium nitrite + sodium thiocyanate
After myocardial infarction	Tachyarrhythmia/VF	DC countershock, lidocaine
	Torsade de pointes	Cardioversion, Mg, pacing, isoproterenol, stop potential drug causes
	Tamponade, cardiac rupture	Pericardiocentesis, fluid, surgical repair
	Bradycardia, AV block	Chronotropic drugs, temporary pacing
After trauma	Exsanguination	Fluid/blood administration, consider laparotomy–thoracotomy
	Tension pneumothorax	Physical examination, chest tube placement
	Tamponade	Pericardiocentesis/thoracotomy
	Abdominal compartment syndrome	Measure bladder pressure, decompress abdomen
Burns	Airway obstruction	Intubate, reintubate
	Hypovolemia	Fluid administration
	Carbon monoxide	100% O_2
	Cyanide	Sodium nitrite–thiosulfate

ABG, arterial blood gases; ACE, angiotensin-converting enzyme; AV, atrioventricular; DC, direct current; ECG, electrocardiogram; ET, endotracheal; PEEP, positive end-expiratory pressure; VF, ventricular fibrillation.

are revived in less than 10 min. To this end, first responders should summon help and begin effective chest compression. If the cardiac rhythm can be monitored and is VT or VF, maximal energy unsynchronized direct current (DC) cardioversion should be delivered as quickly as possible. If these initial actions are unsuccessful, institution of more prolonged, "advanced" resuscitation measures may be indicated.

The primary activities of resuscitation include (i) team direction, (ii) circulatory support, (iii) cardioversion/defibrillation, (iv) airway management and ventilation, (v) establishing intravenous access and administering drugs, and (vi) performance of specialized procedures (e.g., pacemaker and chest tube placement). Managing a cardiopulmonary arrest usually requires five persons. Additional personnel may be needed for particular tasks such as documentation, chart review, and communication with the laboratory or other physicians, but limiting the number of people involved to the minimum required avoids pandemonium.

Principle 1: Define the Team Leader

A single person must command the resuscitation team because chaos often surrounds the initial response. This person should attempt to determine the cause of the arrest, confirm the appropriateness of resuscitation, and establish treatment priorities. The leader should also monitor the electrocardiogram (ECG), order medications, and direct the actions of the team members but must avoid distraction from the command role by performing other functions.

Principle 2: Establish Effective Artificial Circulation

Blood flow during closed-chest CPR likely occurs by two complementary mechanisms: cardiac compression and thoracic pumping. First, compressions generate positive intracardiac pressures, simulating cardiac muscle contraction with the heart valves establishing forward flow. In addition, as the chest is compressed, a positive intra-arterial pressure relative to extrathoracic structures is created propelling flow forward. Retrograde venous flow is prevented by jugular venous valves and functional compression of the inferior vena cava at the diaphragmatic hiatus. On relaxation of chest compression, falling intrathoracic pressure promotes blood flow into the right heart chambers and pulmonary arteries, filling these structures for the next compression.

Regardless of mechanism, ideally performed closed-chest compression provides only one third of the usual output of the beating heart. Thus, when CPR is performed for more than 10 to 15 min, hypoperfusion predictably results in tissue acidosis. If performed improperly, CPR is not only ineffective but potentially injurious. Several points of technique deserve emphasis. Maximal flow occurs when approximately 60% of the cycle is in the compression phase with a compression rate near 100 beats/min. Current recommendations have increased the ratio of compressions to breaths in an attempt to maximize flow. For the same reason, current protocols suggest continuing CPR for several minutes after shock attempts. To optimize cardiac output, it is important to adequately compress the chest. Ideally, the chest is compressed by at least one third of its anterior–posterior diameter. Short-duration "stabbing" chest compressions simulate the low stroke volume of heart failure, whereas failure to fully release compression simulates pericardial tamponade or excessive levels of positive end-expiratory pressure (PEEP). Open chest cardiac compression may provide double the cardiac output of the closed chest technique but presents obvious logistical problems and has not been demonstrated to improve survival.

During CPR, it is difficult to determine whether blood *flow* is adequate, because pulse amplitude, an index of pressure, does not directly parallel flow and each organ derives optimal flow at different pressures. For example, brain flow is determined by differences between mean aortic pressure and right atrial pressure, assuming normal intracranial pressure. Therefore, increasing right atrial pressure will decrease brain blood flow when mean arterial pressure is held constant. A similar situation exists for the heart, in which the driving pressure for myocardial blood flow is best reflected by the diastolic aortic to right atrial pressure gradient. For this reason, vasoconstrictive drugs (i.e., epinephrine, vasopressin) are recommended to raise the mean aortic pressure. Although both epinephrine and vasopressin augment initial resuscitation rates,

neither has been shown to reduce the risk of neurological damage or improve the probability of hospital discharge.

Principle 3: Establish Effective Oxygenation and Ventilation

Establishing an airway and oxygenating the patient is essential if the primary problem was respiratory in origin, or when resuscitative efforts are performed for minutes. Except in unusual circumstances, ventilation can be accomplished with mouth-to-airway or bag-mask ventilation. Because position, body habitus, and limitations of available equipment often compromise either upper airway patency or the seal between the mask and face, effective use of bag-mask ventilation often requires two people. When the airway is patent, the chest should rise smoothly with each inflation. Although cricoid pressure (Sellick maneuver) may help seal the esophagus, gastric distention and vomiting may still occur if inflation pressures are excessive. Inflation pressures generated by bag-mask ventilation are sufficient to cause barotrauma and impede venous return; to minimize these risks, breaths should be delivered slowly, avoiding excessive inflation pressures and allowing complete lung deflation between breaths.

In most cases after effective chest compression and ventilation have been achieved, an experienced person should intubate the airway (see Chapter 6). As a rule, intubation attempts should not interrupt ventilation or chest compression for longer than 30 s. Therefore, all materials, including laryngoscope, endotracheal (ET) tube, and suction equipment, should be assembled and tested before any attempt at intubation. Inability to establish effective oral or bag-mask ventilation signals airway obstruction and should prompt an immediate intubation attempt. When neither intubation nor effective bag-mask ventilation can be accomplished because of abnormalities of the upper airway or restricted cervical motion, temporizing measures should be undertaken while preparations are made to create a surgical airway. The laryngeal mask airway (LMA) is an easily inserted, highly effective temporizing device. Alternatively, insufflation of oxygen (1 to 2 L/min) via a large-bore (14 to 16 gauge) needle puncture of the cricothyroid membrane can temporarily maintain oxygenation in this critical situation. Phasic delivery of higher flows of oxygen by the transtracheal route also can promote CO_2 clearance, but CO_2 removal is of much lower priority.

In the arrest setting direct visualization of the tube entering the trachea, symmetric chest expansion and auscultation of airflow distributed equally across the chest (without epigastric sounds) are the most reliable clinical indicators of successful intubation. Colorimetric CO_2 detectors attached to the ET tube may support impressions of proper tracheal tube placement; however, because circulation is severely compromised during CPR, detectors fail to change color on as many as 25% of properly placed tubes. (Esophageal intubation can produce a temporary false-positive color change if carbonated beverages are present in the stomach.)

During CPR, ventilation should attempt to restore arterial pH to near-normal levels and provide adequate oxygenation. Unfortunately, the adequacy of ventilation and oxygenation is difficult to judge because blood gas data are rarely available in a timely fashion. Furthermore, blood gases alone are poor predictors of the outcome of CPR, making their use in decisions to terminate resuscitation of questionable value. The cornerstone of pH correction is adequate ventilation during effective circulation—not $NaHCO_3$ administration. CO_2 in mixed venous blood returned to the lung during CPR freely diffuses into the airway for elimination; however, reductions in pulmonary blood flow profoundly limit the capacity for CO_2 excretion. Consequently, hypocapnia seldom is produced at the tissue level during ongoing CPR. Conversely, excessive $NaHCO_3$ administration can produce hyperosmolality and paradoxical cellular acidosis. Because end-tidal CO_2 measurements integrate the effectiveness of both ventilation and circulation during CPR, they predict outcome. Higher end-tidal levels of CO_2 (>17 mm Hg) indicate good perfusion and portend a better prognosis, whereas persistently low end-tidal CO_2 concentrations (<7 mm Hg) portend a dismal prognosis. Failure of a colorimetric CO_2 detector to change color during CPR carries a similarly poor prognosis.

Principle 4: Establish a Route for Medication Administration

Access to the circulation must be established rapidly during CPR. Existing peripheral IV catheters are perfectly acceptable for medication administration. When medications are given through peripheral IV lines, they should be followed by at least 20 mL of fluid to facilitate drug entry into the circulation and to prevent mixing incompatible drugs. Central venous catheters (CVCs) reliably deliver drugs

directly to the heart but valuable time should not be wasted inserting a CVC if a peripheral venous catheter exists. (There is also a theoretical concern of delivering very high drug concentrations close to the heart when using a CVC.) Femoral access is less desirable than a jugular or subclavian route because of the higher risk of infection, but is certainly easier to establish without interrupting CPR.

Insertion of a stout needle into a long bone, typically the proximal tibia, can be used as an effective route for drug administration in children and adults who do not have IV access. The luxuriant venous plexus of bones provides an efficient conduit to the circulation. There are currently several commercially available stylet/needle devices to rapidly achieve intraosseous (IO) access. Typically, the needle is inserted through soft tissue until bone is encountered; then the cortex is penetrated using a screwing motion until resistance fades. After removal of the stylet, IO positioning is confirmed by aspiration of a small amount of marrow and the ability to gravity-infuse fluid at a slow rate. Major advantages of the IO route include a high success rate for cannulation (>80%); quick insertion (<2 min); avoidance of CVC related complications; and rapid delivery of drug to the circulation. (In experimental models, IO administered drugs reach the heart in <30 s.) Risks are uncommon and predictable and include nerve or vessel injury, extravasation of drug into soft tissue with necrosis, compartment syndrome, and osteomyelitis.

The intratracheal (IT) route may be used to produce therapeutic drug levels rapidly during resuscitation. Drugs given via the IT route must be delivered in at least 10 to 20 mL of liquid to permit most of the dose to access the alveolar compartment, where absorption occurs. The doses of all drugs given by the IT route should be increased at least 2 to 2.5 times that used with IV dosing. The IT route has been demonstrated to be effective for administration of naloxone, atropine, vasopressin, epinephrine, and lidocaine, easily remembered as by mnemonic "NAVEL." Some commonly used drugs (e.g., norepinephrine and $CaCl_2$, $NaHCO_3$) should not be given via the IT route. The former two can cause lung necrosis and the third depletes surfactant.

Intracardiac injections, although dramatic, are rarely necessary, often unsuccessful, and offer no greater likelihood of successful resuscitation. In addition, intracardiac injections are fraught with complications including coronary laceration, pneumothorax, and tamponade. Intramural drug injection may expose the myocardium to massive concentrations of vasoactive drugs, provoking intractable ventricular arrhythmias. Therefore, intracardiac injection should be used only as a last resort.

Principle 5: Create an Effective Cardiac Rhythm

5 Conceptually, cardiac electrical activity during the arrest can be thought of in two broad categories useful to guide treatment. The first is the combination of ventricular tachycardia and ventricular fibrillation (VT/VF), the second group consists of asystole and pulseless electrical activity (PEA).

Ventricular Tachycardia and Ventricular Fibrillation

VT and VF are the most common rhythms discovered in victims of sudden cardiac death. Although VF may the original arrhythmia, in many cases the first rhythm is VT which deteriorates to VF as the heart becomes progressively hypoxic. VT has been subclassified as being either monomorphic or polymorphic because there are potential treatment implications for the polymorphic variety. Monomorphic VT is typically a monotonous appearing wide complex tachycardia with a constant axis. *Torsades de pointes* is the name given to a unique appearing form of polymorphic VT that is frequently associated with baseline prolongation of the QT interval. *Torsades* is characterized by a constantly changing QRS axis that produces an apparent "twisting of points" about the isoelectric axis (Fig. 20-3). A host of reversible precipitating factors has been identified, including hypokalemia, hypomagnesemia, tricyclic antidepressants, haloperidol, droperidol, and type Ia antiarrhythmics (e.g., quinidine, procainamide, and disopyramide), astemizole, and quinolone antibiotics (see Chapter 4). Both VT and VF can be converted with electrical shock but VF tends to be more resistant. With VF the success of cardioversion is influenced by the amplitude of the electrical signal, which correlates inversely with the duration of fibrillation. Success rates vary from less than 5% when low amplitude

VF is the initial rhythm to greater than 30% when coarse VF is the rhythm. When fine VF is shocked, the most likely resulting rhythm is asystole, whereas coarse VF is more likely to be converted to a supraventricular tachycardia or sinus rhythm.

Regardless of whether the initial rhythm is VF, or monomorphic or polymorphic VT, maximal intensity (360 J) unsynchronized monophasic shock should be administered as quickly as possible. (Equivalent lower intensity biphasic [200 J] shocks are equally effective.) For patients receiving open chest defibrillation, epicardial shocks of 10 to 20 J are almost always sufficient. The goal of cardioversion is to abolish all chaotic ventricular activities, allowing an intrinsic pacemaker to emerge. Many defibrillators allow a "quick look" at the rhythm before shock is attempted, but careful inspection of the rhythm is not mandatory before proceeding. Blind cardioversion will not harm adult patients with agonal bradyarrhythmias or asystole and may benefit those with pulseless tachycardias or VF. Previous guidelines recommended a series of rapidly delivered, incremental intensity shocks based upon the observations that thoracic impedance declines with multiple defibrillations, and that using a lower electrical dose might reduce defibrillation-induced cardiac damage. While both these rationale have merit, it is clearly more important to restore a circulating rhythm rapidly than to be concerned about potential cardiac electrical injury.

Defibrillators are typically calibrated to discharge through impedance less than that of the adult chest. Therefore, the *delivered* energy usually is lower than is indicated by the nominal machine settings. This is particularly true in situations which increase the distance between the paddles and the heart, like morbid obesity and conditions producing high lung volumes (e.g., COPD, large tidal volumes, high PEEP). (Defibrillation at end-expiration may be more successful because thoracic impedance is at its lowest.) Improper paddle positioning dissipates energy and reduces the rate of successful defibrillation. Using the anterolateral technique, paddles are placed at the cardiac apex and just below the clavicle to the right of the sternum. Because bone and

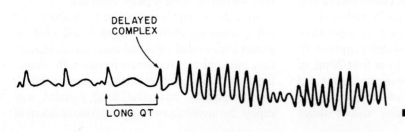

DELAYED COMPLEX

LONG QT

■ **FIGURE 20-3** Torsades de pointes.

cartilage are poor conductors of electricity, paddles should not be located over the sternum. For some patients, anterior–posterior paddle placement delivers energy to the heart more efficiently than the anterior–lateral approach. Defibrillator paddles should not be placed over ECG monitor leads, implanted pacemakers or defibrillators, or transcutaneous drug patches, because of the possibility of electrical arcing, equipment damage, and explosion. Contact between the defibrillator and chest wall should be maximized by use of conducting gels or pads. (Note: Ultrasound gel is a poor electrical conductor.) Standard-sized (8 to 13 cm diameter) paddles on adult defibrillators provide optimal impedance matching between machine and chest wall. If for some reason the defibrillator fails to discharge, ensure that the defibrillator is energized, connected, and correctly set. One rather common reason for failure to discharge during VF is for the machine to be set in the synchronized cardioversion mode. (In the absence of a QRS complex, there is no signal to trigger a "synchronized" discharge of the defibrillator.)

The availability of AEDs has changed defibrillation from an often delayed procedure performed by an expert in a hospital or ambulance to one rapidly accomplished by a novice in a public location. Fortunately, considerable standardization of AEDs has occurred so that regardless of manufacturer, the same basic steps are always used: power on the defibrillator, attach the pads and connect the cables using the illustrations provided, wait for the device to analyze the rhythm and charge, make sure all people are clear of the patient, and then discharge the device if instructed.

VT/VF resistant to cardioversion, after several minutes of effective CPR, predicts a poor outcome. If initial attempts at cardioversion prove unsuccessful, "coarsening" the rhythm and increasing the vascular tone with epinephrine (1 mg IV, q 3 to 5 min) or vasopressin (40 U IV, given once) may be helpful. All the while, effective ventilation and chest compression should be maintained. After epinephrine or vasopressin is given, maximum current defibrillation should be repeated. When the preceding measures fail, a trial of the antiarrhythmics amiodarone (300 mg IV) or lidocaine (1.5 mg/kg IV) may help convert the rhythm when followed by additional shocks.

The small subgroup of patients with *torsades* deserves special mention. While *torsades* is not particularly resistant to cardioversion, the arrhythmia frequently recurs within a short time. For long-term control, discontinuation of potentially precipitating drugs and correction of electrolyte abnormalities are indicated. For patients with a previously normal QT interval, coronary ischemia is a common precipitant amenable to standard treatment. β-Blockers, lidocaine, and amiodarone have all been tried for refractory *torsades* without any one emerging as a clearly superior agent. For patients known to have prolonged baseline QT interval, $MgSO_4$ may be helpful but the most effective measures shorten the QT interval, usually by increasing the heart rate (i.e., pacing or catecholamine infusion). In patients with QT prolongation, phenytoin and lidocaine may be tried if the rhythm is refractory to magnesium and cardioacceleration. Type 1a antiarrhythmics are unlikely to be helpful because of their QT prolonging properties.

Regardless of the initial rhythm, if cardioversion consistently produces any bradycardic rhythm that degenerates to VF, increasing the heart rate with epinephrine, atropine, pacing, or isoproterenol can prove useful. (In this situation, overdose of digitalis, calcium channel blocker, or β-blocker should also be considered.) If countershock returns any tachycardia that repeatedly degenerates to VF or VT, consider the possibility of excessive catecholamine stimulation and decrease infusion rates of adrenergic agents, and/or try administering antiarrhythmics (amiodarone 300 mg IV bolus, procainamide 50 mg/min IV infusion-maximum 1 gm, lidocaine 1 to 1.5 mg/kg IV bolus). Hypokalemia, a frequent contributor to refractory or recurrent VT/VF, is found in approximately one third of all patients suffering sudden death. In this desperate setting, up to 40 mEq of potassium may be administered rapidly. In some cases the low toxicity compound $MgSO_4$ may help stabilize refractory VT/VF, but Mg^{3+} levels are unlikely to be measured during the time span of a resuscitative effort and do not correlate well with effects. Thus, it is reasonable to administer $MgSO_4$ empirically (1 to 2 g over several minutes).

Asystole, Bradycardias, and Pulseless Electrical Activity

For purposes of resuscitation asystole, profound bradycardias and PEA are also conveniently grouped together. Almost any rhythm is better than asystole, the complete absence of electrical activity (a flat ECG) but some rhythms (i.e., pulseless slow bradycardia or ventricular escape beats) are not much better. Therefore, a key aim in asystole is to stimulate some electrical activity and then modify that activity to a rhythm with a pulse. Because asystole usually indicates extended interruption of perfusion and carries a grave prognosis, its discovery should prompt serious consideration of whether resuscitative efforts should even begin. It makes little sense to countershock the truly asystolic patient because there is no "rhythm" to modify. However, low-amplitude VF may go unrecognized unless sought using several leads. VF is best distinguished from "asystole" in leads II and III. Epinephrine (1 mg IV, q 3 to 5 min) and atropine (1 mg IV, q 3 to 5 min to a total dose of 2 to 4 mg) sometimes can restore a vestige of electrical activity, even if disorganized. Manipulation of electrolyte balance (Ca^{2+}, K^+) also may be useful in specific cases. If it is to be tried at all, transcutaneous pacing should be instituted early; however, results in clinical trials have been disappointing (see also Chapter 4). $NaHCO_3$ may be useful if severe acidosis, hyperkalemia, or tricyclic antidepressant overdose is the cause of asystole.

Bradyarrhythmias that cause sudden death have a similarly bad prognosis. In adults, these are often a manifestation of prolonged hypoxemic, hypercarbic respiratory failure, and incipient asystole (Table 20-2). Indeed, the most important measure to undertake first in treating a patient with hypotensive bradycardia is ensuring adequate oxygenation—not administering sympathomimetic or vagolytic drugs. In general, the slower the rate and the wider the ventricular complex, the less effective the myocardial contraction. The vagolytic action of atropine is most useful in narrow complex bradycardias resulting from sinoatrial node failure or type II or III AV block. Doses of at least 1 mg of atropine should be administered and can be repeated every 3 to 5 min to a total dose of 2 to 4 mg. Epinephrine, dopamine, or isoproterenol may be helpful for their chronotropic actions. (Isoproterenol is now rarely

TABLE 20-3 CAUSES OF PEA

Hypovolemia	Tamponade
Hypoxemia	Tension pneumothorax
Hydrogen ions (severe acidosis)	Thrombosis (pulmonary, coronary)
Hyperkalemia or hypokalemia	Trauma
Hypoglycemia	Toxic overdose
Hypothermia	Digitalis
Hyperinflation (auto-PEEP)	β-blockers
	Calcium channel blockers
	Tricyclic antidepressants

used and may be counterproductive because of its peripheral vasodilating properties.) If available, transthoracic pacing can sometimes provide temporary support until definitive transvenous pacing is established or pharmacologic cardioacceleration is achieved. Although useful for symptomatic bradycardia, transvenous ventricular pacing is difficult to achieve in the arrest situation and rarely proves effective in asystole due to massive myocardial infarction.

PEA, also known as electromechanical dissociation (EMD), is characterized by the inability to detect a pulse despite coordinated ECG complexes. The more common causes of PEA can be easily recalled as a list of conditions beginning with the letters "H" and "T" (Table 20-3). When cardiac in origin, PEA carries a dismal prognosis because it usually is a sign of massive pump infarction or free wall rupture. A hint to the origin of the problem (cardiac vs. noncardiac) can be gleaned from the width of the QRS complex. Narrow complexes are more likely the result of a noncardiac cause. Mechanical obstruction to the normal transit of blood through the heart may also cause PEA. Hence, atrial myxoma, mitral stenosis, and critical aortic stenosis may be potential causes. Other reversible conditions that can produce this syndrome include (a) hypovolemia, particularly from acute blood loss (vasopressors are ineffective with uncorrected hypovolemia); (b) pericardial tamponade suspected on the basis of venous engorgement, a history of chest trauma, or preexisting pericardial disease; (c) tension pneumothorax; (d) dynamic hyperinflation (auto-PEEP) from overly zealous ventilation; and (e) massive pulmonary embolism by clot or air. Thromboembolism may fragment and migrate during CPR, opening the central pulmonary artery and reestablishing effective output. Air embolism can be treated by positioning the patient (left side down,

TABLE 20-2 COMMON CAUSES OF BRADYCARDIA

Hypoxemia
Intense vagal stimulation
β blockade
Sinus/atrioventricular node ischemia
Calcium channel blocker use
Drug overdosage (cholinergic effects)
Digitalis
Increased intracranial pressure
Sedative agents (e.g., propofol, dexmetatomidine)

Trendelenburg position) and/or transvenously aspirating air from the right heart; and (f) hyperkalemia; and/or (g) metabolic acidosis.

Pharmacologic therapy of PEA includes epinephrine or atropine in doses identical to those used for asystole. Controversy exists regarding the use of calcium in PEA. Calcium benefits very few patients (perhaps those with marked hypocalcemia, calcium channel blocker overdose, or extreme hyperkalemia), hence its use should probably be restricted to these conditions. On the rare occasion where a toxic overdose results in PEA, a specific therapy may be available (see Chapter 33). Even though it is becoming much less common, digitalis toxicity deserves mention. A wide variety of arrhythmias are associated with digitalis toxicity including high-grade AV block with bradycardia, junctional tachycardias, and even asystole. Treatment begins by stopping the drug and correcting hyperkalemia and hypomagnesemia. Ca^{2+} exacerbates the toxicity and should be avoided. Cardioversion (with the lowest effective wattage) is indicated if ventricular arrhythmias cause symptomatic hypotension. Phenytoin, lidocaine, and procainamide are useful pharmacologic treatments. Pacing usually is required for high-grade AV block. Use of specific digitalis neutralizing Fab antibody fragment preparations is safe and highly effective if renal function is maintained. Because the Fab–digitalis complex is cleared by the kidney, dialysis may be needed for the patient with renal insufficiency (see Chapter 33).

Principle 6 : Evacuate the Patient to the ICU as Soon as Practical

When cardiac arrests occur outside an ICU, facilities, equipment, and personnel for resuscitation are less than ideal. On general wards and in public hospital areas, it is often difficult to access the patient, especially if they have fallen alongside a bed or are in a bathroom or elevator. Simply getting emergency equipment to the patient's side can be a challenge in cramped quarters. There is often a crush of unhelpful bystanders and distraught family members, and even the patient's primary caregiver's effectiveness is hindered by their shock from an unexpected arrest. Electrical access and suction capabilities are commonly limited and specialized equipment, especially for airway management, is not always available. However, the most important limitation of performing resuscitation outside the ICU, especially in a remote part of the hospital (e.g., CT scanner), is that many of the personnel available

to help have little experience performing real resuscitations. Preparation of emergency medications and assistance with procedures that are second nature for ICU personnel are often unfamiliar to non-ICU workers. For all these reasons it makes sense to do the absolute minimum required to establish ventilation and a rhythm that produces a pulse then transport the patient to the ICU.

Principle 7: Reevaluate and Stabilize

After arriving in the ICU with a perfusing rhythm with adequate oxygenation and ventilation, it is important to rethink the cause of the arrest, take measures to prevent recurrence, and to search for resuscitation complications. Tubes and catheters inserted during resuscitative efforts are often suboptimally positioned or are inserted with less than ideal sterile technique. Any intravenous catheter not known to be inserted in a sterile manner should be removed altogether or if still needed, replaced at a new site using sterile technique. It may be wise to administer a single dose of antibiotic that provides coverage of commonly encountered skin flora (e.g., cefazolin) even though this practice is not evidence based. The position of the ET tube and any chest tubes or CVCs should be confirmed radiographically. (It is extremely common that emergently inserted ET tubes are placed in the right mainstem bronchus.) The chest radiograph should also be examined for evidence of resuscitation or procedural injury (e.g., hemothorax or pneumothorax, or rib or sternal fractures) and for clues to the cause of the original arrest (mediastinal widening of aortic injury, enlarged cardiac silhouette of pericardial tamponade, pneumothorax) (Table 20-4). The chest film should also be evaluated for the presence of aspiration or pneumonia that may have precipitated the arrest or resulted from it. If there is a suspicion of hemothorax, or hemoperitoneum, or retroperitoneal hematoma, chest and abdominal CT scans are usually diagnostic. However, careful consideration should be given to transporting a recently

TABLE 20-4 COMPLICATIONS OF CPR

Rib fractures and cartilage separation
Bone marrow emboli
Fractured sternum
Mediastinal bleeding
Liver laceration
Subcutaneous emphysema
Mediastinal emphysema

resuscitated patient outside the ICU; potential benefits should clearly outweigh the risks. If there is suspicion that the arrest may have been precipitated by a neurological event (e.g., ischemic stroke, hemorrhage, tumor, new seizure), it is prudent to obtain an uncontrasted head CT scan with the same caveats regarding transport safety. For patients who are not fully awake after resuscitation, the prospect of ongoing seizures should be considered. If a seizure is a reasonable possibility, an electroencephalogram (EEG) should be obtained.

Acid–base and electrolyte abnormalities are so common after resuscitation that it makes sense to evaluate a full panel of electrolytes, especially Na^+, K^+, Ca^{2+}, Mg^{3+}, and an arterial blood gas. Because hypoglycemia can cause cardiac arrest, and postarrest hypoglycemia and hyperglycemia can cause or exacerbate brain injury, a rapid determination of blood glucose should be done. If there is suspicion that the cause of the arrest could be medication or toxin ingestion, obtaining a urine or plasma drug screen and specific drug levels (e.g., digitalis, lidocaine, phenytoin) may be enlightening. Although troponin and creatine phosphokinase (CPK) levels are frequently modestly elevated, they rarely provide a definitive diagnosis. Noteworthy elevation of the myocardial band (MB) isoenzyme of CPK is unusual unless repeated high-energy electrical shocks have been delivered. Similarly, after resuscitation, impressive elevation of hepatic (and/or skeletal muscle) enzymes is common but of uncertain significance because frank ischemic necrosis and failure of the liver rarely occur. It is smart to obtain a hemoglobin concentration to search for occult bleeding (e.g., hemothorax from rib fractures or arterial injury, hemoperitoneum from liver or spleen laceration) and to detect anemia that might warrant transfusion. Although elevations of white blood cell counts are routine, they are nonspecific and by themselves should not drive antibiotic use. A decision to obtain lung, blood, or urine cultures should be made on an individual basis, depending on the level of suspicion the role of infection played in the arrest.

It is prudent to obtain a 12-lead ECG in all patients after stabilization to evaluate the rhythm and to look for signs of infarction, ischemia, and electrolyte abnormalities, conduction defects, and preexcitation pathways. The use of antiarrhythmic therapy should be based on an evaluation of the current rhythm and the likelihood of stability (see Chapter 4). If there are questions about valvular competence or stenosis, pericardial fluid, or wall motion abnormalities, an echocardiogram is quite helpful.

While the primary focus must be on caring for the patient, it is important not to ignore the family and visitors, especially if they witnessed the arrest. Dispatching *any* free staff member to update the family during the resuscitation and postresuscitation processes can be very effective in allaying fears. In recent years, there has been substantial discussion regarding having family present during resuscitative efforts. This is a very complicated topic but it is clear that this practice should neither have a blanket prohibition nor absolute requirement. Some family members derive comfort from knowing, by seeing, that all that could be done for their loved one was tried. Other family members suffer terror and revulsion seeing the resuscitation process which is often unavoidably undignified, unlike stylized popular media portrayals. For these families, a lasting memory of a violent death endures. Unfortunately, there is no reliable way to know how any particular person will react.

Principle 8: Preserve the Brain

Because neurological outcomes in survivors of cardiopulmonary arrest are poor, there has long been interest in methods for cerebral preservation. It should go without saying that maintaining a reasonable perfusion pressure and hemoglobin concentration and saturation are prerequisites for optimal cognitive recovery. The association of worse outcomes associated with hypoglycemia and hyperglycemia suggests that maintaining a normal range of glucose might be helpful. There is no evidence to support the routine administration of anticonvulsants, anticoagulants, barbiturates, benzodiazepines, or neuromuscular blockers. One recent small randomized study suggests a potential benefit of a single dose of 40 mg of methylprednisilone given with vasopressin during CPR. Although unproven for this purpose, prevention of excessive cerebral metabolic demand (e.g., suppression of high fever, seizures) makes sense and is safe and inexpensive. The use of mild therapeutic hypothermia has shown benefit for patients with out-of-hospital VF arrest, but benefits for out-of-hospital non-VF arrests and for in-hospital arrests are less certain. Potential candidates should not have active bleeding or significant bradycardia since hypothermia may exacerbate both, as well as cause other complications (see Chapter 28). Therapeutic hypothermia is difficult if not impossible to achieve

7

without deep sedation and usually therapeutic paralysis to prevent the inevitable, heat-generating shivering. Invasive and external methods of cooling have been tried but as yet there is no clear superior method. Regardless of method, the target is a core temperature of 32°C to 34°C for 12 to 24 h, with subsequent slow rewarming over 6 to 8 h.

Controversies in Resuscitation

Over the years, the role of $NaHCO_3$ and calcium in the resuscitation of arrest victims has waxed and waned; currently, both are assigned low importance. Despite effective artificial support measures, progressive acidosis is an inevitable result of prolonged CPR and when severe, acidosis can render the heart more resistant to defibrillation. However, ventilation is key to pH correction. $NaHCO_3$ is rarely necessary if circulation and ventilation are restored promptly and no data support its early routine use to improve defibrillation or survival rates. The inability to restore pH toward normal is an ominous sign indicating some combination of failed ventilation and circulatory support. When used, $NaHCO_3$ should be administered cautiously, guided by blood gas analysis. An arterial pH ≥7.00 usually is adequate for cardiovascular function. However, the appropriate pH target for the arrested circulation is highly controversial. Previously recommended doses of $NaHCO_3$ (1 mg/kg) may produce unwanted side effects, including (a) arrhythmogenic alkalemia, (b) increased CO_2 generation, (c) hyperosmolarity, (d) hypokalemia, (e) paradoxical central nervous system (CNS) and myocardial intracellular acidosis, and (f) a leftward shift in the oxyhemoglobin dissociation curve, limiting delivery of O_2 to tissues. Even though the use of $NaHCO_3$ has fallen out of favor, in specific settings (e.g., hyperkalemia with metabolic acidosis, tricyclic antidepressant or aspirin overdose) it can be a useful medication.

Because excessive calcium exacerbates digitalis toxicity and the arrhythmic tendency of unstable ischemic myocardium, enhances coronary artery spasm, impairs cardiac relaxation, and may hasten cellular death, its use should be restricted to patients with known hypocalcemia, calcium channel blocker or β-blocker overdose, and hyperkalemia. The use of calcium during resuscitation is associated with decreased survival to discharge but a cause and effect relationship has not been established. Calcium forms insoluble precipitates when administered with $NaHCO_3$, hence the two compounds should not be commingled.

■ DECIDING WHEN TO FORGO OR TERMINATE RESUSCITATION

Certain clinical disorders are associated with a virtually hopeless short-term prognosis (e.g., refractory widely metastatic carcinoma, end-stage acquired immunodeficiency syndrome, unremitting multiple organ failure following bone marrow transplantation or severe sepsis), and in such cases, it often is appropriate to forgo CPR. Each case must be considered individually with regard for the physical condition of the patient, the wishes of the patient and family (if known), and the likelihood that resuscitation can succeed if performed. CPR is rarely successful if cardiac arrest ensues as the final manifestation of days or weeks of multiple organ failure. The importance of clarifying the "code status" of all seriously ill patients early in the course of an illness should be emphasized. Ideally, the code status is included as part of the admission order set to the ICU. When doubt exists regarding the propriety of resuscitative efforts, CPR should be initiated. A single set of guidelines regarding termination of effort cannot be applied to all clinical situations.

During CPR, neurologic signs and arterial blood gases are unreliable predictors of outcome and should not be used in the decision to terminate resuscitative efforts. With that caveat, however, resuscitation seldom is successful when more than 20 min is required to establish coordinated ventricular activity. With rare exceptions, failure to respond to 30 min of advanced life support predictably results in death. Best results occur when sudden electrical events are corrected promptly with cardioversion. Prolonged resuscitation with a good neurologic outcome may occur, however, when hypothermia or profound pharmacologic CNS depression (e.g., barbiturates) precipitates the arrest.

■ PROGNOSTICATION

CPR usually fails to deliver the desired result-discharge alive with normal neurological function. Resuscitation initially returns circulatory function in approximately 50% of patients to whom it is applied. (The fraction is lower in out-of-hospital cardiac arrests and higher in hospitalized patients, especially those who suffer arrest in the ICU.) Of these early "successes," approximately 50% survive for 24 h, but at best, only 25% to 50% of these 24-h survivors live to hospital discharge, and many of these survivors suffer neurologic impairment. Downtime greater than 4 min before beginning resuscitation, initial rhythms of asystole or bradycardia, prolonged resuscitative efforts, a low exhaled CO_2 concentration, and the need for vasopressor support after resuscitation all are poor prognostic factors. Likewise, poor prearrest health (e.g., severe sepsis, CHF, renal failure), out-of-hospital arrest, and presence of hyperglycemia all are associated with a poor outcome. Interestingly, age alone is not a good predictor of the success of CPR. Long-term survival of severe anoxia is unusual in patients with underlying vital organ dysfunction, perhaps because further organ injury occurs or because neural centers critical to autonomic control and maintenance of protective reflexes are damaged by the event.

The probability of awakening after cardiac arrest is greatest in the first day after resuscitation and declines exponentially thereafter to a very low stable level. (Almost all awakening occurs within 96 h of resuscitation. Nonetheless, recovery from comatose or vegetative states has been reported after 100 days.) Surprisingly, the clinical examination is a better predictor of neurologic recovery than any imaging or laboratory test. Absence of pupillary and corneal responses at or beyond 72 h, especially if there is no motor response or extensor posturing, is a powerful predictor of a poor outcome. Similarly, myoclonus or status epilepticus within the first day following arrest predicts poor outcomes. Although an EEG is very useful for care if it

demonstrates seizures, EEG activity is suppressed by sedatives, anticonvulsants, and hypothermia making the test an insensitive predictor of outcome. CT or MRI of the head may show perfusion-related abnormalities or cerebral edema following CPR but is also poor predictor of outcome. Likewise, somatosensory evoked potentials and serum neuron-specific enolase have been investigated as prognostic features but do not appear to be reliable enough for widespread clinical use.

■ SUGGESTED READINGS

2005 American Heart Association guidelines for cardiopulmonary resuscitation and emergency cardiovascular care. *Circulation.* 2005;112:IV-58–IV-66.

Aung K, Htay T. Vasopressin for cardiac arrest: A systematic review and meta-analysis. *Arch Intern Med.* 2005;165(1):17–24.

Desai AS, Fang JC, Maisel WH, et al. Implantable defibrillators for the prevention of mortality in patients with non-ischemic cardiomyopathy: A meta-analysis of randomized controlled trials. *JAMA.* 2004; 292(23):2874–2879.

Diamond LM. Cardiopulmonary resuscitation and acute cardiovascular life support-A protocol review of the updated guidelines. *Crit Care Clin.* 2007;23:873–880.

Holzer M, Bernard SA, Hachimi-Idrissi S, et al. Hypothermia for neuroprotection after cardiac arrest: Systematic review and individual patient data meta-analysis. *Crit Care Med.* 2005;33(2):414–418.

Mentzelopoulos SD, Zakynthinos SG, Tzoufi M, et al., Vasopressin, epinephrine, and corticosteroids for in hospital cardiac arrest. *Arch Intern Med.* 2009;1669:15–24.

Saxon LA. Sudden cardiac death: Epidemiology and temporal trends. *Rev Cardiovasc Med.* 2005;6(Suppl. 2):S12–S20.

Wijdicks EFM, Hijdra A, Young GB, et al. Practice parameter: Prediction of outcome in comatose survivors after cardiopulmonary resuscitation (an evidence-based review): Report of the Quality Standards Subcommittee of the American Academy of Neurology. *Neurology.* 2006;67(2):203–210.

Acute Coronary Syndromes

Coauthored by Shailesh Shetty

■ **NON-ST ELEVATION ACUTE CORONARY SYNDROMES: UNSTABLE ANGINA AND NON-ST ELEVATION MYOCARDIAL INFARCTION**

Definitions and Pathophysiology of Acute Coronary Syndrome

Unstable angina (UA) and non-ST segment elevation myocardial infarction (NSTEMI) are now grouped under the heading of non-ST elevation acute coronary syndromes (NSTE-ACSs). Because they share a common underlying pathophysiology, the management of these two conditions is quite similar. UA is synonymous with the terms *preinfarction angina, crescendo angina, intermediate coronary syndrome,* and *acute coronary insufficiency.* NSTEMI implies non–Q wave myocardial injury. The main difference between UA and NSTEMI is that biomarkers of myocardial necrosis are elevated in the latter (e.g., creatine kinase–myocardial band [CK–MB], troponin-I, troponin-T).

Myocardial ischemia results from an imbalance **1** between oxygen supply and demand. Anginal chest pain is the clinical expression of this imbalance. Because the left ventricle (LV) comprises most of the cardiac muscle mass and faces the greater afterload, it is at higher risk for ischemia. Myocardial oxygen delivery may be limited by (a) coronary atherosclerosis, (b) plaque rupture with thrombosis, (c) coronary artery spasm, (d) anemia, (e) hypoxemia, (f) limited diastolic filling time (tachycardia), and (g) hypotension.

Four major factors increase cardiac oxygen demand: (a) tachycardia and/or increased systemic metabolic demands for cardiac output; (b) heightened LV afterload causing increased transmural wall tension (e.g., hypertension, LV cavity dilatation, aortic stenosis); (c) increased LV mass (hypertrophy); and (d) increased contractility. Despite the predisposition of the LV to ischemia, conditions that cause hypertrophy, dilatation, or increased afterloading of the right ventricle (RV) also can put its muscle mass at risk. For example, pulmonary embolism may precipitate RV ischemia—a phenomenon that is most common in patients with underlying right coronary artery (RCA) narrowing or *cor pulmonale*.

An unstable coronary atherosclerotic plaque is the key to the pathophysiology of ACS. Histologic studies of coronary vessels have shown that atherosclerotic plaques are intimomedial in location. In general, there two types of coronary plaques: (a) stable plaque with small lipid core and thick fibrous cap and (b) unstable plaque with large lipid core and thin cap. The former generally causes stable angina pectoris if it causes significant obstruction of the vessel (>50% to 70% of the vessel lumen diameter). The bulky, soft, lipid-laden plaques are more prone to rupture and ACS. Many of these plaques do not cause significant obstruction of the lumen of coronary vessels before the onset of the ACS. Hence, the patient may not have experienced any cardiac symptoms prior to the onset of ACS.

Acute instability and rupture of one or more coronary plaques with superimposed thrombosis play a central role in the pathophysiology of ACS. This clot, composed of platelets and thrombin, not only produces a fixed vessel occlusion but also promotes reversible vasoconstriction. The resulting sudden coronary artery occlusion, which may be total or subtotal, causes acute myocardial ischemia or infarction. UA represents a high-risk transition period during which most patients undergo accelerated myocardial ischemia. If unchecked, this transition culminates in acute myocardial infarction (AMI) or sudden cardiac death (SCD) in up to 15% of patients within just a few weeks. Coronary angiography in many of these patients demonstrates complex coronary plaque lesions with varying degrees of superimposed thrombosis. Intravascular ultrasonic examination of coronary vessels (IVUS) is another useful tool that has helped shed considerable light, not only on the pathophysiology but also on the management of coronary artery disease, particularly in the setting of ACS.

The role of platelets in the pathophysiology of ACS has undergone considerable review in the past decade or so. Platelet activation and aggregation play a significant role in the formation and propagation of a platelet-rich or "white" clot over a ruptured atherosclerotic plaque in patients with UA and NSTEMI. This is contrast to the fibrin-rich or "red" clot seen in the coronaries of patients with STEMI. The current recommendations on the use of antithrombin and antiplatelet therapies in NSTEMI and that of fibrinolytic therapy in patients with STEMI derive not only from the pathophysiology of these conditions, but also from the results of various clinical trials performed within the last decade.

Diagnosis

History and Physical Examination

The term *UA* denotes new pain or a departure from a previous anginal pattern. UA occurs at rest or with less provocation than stable angina. Pain lasting longer than 15 min also suggests UA. Angina occurring in the early post-MI period or within weeks of an interventional coronary procedure also is best termed "unstable." Commonly, the pain is described as a "tightness," "heaviness," or "squeezing" in the substernal region. UA may awaken patients from sleep or present as pain at a new site such as the jaw or arm. Autonomic manifestations (nausea, vomiting, or sweating) also favor "instability." Blood pressure frequently rises before the onset of pain, even in resting patients. Rising blood pressure boosts afterload, increasing wall tension and myocardial O_2 consumption. Less commonly, the onset of congestive heart failure (CHF) may be the only manifestation of UA.

Data Profile

Electrocardiographic Changes

During episodes of ischemic chest pain, electrocardiogram (ECG) features may include (a) ST-segment elevation or depression, (b) T wave flattening or inversion, (c) premature ventricular contractions (PVCs), or (d) conduction disturbances, including bundle branch block (Fig. 21-1). Reversible ST depression or T wave inversion is seen in most patients if continuous ECG monitoring is used, a finding that may not emerge during a single 12-lead ECG. Even with intensive monitoring, ECG findings are absent in up to 15% of symptomatic patients with UA. Therefore, a normal ECG does not exclude a diagnosis of UA or MI. Conversely, up to 70% of all ECG-documented episodes of ischemia are clinically silent.

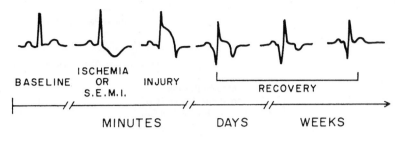

■ **FIGURE 21-1** Electrocardiographic evolution of AMI. SEMI, subendocardial (nontransmural) MI.

Cardiac Enzyme Markers

Elevated total CK (including the CK–MB fraction) and cardiac troponins (I and T) are markers of myocardial necrosis and indicate an MI, even in the absence of convincing ST segment–T wave changes. Troponins (I/T) are more sensitive and specific in making the diagnosis of an AMI than CK-MB. Troponin elevation in NSTE-ACS correlates with adverse prognosis. These are also patients who are likely to benefit from Glycoprotein 2b/3a (Gp2b/3a) receptor antagonist therapy and from early coronary angiography and revascularization. Highly sensitive C-reactive protein (hs-CRP) levels are also increased in patients with ACS. ACS patients with the highest levels of hs-CRP and troponins have the worst prognosis.

Prognostic Factors

Patients with UA have a lower short-term mortality rate (2% to 3% at 30 days) compared to those with acute NSTEMI (5% to 7% at 30 days). The in-hospital or short-term mortality of patients with STEMI is higher compared with those with NSTEMI (6% to 9% vs. 5% to 7% at 30 days). However, the long-term mortality in NSTEMI (10% to 12%) is similar to or greater than that associated with STEMI (9% to 11%), likely due to their greater incidence of multivessel coronary artery disease.

Thrombolysis in Myocardial Infarction Risk Score

Several risk variables have been identified in patients with NSTE-ACS. A value of 1 has been assigned to each risk variable, and the total score has been shown to bear a linear relationship with risk of adverse events (death, MI, recurrent ischemia, and need for urgent revascularization) in the short term. The variables are (a) age greater than or equal to 65 years, (b) prior coronary stenosis greater than or equal to 50%, (c) presence of greater than or equal to three coronary risk factors, (d) ST segment deviation on admission ECG, (e) elevated cardiac biomarkers, (f) greater than or equal to two anginal episodes in last 24 h, and (g) prior use of aspirin (marker for vascular disease). The adverse event rate is 4% to 5% for thrombolysis in myocardial infarction (TIMI) risk score of 0 to 1 but approaches 40% for those with score of 6 to 7. Elevated levels of hs-CRP indicate a worse prognosis in each TIMI scoring category.

Management of NSTE-ACS

Patients with NSTE-ACS should be monitored closely and should receive aggressive antithrombotic, antiplatelet, and antianginal treatments (Fig. 21-2). Most patients with UA can be stabilized with appropriate medical therapy. Coronary angiography and revascularization procedures have become increasingly popular in these patients over the course of the last decade. Although emergent coronary angiography and revascularization procedures are uncommon in NSTE-ACS patients, most need to undergo coronary angiography and possible revascularization within a few days of admission to the hospital. Coronary revascularization procedures include either percutaneous coronary interventions (PCIs) (PTCA and stenting) or coronary artery bypass graft (CABG) surgery. Only patients with contraindications for invasive cardiac procedures are treated with noninvasive medical management. The *two basic principles* in the treatment of UA are to reduce myocardial O_2 demand and improve O_2 supply.

Reducing Myocardial Oxygen Consumption

The principal measures to decrease myocardial oxygen consumption are to limit heart rate and afterload. These goals are immediately accomplished by curtailing physical activity with bedrest. Exercise stress-tests are contraindicated in unstable patients since frank infarction may ensue. Arrhythmias like atrial fibrillation (AF) and ST should be controlled, both to reduce O_2 consumption and to optimize diastolic filling time, thereby maximizing

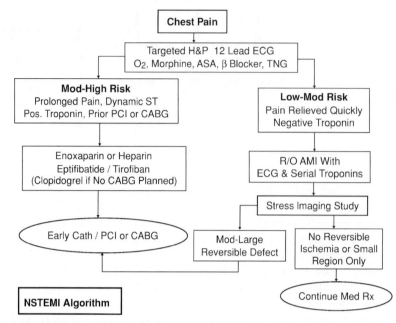

FIGURE 21-2 Non-ST Elevation MI (NSTEMI) management algorithm. ECG, electrocardiogram.

2 the sufficiency of coronary perfusion. Controlling hypertension and CHF decreases myocardial wall tension and therefore facilitates perfusion (see Chapter 22). Situations that increase heart rate (anxiety, use of short-acting nifedipine) or both heart rate and total body oxygen consumption (e.g., thyrotoxicosis, alcohol withdrawal, stimulant drug intoxication, anxiety, agitation, infections, etc.) should be promptly recognized and corrected. β-Blockers effectively reduce myocardial oxygen consumption by decreasing heart rate and cardiac contractility and improve O_2 supply by lengthening diastolic filling time. β-Blocking drugs are particularly useful in reducing oxygen consumption in the tachycardic and hypertensive patient with UA but are contraindicated in acute heart failure, coronary artery spasm, or severe bronchospasm. β-Blocking agents also reduce risk of tachyarrhythmias in patients with ACS.

Increasing Myocardial Oxygen Supply

3 The most important treatment under this category are the strategies for myocardial revascularization which include percutaneous coronary angioplasty, coronary stenting, and coronary artery bypass surgery (will be dealt with later in this chapter). Myocardial oxygen supply can also be increased simply by boosting hemoglobin saturation or elevating hemoglobin concentration to levels higher than 9 or 10 gm/dL, in severely anemic patients.

Pharmacotherapy is also necessary to optimize myocardial perfusion. Nitroglycerin (NTG) is used commonly and may be administered sublingually, orally, transcutaneously, or intravenously. (For unstable patients, the intravenous route is most reliable.) In addition to dilating coronary vessels, NTG also decreases wall tension of the LV by reducing preload and, to a lesser extent, afterload. Acting through these mechanisms, NTG also reduces the risks of life-threatening arrhythmias in acute ischemia. Nitrates are effective both for classical and variant angina because of their direct coronary vasodilating properties. NTG is titrated to relieve chest pain or to reduce blood pressure by 10% to 20%. Usually, intravenous doses of 0.7 to 2.0 μg/kg/min suffice. Intravenous NTG usually is begun at 5 to 15 μg/min and titrated upward as necessary in increments of 5 μg/min every 5 min up to a maximum dose of 200 μg/min. Headache is a common side effect but usually responds to simple oral analgesics. When the dose is excessive or the patient is dehydrated, hypotension and reflex tachycardia result from NTG-induced vasodilatation. These adverse effects usually can be offset by volume expansion or α-agonist therapy. Because ethanol is used as a vehicle for NTG infusions, violent adverse reactions may occur in patients taking Antabuse. Obviously, use of high doses of NTG for prolonged periods may also produce alcohol intoxication. Within 48 to 72 h of initiating NTG therapy, tolerance is often observed, necessitating higher infusion rates. Rare problems induced by NTG therapy include increased intraocular and intracranial (IC) pressures and methemoglobinemia.

Coronary spasm, a major contributor to myocardial ischemia in certain settings, may be ameliorated by nitrates or calcium channel blockers. Blockers of slow calcium channels (e.g., nifedipine, nicardipine, and amlodipine) can be rapidly effective in reversing coronary spasm. In UA, these drugs should be viewed as adjuncts to nitrate, β-blocker, and antithrombotic therapy. Because calcium antagonists have vasodilating, negative inotropic, and positive chronotropic actions, they may have detrimental effects for certain patients. If coronary vasodilating effects predominate, the myocardial oxygen supply–demand balances benefits. Conversely, if systemic vasodilatation, hypotension, and reflex tachycardia predominate, myocardial oxygen demand can outstrip supply and ischemia can worsen. Therefore, caution must be exercised to avoid hypotension or excessive tachycardia when using calcium channel antagonists.

Antiplatelet Therapy

Aspirin

Most patients with NSTE-ACS have an ulcerated atherosclerotic plaque covered by a subocclusive accumulation of platelets, thrombin, and red blood cells. Typically, these patients have platelet-rich or "white-clot." Therefore, aggressive antiplatelet therapies are effective in stabilizing patients with ACS. Aspirin (162 to 325 mg daily) should be initiated immediately for all patients with ACS unless compelling contraindications exist. Cyclooxygenase-1 (COX-1) mediated platelet aggregation is inhibited within 15 min of aspirin administration, if nonenteric coated tablets are chewed and swallowed. Aspirin reduces synthesis of both thromboxane A2 (TXA-2) as well as prostacyclin. TXA-2 is a powerful promoter of platelet aggregation. Prostacyclin, on the other hand, promotes vasodilatation and inhibits platelet aggregation. Low-dose aspirin preferentially inhibits TXA-2 synthesis, and endothelial prostacyclin synthesis is inhibited by high-dose aspirin. In the VA cooperative study, Canadian multicenter trial, and RISC trial, aspirin was found to reduce the risk of death and AMI by approximately 50% in patients with NSTE-ACS. In a large metaanalysis by the antithrombotic trialist collaboration, aspirin reduced risk of death, MI, and stroke by about 46%. The benefits of aspirin may persist for years with continued therapy. The risk of recurrent

events is reduced by at least 25%. The risk of coronary reocclusion after PCIs is reduced by about 50% with use of aspirin. At the low doses (75 to 150 mg) needed for platelet inhibition, few hemorrhagic or gastrointestinal side effects occur. At a lower dose, aspirin caused 2.5% major bleeds with 1% requiring transfusions. Aspirin resistance is seen in about 5% to 10% of patients, and these individuals are at increased risk for cardiovascular events. Although inhibition of platelet aggregation may complicate subsequent coronary artery surgery, aspirin-related clotting defects are reversible with platelet transfusions. Dipyridamole does not enhance the protective effect of aspirin in coronary ischemia, but clopidogrel and ticlopidine do complement the anti-ischemic effect of aspirin.

Clopidogrel, Ticlopidine, and Prasugrel

These agents belong to the thienopyridine class. They prevent platelet aggregation by noncompetitive inhibition of the adenosine diphosphate (ADP) binding to the type 2 purinergic ($P2Y_{12}$) receptor, thereby inhibiting the activation of the glycoprotein IIb/IIIa receptor complex. Ticlopidine requires 3 to 6 days of therapy for full antiplatelet effect and carries a small risk of neutropenia (2.5%) and thrombotic thrombocytopenic purpura–hemolytic uremia syndrome (TTP–HUS). TTP–HUS occurs in the frequency of 1 in 1,500 to 5,000 patients taking ticlopidine. Both these life-threatening complications are most often seen within the first 12 weeks of therapy and necessitate immediate withdrawal of the drug. Patients with TTP–HUS may also need plasmapheresis. The usual dosage of ticlopidine is 250 mg by mouth twice daily. Ticlopidine has largely been replaced by clopidogrel.

Clopidogrel has been extensively studied in patients with ACS and in those who have received intracoronary stents. The life-threatening adverse effects seen with ticlopidine are far fewer with clopidogrel. In the CURE trial, clopidogrel use in ACS was found to significantly reduce risk of cardiovascular events (mostly reinfarctions) compared to aspirin alone. The usefulness of clopidogrel as an agent in reducing risk of cardiovascular events in patients who have received coronary stents has been clearly demonstrated in the PCI-CURE and CREDO trials. Clopidogrel is usually given as an oral bolus of 300 mg, followed thereafter at a dose of 75 mg once daily. Unlike ticlopidine, the antiplatelet effects of clopidogrel are seen within hours. Significant blood levels may be achieved sooner with a larger bolus dose of the medication (600 or 1,200 mg).

Along with ASA (81 mg once daily), it is given for a month after the implantation of bare-metal coronary stents and for at least 3 to 6 months after insertion of drug-eluting coronary stents. In patients with ACS, clopidogrel can be continued for 9 to 12 months. In some individuals at high risk for future cardiovascular events, clopidogrel with low-dose aspirin may be continued indefinitely if there are no contraindications and if cost is not an issue. There is a slight but significant increase in risk of bleeding with combination of clopidogrel and aspirin (3% to 5% risk of major bleeding), particularly in the elderly population.

Prasugrel is the latest of the oral thienopyridine ADP-receptor antagonists available for patients with ACS. It is more a powerful antiplatelet agent as compared with clopidogrel and ticlopidine.

The TRITON-TIMI 38 study compared combination of prasugrel and aspirin to combination of clopidogrel and aspirin in patients with ACS undergoing percutaneous coronary intervention. There were over 13,000 patients in this study and the primary endpoint was reduction of cardiovascular death, nonfatal stroke and nonfatal MI over 6 to 15 month follow-up period. The major safety endpoint was major bleeding. There was a significant reduction in primary endpoints with prasugrel compared with clopidogrel, including significant reduction in death, target vessel revascularization, and stent thrombosis. The risk of stent thrombosis was reduced by nearly over 50%. However, there was a significant increase in risk of serious bleeding (both fatal and nonfatal), which somewhat offsets the benefits. This drug is not yet being routinely used, but is likely to become more popular as the role for drug-eluting stents (DES) begins to expand. This may be a good agent for those who present with stent thrombosis with clopidogrel, in those with multiple DES, and in those at less risk of bleeding (like younger patient population).

Glycoprotein 2b/3a Receptor Inhibitors

Gp2b/3a receptor inhibitor agents are the most powerful intravenous form of antiplatelet agents available. The Gp2b/3a receptor binds to fibrinogen, which actually forms the molecular link that bridges adjacent platelets in the process of platelet aggregation. By binding to the Gp2b/3a receptors, these agents inhibit binding of fibrinogen to this receptor and thus inhibit platelet aggregation. The use of these agents in the management of ACS has increased significantly in the last 8 to 10 years, with a positive impact on patient outcomes. There are two broad classes of these agents: (a) large-molecule agents like abciximab (ReoPro) and (b) small molecule agents (peptidelike eptifibatide [Integrilin] and non-peptide-like tirofiban [Aggrastat]). Because abciximab molecules bind *irreversibly* to the Gp2b/3a receptor and produce permanent noncompetitive platelet inhibition, the clinical effects of the medication can last for 7 to 10 days. Severe uncontrolled bleeding associated with abciximab should be addressed by stopping the medication and transfusing platelets. The small molecule agents bind *reversibly* to the Gp2b/3a receptor to produce competitive platelet inhibition. The antiplatelet effects usually reverse within 4 to 6 h of stopping the medication. Platelet transfusions should not be given for bleeding with small-molecule Gp2b/3a receptor antagonists, as their presence also inhibits new platelet formation.

There have been a number of studies that have proven the efficacy of these agents in reducing the risk of cardiovascular events (death, recurrent ischemia, MI) in patients with ACS. Their beneficial effects have also been proven in the setting of PCIs, both in the patients with ACS and in those with stable coronary artery disease undergoing elective PCI procedures. Typically, small-molecule agents like tirofiban or eptifibatide are used along with aspirin, heparin, and other usual medications for initial stabilization of patients with NSTE-ACS. Tirofiban and eptifibatide are given as a bolus, followed by infusion of the drug lasting for 24 to 72 h. These agents are most beneficial in reducing cardiovascular events of those ACS patients at greatest risk, like those with ST-T abnormalities on ECG, elevated troponins, diabetes mellitus, and those with higher TIMI risk scores. The maximum benefit from use of Gp2b/3a receptor antagonists is seen in those individuals who undergo PCI during their hospital stay. The agents are of questionable benefit in those at low risk (lower TIMI risk score) and those who do not undergo PCI. The majority of high-risk patients undergo coronary angiography and PCI while receiving these agents. The drug infusions are usually continued for 12 to 24 h after the coronary intervention. If patients need coronary bypass surgery, then the medication infusion is stopped for at least 4 to 6 h before proceeding with surgery to minimize risk of bleeding.

Abciximab, on the other hand, is the preferred Gp2b/3a receptor antagonist during PCI in patients with STEMI. However, most centers use the small-molecular weight agents even in patients with STEMI. Abciximab intravenous infusion is continued for 12 h after PCI. If patients on abciximab need emergent bypass surgery, then the medication is stopped and the patients are given a 6- to 12-unit platelet transfusion before coming off the cardiopulmonary bypass pump.

The risk of major bleeding with Gp2b/3a receptor antagonists is 2.5% to 4.0%. Most of the bleeding experienced from these agents is from vascular access sites after PCI. Severe thrombocytopenia with counts less than 50,000/mm^3 is seen in 0.5% to 1.5% of patients who receive abciximab. Because thrombocytopenia can develop within hours of initiating an abciximab infusion, it is prudent to check platelet counts within 4 h of starting the infusion and again at the end of the infusion. Severe thrombocytopenia is rare with small-molecule agents (tirofiban and eptifibatide). There is also a small chance (0.5% to 1.0%) of developing serious pulmonary hemorrhage with abciximab therapy. This is potentially fatal condition and is rarely if ever encountered with the small-molecular weight Gp2b/3a receptor antagonists. The reasons have made the small-molecular weight agents popular with the cardiologists.

Antithrombotic Therapy

Unfractionated Heparin

Adequate doses of intravenous heparin given urgently along with oral aspirin reduce mortality and morbidity in patients with ACS severalfold by immediately interrupting the process of clotting on the coronary endothelium. The combination of heparin and aspirin is superior to aspirin alone in preventing the early complications of UA. Superiority of the combination probably results from the different mechanisms of the two treatments: heparin inhibits soluble clotting factors and thrombin-mediated platelet aggregation, whereas aspirin inhibits COX-mediated platelet aggregation. Even though the addition of heparin to aspirin raises the bleeding incidence slightly, the risk–benefit ratio almost always favors combination therapy. The goal of heparin therapy is to rapidly achieve and maintain a partial thromboplastin time (PTT) of 1.5 to 2.0 times the patient's baseline or laboratory control value. This goal is best achieved using an intravenous bolus (60 units/kg, with a maximum dose of 4,000 units), followed by a continuous intravenous heparin infusion at a rate of 12 units/kg/h (maximum 1,000 units/h). The heparin infusion should be continued until coronary revascularization. Today, most of the ACS patients receive an intravenous infusion of a Gp2b/3a receptor antagonist for 12 to 24 h after PCI. They are also typically on aspirin and clopidogrel long term after PCI. In patients who are candidates for coronary bypass surgery, heparin and aspirin should be continued until surgery. In patients who are not candidates for coronary angiography and revascularization, heparin should be continued for 3 to 5 days. There is a risk of rebound angina when the heparin infusion is stopped. Thereafter, long-term use of aspirin alone can result in a 50% reduction in the incidence of angina recurrence.

Unfractionated heparin (UFH) is a heterogenous mixture of polysaccharides with molecular weights ranging from 3,000 to 30,000. There are several disadvantages with UFH. The antithrombin binding sites of heparin can be bound by a number of other plasma proteins, by platelet factor 4 and also by endothelial cells, thereby diminishing its therapeutic effect. Furthermore, heparin does not bind to clot-bound thrombin and to factor-Xa bound to platelets inside a clot. Thus, there is the possibility of clot propagation while the patient is receiving heparin. Heparin-induced thrombocytopenia (HIT) is another serious adverse effect.

Low-Molecular-Weight Heparins

These are homogenous glycosaminoglycans with molecular weight ranging from 4,000 to 6,000. Low-molecular-weight heparins (LMWH) have greater anti-factor Xa activity and less anti-factor IIa activity as compared to UFH. They act mainly by preventing thrombin generation and have lesser effect on a PTT as compared to UFH. Assays measuring anti-factor Xa activity are becoming available but are not yet in widespread use. Enoxaparin is the most popular of all LMWH that has been shown to be efficacious in patients with NSTE-ACS, as in acute pulmonary embolism and deep venous thrombosis. In the ESSENCE and TIMI 11B trials, enoxaparin has been demonstrated to have an advantage over intravenous heparin in reducing cardiovascular events in patients with NSTE-ACS. In a metaanalysis of these two trials, the risk of death, recurrent ischemia, and MI is reduced by about 20% by the use of enoxaparin as compared to UFH. In the ESSENCE trial, the benefit persisted for over a year. Similarly, dalteparin fared better than intravenous heparin in the FRISC trial in patients with ACS. The benefit was more pronounced in patients with high-risk features like troponin elevation and those with higher TIMI risk scores.

In patients with ACS who have creatinine clearance greater than 30 mL/min, enoxaparin is used in the dosage of 1 mg/kg subcutaneously twice daily. There is no need to monitor the clotting parameters because the therapeutic effect is quite consistent and predictable. The anticoagulant effect with enoxaparin is consistent because of very little binding to plasma proteins, endothelial cells, and macrophages. With newer assays being made available, one may soon be able to monitor anti-factor Xa activity when using enoxaparin. Enoxaparin's risk of thrombocytopenia is quite low. Major bleeding is also uncommon with enoxaparin, but the risk may be higher in the elderly and those with renal failure. In patients requiring CABG, the drug should be stopped 12 to 24 h prior to the operation. In patients undergoing cardiac catheterization and PCI, there is always a concern for bleeding because of concomitant use of UFH, Gp2b/3a receptor antagonists, and clopidogrel. The following rule of thumb can be used for heparin dosing in patients needing PCI: within 8 h of having received a dose of enoxaparin, no additional UFH is needed for PCI; between 8 and 12 h, use UFH at dose of 25 to 50 units/kg; and if greater than 12 h after receiving enoxaparin, use 50 to 70 units/kg of UFH. Despite its proven efficacy, only about 15% of patients in North America and 50% of patients in Europe receive LMWH for ACS.

Direct Thrombin Inhibitors

The direct thrombin inhibitor (DTI) agents available are hirudin, lepirudin (recombinant hirudin), argatroban, and bivalirudin. These agents are substantially more expensive than UFH and enoxaparin. They are powerful anticoagulants and their anticoagulation effect is consistent and predictable. DTIs do not depend on antithrombin III for their activity. They bind to thrombin (factor IIa) and thus inhibit coagulation process. Because thrombin is also a powerful platelet activator, DTIs also inhibit platelet activation. In a large metaanalysis, DTIs were shown to reduce rates of recurrent ischemia and infarctions as compared to heparin in patients with NSTE-ACS, but their use was associated with increased incidence of major bleeding requiring blood transfusions. DTIs are currently only recommended for those with HIT. However, the use of Bivalirudin in the setting of coronary intervention is increasing, ever since the REPLACE-2 trial showed significantly reduced procedure associated bleeding rates compared with heparin and Gp2b/3a receptor antagonists.

This drug although expensive has become more popular with interventional cardiologists.

Fibrinolytic Therapy

There is no proven benefit of fibrinolytic therapy in NSTE-ACS. This is probably because a completely occlusive coronary thrombus is present in fewer than 50% of patients, and also because platelet-rich thrombi which predominate in coronary vessels of patients with NSTE-ACS are resistant to dissolution with fibrinolytic therapy. Fibrinolytic agents have not been demonstrated to be effective in reducing the risk of MI or death in NSTE-ACS and in fact may be deleterious. This is in stark contrast to STE-MI-ACS, where the benefit of fibrinolytic therapy is proven. Therefore, fibrinolytics are contraindicated in NSTE-ACS.

Invasive Strategy of Coronary Angiography and Percutaneous Coronary Intervention

Several recent studies have demonstrated benefit **4** with early invasive strategy in patients with NSTE-ACS as compared to conservative treatment strategy. In the early invasive strategy, patients undergo coronary angiography and revascularization within 12 to 48 h of presentation to the hospital with ACS. In the conservative strategy, patients underwent coronary angiography only for significant recurrent ischemia or ischemia demonstrated by stress testing. The early invasive strategy results in less short-, intermediate-, and long-term major cardiac event rates (death, MI, recurrent ischemia, and revascularization rates) and shorter lengths of stay in the hospital. This is particularly true in patients with high-risk characteristics like elevated serum cardiac biomarkers (like troponins), ongoing chest discomfort, and dynamic ST-T changes on ECG. In intermediate-risk patients, a conservative strategy may be as good as an early invasive strategy. In low-risk patients, a conservative strategy is preferred.

It has been shown that use of aggressive medical regimens including "upstream" use of Gp2b/3a receptor antagonist (tirofiban or eptifibatide) for 12 to 24 h before PCI reduces the risk of MI or death after PCI by at least 30% to 40%. The majority of patients with NSTE-ACS will be candidates for PCI after coronary angiography (70% to 80%). Compared to balloon angioplasty, coronary stenting appears to substantially reduce recurrent ischemia and infarction. Restenosis in 3 to 6 months is a major limitation with bare-metal stents and occurs because of intimal hyperplasia reaction to the vessel wall injury. Since 2003, there has been a widespread use of DES in the United States, which reduces long-term restenosis and repeat revascularization rates by 50% to 70%. However, these patients have to remain on long-term clopidogrel and asprin therapy.

Emergent cardiac catheterization and revascularization in NSTE-ACS is needed less commonly. The indications include pulmonary edema, hypotension, and malignant ischemic ventricular arrhythmias. Most of the other high-risk patients can be stabilized with medical management for 12 to 48 h before angiography and revascularization.

Coronary Bypass Graft Surgery Versus Stenting

The mortality risk with urgent CABG in NSTE-ACS patients is around 4% to 5%. The other complications of bypass surgery include stroke and cognitive abnormalities. This is mainly due to cross-clamping of the aorta and the use of cardiopulmonary bypass. This should be borne in mind especially while operating on elderly patients. The complications and recovery times have improved over the course of the two decades because of refinement in surgical techniques and postoperative care. The advent of left internal mammary artery grafting to the left anterior descending artery was a major advance in bypass surgery since the 1980s. The use of off-pump bypass surgery may reduce the risk of stroke in elderly patients.

The usual length of stay in the hospital is 5 to 7 days, but it may take upto 2 to 3 months for the patients to recover back to their usual baseline.

Only 20% to 30% of NSTE-ACS patients need urgent CABG. The classical indications for CABG include (a) significant left main coronary stenosis, (b) multivessel coronary artery disease (CAD) with left ventricular ejection fraction (LVEF) less than 40%, (c) CAD with significant valvular disease (aortic stenosis and mitral insufficiency), (d) diabetes mellitus with multivessel CAD, (e) coronary anatomy unsuitable for PCI, and (f) failed PCI. It is preferable to stabilize these patients with medical management prior to CABG. Sometimes an intraaortic balloon pump (IABP) may be needed for prior stabilization in patients with hypotension, CHF, and LV dysfunction. However, with the ever-expanding horizons of interventional cardiology many of the patients who previously would have gone for bypass surgery are now receiving DES. The debate of which is better (bypass surgery or stenting) in patients with complex coronary disease (multivessel CAD, total occlusions, left main coronary artery disease, etc.) continues.

The recent SYNTAX trial has compared use of DES (paclitaxel-eluting) to CABG surgery in patients with over 1,800 patients with complex coronary artery disease who were randomized to either bypass surgery or multivessel stenting. The combined endpoint of death, repeat revascularization, stroke, and MI at 1 year favored bypass surgery. The differences were driven mainly by higher repeat revascularization rates in the stent arm of the trial. The risk of death or MI was no different in the two arms. The risk of stroke was more than three times higher in the surgical group. This trial although providing some clear insights has by no means put to rest the raging debate. The recommendation therefore is to individualize therapy after taking into considerations the following factors: (a) coronary anatomy; (b) LV function; (c) comorbid conditions; (d) age of the patient; and (e) patient's wishes.

Intraaortic Balloon Pump

An IABP may prove useful for hemodynamic stabilization while awaiting PTCA or CABG, particularly for patients with LV dysfunction, CHF, hypotension, or acute mechanical defects (e.g., mitral regurgitation [MR] or ventricular septal defect [VSD]). Balloon inflation during diastole augments coronary perfusion and deflation during systole decreases LV afterload. Unless a rapidly correctable mechanical defect is present, the use of IABP does not improve outcomes.

Risk Factor Modification

For the patient who has been stabilized medically or following revascularization procedures, risk factor modification is essential in preventing recurrent ischemia, infarction, and sudden death from progression of CAD. Smoking cessation, control of diabetes mellitus and hypertension, correction of abnormal lipid patterns, and weight reduction are critical elements in risk factor modification. Most should remain on aspirin, β-blockers, statins, and angiotensin-converting enzyme inhibitors (ACEI). Establishing a regular program of exercise is pivotal in achieving these goals and improving exercise tolerance. Patients with good exercise capacity are known to have fewer cardiovascular events and seem to tolerate them better.

■ ACUTE CORONARY SYNDROMES: ST ELEVATION MYOCARDIAL INFARCTION (ACS-STEMI)

Mechanisms

STEMI results from plaque rupture and formation of superimposed thrombus. The thrombus that causes complete occlusion of a major coronary artery is usually rich in fibrin and red blood cells ("red-clot"). This is in contrast to the thrombus seen with NSTE-ACS, which is characterized by formation of a platelet-rich thrombus ("white-clot"). A wave of myocardial necrosis spreads from the endocardium to the epicardium with complete coronary occlusion. The process of infarction is usually completed in 24 h, and it is called a "full-thickness" or completed infarction. Q waves are typically seen in the ECG with a completed or full-thickness infarction. If angiography is performed promptly, a fresh occlusive coronary thrombus may be demonstrated in most cases (approx. 90%). Nonthrombotic spasm of the coronary arteries in an area of atherosclerosis is responsible for a small fraction of AMIs. Rarely, coronary flow may be interrupted by embolism in patients with endocarditis, prosthetic valves, or rheumatic valvular disease. Only 5% to 10% of patients sustaining an MI have normal coronary arteries. (Although spontaneous thrombolysis of clot is suspected, the mechanism of infarction in these cases usually remains unknown.) Cocaine is responsible for an alarming number of MIs. Because cocaine enhances platelet aggregation, causes vasoconstriction, and increases heart rate through catecholamine-mediated mechanisms, it can produce infarction even in patients with normal coronary arteries.

Diagnosis

History

(1) **Classical Presentation** The typical presentation is one characterized by the abrupt onset of left-sided or retrosternal chest, neck, and jaw discomfort, which has been described as burning, squeezing, or pressurelike sensation lasting for more 30 min. The discomfort may radiate to the arms, neck, back, or jaw. It must be emphasized that the pain description may be highly atypical (burning, stabbing, sharp) or may be localized only to the arm or neck. Autonomic symptoms (nausea, vomiting, sweating) are more common than in UA. Up to 20% of MIs are painless (more likely in diabetics and

the elderly). Young age, paucity of classic risk factors, and atypical chest pain character are more common in patients with cocaine-induced infarction.

(2) **Atypical Presentation** Patients may describe pain as being sharp or stabbing. The pain may be localized to the arm, shoulder, or neck. Symptoms may mimic gastroesophageal reflux, cholecystitis, or an acute abdomen. Acute onset of shortness of breath, heart failure, dizziness, syncope, and weakness have all been described as atypical manifestations of an AMI. Atypical presentations are seen in women, diabetics, elderly, and cocaine and other drug overdose states.

(3) **Silent MI** Clinically silent infarcts are detected incidentally on an ECG, echocardiogram, or nuclear scan. Silent MI is usually seen in diabetics with autonomic dysfunction.

Physical Examination

Blood pressure and pulse rate usually are mildly increased. (Tachycardia is more common in anterior or lateral MI than in inferior or posterior MIs, in which bradycardia is more likely.) Fever may accompany uncomplicated MI but rarely exceeds 101°F or persists beyond 1 week. An S4 gallop is very common, whereas an S3 suggests congestive failure, especially if accompanied by pulmonary rales. A paradoxically split S2 indicates increased LV ejection time or may be from a left bundle branch block (LBBB). A systolic murmur should raise the suspicion of acute papillary muscle dysfunction, especially if the patient has presented late (typically, a few days after onset of symptoms). A pericardial friction rub commonly appears in the first 48 h after MI and may be easily confused with a murmur. Although also possible in a classic MI, findings of a hyperadrenergic state (mydriasis, agitation, hypertension, diaphoresis, and/or tachycardia) should raise suspicion of cocaine-induced infarction.

Electrocardiogram

(1) **ST Segment Deflection** ST elevation greater than or equal to 1 mm in two or more contiguous leads is highly suggestive of STEMI. ST elevation has a high localizing value (Table 21-1). The typical ST elevation seen with STEMI has an outward convexity. The ST segment elevations usually return to baseline with myocardial reperfusion and can be used to monitor reperfusion

TABLE 21-1 ANATOMIC PATTERNS OF MYOCARDIAL INJURY

LOCATION OF INJURY	AFFECTED LEADS
Inferior	II, III, F
Anterior/septal	V_2–V_4
Anterolateral	V_3–V_6
Lateral	I, AVL, occasionally V_6
Apical	II, III, F, V_5–V_6
Posterior[a]	V_1 and V_2

[a]ST segment depression with R waves; T wave is inverted initially and then becomes upright.

therapies. The differential diagnosis includes hyperkalemia, acute central nervous system (CNS) injury, acute myocarditis, acute pericarditis, left ventricular hypertrophy, apical cardiomyopathy, Wolff–Parkinson–White syndrome, early repolarization abnormalities, and LV aneurysm. Some of these may mimic an AMI and hence have been termed "pseudoinfarct" pattern.

(2) *Evolution of ECG Changes*   A series of repolarization changes are seen on ECG with complete coronary artery occlusion. The first transient abnormalities seen are the hyperacute T waves (tall, peaked, and symmetrical T waves). Hyperacute T waves are usually gone by the time of initial presentation for emergency care. This is followed by convex, upward ST elevation, which is a sign of transmural myocardial ischemic injury. The number of leads showing the abnormality has a bearing on the size of the infarction and prognosis. T wave inversions are seen with persistent transmural ischemia. By this time, the ST elevations have begun to subside. Q waves are a sign of completion of the infarction and may take hours to days to develop. Persistent ST elevation beyond 3 to 4 weeks is sign of an LV aneurysm.

(3) *Posterior MI*   This manifests as ST depression (≥ 2 mm) in leads V_1 to V_3. It is usually seen along with an inferior wall MI, but can present on its own as a true posterior infarction. This is seen with either left circumflex or distal RCA occlusion.

(4) *RV Infarcts*   Seen in about 30% of the inferior wall infarctions, RV infarcts manifest on ECG as greater than or equal to 1 mm ST elevations in right-sided chest leads, particularly V_3R and V_4R. Pure RV infarcts resulting from occlusion

of RV marginal branch vessels may sometimes mimic an anterior MI by presenting as ST elevations in leads V_1 and V_2.

(5) *New LBBB*   New LBBB is typically seen with large MIs and carries an in-hospital mortality rate of 20% to 25%. There is a substantial benefit from reperfusion therapy (21% reduction in mortality at 7 weeks, which translates into 49 lives saved per 1,000 patients treated). However, an MI may be missed in a significant number of individuals with new complete LBBB, and therefore, they are less likely to get reperfusion therapies than STEMI patients. Criteria for diagnosis of MI in the presence of LBBB is based on ST segment concordance or discordance: (a) greater than or equal to 1 mm concordant elevation, (b) greater than or equal to 5 mm discordant elevation, and (c) greater than 1 mm ST segment depressions in leads V_1 to V_3. Presence of one or more of these criteria makes a diagnosis of AMI more likely with LBBB.

(6) *Normal ECG*   ECG may be normal in high lateral wall infarctions, as this area may be electrocardiographically "silent."

Cardiac Enzymes

Creatine Kinase

Total CK and MB fractions begin to rise by 4 to 8 h of onset of an MI, reach a peak by 18 to 24 h, and return back to baseline by 48 to 72 h. CK peaks earlier in non–Q wave infarctions and in patients who have received thrombolytic therapy to abort an acute infarction. The rapid washout of CK associated with thrombolysis may produce peak enzyme levels as early as 30 min after reperfusion. Peak CK activity correlates with the extent of muscle loss.

Levels are checked every 8 h, and three negative CK–MB levels are used to rule out an AMI. CK–MB levels greater than 3% of total CK levels are used to make a diagnosis of an AMI. The sensitivity and specificity of CK–MB in the diagnosis of an AMI are lower than that of troponins. Thus, one may have a small infarct with normal CK–MB but slightly elevated troponins. Total CK may be mildly elevated by trivial skeletal muscle injury (e.g., severe exercise or intramuscular injection). Even though CK–MB is relatively specific for cardiac muscle, it may be released during massive skeletal or smooth muscle damage (e.g., rhabdomyolysis, polymyositis, small bowel surgery).

Cardiac Troponins

There are two types of cardiac troponin assays available (T and I). Both are cardiac-specific regulatory proteins; troponin-I is in more widespread use. Highly sensitive and specific in making a diagnosis of AMI, their levels elevate within 6 to 8 h of onset of an AMI, peak by 3 to 5 days, and generally last for 7 to 12 days. Renal insufficiency slows their clearance. Thus, they are helpful in making diagnosis of a remote MI. They are also helpful in making a diagnosis of an MI in certain situations like rhabdomyolysis, polymyositis, and renal failure where the CK–MB levels may be elevated.

Although sensitive, the serum aspartate aminotransferase is not sufficiently specific for diagnosis. Similarly, total lactic dehydrogenase (LDH) rises in most cases of MI but has a low specificity. Levels of the LDH-2 isoenzyme normally exceed those of the LDH-1 isoenzyme. Reversal of the ratio suggests MI. LDH begins to rise 12 to 24 h after coronary occlusion, peaking at 2 to 4 days and resolving in 7 to 10 days. Because LDH rises later than creatine phosphokinase (CPK), it may be used to diagnose infarction in patients presenting more than 24 h after onset of symptoms. Initial experience with troponin-I suggests it to be a sensitive and specific serum marker of myocardial damage.

Echocardiography

Although echocardiography cannot be considered a definitive test for ischemia, it is a helpful adjunctive technique. Echocardiography offers information that can help make a diagnosis of ischemia or infarction. A focal wall motion abnormality seen on the echocardiogram in the proper clinical setting can help make the diagnosis of acute ischemia or infarction, especially when the ECG is not helpful. Echocardiography can also help in providing an explanation for hypotension or congestive symptoms in patients with an AMI (e.g., LV or RV dysfunction, pericardial effusion, free wall or septal perforations, acute mitral insufficiency, or aortic dissection). Apart from its value in risk stratification, echo is also instrumental in diagnosing complications of infarction (e.g., chordal disruption, papillary muscle dysfunction, septal perforation, pericardial effusion, free wall rupture, ventricular aneurysm, mural thrombus). The addition of transesophageal echocardiography to the diagnostic armamentarium has substantially increased the ability to detect subtle MR, small ventriculoseptal defects (VSDs), papillary muscle damage, and posterior wall infarction (see Chapter 2).

Treatment

During the last 30 years, advances in coronary care—aggressive treatment of coronary ischemia and arrhythmias—have reduced the mortality of AMI from 30% to less than 10% (Fig. 21-3). Recently, the major therapeutic goal has been to limit infarct size, primarily by achieving early reperfusion. Reperfusion is achieved by pharmacologic or mechanical means and is performed in conjunction with measures to minimize myocardial oxygen demand. The early therapy of AMI has now evolved to a five-armed attack: (a) relieve pain and anxiety; (b) achieve reperfusion using thrombolytic therapy or PTCA in appropriate candidates; (c) improve the balance between myocardial oxygen supply and demand by using supplemental oxygen, nitrates, and β-blockers; (d) initiate antithrombotic therapy (aspirin and heparin) to prevent reformation of a second occlusive thrombus; and (e) limit infarct expansion, prevent adverse ventricular remodeling, and improve ventricular function. These initial steps are followed by critically important secondary prevention efforts, which include continued use of aspirin, β-blockers, statins and clopidogrel, and modification of cardiac risk factors.

Initial Steps

Patients with a chest pain history suggestive of AMI should be placed on bed rest, undergo immediate ECG testing, receive oxygen (2 to 3 L nasal cannula), and have two peripheral intravenous catheters inserted, at which time blood samples should be drawn for electrolyte, hemoglobin, and CPK enzyme analysis. Whenever possible, central venous catheters and arterial punctures should be avoided during antithrombolytic therapy. (Oxygenation usually can be sufficiently assessed by oximetry without arterial blood gases.) If the ECG is suggestive and the history is compatible with MI, aspirin and nitrates should be administered to almost all patients while thrombolytic therapy is prepared. Unless presentation to medical care is seriously delayed following the onset of chest pain or a clear contraindication exists, thrombolytic therapy is administered to all suitable AMI victims within 1 h of diagnosis. Morphine and/or benzodiazepines should be considered for control of pain and anxiety. Unless contraindications exist, β-blockers should be administered to most patients with AMI.

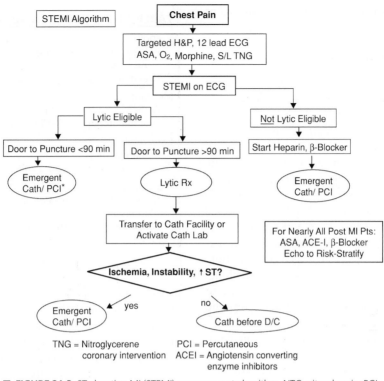

■ **FIGURE 21-3** ST elevation MI (STEMI) management algorithm. NTG, nitroglycerin; PCI, percutaneous coronary intervention; ACEI, angiotension converting enzyme inhibitor.

Aspirin

Because it is safe, fast, and effective at preventing recurrent thrombosis, aspirin (160 to 325 mg) should be given promptly to all patients with AMI without contraindications (e.g., history of aspirin allergy) and should be continued on a daily basis. Aspirin alone achieves an average 20% reduction in mortality, and when combined with thrombolytic agents, an amazing 40% reduction in death rate is observed. For patients who are allergic to aspirin, clopidogrel, which is an ADP-receptor inhibitor, is a good alternative. Regardless of the suitability of the patient for thrombolytic therapy or angioplasty, an aspirin tablet once or twice daily reduces mortality risk and reinfarction rates for essentially all subgroups of patients with MI. Aspirin can be continued safely for years while providing continued benefit. Aspirin alone is as effective as its combination with sulfinpyrazone or dipyridamole.

Nitrates

Unless contraindicated, NTG should be tried in nearly every patient with acute ischemic symptoms and an ECG suggesting MI. If a portion of the affected coronary artery remains patent, nitrates can promote flow through the narrowed segment. If the coronary occlusion is complete, however, nitrate therapy is unlikely to offer much, if any, boost in flow. Nitrates improve myocardial oxygen supply by reducing preload and afterload and by directly dilating coronary arteries. Intravenous nitrates may reduce infarct size and probably reduce mortality of AMI by 10% to 30%. Except for hypotension or profound tachycardia, few contraindications to nitrate therapy exist. Nitrates should be used cautiously in inferior MI because of the potential to aggravate bradycardia and with great caution for patients with RV infarction, in whom small reductions in venous return can produce profound hypotension. Initially, sublingual dosing makes sense because it is fast, is titrated easily, and can help alleviate symptoms while definitive reperfusion therapy is prepared and administered. If pain relief is achieved temporarily with sublingual NTG, administration by continuous intravenous infusion often proves useful for longer relief. Long-acting oral nitrates should be avoided because of the inability to easily reverse or titrate their effects. Headache is common but easily treated with acetaminophen. Alcohol intoxication (from the intravenous preparation) and methemoglobinemia are uncommon complications of prolonged intravenous infusion therapy.

Analgesia and Anxiolysis

Relief of pain and anxiety are important in the treatment of AMI. Ideally, ischemic pain is reversed by achieving reperfusion of the hypoxic cardiac muscle; however, direct analgesia may be necessary. Morphine, given in carefully measured doses, is the drug of choice. In addition to providing direct pain relief, morphine serves to reduce preload and, to a lesser degree, afterload—both potentially improving the balance in myocardial oxygen supply/demand. Furthermore, morphine inhibits anxiety-induced catecholamine release, further reducing myocardial oxygen consumption. Despite fears on the part of physicians, morphine-induced bradycardia and hypotension occur rarely; when they do occur, they usually respond promptly to fluids and/or atropine. When analgesic range doses of morphine (2 to 10 mg) are given slowly, the risk of respiratory depression or any other complication is minimized. For the extremely anxious patient, especially one experiencing MI from cocaine use, benzodiazepines are very useful anxiolytic agents.

β-Blockade

Intravenous β-blockade given soon after the onset of MI reduces infarct size and lowers the risks of cardiac arrest, reinfarction, and death. These benefits are achieved predominantly by lowering myocardial oxygen consumption through reductions in heart rate, blood pressure, and contractility; however, β-blockers also provide independent antiarrhythmic effects. In addition to the early protective effects, continued therapy also lowers the long-term risk of SCD for as long as 1 to 2 years. With these proven benefits, it is curious that so few patients with MI uncomplicated by overt systolic dysfunction receive β-blocker therapy. Possibly, concerns over the potential side effects of therapy or lack of enthusiasm over a "low-tech" treatment are responsible.

Prompt administration of metoprolol or atenolol, first intravenously and then orally, provides benefit. (Suggested dosing regimens are listed in Table 21-2.) Absolute contraindications to β-blockade include known drug hypersensitivity, severe active bronchospasm, type I or type II second-degree atrioventricular (AV) block, complete heart block, sinus bradycardia (pulse < 60),

TABLE 21-2 β-BLOCKER REGIMENS

Atenolol
IV load: 5 mg repeated once after 10 min if pulse rate > 60
Oral maintenance: 50 mg b.i.d or 100 mg daily

Metoprolol
IV load: 5 mg every 5 min, to total dose of 15 mg
Oral maintenance: 50–100 mg b.i.d

Carvedilol
IV load: 2.5 mg
Oral maintenance: 12.5–25 mg b.i.d

Propranolol
IV load 0.1 mg/kg up to three times at 15-min intervals (hold for pulse <50–60)
Oral maintenance: 10–80 mg p.o. every 6 h

hypotension (systolic blood pressure < 100 mm Hg), or overt LV failure (i.e., cardiogenic shock or pulmonary edema). Relative contraindications include insulin-dependent diabetes, concurrent use of a calcium channel antagonist, a history of obstructive lung disease, bibasilar rales, heart rates of approximately 60 beats/min, systolic blood pressure near 100 mm Hg, and a wedge pressure higher than 20 mm Hg. If the blood pressure is marginal or if the history or physical examination suggests that the patient is prone to complications of β-blocker therapy, a short-acting intravenous agent such as esmolol (0.5 mg/kg load followed by 0.05 mg/kg/min infusion) can be tried and terminated rapidly should adverse response occur. Despite the benefits of β-blockers, many patients are unable to tolerate their most common side effects: bronchospasm, heart failure, and conduction system disturbances. Potential side effects must be monitored closely and the drug must be discontinued if they develop.

Insulin Infusion

Hyperglycemia is quite common in patients with complicated AMI, as is the case with most acutely ill intensive care unit (ICU) patients. The DIGAMI trial showed improved survival at 1 year in patients with AMI who were given intensive insulin therapy. Trials done on acutely ill patients in the surgical ICU have also shown improved outcomes with the insulin infusion. The current recommendation is to start all STEMI patients with a complicated course having hyperglycemia on an insulin infusion, maintaining blood sugars around 100 to 140 mg/dL.

Magnesium Infusion

The ISIS-4 trial and MAGIC trials have not demonstrated benefit with routine infusion of magnesium in STEMI patients. Hypomagnesemia occurs in 30% to 40% of patients with AMI and should be corrected with intravenous and/or enteral therapies. The level is kept greater than 2 mmol/L to minimize risk of polymorphic ventricular tachycardia (VT) and ventricular fibrillation (VF).

Reperfusion Therapies

Fibrinolytic Therapy

Mechanism of Action and Choice of Agent
Eighty-five to ninety percent patients sustaining AMI have coronary thrombosis. Fibrinolytics have been shown to limit infarct size, improve LV function, and reduce the mortality of certain patients with AMI by dissolving an intracoronary clot and restoring myocardial blood flow. The thrombolytic agents available for clinical use are (a) streptokinase (SK), (b) tissue plasminogen activator (t-PA or alteplase), (c) recombinant plasminogen activator (r-PA or retavase), and (d) TNK-tPA (tenecteplase). All four agents accelerate conversion of plasminogen to plasmin, an enzyme that attacks fibrin and breaks down fibrin-rich or "red clot." SK binds to plasminogen to form an activator-complex. TNK-tPA and t-PA are fibrin-specific agents that act on clot-bound plasminogen and therefore, do not cause a systemic "lytic" state. SK and to some extent r-PA cause a systemic "lytic" state. This systemic action usually produces a hypocoagulable state by reducing circulating levels of fibrinogen and most clotting proteins, like factors V and VIII, increasing levels of fibrin-degradation products. Unfortunately, none of these drugs can distinguish a "good" from a "bad" clot; therefore, all are associated with some increased risk of hemorrhage. The risk of bleeding is probably highest with r-PA and lowest with SK. Of all the available agents, the fibrin-specific agents are most effective in achieving a patent infarct-related vessel (80% with fibrin-specific agents compared to 50% to 60% with SK). Unfortunately, the accelerated t-PA regimen followed by an intravenous heparin infusion is associated with higher risk of major bleeding (including IC hemorrhage) than is SK. The rates of achieving a patent vessel are similar among t-PA, r-PA, and TNK-tPA. The bleeding risk is lower with TNK-tPA, as compared to the other fibrin-specific agents. TNK-tPA and r-PA are administered as bolus doses and are therefore, much easier to administer compared to accelerated t-PA regimen. Therefore, the agent of choice (in the United States) is TNK-tPA, but SK continues to be popular in Europe and Asia, mainly because of lower costs. SK may also be preferable in older patients (>75 years of age), particularly for small-sized women, if PCI is not available.

Patient Selection and Important Facts of Fibrinolytic Therapy

- See Tables 21-3 and 21-4 for indications and contraindications of fibrinolytic therapy.

TABLE 21-3 INDICATIONS FOR THROMBOLYTIC THERAPY

ANGINOID CHEST PAIN OF LESS THAN 12-h DURATION

PLUS one or more of these:
- ST elevation ≥1 mm in at least two contiguous limb leads
- ST elevation ≥2 mm in at least two contiguous chest leads
- New LBBB

ST, sinus tachycardia; LBBB, left bundle branch bolus.

TABLE 21-4 CONTRAINDICATIONS TO THROMBOLYTIC THERAPY

Absolute contraindications
 Active internal bleeding
 History of CNS disease (stroke, arteriovenous malformation, surgery, tumor, or head trauma) within 6 months
 Hemorrhagic CVA anytime in past
 Suspected aortic dissection
 Underlying coagulopathy, including thrombocytopenia
 Ongoing warfarin therapy with INR > 2.5
 Severe diastolic hypertension (diastolic blood pressure > 110 mm Hg)
 Recent (2–4 weeks) trauma, deep tissue biopsy, or operation
 Pregnancy

Relative contraindications
 Systolic blood pressure > 180 mm Hg
 Remote history of stroke or transient ischemic attack
 Recent prolonged (>10 min) cardiopulmonary resuscitation
 Needle puncture of a noncompressible vessel
 Intracardiac thrombus

CNS, central nervous system.

- All STEMI patient subgroups (age, gender, comorbid conditions) and infarct locations seem to benefit from fibrinolytic therapy.
- Proportionately, the greatest benefits are experienced by patients at greatest risk: those with larger and anterior infarctions, those with new LBBB, and those in CHF.
- In the GISSI-1 trial, fibrinolytic therapy saved 20 more lives per 1,000 patients treated compared to placebo at 6 weeks, and this benefit was preserved at 10 years. In the GUSTO-1 trial, accelerated t-PA regimen saved 10 more lives per 1,000 patients treated compared to standard SK regimen.
- The benefit with fibrinolytic therapy is *time-dependent*. For every 1,000 patients treated with fibrinolytics (compared to placebo), 65 lives were saved if treated within first hour of onset of symptoms, 26 lives if treated within 1 to 3 h of onset of symptoms, and 18 lives if treated within 6 to 12 h of onset of symptoms.
- In the metaanalysis by the fibrinolytic therapy trialists (FTT) collaborative group, there was approximately *30% reduction in mortality* with fibrinolytic therapy in STEMI patients. Overall, fibrinolytic therapy reduces mortality rates by 20% to 50%, and as might be expected, the greatest benefits are observed in patients treated within 1 to 3 h of the onset of pain.
- Fibrinolytic therapy should be given to STEMI patients without contraindications within 12 h of the onset of chest pain and if the *estimated door-balloon time is greater than 90 min* (absence of immediate PCI availability). Patients seen within 12 to 24 h of onset of chest pain and with ongoing chest pain and persistent ST elevations may also considered for fibrinolytic therapy if PCI is unavailable, but the magnitude of benefit is significantly lower. Fibrinolytic should not be used in STEMI patients presenting greater than 24 h of onset of symptoms. Fibrinolytic therapy should be given within 30 min of arrival in the emergency room (door-to-needle time of ≤30 min), once a decision for their use has been made. It is also recommended that patients receiving fibrinolytic therapy should be transferred to a facility with PCI availability as soon as possible. Such transfer has been shown to be safe.
- Antithrombotic therapy with fibrinolytic therapy: UFH is used with fibrin-specific agents (t-PA, TNK-Tpa, and r-PA). It is generally not recommended with SK. It is given in a bolus dose of 60 units/kg (4,000 units maximum), followed by an infusion of 12 units/kg/h (1,000 units/h maximum). The dose of the infusion should be adjusted to keep PTT 1.5 to 2.0 times the upper limit of normal. The infusion is usually continued for 48 h postfibrinolytic therapy. Heparin infusion should be continued beyond 48 h if patients are at high risk for venous or systemic thromboembolic events (large anterior MI, severe LV dysfunction, CHF, thrombi in the LV, AF). Patients must be started on warfarin, and the heparin should be discontinued only once INR is greater than 2.
- Gp2b/3a receptor antagonists can be used with half dose r-PA or TNK-tPA in patients below 70 years of age. In older patients, this combination increases the risk of bleeding.
- The *limitations* of fibrinolytic therapy: (a) 20% to 30% patients have contraindications for thrombolytic therapy; (b) 50% to 70% patients have successful reperfusion; (c) recurrent ischemia or reinfarction is seen in 15% to 30% patients who experienced successful reperfusion; (d) 4% to 5% patients experience major bleeding, including 0.7% to 1.5% risk of intracerebral hemorrhage (which has a high fatality rate).
- Indicators of successful reperfusion: significant improvement or complete disappearance of chest pain along with greater than 50% resolution of ST segment elevation on ECG within 90 min of administration of fibrinolytic therapy. The greater the degree of improvement of ST segment change, the better the long-term outcome.

Complications of Fibrinolytics

(1) **Hemorrhage** Four to five percent of patients experience major bleeding (usually GI) and about 0.5% to 1.5% experience an IC bleed. Factors that predict risk of major bleeding are advanced age (>70 years), female gender, low body weight, hypertension at presentation, bleeding diathesis, IC neoplasms, and previous stroke. Fibrin-specific agents are more prone to cause bleeding than SK. IC bleeds are heralded by mental obtundation, focal CNS deficits, and intense headaches. With onset of these symptoms, one must stop the fibrinolytic therapy, heparin, and all antiplatelet agents including aspirin. A stat CT scan of the head will help confirm the diagnosis. The treatment consists of packed red blood cell transfusions (if hematocrit

drops below 25% and there is associated hypotension), cryoprecipitate infusion (approx. 10 units), and fresh frozen plasma infusion if there is continued bleeding (2 to 6 units). Intravenous protamine (25 to 50 mg after a small test dose) may be needed to reverse the effect of heparin. Platelet transfusions (6 to 12 units) may be needed for continued bleeding, especially if the patient has received abciximab, clopidogrel, and aspirin. Patients with thrombocytopenia (<100,000/mm³) have an 8- to 10-fold risk of bleeding with fibrinolytic therapy.

(2) **Anaphylaxis** Encountered rarely, primarily with SK. Prompt recognition, stopping the drug, airway maintenance, intravenous epinephrine (1 to 5 cc of 1:10,000 solution), intravenous fluid boluses, intravenous hydrocortisone, and methylprednisone are the cornerstones of therapy. Less commonly, intravenous dopamine, phenylephrine, or norepinephrine infusion and inhaled albuterol aerosol may be necessary for persistent hypotension.

(3) **Hypotension** Occurs in 10% to 15% patients with SK. Slowing the infusion rate and giving intravenous fluids usually suffices, but occasionally the drug infusion may have to be stopped temporarily until the blood pressure improves.

(4) **Arrhythmias** The usual reperfusion arrhythmias seen with fibrinolytic therapy are runs of idioventricular rhythm (IVR) (rate 90 to 120 beats/min) and VT. These rhythm disturbances are usually transient and do not need any other treatment besides β-blocker therapy. VF can also occur occasionally with reperfusion and this usually responds promptly to defibrillation. With inferior wall MI with dominant RCA occlusion, one may see transient, third-degree AV block with reperfusion.

(5) **Miscellaneous** Fever, skin rash, and rigors. All these are more common with SK. Skin rash necessitates stopping infusion and considering t-PA or PCI. Benadryl and hydrocortisone given by intravenous route seem to help.

Primary Percutaneous Coronary Intervention (PCI—PTCA and Stenting)

- Primary PCI of the infarct-related vessel is today *the preferred method* of reperfusion in patients with STEMI. When performed soon enough, PTCA achieves TIMI-3 flow in the infarct-related vessel in approximately 90%, compared to 50% to 60% TIMI-3 flow rates with the best fibrinolytic regimen. Mechanical reperfusion with PTCA and stenting has been shown to be superior to fibrinolytic therapy.

- The improved rate of establishing infarct vessel patency with PCI has translated into better clinical outcomes, compared to fibrinolytic therapy. In a metaanalysis of all trials comparing primary PTCA to fibrinolytic therapy, there was a 30% to 50% reduction of death, reinfarctions, and stroke at 1 and 6 months. Improvement in rates of stroke and reinfarction are responsible for most of the benefit seen with PCI. PCI has been shown to save 21 more lives than fibrinolytic therapy for every 1,000 patients treated.

- Although "sooner the better" definitely applies, PCI in STEMI is not as time dependent as fibrinolytic therapy. Primary PTCA reduced 30-day rates of major cardiac events (death, reinfarction, CVA) by 54% in patients presenting within 2 h of onset of symptoms, 39% for those presenting within 2 to 4 h of symptom onset, and 21% for those presenting after 4 h. This is not the case with fibrinolytic therapy, where the benefit diminishes exponentially with each passing hour after onset of symptoms.

- The risk of intracerebral hemorrhage is about 0.1% with primary PCI, which therefore is particularly a good option for those beyond 70 years of age, in whom fibrinolytic therapy significantly increases the risk of bleeding.

- High-volume centers are those that perform greater than 200 to 300 PCI procedures per year. Data from the National Registry for MI (NRMI) shows that there is a 37% reduction in death in STEMI patients treated with PCI at high-volume centers and no change in mortality when treated at low-volume centers. However, a 64% reduction in risk of CVA was seen with PCI at both low- and high-volume centers, which is clearly an advantage compared to fibrinolytic therapy. Therefore, primary PCI is the preferred mode of reperfusion for STEMI patients if access to a high-volume cardiac catheterization laboratory is available and if PCI can be performed in a timely fashion. The ideal door-to-balloon time should be less than 90 min.

- **On-site** fibrinolytic therapy versus transfer of patients for PCI: When patients with STEMI arrive at a hospital without a cardiac catheterization laboratory, the question arises as to whether these patients are better off with on-site fibrinolytic therapy or with transfer for PCI to a larger center with cardiac catheterization facilities. The recent DANAMI-2 and PRAGUE-2 trials have both shown benefit of transferring patients for primary PCI over on-site fibrinolytic therapy, if the transfer of patients can be achieved within 2 h. In the DANAMI-2 trial there was a 40% reduction in reinfarction, death, and CVA at 30 days, compared to fibrinolytic therapy. The transferred patients have outcomes with PCI comparable to those who presented directly to the invasive treatment center. Transfer of patients was found to be safe, with very few adverse events during transportation. Thus, establishment of primary-PCI centers with 24/7 cardiac cath-lab facilities and efficient patient transfer protocols is key to improving outcomes in patients with STEMI. The door-to-balloon time for transfer patients was about 100 min in the DANAMI-2 trial. However, the door-to-balloon time is approximately 3 h in the United States for patients with STEMI transferred for PCI (time of entry to the first emergency room to the time of balloon inflation at the PCI). Therefore, the prevailing guidelines in the United States would favor the administration of fibrinolytic therapy for lytic-eligible patients—if the door-to-balloon time is likely to exceed 90 min. These patients must be transported to a PCI center soon after administration of fibrinolytic therapy, so that if they fail to achieve reperfusion then they could still undergo PCI and mechanical reperfusion in an expeditious manner. For patients with contraindications for fibrinolytics (lytic ineligible) and in situations where the door-to-balloon time is likely to be less than 90 min, quick transfer to another hospital for primary-PCI is the best approach.

- **PTCA versus intracoronary stenting in AMI:** Stents have been shown to improve long-term outcome compared to PTCA. Metaanalysis of all the stent-versus-balloon angioplasty trials shows 46% reduction in composite endpoint of death, reinfarction, and target vessel revascularization at 6 months with stents compared to PTCA. This difference was mainly due to reduced restenosis and recurrent ischemia in the unstented group.
- **DES versus bare metal stents:** Bare-metal stents have been in clinical practice in the United States since 1994. In 2003, the FDA approved Sirolimus (Rapamune) and paclitaxel (Onxol, Taxol) DES for clinical use. Recently zotarolimus and everolimus-eluting stents have also been approved

by the FDA. These stents are made of stainless steel and are covered with a polymer which elutes an antiproliferative drug. The stents usually elute the drug for a period of 3 to 6 weeks from the time they are deployed in the artery. The main advantage of DES as compared with the older bare-metal stent is reduction of restenosis from excessive neointimal proliferation. Neointimal proliferation occurs as a result of intimomedial injury caused by the stent. The antiproliferative agent eluted by the stent prevents neointimal proliferation in the artery. These devices are being used quite extensively in patients with CAD, including in those with AMI. The use of DES has reduced clinical restenosis rates quite dramatically compared to those receiving bare-metal stents (5% to 9% vs. 20% to 40%). Today, in the United States about 75% of all stents used are DES. DES has been shown to have superior clinical outcomes in all subsets of patients, including AMI. The major disadvantage of stents, particularly DES, is stent thrombosis which can cause catastrophic MI or death. Patients who receive bare-metal stents should remain on dual antiplatelet therapy (clopidogrel and ASA) for a minimum of 1 month. The recommendation is minimum 12 months of dual antiplatelet therapy for patients with DES. However, over the course of the last few years it has become apparent that a small group of patients with DES will suffer from the phenomenon of *late-stent thrombosis,* especially with discontinuation of clopidogrel therapy. That is the reason why most patients who receive DES remain on dual antiplatelet indefinitely.

- **Role of thrombus aspiration:** Thrombus aspiration with an aspiration catheter from the occluded vessel prior to balloon PTCA or stenting had been long felt to improve TIMI-3 flow, myocardial blushing and thereby, myocardial salvage. Myocardial blushing is perhaps a better indicator of clinical outcomes like resolution of ST elevation on ECG and myocardial salvage than angiographic TIMI flow rates which have been described earlier this chapter. Myocardial blushing on contrast angiography corresponds to flow of contrast within the coronary microcirculation and thereby, is an indicator of myocardial perfusion. Myocardial blush Grade 0 to 1 = no or very little blush, 2 = moderate blush, and 3 = normal blush, indicating no or minimal, moderately reduced, and normal myocardial perfusion, respectively. The TAPAS trial which randomized more than 1,000 patients with STEMI, compared efficacy of standard practice of balloon angioplasty plus stenting to thrombus aspiration plus stenting, in terms of improvement in myocardial blushing. Thrombus aspiration followed by stenting was superior to standard practice of PTCA and stenting in improving myocardial perfusion. This is mainly because thrombus aspiration reduces the risk of the clot breaking loose and occluding up the distal coronary microcirculation. The 30-day event rate (death and nonfatal MI) was statistically no different between the two groups, but the 1-year follow-up data showed a clinical trend that favored thrombus aspiration.

- **Door-to-balloon (or device) times and prehospital cardiac cath-lab activation:** The standard recommendation for door-to-balloon time in STEMI patients is less than 90 min for both direct admits and for patients being transferred for PCI (door time = time of initial patient arrival in the ER; balloon or device time = time of first balloon inflation or device use [like aspiration catheter] in the patients artery. Some cardiac hospitals have developed protocols where the paramedics activate the cath lab from the field after performing a prehospital ECG. The patient is usually brought in directly to the cath lab bypassing the emergency room, thereby reducing delays. This system has helped reduce door-to-balloon times significantly at these institutions. However, there are times when patients with NSTEMI situations end up arriving in the cath lab (those with LVH, pericarditis, early repolarization, etc.) with this arrangement. The AMI protocol has also been refined significantly in many of the emergency rooms across the nation through joint collaboration between the emergency room physicians and the cardiologists. The usual rule is to get the first ECG within 10 min of a patient with chest pain presenting to the ER. Having an AMI protocol streamlines care and reduces delays significantly. The on-call cath-lab team including the interventional cardiologist should be living within 15 to 20 min of the hospital. Most often the patient gets a chest X-ray and after an aortic dissection is ruled out, gets started on heparin and a Gp2b/3a receptor antagonist, before the cath-lab team takes the patient to the cath lab for PCI.

- **Facilitated PCI:** In the PACT study, administration of a 50 mg t-PA bolus prior to angiography demonstrated better TIMI-3 flow rates compared to heparin alone, but this did not have any bearing on the eventual result of the PCI, on LV function, or on the clinical outcome. In the PRAGUE trial,

t-PA administration at time of transport for PCI was associated with higher mortality and CVA at 30 days, as compared to those who underwent PCI without preprocedural t-PA. In small, nonrandomized single institution studies, there appeared to be some benefit from use of half-dose lytic therapy in patients being transferred for PCI. There were reports of improved TIMI-3 flow with this strategy. However, the recently published large randomized trial (FINESSE) looking into this matter failed to show any benefit with half-dose lytic theapy prior to angioplasty and therefore, is no longer recommended.

- **Rescue PCI:** In patients who fail to achieve reperfusion with fibrinolytic therapy should be transferred to a hospital for emergent PCI. This has a higher mortality than primary PTCA (5% to 10%) and if rescue PCI fails to establish adequate myocardial perfusion, the mortality is as high as 35% to 40%. The poor outcomes are caused by occlusion of the distal coronary microcirculation by edema, leukocytes, platelet aggregates, and distal embolization of thrombus or plaque debris. The results of rescue PCI have improved over the course of the last decade with the use of intracoronary stents and Gp2b/3a receptor antagonists like abciximab during PCI. Patients with persistent ST elevation and chest pain 90 min after administration of fibrinolytic agent and those with hemodynamic instability should be considered for emergency angiography and rescue-PCI.

- **Immediate or adjunctive-PCI:** Coronary angiography and PCI that is performed routinely within hours or days after successful reperfusion with fibrinolytics is called immediate or adjunctive-PCI. After successful fibrinolysis, there usually is a significant residual plaque in the infarct-related vessel which potentially can cause recurrent ischemia or reinfarction. Recent trials, like SIAM III and GARCIA, have shown significant reduction in recurrent ischemia. Retrospective analyses of trials like InTIME-II and TIMI have also shown significant reduction in mortality with adjunctive-PCI performed routinely after fibrinolytic therapy. Adjunctive-PCI has, therefore, become quite a routine in clinical practice in the United States. There are, however, certain specific indications for postfibrinolytic cardiac catheterization and revascularization: (a) previous history of MI, CAD, PCI, or bypass surgery; (b) LV dysfunction with LVEF less than or equal to 40%; (c) recurrent ischemia (either spontaneous or by stress testing); (d) ventricular tachyarrhythmias with hemodynamic instability; and (e) VT after the first 48 h of reperfusion.

- **Delayed PCI:** Delayed PCI several days after fibrinolysis is fully justified for recurrent ischemia, reinfarction, heart failure, or significant ventricular arrhythmias. With successful PCI, ventricular remodeling and LVEF are improved and these patients may tend to have fewer ventricular arrhythmias. Thus, it may be worthwhile attempting late revascularization (PCI or CABG surgery) in occluded coronary vessels if there is evidence of myocardial viability and especially if a large area of myocardium is in jeopardy.

- **Antithrombotic therapy in primary PCI:** Patients undergoing primary PCI for STEMI should receive UFH (50 to 70 units/kg bolus followed by an infusion at rate of 12 to 15 units/kg/h). Heparin should be started while the patient is waiting to be transferred to the cardiac catheterization laboratory. The ACT in the cardiac catheterization laboratory must be kept 200 to 250 s with concomitant use of a Gp2b/3a receptor antagonist and greater than 300 s if heparin is used alone. An infusion of heparin after the procedure is unnecessary, unless an IABP is used or if the result is unsatisfactory and there is ongoing ischemia postprocedure. The vascular sheaths are generally removed 3 to 6 h after heparin dosing (typically when the ACT is below 170 s). Enoxaparin can be used as an alternative to heparin in the dose of 1 mg/kg subcutaneously twice daily. There is no need to monitor ACT or for additional antithrombotic therapy if PCI is done within 8 h of enoxaparin dose. The vascular sheaths can be removed 8 to 12 h after the last dose of enoxaparin.

- **Bivalirudin in STEMI:** Bivalirudin is a DTI. Recent HORIZONS-AMI trial showed lower cardiac death and bleeding rates at 30 days with bivalirudin compared to standard treatment of heparin combined with Gp2b/3a receptor antagonists in STEMI patients undergoing emergent PCI. The drug although becoming more popular with interventional cardiologists has not yet achieved universal acceptance, mainly because of the costs.

- **Gp2b/3a receptor antagonists in primary PCI:** Gp2b/3a receptor antagonist agents are routinely used in patients with AMI. Abciximab has been shown to be beneficial in STEMI patients and as an adjunctive pharmacological therapy for primary PCI. Many interventional cardiologists use this agent routinely in almost all STEMI patients. Others would use it selectively in those with large thrombus burden, diabetic patients, and

complications like distal embolization and dissections. Many hospitals are now using one or the other small molecule agents (eptifibatide and tirofiban) for patients with STEMI, since the incidence of dangerous bleeding, thrombocytopenia, and pulmonary hemorrhage are lower with these agents as compared with abciximab. For best results, the medications should be started prior to the start of the PCI procedure.

- **Clopidogrel:** This is given as a 300 to 600 mg bolus at the completion of the acute-infarct PCI, particularly in those who receive intracoronary stents. The medication is generally continued for a minimum of 12 months in AMI patients receiving DES.

Indications for CABG in STEMI

- Urgent or emergent CABG may be necessary in up to 5% to 8% of patients with STEMI undergoing emergent PCI. The usual indication for emergent CABG is failure of reperfusion with PCI, a large area of jeopardized myocardium, a coronary anatomy suitable for CABG, especially if the patient is within 6 to 12 h of an acute infarction.

- Patients with mechanical complications of an MI, such as acute MR, acute VSD or wall ruptures, are also candidates for emergent surgery. Patients with certain coronary anatomies may benefit from emergent or urgent CABG: severe left main disease (>70% stenosis) and severe proximal multivessel disease (especially those with CHF or cardiogenic shock).

- The mortality is 10% to 15% in STEMI patients undergoing emergent CABG within the first few hours of infarction. However, this may be the only way to salvage myocardium in some patients with STEMI who fail PCI. Improvement in techniques for myocardial preservation (like use of blood cardioplegia) during CABG has certainly improved outcomes with emergent surgery. Also, it is important to keep bypass pump time short in these patients. In fairly stable patients, one should try to graft the left internal mammary artery (LIMA) to the left anterior descending (LAD) artery (wherever applicable), but in unstable patients vein grafts are preferred, as this shortens the time on the bypass pump.

- In patients with cardiogenic shock who are less than 75 years of age, emergent bypass surgery should be considered as soon as possible if they are not candidates for PCI or if they fail PCI. Stabilization with IABP counterpulsation and vasopressors is necessary before and after surgery in most of these patients. In patients with STEMI presenting late (>12 to 24h) and in the need for CABG, it may be advisable to wait for few days to a week before surgery, especially they are not showing any signs of acute ischemia and are relatively stable. The surgical mortality in stabilized STEMI patients is lower than in those who undergo emergent surgery within the first 24h of infarction.

- In patients needing emergent CABG, use of Gp2b/3a receptor antagonist and clopidogrel before surgery will increase risk of bleeding.

These agents must be stopped right away when the decision to operate on these patients is made. Cautious dosing of heparin based on ACT while going on bypass pump may also reduce the risk of bleeding in these patients, many of whom would have also received Gp2b/3a receptor antagonists. For patients who have received abciximab and/or clopidogrel, infusion of 6 to 12 units of platelets while coming off pump will serve to reduce postoperative bleeding (Fig. 21-4).

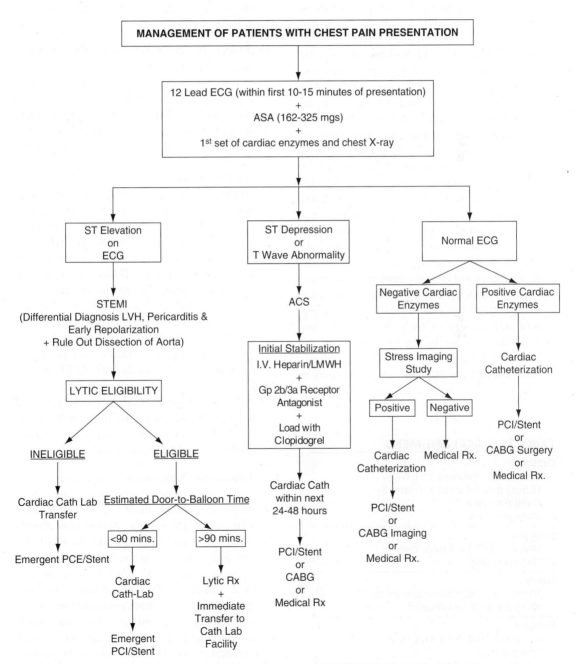

■ **FIGURE 21-4** Management of patients with chest pain presentation algorithm.

Medical Treatment of STEMI Patients after Reperfusion Therapy:

(1) *Antiplatelet Therapy* Aspirin (81 to 162 mg per day) should be given indefinitely to all patients with history of MI or CAD. Clopidogrel is routinely given for all those who receive stents for a duration of 6 to 12 months or longer.

(2) *Angiotensin-Converting Enzyme Inhibitors* ACEI favorably influence ventricular remodeling after AMI, thereby reducing the risk of dilated cardiomyopathy, CHF, and death. The benefits of ACEI therapy in post-MI patients have been shown in several large trials, including GISSI-3 and ISIS-4. The greatest benefits have been observed in patients at highest risk (e.g., patients with large anterior wall infarctions, patients who are older than 70 years of age, and women). Ideally, an oral ACEI is started within 24 to 48 h of the onset of the infarction. Intravenous dosing and use of "loading doses" are not only unnecessary but may prove harmful. Several examples of potential ACEI regimens are presented in Table 21-5. Contraindications to ACE therapy include known hypersensitivity, cardiogenic shock, renal failure, and bilateral renal artery stenosis. Renal insufficiency is not a contraindication for ACEI therapy, but one should monitor creatinine and potassium closely. In patients at low risk, there may not be any benefit beyond the first 3 to 6 months of an AMI. By contrast, high-risk patients (such as those with ejection fractions below 40%, overt heart failure, or clinical evidence of a large infarction) benefit from long-term (potentially permanent) therapy. As a matter of practicality, all patients with MI once started on an ACEI continue the medication indefinitely. Large trials have failed to substantiate fears that ACEI could worsen outcome by precipitating hypotension.

(3) *Angiotensin-II Receptor Blocker Antagonists* alsartan or candesartan can be used instead of ACEI in post-AMI patients who are intolerant to ACEI and have LVEF less than 40% and/or CHF.

(4) *β-Blockers* β-Blockers have been shown to reduce risk of recurrent MI and sudden death in patients with previous MI. They also may help prevent adverse LV remodeling after an MI (along with ACEI therapy) and risk of ventricular arrhythmias. Long-term β-blocker therapy with either metoprolol or atenolol (β_1 receptor antagonists) is recommended. Carvedilol can also be used in patients with severe LV dysfunction and heart failure. In this patient population, it has been shown to significantly reduce mortality. Far more expensive than metoprolol or atenolol, carvedilol blocks β_1-, β_2-, and α-receptors and has also been shown to have antioxidant properties. β-Blockers have been shown to improve survival in all patient subgroups, including those in whom they are traditionally considered as relatively contraindicated (diabetics, chronic obstructive pulmonary disease [COPD], heart failure, and peripheral vascular disease). Just as with ACEI therapy, β-blockers should be started in small dosage and gradually increased as tolerated. They must be used with caution in those with severe COPD or bronchospasm, overt CHF, bradyarrhythmias, and brittle diabetes.

(5) *Aldosterone-Antagonists* Eplerenone (an aldosterone receptor antagonist) has been shown to reduce mortality in post-MI patients with severe LV systolic dysfunction already taking ACEI and β-blockers in the EPHESUS trial. Spironolactone is another agent with similar action that could potentially be used in these patients. Although cheaper in cost, spironolactone has more unpleasant endocrine side effects compared to eplerenone. These include hirsutism in women and painful gynecomastia in men. Therefore, all post-MI patients with LVEF less than 40%, symptomatic CHF, or

TABLE 21-5 ACEI REGIMENS

Captopril
  6.25 mg p.o., followed 2 h later by
  12.5 mg p.o., followed 12 h later by
  25 mg p.o., then
  50 mg p.o. b.i.d

Lisinopril
  5 mg p.o. daily for 2 days, then
  10 mg p.o. daily

Enalapril
  2.5 mg p.o. b.i.d. titrated upward to
  10 mg p.o. b.i.d. as tolerated

Ramipril
  2.5 mg p.o. b.i.d. for 2 days, then
  5 mg p.o. b.i.d

diabetes mellitus and without renal failure (creatinine < 2.5 mg%) or hyperkalemia (potassium > 5.0 mmol/L) should be considered for an aldosterone-antagonist if they are already on an ACEI. The preferred agent is spironolactone at a dose of 25 mg per day, but may be switched to eplerenone (25 mg per day) in the event of side effects. Creatinine and potassium must be monitored closely in all these patients.

5 (6) *Statin Therapy*   Multiple, secondary prevention trials have all shown reduction of reinfarction and death in post-MI patients. The previous trials like CARE have shown benefit in those with LDL-c greater than 125 mg per dL, but the more recent PROVE IT trial and the Heart Protection Study have shown benefit even in those with LDL-c less than 100 mg/dL. It now appears that aggressive LDL-c reduction in this patient population to levels less than 70 mg/dL would significantly reduce risk of recurrent AMI or death. Thus, the current guidelines suggest achieving a goal LDL-c level less than 70 mg/dL in these patients, with use of powerful statin drugs like atorvastatin or simvastatin. One must monitor these patients periodically for side effects like myalgias, myositis, and drug-induced hepatitis. Statin therapy should be continued indefinitely if well tolerated. If the patient experiences side effects, lower doses or a switch to a less-powerful statin like pravastatin seems indicated.

(7) *Antiarrhythmic Agents*   Routine use of prophylactic antiarrhythmic therapy is not necessary in patients with AMI. Even though PVCs and nonsustained VT are markers of increased risk of SCD, especially in the setting of decreased LV systolic function, their suppression with antiarrhythmic agents may actually result in increased mortality because of proarrhythmic phenomena (CAST trial findings). The best way to reduce risk of SCD in these patients is by means of quick reperfusion, use of β-blockers and ACEI. β-Blockers and ACEI have been shown to reduce SCD in the long-term through positive ventricular remodeling, which also ensures electrical stability. Antiplatelet agents (aspirin, clopidogrel) and statins have also been shown to reduce SCD long-term in post-MI patients. There is epidemiological evidence supporting use of fish oils rich in omega-3 fatty acids, which have been shown to reduce to risk of SCD. In patients with STEMI resuscitated from VF arrest and in those with symptomatic sustained VT, one may consider amiodarone, which is not only very effective in suppressing ventricular and supraventricular arrhythmias, but also one of the safest antiarrhythmic agents from the standpoint of proarrhythmia. It may also be indicated for prophylaxis against recurrent AF, in which case it is usually given for 8 to 12 weeks. In dire emergencies like resuscitated VF arrest, sustained VT, and symptomatic supraventricular tachycardia (SVT) including AF, it is usually given intravenously in the dose of 150 mg bolus followed by infusion of 1 mg per min for 6 h, followed by infusion of 0.5 mg per min for 18 h. This is usually followed by oral amiodarone therapy lasting for 3 to 6 months or longer.

(8) *Calcium Channel Blockers*   Although they are effective for controlling acute hypertension, reversing coronary spasm, and relieving pain of coronary thrombosis, calcium channel antagonists have not improved survival in several clinical trials; in at least one study, short-acting nifedipine adversely affected survival. Therefore, the routine use of calcium channel antagonists cannot be advocated. In the event of severe hypertension complicating AMI or UA, however, diltiazem or amlodipine may be used along with the use of ACEI agents and β-blockers.

(9) *Warfarin*   Chronic systemic anticoagulation is indicated in those at risk for systemic or venous thromboembolism, like those with large anterior MI with akinetic apex, severely reduced LV function, AF, and presence of LV thrombus on echocardiography. In patients with large anterior MI, warfarin may be continued for 3 to 6 months.

General Support

Close monitoring for electrical and mechanical complications and direct control of pain and stress are basic measures applied for all MI victims. A liquid diet usually is provided for 24 h after infarction. Temperature extremes of foods are avoided in an attempt to minimize the risk of arrhythmias. Sedation and stool softeners to prevent anxiety and straining also may decrease the risk of arrhythmias. When systemic anticoagulation is not performed, subcutaneous heparin (7,500 units SQ b.i.d) or enoxaparin (40 mg SQ, once daily) is indicated for the prevention of deep venous thrombosis for patients with MI on strict bed rest. Once adequately reperfused, ambulation within the next day or so is advisable. Cardiac rehabilitation personnel should make an initial evaluation, preferably soon after reperfusion therapies. Despite numerous large-scale clinical trials, several commonly used therapies remain of unproven benefit (Tables 21-6 and 21-7).

Outcome of Myocardial Infarction

Overall, MI carries a mortality of approximately 15% to 20%. Most of the deaths occur within the first hour or two of infarction and are the result of prehospital ventricular arrhythmias, which, to a large degree cannot be prevented. The in-hospital death rate is around 5% to 9%, which has improved significantly over the last 3 to 4 decades, because of advances in reperfusion therapies. In contrast to prehospital mortality, most of the deaths in patients reaching the hospital occur from refractory pump failure. Therefore, survival is maximized by limit-

ing infarct size and by promptly treating mechanical and electrical complications. Survival is best predicted by the patient's age, preinfarction physical fitness, degree of left ventricular impairment (a reflection of the mass of lost myocardium), and comorbid conditions.

Complications of Myocardial Infarction

Half of all patients sustaining MI have no significant complications. Of those with a complicated course, most serious events occur within the first 5 days. Complications generally fall into one of two categories—electrical or mechanical. With the advent of specialized coronary care units able to immediately treat arrhythmias, mechanical complications have assumed greater importance.

Electrical Complications

A detailed discussion of arrhythmias, heart block, and the use of cardiac pacing is presented in Chapter 4. Tachyarrhythmias are very common within the first 3 days after MI as a result of the electrical instability from ischemic or dying cells. Fortunately, most early tachyarrhythmias are self-limited. These early arrhythmias have little prognostic import if they receive appropriate treatment when symptomatic. A major change in the philosophy of caring for patients with MI has occurred in the practice of tachyarrhythmia treatment. Whereas essentially all patients with MI once received prophylactic antiarrhythmic therapy (lidocaine) to suppress ventricular tachyarrhythmias, the use of routine arrhythmia prophylaxis is now rare. Amiodarone is now favored (over lidocaine) in those with sustained symptomatic VT and in those who have survived VF. Although effective in suppressing ventricular tachyarrhythmias, lidocaine can increase risk of asystole.

Premature Ventricular Contractions

PVCs occur in almost all patients with MI, but their incidence declines rapidly with time. (Baseline rates are usually restored within 24 to 72 h.) Isolated unifocal PVCs are of little importance. However, in the setting of acute infarction, consideration should be given to treating PVCs only if they are frequent and precipitate angina or hemodynamic instability. Besides myocardial reperfusion, use of β-blockers and correction of electrolyte imbalances (keep potassium > 4 mmol/L and magnesium > 2 mmol/L)

TABLE 21-6 UNPROVEN INTERVENTIONS IN ACUTE MI

Antiarrhythmic agents
Calcium channel antagonists
Magnesium sulfate therapy

TABLE 21-7 THERAPY OF ACUTE MI

Acute therapy
Aspirin, 325 mg p.o.
Sublingual TNG p.r.n. for pain
Morphine sulfate, 2–10 mg IV p.r.n. for pain
Oxygen 2–3 L by nasal cannula
IV β-blocker
Consider thrombolytic therapy, PTCA
Continue ECG monitoring, daily aspirin, and
  β-blocker

Day 1
Oral ACEI for high-risk patients
Begin risk factor modification

During hospitalization
Consider starting ACEI and β-blocker if not
  started on admission

6-Weeks postdischarge
Discontinue ACEI for low-risk patients with
  ejection fraction > 40%, without CHF

1-Year postdischarge
Discontinue β-blocker if low risk and no other
  indications exist for its use

Indefinitely
Continue aspirin and risk factor modification

will help a great deal. Less commonly, intravenous followed by oral amiodarone may be used if the patient continues to have troublesome ventricular arrhythmias. Although expensive, intravenous amiodarone has replaced lidocaine as the drug of choice for ventricular arrhythmias because of its effectiveness and safety profile. If used at all, lidocaine should probably be reserved for young patients with good pump function. For patients with hepatic disease, poor LV function, and high-grade AV block and for elderly patients, the risks of prophylactic lidocaine usually exceed the benefits. In the skillfully monitored critical care unit, the development of early VT or VF is of little importance because it is corrected rapidly by electrical cardioversion.

Ventricular Tachycardia

For patients with acute ischemia, sustained VT occurs commonly within the first 48 h and usually needs suppression. During an episode of VT, if the patient becomes unstable, immediate DC-cardioversion should be performed. If the rate is less than 150/min and patient relatively stable, antiarrhythmic therapy should be tried. Amiodarone is the drug of choice for control, initially given as a 150 or 300 mg bolus, followed by an infusion of 1 mg per min for 6 h and 0.5 mg per min for 18 h. Oral amiodarone is usually overlapped with intravenous form of the medication and should be continued for 3 to 6 months. Lidocaine infusion can also be used in this situation. It is given in bolus of 75 mg intravenously, followed by 50 mg every 5 min × 3 (for a total of 225 mg). The bolus doses achieve rapid therapeutic concentration. It is important to use lean body weight in calculating lidocaine doses to avoid toxicity. After loading, a continuous infusion of 1 to 2 mg per min is used for continued control. Because lidocaine is eliminated by the liver, patients with hepatic disease, CHF with passive hepatic congestion, and advanced age can have a reduced rate of clearance. In such patients the loading dose should be lowered to 75 to 125 mg and the infusion rate to 0.5 to 1 mg per min. Toxicity usually is manifest as either a CNS alteration (e.g., agitation, somnolence, seizures, confusion, muscle twitching) or cardiac effect (hypotension, bradycardia, sinus arrest). Plasma lidocaine levels probably should be monitored on a daily basis in patients at highest risk for lidocaine toxicity and should be spot checked in all patients who exhibit CNS alterations compatible with lidocaine toxicity. For patients who are refractory to the effects of lidocaine in therapeutic doses, procainamide is given in an intravenous infusion at a dose of 20 mg per min loading dose until arrhythmia is suppressed, a total of 17 mg/kg is administered, hypotension occurs, or if QRS duration increases beyond 50%. Following the bolus, it is continued as an infusion at a dose of 1 to 4 mg per min. Procainamide can induce *torsades de pointes* in patients with hypokalemia, hypomagnesemia, LV dysfunction, and renal failure. Continuous monitoring of BP and ECG is necessary during procainamide infusion.

Prompt myocardial reperfusion, β-blocker therapy, and correction of electrolyte and metabolic abnormalities are vital in ensuring electrical stability in these patients.

One particular form of VT, IVR, deserves special mention. Usually self-limited, IVR is a series of wide QRS complexes of ventricular origin. When IVR occurs at a rate of 60 to 100 beats/min, it is termed "accelerated." This rhythm most commonly occurs after reperfusion of ischemic myocardium or as an escape mechanism for patients with high-grade AV block. If perfusion is adequate, no treatment is indicated. Indeed, suppression may cause asystole.

VT that occurs within the first 48 h has no long-term impact on patients' mortality. However, that which occurs afterward usually does so in the setting of LV dysfunction and carries increased risk of mortality. These patients must all be revascularized appropriately and considered for defibrillator implantation.

Ventricular Fibrillation

VF occurs in up to 10% of all cases of MI and is responsible for 65% of all deaths. Most deaths occur in the prehospital phase of care, usually within the first hour of ischemia. An additional 15% to 20% of patients suffer VF after hospitalization. If applied promptly, DC-cardioversion can correct more than 50% of episodes of acute VF due to AMI. Defibrillation is successful in less than 25% if applied after 4 min of onset of VF. VF carries little prognostic import if defibrillation is successful and if the disturbance occurs as an isolated electrical event early in the course of an MI (within first 24 to 48 h). VT or VF after the first 48 h of an MI usually occurs in the setting of poor LV systolic function and carry a poor long-term prognosis. These patients must be considered for implantable cardioverter–defibrillators (ICD). Reversible factors increasing the risk of VF should be addressed promptly, and these include ongoing ischemia, electrolyte imbalances, anemia, hypoxemia, excessive catecholamine stimulation, or presence of pulmonary artery catheters or pacemakers in the heart. For refractory or recurrent VF, intravenous amiodarone or lidocaine can be used after the initial resuscitation. Intravenous procainamide can be given in rare situations where the arrhythmia is refractory to lidocaine or amiodarone. Magnesium sulfate (1 to 2 gm intravenously) has been advocated as a safe, prophylactic antiarrhythmic agent. It can be used in patients with polymorphic VT or hypomagnesemia. Although magnesium is almost certainly safe in patients with normal renal function, commonly used doses are of questionable efficacy.

Bradycardia

Bradyarrhythmias occur more commonly in inferior and posterior MIs because of intense vagal stimulation and a higher incidence of sinoatrial (SA) and AV nodal ischemia resulting from occlusion of the right or circumflex coronary arteries. AV block and use of pacemakers are described in detail in Chapter 4. Bundle branch blocks and infranodal high-grade AV blocks that occur in the setting of an anterior MI carry poor prognosis because of the extent of myocardial damage and usually need permanent pacing if the patient survives. Acute right bundle branch block (RBBB) occurs in about 5% of acute infarctions and is associated with increased mortality. Transcutaneous or transvenous pacing may be needed if there is symptomatic bradycardia. Acute LBBB, which complicates 1% to 5% of acute infarcts, is associated with a 25% rate of in-hospital mortality and pacing may be needed in these patients as well.

AF is not uncommon and is usually of acute onset. Acute and rapid AF can precipitate heart failure. The patient must be anticoagulated with IV heparin or enoxaprin (1 mg/kg SQ b.i.d). Initially, the ventricular rate can be controlled with beta-blockers or calcium-channel blockers. The patient should be cardioverted with IV amiodarone or by electrical means in situations of acute AF. The patient may need to stay on oral amiodarone for 6 to 8 after cardioversion if amiodarone had been used.

Mechanical Complications

Pericarditis/Tamponade

Post-MI pericarditis can be divided conveniently into two distinct types: acute early pericarditis and delayed pericarditis (Dressler syndrome). The pain of pericarditis may be distinguished from that of continued or recurrent myocardial ischemia by its failure to radiate to distant sites, its poor response to antianginal therapy, the presence of a friction rub, and its sharp, pleuritic, or positional nature. The ECG usually exhibits diffuse ST segment elevation not typically seen after occlusion of a major coronary artery. Histologic evidence of pericarditis occurs in almost all transmural MIs but usually is mild and clinically insignificant. Symptoms typical for pericarditis occur in only a small proportion of such cases. In the 10% of patients affected by acute pericarditis, symptoms usually emerge 2 to 4 days after the MI. Nonsteroidal anti-inflammatory drugs (e.g., aspirin and/or indomethacin) are helpful in controlling the inflammation and pain. Although effective as analgesic/anti-inflammatory agents, corticosteroids increase the risk of free ventricular wall rupture. Large pericardial fluid accumulations occur in fewer than 10%. Rarely, pericardial fluid may become hemorrhagic and accumulate sufficiently to cause tamponade in anticoagulated patients.

Delayed episodes of immunologically mediated febrile pleuropericarditis (Dressler syndrome) may complicate either MI or pericardiotomy any time within 3 months. Dressler syndrome is much less common than acute pericarditis, occurring in only 1% to 3% of patients with MI. Leukocytosis and an elevated sedimentation rate are associated laboratory features. Pleural effusions are common in Dressler syndrome but rare in acute pericarditis. Because there is substantial risk of hemorrhagic pericarditis and tamponade in Dressler syndrome, anticoagulants are contraindicated. Indomethacin, with or without colchicines, may be used in the treatment of this condition.

Pump Failure with Cardiogenic Shock

Most in-hospital deaths from MI occur within 96 h of admission secondary to shock resulting from LV failure. Clinical evidence of heart failure develops when more than 20% of the LV sustains damage. (Persistent ST may be a hint of incipient heart failure if present longer than 48 h after infarction.) Fatal pump failure usually ensues when more than 40% of the LV mass is infarcted or dysfunctional. The muscle mass lost during infarction is a much more powerful determinant of outcome than the anatomic location of the infarct. Therefore, rapid myocardial reperfusion is the key to an optimal outcome. Contractility of ischemic but salvageable muscle may return after a period of hours to days ("stunned myocardium"). Ischemia-induced decreases in LV compliance usually require increased filling pressures to maintain stable cardiac output. Under most circumstances, a pulmonary capillary wedge pressure near 18 mm Hg is optimal.

Pulmonary edema should be treated with oxygen, mechanical ventilation, diuretics, and inotropic drugs, as dictated by hemodynamics and ventilatory parameters. Coronary angiography with prompt revascularization by PCI or emergent coronary bypass surgery may be the only hope for most of these patients. Revascularization therapy may be particularly beneficial in those less than 75 years of age. Initial stabilization with IABP support is helpful. IABP counterpulsations not only reduce afterload, but also improve coronary blood flow. Because a substantial portion of the limited cardiac output must be diverted to the respiratory pump, mechanical ventilation can boost oxygen delivery to deprived vital organs and should be considered whenever respiratory distress becomes evident. Treatment of severe heart failure and cardiogenic shock are detailed in Chapter 3. Unfortunately, the prognosis for cardiogenic shock remains dismal, with in-hospital mortality of 50% to 80%.

Right Ventricular Infarction

Some degree of right ventricular (RV) infarction is seen in up to 30% to 40% of all inferior MIs. Hypotension, jugular venous distention, the Kussmaul sign, and clear lung fields are key diagnostic characteristics. An important feature distinguishing RV infarct from pulmonary embolism is the rarity of dyspnea in the former condition. RV infarction may be confirmed electrocardiographically by ST segment elevation in right precordial leads (V_3R and V_4R). Pulmonary artery catheterization may be confirmatory when right atrial pressures are disproportionately elevated in relation to a wedge pressure. (Hemodynamic monitoring is also useful to exclude the presence of pericardial tamponade or constriction, which may have similar clinical appearance.)

RV infarction, usually the result of RCA occlusion, rarely occurs as an isolated event. Inferior LV infarction almost always accompanies an RV infarct because LV wall thickness and afterload exceed those of the RV and because the RV, posterior interventricular septum, and inferior LV wall share a common blood supply.

The physiologic derangements of RV infarction closely parallel those of constrictive pericarditis and tamponade. As the RV fails, it dilates, restricting LV filling. This combination of reduced RV systolic function, RV dilation, and limited LV filling, which occurs within the poorly distensible pericardial sac, dramatically reduces cardiac output. The presenting symptom of RV infarction is hypotension—not pulmonary edema. Therefore, the treatment of the RV infarct differs in several important respects from symptomatic LV infarction. As a priority, the filling pressure of the RV must be optimized. This may require mean right atrial pressures higher than 20 mm Hg to maintain an acceptably high wedge pressure and cardiac output. Once adequate RV filling has been ensured, cautious trials of inotropic drugs and/or afterload reduction also may prove helpful.

Conduction disturbances are very common in RV infarction and are often refractory to ventricular pacing. Because of the difficulty in achieving successful ventricular pacing and because of the substantial contribution of the atria to cardiac output during RV infarction, *sequential* AV pacing is often more successful than ventricular pacing alone. AF occurring during RV infarction is particularly detrimental because of reduced ventricular compliance and should be treated aggressively with electrical or chemical cardioversion.

Atrial infarction occurs rarely, usually in combination with infarction of the inferior wall of the LV. Fed by branches of the RCA, the right atrium is the most commonly affected chamber. Ischemia of the SA node and conduction pathways accounts for its most common manifestations: bradycardia, atrial arrhythmias, and heart block. Thrombi formed within the infarcted right atrium may embolize to the pulmonary artery.

Acute Mitral Regurgitation

Papillary muscle dysfunction or rupture is the most common mechanical complication of MI. In most cases, mild and transient MR is the result of papillary muscle ischemia or changes in LV geometry. MR has a wide range of presentations, from minimal malfunction to frank rupture. MR most commonly results from malfunction of the posterior papillary muscle because it is fed by the single posterior descending artery, whereas the anterior papillary muscle is supplied by branches of both the left anterior descending and circumflex arteries. Frank papillary muscle rupture is a rare but highly lethal event that carries a 24-h mortality rate near 70%. MR typically occurs 2 to 10 days after posterior or inferior MI and should be suspected in any patient with MI developing a new murmur (often at the cardiac apex).

The murmur of MR is often unimpressive; therefore, a high degree of suspicion should be maintained anytime a patient rapidly develops symptoms of left ventricular failure, especially when normal systolic function seems preserved. Regurgitant flow is greatest after papillary muscle rupture and less intense when dysfunction is caused by ischemia without structural damage. The diagnosis may be confirmed by echocardiography or pulmonary artery catheterization. Echocardiography (especially transesophageal studies) may reveal a hyperdynamic (unloaded) LV and flail mitral leaflet. (The surface echocardiogram may fail to detect small valvular defects.) Doppler studies may demonstrate the regurgitant left atrial jet. Invasive monitoring is indicated in almost all patients with MI who develop a new murmur, particularly if pulmonary congestion is present. Although pulmonary artery pressure tracings usually reveal large V waves produced by retrograde flow of blood across an incompetent mitral valve, V waves are much more sensitive than specific. VSD, mitral stenosis, or severe heart failure occasionally mimics MR by producing large V waves.

The primary objective in treating acute MR is to reduce left ventricular impedance (afterload). For stable patients with mild MR, LV afterload reduction may be sufficient. However, when florid pulmonary edema follows papillary muscle rupture, vasodilators (nitroprusside, nicardipine, or NTG) and intraaortic balloon pumping should be followed immediately by surgery.

Ventricular Septal Defect

The ventricular septum ruptures in approximately 2% of all MIs. Predisposing factors for postinfarction VSD include an anterior–septal MI, hypertension, female gender, advanced age, and first infarction. VSD-related, left-to-right shunting reduces effective output and causes pulmonary edema. The anterior portion of the interventricular septum is supplied predominantly by a single vessel (the left anterior descending), whereas the posterior portion is fed collaterally by several sources. Therefore, postinfarction VSD usually is a consequence of an anterior MI that involves the LAD. Conversely, VSD developing after a (true) posterior MI is a marker of diffuse multivessel disease and carries a worse prognosis.

For most patients, physical examination reveals biventricular heart failure and a new murmur. The new murmur usually is loud, harsh, holosystolic, and of maximal intensity at the left lower sternal border. An accompanying thrill is common. Pulmonary artery catheterization demonstrates a step-up in hemoglobin saturation between the right atrium and pulmonary artery (usually > 10%). Diagnosis also can be made by left heart catheterization demonstrating movement of contrast from the LV to the RV. Hemodynamic compromise and magnitude of the left-to-right shunt parallel the size of the defect. Echocardiography may demonstrate a VSD, particularly if Doppler techniques and transesophageal imaging are used. A "bubble" echocardiogram (with agitated saline or optisonic contrast) occasionally shows bidirectional ventricular flow.

Therapy for a VSD depends on systemic and pulmonary capillary wedge pressures. Hypotensive patients with a low wedge pressure should receive fluids initially. If the blood pressure is maintained adequately and the wedge pressure is lower than 18 mm Hg, semielective surgical repair should be undertaken. Vasodilators may be useful if blood pressure remains adequate despite a low cardiac output and an elevated wedge pressure. If the patient is hypotensive with a high wedge pressure, temporary support by balloon pumping, ionotropes, and vasodilators should precede immediate surgical correction.

There are currently devices (AMPLATZER, CARDIOSEAL) that are available for percutaneous closure of a VSD. This is alternative to surgery, especially in sick patients where the surgical risk is quite high.

The outcome of post-MI VSD is very poor, with mortality mounting to approximately 90% at 2 months. However, the long-term results in patients undergoing successful early repair are excellent. Therefore, surgical repair at the earliest possible time after hemodynamic stabilization is desirable.

Free Wall Rupture

Almost invariably, rupture of the ventricular free wall proves rapidly fatal, as the patient succumbs to tamponade physiology. Although unusual (incidence between 2% and 8%), ventricular rupture occurs more commonly than either papillary muscle rupture or VSD; 10% of MI deaths result from free wall rupture. Most myocardial ruptures are early events; half occur within 4 days and almost all occur within 2 weeks after AMI. Hypertension accentuates wall stress and contributes to muscle disruption at the border of the normal and infarcted tissue. Ventricular rupture is most likely in elderly patients with extensive transmural damage and little collateral flow. Use of late fibrinolysis may hasten the occurrence of perforation. The clinical presentation of wall rupture usually is one of recurrent chest pain rapidly followed by neck vein distention, paradoxical pulse, shock, and death. ECG may show recurrent ST elevation or may not show any change at all. Differential diagnosis includes pericardial tamponade, tension pneumothorax, and massive muscle damage. Immediate thoracotomy must follow temporary stabilization with volume expansion, transfusion, and pericardiocentesis. Echocardiography may visualize a defect of the LV wall, free pericardial fluid, and diastolic right-sided cardiac collapse. Cardiac catheterization is not feasible for most patients and delays definitive surgical therapy, which is perhaps the only hope in many patients with this condition.

Systemic Embolism

The incidence of mural thrombi and arterial embolism may reach 30% in selected subsets of patients with MI. Large infarctions, particularly those involving the anterior and apical segments of the LV, predispose systemic embolism. Systemic embolism is less common now that many patients receive heparin and aspirin (with or without thrombolytic therapy) for AMI therapy. Patients with large infarctions, mural thrombi, or overtly dyskinetic segments on echocardiography should be anticoagulated, unless compelling contraindications exist.

Role of ICD in Myocardial Infarction

Patients who demonstrate sustained or nonsustained VT after the first 48 h of AMI are at increased risk of SCD during and after discharge from hospital. Severe LV systolic dysfunction is also a marker of risk for SCD. An ICD device is implanted just like a pacemaker, and in fact, most of the currently available ICD models can also pace the heart for bradycardia. The ICD device monitors the rhythm, and if the patient goes into rapid VT, it is programmed to perform antitachycardia pacing, followed by delivery of DC shock if needed. If the patient drops into VF, it will deliver a shock immediately. The risk of SCD can be reduced significantly after revascularization and with use of adequate medical therapies (β-blocker, antiplatelet agents [clopidogrel and aspirin], statin, ACEI, and possibly also fish oils). The MADIT-1, MADIT-2, and MUSTT trials have helped form some guidelines for ICD implantation in post-MI patients.

The following are the guidelines for use of an ICD device following an MI:

1. Resuscitated VT/VF arrest after the first 48 h of an MI.
2. LV ejection fraction less than 35%, nonsustained VT on monitor, and inducible, nonsuppressible VT on EP study.
3. LV ejection fraction less than 30% on echocardiography 1 month after MI, especially if the QRS duration is greater than 0.12 s.

Patients with incessant VT/VF episodes, those with class IV CHF, those with other severe comorbid conditions (terminal cancer, lung or liver disease) are considered contraindications for the ICD. Those with ischemic cardiomyopathy should ideally undergo revascularization procedures first (if they are candidates) and later be reevaluated for ICD. Patients who have suffered a large MI should undergo repeat echocardiography and possibly also 24- or 48-h Holter monitoring 1 to 3 months after the event.

■ SUGGESTED READINGS

Antman EM, Van de Werf F. Pharmacoinvasive therapy: The future of treatment for ST-elevation MI. *Circulation*. 2004;109(21):2480–2486.

Fox KA. Management of acute coronary syndromes: An update. *Heart* 2004; 90(6):698–706.

Gluckman TJ, Sachdev M, Schulman SP, et al. A simplified approach to the management of non-ST-segment elevation acute coronary syndromes. *JAMA*. 2005;293(3):349–357.

Rebeiz AG, Roe MT, Alexander JH, et al. Integrating antithrombin and antiplatelet therapies with early invasive management for non-ST-segment elevation acute coronary syndromes. *Am J Med*. 2004; 116(2):119–129.

Roe MT, Ohman EM, Pollack CV Jr, et al. Changing the model of care for patients with acute coronary syndromes. *Am Heart J*. 2003;146(4): 605–612.

Hypertensive Emergencies

■ DEFINITIONS

Historically, the term "malignant hypertension" was defined by severe elevations of blood pressure (BP) and advanced retinopathy and papilledema. For patients meeting this definition, accompanying organ dysfunction was common but not universal. Similarly, "accelerated hypertension" was traditionally defined by comparable elevations of BP with lesser degrees of retinopathy in patients not exhibiting other organ damage. Unfortunately, this distinction is artificial and not very clinically useful.

A simpler and more useful approach is to classify hypertensive crises by the presence or absence of life-threatening organ damage and hence, the urgency for treatment. When organ failure accompanies severe hypertension, interventions to reduce BP toward normal should be accomplished within minutes to hours, whereas in cases of hypertension without organ failure, more gradual BP reduction over hours to days is prudent.

■ PATHOPHYSIOLOGY

Organ damage in hypertension is caused largely by a small vessel (arteriolar) necrotizing vasculitis that results in platelet and fibrin deposition and loss of vascular autoregulation raising systemic vascular resistance (SVR). In most patients, the pathophysiology of a hypertensive emergency is elevated SVR, not volume overload or elevated cardiac output. In reality, absent renal failure, ongoing hypertension results in natriuresis and intravascular volume *contraction*. Therefore, the most efficacious hypertension treatments reduce afterload, not preload and in some cases, intravenous volume expansion may even be necessary.

Although hypertension with a specific etiologic cause is rare in the general population, as many as half of all patients presenting for the first time with hypertension-induced organ failure are discovered to have an identifiable cause of hypertension. Young patients (<30 years of age) and those of African descent are more likely to have one of these secondary (usually, renovascular or endocrine) causes. Most hypertensive crises seen in the intensive care unit (ICU) are not, however, these newly discovered patients with secondary hypertension but rather patients, more commonly men, with **1** known "essential" hypertension noncompliant with previously effective medical therapy. Oftentimes, these days cocaine use is a contributing factor. Regardless of the etiology, hypertension-induced organ failure is a serious problem. Historically, more than 90% of patients presenting with organ failure from hypertension were dead within a year of the diagnosis. Although the causes of death from hypertension have not changed, (heart failure, myocardial infarction, stroke, and renal failure) mortality rates are now less than 10% provided the patient will simply take prescribed medications.

■ HISTORY AND PHYSICAL EXAMINATION

The goals of the history and physical are to distinguish hypertension that requires immediate treatment from that to be corrected more gradually and to define the reason for the crisis. Obtaining a history of long-standing hypertension, antihypertensive drug use, or illicit or over-the-counter drug use is critical. Knowledge of preexisting organ failures also helps define the urgency of therapy. (Patients with well-established chronic renal failure do not require the same haste for BP control as patients acutely developing a similar elevation in serum creatinine.) Most patients with hypertensive crises are symptomatic but have nonspecific complaints. Headache occurs in approximately 85% of patients and blurred vision occurs in more than 50%. Cardiac symptoms (e.g., angina, congestive heart failure) and dyspnea are frequent, whereas nausea, vomiting, and focal neurological deficits are distinctly uncommon.

BP should be measured in all four limbs using an appropriate-size cuff. Failure to compare upper to lower extremity BP risks missing aortic coarctation or distal dissection, whereas failure to detect asymmetrical arm BP risks missing proximal aortic dissection. Surprisingly, many patients presenting with severe hypertension exhibit orthostatic symptoms because of pressure-induced diuresis. Physical examination should devote special attention to inspection of the ocular fundus and to examination of the neurologic and cardiopulmonary systems. Retinopathy is a sensitive indicator of hypertension-induced organ injury. Papilledema, exudates, flame hemorrhages, and arteriolar constriction characterize the retinopathy traditionally associated with "malignant hypertension" and correlate well with renal involvement. After control of BP, retinal hemorrhages and papilledema resolve or heal over weeks to months. Confusion can be an important sign of hypertensive encephalopathy or ischemic or hemorrhagic stroke. Examination of the heart can reveal enlargement and a fourth heart sound with long-standing hypertension and a third heart sound in the presence of left ventricular decompensation. Murmurs of aortic or mitral insufficiency are important to identify as potential causes of pulmonary edema. Detection of an abdominal bruit, suggestive of renal artery stenosis, is an uncommon but critical physical finding.

Laboratory examination should include urinalysis, electrocardiogram, chest radiograph, blood smear, and determinations of electrolytes and creatinine. Evidence of left ventricular or atrial enlargement is common, occurring in about a quarter of patients. Renal insufficiency (i.e., serum creatinine > 3.5 mg/dL) is also present in about one fourth of cases. In patients with an elevated creatinine, urinalysis commonly shows proteinuria, hematuria, and red cell cast formation. The peripheral blood smear may demonstrate microangiopathic hemolysis. Hypokalemic alkalosis frequently occurs as a result of secondary hyperaldosteronism consequent to diuretic usage, but could be a clue to primary hyperaldosteronism.

■ TREATMENT PRINCIPLES

Hypertension with Organ Failure (Hypertensive Emergency)

The aggressiveness of therapy should be guided by **2** chronicity of the condition and evidence for organ damage, not by BP values alone. In fact, most patients with "severe hypertension" defined as a systolic BP greater than 160 mm Hg or a diastolic BP greater than 100 mm Hg have no acute organ dysfunction, and it is uncommon to see organ injury until the values exceed 220/130 mm Hg. A significant exception to this rule is the pregnant patient, in whom end-organ effects may be seen with diastolic values as low as 100 mm Hg. (Children can also have noteworthy end-organ damage at seemingly low BPs.) Patients requiring immediate treatment should be admitted to an ICU for closely monitored therapy. If there are doubts regarding the accuracy of noninvasive measurements, an arterial catheter can be inserted, but one is not routinely necessary.

Surprisingly, given the incidence of severe hypertension, there are no studies which demonstrate superiority of one drug class over another with regard **3** to organ protection or survival. Given lack of proven advantage of a particular treatment, drug selection is typically made based on patient characteristics, drug cost, and physician preference. The ideal emergency antihypertensive would be potent, titratable, intravenous, rapid but short-lived, and would act by reducing afterload. Sodium nitroprusside, nicardipine, and to a lesser degree, nitroglycerin best fit this description. The advantages and disadvantages of commonly used drugs for severe hypertension treatment are shown in Table 22-1. Whenever possible, oral

TABLE 22-1 PARENTERAL DRUG THERAPY FOR SEVERE HYPERTENSION

DRUG	TYPICAL DOSING	SITE OF ACTION	ADVANTAGES	SIDE EFFECTS/PROBLEMS
Clevidipine	Begin 2 mg/h Increase in 2 mg/h increments every 5–10 min	L-type Ca^{2+} blocker, arterial dilator	Rapid onset Rapid offset Plasma metabolism	Vomiting Time-limited refrigerated emulsion Expensive
Diazoxide	Begin with 1–2 mg boluses Increase to 5 mg bolus in 1 mg increments	Direct dilator (arterial and venous)	Rapid onset Not sedating	Imprecise dosing Reflex tachycardia Hyperuricemia Hyperglycemia
Esmolol	Begin 500 μg/kg load with 25–50 μg/kg/min infusion Increase in 25 μg/kg/min increments every 10 min	β-blocker	Rapid onset Antiarrhythmic Rapid offset	Exacerbates CHF and asthma Cardiac conduction block Nausea
Enalaprilat	Begin 1.25 mg every 4–6 h Increase by 1.25 mg increments with each subsequent dose	Angiotensin converting enzyme (ACE) inhibitor	Effective in high-renin states	Hypotension in volume depleted May exacerbate renal failure Headache Contraindicated in pregnancy
Fenoldopam	Begin 0.1 μg/kg/min infusion Increase in 0.1 μg/kg/min increments every 5–10 min	Dopamine 1 agonist	Increased renal blood flow	Expensive
Hydralazine	Begin 5–10 mg bolus every 15–20 min	Direct dilator (arterial > venous)	No CNS effects	Reflex tachycardia Overshoot hypotension Headache Vomiting

Drug	Dosing	Type	Advantages	Side Effects
Labetalol	20 mg boluses at 15-min intervals as needed or 20 mg bolus followed by 2 mg/min infusion. Increase in 2 mg/min increments every 10–15 min	α- and β-blocker	No "overshoot" hypotension. Preserved cardiac output	Exacerbates CHF and asthma. Cardiac conduction block. Tolerance with prolonged use
Nicardipine	Begin 5 mg/h. Increase in 2.5 mg/h increments every 10–15 min	Ca^{2+} blocker. Arterial dilator	Rapid onset. Easy to titrate. Coronary dilator	Reflex tachycardia. Headache
Nitroglycerin	Begin 5 μg/min. Increase in 5–10 μg/min increments every 5–10 min	Direct dilator (venous > arterial)	Coronary dilator. Rapid onset	Weak arterial dilator. Headache. Ethanol vehicle. Absorbed by some IV tubing
Nitroprusside	Begin 0.5 μg/kg/min. Increase in 1 μg/kg/min increments every 5–10 min. Caution at dose above 3–4 μg/kg/min	Direct dilator (balanced)	Rapid onset. Easy to titrate. Nonsedating. Rapid offset	Thiocyanate/cyanide toxicity. Reflex tachycardia. Vomiting. Light sensitive
Phentolamine	1–5 mg boluses	α-blocker + direct vasodilator	Excellent for adrenergic crisis. Rapid onset	Tachycardia. Angina. Vomiting. Tachyphylaxis
Trimethaphan	Begin infusion 0.3 mg/min. Increase dose in 0.3–0.6 mg/min increments every 10–15 min	Ganglionic blocker (balanced)	Aortic aneurysm. No CNS effects	Anticholinergic effects. Decreased cardiac output. Cycloplegia—blurred vision

4 therapy should be initiated concurrently to minimize the duration of IV therapy and ICU stay.

As a general rule, when acute myocardial infarction, aortic dissection, pulmonary edema, cerebral hemorrhage, or hypertensive encephalopathy **5** complicates severe hypertension, the goal should be to reduce diastolic BP by roughly 15% to 20% or achieve a diastolic BP near 110 mm Hg as quickly as possible (typically, within an hour). Slowly progressive renal insufficiency or mild left ventricular failure present less-threatening problems and mandate less-urgent treatment. In such cases, the goal should be to reduce the BP more gradually.

Hypertension Without Organ Failure (Hypertensive Urgency)

Although important, hypertension occurring in the absence of organ failure does not present the same urgency as that when organ failure is present. In this setting, a reasonable goal is also reduction in mean arterial BP by approximately 15% to 20%, usually to a diastolic value near 110 mm Hg but over a longer (24 to 48 h) period. Subsequent normalization of BP over days to weeks is safe and averts complications associated with rapid or excessive reductions.

An elevated BP alone does not necessarily require invasive monitoring or parenteral treatment. In fact, when hypertension is the result of cocaine, amphetamine, or phencyclidine ingestion, antihypertensive drugs may not even be needed; withholding the offending agent and providing judicious benzodiazepine sedation often suffices. In hypertensive urgencies, oral therapy can be successfully used (Table 22-2). Because many of these cases are the result of noncompliance with a previously effective regimen, merely restarting the patient's outpatient medications is often effective. It is important to identify the reasons for noncompliance for if it is due to prohibitive drug costs or intolerable side effects (e.g., sedation, fatigue, or impotence), the problem is likely to be repeated. Currently, as there are so many choices for antihypertensive treatment, such problems can almost always be surmounted. In previously untreated patients, oral clonidine and nifedipine have been used as initial treatment. Of the two, clonidine reduces BP more gradually (over 30 to 120 min) and is less likely to result in hypotension. However, many physicians are reluctant to use clonidine because of its propensity to cause sedation and potential for bradycardia and high-grade atrioventricular block. Short-acting nifedipine should be used very cautiously if at all. Patients with the highest BP usually show the largest declines, and occasionally disastrous results occur when BP plummets to dangerous levels.

■ SPECIFIC HYPERTENSIVE PROBLEMS

A summary of preferred therapy for various hypertensive emergencies is presented in Table 22-3; however, a brief discussion of the most common hypertensive situations below will emphasize the unique aspects of pathophysiology and treatment.

Hypertensive Encephalopathy

Hypertensive encephalopathy is diffuse brain dysfunction caused by cerebral edema resulting from the loss of central nervous system (CNS) vessel autoregulation. The rate at which the BP increases probably is as important as the absolute level achieved. In chronic hypertension, changes in cerebral autoregulation tend to reduce the risk of hypertensive encephalopathy, even with marked elevations in BP. By contrast, an acute BP rise during pregnancy or an episode of glomerulonephritis may cause encephalopathy with a BP as low as 160/100 mm Hg.

TABLE 22-2	ORAL REGIMENS FOR MODERATE HYPERTENSION		
DRUG	**INITIAL DOSE**	**SUBSEQUENT DOSES**	**DURATION**
Clonidine	0.1–0.2 mg orally	0.1 mg every 1 h to maximum dose of 0.7 mg	8–12 h
Nifedipine[a]	10 mg orally	10–20 mg every 15 min	3–6 h
Captopril[a]	12.5–25 mg	25 mg every 8 h	6–8 h

[a]Use with extreme caution.

TABLE 22-3 ANTIHYPERTENSIVE CHOICES IN SPECIFIC CONDITIONS

CONDITION	PREFERRED DRUGS	DRUGS TO AVOID
Dissecting aneurysm	Nitroprusside + β-blocker Nicardipine ± β-blocker Labetalol Trimethaphan	Direct vasodilators alone (nitroprusside diazoxide, hydralazine)
Pulmonary edema	Nitroprusside Nitrates Nicardipine Fenoldopam Diuretics	β-Blockers[a] Trimethaphan Labetalol
Angina/MI (without CHF)	β-Blockers Nitrates Nicardipine Calcium blockers Labetalol	Direct vasodilators alone (nitroprusside diazoxide, hydralazine) Phentolamine
Cerebral hemorrhage	No treatment (?) Nitroprusside Nicardipine	Trimethaphan Methyldopa Clonidine Diazoxide
Hypertensive encephalopathy	Nitroprusside Nicardipine Labetalol Fenoldopam	Methyldopa Clonidine Reserpine β-Blockers
Catecholamine excess	Phentolamine Trimethaphan Nicardipine Nitroprusside + β-blocker Benzodiazepine as adjunct	β-Blockers alone Diazoxide Labetalol
Postoperative HTN	Nitroprusside Nicardipine Esmolol	Long-acting agents
Preeclampsia	Labetalol Nicardipine	Angiotension converting enzyme inhibitors

[a]Exception: β-Blockers useful in pulmonary edema from diastolic dysfunction.

Hypertensive encephalopathy must be distinguished from the much more common mental-status-altering disorders, including ischemic or hemorrhagic stroke, hypoglycemia, subarachnoid hemorrhage, meningitis, encephalitis, brain tumors, and seizures. The distinction may be difficult because many of these conditions may be accompanied by secondary elevations of BP. Headache is the most common complaint, followed by nausea, vomiting, blurred vision, and confusion. Focal neurological deficits, including hemiparesis and cranial nerve palsies (particularly of the facial nerve), may occur but are uncommon. Arteritis of the vessels nourishing the optic nerve (not increased intracranial pressure) produces the papilledema seen in most cases of hypertensive encephalopathy. There are no specific laboratory findings in hypertensive encephalopathy; the electroencephalographic features are nondiagnostic, and although the opening pressure recorded during a lumbar puncture may be elevated, the fluid analysis usually is unremarkable.

The *sine qua non* of hypertensive encephalopathy is mental clearing within hours of BP control. Therefore, the goal of therapy is to lower the BP to "safe" levels as quickly as possible with nitroprusside, nicardipine, fenoldopam, or trimethaphan (now rarely used). A diastolic BP of 100 to 110 mm Hg is an appropriate initial target that must not be undershot. Normally, cerebral blood flow (CBF) is autoregulated to maintain constant perfusion over a wide range of mean arterial pressures (Fig. 22-1).

6

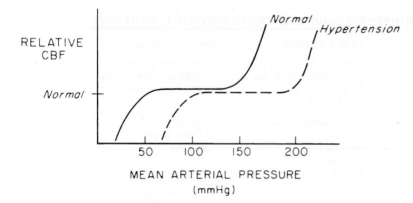

■ **FIGURE 22-1** Effects of mean arterial pressure on CBF. Although CBF normally is autoregulated in the range of 50 to 150 mm Hg, chronic hypertension shifts this curve rightward and necessitates a higher minimal pressure for adequate flow.

Failure of cerebral autoregulation may allow excessive perfusion (resulting in cerebral edema) or transient periods of hypoperfusion and ischemia. Normal regulatory mechanisms are modified by the presence of chronic hypertension, making higher mean arterial pressures necessary for adequate cerebral perfusion. Therefore, it is important not to lower perfusion pressure excessively in any hypertensive CNS syndrome.

Cerebral Ischemia and Hemorrhage

Hypertension predisposes to three specific "stroke syndromes": bland cerebral infarction, subarachnoid hemorrhage, and intracerebral hemorrhage. Sudden onset of focal neurologic deficits, obtundation, headache, and vomiting are the most frequent symptoms of these disorders. (Focal deficits are less common with subarachnoid hemorrhage.) In all three situations, vascular autoregulation is lost in areas of acute bleeding or infarction and typically in the period surrounding a stroke, BP rises probably as a putative protective mechanism against ischemia. Although the mechanism is uncertain, it is clear that transient hypertension often resolves within 7 to 10 days of the event and this modest hypertensive response is not harmful.

BP manipulation in patients with stroke remains controversial. (see Chapter 34). Current expert recommendations are that unless thrombolytic therapy is planned, the BP is greater than 220/120 mm Hg; or if there is evidence of extracerebral organ damage, BP should not be reduced. Opposing this advice are data suggesting that reducing BP greater than 180/110 mm Hg may decrease the risk of transforming ischemic to hemorrhagic strokes. It is clear that excessive or very rapid reductions in BP may worsen CNS deficits. Therefore, cautious lowering of the diastolic BP to the 100 to 110 mm Hg range is a reasonable goal.

Without a predisposing anatomic abnormality, hypertension rarely results in subarachnoid hemorrhage. In clinical trials of antihypertensive therapy in subarachnoid bleeding, mixed results have been observed. BP reductions halve the risk of rebleeding but increase the risks of ischemic infarction. Hence, therapy is usually withheld unless the diastolic BP is greater than 120 mm Hg. Arterial vasospasm, a process that further reduces perfusion, is common several days to a week after subarachnoid hemorrhage. Use of the calcium channel blocker nimodipine is efficacious in subarachnoid hemorrhage even in the absence of BP reductions. Among patients with a mechanically repaired aneurysm and prominent vasospasm, if neurological deficits worsen with lower BPs, so-called hypervolemic hypertensive therapy has been used with some success. In this strategy, a combination of volume expansion and vasopressor therapy is used to raise BP to levels about 20% above baseline while monitoring for neurological improvement.

In contrast to subarachnoid hemorrhage, hypertension is a major predisposing factor for intracerebral hemorrhage, especially in patients receiving systemic anticoagulation. In patients with parenchymal bleeding, blood often enters the subarachnoid space (mimicking subarachnoid hemorrhage) by dissecting through the internal capsule or putamen into the lateral ventricles. Although it makes sense to reduce BP, the benefits are unproven unless diastolic pressures exceed 130 mm Hg.

When a reduction in BP is indicated in any of these three conditions, the short-acting agents, nitroprusside, nicardipine, and labetalol, are the drugs of choice. The sedative effects of clonidine, methyldopa, and reserpine impair monitoring of mental status and should be avoided. Nifedipine, hydralazine, and angiotensin converting enzyme (ACE) inhibitors are not good choices because of the difficulty in controlling response.

Aortic Dissection

Aortic dissection should be suspected in the setting of profound hypertension when patients have chest or back pain; an arm/leg BP difference; absent pulses in the lower extremities, or asymmetry in BP between arms. A history of cocaine use should heighten suspicion of dissection even in young patients. Artifactual hypotension may result if BP is checked only in the left arm of a patient with aortic dissection as blood flow to the left subclavian artery is compromised. The diagnosis of aortic dissection is supported by finding a widened mediastinum on chest radiograph. Confirmation comes from computed tomography (CT), magnetic resonance imaging (MRI), or aortography. The goal is to immediately decrease both mean BP and the rate of increase in systolic pressure (ejection velocity) while preserving vital organ perfusion. A target diastolic BP of approximately 100 mm Hg usually is appropriate. Ganglionic blockade with trimethaphan is very effective at lowering BP and ejection velocity but most physicians are unfamiliar with the drug making therapeutic misadventures common. β-blockade is quite effective at reducing ejection velocity but unfortunately β-blockers alone usually do not provide a sufficiently rapid reduction in BP. Because direct vasodilators alone (e.g., hydralazine, nitroprusside, and diazoxide) increase heart rate, cardiac output, and ejection velocity, they represent suboptimal choices for therapy. Therefore, β-blockers often are used in conjunction with a vasodilator like nitroprusside or nicardipine. Alternatively, a combined α- and β-blocker like labetalol can be used. Vascular surgery consultation is prudent even though many cases are now managed with percutaneous graft placement. In proximal dissection, after BP is controlled, surgical intervention is indicated and although surgery is not necessary in most cases of distal dissection, compromise of blood flow to a limb or leakage may require surgical intervention.

Renal Failure

Renal disease may be the cause of hypertension as with glomerulonephritis, vasculitis, or renal artery stenosis or may be the result of damage from a hypertensive crisis. When hypertension is the cause of kidney injury, reversible perfusion-related increases in creatinine and blood urea nitrogen (BUN) frequently follow BP reduction. Nevertheless, reestablishing a safe BP is the main priority. Although other reversible causes of renal insufficiency (volume depletion, renal artery occlusion, lower tract obstruction) should be considered, an increasing BUN or creatinine should not deter the clinician from continuing antihypertensive therapy. For patients presenting with a serum creatinine greater than 3.5 mg/dL, progressive acute kidney injury is a likely and often unavoidable consequence of therapy. In renal insufficiency, nitroprusside is a good drug for BP control, even though thiocyanate toxicity is a concern, if patients are quickly transitioned to oral therapy it is rarely a problem. Labetalol, nicardipine, and fenoldopam represent good alternatives.

Pulmonary Edema

In most cases of severe hypertension, pulmonary edema is primarily the result of excessive left ventricular afterload, not excessive circulatory volume, and usually responds rapidly when SVR is lowered. An exception to this rule is the patient with dialysis-dependent renal failure who may have volume-dependent hypertension. Heightened afterload is most likely to cause pulmonary edema in patients with preexisting left ventricular dysfunction (including diastolic dysfunction) or aortic or mitral insufficiency. Effective therapy focuses on reduction of afterload, making nitroprusside, nicardipine, and perhaps fenoldopam, the most useful agents. Nitroglycerin, is particularly useful in hypertensive patients with volume overload and myocardial ischemia. In clearly volume-overloaded patients, morphine sulfate, diuretics, and hemofiltration are useful adjuncts.

Angina and Myocardial Infarction

During acute myocardial ischemia, reductions in BP preserve endangered myocardium by reducing afterload, decreasing wall stress, and increasing myocardial perfusion. In severe hypertension with cardiac ischemia, unopposed use of arterial vasodilators that produce tachycardia and thereby increase myocardial oxygen consumption (e.g., hydralazine, diazoxide, minoxidil) should be avoided. Caution also should be exercised when using nitroprusside, a drug that tends to divert blood away from the most ischemic areas of heart. Labetalol, nicardipine, and β-blockers are attractive therapeutic options because they improve the ratio of oxygen supply to demand. Nitroglycerin is much more a venodilator than arterial dilator, hence, alone it is rarely sufficient to control BP. Nevertheless, at high end doses it dilates both peripheral and coronary arteries, thereby reducing preload, decreasing BP, and increasing myocardial blood flow.

Catecholamine Excess

Conditions resulting in catecholamine-induced hypertension include (a) pheochromocytoma, (b) sympathomimetic drugs (cocaine, lysergic acid diethylamide [LSD], phencyclidine, and amphetamines), (c) monoamine oxidase inhibitor (MAOI) crisis, and (d) antihypertensive withdrawal (rebound) syndrome. Patients with these disorders commonly present with tachycardia, diaphoresis, pallor, pounding headache, and vomiting.

Pheochromocytoma is a rare cause of hypertensive crisis but should be considered in patients with hypertension induced by performance of angiography or the induction of anesthesia and in patients with a history of hyperparathyroidism or a family history of pheochromocytoma. MAOI crisis is also rare, occurring when tyramine-containing foods (cheese, beer, wine, chocolate) or other sympathomimetic agents are ingested by patients receiving MAOI antidepressants. (The antibiotic linezolid also has MAOI properties.) The problem of rebound hypertension is especially common in postoperative patients and those in the ICU after abrupt discontinuation of antihypertensive drugs. Although this syndrome is most frequently associated with the centrally acting α-agents (e.g., clonidine and methyldopa), withdrawal of β-blockers also may produce rebound hypertension. When a sympathomimetic drug is the cause of hypertensive crisis, control of agitation with a benzodiazepine and tincture of time are often the only needed treatments.

If treatment of any of these syndromes is required, α-adrenergic blockers (e.g., phentolamine) or direct vasodilators (e.g., nitroprusside) are the mainstays of therapy. Nicardipine and fenoldopam are useful alternatives. Used alone, β-blockers are contraindicated in catecholamine excess because unopposed α-adrenergic effects may paradoxically worsen hypertension. The same problem may also be encountered with labetalol because its β-blocking effects are substantially more prominent than its α-blocking actions.

Preeclampsia/Eclampsia

Eclampsia is defined as the occurrence of hypertension, edema, proteinuria, and seizures in the last trimester of pregnancy. (Lacking seizures, the syndrome is termed preeclampsia.) Although the specific cause of eclampsia is unknown, the syndrome responds to delivery of the infant. Most patients have significant elevations in SVR, and intravascular volume depletion with hemoconcentration (even patients with edema). Based upon very limited data, a target BP of 140 to 160/90 to 105 mm Hg is recommended. In addition to magnesium (4 to 6 gm IV over 1 h followed by 1 to 2 gm/h IV), specific antihypertensive therapy should be initiated. There are no good data on the comparative safety or effectiveness of antihypertensives in pregnancy, although it is generally accepted that ACE inhibitors should be avoided. Hydralazine and alpha-methyldopa have been traditional therapeutic choices but neither is ideal because of difficulty in titrating the response and the frequency of side effects. Calcium channel and β-blockers have also been generally considered safe. For severe hypertension, labetalol, nicardipine, or nitroprusside are effective. (Because of its chemical composition, there is substantial emotion regarding the use of nitroprusside in pregnancy but little data to suggest that the drug is unsafe.) Diuretics can be used if there is convincing evidence of intravascular volume expansion. As is always the case in pregnancy, the risks of any chosen therapy must be weighed against benefits and potential alternatives.

■ THERAPY FOR HYPERTENSIVE EMERGENCIES

Commonly Used Agents

Diuretics

Because most patients with severe hypertension have normal or reduced circulating blood volume, diuretics should be avoided in the emergency setting unless overt signs of heart failure, pulmonary edema, or fluid overload are present. Although not intuitive, volume supplementation with isotonic saline often is necessary when using potent vasodilators to correct hypertensive crises. (With more chronic use, however, most antihypertensive agents tend to cause sodium retention and, thus, should be used in conjunction with a diuretic.) IV furosemide is the most commonly used diuretic because it is potent, rapidly acting, inexpensive, and provides mild vasodilation. Bumetanide is essentially equivalent.

Nitroprusside

Nitroprusside is a direct-acting arteriovenous dilator with an immediate onset of action (usually <1 min) and the potential for rapid termination of action (1 to 3 min). Nitroprusside's effects are mediated by the vascular release of the endogenous vasodilator, nitric oxide. The photoinstability of nitroprusside mandates frequent changes of solutions and use of light-protected containers. Infusion, typically, is initiated at a dose of 0.5 μg/kg/min and titrated upward at 5- to 10-min intervals to produce the desired BP. Doses required for hypertension often are higher than those needed for the treatment of congestive heart failure but generally do not exceed 10 μg/kg/min. Because of its potency, controlled administration by infusion pump is mandatory. At low dosage rates, reductions in SVR are offset by increases in cardiac output. Therefore, BP may remain stable initially despite a beneficial action; reduction of BP often requires higher range dosing. The effects of nitroprusside are most pronounced in patients taking multiple other antihypertensive drugs and those who are volume depleted.

Nitroprusside (which is approx. 40% cyanide) is metabolized hepatically to cyanogen and then by the enzyme thiosulfate sulfurtransferase to thiocyanate, which is then cleared by the kidney. Therefore, hepatic failure may result in cyanide toxicity, and renal failure may lead to thiocyanate toxicity. Cyanide levels higher than 10 mg/dL may cause hepatic failure, metabolic acidosis, dyspnea, and vomiting. Nevertheless, both toxicities are very rare when nitroprusside is administered at the usual doses of less than 3 μg/kg/min for less than 72 h. Nitrates, cyanocobalamin (vitamin B$_{12}$), and thiosulfate are useful in the treatment of thiocyanate toxicity (see Chapter 38).

Calcium Channel Blockers

Calcium channel blockers produce systemic and coronary vasodilation by inhibiting slow calcium channels. Verapamil, the first parenteral calcium channel blocker, causes myocardial depression and conduction blockade in a substantial number of patients, even though it promptly but briefly lowers BP after a single IV dose. Because of its negative inotropic action and because cardiac conduction is so often impaired, resulting in a slower heart rate, increased PR interval, and occasionally second-degree and third-degree atrioventricular blocks, verapamil represents a relatively poor choice for acute hypertension treatment. Because nifedipine is not available IV and oral use often results in precipitous, dangerous declines in BP, it should not be used in hypertensive crises.

Nicardipine, a parenteral calcium channel blocker, rapidly (within 5 to 15 min) reduces BP when administered by continuous infusion at rates of 5 to 15 mg/h. Unlike its predecessor, verapamil, cardiac contractility and conduction rarely are adversely affected. Increases in ejection fraction and stroke volume are responsible for the rises in cardiac output observed in most patients. Reflex tachycardia stemming from vasodilation rarely is a problem, making this drug an excellent alternative to nitroprusside in cases of hypertension associated with myocardial ischemia or congestive heart failure.

Clevidipine is the newest IV calcium channel blocker. It is an arteriolar dilator with the theoretical advantage of being metabolized by plasma esterases, hence not subject to changes in hepatic or renal function. Although little data support use in hypertensive crises, the drug does appear to be effective in postoperative hypertension. Clevidipine does not have sufficient advantages over nicardipine to justify its incremental cost.

β-Blockers

Esmolol is a β-blocker with a very short duration of action due to its rapid hydrolysis in blood. Because esmolol begins to act within 1 min and lasts only 10 to 20 min after stopping infusion, it is a nearly ideal agent for control of supraventricular arrhythmias and hypertension, provided β-blockade is not contraindicated. An initial loading dose of 250 to 500 μg/kg is followed by a constant infusion of 25 to 50 μg/kg/min titrated upward every 10 to 20 min until control is achieved. It is rare to require infusions above 300 μg/kg/min. Toxicity is related to β-blockade (e.g., bradycardia, conduction abnormalities, and low cardiac output).

Labetalol is a combined α- and β-blocker with rapid onset but a long and variable duration of action (1 to 8 h). The β-blocking properties of labetalol are substantially more potent than its α-blocking effects, occasionally resulting in paradoxical hypertension in high catecholamine states. Advantages of labetalol are the rarity of "overshoot hypotension," or impairment of cardiac output. An initial bolus of 20 mg is almost always effective in lowering BP within 2 to 5 min, whereas doses of 20 to 80 mg at 20- to 40-min intervals provide continued BP control. An alternative to repeated boluses is a continuous infusion of 1 to 2 mg/min. Labetalol also is available orally, facilitating conversion from IV dosing. The primary disadvantages of labetalol lie in its potential to exacerbate heart failure and bronchospasm and its long duration of action.

Fenoldopam

Fenoldopam is a short-acting, hepatically cleared, dopamine receptor 1 agonist that lowers BP and increases renal blood flow causing naturesis. An initial dose of 0.1 μg/kg/min followed by an initial infusion of 0.05 to 0.1 μg/kg min titrated upward usually controls BP over 1 to 3 h. Initial antihypertensive effects occur within 5 to 10 min. Reflex tachycardia is common. Fenoldopam has seen only limited use for treatment of hypertensive crises, hence the best niche for this agent remains unclear.

Nitrates

Nitroglycerin is primarily a venodilator having an immediate onset but brief duration of action. Because patients with hypertensive crises are often volume depleted, and venodilation is much more prominent than peripheral arterial dilation, nitroglycerin often causes cardiac output to decline. Because it is not a potent arterial vasodilator, nitroglycerine must usually be combined with other classes of drugs like β-blockers or calcium channel blockers for effect. Nitroglycerin is particularly useful in the setting of hypertensive myocardial ischemia with congestive heart failure, or pulmonary edema. Initial doses of 5 to 10 μg/min are reasonable. Liver disease reduces the hepatic metabolism of nitrates potentiating their effects. The side effects of nitrates include headache, tachycardia, and flushing, but rarely are dose limiting.

Angiotensin-converting Enzyme Inhibitors

Angiotensin-converting enzyme (ACE) inhibitors prevent conversion of angiotensin I to the extremely potent vasoconstrictor angiotensin II. Reductions in SVR with stable pulmonary capillary wedge pressures and cardiac outputs usually are usually seen after ACE administration, although patients with congestive heart failure may have a fall in filling pressures and a rise in cardiac output. There are a host of oral ACE inhibitors but captopril, enalapril, and lisonpril are inexpensive generics that are absorbed within 30 to 90 min, providing BP reduction for 8 h for the former and 24 h for the latter two. Few side effects are associated with these drugs if their dose is reduced in renal insufficiency and if they are not given to profoundly volume-depleted patients. Hyperkalemia may be seen in patients with renal artery stenosis and those receiving potassium supplements or nonsteroidal anti-inflammatory drugs. For patients who cannot tolerate ACE inhibitors, angiotensin receptor blockers (ARBs) offer a similar mechanism of action albeit at higher cost.

The parenteral preparation, enalaprilat, is an active form of enalapril that produces rapid (within 15 min) BP reduction by inhibiting angiotensin II formation. Initial doses of 1.25 mg IV every 6 h are usually effective; however, higher doses (up to 5 mg every 6 h) may be necessary. Enalaprilat may produce severe hypotension in volume-depleted patients. Equally potent hypotensive effects are observed at almost all doses; increasing the dose only extends the duration of action. A long duration of action (nearly 24 h) represents a potential disadvantage in cases of overshoot hypotension. ACE inhibitors should not be given in pregnancy.

Rarely Used Agents

Diazoxide, a direct arteriolar vasodilator, frequently induces hypotension when given rapidly in large (5 mg/kg) doses. Use of smaller IV boluses of 1 to 2 mg/kg (given at 10-min intervals) or a constant infusion (at rates of up to 15 mg/min) are alternative methods of administration that reduce the risk of hypotension. With an onset of action of 1 to 2 min and a mean duration of action of 8 h, diazoxide maybe useful for patients who cannot be monitored on a minute-to-minute basis. Nausea and vomiting are common side effects of diazoxide, limiting its usefulness in patients with altered levels of consciousness. Furthermore, cerebral perfusion may be reduced disproportionately to BP by this drug. Reflex increases in heart rate make it alone a poor choice for patients with ischemic heart disease or aortic aneurysm. The potent, fluid-retaining properties of diazoxide almost always require the concurrent use of diuretics after BP has been controlled. Hyperglycemia, hyperuricemia, and potentiation of warfarin anticoagulation are other common side effects.

Trimethaphan, a ganglionic blocker, exerts direct peripheral vasodilating effects. Although its rapid onset (1 to 2 min) is desirable, the sustained (10-min) duration of action may be problematic for patients who develop hypotension in response to an excessive dose. Customary initial infusion rates are 0.5 to 1 mg/min and can be titrated upward to maximum doses of 15 mg/min for BP control. Severe orthostatic hypotension is seen in almost all patients receiving the drug, and positional sensitivity should be considered when difficulty is encountered in obtaining precise BP control. Tachyphylaxis limits its efficacy to 3 to 4 days. Trimethaphan routinely reduces cardiac output and renal blood flow and rarely causes apnea. Furthermore, parasympathetic blockade may result in such distressing symptoms as dry mouth, blurred vision, constipation, and abdominal distention. With the possible exception of dissecting aortic aneurysm and catecholamine excess, equally efficacious and less-toxic alternatives have generally supplanted the use of trimethaphan.

Hydralazine, is a direct vasodilator, that begins acting within 10 min if given IV and within 30 min if given intramuscularly. Unfortunately, its prolonged duration of action (3 to 6 h) may cause persistent overshoot hypotension. Because hydralazine is not consistently effective at lowering BP, it is a poor choice for acute treatment of life-threatening hypertension. Unless counteracted by a β-blocker, the arteriolar dilating effects of hydralazine often result in reflex tachycardia and enhanced contractility, thereby worsening coronary ischemia and aortic dissection. By reducing its clearance from the body, renal failure potentiates the effects of hydralazine.

Methyldopa is a long-acting central sympatholytic with a delayed onset of action (2 to 4 h). Its delayed action and tendency to cause sedation make it undesirable for use in hypertensive emergencies; however, for patients with non–life-threatening hypertension, methyldopa has the advantage of lowering BP gradually (over several hours). Overshoot hypotension is uncommon, but long-term use is associated with drug-induced fever, hepatocellular inflammation, and hemolytic anemia. Methyldopa is rarely used because other less side-effect-laden choices are available.

Phentolamine is an α-adrenergic blocking drug with an abrupt onset of action (1 to 2 min). Its twin effects of α-blockade and non–α-mediated vasodilation precipitate hypotension, tachycardia, nausea, and vomiting in a large percentage of patients who receive it. Unfortunately, reflex tachycardia induced by phentolamine may worsen coronary ischemia, even when beneficial reductions in afterload are achieved. Again, because of the development of equally effective and less-toxic therapies, phentolamine use has largely fallen out of favor. Repeated boluses of 1 to 5 mg IV to a maximum dose of 15 mg provide control.

■ **SUGGESTED READINGS**

Abdelwahab W, Frishman W, Landau A. Management of hypertensive urgencies and emergencies. *J Clin Pharmacol.* 1995;35(8):747–762.

Blumenfeld JD, Laragh JH. Management of hypertensive crises: The scientific basis for treatment decisions. *Am J Hypertens.* 2001;14 (11 Pt 1):1154–1167.

Ghandi SK, Powers JC, Nomeir AM, et al. The pathogenesis of acute pulmonary edema associated with hypertension. *N Engl J Med.* 2001; 344:17–22.

Perez MI, Musini VM. Pharmacological interventions for hypertensive emergencies. *Cochrane Database Syst Rev.* 2008;23(1):CD003653.

Rodriguez G, Varon J. Clevidipine: A unique agent for the critical care practitioner. *Crit Care Shock.* 2006;9:9–15.

Tumlin JA, Dunbar LM, Oparil S, et al., Fenoldopam a dopamine agonist for hypertensive emergency: A multi center randomized trial. *Acad Emerg Med.* 2000;7:653–662.

Varon J, Marik PE. Hypertensive crises: Challenges and management. *Chest.* 2007;131(6):1949–1962.

Venous Thromboembolism

KEY POINTS

1 Because venous thromboembolism is so common and in large part preventable, essentially all hospitalized adults with risk factors should be strongly considered for prophylaxis.

2 Because of its safety, availability, and diagnostic power, the best first diagnostic test when venous thromboembolism is seriously considered is leg ultrasound.

3 Pulmonary emboli are often difficult to diagnose. Usually, a chest imaging study should be undertaken only after developing a high clinical suspicion, excluding alternative diagnoses, and searching for deep venous thrombosis.

4 Most ventilation perfusion scans are nondiagnostic and require either a pulmonary arteriogram showing pulmonary embolism or leg study showing deep venous thrombosis for confirmation. A normal ventilation perfusion scan or a high-probability scan probably is sufficient for clinical decision making. A contrasted spiral CT scan can often reveal central emboli in those who cannot undergo angiography.

5 Full-dose anticoagulation with some form of heparin or fondaparinux should be started empirically for almost all patients suspected of having venous thromboembolism, unless bleeding risk is prohibitive.

6 The risk of pulmonary embolism recurrence is in part a function of the duration of time unanticoagulated; therefore, early and aggressive anticoagulation is indicated. Either weight-based SC low molecular weight heparin or fondaparinux, or IV unfractionated heparin adjusted every 4 to 6 h until the activated partial thromboplastin time is in the therapeutic range should be used.

7 There is a much less certain relationship between a high activated partial thromboplastin time and bleeding than there is between a low activated partial thromboplastin time and thrombosis.

8 Thrombolytic or surgical therapy is rarely needed for venous thromboembolism.

■ MECHANISMS

Pulmonary embolism (PE) results when any insoluble substance gains access to the systemic veins. Because blood filtering is a natural function of the lung, small and asymptomatic emboli occur periodically, even in healthy persons. Distinctive syndromes have been described for embolism of air, fat, tumor cells, amniotic fluid, and foreign matter, as well as for bland and infected clots. In critical care, air, fat, amniotic fluid, and septic and bland thrombotic emboli are the major syndromes of interest. Air embolism is discussed in Chapter 8.

Fat embolism, almost always results from trauma to long bones; rarely vertebral fractures are to blame. Fat emboli do not substantially impede blood flow. Instead, symptoms develop because fatty acid products of lipid digestion produce bronchoconstriction, vasoconstriction, and vascular injury with capillary leak and pulmonary edema (acute respiratory distress syndrome [ARDS]) (see Chapter 24).

Amniotic fluid embolism is a rare peripartum condition in which amniotic fluid and fetal cells enter the pulmonary circuit. Like fat embolism, the syndrome is more inflammatory than obstructive. The classical risk factors of premature rupture of membranes, older maternal age, and fetal death have been questioned in recent studies. The syndrome is characterized by abrupt dyspnea and pulmonary edema followed by sudden cardiovascular collapse. Disseminated intravascular coagulation is common among survivors of the initial crisis. Therapy is supportive along with timely delivery of the child.

Similarly, the major threat to life in septic embolism is not vascular obstruction but septic physiology. Small, friable fragments of infected material embolize to cause fever, toxicity, and a characteristic radiograph: multiple ill-defined infiltrates or nodules (especially lower lobe) of varied sizes that frequently cavitate and usually display soft, irregular outlines. Perfusion defects on lung scan are typically unimpressive compared to the radiograph. Pelvic veins, venous catheters or right-sided heart valves, and nonsterile injections (related to drug abuse) are common sources of infected material. After identification, the source must be isolated surgically or removed and the infection treated vigorously with antibiotics directed at the offending organism(s).

The remainder of this chapter will focus on classical venous thromboembolism (VTE), one the most frequent and preventable causes of death in hospitalized patients. The term VTE will be used collectively for deep venous thrombosis (DVT) and PE because the link between the conditions is strong. An analogy to cancer treatment is apropos in which DVT represents the primary tumor and PE the metastases. In this comparison, preventing the primary problem negates spread of the disease. Also in line with the cancer analogy, discovering either the primary tumor (DVT) or metastases (PE) mandates treatment and in most cases finding metastases make a search for the primary superfluous. Similarly, on rare occasion no primary can be found despite clear metastatic disease. Finally, both VTE and neoplasia are treated with systemic "chemo" therapy; in the case of VTE, it is anticoagulation.

■ DEEP VENOUS THROMBOSIS

Risk Factors

1 In the United States, each year more than five million patients develop DVT with more than 10% of these patients experiencing PE. It is estimated that as many as 250,000 deaths can be attributed to clot annually. VTE rarely occurs among healthy ambulatory people. Essentially, all victims have easily identified risk factors falling into one of three general categories: stasis of venous blood, injury to the venous intima, and/or hypercoagulability. Thus, increasing age, reduced mobility, pregnancy, previous DVT, trauma (especially to the legs), surgery, severe sepsis, cancer, indwelling venous catheters, chronic obstructive pulmonary disease, and heart failure are common predisposing conditions. The more risk factors present, the higher the likelihood of VTE. In the absence of prophylaxis, some patient groups are at amazingly high risk. For example, VTE incidence is greater than 60% following hip or

knee replacement or fracture repair; nearly 40% among ICU patients; 30% in general surgical patients; and at least 15% among general medical patients.

Because it is hard to believe that such a common and important condition could result from such mundane causes, great interest exists in the role of the half a dozen or so, well-characterized thrombophilic (procoagulant) disorders (e.g., factor V Leiden, prothrombin 20210 mutation, anticardiolipin antibodies, homocystinuria or deficiencies of antithrombin, or proteins C or S). Together, the two most common factor V Leiden (activated protein C resistance) and the prothrombin 20210 mutation can be identified in 5% to 10% of the white population. Despite their high prevalence, VTE risk among those affected is low without additional risk factors. Controversy exists regarding the importance of diagnosing thrombophilia, particularly in asymptomatic individuals, and the optimal course of action if diagnosed. Traditional teaching encourages a search for thrombophilia in patients who develop VTE in the absence of other risk factors, especially if young, or when history shows a personal or family history of recurrent thrombosis. Because testing is complex, expensive, and holds lifelong implications for the patient labeled with an "incurable" genetic disease and their family, evaluation should almost certainly be left to a coagulation specialist probably in conjunction with a genetic counselor. Fortunately, there is never an urgency to evaluate patients for these conditions, and their diagnosis does not change the acute VTE treatment. At this time, routine screening of patients with VTE for thrombophilia is not indicated (see Chapter 30).

Clot Sources

Traditional teaching holds that near 90% of PEs result from lower extremity DVTs and that the arms and neck are rarely if ever a clot source. However, changes in practice have altered the epidemiology of the disease; now hospitalized patients routinely have upper extremity sources of clot. For example, central venous catheters (including peripherally inserted central lines) are more common than ever and provide a nidus for thrombus formation. Embolization is particularly likely upon catheter removal, as the encasing thrombus is stripped away. It is now estimated that perhaps as many as 30% of fatal PEs stem from catheters. Heparin-bonding may protect temporarily until the anticoagulant is leached out of the catheter over 24 to 36h. In contrast to disease of the deep veins, superficial thrombophlebitis manifest by erythema, tenderness, and a palpable "venous cord" poses a low VTE risk and can usually be treated symptomatically. On rare occasions, extension into the deep veins occurs.

The natural history of leg DVT is well characterized. Most clots begin as asymptomatic calf thrombi, hence many physicians regard them as having little importance. Unfortunately, 30% to 50% of these clots propagate above the knee and 30% to 50% of proximal DVTs eventually produce PE. Therefore, between 10% and 25% of untreated patients with calf thrombi develop PE. Surprising to many clinicians is the fact that during life, most acute thrombi in the legs *and* lungs are asymptomatic and therefore go undiagnosed.

Prevention

Prevention is the most important treatment of VTE. In fact, deterrence is so important and so often overlooked that it makes sense to institute hospital-wide prophylaxis programs for patients at risk. Fortunately, nearly 90% of United States ICU patients now receive some form of effective prophylaxis compared to just 30% a few years ago. Rates of protection are profoundly lower for hospitalized patients outside the ICU.

Although benefit is unproven for the hospitalized patient, DVT risk might be reduced by ambulation. A corollary is that avoidance of excessive sedation and unnecessary paralysis could reduce risk by shortening periods of immobility. Unfortunately, walking is "ordered" for hospitalized patients far more often than performed, and activity never reaches normal levels. Furthermore, ICU patients rarely walk although it is possible to have selected intubated patients ambulate with portable ventilators. However, even if frequent vigorous walking were conducted, doing so would reverse only one of the numerous VTE risk factors present in most hospitalized patients.

Because of its superior effectiveness, pharmacologic prophylaxis should be provided to inpatients with VTE risk factors unless there is a contraindication to use. Fixed-dose subcutaneous (SC) unfractionated heparin (UFH) reduces DVT risk by as much as 66% in general medical and surgical patients when given thrice daily. Unfortunately, higher risk patients (i.e., critically ill, multitrauma, hip or knee replacement or intra-abdominal or pelvic cancer surgery) do not enjoy the same protection. Those at highest risk should receive an appropriate dose of a low-molecular-weight heparin (LMWH) or fondaparinux; UFH in a dose adjusted to prolong the activated partial thromboplastin time (aPTT) (typically 7,500 to 10,000 units SC every 8 h); or oral warfarin given in a dose and a time frame sufficient to prolong the prothrombin time (PT). Surprisingly, little data support the common practice of administering 5,000 units of UFH every 12 h, even to the so-called low-risk patients. When used in fixed prophylactic doses, UFH and LMWH do not prolong the aPTT or increase serious hemorrhagic complications; however, all heparins and fondaparinux tend to accumulate when glomerular filtration rate falls below 30 mL/min, increasing the likelihood of bleeding (see Chapter 30).

LMWHs equal or surpass the effectiveness of UFH for VTE prophylaxis and have a lower incidence of bleeding and heparin-induced thrombocytopenia (HIT). Overall, LMWHs provide greater than 75% relative risk reduction for DVT formation. High bioavailability (approx. 90%) and longer half-life (4 to 5 h) allow single daily injections for most indications. (After total knee replacement, twice daily injections may be optimal, and there is debate regarding the need for twice daily therapy in the critically ill and obese patient.) Because each LMWH has different pharmacological properties and few head-to-head comparisons have been conducted, LMWHs should not be considered interchangeable. There is little financial incentive to choose one over another, as differences in cost among brands is trivial. To avoid confusion regarding dose and frequency and to control costs, it makes sense to limit the number of prophylactic agents on the formulary. As a result, many institutions select one LMWH with a broad range of indications. The higher costs of LMWHs compared to UFH for prophylaxis seems well worth the investment, given the superior effectiveness, lower incidence of HIT, and reduced number of injections required. The price differential has also dramatically narrowed with recent increases in UFH cost associated with contamination related shortages.

For some orthopedic procedures (e.g., hip or knee replacement), specific protocols using preoperative warfarin have been shown to reduce VTE risk, but rarely in practice are the proven protocols followed. The custom of administering the first warfarin dose the night before, or day of, surgery does not provide effective perioperative prophylaxis—prevention requires an international normalized ratio (INR) greater than 2, a target which typically requires 5 days to achieve.

Fondaparinux is a synthetic factor Xa inhibitor which has been shown to be effective prophylaxis for patients undergoing abdominal, knee, and hip surgery. High bioavailability is advantageous but lack of reversibility, dependence on renal clearance, and the extremely long half-life approximately 17 h are disadvantages. Fondaparinux should not be used in patients with renal insufficiency. Optimism that fondaparinux might not be associated with thrombocytopenia has been undermined by a recent report of HIT. Studies comparing this drug to LMWH demonstrate a slightly higher bleeding risk, but a slightly lower DVT risk (with a low overall clot risk for both agents) results that are not surprising, given that fondaparinux was administered closer to the time of surgery. There does not appear to be a convincing advantage of fondaparinux over an appropriately selected LMWH.

Dextran, aspirin, and other NSAIDs, and dipyridamole should be avoided because they have not been shown to be as effective as UFH, LMWH, fondaparinux or warfarin prophylaxis, and in the case of dextran, a higher risk of bleeding is seen.

Custom-fitted, elastic, graded compression stockings and pneumatic compression devices are options for patients at unacceptable risk for bleeding if given anticoagulants (e.g., coagulopathy, trauma, or neurosurgery). Interestingly, the mechanism of action of these mechanical devices is probably not the mere squeezing of blood from the legs, but in part an antithrombotic and profibrinolytic effect induced by vascular endothelial compression. Alone, each device has been shown to reduce the risk of DVT, with even lower rates observed when they are used concurrently. At a 30% relative risk reduction for custom-fitted elastic stockings and a 50% relative risk reduction for pneumatic compression devices, neither is as effective as pharmacologic prophylaxis. Because of patient discomfort or through sheer forgetfulness, these devices are often not worn at all or are applied inconsistently. Furthermore, elastic stockings often fit poorly because they are rarely custom manufactured. Obviously, if malfitting or not worn, neither device offers protection. In addition, the effectiveness of *lower* extremity mechanical devices to reduce the risk of *upper* extremity (often catheter related) DVT is questionable.

Diagnosis

The signs of DVT relate to venous inflammation and obstruction. Unilateral lower-extremity erythema, warmth, swelling, edema, and pain suggest DVT. The Homans sign is a nonspecific indicator of calf inflammation seldom present in documented DVT. Unfortunately, the physical examination is poor for detecting DVT and distinguishing it from common mimics.

Several common conditions mimic DVT. A ruptured Baker's cyst presents as a mass in the calf with pain and erythema, usually in patients with rheumatoid arthritis. An accurate diagnosis must be made to avoid the use of potentially dangerous therapies (e.g., thrombolytic drugs) that could provoke bleeding into the cyst. Rupture of the plantaris tendon also may mimic DVT on examination, but the history is key, revealing recent exertion with the acute onset of pain. Crystalline arthritis (gout or pseudogout) may produce intense joint space inflammation that extends into the calf. Cellulitis, especially that seen in the setting of direct trauma or chronic fungal infection of the feet or after coronary bypass surgery, often is confused with DVT. It is frequently so difficult to distinguish DVT from cellulitis that concomitant antibiotic and anticoagulation therapy are begun empirically until DVT is confirmed or excluded. Although sometimes confused with DVT, pulmonary osteoarthropathy presents with pain, tenderness, and swelling over the *anterior* tibia, with or without clubbing, and can be confirmed radiographically. In patients with hemophilia or those taking anticoagulants, hematoma formation in the calf muscles also may produce a syndrome clinically similar to DVT. Postphlebitic syndrome (deep venous insufficiency) develops to some degree in nearly half of all patients after a DVT. The syndrome, which typically becomes fully manifest over 3 to 5 years, can be a particularly confounding problem because the recurrent discomfort and swelling that occurs often prompts frequent DVT reevaluations.

Diagnostic Testing

Because the physical examination is insensitive and nonspecific, a confirmatory study is necessary in essentially all cases. Although immensely popular, the d-dimer is of little or no diagnostic value in hospitalized patients because its concentration is increased by essentially every critical illness (e.g., stroke, severe sepsis, trauma, surgery, pregnancy, liver failure, myocardial infarction). This differs from the outpatient setting where a negative d-dimer is common, and when a negative result is paired with a low validated risk score (e.g., Wells criteria) the likelihood of clot is so small no additional testing is indicated.

2   Ultrasound (US) is capable of imaging veins and probing venous flow. When noncompressible clot is imaged, the diagnosis is all but certain. Doppler studies can reliably confirm obstruction, unless flow is compromised by low cardiac output or high intra-abdominal or central venous pressures. In such cases, low flow may be reported but clot will not be seen. US is not as sensitive as contrast venography for detecting calf clot and may miss some clots restricted to the pelvis. Portability, low cost, and unquestioned safety make US the preferred first test in the ICU population despite these limitations.

The contrast venogram is simultaneously the most sensitive, definitive, time-consuming, and potentially injurious method for detecting DVT. An advantage to venography is its ability to visualize thrombus from the feet to the vena cava. Venography also occasionally helps distinguish acute thrombosis from chronic thrombosis based on appearance of the clot and is immune to false positive results brought about by low flow states. Because contrast may precipitate renal insufficiency and cause allergic reactions and phlebitis, venography is most appropriate when US is technically limited.

In up to one third of cases of angiographically proven PE, studies for DVT are negative. This situation could be because all leg clots have embolized to the lung or the legs were not the source of the PE. Although a negative leg US or venogram does not exclude a diagnosis of PE, in almost all cases a positive study permits VTE treatment to be initiated without additional testing.

■ PULMONARY EMBOLISM

Natural History

PE is a complication of the root disease DVT, hence prophylaxis for DVT decreases PE rates. Between 30% and 50% of patients with proximal DVT can be shown to have a PE, even though the vast majority has no respiratory symptoms. Tragically, the very first symptom of PE in the hospitalized patient is *usually* sudden fatal cardiovascular collapse. When symptoms lead to a diagnosis of PE during life and effective treatment is begun, the outcome is generally good with mortality rates less than 10%. Subgroups at highest risk for death include patients with shock and refractory hypoxemia. The utility of echocardiography and biochemical testing (e.g., troponin, creatine phosphokinase, or natriuretic peptides) to identify higher risk patients remains experimental.

Symptoms and Signs

Signs and symptoms of PE are modified in severity and duration by underlying cardiopulmonary status. No symptom or physical finding is either universal or specific. Therefore, when PE is suspected, the patient should be anticoagulated empirically until the diagnosis of VTE is refuted or confirmed by objective testing. (The obvious exception would be patients who are hemorrhaging or at very high risk to bleed.) For most patients, the symptoms of PE spontaneously improve within the first few hours or days after the event. Signs disappear more slowly. Among patients with large emboli, the following signs and symptoms are observed: dyspnea and tachypnea (90%); pleuritic pain (70%); apprehension, rales, and cough (50%); and hemoptysis (30%). Tachycardia (>100/min) and fever occur in a significant minority of cases. When syncope occurs, it usually is the result massive embolism. It is important to note that for sedated, mechanically ventilated patients, the only clues to the disease may be worsening of baseline tachycardia and an increase in minute ventilation.

Pulmonary artery pressures do not rise markedly unless the embolism obstructs more than 50% of the capillary bed or the circulation was previously compromised. Therefore, a right-sided gallop, increased pulmonic component of the second heart sound (P_2), or pulmonary hypertension documented by echocardiography or pulmonary artery catheterization signify massive acute obstruction or lesser obstruction in a patient with underlying pulmonary vascular disease. Detection of a pleural effusion may be helpful: Among patients with pleuritic chest pain, PE is a more likely diagnosis than infection when effusion is present.

Routine Diagnostic Tests

Routine diagnostic tests (chest X-ray [CXR], electrocardiogram [ECG], blood gases, leukocyte count) are most useful to exclude alternative diagnoses (e.g., pneumonia, pneumothorax, myocardial infarction, and pulmonary edema) rather than to confirm a diagnosis of PE.

Electrocardiogram

The ECG is sensitive but nonspecific. Even in patients without prior cardiopulmonary disease, the ECG is normal in only a small proportion (approx. 10%). Nonspecific ST and/or T wave changes occur in most patients. Except for moderate sinus tachycardia, rhythm disturbances are unusual. Atrial fibrillation and flutter seldom occur in patients without preexisting cardiovascular compromise. Similarly, bundle branch block is highly unusual but when it occurs, left and right tracts are affected equally often. ECG evidence of acute cor pulmonale (S_1, Q_3, T_3 pattern or acute right bundle branch block) appears rarely (<10%) and then only in patients with severe vascular obstruction.

Blood Studies

Although hypoxemia is the rule, emboli frequently are found in patients with normal values for PaO_2, $PaCO_2$, and A-a gradient. Even a normal arterial blood gas (ABG) result does not exclude the diagnosis of PE; young, otherwise healthy patients have normal results up to 40% of the time. As a general rule, the more profound the underlying cardiovascular disease, the less likely the ABG is to be normal when a PE occurs.

Fibrin-degradation-product assays (e.g., d-dimer) are essentially never helpful in hospitalized patients. Although a negative *sensitive* d-dimer assay can be helpful in refuting a VTE diagnosis in low-risk outpatients, the test is almost uniformly positive in inpatients, which limits its utility. (Severe sepsis, renal failure, surgery, pregnancy, and trauma all increase the d-dimer levels even in the absence of clot.) It is important to know which d-dimer test is used in a given institution; several assays are available, some of which have dismal sensitivity and specificity. It is not prudent to bet an inpatient's life on a negative d-dimer (or any other single study) without confirmatory clinical, radiographic, or laboratory data. VTE is a sufficiently difficult diagnostic problem; it is unlikely that any single laboratory test will ever make or exclude the diagnosis.

Chest Radiograph

Nonspecific findings, including cardiomegaly, pleural effusion, an elevated hemidiaphragm, consolidation, and atelectasis, are common. Indeed, the CXR remains unchanged from the pre-event film in less than one quarter of all patients. Small or moderate-sized effusions occur in approximately one fourth of all cases; most (but not all) are exudative. Embolic effusions tend to appear early and unilaterally. A bloody effusion found before anticoagulation suggests infarction or an alternative diagnosis (tuberculosis, malignancy, and trauma). More specific features, including segmental oligemia (the Westermark sign) and Hampton's hump (a wedge-shaped peripheral density resulting from pulmonary infarction), are unusual.

Infiltrate may represent parenchymal hemorrhage (resolving rapidly without effusion) or infarction (resolving slowly, often accompanied by a bloody effusion). Fresh infarcts always are pleural based and cavitate frequently. Because the dual parenchymal blood supply usually protects against tissue ischemia, infarction occurs most commonly in patients with preexisting cardiopulmonary disease. When resolving, the infiltrate often rounds up to form a spheroid "nodule." Multiple, widely scattered, cavitating infiltrates that develop acutely suggest septic emboli.

Specialized Diagnostic Tests

Clinical judgment plays an indispensable role in the diagnosis of PE. Special diagnostic studies should only be ordered only for patients considered to have a "high clinical likelihood" of having a PE. Formal scoring systems like the Wells score help assess VTE probability. Because ventilation–perfusion (VQ) scans and contrasted CTs are noninvasive and are perceived to offer little risk, there is often a low threshold to order them for patients with dyspnea or chest pain. However, both studies are expensive (>$1,000) and expose patients to radiation, and the CT has the added risk of contrast exposure. Casual ordering frequently creates a dilemma when the result of a VQ or CT scan is at odds with the clinical situation. The situation most often encountered is one in which an "indeterminate" VQ scan result is obtained in a patient with a low clinical probability of PE. A consultant is then summoned to explain the results. Such patients are often unnecessarily subjected to angiography or alternatively anticoagulation with an uncertain diagnosis. The best strategy is not to perform a VQ or CT scan unless (a) the clinical likelihood of PE is high and (b) if the VQ or CT scan proves nondiagnostic, there is a commitment to pursue the diagnosis to certainty or exclusion.

Ventilation–Perfusion Scans

A perfusion (Q) scan is performed by injecting radioactive macroaggregated albumin, a compound with a particle size exceeding the diameter of the alveolar capillary. The albumin is then trapped in perfused lung areas. Areas devoid of perfusion are suspect for PE but also can result from tumor, obstructive lung disease, or hypoxic vasoconstriction induced by airspace disease. Therefore, atelectasis, emphysema, and pneumonia all can induce perfusion defects. In an attempt to exclude airspace disease as a cause of a perfusion defect, a CXR is performed routinely. Because infiltrates can change rapidly in hospitalized patients, the comparison CXR should be obtained within hours of the scan. The diagnosis of PE is more likely when the perfusion scan defect occurs in an area without apparent disease on CXR.

To further increase the specificity of the perfusion scan, a ventilation (V) scan can be added to the diagnostic package. Because not all airspace disease is apparent on plain CXR, the ventilation scan is used to identify poorly ventilated areas that could cause regional reductions in perfusion. When a large perfusion defect occurs in a normal area on plain CXR that also is normally ventilated on VQ scan, PE is likely. The ventilation scan (xenon or diethylenetriamine penta-acetic acid) improves specificity for embolism; gross VQ mismatching often allows a diagnosis to be made with confidence. However, matching VQ abnormalities sometimes occur in PE because of bronchoconstriction, atelectasis, or secretion retention. Conversely, mismatching can occur when no embolus is present. A major limitation of this strategy is the inability to obtain the ventilation portion of the study in mechanically ventilated patients.

Criteria for "high-probability" and "low-probability" scans vary with the interpreter but generally depend on the size, number, and distribution of perfusion defects, as well as their relationship to CXR and ventilation scan abnormalities. A perfusion defect larger than a corresponding density on chest film suggests embolism; a perfusion defect equal to or smaller than the radiographic abnormality suggests that embolism is less likely. A similar rule applies even more strongly to areas of VQ mismatching. Experts often disagree among themselves in interpretation of VQ scans; consequently, the false-positive rate may be very high in some centers. Classically, scans are interpreted as falling into one of four categories: (a) normal, (b) low probability, (c) intermediate probability, and (d) high probability. However, a more practical scheme is to classify scans as only normal, high probability, or *indeterminate*.

The most useful of all scans, a perfectly normal perfusion study, effectively rules out a clinically significant PE. The single rare exception to this rule may be submassive PE confined to the pulmonary outflow tract, producing symmetric reduction in flow as a result of central obstruction. (Contrasted CT scans often detect such clots.) The second most useful VQ result is the finding of multiple mismatched VQ defects of segmental or greater size. Such a result in a patient with a high clinical probability is associated with at least a 90% likelihood of a PE.

Unfortunately, most scans (nearly 70%) are interpreted as low or intermediate probability (i.e., indeterminate), which is unhelpful. A "low-probability" or indeterminate scan should not be confused with a normal scan. A substantial fraction (up to 15%) of patients with low probability scans (matched subsegmental defects) have angiographically demonstrable PE. Similarly, up to 50% of patients with indeterminate scans (matched or mismatched segmental defects) have PE. Therefore a low-probability or indeterminate scan almost always requires additional diagnostic testing if the clinical suspicion of PE is high.

The problem of a false-positive scan is common for the ICU patient in whom the prevalence of underlying cardiopulmonary disease is high. In general, perfusion defects in patients with proven PE are multiple and bilateral. Hence, the diagnosis of PE should be suspect when abnormalities are single or unilateral. Complete unilateral absence of perfusion with a normal contralateral lung probably is more likely to be the result of a mediastinal tumor, central mucous plug, bronchial cyst, or congenital pulmonary artery defect than PE. Emboli isolated to the upper lobes are unusual in ambulatory patients whose blood flow, when upright, distributes preferentially to the bases—this rule is often violated in bedridden patients in the ICU.

Contrasted CT Scanning

The contrasted CT scan, often redundantly called a "spiral CT," has become a popular diagnostic test, in large part because it is often easier and faster to obtain than VQ scan. When ordering a CT scan for suspected PE, it is important to communicate that fact to the radiology staff so optimal technique is used. The speed with which the scan is obtained (largely determined by the number of rows of detectors); the direction of scanning (foot to head or vice versa); the amount of, infusion rate and gating of contrast; width of the CT slice, and the reconstruction method all impact ability to see emboli. Another factor contributing to the popularity of CT is the *apparent* simplicity of interpretation compared to the VQ scan. This is translated into the common belief that there is never uncertainty and CT scans are only "positive" or "negative." However, studies using expert readers, and optimal equipment and injection technique, indicate that CT sensitivity and specificity ranges from 60% to

100% and 80% to 100%, respectively. These results mean that under ideal circumstances, the CT is comparable to the VQ scan. In addition, up to 15% of CT scans are "indeterminate" because of morbid obesity, motion artifact, or suboptimal contrast technique. The perceived simplicity in reading CTs can be seductive; the inexpert reader may interpret "streaming artifact" from poor contrast injection or low cardiac output as PE. Likewise, false-positive CTs can result from pulmonary artery compression from mediastinal lymphadenopathy, fibrosis, or tumor. Nevertheless, when a technically adequate CT demonstrates one or more luminal filling defects, especially if bilateral, PE is near certain. By contrast, a "negative CT" does not mean absence of PE; clot at the subsegmental level and beyond is routinely missed as is chronic thromboembolic disease.

CT has some clear disadvantages. In all cases, contrast is needed making the CT less attractive than the VQ scan in patients at risk for kidney injury. There is also a growing awareness of the dangers of diagnostic radiation exposure from CT. Another major drawback of the CT is the need to breath-hold during scanning—a difficult task for the dyspneic patient. Failure to remain motionless can result in false-negative studies. A final limitation of the CT is the relatively poor ability to visualize clots in vessels paralleling the CT beam track, especially when small.

So, given the characteristics of both studies, how does one decide between the VQ and CT? Obviously, in hospitals without nuclear medicine capabilities the choice is easy—after leg US is negative, if PE is suspected, contrasted CT is next. The choice is also easy for patients in shock; the CT is preferable because if the cause is PE, it will be large, centrally located, and easily seen (i.e., chances of a false-negative CT are near zero). In addition, if the catastrophe is not PE, the CT can identify a leaking aorta or large pericardial effusion. The CT is also probably the preferred imaging study for patients with profoundly abnormal CXRs (infiltrates or emphysema) in whom the VQ scan can be particularly difficult to interpret. In all other situations, the VQ scan is the preferred test.

Echocardiography

Transthoracic and transesophageal echocardiographies are sometimes diagnostic and are both useful adjuncts in the care of patients with PE. For example, in an ICU patient who develops unexplained hypoten-sion, an echocardiogram showing *new* right ventricular (RV) dilation and hypokinesis, and tricuspid regurgitation, with normal left ventricular (LV) function is suggestive of acute PE. Suspicions of PE are confirmed when on rare occasion, clot is visualized in the right heart or pulmonary outflow tract, the so-called clot in transit. Alternatively, that same study could reveal non-PE causes of hypotension: a large pericardial effusion, isolated poor LV contractility suggesting ischemia or infarction, or normal ventricular contractility and inspiratory vena cava collapse suggesting intravascular volume depletion. Although study continues, at this time, echocardiographic findings do not appear to carry sufficient weight to dictate the type of treatment. Specifically, RV dilation is so common a finding in patients with nonhemodynamically significant PE, it does not mandate thrombolytic therapy nor surgical or radiological intervention.

Angiography

Angiography is the definitive test for PE and is capable of yielding alternative diagnoses. In most cases, it is prudent to perform a VQ or CT scan before an angiogram. If the VQ scan is normal, angiography is unnecessary; if it shows perfusion defects, it guides the angiographer to the site for safe selective injections. A diagnostic CT also precludes need for angiography. Measurement of intracardiac and pulmonary artery pressures and cardiac output should be obtained with each arteriogram. Such measurements confirm alternate diagnoses (e.g., primary pulmonary hypertension, mitral stenosis) if the angiogram fails to show PE. When a contrasted CT is nondiagnostic and the clinical suspicion remains high, angiography is also appropriate because CT scanning may miss smaller emboli. Concern about the potential for "false-negative" angiograms if obtained hours or days after the onset of symptoms is unwarranted—the angiogram usually remains positive long (days to a week) after the embolic event. Criteria for an angiographic diagnosis must include an intraluminal filling defect or an abrupt convex "cutoff." (Oligemia and vessel tortuosity are nondiagnostic.) In the absence of DVT, a negative angiogram, carefully performed within 48 h of the onset of symptoms, indicates a negligible risk of clinically significant PE. Angiograms performed without "cut films," selective injections, multiple views, and magnification may miss a small emboli.

Risks of arteriography have been greatly over-stated—the overall mortality rate is lower than 0.01%. Likewise, there is a low risk of allergic dye reaction and vascular damage (right ventricular or pulmonary artery perforation). Catheter-induced arrhythmias usually are self-limited or easily treated. The greatest risks are incurred during contrast injection in patients with severe pulmonary hypertension, but even then, patients can safely undergo selective angiography with nonionic contrast media. If subsequent thrombolytic therapy is contemplated, punctures of noncompressible vessels should be avoided.

Bedside arteriography using a balloon flotation catheter has been tried in patients too unstable to leave the ICU. Unfortunately, bedside injections are much less sensitive and specific than studies performed in the angiography suite. Therefore, this test is helpful if positive but cannot confidently exclude emboli.

VTE Diagnostic Plan

No universally applicable diagnostic protocol can **4** be recommended; however, one rational strategy is suggested in Figure 23-1 and explained below. Usually, the best first diagnostic test is bilateral

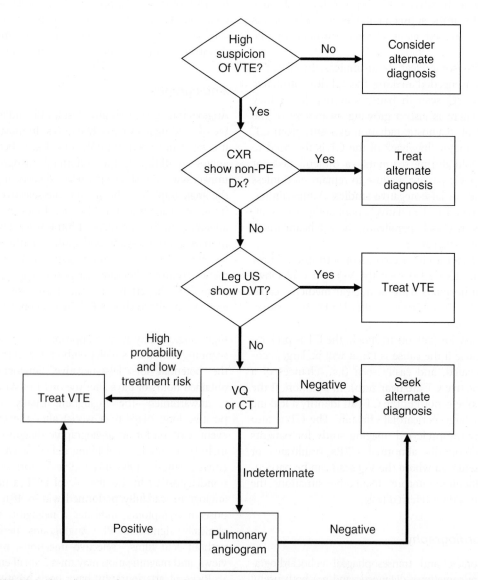

■ **FIGURE 23-1** Flow diagram of one strategy for evaluating inpatients with suspected PE. US, ultrasound; VTE, venous thromboembolism; DVT, deep venous thrombosis; VQ, ventilation–perfusion lung; CXR, chest X-ray; CT, computed chest tomogram; PE, pulmonary embolism.

lower-extremity US. If positive, the need for anticoagulation is established and information is provided as to the extent of clot and potential for subsequent PE. A negative study makes placement of an inferior vena cava (IVC) filter superfluous, even if PE is present because there is no "at-risk" thrombus. Although lower-extremity US will be negative in many cases of PE, safety, low cost, and portability make it an excellent first choice. In cases where a VQ or chest CT was chosen as the first diagnostic test but results are equivocal, a positive US establishes the need for treatment without resorting to angiography.

Controversy exists with regard to the second diagnostic test in suspected PE. Even though the VQ scan has limitations, it remains the next best study for hemodynamically stable patients without profoundly abnormal CXRs. By contrast, for the patient in shock or whose CXR is highly abnormal by virtue of diffuse infiltrate or emphysema, the contrasted CT is a better option. For the hypotensive patient, the CT will almost certainly visualize clot if it is the cause of shock and may give an alternative explanation (e.g., dissecting aneurysm).

A negative angiogram rules out clinically significant PE but does not exclude the possibility of DVT. It also is clear that a normal VQ scan rules out the need for angiography. Between these limits, the decision to perform or withhold angiography is based, in large part, on the need for diagnostic certainty and the perceived reliability of VQ or CT scan results. Many clinicians use the VQ scan only to exclude PE or as a map for selective angiography. Others rely heavily on patterns of scan defects for guidance. Because the therapy of DVT and PE usually is identical, demonstrating a DVT obviates the need for a pulmonary arteriogram. Indeed, one third or more patients with nondiagnostic VQ scans may avoid arteriography by performing a study for DVT.

Given all these considerations, an angiogram is probably indicated: (a) when thrombolytic therapy or interventional radiology or surgical embolectomy is contemplated; (b) when paradoxical embolism is suspected (to document right-to-left shunt or PE); and (c) when there is a high clinical suspicion of PE but leg US is negative and VQ or CT scan is nondiagnostic. PE is unlikely and hence an angiogram is probably not needed if the clinical probability of PE is considered to be low, leg US is negative and (a) chest CT or VQ scan is normal, (b) the VQ perfusion defect is smaller than CXR abnormality, (c) the VQ ventilation defect is much larger than perfusion defect, and (d) few matched subsegmental defects are observed on VQ scan. PE is very likely and an angiogram is probably not necessary when the clinical suspicion is high and VQ scan shows more than one lobar or more than two segmental mismatched defects with a CXR showing no acute changes in involved areas.

Prognosis and Rate of Resolution

A significant percentage of patients with massive PE die before the diagnosis is made, usually within hours of embolization. Adequately, anticoagulated patients who survive for several hours have an excellent prognosis. If anticoagulation with an antithrombin agent is not begun, clinically significant PE occurs in at least one third of cases. This risk falls to less than 10% with full effective anticoagulation. Whether or not VTE is treated, subclinical recurrence of PE (new lung scan defect) occurs in approximately 5% of patients, most within the first several days of initiating therapy. For well-anticoagulated patients, such early episodes represent embolization of preformed thrombus, not additional thrombus proliferation and thus, do not represent "anticoagulation failure." Because the thrombus is already formed, vena caval filtering may be the only therapy that might lower the incidence of PE.

Hemodynamic and gas exchange abnormalities usually reverse rapidly in patients who survive long enough for treatment to be started. Distal migration or shrinkage or fragmentation of clot certainly plays a role in this improvement, but vasoactive mediators (e.g., thromboxane and prostacyclin) are also operative. Angiographic findings can improve within 12 to 48 h but usually require 2 to 3 weeks or longer for complete resolution. Likewise, perfusion scan defects may disappear quickly (over days), but most resolve over weeks to months. Most (approx. 85%) of all perfusion defects resolve within 3 months; defects persisting at that time are likely to be permanent. Repeat VQ scanning at 6 to 12 weeks can document resolution of clot. Prospective studies suggest that chronic thrombotic pulmonary hypertension develops in 3% to 4% of PE victims, although it is not clear if in situ thrombosis, recurrent silent emboli or clot triggered vascular remodeling is to blame. The problem of chronic thrombotic pulmonary hypertension can be vexing unless the patient is generally healthy and the clot is amenable to thromboendarterectomy.

DVT and PE Treatment

Acute Anticoagulation

5 The treatments of DVT and PE rarely differ; therefore, making the diagnosis of either usually obviates the need to search for the complementary condition. The goals of treatment are to prevent clot extension, preserve venous architecture, and relieve pain. Because anticoagulation does not dissolve clot, even optimal therapy does not guarantee that PE will not occur in patients with established DVT. Although bed rest may reduce swelling and discomfort in the legs of patients with DVT, the need for bed rest to prevent dislodging clots is disproven. In fact, patients with DVT treated outside the hospital with unrestricted activity have lower rates of embolization than those confined to bed. In practice, many physicians confine patients to bed for the first 24 to 48 h of therapy as much to improve comfort as to reduce the risk of embolization. For patients with DVT, the application of graded compression stockings as soon as possible and continued for 6 to 12 months helps deter development of postthrombotic venous insufficiency.

VTE can be treated using weight-based intravenous (IV) or SC UFH adjusted by aPTT monitoring; or weight based subcutaneous LMWH or fonda-
6 parinux. Unless a dosing protocol is used, the likelihood of prompt therapeutic success with UFH is low (typically <50% over the first few days). All the while, the underanticoagulated patient remains at risk for clot propagation and PE. Key elements of an UFH protocol are (a) empiric anticoagulation while awaiting a confirmatory diagnostic test (unless the patient is bleeding); (b) weight-based dosing; (c) use of a large initial UFH bolus (approx. 80 to 100 units/kg); (d) using a higher than customary UFH infusion rate (18 to 20 units/kg/h); (e) performing a 6-h postbolus aPTT to prove adequate anticoagulation intensity; (f) frequent (typically every 6 h) monitoring until a therapeutic aPTT is achieved then at least daily aPTT check; and (g) rapidly achieving a "target" aPTT of 1.5 to 2.5 times the laboratory control or the patient's baseline aPTT if known.

Reasons for these protocol elements follow. Empiric anticoagulation is important because even in efficient hospitals there is often substantial delay (8 to 12 h) between the times a diagnostic test is ordered and the results are conveyed to the clinician. Indexing UFH therapy to weight has been shown to substantially improve the rate at which a therapeutic aPTT is reached. A large UFH bolus is required to overcome the nonspecific binding of UFH to numerous plasma and platelet proteins. The first aPTT after initiating heparin should be done at 6 h. If done sooner, it reflects residual bolus effect, not steady state, and may prompt inappropriate dose reductions because of worries over a "high" aPTT. If done later and subtherapeutic, the patient has been exposed to a prolonged period of underanticoagulation. Prompt success is important; failure to achieve anticoagulation within the first 24 h is associated with a substantially higher risk of recurrence. Because UFH clearance varies considerably among patients and over time in an individual, the rate of administration must be adjusted to maintain a target aPTT of 1.5 to 2.5 times normal. The aPTT often oscillates around the target value, seemingly without regard to dosing. Instead of "chasing" the aPTT with large changes in dose, a better strategy is to make modest changes in dosing and then reassess the effect. When the aPTT is below target, an UFH bolus (5,000 to 10,000 units) and an increase in the infusion rate of approximately 20% usually bring the aPTT into range. Dosing changes should be followed by an aPTT in 6 h. The half-life of UFH averages 60 to 90 min in patients with active thrombosis (absent renal failure). Therefore, unless the aPTT exceeds 2.5 to 3.0 times the control value or the patient is bleeding, it is unwise to completely stop an UFH infusion; to do so results in a subtherapeutic aPTT approximately half the time. A better strategy is to reduce the infusion rate by 20% to 25% and recheck the aPTT in 6 to 12 h. Early on, it is often necessary to measure the aPTT every 6 h until therapeutic levels are established. However, once two consecutive therapeutic aPTTs have been achieved, it is reasonable to reduce the frequency of aPTT sampling to once daily. Therapeutic aPTT values are much more likely to be achieved with the strategy outlined, but sometimes even with high UFH infusion rates, targets are not reached. In such patients, antiheparin antibodies and deficiencies of antithrombin or protein C or S should be suspected. High levels of factor VIII can also deter aPTT prolongation even though UFH blood levels are adequate. Because heparin resistance is a complex problem, an expert consultant in coagulation should be sought when the problem is encountered. Most "heparin failures" occur in patients who *consistently* have not been kept anticoagulated. Conversely, the risk of embolization because of an isolated subtherapeutic aPTT is minuscule.

Excessive prolongation of the aPTT (>100 s) may **7** increase the risk of bleeding, but the relationship between lesser aPTTs and bleeding is less clear. Overall, approximately 1% of anticoagulated patients will suffer some bleeding complication each day of treatment, accounting for the overall 10% incidence of hemorrhage during hospital-based UFH therapy. Spontaneous hemorrhage is rare in the absence of breached vascular integrity, renal insufficiency, impaired platelet function, or massive UFH overdose. Therefore, bleeding is most common among alcoholics, elderly patients, postoperative patients, and patients receiving drugs that impair platelet function. If serious bleeding occurs on UFH, the drug should be stopped and its anticoagulant effect will wane in roughly 8h. Reversal of UFH can be accelerated by using protamine sulfate; however, in practice, this is rarely done because of uncertainty of the correct protamine dose and because of the risk of anaphylactoid "protamine reactions." (Each milligram of protamine neutralizes approx. 100units of heparin.)

Although suboptimal because of discomfort to the patient and complexity of monitoring, UFH can also be given SC (approx. 7,500 to 10,000 units every 6h) if venous access is problematic. When given in this manner, dosage must also be guided by aPTT measurements.

LMWHs are replacing continuous infusion UFH because of their superior efficacy, ease of administration, and the reduced total cost of therapy. In comparative studies versus UFH, LMWHs are associated with fewer bleeding complications and perhaps as much as a 10-fold lower risk of HIT. Intermittent SC LMWH injections without aPTT monitoring reduce costs and shorten hospital stay. Many reliable patients with DVT with or without PE are now being treated at home if they are hemodynamically stable and do not require oxygen. Not all LMWHs can be considered equivalent; in the United States only two (enoxaparin and tinzaparin) are approved for VTE treatment. When serious bleeding develops in a patient receiving therapeutic doses of a LMWH, the drug should be stopped. Because of their longer half-lives, the majority of the anticoagulant effect of LMWHs disappears over 12 to 16h instead of the 8h for UFH. Protamine can be used to partially reverse the effects of LMWH.

Fondaparinux is a rapidly absorbed synthetic factor Xa inhibitor. Because of the compounds long half-life, once daily weight-based SC doses can be used for VTE treatment. (Because of uncertainty of the proper dose, patients less than 45kg should not be given the drug.) Recurrence and bleeding rates during VTE treatment are comparable to UFH and LMWHs in comparative trials. The hope that the smaller, synthetic fondaparinux molecule would completely avoid the problem of HIT has not been borne out as case reports have surfaced. Although there are no comparative trials of anticoagulants for HIT, the association of fondaparinux with the syndrome should probably discourage its use for this purpose.

Acute anticoagulation in special populations deserves comment. Caution should be exercised when giving *any* type of heparin to patients with renal insufficiency (i.e., GFR < 30 mL/min) because all varieties accumulate, enhancing bleeding risk. In patients with renal insufficiency, bleeding may be more common with LMWH compared to UFH for two reasons: First, UFH is typically monitored with an aPTT and hopefully doses are adjusted downward as the aPTT climbs, whereas in vitro monitoring is not usually performed with LMWHs. Anti-Xa assays can be done, but doing so removes many of the cost and convenience advantages of LMWHs. (When anti-Xa assays are performed, it is often found that reducing the LMWH dose by roughly 50% achieves an appropriate degree of anticoagulation.) Second, the longer half-lives of LMWHs may disproportionately predispose to drug accumulation. Thus, when dialysis-dependent patients require full anticoagulation, for now, it is probably best to use UFH. Because fondaparinux has no antidote, is exclusively cleared by the kidney, and has a half-life of 17h even when renal function is normal, it should not be given to patients with renal insufficiency.

For the morbidly obese patient, appropriate doses of UFH, LMWH, and fondaparinux are uncertain but the limited data that are available suggest that for patients up to approximately 160kg, enoxaparin at 1mg/kg every 12h is a reasonable choice. Pharmacokinetic studies using anti-Xa levels suggest that for patients greater than 160kg, dosing should be 1mg/kg of *actual* body weight. Alternative course of action is to use UFH monitored by aPTT or to monitor LMWH dosing with the anti-Xa assay.

Regardless of the form of heparin used, measuring hematocrit and platelet count approximately every 3 days is reasonable to detect asymptomatic anemia or thrombocytopenia. Heparins are typically continued for 5 to 7 days, while awaiting 2 to 3 days of proven warfarin-induced PT (INR) prolongation.

Thrombolytic Therapy

8 Unquestionably, thrombolytic agents accelerate the rate of clot resolution, sometimes dramatically. Unfortunately, these drugs have not been shown to decrease morbidity or mortality from PE, and the incidence of adverse effects is considerable. Most problematic is the risk of hemorrhage, especially intracranial bleeding (approx. 10% of patients have a serious bleeding complication with 1% to 2% experiencing intracranial hemorrhage). Therefore, contraindications include any condition that predisposes to serious bleeding (especially brain or spinal cord conditions). Puncture of noncompressible venous sites (e.g., subclavian) should be avoided while thrombolytics are administered. The potential for devastating hemorrhage and absence of demonstrated mortality benefit makes many physicians question the role of thrombolytic agents in the treatment of PE and certainly in DVT. By weighing the risk–benefit ratio, it seems reasonable to reserve thrombolytic drugs for patients with proven massive PE (a) with shock, (b) with refractory hypoxemia, or (c) for those with limb-threatening leg swelling from DVT. When used, these drugs should be initiated as soon as possible after the thrombotic event has been confirmed. No comparative trials provide the optimum dosing regimen for thrombolytic agents but currently, accelerated (1 to 2 h) administration of tissue plasminogen activator is the most popular approach. In dire circumstances, faster administration is often performed. Antithrombin therapy is begun as thrombin time and aPTT fall to approximately 1.5 times normal. Warfarin can be initiated simultaneously with UFH or LMWH. Aminocaproic acid can be used topically to stop local oozing or systemically to counteract thrombolysis if serious bleeding occurs. Reversal of the coagulation disorder also can be accomplished with fresh frozen plasma or cryoprecipitate.

Caval Interruption and Embolectomy

Percutaneous IVC filter placement, under X-ray or US guidance, can block passage of large clots from the legs and pelvis to the lungs. Amazingly, very limited data are available on the effectiveness of IVC filters and no data to indicate lifesaving benefit. The single well-done randomized clinical trial indicates that IVC filter insertion reduces the risk of recurrent embolization by 3% to 4% during the first 14 days after placement, but results in doubling of the risk of DVT recurrence (from 10% to 20%) in the next 2 years. Long-term follow-up shows that filter placement is associated with an astoundingly high risk of postthrombotic venous insufficiency. It is these long-term complications that spurred development of temporary filters which can be inserted acutely when anticoagulation is contraindicated and then be removed later when anticoagulation becomes safe. (All temporary filters are approved for permanent installation.) Although the concept of a removable filter is rational, in practice the vast majority of filters are never removed, and ironically when extraction is performed, it often causes DVT at the site of withdrawal. Despite limited data, it is reasonable to perform caval filtration for patients who have proven residual pelvic or lower extremity clot and (a) recurrent life-threatening PE despite adequate anticoagulation, (b) cannot receive thrombolytic therapy or anticoagulation safely, (c) suffer massive embolism or paradoxical emboli, (d) develop septic embolism from the lower extremities, or (e) clearly cannot withstand the hemodynamic effects of another embolism. Obviously, IVC filters have no effect on embolic risk if the source is in the upper extremities.

In experienced hands, serious insertion related complications are rare. Caval perforation happens more commonly than one might expect but fortunately it is not often problematic. Rarely, filters perforate the IVC causing retroperitoneal bleeding or migrate to the heart or pulmonary outflow tract—potentially lethal events. The filtered cava eventually clots off in one third or more of cases within the first 2 years. Large collaterals eventually may develop, but reports suggest that the risk of clinically important embolization through these vessels is low.

Because the procedure must be accomplished rapidly and requires cardiopulmonary bypass, emergent embolectomy is rarely successful. In most successful cases, the patient was already in the operating suite for another reason and was fortunate enough to have a thoracic surgical team and bypass setup available within minutes. Fortunately, most patients surviving long enough for the diagnosis of PE to be made will respond to thrombolytic or anticoagulant therapy. It is only in those patients who are gravely ill and deteriorating despite treatment that surgical therapy should be considered. On the other hand, a surgical approach to chronic, persistent central emboli may offer the only chance of relieving disability and potentially lethal pulmonary hypertension. For patients with suspected chronic thrombotic pulmonary hypertension, a VQ scan should demonstrate abnormalities that can then be confirmed by pulmonary angiography. Although less risky than an acute procedure, embolectomy for chronic thrombotic pulmonary artery disease remains hazardous and candidates must be carefully selected.

Long-Term Therapy

Regardless of the acute treatment chosen, at least 3 months of anticoagulation (usually with warfarin) is indicated. The goal in long-term therapy is to deter clot recurrence by maintaining an INR of 2 to 3. Patients with inherited thrombophilias may require more intense anticoagulation. For example, patients with anticardiolipin antibody syndrome often require INRs greater than 3. The INR should be in the therapeutic range for 2 to 3 days before heparin is stopped. Typically a 5-day overlap is necessary because initial prolongations of the PT (due to factor VII depletion) occur well before all components of the vitamin K-dependent pathway are depleted, during which time clotting is still possible. Most of the time a patient spends in the hospital is waiting for warfarin effect, and no credible evidence indicates that patients must receive a fixed period of heparin before warfarin can be safely initiated. Thus, it makes sense to start warfarin simultaneously with heparin. Although controversial, initial warfarin doses of 10 mg are safe and reduce the time to therapeutic effect compared to the commonly used 5-mg dose. However, even larger "loading" doses of warfarin do not prolong the PT more rapidly than these conventional doses and are not indicated.

The duration of warfarin anticoagulation must reflect not only the risk for recurrence and its potential physiologic consequences but also the risk of the therapy. Because the rate of recurrence falls rapidly with time from embolization, full anticoagulation for ≥3 months has become the standard in most situations. However, each time the duration of anticoagulation has been studied it appears that longer periods are associated with a substantially reduced risk of recurrence but only a slightly higher bleeding risk. Patients at continued high risk of recurrence, including those with genetic thrombophilias, anticardiolipin antibodies, uncured cancer, and patients, who have two or more thrombotic episodes, should probably be anticoagulated indefinitely, unless bleeding risk is prohibitive.

■ SUGGESTED READINGS

Geerts WH, Bergqvist D, Pineo GF, et al. Prevention of venous thromboembolism. *Chest.* 2008;133:S381–S453.

Kearon C, Kahn SR, Agnelli G, et al. Antithrombotic therapy of venous thromboembolism. *Chest.* 2008;133:S454–S545.

Kyrle PA, Eichinger S. Deepveinthrombosis. *Lancet.* 2005;365(9465): 1163–1174.

Prandoni P, Bernardi E. Upper extremity deep vein thrombosis. *Curr Opin Pulm Med.* 1999;5(4):222–226.

Streiff MB. Vena caval filters: A review for intensive care specialists. *J Intensive Care Med.* 2003;18(2):59–79.

Tooher R, Middleton P, Pham C, et al. A systematic review of strategies to improve prophylaxis for venous thromboembolism in hospitals. *Ann Surg.* 2005;241(3):397–415.

Oxygenation Failure, ARDS, and Acute Lung Injury

KEY POINTS

1 Six mechanisms may contribute to arterial oxygen desaturation: (a) inhalation of a hypoxic gas mixture, (b) alveolar hypoventilation, (c) impaired diffusion of oxygen across the alveolus, (d) $\dot{V}/\dot{Q}$ mismatching, (e) shunting of systemic venous blood to the systemic arterial circuit, and (f) abnormal desaturation of systemic venous blood in the presence of a $\dot{V}/\dot{Q}$ abnormality or shunt.

2 Clues to the nature of an oxygenation crisis are offered by radiographic appearance. Lung collapse (atelectasis), diffuse or patchy parenchymal infiltration, fluid overload, localized or unilateral infiltration, and a clear chest radiograph are distinct patterns that suggest specific etiologies and approaches to the treatment. Chest CT provides invaluable information to resolve overlapping shadows of lung parenchyma, pleural space, and chest wall.

3 Atelectasis is perhaps the most common cause of hypoxemia for the bedridden, critically ill, and postoperative patient. Potential consequences are worsened gas exchange, pneumonitis, and increased work of breathing. Mobilization, continuous positive airway pressure, and assiduous bronchial hygiene are keys to successful prevention and management.

4 Acute lung injury and acute respiratory distress syndrome are characterized by a delay between a characteristic precipitating event and the onset of dyspnea, impaired respiratory system compliance that results primarily from the loss of functional lung units, markedly reduced aerated lung volume, hypoxemia refractory to modest concentrations of inspired oxygen, and diffuse pulmonary infiltrates. The associated high-protein edema resolves more slowly than hydrostatic edema and is more likely to generate a patchy distribution and detectable air bronchograms.

5 Basic therapeutic principles in treating an oxygenation crisis are to minimize the risk:benefit ratio of ventilation by accepting hypercapnia in preference to high tidal volumes and ventilating pressures, to adequately recruit the lung, and to minimize tissue oxygen demand and ventilation requirements (e.g., by sedation).

6 Shifts of body position alter the regional distributions of ventilation and perfusion and may be associated with changes in tidal and end-expiratory volumes. Prone positioning clearly alters the regional distribution of transpulmonary pressure and may dramatically improve the efficiency of arterial oxygenation associated with an unchanging ventilatory pattern and level of applied positive end-expiratory pressure.

7 Manipulation of peak, mean, and end-expiratory alveolar pressures plays a crucial role in achieving adequate arterial oxygenation at an acceptable FiO_2. Moderately high pressures may be needed during a recruiting maneuver to increase the transpulmonary pressure enough to open refractory lung units, especially those in dependent zones. End-expiratory alveolar pressure (total positive end-expiratory pressure, the sum of positive end-expiratory pressure and auto-positive end-expiratory pressure) helps maintain patency of alveolar units at risk for collapse. Under conditions of passive inflation, mean airway pressure reflects average lung size and correlates with oxygenation efficiency.

8 High tidal volume/low positive end-expiratory pressure strategies may extend alveolar injury or retard healing of the already-injured tissues. In the early phase of acute respiratory distress syndrome, avoiding excessive transpulmonary stretching pressures and inspiratory flow rates during tidal inflation while maintaining sufficient end-expiratory transpulmonary pressure is a rational ventilatory strategy. This approach often results in low tidal volumes (depending on lung compliance) and the need to accept CO_2 retention (permissive hypercapnia).

9 Many choices for ventilatory mode are equally defensible, as long as the practitioner ensures adequate oxygen delivery, follows similar guidelines for lung protection, and remains alert to the potential shortcomings and complications of the mode in use.

10 The essential elements of a lung-protective approach to ventilating acute respiratory distress syndrome are (a) to minimize oxygen and ventilation demands, (b) to apply sufficient end-expiratory and end-inspiratory pressures to maintain nearly complete recruitment of functional alveoli, (c) to avoid overstretching the lung, (d) to accept hypercapnia unless there is a serious neurologic or cardiovascular contraindication, (e) to implement prone positioning in the difficult-to-oxygenate patient, and (f) to consider the potential benefits of avoiding fluid excess and of using adjunctive ventilatory aids (such as inhaled prostacyclin).

■ OXYGENATION FAILURE

Definitions

Respiratory failure may be considered a problem in one or more of the steps necessary to sustain mitochondrial energy production. Dysfunction may occur in ventilation (the movement of gases between the environment and the lungs; see Chapter 25), in intrapulmonary gas exchange (the process in which mixed-venous blood releases CO_2 and becomes oxygenated), in gas transport (the delivery of adequate quantities of oxygenated blood to the metabolizing tissue), or in tissue gas exchange (the extraction or use of O_2 and release of CO_2 by the peripheral tissues).

The latter two steps in this process may fail independently of the performance of the lung or ventilatory pump. Tissue O_2 delivery depends not only on the partial pressure of arterial oxygen (PaO_2) but also on the nonpulmonary factors—

cardiac output, hemoglobin (Hgb) concentration, and the ability of Hgb to take up and release O_2. Cardiogenic shock, severe anemia, and carbon monoxide poisoning provide clinical examples of O_2 transport failure (see Chapter 38). Laboratory abnormalities characteristic of such conditions are lactic acidosis and reduced O_2 content of mixed-venous blood (even in the face of adequate arterial oxygen tension).

Failure of O_2 uptake refers to the inability of the tissue to extract and use O_2 for aerobic metabolism. The clearest clinical examples of a derangement in this terminal phase of the oxygen transport chain are septic shock and cyanide poisoning, in which cellular cytochromes (key enzymes in the electron transport process) are inhibited. During sepsis, there is failure of an often generous cardiac output to distribute appropriately and/or an inability of the tissues themselves to make use of the O_2 available. Unlike transport insufficiency, failure of tissue uptake implies insufficient O_2 *extraction* and, therefore, may be associated with normal or even high values for mixed-venous oxygen tension, saturation, and content. Some indices that are helpful in other forms of oxygenation failure (i.e., cardiac output, arterial O_2 tension, and mixed-venous O_2 saturation [SvO_2]) may not reflect the impaired tissue O_2 uptake reliably; lactic acidosis may be the sole laboratory indicator. Therapy directed at failure of the O_2 transport mechanism is discussed in detail elsewhere (see Chapters 1 and 3). The following discussion focuses on the problems that bear on the performance of the lung in oxygenating the arterial blood and in ventilatory failure.

■ MECHANISMS OF ARTERIAL HYPOXEMIA

Six mechanisms may contribute to arterial oxygen **1** desaturation (Table 24-1):

TABLE 24-1 MECHANISMS OF ARTERIAL HYPOXEMIA

Low inspired FiO_2
Hypoventilation
Impaired diffusion
$\dot{V}/\dot{Q}$ mismatching
Shunt
Desaturated mixed-venous blood[a]

[a]In the presence of other mechanisms for hypoxemia.

1. Inhalation of a hypoxic gas mixture or ascent to altitude
2. Hypoventilation
3. Impaired alveolar diffusion of oxygen
4. Ventilation–perfusion ($\dot{V}/\dot{Q}$) mismatching
5. Shunting of systemic venous blood to the systemic arterial circuit
6. Abnormal desaturation of systemic venous blood in conjunction with cause 3, 4, or 5

Low Inspired Oxygen Fraction

A decrease in the partial pressure of inhaled oxygen occurs in toxic fume inhalation, in closed-space fires that consume O_2 in combustion, and at high altitudes because of reduced barometric pressure. In this "low fraction of inspired oxygen (FiO_2)" context, it should not be forgotten that very rarely, unsuspected disconnection from supplemental oxygen precipitates hypoxemia.

Hypoventilation

Hypoventilation causes the partial pressure of alveolar oxygen (PAO_2) to fall when alveolar oxygen is not replenished quickly enough in the face of its ongoing removal by the blood. Although PaO_2 may fall much faster than $PaCO_2$ rises during the initial phase of hypoventilation or apnea, the steady-state concentration of PaO_2 is predicted by the simplified alveolar gas equation:

$$PAO_2 = PiO_2 - PaCO_2/R$$

In this equation, PiO_2 is the partial pressure of the inspired oxygen at the tracheal level (corrected for water vapor pressure at body temperature), and R is the respiratory exchange ratio (i.e., the ratio of CO_2 production to oxygen consumption at steady state). Transiently, R can fall to very low values because oxygen is taken up faster than CO_2 is delivered to the alveolus. Such a mechanism explains posthyperventilation hypoxemia and may contribute to hypoxemia that accompanies hemodialysis.

Impaired Diffusion

Impaired diffusion of oxygen prevents complete equilibration of alveolar gas with pulmonary capillary blood. Although this mechanism has uncertain clinical importance, many factors that adversely influence diffusion are encountered clinically: increased distance between alveolus and erythrocyte, decreased O_2 gradient for diffusion, and

shortened transit time of the red cell through the capillary (high cardiac output with limited capillary reserve).

Ventilation–Perfusion Mismatching

$\dot{V}/\dot{Q}$ mismatching is the most frequent contributor to the clinically important O_2 desaturation. Lung units that are poorly ventilated in relation to perfusion cause desaturation; high $\dot{V}/\dot{Q}$ units contribute to physiologic dead space but not to hypoxemia. The relationship of O_2 content to PaO_2 is curvilinear. At normal barometric pressure, little additional O_2 can be loaded onto blood with already saturated Hgb, no matter how high the O_2 tension in the overventilated alveolus may rise. Because samples of blood exiting from different lung units mix gas contents (not partial pressures), overventilating some units in an attempt to compensate for others that are underventilated does not maintain PaO_2 at a normal level. Therefore, when equal volumes of blood from well-ventilated and poorly ventilated units mix, the blended sample will have O_2 content halfway between them but PaO_2 disproportionately weighted toward that of the lower $\dot{V}/\dot{Q}$ unit. Even though minute ventilation (V_E) and cardiac output ($\dot{Q}$) may be absolutely normal, *regional* $\dot{V}/\dot{Q}$ mismatching will cause PaO_2 to fall.

A high concentration of inspired O_2 will correct hypoxemia when $\dot{V}/\dot{Q}$ mismatching, hypoventilation, or diffusion impairment is the cause. (The PAO_2 of even poorly ventilated nonshunt units climbs high enough to achieve full saturation.) After breathing 100% O_2 for a sufficient period of time, only perfused units that are totally unventilated (shunt units) contribute to hypoxemia. However, when hypoxemia is caused by alveolar units with very low $\dot{V}/\dot{Q}$ ratios, relatively concentrated O_2 mixtures must be given before a substantial change in the PaO_2 is observed (see Fig. 5-2 in Chapter 5).

Shunting

The term *shunt* refers to the percentage of the total systemic venous blood flow that bypasses the gas-exchanging membrane and transfers venous blood unaltered to the systemic arterial system. Changes in FiO_2—either upward or downward—have very little influence on PaO_2 when the true shunt fraction, as measured on pure oxygen, exceeds 30% (Fig. 24-1). In contrast, venous admixture of similar magnitude is variably responsive, to the extent

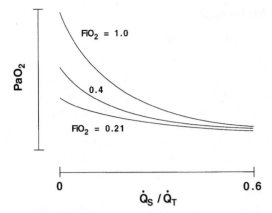

■ **FIGURE 24-1** Relationship of arterial oxygen tension (PaO$_2$) to true shunt fraction ($\dot{Q}_S/\dot{Q}_T$) for three values of inspired oxygen fraction (FiO$_2$). Variations of FiO$_2$ exert negligible effects on PaO$_2$ when true shunt exceeds 30%.

that low $\dot{V}/\dot{Q}$ units account for the hypoxemia. Shunt can be cardiovascular, as in cyanotic right-to-left congenital heart disease, the opening of a patent foramen ovale due to right ventricular overload, or the passage of blood through abnormal vascular channels within the lung (pulmonary arteriovenous malformations). However, by far the most common cause of shunting is pulmonary disease characterized by unventilated alveolar spaces that cannot respond to oxygen therapy. After an extended exposure to an FiO$_2$ of 1.0, all alveoli that remain open are filled with pure oxygen. (Some absorption atelectasis may occur in very low $\dot{V}/\dot{Q}$ areas when pure oxygen is breathed, adding to the measured shunt. In the clinical setting, however, the magnitude of this artifact usually is small.) The fraction of blood shunted across the lung from all sources (Q_S/Q_T) can be calculated from the following formula:

$$Q_S/Q_T = [(CcO_2 - CaO_2)/(CcO_2 - CvO_2)]$$

In this equation, C denotes content, and the lower case letters c, a, and v denote end-capillary, arterial, and mixed-venous blood, respectively. In making such calculations, end-capillary and calculated alveolar oxygen tensions are assumed equivalent. For a patient breathing pure O$_2$, shunt percentages lower than 25% can be estimated rapidly by dividing the alveolar to arterial O$_2$ tension difference (approx. 670—PaO$_2$) by 20, assuming also that the PaCO$_2$ and CvO$_2$ are normal. For example, if measured PaO$_2$ is 270 mm Hg, estimated shunt is 400/20, or 20%.

At inspired oxygen fractions lower than 1.0, true shunt cannot be estimated reliably by an analysis of oxygen contents, but "venous admixture" or "physiologic shunt" can. (Many publications

erroneously refer to venous admixture from all causes as "shunt.") Any degree of arterial O$_2$ desaturation can be considered as if it all originated from true shunt units. To calculate venous admixture, CcO$_2$ in the shunt formula is estimated from the ideal alveolar PO$_2$ at that particular fraction of inspired oxygen (FiO$_2$).

Many indices have been devised in an attempt to characterize the efficacy of oxygen exchange across the full spectrum of FiO$_2$ values. Although no index is completely successful, the PaO$_2$:PAO$_2$ ratio and the alveolar to arterial oxygen tension difference (A–a)O$_2$ are often used (see Chapter 5). Both, however, are affected by changes in S$\bar{v}$O$_2$, even when the lung tissue itself retains normal ability to transfer oxygen to the blood. Another imprecise but commonly used indicator of oxygen exchange is the PaO$_2$:FiO$_2$ ratio (the P:F ratio). In healthy adults, this ratio normally exceeds 400, whatever the FiO$_2$ may be. Hypoventilation and changes in the inspired O$_2$ concentration minimally alter these ratios in the absence of FiO$_2$-related absorption atelectasis or cardiovascular adjustments.

Abnormal Desaturation of Systemic Venous Blood

The admixture of abnormally desaturated venous blood is an important mechanism acting to lower the PaO$_2$ in patients with impaired pulmonary gas exchange and reduced cardiac output. CvO$_2$, the product of Hgb concentration and S$\bar{v}$O$_2$, is influenced by cardiac output (Q), arterial oxygen saturation (SaO$_2$), and oxygen consumption (VO$_2$):

$$S\bar{v}O_2 \approx SaO_2 - [VO_2/(Hgb \times Q)]$$

It is clear from this equation that S$\bar{v}$O$_2$ is directly influenced by any imbalance between VO$_2$ and oxygen delivery. Thus, anemia that is inadequately compensated by an increase in cardiac output or a cardiac output too low for metabolic needs in a nonanemic patient can cause both S$\bar{v}$O$_2$ and PaO$_2$ to fall when the venous admixture percentage is abnormal.

Fluctuations in S$\bar{v}$O$_2$ exert a more profound influence on PaO$_2$ when the shunt is fixed, as in regional lung diseases (e.g., atelectasis), than when the shunt varies with changing cardiac output, as it tends to do in diffuse lung injury (acute respiratory distress syndrome [ARDS]) (Fig. 24-2). Even when S$\bar{v}$O$_2$ is abnormally low, PaO$_2$ will remain

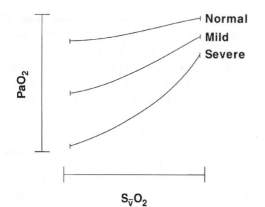

■ **FIGURE 24-2** Influence of mixed venous oxygen saturation (S$\bar{v}$O$_2$) on PaO$_2$ in patients with mild and severe lung disease. Variations in S$\bar{v}$O$_2$ related to an oxygen consumption/delivery imbalance have minimal effects on PaO$_2$ in normal subjects but may profoundly affect PaO$_2$ in patients with extensive lung disease.

unaffected if all mixed-venous blood gains access to well-oxygenated, well-ventilated alveoli. (A marked decline in S$\bar{v}$O$_2$ without arterial hypoxemia routinely occurs during heavy exercise in healthy subjects.) Therefore, abnormal $\dot{V}/\dot{Q}$ matching or shunt is necessary for venous desaturation to contribute to hypoxemia.

■ DISEASE-INDUCED HYPOXEMIA

2 Oxygenation disorders can be categorized by their radiographic appearances, which give important clues to the appropriate management approach. Lung collapse (atelectasis), diffuse or patchy parenchymal infiltration, hydrostatic edema, localized or unilateral infiltration, and a clear chest radiograph are common patterns (Fig. 24-3).

Atelectasis

Variants of Atelectasis

There are several morphologic types and mechanisms of atelectasis. Regional microatelectasis develops spontaneously in a healthy lung during shallow breathing when it is not periodically stretched beyond its usual tidal range. Platelike atelectasis may be an exaggeration of this phenomenon because of regional hypodistention (e.g., secondary to pleural effusion or impaired diaphragmatic excursion). Both microatelectasis and platelike atelectasis occur most commonly in dependent regions. Lobar collapse usually results from gas absorption behind an airway plugged by retained secretions, a misplaced endotracheal tube, bronchial compression by the heart or pleural effusion, or a large airway mass. Microatelectasis and platelike atelectasis occur routinely in patients on prolonged, uninterrupted bedrest and in postoperative patients who have undergone upper abdominal incisions.

Potential consequences of acute atelectasis are worsened gas exchange, pneumonitis, and increased work of breathing. PaO$_2$ drops precipitously to its nadir within minutes to hours of sudden bronchial occlusion, but it then improves steadily over hours to days as hypoxic vasoconstriction and mechanical factors increase pulmonary vascular resistance through the affected area. Whether an individual patient manifests hypoxemia depends heavily on the vigor of the hypoxic vasoconstrictive response, the abruptness of collapse, and the tissue volume involved. If small areas of atelectasis develop slowly, hypoxemia may never surface as a clinical problem.

Diffuse microatelectasis may be radiographically silent but detectable on physical examination by

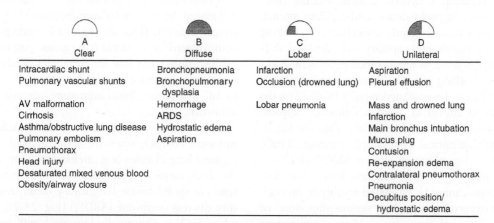

A Clear	B Diffuse	C Lobar	D Unilateral
Intracardiac shunt	Bronchopneumonia	Infarction	Aspiration
Pulmonary vascular shunts	Bronchopulmonary dysplasia	Occlusion (drowned lung)	Pleural effusion
AV malformation	Hemorrhage	Lobar pneumonia	Mass and drowned lung
Cirrhosis	ARDS		Infarction
Asthma/obstructive lung disease	Hydrostatic edema		Main bronchus intubation
Pulmonary embolism	Aspiration		Mucus plug
Pneumothorax			Contusion
Head injury			Re-expansion edema
Desaturated mixed venous blood			Contralateral pneumothorax
Obesity/airway closure			Pneumonia
			Decubitus position/ hydrostatic edema

■ **FIGURE 24-3** Radiographic patterns associated with hypoxemia.

dependent (posterior or basilar) end-inspiratory rales, which improve after several sustained deep breaths (sighs) or coughs. Plate atelectasis yields similar physical findings plus tubular breath sounds and egophony over the involved area. Lobar atelectasis gives a dull percussion note and diminished breath sounds if the bronchus is occluded by secretions, but tubular breath sounds and egophony are heard if the central airway is patent. (The latter findings correlate well with the presence of air bronchograms on chest radiograph.) Plate atelectasis develops most frequently at the lung base above a pleural effusion or above a raised, splinted, or immobile hemidiaphragm. Obesity predisposes to *all* forms of atelectasis. Lobar atelectasis occurs most commonly in patients with copious airway secretions and limited power to expel them. Acute upper lobe collapse occurs less commonly and tends to resolve quickly because of comparatively good gravitational drainage and greater local transpulmonary pressure. Collapse of the left lower lobe is more frequent than collapse of the right lower lobe, perhaps because of its retrocardiac position and its smaller caliber, sharply angulated bronchus. Lobar atelectasis may be complete or partial, but in either case, it is radiographically recognized by opacification in an anatomically geographic distribution, displaced fissures and hilum, compensatory hyperinflation of surrounding tissue, narrowed rib interspaces, and obliterated air/soft tissue boundaries (see Chapter 11). Small amounts of pleural fluid form as an expected consequence of lobar collapse and do not necessarily signify an additional pathologic process.

Management of Atelectasis

Prophylaxis
Effective prevention of atelectasis in high-risk patients counteracts shallow breathing, maintains adequate transpulmonary pressure by appropriate positioning or airway pressure, and avoids secretion retention. Obesity, chronic bronchitis, impaired airway clearance, neuromuscular weakness, regional chest wall trauma, recent thoracic or abdominal surgery, and advanced age are predisposing factors. Atelectasis is to be expected whenever the patient is prevented from taking a deep breath by pain, splinting, or weakness. Upper abdominal, lateral chest, midline chest, and lower abdominal incisions are associated with the highest incidence of postoperative atelectasis (in that order). Preoperatively, the airways should be maximally dilated and free of

infection. Postoperatively, patients should be encouraged to breathe deeply, to sit upright, and to cough vigorously. Pain should be relieved, but alertness should be preserved. Drainage of excess pleural fluid or ascites deserves consideration. Frequent turning and early mobilization are among the most important prophylactic measures. Continuous positive airway pressure (CPAP) may be helpful, especially for intubated patients. Respiratory therapy (RT) techniques such as airway suctioning, incentive spirometry, and chest vibropercussion (if tolerated) are prophylactically as well as therapeutically effective in well-selected patients (see Chapter 18).

Treatment
Whenever possible, mobilization is a highly effective treatment. Periodic deep breathing effectively reverses platelike atelectasis and microatelectasis. Sustained deep breathing is particularly useful. Whether a higher lung volume is achieved by positive airway pressure or by negative pleural pressure is immaterial, assuming that a similar extent and distribution of distention occurs in both cases. Adequate PEEP or CPAP is accepted as routine in treatment of established collapse. Relief of chest wall pain helps reduce splinting and enables more effective coughing. Intercostal nerve blocks with anesthetic agents such as bupivacaine may be effective for 8 to 12 h. Epidural narcotics also may be effective in certain settings. Retained secretions must be dislodged from the central airways. For the unintubated patient, effective bronchial hygiene is inconsistently accomplished with blind tracheal suctioning alone. Nasopharyngeal airways certainly help, but they are not well tolerated by patients who are awake and are not intended for extended care (see Chapter 6). Vigorous RT initiated soon after the onset of lobar collapse (which may include postural maneuvers and/or vibropercussion) can reverse most cases of atelectasis that are due to airway plugging within 24 to 48 h. As a rule, fiberoptic bronchoscopy should be reserved for patients with symptomatic lobar collapse who *lack* central "air bronchograms" that branch into the collapsed zone and who cannot undergo (or fail to respond to or tolerate) 48 h of vigorous RT. Even whole lung collapse usually merits at least one RT treatment (including stimulated cough and tracheal suctioning) before bronchoscopy is performed. After re-expansion, a prophylactic positioning and RT program should be initiated to prevent recurrence. Adjunctive measures (e.g., bronchodilators, hydration, and

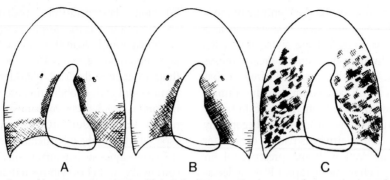

■ **FIGURE 24-4** Radiographic patterns in patients with impaired oxygenation because of congestive heart failure **(A)**, vascular congestion because of volume overload **(B)**, and ARDS **(C)**. Kerley lines, widened vascular pedicle, costophrenic angle sparing, blurred hilar structures, and paucity of air bronchograms help distinguish congestive heart failure from ARDS. (Reprinted from Milne et al. *Am J Roentgenol.* 1985;144:879–894, with permission.)

frequent turning and in some cases, mucolytics and mucus lubricants) should not be ignored.

Diffuse Pulmonary Infiltration

Fluid confined to the interstitial spaces may cause hypoxemia as a result of peribronchial edema, $\dot{V}/\dot{Q}$ mismatching, and microatelectasis; however, very few processes are confined exclusively to the air spaces or to the interstitium. Radiographic signs of extensive alveolar filling include segmental distribution, coalescence, fluffy margins, air bronchograms, rosette patterns, and silhouetting of normal structures. A diffuse infiltrate is said to be largely "interstitial" if these signs are largely absent and the infiltrate parallels the vascular distribution. Computed tomography imaging greatly increases the diagnostic precision, especially when a thickened or diseased chest wall obscures radiographic features of the lung parenchyma. Any diffuse interstitial process will appear more radiodense at the bases than at the apices, in part because there is more tissue to penetrate and because vascular engorgement tends to be greater there. Gravitationally dependent alveoli also are less distended, so the ratio of aerated volume to total tissue volume declines.

The major categories of acute disease that produce diffuse pulmonary infiltration and hypoxemia are pneumonitis (infection and aspiration), cardiogenic pulmonary edema, intravascular volume overload, and ARDS. From a radiographic viewpoint, these processes may be difficult to distinguish; however, a few characteristic features are helpful.

Hydrostatic Edema

Perihilar infiltrates (sparing the costophrenic angles), a prominent vascular pattern, and a widened vascular pedicle suggest volume overload or incipient cardiogenic edema (Fig. 24-4). A gravitational distribution of edema is highly consistent with well-established left ventricular failure (or long-standing, severe volume overload), especially when accompanied by cardiomegaly and a widened vascular pedicle. Patchy peripheral infiltrates that lack a gravitational predilection and show reluctance to change with position suggest ARDS. Interestingly, septal (Kerley) lines and distinct peribronchial cuffing are very seldom seen in ARDS without coexisting volume overload (see following). On the other hand, prominent air bronchograms are quite unusual with purely hydrostatic etiologies but occur commonly in permeability edema (ARDS) and pneumonia. It should be recalled that permeable vessels leak fluid even at normal vascular pressures, so mixed patterns of ARDS and hydrostatic edema are often seen.

Variants of Hydrostatic Edema

Hydrostatic pulmonary edema (HPE) may occur in multiple settings that have differing implications for prognosis and treatment. The most familiar form of HPE accompanies left ventricular failure. In this setting, signs of systemic hypoperfusion and inadequate cardiac output often accompany oxygenation failure. However, HPE can develop even with a normally well-compensated ventricle during transient cardiac dysfunction (ischemia, hypertensive crisis, arrhythmias, etc.). When the myocardium fails to fully relax during diastole (diastolic dysfunction), volume loading or temporary disturbances of left heart contractility (e.g., ischemia), mitral valve functioning, or heart rate or rhythm may cause rapid, transient alveolar flooding known as "flash pulmonary edema." In this setting, an impressive radiographic appearance may both develop and resolve quickly.

Acute Lung Injury and ARDS

Definitions and Categories

For many years after its original description, ARDS signified the "adult" respiratory distress syndrome. In current parlance, however, acute lung injury (ALI) is a general term that is applied to all degrees of radiographically apparent, diffuse hypoxemic lung injury of diverse etiologies, with ARDS being the most severe form of ALI—regardless of age. "Acute respiratory distress syndrome" is an imprecise term that is often applied to any acute diffuse parenchymal infiltration associated with severe hypoxemia and not attributable to HPE. Published definitions are quite liberal and do not specify the characteristics of the acute infiltrates, nor the mechanical properties of the thorax, nor the conditions under which the oxygenation data were gathered. Several published studies document that experts frequently disagree on whether a radiograph is consistent with "ARDS," and others have shown that modifications of PEEP and/or position can move a potential candidate into or out of the accepted PaO_2/FiO_2 criterion. Given these definitional shortcomings, it may not be surprising that few "positive" therapeutic trials in ALI/ARDS have appeared, even though the mortality of patients with similar severity of physiologic impairment has clearly declined over the past decades. The ARDS designation may be most useful when restricted to acute noncardiogenic pulmonary edema with certain characteristic features:

1. Brief delay between the precipitating event and rapidly developing dyspnea
2. Impaired respiratory system compliance
3. Markedly reduced aerated lung volume
4. Hypoxemia refractory to modest levels of inspired oxygen and PEEP
5. Delayed resolution

Primary (Pulmonary) Versus Secondary (Extrapulmonary) Acute Lung Injury

The pathogenesis of permeability edema is almost certain to vary with the inciting event. Despite its many diverse causes, sepsis, pneumonia, aspiration, and multiple traumas account for most cases.

One useful categorization of patients with ALI and ARDS considers that "primary" ARDS, in which lung injury is initiated from the epithelial or pulmonary side (e.g., pneumonia), behaves somewhat differently from ARDS caused by injury to the vascular endothelium ("secondary" or "extrapulmonary" ARDS). There are some data to support this contention, as the lungs of "primary" patients are less likely to recruit effectively than are those of "secondary" patients. Despite such differences, the core pathophysiology of ARDS is sufficiently similar to warrant a common treatment approach.

A prominent feature of all forms of ARDS is injury to the alveolar–capillary membrane from either the gas side (e.g., smoke inhalation, aspiration of gastric acid) or the blood side (e.g., sepsis, fat embolism). Increased membrane permeability allows seepage of protein-rich fluid into the interstitial and alveolar spaces. Such fluids inhibit surfactant, contributing to widespread microatelectasis. Although wedge pressure usually remains normal, increased pulmonary vascular resistance and some degree of pulmonary hypertension are almost invariable in the latter stages of severe disease. Extreme pulmonary hypertension portends a poor prognosis. Occasionally, the development of pulmonary hypertension causes elevated right-sided filling pressure and opening of a patent foramen ovale, with resulting right-to-left shunting through the heart. An echocardiogram with commercial contrast agent or agitated saline (bubble study) is a worthwhile undertaking in cases of hypoxemia refractory to usual measures. Images should be obtained in both upright and recumbent positions, especially when there is a noticeable positional difference in arterial oxygen saturation.

Diffuse pulmonary infiltration with a normal wedge pressure can be seen in other problems, such as flash pulmonary edema and partially treated heart failure. Apart from any difference in capillary pressure, permeability edema differs from hydrostatic edema in that it resists clearance by diuretic therapy and initiates a cellular inflammatory response that may require weeks to recede and even longer to heal.

Rapidly Resolving Noncardiogenic Edema

A few disorders that fall loosely under the heading of ARDS are worth noting because of their fundamentally different pathophysiology and clinical course. In certain settings, transient disruption in the barrier function of the pulmonary capillary can occur without overt endothelial damage. Neurogenic and heroin-induced pulmonary edema, for example, are two problems in which a transiently elevated pulmonary venous pressure is believed to open epithelial tight junctions, forcing extravasation of proteinaceous fluid. However, barrier resealing and resolution of edema occur promptly without widespread endothelial damage or protracted inflammation. A similar process may be seen in settings such as severe metabolic acidosis and cardiopulmonary resuscitation. From the alveolar side, certain inhalational injuries (e.g., limited chlorine or ammonia gas exposure) can produce a dramatic initial picture, only to clear rapidly over a brief period. Pulmonary edema that follows re-expansion of lung compressed by air or fluid may relate partially to the negative pressures developed during the procedure and to the deficiency of functional surfactant that characterizes airless lung.

Hypoxemia with a Clear Chest Radiograph

It is not uncommon for patients to present with new-onset, life-threatening hypoxemia without major radiographic evidence of infiltration. In such cases, occult shunting and severe $\dot{V}/\dot{Q}$ mismatching are the most likely mechanisms (Table 24-1). Despite an unremarkable plain chest film, computed tomography almost invariably shows evidence for "ground glass" infiltration that signifies microcollapse and/or edema. Intracardiac or intrapulmonary shunts, asthma and other forms of airway obstruction, low lung volume superimposed on a high closing capacity (e.g., bronchitis in a supine obese patient), pulmonary embolism, and occult microvascular communications (such as those occurring in patients with cirrhosis) are potential explanations. Hypoxemia is amplified by profound desaturation of mixed-venous blood, by reversal of hypoxic vasoconstriction with therapeutic vasoactive agents (e.g., nitroprusside, calcium channel blockers, and dopamine), and by the severe $\dot{V}/\dot{Q}$ imbalance occasionally encountered after acute head injury.

Unilateral Lung Disease

Unilateral infiltration or marked asymmetry of radiographic density suggests a confined set of etiologic possibilities, most of which occur in highly characteristic clinical settings (Fig. 24-3). Marked asymmetry of radiographic involvement should prompt an especially careful search for an unaddressed and readily reversible cause of hypoxemia. In some cases, especially pneumonitis or airway plugging, precautions also should be taken against generalization of the process—"propagation prevention" (see Chapter 8).

■ TECHNIQUES TO IMPROVE TISSUE OXYGENATION (TABLE 24-2)

Basic Therapeutic Principles

Although atelectasis, fluid overload, and infection often yield to specific measures, the treatment of diffuse lung injury remains largely supportive. The primary therapeutic aims are to maintain oxygen delivery, to relieve an excessive breathing workload, and to establish electrolyte balance while preventing further damage from oxygen toxicity, barotrauma, ventilator-induced lung injury (VILI), infection, and other iatrogenic complications. To these ends, the clinician should keep a few fundamental principles in mind.

Minimize the Risk: Benefit Ratio

Positive airway pressure, oxygen, and vasoactive drugs are potentially injurious. Therefore, frequent reassessment is indicated of the need for current medications as well as levels of PEEP, FiO_2, and the use and intensity of ventilator support. In well-selected cases, an oxygen saturation of 85% may be acceptable if the patient has adequate oxygen-carrying capacity and circulatory reserve without signs of oxygen privation (e.g., lactic acidosis). Similarly, allowing $PaCO_2$ to climb (buffering pH, if necessary, with $NaHCO_3$) may minimize the ventilatory

TABLE 24-2 TECHNIQUES TO IMPROVE TISSUE OXYGENATION

Increase FiO_2

Increase mean lung volume and alveolar pressure
    PEEP/auto-PEEP
    Extend inspiratory time fraction

Decubitus, upright, or prone positioning
Bronchodilation

Improve O_2 delivery/consumption ratio
    Reduce O_2 requirements
    Work of breathing
    Fever
    Agitation
    Increase cardiac output
    Increase Hgb

Remove systemic pulmonary vasodilators (e.g., nitroprusside)

Consider adjunctive support
    Vibration
    Inhaled Nitric oxide or inhaled prostacyclin

requirement and reduce the risk of barotrauma (see Permissive Hypercapnia, following, and Chapter 8). Mean intrathoracic pressure can be reduced by allowing the patient to provide as much ventilatory power as possible, compatible with ventilatory capability and comfort.

Prevent Therapeutic Misadventures

Patients should be kept under direct observation at all times by well-trained personnel. Paralyzed patients must be watched with special care, because ventilation is totally machine dependent. Furthermore, the hands must be restrained in semiconscious, agitated, confused, or disoriented patients who receive mechanical ventilation; ventilator disconnections and extubations in patients with ARDS, for example, can abruptly precipitate lethal arrhythmias, hypoxemia, asphyxia, or aspiration. Special caution is warranted for orally intubated patients who tend to self-extubate more readily (see Chapter 6). In the setting of pulmonary edema, the interruption of PEEP for even brief periods (suctioning, tubing changes, etc.) may cause profound, slowly reversing desaturation as lung volume falls and the airways rapidly flood with edema fluid. The stomach should be actively decompressed in most recently intubated patients with air swallowing, vomiting, or ileus. For mechanically ventilated patients, the clinician must stay alert to the possibility of tension pneumothorax, especially in patients with radiographic evidence of pneumomediastinum or subcutaneous emphysema (see Chapter 8). Because of the very high incidence of tissue rupture, prophylactic chest tubes may be indicated for patients who form tension cysts that evolve on serial films.

Consider ARDS to Be a Multisystem Disease

Intravascular volume must be regulated carefully (see following). Although fluid excess must be avoided to minimize lung water and improve oxygen exchange, severe fluid restriction may compromise the perfusion of gut and kidney. Appropriate levels of nutritional support and prophylaxis for deep venous thrombosis, skin breakdown, and gastric stress ulceration should be considered for all mechanically ventilated or immobile patients (see Chapter 18).

The routine *early* use of corticosteroids is not justified. Adverse changes in immunity, mental status, metabolism, and protein wastage tend to outweigh any potential therapeutic benefit in the first week of the course. However, ARDS-like illnesses caused by documented vasculitis, fat embolism, or allergic reaction are exceptions to this rule. Corticosteroids may also be lifesaving in certain steroid-responsive diseases that mimic ARDS (e.g., bronchiolitis obliterans organizing pneumonia [BOOP], pulmonary hemorrhage syndromes, *Pneumocystis carinii* pneumonia). Moreover, in such life-threatening circumstances, adrenal insufficiency occurs with surprising frequency; if the presentation is compatible, this problem should be pursued diagnostically and stress doses of hydrocortisone given (see Chapter 32). Used in sufficient doses and for appropriate durations, corticosteroids may help resolve the fibroproliferative stage of this illness. Although there is no firm consensus on whether corticosteroids improve eventual mortality, it is clear from a recent large ARDSnet trial that steroids help many patients come off ventilator support more quickly. Despite many attempts to find an effective anti-inflammatory pharmaceutical approach, there remains little unequivocal confirmation from clinical trials of predictable benefit from any tested medication. The imprecision of the current American-European Consensus definition for ARDS may partially explain this failure.

Improving Tissue Oxygen Delivery

In the setting of ALI/ARDS, attention focuses on maintaining an adequate oxygen delivery: consumption ratio while reversing the underlying lung pathology. Oxygen delivery is the product of cardiac output and the O_2 content of each milliliter of arterial blood. Techniques for improving cardiac output are discussed in detail in Chapter 3. The O_2-carrying capacity can be improved by increasing Hgb concentration and optimizing its dissociation characteristics. Increasing Hgb tends to increase mixed-venous oxygen saturation as it reduces the need for any rise in cardiac output compensatory to anemia. Both of these actions (lower cardiac output demand and higher mixed-SvO_2) tend to reduce venous admixture. Hgb performance is improved by reversing alkalemia to facilitate O_2 off-loading. As hemoglobin concentration rises, blood viscosity increases, retarding passage of erythrocytes through capillary networks. Therefore, actual O_2 delivery can be impaired as hematocrit (Hct) rises. Although the optimal target for patients experiencing an oxygenation crisis is unknown, it makes sense to restore

Hgb concentration to 10 to 12 gm/dL. More extensive supplementation increases the risks of transfusion without proven benefit (see Chapter 14).

A very high percentage of the oxygen contained in blood is bound to Hgb; the proportion of oxygen solubilized in plasma is very small (<3%) at ambient pressure. However, in severe anemia, the Hgb-bound fraction is disproportionately small, so the total O_2-carrying capacity is boosted significantly when 100% O_2 is used.

Because extravascular water accumulates readily in the setting of permeability edema, fluids should be used judiciously to keep the lungs from flooding and to discourage water retention, consistent with adequate oxygen delivery. The results of a recent large ARDSnet trial strongly support the superiority of a "dry lung" approach as ventilator and ICU days were less than experienced with a fluid-liberal strategy. Careful use of inotropes and other vasoactive drugs can help to avoid volume excess, especially in certain postoperative or posttrauma settings. Driving the cardiac output to "supraphysiologic" levels, however, does not seem to be routinely helpful for medical patients with ARDS.

Oxygen Therapy

Increasing the FiO_2 improves PaO_2 in all instances in which shunting is not entirely responsible for desaturation. The goal is to increase arterial O_2 saturation to 85% to 90% or greater without risking O_2 toxicity. Oxygen toxicity is both concentration dependent and time dependent. As a rule, very high inspired fractions of oxygen can be used safely for brief periods as efforts are made to reverse the underlying process. Sustained elevations of FiO_2 greater than 0.6 result in inflammatory changes and eventual fibrosis in experimental models; therefore, it seems logical that efforts are made to keep FiO_2 lower than 0.7 during the support phase of ALI.

PEEP, Positioning, and Other Techniques for Raising Lung Volume

PEEP and other techniques (e.g., inverse ratio ventilation) for increasing mean alveolar pressure often succeed in maintaining lung volume recruitment. These topics are reviewed in detail in Chapter 9. Virtually all patients (with or without ALI) benefit from low levels of PEEP (e.g., 5 cm H_2O), which helps compensate for the loss of volume that accompanies recumbency and translaryngeal intubation.

While PEEP inhibits airway flooding, discourages migration of airspace biofluids, and can be shown to inhibit VILI, as yet there is little clinical evidence that PEEP protects against the onset of ARDS. Although PEEP may be highly effective in the relaxed subject, its volume-recruiting effects can be negated by patient effort. Vigorous expiratory muscle action forces the chest to a lung volume lower than the equilibrium position. When this happens, relaxing or silencing the expiratory muscles by sedation (and/or paralysis, if needed) can prove very helpful. When infiltration is highly asymmetrical, PEEP may be ineffective in improving oxygenation.

As discussed later and in Chapter 9, shifts from **6** the supine to the prone position often help dramatically in reversing hypoxemia in the early stage of ARDS. Alternating the lateral decubitus positions both stretches and improves the secretion drainage of the uppermost lung. Indeed, the incidence of pulmonary infections may be reduced by such mechanisms. (Because mobile edema characterizes the very first day of ARDS, it is theoretically prudent *not* to prone or reposition aggressively during this initial period unless a relatively high level of PEEP is maintained to retard the extension of inflammation to healthy units via the airways.) Several types of specialized beds perform this function automatically, but generally speaking, the rotation angles (maximally 35 to 40 degrees from horizontal) do not closely approach that of the full decubitus positions. When one lung is affected differentially, oxygenation occasionally improves—sometimes dramatically—with the good lung in the dependent position, but this is not observed reliably. Again, care should be taken to ensure that secretions from the infiltrated lung are not aspirated into the airway of the dependent viable lung during this process.

Recruiting Maneuvers and PEEP Selection

The principles of avoiding VILI are discussed in **7** Chapter 8. It must be remembered that, assuming that peak inflation pressure does not also rise, PEEP itself does not recruit atelectatic lung units but only keeps recruited units from recollapsing. To accomplish optimal recruitment (and thereby improve oxygenation and reduce potentially damaging lung stresses), sufficient pressure must first be applied to exceed the opening pressures of most recruitable units and then to maintain a total PEEP sufficient to exceed their closing pressures (Fig 24-5). Brief

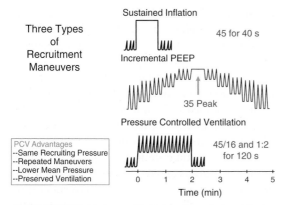

Three Types
of
Recruitment
Maneuvers

Sustained Inflation

45 for 40 s

Incremental PEEP

35 Peak

Pressure Controlled Ventilation

45/16 and 1:2
for 120 s

PCV Advantages
--Same Recruiting Pressure
--Repeated Maneuvers
--Lower Mean Pressure
--Preserved Ventilation

Time (min)

■ **FIGURE 24-5** Lung recruiting maneuvers. Lung units can be effectively opened and prevented from recollapsing by elevating PEEP while maintaining a prudent driving pressure (e.g., PCV) or tidal volume (ACV). If successful, a higher than original PEEP is usually needed to sustain the benefit after the RM has been completed.

applications of high airway pressure do not cause VILI, especially when achieved by elevating PEEP with a fixed and modest driving pressure. Recruitment maneuvers are integral to rational PEEP setting when potentially hazardous plateau pressures (>25 cm H_2O) are needed. It stands to reason, therefore, that "recruiting" maneuvers with relatively high pressure may be required after airway suctioning, following brief disconnections of the ventilator circuit, or perhaps periodically to achieve and sustain optimal arterial oxygenation when small tidal volumes are used for patients with acute oxygenation failure, as they often are in ARDS. Methods for accomplishing lung recruitment and selecting PEEP are described in Chapter 9.

Secretion Management and Bronchodilation

Although ARDS often is regarded as a problem of parenchymal injury, airway edema and secretion retention often contribute to hypoxemia, especially in "primary" ARDS. Retained secretions pose an overlooked problem that increases endotracheal tube resistance, infection risk, hazard of barotrauma, and the maldistribution of ventilation. For some patients with diffuse lung injury, profound bradycardia develops during ventilator disconnections and/or airway suctioning. Although hypoxemia occasionally contributes, this bradycardia usually is reflex in nature and responds to prophylactic (parenteral) atropine or prompt reapplication of positive airway pressure. The now ubiquitous closed circuits that do not interrupt tidal breath delivery or PEEP during suctioning may offer some advantage.

Importance of Reducing Oxygen and Ventilation Requirements

Lung-protective ventilation strategies usually focus on the "supply side" components of the tidal cycle—tidal volume, plateau pressure, and PEEP. Much less clinical attention has been directed at the "demand" side of the equation, i.e., at reducing the need to apply potentially damaging airway pressures and to push high vascular flows through the damaged lung. The drivers of these needs are minute ventilation and cardiac output. Both are potentially modifiable, and doing so in the first days of ALI/ARDS may dramatically reduce the iatrogenic potential of ventilatory support.

Fever, agitation, overfeeding, vigorous respiratory activity, shivering, sepsis, and a host of other commonly observed clinical conditions can markedly increase VO_2, the need for O_2 delivery, and the extent of mixed-venous and arterial O_2 desaturation. Fever reduction may have therapeutic value, but shivering must be prevented. When possible, correction of metabolic acidosis reduces the ventilation need. Sedation and the use of antipyretics in preference to cooling blankets often make good therapeutic sense. (Although phenothiazines may prevent shivering, their use may inhibit the cutaneous vasodilation necessary for rapid heat loss.)

Enforced acceptance of respiratory acidosis (and of a lower V_E)—"permissive hypercapnea"—can be achieved in the ventilated patient by suppressing the drive to breathe and/or by preventing contraction of the respiratory muscles. A good argument can be made to encourage gentle, spontaneous efforts whenever feasible to do so. Nonetheless, for the first 24 to 48 h of treatment, deep sedation, coupled with pharmacoparalysis if necessary, remains a valuable adjunct to reduce oxygen consumption and improve PaO_2 in patients who are severely ill, remain agitated, or fight the ventilator despite more conservative measures. It is prudent to target lower minute ventilation in the first days of ARDS therapy when the lung is most recruitable and at risk for VILI (Table 24-3). Although paralysis is often helpful during this initial period of machine support, protracted paralysis must be avoided for several reasons. Paralysis places the entire responsibility of achieving adequate oxygenation and ventilation on the medical team. Furthermore, the patient is defenseless in the event of an unobserved ventilator disconnection. Paralysis also silences the coughing mechanism and creates a monotonous breathing pattern that encourages

TABLE 24-3 CONDITIONALLY IMPORTANT TO VILI DURING HIGH STRESS VENTILATION

- $PaCO_2$ and pH
- Frequency
- Position
- Vascular pressures
- Temperature
- Minute ventilation and flow
  - dp/dt (Inspiratory flow)
  - I:E ratio (Adverse tension-time product)

secretion retention in dependent regions. Finally, protracted and unmonitored paralysis may cause weakness or devastating neuromyopathy (see Chapter 17).

Mechanical Ventilation of Acute Lung Injury and ARDS

Traditional Approach

The basic principles of managing ALI are widely accepted. The primary objective is to accomplish effective gas exchange without iatrogenic damage by inspired oxygen or airway pressure. Nonetheless, although the principles of VILI prevention are increasingly well understood (see Chapter 8), the relative hazards of oxygen therapy, high-pressure ventilatory patterns, and abnormal target values for arterial blood gases, pH, and cardiac output are still actively debated (Table 24-4).

Most traditional ventilatory strategies used in intensive care evolved directly from anesthetic and surgical postoperative practice. When the lungs are uninjured and their capacity to expand remains normal (as is common in the perioperative period), large tidal volumes (V_T) of 12 to 15 mL/kg generate only modest end-inspiratory transalveolar pressures. In fact, large tidal volumes prevent the microatelectasis that accompanies monotonous shallow

TABLE 24-4 APPROACHES TO ARDS VENTILATION

CONVENTIONAL	"LUNG PROTECTIVE"
Large tidal volume	Small tidal volume
Minimum PEEP	"Sufficient" PEEP
Normalize $PaCO_2$	Permissive hypercapnia
Unrestrained P_{aw}[a]	Pressure limitation

[a]Airway pressure.

breathing and are needed by many spontaneously breathing patients to satisfy high ventilatory demands (e.g., metabolic acidosis). Postoperatively, the mandatory respiratory rate usually is adjusted to "normalize" pH and/or $PaCO_2$, and sufficient PEEP is used to achieve acceptable O_2 delivery at what is assumed to be a nontoxic FiO_2. (An FiO_2 < 0.70 is commonly targeted.) Typically, airway pressures are monitored but not rigidly constrained.

With few modifications, this high tidal volume, normoxic, normocapnic ventilation paradigm was developed as the standard approach to supporting most critically ill patients as well. Consequently, tidal volumes that exceed 800 mL and end-tidal (plateau) alveolar pressures approaching 50 cm H_2O—values that violate currently understood principles of lung protection—are still applied by some practitioners who treat ARDS. How best to select "optimal" PEEP remains controversial, and machine settings that achieve all important clinical objectives do not invariably coincide. A growing number of practitioners are now shifting first priority from optimizing gas exchange, oxygen delivery, or respiratory system compliance to a strategy that minimizes the potentially injurious effects of mechanical ventilation.

Ventilator-Induced Lung Damage

Implications of Evolving Histology

Histologic findings evolve continuously (but heterogeneously) over the course of ALI (Table 24-5). It is reasonable to assume that all lung regions sustain the initial insult more or less simultaneously and that, in the most severe cases, proliferation, organization, remodeling, and fibrosis sequentially follow an initial phase of edema and atelectasis. Although parenchymal damage is widespread, the nature, severity, pace of evolution, and perhaps even the stage of injury vary from site to site within the damaged lung. Early in the course of ARDS, airspace fluids are edematous and mobile. Gravitationally dependent areas are extensively consolidated and atelectatic, whereas nondependent regions tend to aerate best. Regional blood flows and vascular pressures also vary (Fig. 24-6). Changes of body position alter the lung (or chest wall) mechanics, influence the radiographic findings, and affect the gas exchange. Although counterexamples occasionally occur, perhaps 60% to 70% of patients respond to prone positioning by improving PaO_2 significantly during this early phase of ARDS (see later). The efficacy of PEEP in

TABLE 24-5 CHARACTERISTICS OF EARLY- AND LATE-PHASE ARDS

	EARLY PHASE (0–3 DAYS)	LATE PHASE (>7 DAYS)
Structural collagen	Strong	Degraded
Atelectasis	Prevalent	Less prevalent
Edema	Prevalent	Less prevalent
Mechanics	Heterogeneous	Less heterogeneous
Ventilator lung injury	Edema and hemorrhage	Pneumothorax solidus Cystic barotrauma

ARDS, acute respiratory distress syndrome.

improving oxygen exchange relates directly to the reversal of atelectasis and the redistribution of lung water. It is not surprising, therefore, that recruitability and PEEP's effectiveness in improving oxygen exchange tend to decline as time passes. Whereas initially a large proportion of the lung can be aerated if sufficient pressure is used or fluid resuscitation is exuberant, recent studies suggest that only a small percentage of the infiltrated lung remains so after the first few days of ARDS onset.

The collagen framework of the normal lung remains relatively intact during the first days of injury but later weakens as inflammation gradually degrades the structural protein and nonuniformly remodels the lung's architecture. Therefore, the same pressures that were withstood acceptably well initially may cause alveolar disruption after the disease is well established. This may explain the tendency for radiographically detectable barotrauma to occur late in the course of the disease—often well after gas exchange abnormalities have noticeably improved and ventilatory pressures have declined.

Tidal Volume, PEEP, and VILI (see Chapters 5 and 8) (Table 24-6)

Only a portion of the lung remains accessible to gas after injury; in severe cases, no more than one third of all alveoli are patent. Considering that well-ventilated lung units may retain nearly normal elastance and fragility, the apparent "stiffness" of the lung in the early phase of ALI is better explained by fewer functioning alveoli than by a generalized increase in recoil tension. Increased tissue recoil contributes more significantly later on, when cellular infiltration is intense, edema has been reabsorbed or organized, atelectasis is less extensive, and fibrosis is under way. Because the lung's reduced functional compartment must accommodate the entire tidal volume, large (traditional) tidal volumes may cause overdistention, local hyperventilation, and inhibition or depletion of surfactant. Moreover, during repeated and abrupt inflations to high trans-alveolar pressures, intense shearing forces may develop at the junctions of structures that are mobile (aerated lung units) with

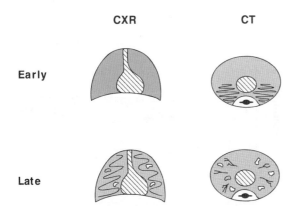

CXR   CT

Early

Late

■ **FIGURE 24-6** Chest radiographic (CXR) and computed tomographic (CT) appearances of the chest in early and late phases of ARDS. The lung seems to be diffusely and uniformly affected in the early stage. However, CT demonstrates a preponderance of atelectasis in the dependent (dorsal) regions. Later, infiltrates are more widely distributed, and cystic spaces often form. In this stage, atelectasis is less prevalent, and infiltrates are more evenly distributed in the transverse plane of the CT.

TABLE 24-6 MODIFIABLE DETERMINANTS OF VILI

- Trans-lung pressure
  - Tidal volume
  - PEEP
- Driving pressure
- Minute ventilation and inspiratory flow rate
- Conditional co-factors
  - Position
  - Vascular pressures and flows
  - Body temperature
  - Airway spread of inflammatory edema

those that are immobile: collapsed or consolidated alveoli, and distal conducting airways (see Chapter 8). It is recommended that tidal volumes are kept within the range of 4 to 8 mL/kg predicted body weight, depending on the PEEP used and the resulting plateau pressure, which should not exceed 30 cm H_2O.

8

Tidal pressures within the alveolus must neither rise too high at any time during the disease course nor fall too low, especially during the first 3 to 5 days of treatment. Structural (tearing, ripping, etc.) damage to the parenchyma and more subtle mechanosignaling of inflammation have been shown to result from high alveolar and driving pressures, especially when flow rate is high. The peak inflation pressure is not itself the stretching pressure that correlates with VILI; instead, peak *transalveolar* pressure (roughly approximated by the difference between alveolar and pleural pressures) is the relevant variable. When ventilation is passive, the plateau pressure is perhaps the best clinical correlate of peak alveolar (but not necessarily transalveolar) pressure. The severity of "stretch injury" seems greatest when these maximum transalveolar pressures are high and insufficient PEEP fails to keep unstable lung units fully recruited. The difference between plateau pressure and PEEP is known as the "driving pressure," and this difference determines the tidal volume. Unsupported by PEEP, certain collapsible alveoli may wink open and close with every tidal cycle, generating shearing stresses within junctional tissues and tending to deplete surfactant. Increases in cycling frequency and duration of exposure to adverse ventilatory patterns accentuate any tendency for damage. The magnitude of blood flow in these stressed areas also may play an important role.

Bronchiolar dilatation, cystic changes, and/or microabscesses can be demonstrated in most patients with ALI ventilated for lengthy periods with peak airway pressures considered modest by traditional clinical standards. Such airway damage not only impairs gas exchange but also predisposes secretion retention and pulmonary infection.

Importance of Cycling Frequency (Table 24-7)

At levels of minute ventilation and tidal volume that are traditionally accepted, the ventilator may cycle in excess of 30,000 times per day (20 cycles/min, 60 min/h, 24 h/day). Even if each tidal pressure profile is only slightly damaging, the cumulative

TABLE 24-7   POTENTIAL IMPORTANCE OF OXYGEN DEMAND FOR VILI EXPRESSION
• Cardiac output
– Pulmonary blood flow
– Microvascular pressure gradient
• Ventilation requirement
– Cycling frequency
– Ventilation pressures
• Static
• Dynamic

effect might be severe. It is very important to reduce V_E requirements and cycling frequency whenever high cycling pressures are in use. Raised frequency is much less damaging when parenchymal stresses remain within the acceptable bounds, as during high-frequency ventilation (HFV).

P_{flex} and the Choice of PEEP (see Chapter 9)

Although it is now widely recognized that chest wall compliance differences as well as inherent variability in the aeratable capacity of the lung to accept volume invalidate firm numerical guidelines for PEEP or tidal volume selection, the widely discussed and empirically derived pressure–volume display may fare little better. As a composite of the behaviors of all alveoli within the heterogeneous lung, the contours of the static pressure–volume loop (comprised of two quite different inspiratory and expiratory limbs) (Fig. 24-7) obscure very

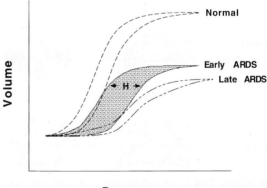

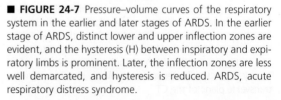

■ **FIGURE 24-7** Pressure–volume curves of the respiratory system in the earlier and later stages of ARDS. In the earlier stage of ARDS, distinct lower and upper inflection zones are evident, and the hysteresis (H) between inspiratory and expiratory limbs is prominent. Later, the inflection zones are less well demarcated, and hysteresis is reduced. ARDS, acute respiratory distress syndrome.

important regional differences. Alveoli in dependent regions are most susceptible to collapse, and those in nondependent regions are vulnerable to overdistention. This variability of opening pressures helps account for the *zones* (rather than *points*) of lower and upper inflection. In fact, as detailed in Chapter 9, recruitment and overdistention coexist at virtually all lung volumes across the inspiratory capacity range. The proportions of each are likely to account for such topographical features of the passive inflation curve as the lower inflection point (P_{flex}), which is no longer considered a theoretically valid guide to PEEP selection. Nonetheless, clinical trials have demonstrated better outcomes in the group using P_{flex} to guide PEEP selection than those assigned to least acceptable PEEP. Although the *expiratory* curve contours have more appeal, there currently exists little evidence that they will prove to be the long-sought clinical tool for identifying the "optimum recruitment" point. At present, an empirical approach that incorporates multiple indicators of response and the recruitment maneuver in PEEP selection appears most rational (see Chapter 9). Recently published clinical trials strongly suggest improved outcomes for ventilating strategies geared to avert widespread alveolar collapse during tidal breathing while keeping the plateau pressure beneath a ceiling of approximately 30 cm H_2O. That is not to say that all patients should be ventilated with high PEEP, especially not those who have low plateau pressures and adequate oxygenation, but many severely ill patients will need initial PEEP levels greater than 12 to 15 cm H_2O. This should come as little surprise, as even normal patients require 5 to 10 cm H_2O simply to offset the functional residual capacity (FRC) reduction that occurs with recumbency.

Implications of Pressure Limitation for Tidal Volume

Based on the results from the NIH-sponsored trial of tidal volumes, a reasonable starting tidal volume target for patients with ARDS is 6 mL/kg of lean body weight. However, this rather arbitrary value may not suit all patients because of comfort issues, high-ventilation requirements, oxygenation concerns, or pressure limitations imposed by a lung protective strategy. Therefore, V_T should be adjusted with guidance by plateau pressure and the response of oxygen exchange to changes of tidal volume.

Modes of Mechanical Ventilation in ARDS

Something of a mystique has developed around the topic of mode selection in ARDS. Although many would disagree, we believe that many choices are equivalent, as long as the practitioner ensures adequate O_2 delivery at a safe FiO_2, follows similar guidelines for lung protection, and remains alert to the potential shortcomings and complications of the mode in use. As a rule, spontaneous ventilation should be encouraged, except when oxygenation is marginal, heart function is seriously compromised, or ventilatory efforts are labored. It has been argued that newer techniques such as pressure control, high-frequency oscillation, pressure-regulated volume control, inverse ratio ventilation, and airway pressure release ventilation confer advantages over the more traditional approaches, but none has yet been shown in a fair comparison to be consistently superior to its alternatives. The general concepts of effective and safe ventilation are outlined elsewhere (see Chapter 7). The important difference in managing patients with ARDS is that the choices of maximum allowed tidal pressure and chosen level of PEEP may be crucial to safe ventilatory support. What is often forgotten is the need to reduce unnecessary ventilation and oxygenation requirements to reduce the patient's need to be exposed to high-pressure breathing cycles.

Permissive Hypercapnia

Carbon dioxide retention is often an inevitable consequence of a "lung-protective" strategy that tightly restricts applied pressure and maintains a certain minimum (end-expiratory) lung volume (see Chapter 7). Maintaining normocapnia is not appropriate if the cost is an impaired lung healing and a heightened risk of extending tissue damage. "Permissive hypercapnia," a strategy that allows alveolar ventilation and peak ventilatory pressures to fall and $PaCO_2$ to rise, may reduce barotrauma and enhance survival in status asthmaticus and ALI. The basis for any possible survival advantage has not yet been determined. However, lungs damaged by stretch injury are susceptible to pneumonia and may be a source of inflammatory mediators that are transferred to the systemic circulation to incite dysfunction elsewhere. Disruption of the lung's architecture also may promote bacteremia or even gas microembolism. Apart from reducing the need for the lung to undergo damaging stress and strain, acute hypercapnia holds the potential for reducing

TABLE 24-8 CONSEQUENCES OF HYPERCAPNIA

SYSTEM	EFFECT[a]
Respiratory	Reduced alveolar PO_2 Rightward shift of Oxy-Hgb curve Impaired diaphragm function Pulmonary vasoconstriction Worsened $\dot{V}/\dot{Q}$ mismatching
Renal	Enhanced bicarbonate reabsorption
CNS	Cerebral vasodilation Increased intracranial pressure Depressed consciousness Biochemical changes
Cardiovascular	Reduced cardiac contractility[b] Stimulation of sympathoadrenal axis Lower systemic vascular resistance

[a]Most effects wane with time as cellular and extracellular pH readjust.

[b]Only if not offset by adrenergic reflex compensation.

TABLE 24-9 CAUTIONS AND CONTRAINDICATIONS TO PERMISSIVE HYPERCAPNIA

Intracranial hypertension
    Head trauma
    Hemorrhage
    Severe systemic hypertension
    Space-occupying lesions
Cardiovascular instability

Cor pulmonale
β-Blockade
Severe, uncorrected metabolic acidosis

oxidative injury—a protective effect of respiratory acidosis. Despite these advantages, acute hypercarbia raises concerns as well.

Physiologic Effects of Hypercarbia

The physiologic effects of CO_2 retention are determined by the severity of hypercapnia and the rate of its buildup (Table 24-8). Except in the most severe cases or those complicated by extraordinary CO_2 production, the CO_2 retention that results from the pressure-targeted ventilation itself is usually modest ($PaCO_2 < 70$ mm Hg). Chronic hypercapnia of this magnitude seems to have few notable side effects, other than the reduction in ventilatory drive attendant to compensatory metabolic alkalosis. Respiratory acidosis may even reduce the intensity of inflammation or limit the expression of VILI.

Although gradual elevations of $PaCO_2$ (2 to 5 mm Hg increases per hour) are often tolerated remarkably well, abrupt increases are ill advised. *Acute* elevations in $PaCO_2$ not only promote dyspnea but also increase the sympathetic activity, raise cardiac output, heighten pulmonary vascular resistance, alter bronchomotor tone, impair skeletal muscle function, dilate cerebral vessels, and impair central nervous system function. Allowing hypercapnia may not be a viable option for all patients with ALI (e.g., patients with coexisting head injury, recent cerebral vascular accident, or significant cardiovascular dysfunction [Table 24-9]). Carbon dioxide retention may be tolerated poorly by patients with autonomic insufficiency, β-blockade, or other conditions interfering with sympathetic tone and compensatory mechanisms.

When achieved quickly, arterial pH may not closely reflect the pH of the intracellular environment in which key cellular enzymes operate. The magnitude of any intracellular acidosis resulting from permissive hypercapnia, however, is almost certain to be less than the profound intracellular pH changes produced by ischemia. Because CO_2 affects cardiac output and influences vascular and bronchomotor tone, it is uncertain if hypercapnia disturbs $\dot{V}/\dot{Q}$ matching or modulates the extent of lung injury and edema during the course of mechanical ventilatory support. Initially, the implementation of permissive hypercapnia often requires deep sedation and/or paralysis, a requirement that may be associated with serious side effects: impaired secretion clearance, fluid retention, and residual muscle weakness. Moreover, permissive hypercapnia may not be advisable (or even possible to implement safely) in the setting of a coexisting metabolic acidosis or an uncorrected hypoxemia.

Alternative Ventilatory Strategies and Adjuncts to ARDS Ventilation

Recently, there has been renewed interest in devising ways in which to accomplish effective arterial oxygenation and ventilation without inflicting further damage on the injured lung. Some of these innovations modify the fundamental nature of ventilatory support (HFV), whereas others provide gas exchange external to the lungs (extracorporeal or intra–vena caval gas exchange), alter body position (prone positioning), or administer therapeutic agents designed to aid $\dot{V}/\dot{Q}$ matching (nitric oxide, aerosolized prostacyclin, etc.). One technique modifies the nature of the gas-carrying medium itself (partial liquid ventilation). A few of these adjuncts are at the margin or just beyond the perimeter of routine clinical practice.

High-Frequency Ventilation

In its various forms, HFV has been investigated and clinically applied for more than a quarter century. Such attention is understandable; when conducted at an appropriate lung volume and frequency, HFV seems well aligned with current principles of lung protection and has a clear rationale (see Chapter 7). Inherently, small tidal volumes confine the maximum pressures applied to the damaged lung to the range advocated, and inherently high end-expiratory pressures have the potential to prevent widespread collapse. Moreover, with the advent of the adult oscillator, perhaps the most promising of several HFV variants, implementation of HFV has become a viable option for clinical practice. Although limited, published experience using HFO as a salvage technique for ARDS patients failing more conventional approaches appears quite favorable and suggests that this approach might be advisable at a much earlier point in the life support process. To this point, however, its superiority has been neither shown nor disproved.

Extrapulmonary Gas Exchange

Partial substitution for the lung's gas exchanging function reduces the requirement for ventilating pressure. Like HFV, extrapulmonary gas exchange has a long history and diminishing appeal now that strategies for lung protection and acceptance of abnormal blood gas tensions are increasingly implemented. Nonetheless, for the critically ill with very severe lung damage, such technologies offer the only slim hope of survival. Methods for assisting in the process of exchanging respiratory gases include extracorporeal membrane oxygenation (ECMO), extracorporeal CO_2 removal ($ECCO_2R$), and intra–vena caval gas exchange. All are highly technical methods best undertaken by an experienced and dedicated team. Each has a good rationale, and laboratory experience and various clinical reports have been encouraging. Unfortunately, none has yet been confirmed by well-controlled trials to add consistently to the routine measures. Although experience to date with these exotic techniques has been frustrating, developmental advances continue, and well-selected patients may benefit. For example,

extracorporeal access can now be provided by large catheters placed percutaneously, lower clotting risk has allowed less-aggressive anticoagulation, and blood product needs are now markedly lower. In at least one center experienced in $ECMO/ECCO_2R$ technique, extracorporeal support has been continued for longer than a month in several patients, with ultimate survival. It appears that membrane oxygenation may be the only hope of salvage in patients who are the most difficult to oxygenate.

The potential to implement extrapulmonary gas exchange without the heroic investment of equipment and personnel that characterize $ECMO/ECCO_2R$ techniques has recently been realized by simpler devices, including passive and pump-driven venovenous gas exchangers (e.g., Novalung, Hemolung). Relative simplicity is attractive but clinical experience has been very limited. Whether they improve prognosis with acceptable complication rates has yet to be determined.

Catheters that can accomplish the gas exchanging function of the lung in the vena cava offer the prospect of reducing ventilation requirements, boosting oxygenation, and perhaps reducing pulmonary hypertension by releasing hypoxic pulmonary vasoconstriction. In principle, the many tightly packed, hollow, gas-permeable fibers contained within a catheter bundle are deployed in the vena cava and are swept continuously under negative pressure by an oxygen stream, allowing a sizeable portion of oxygen and CO_2 exchange to occur before the lung contacts. Whereas the first units tested (IVOX) were prone to clotting, required a surgical procedure to implant, and were disappointingly inefficient, the next generation (e.g., Hattler) catheters have addressed these shortcomings by heparin bonding to superior materials and countercurrent agitation (to enhance gas exchange) provided by a vibrating balloon core. Again, whether these latest innovations bring effective extrapulmonary gas exchange closer to reality remains uncertain.

Tracheal Gas Insufflation

An alternative to allowing extreme or rapidly developing hypercapnia or to using extrapulmonary techniques for gas exchange in ARDS is to enhance the efficiency of CO_2 elimination at low V_T and cycling pressures by the tracheal insufflation of fresh gas during expiration (tracheal gas insufflation [TGI]). Only a modest flow (6 to 10 L/min) is required. Moreover, fresh gas can be injected selectively during expiration through a

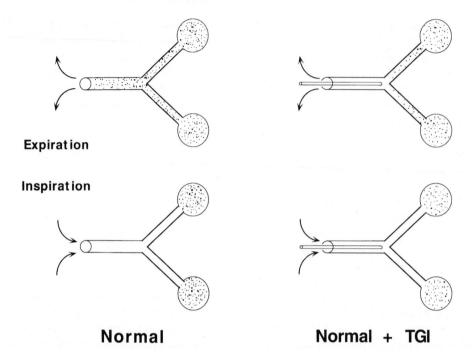

Expiration

Inspiration

Normal   **Normal + TGI**

■ **FIGURE 24-8** Tracheal gas insufflation (TGI). CO_2-laden gas that fills the central airways at end-expiration is recycled to the alveolus with the subsequent inspiration. Expiratory flushing of CO_2 from the central airway by fresh gas helps improve CO_2 elimination and reduces dead space. The effectiveness of TGI is reduced when a high alveolar dead space lowers the end-expiratory tracheal CO_2 concentration but is enhanced when hypercapnia raises the concentration of CO_2 in the central airways during expiration.

channel within the endotracheal tube wall without significantly impeding exhalation or raising the airway pressure significantly. This minimally invasive approach reduces the effective series (anatomic) dead space by bypassing the airway proximal to the carina during inspiration, by washing out the PCO_2 of this same region during expiration, or by both (Fig. 24-8). Because much lower concentrations of CO_2 are delivered to the central airway as the lungs deflate, TGI loses its effectiveness when there is a large amount of alveolar (as opposed to anatomic and apparatus) dead space. ARDS is a typical example of such a condition. Conversely, hypercapnia boosts the expiratory CO_2 concentration within the trachea, improving the effect of TGI. Because of its potential to moderate the rate and extent of CO_2 retention, TGI would appear particularly well suited to serve as an adjunct to a pressure-targeted, lung-protective ventilatory support for ARDS.

Prone Positioning

Frequent changes of body posture are integral to normal activity, but normal positional variation is forgone for lengthy periods in the bedridden, critically ill patient. By tradition, the patient is cared for in the supine position, which allows more direct eye contact with the caregivers, family, and visitors, as well as better access to the vascular system and vital structures, thereby facilitating nursing care. Cardiopulmonary resuscitation must be conducted in the supine position. Despite these undeniable advantages, there is good reason to question our current practice of using only the supine orientation. A growing interest in therapeutic positioning has been stimulated by the observation that the prone position improves oxygen exchange significantly in 50% to 70% of patients treated in the early phase of ARDS, allowing the physician to reduce both FiO_2 and PEEP. Moreover, prone positioning confers a lung-protective advantage in experimental models of VILI. Although four clinical trials of proning in ARDS failed to show a consistent survival advantage for all patients, proned patients in the most severely affected cohorts of each study have fared impressively better. This benefit has also been reported for those at highest risk for VILI and in those who experience improved CO_2 exchanging efficiency (suggesting recruitment) at first proning (Table 24-10). Airways serving the expansive dorsal regions generally are better drained in this position as well. Although helpful later on in removing the

---

TABLE 24-10 ADVANTAGES OF PRONE POSITIONING IN ARDS

- "Regional" PEEP in well-perfused dorsal zones
- Reduced gravitational gradient of pleural pressure
  - Improved *V/Q* matching
- Improved airway drainage
- Reduced LLL compression
- Improved distribution of inhaled medications
- Better venous/lymphatic drainage (?)

---

retained secretions, in the first 24 to 48 h, proning carries the attendant potential for injury propagation as mobile inflammatory biofluid is encouraged to migrate to previously unaffected anterior zones. (Adequate PEEP may counter this tendency.)

Practical Points in Prone Positioning (Table 24-11)

Although hemodynamic parameters tend to remain unchanged, hypotension, desaturation, and arrhythmias may occur during the process of turning from the supine to the prone position. These transient problems generally do not persist and can be minimized by using sedation, prior airway suctioning, and 100% oxygen during the maneuver. Continuous arterial pressure monitoring, electrocardiography, and pulse oximetry are strongly advised. Deep sedation and occasionally paralysis will be required to secure patient compliance. Attention also must be given to preserving the position and patency of intravascular lines and endotracheal tubes during the turning process. Use of a soft (air-cushioned) bed is all but mandatory for comfort. Pillows must be used to support the hips, pelvis, shoulders, and head. Patients with tracheostomies present a particular challenge. The

---

TABLE 24-11 PRACTICAL POINTS FOR PRONE POSITIONING IN ARDS

Soft bed
Secure endotracheal tube and all lines before transition
Sedate and preoxygenate before turning
Monitor carefully during transitions
Support shoulders and hips
Adjust PEEP and tidal volume after positioning
Protect eyes, facial areas
Exercise special caution if bronchopleural fistula present
Flip one to three times daily

---

compliance of the respiratory system generally changes little in shifting to the prone position. This is variable, however; tidal volume should be monitored (and adjusted if necessary) during pressure-controlled ventilation, which is influenced by any position-related changes in chest wall compliance. Furthermore, for the same plateau pressure, peak pressures may change if flow-controlled volume-cycled ventilation is used. For similar reasons, a given level of PEEP may be more or less effective in one position versus the other. Although the optimal frequency of supine–prone interconversions is not clear, in current practice, most experienced centers maintain the prone position for approximately 20 h when it shows an oxygenation advantage and "flip" patients supine once daily for about 4 h to allow cleanup, nursing care, catheter placement, and imaging studies. Supine repositioning allows certain nursing procedures (washing, line dressing changes, etc.) to be delivered and helps resolve facial edema. It seems reasonable to assign the relative duration of each position in proportion to the gas exchange response. (For example, equal times would be assigned if only a minor gas exchange difference is observed between positions.) Prone repositioning should be reevaluated often in the first 3 to 5 days of illness, after which time its efficacy begins to wane.

Inhaled Nitric Oxide and Prostacyclin

Nitric oxide (NO) is a key biologic mediator of smooth muscle relaxation. When inhaled, NO has the therapeutic potential to dilate the pulmonary vasculature in well-ventilated regions, tending to reduce pulmonary hypertension and improve the matching of ventilation and perfusion in an unevenly damaged lung. Inhaled NO is only active locally, as it is quenched immediately on exposure to Hgb. Extremely low concentrations of NO achieve nearly full effect. The physiologic effects of NO in ARDS are highly variable—sometimes dramatic, but often quite modest. Although the onset and offset of the effects of NO are extremely rapid and its benefit remains durable over time, gradual accommodation to its beneficial vasodilatory effects can result in rebound vasoconstriction when it is terminated abruptly. High concentrations of NO and minute quantities of its associated oxides, NO_2^{-1} and NO_3^{-2}, are histotoxic and must be avoided. Other hypothetical concerns relate to its potential for immune suppression, potential for mutagenicity, and the tendency for high NO concentrations to generate methemoglobin. Conversely, other reported effects might prove salutary—antiplatelet, antipermeability, and anti-inflammatory properties could yield benefit in ALI. No trial has yet shown a convincing benefit of inhaled NO regarding mortality and from a logistical standpoint, NO delivery is somewhat cumbersome and extremely expensive. Thus, current enthusiasm is muted, and the eventual place of NO in the management of ARDS has not yet been settled. At present, it seems most likely to benefit those cases in which life-threatening hypoxemia is refractory to other measures or when hypoxic vasoconstriction accentuates symptomatic pulmonary hypertension.

Vasodilating aerosols, of which inhaled prostacyclin (e.g., epoprostenol or Flolan) is the most frequently used, operate by the same principle of selectively increasing perfusion to well-ventilated regions and appear to offer similar efficacy. Delivery and monitoring of inhaled prostacyclin are less complicated than NO, and expense is considerably less. Like NO, the physiologic effects of inhaled prostacyclin on oxygenation and pulmonary arterial pressure can occasionally be dramatic, but its routine clinical benefit has yet to be demonstrated.

Surfactant

Because ARDS is characterized in part by microatelectasis, inflammation, and deficiency of viable surfactant, the exogenous replacement of this important biologic substance has a clear rationale. Beyond doubt, surfactant replacement has had a beneficial impact on the care of premature infants in respiratory distress. To date, however, results of multiple clinical studies of surfactant replacement in adults have been profoundly disappointing. Whether inefficacy relates to the method of delivery, type of formulation, inherent nature of the disease, imprecisely defined study populations, or timing of administration is unclear. Without substantiation of its benefit, surfactant cannot be recommended for this clinical application.

A Lung-Protective Approach to Ventilating ALI and ARDS

Although definitive clinical data are needed to confirm the wisdom of adopting a pressure-targeted approach, a rational strategy for ventilating patients with ALI can be formulated based on firm theoretical and experimental grounds (Table 24-12 and Fig. 24-9). Such a strategy recognizes that several mechanically distinct alveolar populations coexist

TABLE 24-12 A LUNG-PROTECTIVE STRATEGY FOR VENTILATING ARDS
Tailor ventilatory strategy to the phase of the disease (generous PEEP in early stage; withdraw PEEP later)
Minimize oxygen demands
Hold $FiO_2 < 0.65$
Minimize pulmonary vascular pressures
Control alveolar pressure, not $PaCO_2$
Maintain full recruitment of unstable alveoli in the early phase
Maintain total end-expiratory P_{alv} (PEEP + auto-PEEP) several cm H_2O above P_{flex}. In general, this will be >7 cm H_2O but <20 cm H_2O
Avoid large V_T and use least P_{alv} required to meet *unequivocal* therapeutic goals
Hold tidal transalveolar pressure < 35 cm H_2O
Consider making necessary increases in mean P_{aw} by changing the inspiratory time fraction
Consider specialized adjunctive measures to improve gas exchange and O_2 delivery[a]

[a]In addition to such standard measures as skillful management of pulmonary vascular pressure, repositioning, recruiting maneuvers, and use of cardiotonic agents, specialized adjunctive measures might include (where available) such experimental methods as $ECCO_2R$, inhaled nitric oxide or prostacyclin, partial liquid ventilation, and intravenous (IVOX) or intratracheal catheter-assisted gas exchange (TGI).

P_{alv}, alveolar pressure; P_{flex}, lower inflection zone of the static pressure volume relationship of the respiratory system.

within the acutely injured lung, that a poorly chosen ventilatory pattern can be damaging, and that the underlying pathophysiology changes over time. This approach gives higher priority to controlling maximal and minimal transalveolar pressures than to achieving normocapnia.

Assuming that oxygen and ventilatory demands have been minimized, that FiO_2 is kept ≤ 0.7, and that fluid balance and cardiac function have been optimized, the essential strategic elements are as follows:

1. Sufficient end-expiratory transalveolar pressure must be used to avert tissue damage resulting from surfactant depletion or stresses associated with repeated opening and closure of collapsible units during the tidal breathing cycle. Improved arterial oxygenation tends to parallel effective

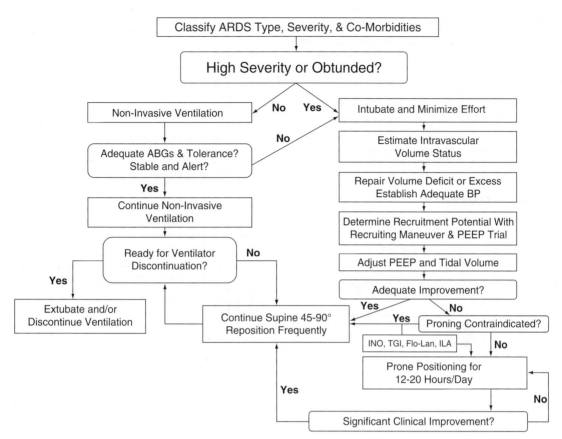

■ **FIGURE 24-9** A management algorithm for acute lung injury and ARDS. INO, inhaled nitric oxide; TGI, tracheal gas insufflation; Flo-Lan, inhaled prstacyclin; ILA, extra-pulmonary gas exchange.

recruitment, and CO_2 retention is a consequence of alveolar overdistension.

2. Because alveolar subpopulations with nearly normal elastic properties may coexist with flooded or infiltrated ones, the clinician must avoid applying tidal *transalveolar* pressures greater than normal lung tissue is designed to sustain at its maximum capacity. When breathing is passive, this pressure generally corresponds to end-inspiratory static airway pressures ("plateau" pressures) less than 30 H_2O, but higher values may sometimes be permissible, depending on the stiffness of the chest wall. Conversely, limiting static airway pressure to 30 cm H_2O (or any other target) does not guarantee safe ventilation when the patient actively triggers breathing and exerts an unknown end-inspiratory pressure on the pleural side of the lung. Any exertion must be limited.

It seems wise to avoid the upper inflexion range of the static pressure–volume curve whenever possible. Incursion into the noncompliant zone is signaled by deterioration of tidal compliance and, for a passively inflated patient, by convexity of the inspiratory airway pressure curve to the horizontal (time) axis during constant flow ventilation. The shaping characteristic of the pressure tracing has been termed the "stress index," with any departure from linearity suggesting a hazardous pattern of ventilation due to either tidal recruitment or overdistention (see Chapter 5).

3. Empirically select an appropriate combination of PEEP and tidal volume, using the principles of initial recruitment, adequate PEEP, and respect for the damaging potential of excessive plateau pressure. (See "Selecting PEEP and Tidal Volume in ARDS," Chapter 9.)

4. When not contraindicated, hypercapnia should be accepted from the onset of therapy in preference to violating the guidelines of controlling alveolar pressure. Deep sedation and/or paralysis may be required. Permissive hypercapnia may be difficult to implement in the presence of metabolic acidosis, when other measures (e.g., dialysis) may be needed adjunctively.

5. The prone position should be considered for patients with severe disease who are difficult to oxygenate. Prone positioning generally offers its greatest oxygenation benefit relatively early in the course of illness.

6. After the first 3 to 5 days of treatment, begin to reduce the PEEP and the frequency of prone positioning as oxygenation allows, seeking to reduce maximum alveolar pressure and prevent alveolar rupture.

■ SUGGESTED READINGS

Borges J, Okamoto VB, Matos GF, et al. Reversibility of lung collapse and hypoxemia in early acute respiratory distress syndrome. *Am J Respir Crit Care Med.* 2006;174:268–278.

Chiumello D, Carlesso E, Cadringher P, et al. Lung stress and strain during mechanical ventilation for acute respiratory distress syndrome. *Am J Resp Crit Care Med.* 2008;178(4):346–355.

Cranshaw J, Griffiths MJ, Evans TW. The pulmonary physician in critical care—part 9: Non-ventilatory strategies in ARDS. *Thorax.* 2002;57(9):823–829.

Gattinoni L, Caironi P, Cressoni M, et al. Lung recruitment maneuvers in patients with acute respiratory distress syndrome. *N Engl J Med.* 2006;354:1775–1786.

Laffey JG, O'Croinin D, McLoughlin P, et al. Permissive hypercapnia—role in protective lung ventilatory strategies. *Intensive Care Med.* 2004;30(3):347–356.

Levy ML. Update in sepsis. *Curr Opin Crit Care.* 2008;29(4):585–747.

Marini JJ. Advances in the understanding of acute respiratory distress syndrome: Summarizing a decade of progress. *Curr Opin Crit Care.* 2004;10(4):265–271.

Marini JJ, Gattinoni L. Ventilatory management of acute respiratory distress syndrome: A consensus of two. *Crit Care Med.* 2004;32(1):250–255.

Marini JJ, Gattinoni L. Propagation prevention: A complementary mechanism for "lung protective" ventilation in acute respiratory distress syndrome. *Crit Care Med.* 2008;36(12):3252–3258.

Messerole E, Peine P, Wittkopp S, et al. The pragmatics of prone positioning. *Am J Respir Crit Care Med.* 2002;165(10):1359–1363.

Pontoppidan H, Geffin B, Lowenstein E. Acute respiratory failure in the adult. [A classic, three part review]. *N Engl J Med.* 1972;287:690–698,743–752,799–806.

The National Heart, Lung, and Blood Institute Acute Respiratory Distress Syndrome (ARDS) Clinical Trials Network. Comparison of two fluid-management strategies in acute lung injury. *N Engl J Med.* 2006;354:2564–2575.

Villar J, Kacmarek RM, Perez-Mendez L, et al. A high positive end expiratory pressure-low tidal volume ventilatory strategy improves outcome in persistent acute respiratory distress syndrome: A randomized, controlled trial. *Crit Care Med.* 2006;34:1311–1318.

Wheeler AP, Bernard GR. Acute lung injury and the acute respiratory distress syndrome: A clinical review. *Lancet.* 2007;369:1553–1564.

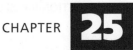

Ventilatory Failure

KEY POINTS

1 Three major mechanisms cause or contribute to ventilatory failure: deficient central drive, ineffective muscular contraction, and excessive breathing workload. Important factors contributing to the minute ventilation requirement include levels of alertness, agitation, pain, body temperature, metabolic stress, ventilatory dead space fraction, nutritional status, and high breathing workload.

2 Although isolated disorders of central ventilatory drive are quite uncommon causes of respiratory failure, they frequently serve as background conditions that lead to acute decompensation when the breathing workload increases or the muscular capability is impaired. Sedatives, sedating antidepressants, psychotropic agents, hypnotics, and opiates must be used very cautiously in elderly patients, patients with chronic sleep deprivation, and patients with subacute or chronic CO_2 retention.

3 An investigation of the cause for ventilatory failure should include systematic evaluation of ventilatory drive, minute ventilation, the pressure required per liter of ventilation, and neuromuscular performance. The electrolyte, chemistry, and medication profile must be carefully reviewed. Therapy to reverse ventilatory failure should be guided by knowledge of the underlying defect.

4 Signs and symptoms suggestive of upper airway obstruction include the following: inspiratory limitation of airflow, stridor, difficulty clearing airway secretions, altered voice or cough, marked accentuation of dyspnea by exertion or hyperventilation, and altered breathing symptoms with position changes or neck movements. Specialized pulmonary function tests (such as complete flow–volume loops) help document upper airway obstruction.

5 The nonintubated patient with upper airway obstruction may benefit from maintaining the head-up position, breathing helium–oxygen mixtures, and receiving positive end-expiratory pressure or continuous positive airway pressure. Glottic edema that occurs postextubation may respond to racemic epinephrine aerosols. Other key measures include decreasing pleural pressure swings by reducing minute ventilation requirements, relieving bronchospasm, and eliminating retained airway secretions.

6 An asthmatic attack may be triggered by a host of provocative stimuli that include bronchial irritation, allergen inhalation, emotion, exercise, sinus drainage, gastroesophageal reflux, and pulmonary venous congestion.

7 Specific danger signs in asthma that warn of the need for urgent intubation include deteriorating mental status, a wide paradoxical pulse, severe hyperinflation, inability to talk in complete sentences, CO_2 retention, acidosis, and cyanosis.

8 Secretion plugging of the airways may be very widespread in status asthmaticus. Appropriate therapeutic interventions include β-adrenergic and anticholinergic aerosols, corticosteroids, and mechanical ventilation. Magnesium sulfate, theophylline derivatives, mucolytics, mucus lubricants, and vigorous respiratory therapy are of less-certain benefit during the acute phase of status asthma.

9 Many patients with chronic obstructive pulmonary disease also have underlying heart disease that complicates their management. This may take the form of *cor pulmonale* or ischemic left ventricular disease. Atrial arrhythmias are unusually common and problematic for these patients. Positive end-expiratory pressure or continuous positive airway pressure often helps to offset auto-positive end-expiratory pressure and improve triggering sensitivity, thereby decreasing the work of breathing in these flow-limited patients.

Respiratory therapy assumes a crucial role in the management of many such patients. In addition to antibiotics and corticosteroids, noninvasive ventilation has an established place in managing acute exacerbations of chronic obstructive pulmonary disease. Response is most likely when the patient is alert, tolerant of the mask interface, and supported early in the hospital course. When intubation is required, care should be taken to avoid overventilating the patient and to maintain adequate nutrition.

10

For patients with neuromuscular diseases, derangements of calcium, magnesium, phosphate, potassium, and pH may impair respiratory muscle function. Other important problems are sleep-disordered breathing, derangements of thoracic configuration (obesity, pleural effusion or pneumothorax, and kyphoscoliosis), excess total body water, and deficits in muscular strength and coordination (diaphragmatic weakness, quadriplegia).

11

■ PATHOGENESIS OF VENTILATORY FAILURE

Definition

Ventilatory failure is the inability to sustain a sufficient rate of CO_2 elimination to maintain a stable pH without mechanical assistance, muscle fatigue, or intolerable dyspnea. Failure to maintain adequate alveolar ventilation usually is recognized by CO_2 retention and acidosis. Although a rise in $PaCO_2$ to a level higher than 50 mm Hg has been suggested as definitive, ventilatory failure can occur even when $PaCO_2$ falls to a value lower than its chronic level (which itself may exceed 50 mm Hg). For example, a modest metabolic acidosis may exhaust the limited ventilatory reserve of a patient with quadriplegia, severe airflow obstruction, or acute respiratory distress syndrome (ARDS). In similar fashion, hypocapnic alkalosis may deteriorate to "normal" values for pH and $PaCO_2$ as ventilatory failure develops in a fatiguing asthmatic patient. Conversely, many patients comfortably maintain $PaCO_2$ levels higher than 50 mm Hg on a chronic basis, without satisfying the aforementioned definitions.

Mechanisms of Ventilatory Failure

To maintain effective ventilation, an appropriate signal must first be sent from the brain to the ventilatory muscles. The muscles must then contract with

TABLE 25-1   CAUSES OF VENTILATORY FAILURE

Airflow obstruction
Upper airway obstruction
  Extrathoracic
  Intrathoracic
  Functional (OSA)
Lower airway obstruction
  Asthma
  COPD
Bronchial stenosis (transplant, trauma, tumor)

Muscular weakness
Skeletal muscles
  Weakness
  Neuromuscular impairment
  Quadriplegia
  Myopathy
Diaphragm paralysis
Functional
  Hyperinflation
  Drugs, electrolytes

Ineffective musculature
Thoracic configuration
Chronic
  Kyphoscoliosis
  Thoracoplasty
Acute
  Pneumothorax
  Pleural effusion
  Flail chest
  Hyperinflation

Inadequate ventilatory drive
Intrinsic
  Congenital
  Chronic loading (obesity, severe airflow obstruction)
    Advanced age
    Endocrine disturbance
Extrinsic
  Drugs/sedatives
  Sleep deprivation
  Metabolic alkalosis
  Nutritional insufficiency

enough force and coordination to generate the fluctuating pleural pressures that drive airflow. The ventilatory power required depends on the difficulty of gas movement and the minute ventilation requirement. Three major mechanisms cause or contribute to ventilatory failure: deficient central drive, ineffective muscular contraction, and excessive workload (Table 25-1). The primary physical signs of ventilatory overstress or fatigue are vigorous use of accessory ventilatory muscles, tachypnea, tachycardia, diaphoresis, and paradoxical motion of the chest or abdomen. The preagonal breathing pattern may be slow, eventually becoming irregular and gasping.

1

General Principles of Managing Ventilatory Failure

2 Ventilatory failure is managed by defining its cause, by correcting reversible problems, and by providing mechanical support when required. If the cause of ventilatory failure is not obvious, bedside measurements intended to determine the mechanisms at work are especially important. Ventilatory workload is reflected in the $\dot{V}_E$ and machine pressures needed to deliver the tidal volume (see Chapter 5). Important factors contributing to the minute ventilation requirement include levels of alertness, agitation, pain or discomfort, body size and temperature, pathologic metabolic stress (sepsis, trauma, burns, etc.), ventilatory dead space fraction, nutritional status, and the work of breathing. The difficulty of chest inflation per liter of ventilation is best gauged by the peak dynamic and static (plateau) inflation pressures as well as by the estimated values for resistance, compliance, and auto-PEEP. Neuromuscular function is evaluated by observing the ventilatory pattern, the tidal volume and breathing frequency, and the actions of the respiratory muscles. At the bedside, the appropriateness of ventilatory drive is often best assessed by examining the pH and $PaCO_2$ in relation to breathing effort. (For example, if $PaCO_2$ is high and pH is low, drive may be deficient, muscular reserve may be inadequate, or both; evidence of patient agitation, dyspnea, or distress argues for primacy of the latter.) Integrative indices of demand and capacity, such as the rapid shallow breathing index or the tidal mouth occlusion pressure ($P_{0.1}$), which is just now coming into clinical use as a quantitative drive index, may be helpful when assessing the continuing need for machine support (see Chapter 10).

Correcting Reversible Factors

3 The quest to determine the cause for ventilatory failure should be guided by a systematic evaluation of ventilatory drive, $\dot{V}_E$, the work of breathing, and neuromuscular performance. In passive ventilated patients, resistance and compliance can be measured during constant flow ventilation (see Chapter 5). Therapy to reverse ventilatory failure should be guided by knowledge of the underlying defect and its severity (Table 25-2). Impedance can be improved by relieving airway obstruction (bronchodilation, secretion clearance, placement of a larger endotracheal tube, etc.), by increasing parenchymal compliance (reduction of atelectasis, edema,

TABLE 25-2 REVERSIBLE FACTORS IN VENTILATORY FAILURE

Excessive ventilation requirement
  Metabolic acidosis
  Increased CO_2 generation
    Fever
    Agitation
    Work of breathing
    Excessive calories
  Increased dead space
    Airway apparatus
    Hypovolemia
    Vascular obstruction

Increased impedance to ventilation
  Secretions
  Bronchospasm
  Airway apparatus
  Pleural air or fluid
  Abdominal distention
  Auto-PEEP
  Pulmonary edema

Impaired muscle strength and endurance
  Nutritional deficiency
  Electrolyte disturbances
    PO_4^{3-}, Mg^{2+}, K^+
  Endocrine disorders
  Inadequate cardiac output
  Myasthenia gravis/Parkinson disease
  Hyperinflation
  Drugs (β-blockers, calcium channel blockers)

Impaired ventilatory drive
  Drugs (sedatives/analgesics)
  Malnutrition
  Sleep deprivation
  Metabolic alkalosis
  Hypothyroidism

and inflammation), and by improving chest wall distensibility (drainage of air or fluid from the pleural space, relief of abdominal distention, muscle relaxation, or analgesia). A common problem overlooked in ventilated patients is a closed circuit suction catheter inadvertently left in an advanced position beyond the wye piece. This partial occlusion dramatically narrows the effective caliber of the endotracheal tube and is easily remedied by withdrawing the catheter to its usual position.

Serum chemistries and medication list must be carefully reviewed for potential suppressants of mental status or muscular strength. Neuromuscular efficiency should be optimized by ensuring alertness, maintaining the patient in an appropriate position (usually as upright as possible), relieving pain, and addressing electrolyte disturbances, nutritional deficiencies, and endocrine disorders.

Elevations of ammonia, an endogenous suppressor of consciousness and drive to breathe, should be addressed by reducing correctable sources of its generation—upper GI bleeding, depakote, etc.—by encouraging its gut elimination (lactulose), or by enhancing the metabolism of ammonia to glutamine and hippurate, by using ornithine or benzoate, respectively. Although Addison disease is rare, adrenal insufficiency (absolute or, more commonly, *relative*) is surprisingly common among critically ill and chronically debilitated patients who undergo major physiologic stress. Measures that improve cardiac output or arterial oxygenation also will improve neuromuscular performance. Treatable neuromuscular disorders (e.g., myasthenia, polymyositis, Parkinson disease) should not be overlooked. Some problems of decreased ventilatory drive are self-limited (e.g., sedative or opiate excess); others improve with nutritional repletion, electrolyte adjustment (metabolic alkalosis), hormone replacement (e.g., hypothyroidism), or recovery of mental status. Very few respond to nonspecific ventilatory stimulants such as progesterone. (Obesity hypoventilation syndrome may be one exception—see following discussion.) Unfortunately, many such problems are refractory to drug manipulation and must be treated by optimizing ventilatory mechanics with the goal of reducing the work of breathing sufficiently to restore compensation.

Mechanical Support

The general principles of intubation, mechanical ventilation with positive pressure, and weaning are presented elsewhere (see Chapters 6 to 8 and 10). Noninvasive ventilation offers an attractive option for many patients with mild to moderate disease with rapidly reversible etiologies for ventilatory failure.

■ SPECIFIC PROBLEMS CAUSING VENTILATORY FAILURE

Airflow Obstruction

Airflow may be obstructed at any level of the tracheobronchial tree. Even in the absence of underlying lung pathology, discrete lesions cause symptomatic airflow obstruction if located at the level of the larynx, trachea, or central bronchi (upper airway obstruction [UAO]). Mediastinal compression because of fibrosis, granuloma, or neoplasia can narrow the trachea or major bronchi.

Diffuse diseases of the airways (asthma, chronic bronchitis, emphysema, etc.) usually limit the flow in peripheral air channels (<2 mm in diameter). For certain patients with asthma, however, the primary problem may center on the larynx and upper airway. Airflow obstruction also can occur with such chronic conditions as bronchiectasis, cystic fibrosis, sarcoidosis, and eosinophilic granuloma (histiocytosis). Aspiration, reflux esophagitis, morbid obesity, retained airway secretions, and congestive heart failure (CHF) routinely contribute to airflow obstruction.

Upper Airway Obstruction

Sedentary patients with low ventilation requirements and UAO may remain relatively symptom free until the airway lumen achieves a surprisingly small diameter. Dyspnea then progresses disproportionately to any further decrements in caliber. The complaints of UAO may be difficult to distinguish from those of lower airway disease and may include cardiovascular as well as pulmonary symptoms.

Signs and Symptoms of UAO

The following signs and symptoms are particularly **4** suggestive of UAO (Table 25-3).

1. *Inspiratory limitation of airflow.*
2. *Stridor.* This shrill, inspiratory sound is particularly common with extrathoracic obstruction. In an adult, stridor at rest usually indicates a very narrow aperture (diameter <5 mm).
3. *Difficulty clearing the central airway of secretions.*
4. *Cough of a "brassy" or "bovine" character.*

TABLE 25-3 SIGNS AND SYMPTOMS OF UPPER AIRWAY OBSTRUCTION[a]

Inspiratory limitation of airflow
Stridor
Impaired secretion clearance
Brassy or bovine cough
Breathy voice
Disproportionate exercise intolerance
Symptom variation with neck movement
Failure to respond to bronchodilators
Rapid reversal of dyspnea upon intubation
Fulminant episodic pulmonary edema
Frequent panic attacks

---

[a]Incidence of these signs will vary with nature, location, and severity of the obstruction.

5. *Altered voice.* Hoarseness may be the only sign of laryngeal tumor or unilateral vocal cord paralysis. (Although not itself responsible, unilateral cord paralysis frequently is associated with processes that do cause obstruction.) Cords paralyzed bilaterally usually meet near the midline, so the voice may be "breathy" or soft but remains audible, despite serious obstruction. Bilateral vocal cord paralysis impairs the ability to generate sound, so the patient must drastically increase airflow for each spoken word. Only short phrases can be spoken before the next breath, and the patient may experience dyspnea when conversing.

6. *Marked accentuation of dyspnea and signs of effort by exertion or hyperventilation.* The explanation of this nonspecific phenomenon is mechanical. During vigorous inspiratory efforts, negative intratracheal pressures and turbulent inspiratory airflow tend to narrow a variable extrathoracic aperture. Exertion is unusually stressful because obstruction worsens rather than improves during inspiration, as it does in asthma or chronic obstructive pulmonary disease (COPD).

7. *Change in breathing symptoms with position changes or neck movement.*

8. *Failure to respond to conventional bronchodilator therapy and/or steroids.*

9. *Unexpected ventilatory failure on extubation or precipitous reversal of ventilatory failure by tracheal intubation alone, without ventilatory support.*

10. *Sudden pulmonary edema.*

During asphyxia and severe choking episodes, very forceful inspiratory efforts markedly lower the intrathoracic pressure, increase the cardiac output, and stimulate the release of catecholamines and other stress hormones. The increased loading conditions of the heart, in conjunction with augmented transcapillary filtration pressures, encourage the formation of pulmonary edema.

Diagnostic Tests

The diagnostic workup of UAO may include routine films, computed tomography (CT) or magnetic resonance imaging (MRI) scans of the neck and trachea, and direct visualization by bronchoscopy or laryngoscopy (mirror, direct, or fiberoptic). Reconstructed or 3-dimensional (3D) CT images are often highly informative. Main bronchial obstruction caused by foreign body, tumor, or mediastinal

---

TABLE 25-4 PULMONARY FUNCTION TESTS SUGGESTING UPPER AIRWAY OBSTRUCTION

Disproportionately reduced peak flow
Maximal midinspiratory flow < maximal midexpiratory flow
Vital capacity well preserved despite severely reduced FEV_1
Specific airway conductance low despite nearly normal FEV_1
MVV^a <30 × FEV_1
End-expiratory flows relatively well preserved
$DLCO/V_A{}^b$ well preserved

[a]Maximum voluntary ventilation (L/min).

[b]DLCO referenced to single-breath lung volume (FRC).

---

fibrosis may give rise to strikingly asymmetric ventilation and perfusion scans. Similar information may be available through a comparison of full inspiratory with full expiratory chest radiographs. In stable, cooperative patients, pulmonary function tests should include inspiratory/expiratory flow–volume loops, maximal voluntary ventilation, and diffusing capacity as well as routine unforced and forced expiratory spirometry (Table 25-4). Typically, UAO impairs inspiratory flow more than expiratory flow, impairs peak flow and airway resistance disproportionately to FEV_1, and responds extraordinarily well to a low-density gas (helium–oxygen) but not well to bronchodilators (unless there is simultaneous bronchospasm). Maximum voluntary ventilation typically is much less than the value predicted from spirometry, whereas vital capacity may be comparatively normal, relative to FEV_1.

Diffuse airway diseases such as asthma and COPD tend to produce a different pulmonary function test profile. However, asthma can have a significant upper airway component, and occasionally, stridor will be a prominent presenting sign. Often, these patients benefit from anxiolytics or psychotropic drugs as well as bronchodilators and steroids. Unlike the diffuse obstructive diseases, which alter lung volume, distribution of airflow, and diffusing capacity, UAO tends to leave the parenchyma unaffected. Diffusing capacity is relatively well preserved.

The flow–volume loop contour depends on (a) the fixed or variable nature of the obstruction and (b) the intrathoracic or extrathoracic location (Fig. 25-1). A fixed lesion inside or outside the thorax blunts the maximal inspiration and maximal expiration to a similar degree,

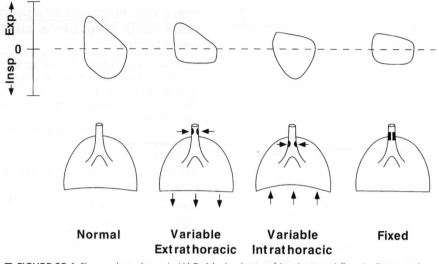

■ **FIGURE 25-1** Flow–volume loops in UAO. Maximal rate of inspiratory airflow is disproportionately curtailed as negative tracheal pressure accentuates resistance through a variable extrathoracic lesion. In similar fashion, the positive pleural pressures generated during forced exhalation selectively limit the airflow across a variable intrathoracic lesion. A fixed lesion at either site limits the maximum flows in both phases.

giving a "squared off" loop contour. A variable *extrathoracic* lesion, surrounded by atmospheric pressure, retracts inward when subjected to negative inspiratory airway pressure but dilates when exposed to positive airway pressure. Conversely, a variable *intrathoracic* lesion, surrounded by a pleural pressure more negative than airway pressure, dilates on inhalation. On exhalation, the lesion is pushed inward to critically narrow the airway. Unilateral obstruction of a main bronchus may not generate such characteristic curves.

Management of UAO

5 The basic principles of managing UAO can be summarized as follows: Patients with symptoms at rest should be kept under continual surveillance and well monitored until the acute crisis resolves. Although certainly indicated, pulse oximetry may give a false sense of security, as O_2 saturation may remain within broad normal limits until the brink of total airway obstruction, physical exhaustion, or full respiratory arrest is reached. Postextubation glottic edema and laryngeal swelling resulting from injury usually peak within 12 to 24 h and then recede over the following 48 to 96 h. Racemic epinephrine aerosols may help reduce glottic edema as they cause topical vasoconstriction and bronchodilate the lower airway to reduce the vigor of breathing efforts. For spontaneously breathing patients not already receiving ventilatory support,

continous positive airway pressure (CPAP) or BiPAP delivered by mask is often helpful. Upright positioning is favored. For unusually labile or otherwise precarious patients, intubation and tracheostomy kits, as well as a 14-gauge needle (for cricothyroid puncture), should be at the bedside for emergent use. In an emergency, oxygen can be insufflated via the needle until an airway is secured (see Chapter 6). Relief of bronchospasm is particularly important in the setting of a UAO. Relief of lower (small) airway obstruction reduces the intrapleural pressure swings and the severity of upper airway (particularly extrathoracic) obstruction. If there is inflammatory obstruction, tactile stimulation of the involved region must be avoided, and steroids may be helpful. Heliox may also be a reasonable option, especially for those who cannot tolerate or do not respond well to pressurized masks and whose oxygen exchange is well preserved. The patient should be kept calm but alert in a head-up posture. Endotracheal intubation or tracheostomy may be needed if ventilatory failure ensues or secretions cannot be cleared. These procedures should be attempted only by experienced personnel. For otherwise stable patients in whom the airway is "high risk" or known to be difficult to intubate, consideration should be given to conducting intubation and/or extubation in an operating environment where the full range of instruments and supporting measures is available.

Care of the Fresh Tracheostomy
(see also Chapter 6)

Inadvertent decannulation of a recent tracheostomy in a patient with UAO may present a genuine emergency. As a prophylactic measure, many surgeons provide exteriorized stay sutures to help locate and elevate the stoma. Others immobilize the tube by suturing it in place. If decannulation occurs, the first priority should be to maintain oxygenation as attempts are made to reestablish the airway. Oxygen should be provided by face mask or over the open stoma until the airway can be resecured. At least one brief attempt to reinsert the original tube usually is warranted, but this occasionally proves difficult. A tracheostomy tube of one size smaller should be kept at the bedside, as well as endotracheal tubes of one and two smaller sizes to serve as a temporary airway until the definitive tracheostomy can be reestablished by the experienced personnel. Whichever airway is selected, proper location must be ensured quickly by the unopposed passage of a suction catheter and effortless manual insufflation and recovery of the tidal volume. If the trachea cannot be entered within the first few minutes, consideration must be given to immediate oral intubation, unless this is contraindicated by spinal injury, aberrant cervical anatomy, or pharyngeal pathology.

Obstructive Sleep Apnea

Although usually considered an "outpatient" problem, obstructive sleep apnea (OSA) or central apnea is observed quite often in the intensive care unit (ICU) environment as an isolated problem, complicating a predisposing disease, or provoked by sedation, analgesia, or postextubation swelling of the laryngopharynx. The prototypical patient with OSA is an obese, middle aged, male or postmenopausal female who is predisposed by pharyngocervical anatomy—but numerous exceptions to these stereotypes are encountered, especially under the provocation of physiologic stress, sedation, and fatigue. The well-monitored patient will demonstrate typical oscillations of the continuous oximeter and pulse tracings during sleep (Fig. 25-2), and the heroic snoring efforts are hard to miss in this closely observed setting. Most (but not all) patients will demonstrate evidence of CO_2 retention during wakefulness as well—a consequence of impaired drive to breathe coincident with or resulting from loaded breathing in a

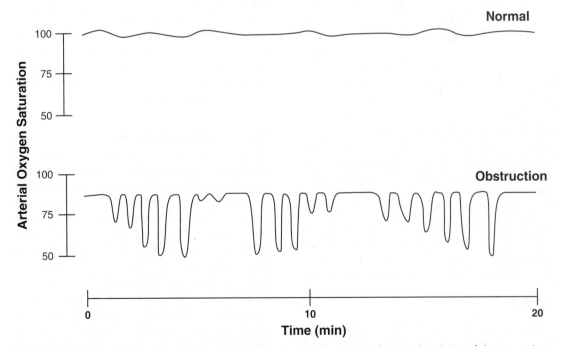

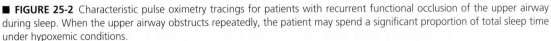

■ **FIGURE 25-2** Characteristic pulse oximetry tracings for patients with recurrent functional occlusion of the upper airway during sleep. When the upper airway obstructs repeatedly, the patient may spend a significant proportion of total sleep time under hypoxemic conditions.

predisposed subject. A tentative diagnosis is made by extended sleep oximetry (with or without electrocardiogram [ECG] and blood pressure recording). As in the outpatient setting, nocturnal noninvasive ventilatory support (e.g., with CPAP or BiPAP, if necessary) is extremely helpful for patients who tolerate this intervention.

Obesity-Hypoventilation Syndrome

The prevalence of morbid obesity has never been higher in the industrialized "first" world. As a consequence, a once unusual problem, obesity-hypoventilation syndrome (OHS) has become increasingly common. OHS is characterized by extreme obesity and alveolar hypoventilation, hypersomnolence, and hypoxemia, with resulting cyanosis, polycythemia, and plethora. OSA is a frequent (but certainly not ubiquitous) accompanying feature. Increased body weight lowers lung compliance and raises the total mechanical work of breathing. If body weight doubles, for example, the mechanical work performed to expand the lungs and chest wall increases by more than two thirds. This increase has been attributed to closure of small airways and to engorgement of pulmonary capillaries with the increased pulmonary blood volume that occurs in massive obesity. Although it is understood that increased breathing workload is an inherent feature of obesity, most morbidly obese patients do not become hypercapnic and, in those who do, there is no correlation between the degree of obesity and the ventilatory abnormalities. Some endogenous impairment of ventilatory drive, therefore, appears to be unmasked by the obesity or by the OSA that accompanies it. Depressed ventilatory drive—an abnormality of respiratory control that is genetically inherent or acquired—is suggested by demonstrating that patients with OHS have decreased respiratory responsiveness to both hypoxemia and hypercapnia. Once hypercapnia is underway, renal compensation for hypercapnia raises the plasma bicarbonate concentration, thereby minimizing the usual fall in arterial pH. Attenuation of hypoventilation and hypercapnia during sleep via nasal BiPAP ventilation returns $PaCO_2$ to more normal levels during wakefulness.

Asthma

Asthma is characterized by airway inflammation, edema, and bronchospasm. The episodic airflow obstruction that results from these processes reverses partially or completely with medication.

The trigger for inflammation and bronchospasm **6** may be (a) an inhaled or ingested allergen; (b) a bronchial irritant causing reflex bronchoconstriction (infection, endotracheal tube stimulation, smoke, fumes and odors, aspirated food, oral secretions, or excessively dry, humid, or cold air); (c) emotion; (d) exercise; (e) sinus drainage; (f) gastroesophageal reflux; or (g) pulmonary venous congestion or cardiac dysfunction. Obese patients often have a disproportionately reduced resting lung volume and correspondingly increased airway resistance. For such patients, relative small changes in airway caliber may cause wheezing and hypoxemia that simulate asthma. Asthma may cause airway obstruction that never remits completely, but unlike emphysema, it does not routinely disrupt the parenchyma.

Exudative Tracheobronchitis

Although rare, it should be kept in mind that exudative laryngotracheobronchitis (e.g., resulting from herpes simplex) can masquerade as refractory asthma. Herpes tracheobronchitis occurs more often in intubated elderly patients with extensive burns or immune compromise. Infiltrates and fever are uncommon. Oropharyngeal signs of herpes often are absent or obscured. The diagnosis is supported by recovery of virus or viral antigen from sputum but must be confirmed by direct inspection. Bronchoscopic findings include an erythematous and friable mucosa that sometimes ulcerates. A fibrinous, pearly white membrane often lines the airway. The problem may prove refractory to corticosteroids and bronchodilators until treated definitively with intravenous acyclovir.

Physical Diagnosis of Asthma

When admitted to the ICU, most patients with exacerbated asthma relate a history of gradually worsening dyspnea. These patients usually require intensive therapy extending over several days before resolution. A subset of asthmatic patients, typically in a young age category, develop life-threatening bronchospasm and ventilatory failure with frightening suddenness—over minutes to hours. In these "sudden asphyxic" asthmatics and for those with other asthma variants, upper airway signs may predominate. Inspissated mucus and edema are less prevalent, whereas emotion, an identifiable provocative agent, and asthmatic stridor often figure prominently in the presentation. Life-threatening airflow obstruction often quickly reverses after intubation, sedation, and appropriate pharmacologic therapy are initiated.

Noncritically ill patients with asthma may report few symptoms despite impressively abnormal examination findings and pulmonary function tests. Rhinitis, sinus congestion postnasal drainage, and cough often coexist. Dyspnea characteristically begins or worsens at night or in the early morning. Hoarseness or gastroesophageal reflux suggests chronic nocturnal aspiration of small volumes of gastric contents. Substernal chest pain developing suddenly in a young patient with asthma suggests associated bronchitis or mediastinal emphysema because of alveolar rupture. A patient who is unable to converse in complete sentences has severe airflow obstruction and/or fatigue. Because wheezing depends on both degree of obstruction and velocity of airflow, it is detectable with forceful breathing in mild obstruction, reaches loud intensity in moderate obstruction, and disappears in very severe obstruction. Wheezing may be audible only when the patient is supine. Wheezes do not necessarily imply asthma. The differential diagnosis includes left ventricular failure (cardiac asthma), pulmonary embolism, UAO, and bronchitis (acute or chronic).

7 Specific Danger Signs

Deteriorating Mental Status   Deteriorating mental status often is a harbinger of physical exhaustion and impending ventilatory arrest. Sleep deprivation, muscle fatigue, sustained catecholamine stimulation, and acute cerebral acidosis (occurring just before arrest) are likely contributing factors. When patients with asthma decompensate, they often do so suddenly. A low threshold should be maintained for intubating a disoriented, lethargic patient.

Arterial Pulsus Paradoxus Exceeding 15 to 20 mm Hg Normally, as arm cuff pressure is reduced, the discrepancy (the "paradox") between the point at which the first intermittent systolic Korotkoff sounds are detected and the arterial pressure at which all are heard is less than 8 mm Hg. The respiratory variation of systolic blood pressure increases as airflow obstruction worsens and is made obvious by tracings from patients with indwelling arterial lines. This phenomenon is believed to result from the wide phasic swings of intrapleural pressure necessary for ventilation, which have several effects:

1. Forceful inspiration effectively "afterloads" the left ventricle. Surrounded by very negative pleural pressure, the left ventricle must, nonetheless, raise intracavitary pressure to systemic levels.

Systolic pressure falls during inspiration, whereas reduced left ventricular afterload occurs during forced exhalation.

2. Although inflow to the right atrium increases during inspiration, preload to the left ventricle decreases simultaneously because a relatively small quantity of blood returns to the left atrium and because of low right ventricular output during the preceding exhalation. Furthermore, the expanded right ventricle impairs left ventricular filling during inspiration because the left and stretched right ventricles share myocardial fibers, the interventricular septum, and the pericardial space.

Severe Hyperinflation   Hyperinflation increases with the severity of obstruction and with $\dot{V}_E$. The increase in resting lung volume is produced by the combined effects of air trapping and the need to hold airways open to minimize the work of breathing. Moreover, in very severe attacks of asthma, many air channels are plugged completely and do not communicate with the central airway at all. When such plugging is extensive, severe hyperinflation is evident on the chest radiograph, but auto-PEEP measured in the intubated patient may be misleadingly low, as it reflects only those pressures within alveoli that communicate with the airway (Fig. 25-3). Considerable regional variation of

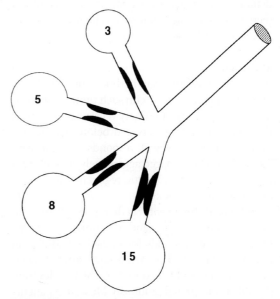

■ **FIGURE 25-3** Regional variation in auto-PEEP. The greatest tendency for airway closure and gas trapping tends to occur in dependent regions. Although end-expiratory airway occlusion reflects the average auto-PEEP among open alveolar units, the highest levels of auto-PEEP are encountered by alveoli cut off from the airway opening.

auto-PEEP values is common, whereas the end-inspiratory alveolar pressures may not differ greatly from site to site. In these cases, therefore, the end-inspiratory *plateau* pressure during flow-controlled volume-cycled ventilation is a much better indicator of gas trapping when tidal volume and PEEP are fixed. Unless otherwise explained, a marked disparity between a high-plateau pressure and a low measurable auto-PEEP (and/or between the appearance of the hyperinflated chest radiograph and auto-PEEP) suggests extensive airway plugging as the basis for gas trapping.

CO₂ Retention/Acidosis/Cyanosis If the patient remains well compensated, an acute attack of asthma usually elicits mild alveolar hyperventilation and mild-to-moderate hypoxemia. (Typically, pH is greater than 7.40, $PaCO_2$ is less than 40 mm Hg, and PaO_2 breathing air generally exceeds 60 mm Hg in a patient without underlying cardiopulmonary disease of another type.) Compensated asthma is unique among the obstructive diseases in promoting alveolar hyperventilation. Significant central cyanosis (implying marked arterial desaturation or *cor pulmonale*), elevated $PaCO_2$, and acidosis are important danger signs. If the patient does not appear fatigued and retains normal mental status, these findings by themselves do not demand intubation and mechanical support. Once appropriate therapy is under way, however, progressive deterioration in pH, $PaCO_2$, muscular strength, or mental status does require mechanical support, almost invariably with intubation.

Management

An attack of asthma may be brief, mild, and self-limited or may continue with such protracted severity as to require extraordinary measures. As a rule, the longer the attack persisted before ICU admission, the more slowly it responds to treatment. Asthma must be managed aggressively, with prompt escalation of the therapeutic regimen if the attack does not "break" quickly.

In-Hospital Treatment Lethargy or disorientation, obvious fatigue, and deteriorating arterial blood gases are grounds for immediate admission to the ICU (Table 25-5). Yet, a single arterial specimen showing mild acidosis or $PaCO_2$ elevation should be interpreted cautiously. Most such patients will require admission to the ICU, but if the patient is alert and both the arterial blood gases and the patient show prompt and marked improvement with treatment, ICU admission is sometimes avoidable. Oxygen, corticosteroids, bronchodilators, and

TABLE 25-5 DANGER SIGNS IN ASTHMA

Deteriorating mental status
Arterial pulsus paradoxus > 15–20 mm Hg
Severe hyperinflation
Increasing CO_2 retention despite R_x
Cyanosis unresponsive to oxygen supplementation
Retained central airway secretions
CHF
Unstable hemodynamics

intravenous fluids are required for virtually all patients. For specific indications, antibiotics and ventilatory support are needed as well. During an established attack, the patient may not seem to improve for days, only to recover rapidly thereafter without a major change in therapy.

Oxygen Oxygen should be administered by nasal prongs or mask to all patients with less than full arterial saturation of hemoglobin.

Inhaled Bronchodilators Although a focus for management, bronchospasm is by no means the entire (or sometimes even the primary) problem for patients with asthma who require intensive care. Termination of the inflammatory response, resolution of mucosal edema, and clearance of airway secretions are perhaps more important, especially in patients who have had respiratory compromise for days before hospitalization. In the setting of status asthmaticus, bronchodilating aerosols do not penetrate deeply into the obstructed airways. (This is especially true for the intubated patient receiving mechanical ventilatory support.) It is generally acknowledged that more frequent dosing of β_2 agonists is required during an acute exacerbation of asthma. In the breathless patient, nebulization is generally superior to metered-dose aerosols. There is no convincing evidence, however, that continuous nebulization is preferable to the same total dose given intermittently. Moreover, intermittent administration encourages the frequent reassessment appropriate to this setting.

It must be remembered that a rapid response to bronchodilators is not to be expected in the patient admitted to the ICU with full-blown status asthma who already has been taking such treatment with deteriorating compensation. Furthermore, there are important costs and hazards associated with frequent administration of high-dose β agonists. Very frequent intermittent dosing may interfere with sleep and/or rest of an exhausted patient. Regardless of dosing method, β agents induce agitation, tachycardia, arrhythmia, or hypokalemia. Such an intense treatment schedule may be counterproductive. These side effects and hazards are even more prevalent when nonaerosolized (enteral or parenteral) β agents are used.

In the hyperacute phase, albuterol can be given every 30 to 120 min unless there are limiting side effects. For most patients with asthma, the anticholinergic agents (e.g., ipratropium, atropine) are no more effective than the β_2 agonists, and usually less so. Because ipratropium is absorbed poorly from the airway mucosa, tachycardias, arrhythmias, and hypokalemia are decidedly less common than with the adrenergic agents; therefore, to reduce side effects, many clinicians elect to use them alternately with the β_2 bronchodilators, especially if the patient has a known or suspected cardiac condition. Ipratropium may be less effective in stable asthma but has a good rationale when tachycardia results from the β_2 bronchodilators, when β_2 tachyphylaxis is suspected, or when irritative (vagally mediated) bronchospasm figures prominently in the pathogenesis (e.g., smoke inhalation, chemical exposure, "cardiac" asthma, acute bronchial infection). Efficacy should be documented individually and should not be administered more often than every 4 to 6 h, for fear of drying secretions, blurring vision, or causing mental status changes. A combination anticholinergic/β_2 inhaled bronchodilator may be a good choice for scheduled treatments, supplemented by interspersed doses of pure β_2 agent, as necessary. When severely ill, many patients prefer a wet nebulizer to a metered-dose canister, even though some comparative studies fail to show a bronchodilating advantage when sufficient number of metered puffs are given. Wet nebulization of more than 10 to 15 mg of albuterol (or its equivalent) may be associated with undesirable cardiovascular stimulation, a fall in serum potassium concentration, or lactic acidosis. Patients predisposed to tachycardia or arrhythmia may benefit from nebulized levalbuterol, a highly selective β_2 agonist, which may stimulate the heart less than the mixed isomeric albuterol on which it is based. If inhaled bronchodilators are prescribed, careful attention should be directed to the duration of effective action, which varies with dosage. For standard doses:

Metaproterenol: 2 to 4 hr

Albuterol: 3 to 6 hr

Levalbuterol: 4 hr

Salmeterol: 8 to 12 hr

Formoterol: 8 to 12 hr

Ipratropium: 4 to 7 hr

Tiotropium: 24 hr

Rapidity of the onset tends to be inversely proportional to the duration of action. Inhaled corticosteroids, cromolyn, and necrodomil aerosols, which are intended for prophylactic use, have no place in the management of hospitalized patients. In fact, their irritant effects actually may worsen symptoms during the acute phase.

Corticosteroids   Virtually every patient hospitalized for asthma should be given corticosteroids promptly and in high doses. Steroids reduce inflammation, help thin secretions, block components of the allergic response, and may enhance responsiveness to β-adrenergic bronchodilators. Whether superhigh doses of steroids (>125 mg of methylprednisolone every 6 h) are preferable to moderately high doses (60 to 100 mg every 6 h) is unknown. The question is not academic; apart from the financial cost, high-dose steroids often interfere with sleep, mood, cooperation, and thinking as well as disturb glucose homeostasis. Although high-dose steroids are generally safe and well tolerated for short periods, profound neuromyopathy, manifest by elevated levels of creatine kinase and protracted weakness, is believed to result from the use of corticosteroids alone or in combination with extended neuromuscular blockade with nondepolarizing agents (see following and Chapter 17). Nevertheless, the danger of uncontrolled asthma clearly outweighs the danger of administering high-dose steroids for a brief period. The therapeutic effects of a single corticosteroid bolus are evident within 4 to 6 h, peaking within 12 to 16 h. There remains considerable disagreement regarding optimum delivery methods, doses, and schedules of administration. One rational recommendation is to administer an initial dose of 1 to 3 mg/kg of methylprednisolone (or equivalent) intravenously, followed by a similar dose every 6 to 12 h until the attack is broken. (For many patients, the oral route is equally efficacious and dramatically more cost effective than parenteral dosing.) Once symptoms have improved considerably, the dosage can be cut back to moderately high doses (0.5 to 1.0 mg/kg twice a day) for a few days before tapering gradually to the prehospital dose over 3 weeks. An inhaled steroid can be added at approximately 10 to 14 days, if indicated. Final tapering to the preattack dose should be performed by the outpatient physician.

Sedation, Paralytics, and Iatrogenic Neuromyopathy Many patients hospitalized with status asthmaticus are so exhausted that they sleep deeply and require little or no sedation during the first few hours of their intubation. Others, however, will require deep sedation and even muscle relaxants to reduce the ventilatory requirement to tolerable levels and to accept the permissive hypercapnia required to apply safe levels of airway and alveolar pressure (see Chapters 7, 24, and following discussion). Neuromyopathy presents a serious risk in the controlled ventilation of the asthmatic patient. During the period of immobilization, myopathy manifests in the short term as an elevation of muscle enzymes and later as a profound weakness requiring weeks to months for reversal. In the great majority of reported cases of neuromyopathy in asthma, high-dose corticosteroids were given. Most myopathic patients also received nondepolarizing paralytic agents uninterruptedly for longer than 48 to 72 h, often without the depth of relaxation monitoring. On the basis of current evidence, it seems advisable to limit the use of muscle relaxants to those who clearly need them and to use only the amounts necessary to accomplish partial paralysis for the shortest possible time. This need for paralysis is best established by attempting to withdraw the muscle relaxant entirely several times per day, thereby also allowing the physician to gauge the adequacy of sedation. "Train of four" monitoring, titrating to a two-twitch response, is also rational when continuous paralysis is targeted. This alternative, however, runs the risk of unnecessarily delaying withdrawal of the paralytic agent and may mask underlying alertness.

Theophylline   Although clearly useful for some patients, theophylline derivatives must be used very cautiously (if at all) in status asthmaticus, with appropriate respect for their low therapeutic index. Failure of the left or right ventricle, hepatic disease, life-threatening illness, and certain drugs (notably ciprofloxacin and histamine-blocking drugs) slow its catabolism. Both efficacy and toxicity of theophylline roughly parallel its blood level; 10 to $20\,\mu g/mL$ is usually a safe therapeutic range but occasionally may cause arrhythmias. As with most bronchodilators, greater effect can be achieved with higher doses, but response relates only logarithmically to dose, and the incidence of toxic effects accelerates at higher serum levels. Theophylline holds a questionable place in the treatment of the patient with acute asthma who is receiving β agonists and corticosteroids simultaneously. Despite its shortcomings, there recently has been a renewed surge of enthusiasm for its carefully monitored use. Some experienced practitioners believe that it improves diaphragmatic function, helps mobilize secretions, and improves cardiac contractility, but these potential benefits are controversial. The weight of current evidence suggests that theophylline seldom adds to the bronchodilating effect of an optimized β-aerosol regimen, and it has little value as a stimulant to respiratory drive.

The warning signs of theophylline toxicity (nausea, abdominal discomfort, etc.) may not be sensed or reported by seriously ill patients; therefore, frequently obtained serum levels are mandatory. Cardiac arrhythmias predictably develop at levels greater than $25\,\mu g/mL$; in predisposed patients, it is likely that theophylline is arrhythmogenic at much lower levels. Central nervous symptoms (agitation, confusion, seizures, etc.) appear routinely at levels greater than $35\,\mu g/mL$ but can be seen in a lower range. Theophylline seizures are problematic because of their resistance to standard anticonvulsants. An intravenous bolus of theophylline (aminophylline) can precipitate profound hypotension or sudden respiratory arrest. After a loading dose is given cautiously, aminophylline is best delivered by continuous pump infusion via a peripheral (not central) intravenous line.

Magnesium Sulfate   As a smooth muscle relaxant, magnesium sulfate possesses mild bronchodilating effects, believed to relate to modulation of calcium ion fluxes in smooth muscle. Studies conflict, however, regarding its value in refractory asthma. Although the toxicity of a 1- to 2-gm dose in patients with normal renal function seems limited to flushing and mild sedation or mild hypotension, most patients given full doses of conventional bronchodilators experience little additional benefit.

Fluids   The patient should be amply hydrated (2 to 3 L of fluid daily) to aid thinning of secretions. Copious fluids are unnecessary and may cause volume overload. Although physiologic saline may help lubricate viscid secretions and facilitate airway suctioning in intubated patients, hydrating aerosols (mist therapy) may exacerbate obstruction because of bronchospasm or cause swelling in situ of retained secretions.

Respiratory Therapy   Secretion retention is a **8** very serious problem in asthma and is caused partly by the unusually tenacious nature of the sputum. Many airways are totally plugged, impeding dislodgment of the mucus. Unfortunately, chest percussion and postural drainage are relatively ineffective and poorly tolerated until a measure of bronchospasm has been relieved (usually the second or third day). Until that point, coaching to cough, bronchodilator inhalation, airway humidification, and oxygen therapy approach the limits of useful respiratory therapy services for the nonintubated patient. Noninvasive ventilation and CPAP are tolerated poorly by most patients with severe disease but are worth attempting in cooperative patients with more moderate illness (see Chapter 7). Iodinated glycerol compounds (e.g., potassium iodide) have little role in the treatment of acute airflow obstruction because their actions are delayed for days to weeks. Mucolytics (such as hypertonic $NaHCO_3$, acetylcysteine, and dornase) may irritate the twitchy airways of the decompensated asthmatic and must be used concurrently with or immediately after an inhaled bronchodilator. Bronchoscopy and lavage of inspissated mucus may be indicated in ventilated patients who fail to improve.

Mechanical Ventilation   Mental status or blood gas deterioration that occurs despite aggressive medical therapy is an important indication for ventilator support. Noninvasive ventilation may be helpful in the fully alert subject who can tolerate it. Although not as clearly helpful as in exacerbated COPD, noninvasive ventilation may help forestall the onset of fatigue while steroids and bronchodilators make headway against the disease itself. Unlike many patients with COPD, patients with asthma tend to sustain adequate alveolar ventilation during attacks until sudden decompensation occurs. Invasive mechanical support may afford the rest needed for recovery and should not be delayed once a firm indication appears. Although most patients with asthma can be disconnected from the ventilator within 3 to 5 days of intubation, others require much longer.

The basic principles of ventilator management during status asthmaticus do not differ greatly from those of other conditions. However, hemodynamic compromise and certain forms of barotrauma (pneumomediastinum, pneumothorax, etc.) are important consequences of gas trapping. Peak alveolar end-inspiratory (plateau) pressure should be monitored closely and kept lower than 30 cm H_2O. For most patients, this will mean the acceptance of hypercarbia and respiratory acidosis (permissive hypercapnia). Deep sedation and, in severe cases, muscle relaxants may be required to impose this gentler breathing pattern.

As a guideline, a tidal volume of 6 to 7 mL/kg, a backup frequency of approximately 12 breaths/min, and a flow setting and waveform that provide a 1:2 I:E ratio are a satisfactory starting point for ventilator settings in a patient who is well sedated. Failure to keep end-inspiratory static plateau pressure less than 30 cm H_2O should prompt reductions of frequency or tidal volume. Intravenous bicarbonate may be advisable if pH is less than 7.20, but this recommendation is controversial. Some physicians allow pH to fall to 7.10 (or even lower) if the patient demonstrates good physiologic tolerance, but this approach cannot be advocated for general use. The degree of dynamic hyperinflation is generated by the severity of airflow obstruction, the tidal volume, and the duration of expiration. The duration of expiration is most effectively extended by decreasing the breathing frequency (and minute ventilation). Very rapid inspiratory flow rates should be avoided during volume-cycled ventilation. For the same inspiratory time, most severe asthmatic patients will have a lower peak airway pressure with a gently decelerating waveform. Strong, spontaneously triggering patients often require "square wave" inspiratory flow or pressure-controlled ventilation to meet their flow demands throughout inspiration.

Positive End-Expiratory Pressure   The place of positive end-expiratory pressure (PEEP) in the management of asthma remains controversial. When resistance is volume dependent and flow limited, as it tends to be in this setting, PEEP may possibly improve bronchodilator penetration. In spontaneously breathing patients, CPAP may help even the distribution of ventilation as well as reduce the triggering threshold and the work of breathing (see Chapter 9). In certain patients, occluded airways may sometimes reopen under its influence. However, if expiration is not flow limited, adding PEEP could simply raise both peak and mean alveolar pressures. As a rule, a low level of PEEP (<8 to 10 cm H_2O) can be added, as long as end-inspiratory static "plateau" pressure does not rise.

Chronic Obstructive Pulmonary Disease

Characteristic Features

The obstructive lung diseases associated with cigarette smoking (primarily emphysema and chronic bronchitis) often coexist but are fundamentally different processes. Emphysema destroys the alveolar surface membrane and blood vessels, reducing elastic recoil and diffusing capacity, leaving the airways collapsible but morphologically intact; emphysematous obstruction of the airway is a functional, not anatomic, problem. Conversely, chronic bronchitis causes airway damage, bronchospasm, and sputum production but leaves the parenchyma minimally affected.

Pure cases of emphysema are clinically distinguishable from those of chronic bronchitis. On the chest radiograph, bullae, hyperlucency, diminished peripheral vascular markings, and increased lung volume are often seen in emphysema. CT is vastly superior for detecting these alterations. Such findings differ from the increased bronchovascular markings and more normal lung volumes of chronic bronchitis. Patients with pure emphysema produce little or no sputum. Conversely, chronic bronchitis is defined as an airway disease in which there is habitual sputum production, especially in the morning. (That characteristic is shared by other airway diseases, such as sinusitis and bronchiectasis.)

Emphysematous patients tend to experience breathlessness with minimal exertion but usually do not enter the hospital with exacerbations of their disease until they near their terminal phase. In contrast, patients with chronic bronchitis often seem less distressed by their symptoms but decompensate more frequently.

The verbal caricatures of patients with emphysema as "pink puffers" and patients with chronic bronchitis as "blue bloaters" are overdrawn. Many—if not most—have elements of both. Emphysema tends to destroy capillaries and alveolar septae in proportion to one another, preserving near-normal arterial blood gases at the cost of elevated minute ventilation. Diffusing capacity is routinely impaired. Bronchitis, on the other hand, produces extensive ventilation–perfusion ($\dot{V}/\dot{Q}$) mismatching and hypoxemia, without impairing the diffusing capacity adjusted for the volume of aerated tissue, and hypercapnia occurs more commonly.

Pulmonary hypertension marks the end stage of both diseases, but for different reasons. In pure emphysema, pulmonary capillaries are destroyed, but normal oxygen saturation of arterial blood is the rule. In chronic bronchitis, pulmonary hypertension develops earlier, as a consequence of persistent alveolar hypoxia. Therefore, cor pulmonale in a patient with bronchitis and hypoxemia may be partially reversed with supplemental oxygen. Cor pulmonale developing in the setting of emphysema is an ominous sign, responding poorly to therapy unless hypoxemia coexists. Despite the aforementioned characteristics, there are many variations of presentation in patients with advanced forms of either chronic obstructive disease.

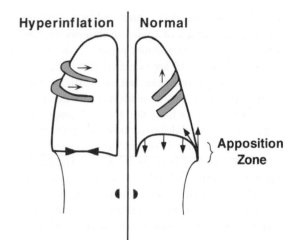

■ **FIGURE 25-4** Respiratory muscle compromise during acute hyperinflation. Normally, the curved hemidiaphragm is positioned optimally to splay the ribs outward by its bucket-handle action and by the positive outward abdominal pressure exerted on the ribs in the zone of apposition. The hyperinflated patient may have a flattened diaphragm with no useful inspiratory force vector, lose the zone of apposition, and inspire against the inward recoil of the horizontal ribs. Simultaneously, the work of breathing is increased (see Chapter 10).

Associated Problems

Hyperinflation helps speed expiratory airflow but increases the elastic work of breathing. More importantly, the inspiratory musculature is placed at a serious mechanical disadvantage (Fig. 25-4).

Poorly ventilated cystic spaces may fill with fluid when the surrounding parenchyma is infiltrated or flooded (bullitis), a problem simulating cavities or lung abscesses but generally less resistant to therapy. Distinction by chest film or CT usually can be made easily, and the prospect for quick resolution is much better than for abscess.

Pneumonia and CHF often complicate COPD but frequently are difficult to recognize as such because the parenchyma is hyperinflated and distorted.

Heart rhythm disturbances—typically atrial fibrillation, atrial flutter, and multifocal atrial tachycardia—are characteristic of decompensated COPD.

Management

Etiology of the Exacerbation The exact cause for many exacerbations of COPD remains unknown. Ischemic heart disease and diastolic dysfunction often coexist. Entry into a rapid atrial rhythm often precipitates dyspnea and altered gas exchange. Cor pulmonale is notoriously difficult to diagnose accurately, especially when a high-quality echocardiogram is not available. Numerous patients with severe disease blame climatic changes for their deterioration. Treatable causes (infection, pneumothorax, pleural effusion, congestive failure, embolism, etc.) must be addressed (see Table 25-2).

Oxygen Therapy   Although it is true that high inspired fractions of oxygen may cause catastrophic blunting of ventilatory drive in susceptible individuals, judicious administration of the correct dose of oxygen can be lifesaving.

Reversal of hypoxemia may diminish hypoxic drive and work of breathing. In symptomatically hypoxic patients, oxygen improves alertness and muscular function and helps relieve cor pulmonale as well. (For this latter reason, oxygen often proves an effective diuretic.)

Although Venturi masks deliver a fixed FiO_2 and should be used when control of the inspired O_2 fraction is crucial, nasal prongs are more comfortable for patients with dyspnea and allow expectoration without interrupting the flow of oxygen.

Most patients respond to relief of hypoxemia by retaining slightly more CO_2 because hypercapneic drive and hypoxic drives are both reduced by supplemental oxygen. Two rules are useful: First, patients at risk to retain excessive CO_2 are those who already manifest some degree of hypercapnia before O_2 therapy is initiated. Second, in otherwise stable patients given "low-flow" oxygen, the rise in $PaCO_2$ generally is less than 10 mm Hg and usually occurs within the first hour of oxygen administration. Therefore, rather than withhold oxygen, the appropriate strategy is to raise PaO_2 to 55 to 60 mm Hg, watch the patient closely for signs of obtundation, obtain blood gases 20 to 30 min after the FiO_2 was increased, and adjust the oxygen flow rate accordingly. The therapeutic endpoint is an acceptable PaO_2, documented by blood gas analysis.

Medication Regimen   Bronchodilator therapy is similar to that already described for asthma. Anticholinergic aerosols, however, may be somewhat more effective in these "irritant" forms of bronchospasm. These include ipratropium (Atrovent) and tiotropium (Spiriva), a very long-acting agent that is increasingly used in the hospital setting. For acutely ill patients, the former is often combined with albuterol, an adrenergic agent of similar duration of action (Combivent MDI or Duo-Neb). The reversible component of bronchospasm in COPD is usually small, and such patients are generally older

and more fragile than those with asthma. Fluid/electrolyte balance, oxygen therapy, and respiratory therapy assume greater importance. Improving nutrition is helpful over the medium and long term.

Thick green or deep yellow sputum with leukocytes and gram-stainable intracellular organisms should be treated with an appropriate antibiotic, whereas sputum eosinophilia suggests the probable utility of corticosteroids. (Both medications are given almost routinely, even in the absence of such data.) The choice of antibiotic should be guided by the sputum smear and by knowledge of the organisms to which these patients are vulnerable (i.e., *Haemophilus influenzae, Streptococcus pneumoniae,* and *Moraxella catarrhalis*) (see Chapter 26). If no organism is seen, a virus or mycoplasma is the likely infectious cause of the exacerbation. In some regions of the country, *Legionella* is a prevalent community-acquired pathogen that is difficult to identify on Gram stain. Practically speaking, antibiotics are usually begun empirically, with amoxicillin, doxycycline, and azithromycin all rational choices as they address the most commonly encountered organisms. Macrolides (erythromycin-like) drugs may have anti-inflammatory as well as antibacterial properties. Selected cephalosporins and fluoroquinolones (e.g., moxifloxacin) are also effective and may offer advantages regarding dosing frequency or convenience, but they are generally more costly. Duration of treatment should be limited to 5 to 7 days unless continued fever and/or infiltrates are worrisome for pneumonia.

A patient who fails to respond despite appropriate initial measures probably should receive a trial of corticosteroids. This recommendation includes the majority of those admitted to the hospital. Although there is some controversy regarding proper dosing and duration, massive doses of corticosteroids similar to those given in asthma should be avoided. Very high doses of steroids disrupt thinking, interfere with sleep, encourage protein wasting, elevate blood urea nitrogen (BUN) and white blood cell count, predispose to infection, and cause fluid retention. Metabolic alkalosis, hyperglycemia, and gut dysfunction or ulceration also are to be expected. A reasonable schedule is to give 0.25 to 0.5 mg/kg of methylprednisolone or its equivalent every 6 h during the first 24 to 48 h of an acute crisis, with conversion to oral prednisone and tapering thereafter to the patient's baseline over a 10- to 14-day period. Given steroids, some patients improve both baseline function and response to bronchodilators. Such persons have been termed "hidden asthmatics."

Respiratory Therapy   Respiratory therapy may assume a crucial role in the management of hospitalized patients with chronic airflow obstruction. Most problems can be reversed by relieving hypoxemia, treating infection or fluid overload, and improving secretion clearance with the respiratory therapy techniques of coughing, deep breathing, and intensified bronchodilator therapy. The patient must be actively stimulated to cough, using endotracheal suctioning and/or vibropercussion of the chest wall or airway if necessary. Chest vibropercussion and postural drainage are often effective when secretions are plentiful and the treatment is well tolerated. However, no physiotherapy technique should be continued unless its efficacy can be documented.

Intubation and Mechanical Ventilation   Whenever possible, intubation and mechanical ventilation must be avoided for the following reasons:

1. Most patients without advanced cor pulmonale tolerate mild-to-moderate hypoxemia and mild acidosis quite well.
2. An effective cough clears the peripheral airways better than endotracheal intubation and suctioning.
3. Patients with COPD are at particular risk for the complications of mechanical ventilation (e.g., infection, hypotension, barotrauma) and can be exceptionally difficult to wean because of the high work/cost of breathing, weakness, and muscular discoordination.
4. When intervention is early enough, some patients may respond well to noninvasive ventilation by nasal cannula or facial mask (see Chapter 7). Even though noninvasive ventilation is of unquestioned benefit for many patients, many centers lack the highly trained and motivated nursing and respiratory care practitioners required to implement this technique safely, effectively, and expeditiously in this challenging setting. Early intervention, careful coaching of the patient, and a high degree of vigilance are essential to a successful outcome (see Chapter 7).

Indications for Intubation   Indications for intubation include deteriorating mental status, loss of effective cough (with retained secretions in central airways), progressive respiratory acidosis despite aggressive medical and respiratory therapy, and unstable hemodynamics.

If mechanical assistance is necessary, care should be taken not to overventilate with respect to the chronically stable state of CO_2 retention, a development signaled by the sudden development of metabolic alkalosis when mechanical assistance is begun.

Throughout the course of ventilatory support, the staff must check periodically for evidence of dynamic hyperinflation (auto-PEEP) and its response to PEEP. Simultaneous airway pressure and flow tracings help greatly in this assessment (see Chapters 5 and 9). The auto-PEEP effect is associated not only with cardiovascular consequences but also with increased work of breathing. Increased air trapping and expiratory effort occur very commonly during spontaneous breathing as well. Weaning must be undertaken as soon as feasible but conducted cautiously to avoid cardiopulmonary decompensation or panic attacks (see Chapter 10).

Treatment of Arrhythmias and Cardiac Dysfunction   Atrial and ventricular arrhythmias of all types occur commonly because of right atrial overdistension, catecholamine release, medication effects, pH and electrolyte disturbances, hyperinflation-related heart–lung interactions, and hypoxemia. The onset of atrial fibrillation can severely impair the efficiency of the ventricular pump and precipitate deterioration. Multifocal atrial tachycardia (chaotic but coordinated atrial contraction originating from at least three pacemaking foci; see Chapter 4) is a characteristic rhythm that often responds only to the relief of metabolic derangement and respiratory failure. In certain cases, a calcium channel blocker (e.g., diltiazem) can effectively slow the rate. Caution is indicated, however, because these agents may possibly worsen $\dot{V}/\dot{Q}$ matching, impair the myocardial performance, or impede the conduction (see Chapters 3, 4, and 22). In such patients, ischemic cardiac disease frequently coexists and may present with atypical signs or symptoms. The clinician should remain vigilant to the possibility of occult ischemia, CHF, and diastolic dysfunction—as well as cor pulmonale.

Nutrition   The ability of the patient with COPD to cope with the respiratory workload depends on the strength and endurance of the ventilatory pump. Reversal of chronic malnutrition cannot be accomplished quickly, but maintaining adequate calorie intake is vital. Diaphragmatic bulk parallels the body weight. Although it is possible to generate excessive CO_2 by overfeeding, this seldom presents a problem for hospitalized patients who are able to eat normally. Instead, attention should focus on providing adequate nutrition (2,000 cal daily). Large meals or brisk enteral feedings may cause abdominal distention, discomfort, and breathing difficulty. Relief and prevention of obstipation are particularly important to breathing comfort but are frequently overlooked.

Neuromuscular Dysfunction

As causes of ventilatory failure, extrapulmonary disorders that involve the central drive mechanism, chest wall, or respiratory muscles typically have relatively well-preserved pulmonary gas exchanging function. Hypoxemia usually presents a secondary problem, and minute ventilation requirements are generally modest. In such a setting of diminished reserve, taking special care to avoid the superimposition of a secondary process (metabolic acidosis, aspiration, etc.) takes on special importance.

Functional Anatomy of the Respiratory Muscles

In healthy individuals, quiet tidal breathing is accomplished by active inhalation and passive deflation. The inspiratory muscle category is composed of the diaphragm (responsible for the major portion of ventilation at all but extreme work rates) and the accessory group, primarily the external and parasternal intercostals, scalenes, and strap muscles of the neck. Normally, expiratory muscle activity is required for expulsive efforts (cough, sneeze, defecation, etc.), for high levels of ventilation (>15 L/min), and for breathing against a significant resistive load (as during an exacerbation of asthma or COPD). An increased workload and impaired pump function often coexist in patients presenting with ventilatory failure. Because maintenance of alveolar ventilation requires a pressure gradient sufficient to overcome resistive and elastic forces, any condition that interferes with the ability to generate negative intrathoracic pressure (e.g., weakness, abnormal thoracic configuration, or muscular incoordination) will stress the system and may lead to ventilatory failure, with or without increased force requirement or derangement of gas-exchanging efficiency.

Components of Pump Efficiency

Muscular Strength Muscular strength depends on the bulk of the muscle, its contractility, the integrity of its innervation, and its loading conditions.

Advanced age and poor nutrition are associated **11** with reduced skeletal muscle mass. Contractility is influenced by the muscle's chemical environment. Derangements of Ca^{2+}, Mg^{2+}, PO_4^{3-}, K^+, CO_2, pH, and perhaps Fe^{2+} are particularly important to correct. The shorter the inspiratory muscle fiber and the greater its velocity of shortening, the less forceful will be the contraction for any specified level of neural stimulation. The greater the "afterload" faced by the muscle (because of resistive or elastic loading), the less effectively will the muscle contraction perform useful external work. Achieving adequate intravascular volume, ensuring optimal cardiac function, and normalizing hemoglobin concentration help to maintain ample O_2 delivery to these metabolically active tissues.

Thoracic Configuration However well individual muscle fibers contract, geometric alignment determines how effectively the force generated accomplishes ventilation. When totally flattened, for example, the diaphragm develops tension that tends to pull the ribs inward in an *expiratory* rather than inspiratory action (see Fig. 25-4). Partially for this reason, acute hyperinflation represents an important impediment to effective ventilation.

Muscular Coordination In generating negative intrathoracic pressure, the inspiratory muscles normally contract synchronously to either displace volume directly or to stabilize the rib cage or abdomen so that the inspiratory actions of complementary muscles work effectively together and are not offset by expiratory activity. Both a stable chest wall and coordinated muscular activity are essential to pump efficiency.

Common Disorders of the Respiratory Pump

Chest Wall Configuration

Obesity and Ascites Massive obesity and ascites are common disorders of chest wall configuration. The stiff chest wall and abdomen afterload the muscles of inspiration. However, although the diaphragm must push against the abdominal contents, impairing diaphragmatic descent, the abdomen can provide a fulcrum around which the diaphragm can flare the rib cage outward, expanding its volume. More extensive rib cage displacement may compensate for the reduced caudal displacement of the diaphragm, so quiet breathing is little compromised. Under the stress of increased ventilation requirements, however, higher tidal volumes are needed, and the elastic work of breathing may increase dramatically. With the abdominal contents thrusting against the diaphragm, the equilibrium position of the chest wall is displaced to a lower volume, so the functional residual capacity (FRC) tends to fall. In comparison to patients without chest wall abnormality, higher levels of PEEP are needed to produce the physiologically effective changes in lung volume that influence oxygenation. This is especially true in the supine position, in which abdominal forces push the underside of the diaphragm cephalad. Airway calibers are reduced commensurately as FRC falls and resistance to breathing increases. Moreover, the tendencies for hypoxemia and positional desaturation are increased because the patient often tends to breathe below the "closing volume" of the lung. In managing the obese, pregnant, or ascitic patient, special attention must be paid to maintaining positions—usually upright—that minimize abdominal pressure and to supplementing inspired O_2 when necessary.

Pleural Effusion and Pneumothorax   Although massive pleural effusion and pneumothorax are not usually considered problems of chest wall configuration, in fact, both can cause dyspnea by this mechanism (see Chapter 8). For example, either may flatten or invert the ipsilateral diaphragm and drive the accessory inspiratory muscles to a hyperinflated position. In this configuration, the individual muscle fibers foreshorten, and the geometry does not permit efficient inspiratory motion. Thus, a major component of the relief of dyspnea after thoracentesis or chest tube placement relates to the recovery of an effective mechanical advantage for the diaphragm. Interestingly, large pleural effusions may not impair the expandability of the lung itself provided that PEEP is applied and the surrounding chest wall (muscle, rib, and cutaneous tissue) is not stiff (see Chapter 8).

Flail Chest   Large or painful, flail segments may dissipate a portion of the force developed by the intact ventilatory musculature or lead to "splinting," secretion retention, hypoxemia, and ineffective ventilation. Reducing minute ventilation requirements, effective bronchial hygiene, adequate analgesia, restoring FRC, and providing ventilatory support form the cornerstones of treatment until the chest wall stabilizes and the pain recedes.

Kyphoscoliosis   Kyphoscoliosis exemplifies a category of distorts of the other component of the thoracic shell, the rib cage. This deforming disorder seriously impairs inspiratory capacity, preventing the deep breaths needed for exertion or coughing. In distinction from parenchymal restrictive diseases like pulmonary fibrosis, FRC and diffusing capacity tend to be comparatively well preserved. Initially, the problem is purely one of configuration, but the inability to ventilate and clear secretions effectively can lead to reduced lung compliance, bronchiectasis, and hypoxemia later in the course. Difficulty increases in proportion to the bony deformity. In scoliosis, for example, serious respiratory problems attributable solely to its mechanical disadvantage are seldom evident until angulation exceeds 100 degree. Muscles that would ordinarily have an inspiratory action can be placed into a neutral or expiratory alignment by bony distortion. In addition, the chest cage becomes difficult to deform with tidal breathing efforts. Severe hypoxemia and cor pulmonale are frequent late complications. For such patients, maintaining the airway free of retained secretions and infection, treatment of hypoxemia, and ensuring appropriate electrolyte balance and nutrition are keys to effective management.

Muscular Strength and Coordination   Many disorders of neuromuscular dysfunction have coexisting elements of secretion retention, atelectasis, aspiration of oral or gastric contents, and sleep-disordered breathing. Nutritional support, assiduous bronchial hygiene, minimization of the breathing workload, avoidance of electrolyte imbalance and consciousness-suppressing drugs, and liberal use of positive airway pressure and ventilation (administered noninvasively, if possible) are general management principles that are applicable across the spectrum of diseases that comprise this category.

Diaphragmatic paralysis and quadriplegia provide complementary but opposing examples of regional muscular weakness. Both disorders present inherent problems of impaired muscular coordination as well as loss of effective muscle bulk and strength.

Diaphragm   Certain events and acute problems observed in the ICU may result in diaphragmatic dysfunction: pneumonia, surgery, radiation, trauma, and anesthetic complications provide common examples. A paralyzed diaphragm tends to rise rather than fall during the inspiratory half-cycle. Acting as a passive membrane, it then moves in accordance with the transmural pressure gradient across it. As intra-abdominal pressure rises and intrathoracic pressure falls, the diaphragm tends to ascend into the chest. In the chronic setting, unilateral diaphragmatic paralysis only modestly impairs ventilatory capability, with vital capacity falling approximately 20% to 30% from its normal value. Quiet tidal breathing is little affected, and many such patients remain relatively asymptomatic throughout life. Symptoms may only surface under periods of stress or in the presence of a comorbid problem. Although causes of permanent unilateral paralysis can sometimes be identified (e.g., tumor, infection, radiation, or surgery), the origin of most remains unknown.

By contrast, bilateral diaphragmatic paralysis is a devastating illness that usually is idiopathic. These patients must take up the entire ventilatory burden using the accessory muscles. When upright, the expiratory muscles can contract to drive the diaphragm high into the chest at end-exhalation. When expiratory tone is released, the falling abdominal pressure sucks the diaphragm caudally, thus aiding inspiration. In the supine position, this gravity-dependent mechanism cannot work, and the abdomen moves paradoxically inward during inspiration. Therefore, these patients experience extreme orthopnea and often present with sleep disturbances and headache related to nocturnal CO_2 accumulation. Vital capacity shows significant positional variation, falling by more than 30% in the transition from the upright to supine orientation. Many such patients can sustain ventilation for many hours when upright but need ventilatory support (invasively or noninvasively) for rest periods, especially during sleep. Although a positive-pressure ventilator is used most commonly for this purpose (with or without airway intubation), a negative-pressure body suit also can be used, without the need for tracheostomy or facial mask. Poor regional ventilation in dependent areas, frequently combined with the need for tracheostomy, causes problems with atelectasis, pneumonitis, and bronchiectasis in basilar regions. Because diaphragmatic function seldom returns, treatment is supportive. Therapy centers on maintaining optimal secretion clearance, keeping the lungs free of infection, and optimizing nutrition.

Skeletal Muscle Weakness and Paralysis   The severity of ventilatory problems relating to spinal cord injury relates to the level of the lesion and, to some extent, to the time elapsed since the injury occurred. Ventilatory effectiveness can improve significantly in the weeks after the injury, as neural function improves, muscle tone alters the compliance of the chest wall, and any functional accessory muscles strengthen. In the usual forms of quadriplegia (levels at or below C5), diaphragmatic

function is well preserved. Unfortunately, some accessory inspiratory muscles may be compromised, and a variable fraction of expiratory power is routinely lost. Quadriplegic patients and those with acute myopathy often maintain excellent ventilation during quiet breathing but have little or no reserve. Expulsive activity may be severely impaired. For some patients, any pneumonia is potentially life threatening; secretions cannot be raised, and the ventilatory requirement is increased. Maintenance of an upright position and the use of PEEP to avert atelectasis are often helpful. Various techniques and devices are available to assist coughing, including manual compression, chest vibration, airway oscillation, and cough amplifiers that use a biphasic (positive–negative) pressure applied at the airway opening.

Paradoxically, some quadriplegic patients breathe more easily in the recumbent position than when upright. Presumably, the enhanced diaphragmatic curvature of the supine position, as well as the larger area of apposition of the diaphragm to the lower rib cage, improves mechanical efficiency. Like diaphragmatic paralysis, the focus should center on reducing the ventilatory requirement and on keeping the lungs free of infection. For patients who do not have an effective cough, secretion retention and mucus plugging are continual risks. Vital measures are maintenance of optimal nutrition, prevention of aspiration, optimized bowel motility, prevention of abdominal distention, and prophylactic respiratory therapy, supplemented by assisted coughing (when feasible, indicated, and not contraindicated by abdominal distention, esophageal incompetence, severe thoracic deformity, spinal fracture, etc.). When some expiratory force can be generated (thoracic cord interruptions), abdominal compression may assist the coughing effort by splinting the abdomen and allowing intrathoracic pressure to build. Marginal patients often benefit from noninvasive nocturnal ventilatory support. Severely compromised patients who cannot effectively clear the airway with noninvasive aids or who have other airway, lung, or chest wall diseases will require tracheostomy and conventional ventilation.

■ SUGGESTED READINGS

Barnes PJ. Chronic obstructive pulmonary disease. *N Engl J Med*. 2000; 343(4):269–280.

Cairns CB. Acute asthma exacerbations: Phenotypes of management. *Clin Chest Med*. 2006;27:99–108.

Hanania NA, Shara F, Khaneh A. Update on the pharmacologic therapy of chronic obstructive pulmonary disease. *Clin Chest Med*. 2007;28: 589–607.

Hurst JR, Wedzicha JA. Chronic obstructive pulmonary disease: The clinical management of an acute exacerbation. *Postgrad Med J.* 2004;80(947):497–505.

Koh Y. Ventilatory management in patients with chronic airflow obstruction. *Crit Care Clin.* 2007;23:169–181.

McCrory DC, Broun C, Gelfand SE, et al. Management of acute exacerbations of COPD: A summary and appraisal of published evidence. *Chest.* 2001;119(4):1190–1209.

National Heart, Lung, and Blood Institute/World Health Organization. The GOLD Workshop Panel. *Global Strategy for the Diagnosis, Management,* *and Prevention of Chronic Obstructive Pulmonary Disease: NHLBI/WHO Workshop Report.* Bethesda, MD: National Heart, Lung, and Blood Institute. 2001. NIH Publication No. 2701.

Phipps P, Garrard CS. Acute severe asthma in the intensive care unit. *Thorax.* 2003;58(1):81–88.

Rodrigo GJ, Rodrigo C, Hall JB. Acute asthma in adults: A review. *Chest.* 2004;125(3):1081–1102.

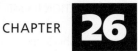

ICU Infections

■ SUSPECTING INFECTION

Infection may be suspected on the basis of localizing signs (e.g., swelling, erythema, wound discharge) or localizing symptoms (e.g., pain, dyspnea, cough) but most commonly is considered because of the presence of fever or leukocytosis. Fever afflicts at least half of all patients during their stay in the intensive care unit (ICU) and often is an important clue to the presence of infection. The magnitude and pattern of fever, typically defined as a temperature exceeding 101°F (38°C) to 101.4°F (38.5°C), are often accorded undue significance; fever characteristics actually have little diagnostic value. It is essential to recognize that not all fever is due to infection. Several diseases as deadly as disseminated infection can induce fever. Prominent among them are heat stroke, neuroleptic malignant syndrome, and the endocrine disorders of hyperthyroidism, adrenal insufficiency, and pheochromocytoma. Noninfectious causes of febrile syndromes are discussed in detail in Chapter 28.

For some patients, diagnosis of infection is difficult because both localizing and generalized signs are unimpressive. Patients infected with human immunodeficiency virus (HIV) often have minimal tissue inflammation when infected. Elderly patients and patients with hypothyroidism and renal failure often have reduced fever responses compared to younger patients. Both neutropenia and immunosuppressive drug therapy tend to reduce the local response to infection, making erythema, pain, swelling, and pus formation less likely.

■ COMMON SCENARIOS

Three categories account for most infections seen in the ICU: primary bacterial infections that prompt admission (e.g., pneumonia, urinary tract infection [UTI], meningitis); nosocomial infections (e.g., catheter-related sepsis, nosocomial pneumonia); and infections of the immune-compromised host. The broad topic of infection cannot be addressed comprehensively in a single chapter of reasonable length; therefore, the discussion that follows focuses on the most common and serious infections occurring in the ICU. Patient characteristics profoundly influence the likely site of infection and the likely organisms responsible. The selection of antimicrobials must take allergies and organ dysfunctions into account. Furthermore, individual hospitals have different spectra of bacteria causing a particular clinical syndrome, and even within a single hospital antibiotic susceptibility can vary widely among units. Therefore, practitioners must have a thorough knowledge of the patient being treated, the likely pathogens, and the antimicrobial susceptibility pattern of the hospital in which they practice.

Antimicrobial options are constantly evolving. In recent years, for example, entirely new antibiotic categories have been exploited and better-tolerated formulations of long-established drugs have been commercially released. In the former category are drugs directed at organisms resistant to most standard agents, such as linezolid, daptomycin, and quinupristin–dalfopristin for methicillin-resistant *Staphylococcus aureus* (MRSA) and vancomycin-resistant *Enterococcus*. Others include new antifungal agents, such as caspofungin for invasive *Aspergillus* and *Candida* infections. Nephrotoxicity of traditional amphotericin desoxycholate has been attenuated by its lipid complex, cholesteryl complex, and liposomal variants. Voriconazole, a modified triazole, now offers a well-tolerated alternative to amphotericin that can be given orally as well as parenterally in the treatment of aspergillosis. Modifications within well-established antimicrobial categories have extended their spectra and/or limited their side effects. For example, fluoroquinolones (e.g., levofloxacin, gatifloxacin, and moxifloxacin) offer potent competition to traditional drugs in the treatment of typical and atypical pneumonia. Although allergic sensitivity, renal insufficiency, hepatic dysfunction, bleeding tendency, or other vital organ dysfunction may restrict the options, almost always, there is more than one potentially effective antimicrobial combination for any given infection. Suggestions that follow for antibiotic therapy are based on the most common pathogens and their usual susceptibility patterns while considering the frequency and severity of side effects and ease and cost of administration. "Broad-spectrum" effectiveness is both a luxury and a liability, as the desire to cover a large number of potential pathogens comes at a high price. Indiscriminate use of broad-spectrum antibiotics is rapidly producing multidrug-resistant bacteria. MRSA and penicillin-resistant *Pneumococcus* are now pandemic. New and menacing pathogens such as multiresistant *Enterococcus* and *Acinetobacter* are recognized with increasing frequency, and unless patterns of antibiotic use

change, it is likely such infections will grow in importance. Antibiotics are the only class of drugs that, when misused, can injure not only the patient being treated but nearby patients and patients admitted to the ICU in the future. For example, the routine use of vancomycin to treat diarrhea or to cover for Gram-positive pathogens may inadvertently "select out" organisms resistant to this useful drug. These highly resistant organisms then lurk in the ICU, ready to infect subsequent patients.

■ URINARY TRACT INFECTIONS

Pathogenesis

The urinary tract is the most common site of ICU infection, accounting for almost 40% of all infections. Although UTIs usually are inconsequential, the mortality rate for a bacteremic UTI approaches 30%. Risk factors for UTI include presence of a urinary catheter, female gender, diabetes, and advanced age. Colonization of urinary catheters occurs at a rate of about 5% to 10% per day, and most ICU-acquired UTIs occur in such colonized patients. Presumably, the colonized catheter permits retrograde passage of pathogenic bacteria into the bladder where they proliferate. Urinary catheter composition (Teflon rather than rubber) may reduce the infective hazard; however, there is no evidence that routine changing of the catheter or external application of antibiotic ointment decreases risk. Keys to preventing nosocomial UTI are sterile catheter insertion, early catheter removal, and maintaining a closed drainage system.

Diagnosis

The diagnosis of UTI is all but certain when greater than 10^5 bacteria/mL are isolated from culture of freshly collected urine. This level of bacteriuria correlates well with the presence of more than one organism per high-power field of unspun urine. Unfortunately, fewer bacteria do not exclude the presence of infection. True infections have been documented with colony counts as low as 10^2/mL. *Escherichia coli,* the most common bacterial isolate, occurs in about 30% of UTIs. *Enterococcus* and *Pseudomonas* are each recovered about 15% of the time in the ICU population. *Klebsiella* and *Proteus* species represent less-common isolates. Contrary to previous teaching, in many cases, pure cultures of *Staphylococcus epidermidis* represent infection, not contamination. In the absence of frank pyuria or quantitative culture data, it is difficult to differentiate colonization from infection in critically ill patients with indwelling catheters. In the tenuous patient with bacteriuria, it is probably best to err on the side of brief, organism-directed antibiotic therapy. For more resilient patients in the ICU, treatment of asymptomatic bacteriuria may be deferred safely.

Recovery of *Candida* species in urine is a common event. The choice of therapy for isolated candiduria should be based on a clinical judgment regarding whether the patient is "colonized" or "infected." Unfortunately, there are few reliable signs to distinguish these conditions. A clinical picture of sepsis, with recovery of *Candida* from blood cultures as well as urine, suggests disseminated infection that should be treated with intravenous antifungals such as amphotericin B, fluconazole, or caspofungin. Conversely, finding small numbers of yeast in an asymptomatic patient with an indwelling urinary catheter rarely requires systemic treatment (except expedited removal of the catheter). The most difficult situation occurs when large numbers of yeast or clumps of hyphal forms are found in the urine of an asymptomatic patient or a patient with only modest fever. Although suggestive of invasive infection, such patients usually respond promptly to fluconazole (oral or intravenous), especially if the urinary catheter can be removed. Without evidence of infection elsewhere, parenteral amphotericin B probably should be reserved for immunocompromised patients or those with limited physiologic reserves. Bladder irrigation with amphotericin B is time consuming, expensive, of uncertain benefit, and confounding to accurate assessment of urine output. Fluconazole has all but eliminated bladder irrigation.

Pyocystis, an invasive infection of the bladder wall, may complicate oliguria or anuria, especially in patients requiring hemodialysis. In this setting, reduced urine flow allows bacteria to proliferate to massive numbers within the bladder. For oliguric patients with obscure fever, the bladder should be catheterized and the urine sediment should be examined. In the appropriate setting, murky, turbid, culture-positive urine establishes the diagnosis.

Treatment

The aggressiveness of therapy should parallel the clinical severity of the acute syndrome and the underlying illness. As a rule, presumed UTIs should be treated aggressively because patients in the ICU often have impaired immunity (diabetes, HIV infection, immunosuppressive therapy); numerous indwelling devices (e.g., vascular catheters, prosthetic heart valves, pacemakers); and marginal physiologic reserves. The treatment of UTI includes the promotion of urine flow and drainage, removal of urinary catheters (when feasible), and antibiotic therapy. Not all patients with bacteriuria require prolonged courses of expensive, broad-spectrum, intravenous antibiotics. Otherwise stable immunocompetent patients can be treated successfully using enteral antibiotics (e.g., ampicillin, trimethoprim-sulfamethoxazole, quinolones). Oral therapy is not appropriate for septic patients or patients with obstructive uropathy or a focal complication (e.g., renal abscess). The need for two drug coverage of pseudomonal infections in non-immunocompromised patients is uncertain, but two drugs effective against *Pseudomonas* should be given to patients with abnormal immunity. (These include intravenous aminoglycosides and antipseudomonal penicillins, fluoroquinolones, or third-generation cephalosporins.) If *Enterococcus* or *Staphylococcus* is deemed likely (based on the urine Gram stain or culture), vancomycin probably should be first-line therapy. Rarely, when the infection is life threatening and the possibility of vancomycin resistance is high, linezolid is an appropriate choice. Urine concentrations of renally excreted antibiotics often are dramatically higher than those used in sensitivity testing; therefore, UTIs often can be cured using an antibiotic to which the bacteria are found to be "resistant" in vitro. Because drainage bags provide important pathogen reservoirs, manipulations of the closed drainage system should be undertaken only when necessary and conducted with sterile technique. Furthermore, drainage bags should not be raised above the level of the bladder, as often occurs during patient transport. Doing so, even briefly, produces urinary stasis and retrograde flow of potentially highly contaminated urine.

■ PNEUMONIA

Pathogenesis

Pneumonia-producing organisms usually enter the lower respiratory tract in aspirated upper airway secretions. Hematogenous seeding is a much less-common mechanism. Unless the inoculum is very large, glottic closure, cough, and mucociliary clearance normally provide an effective mechanical defense (Table 26-1). Even when mechanical barriers fail, infection usually is averted by

TABLE 26-1 CONDITIONS PROMOTING LUNG INOCULATION

Aspiration
   Depressed consciousness
   Swallowing disorders
   Nasogastric and tracheal tubes

Hematogenous
   Bacteremia

Infected aerosol
   Contaminated ventilator tubing and humidifiers

effective cellular (neutrophil and macrophage) and humoral immunity (antibody secretion). Unfortunately, both mechanical and immune defenses are jeopardized commonly in critically ill patients, even in those without a recognizable immune deficiency. Common conditions that allow proliferation of organisms leading to pneumonia are listed in Table 26-2. The organism causing pneumonia is highly dependent on where the infection was acquired and on individual patient characteristics.

Diagnosis

In the community, a patient with acute onset of fever, dyspnea, chest discomfort, and cough productive of purulent sputum is likely to be suffering from bacterial pneumonia. Leukocytosis with a predominance of neutrophils and distinct (new) infiltrate(s) on chest radiograph are strong supporting data. Sputum that demonstrates an

TABLE 26-2 CONDITIONS ALLOWING PROLIFERATION OF MICROORGANISMS IN LUNG

Impaired immunity
Parenchymal necrosis
Malnutrition
Steroids/cytotoxic drugs
Alcohol
Diabetes
Secretion retention
Atelectasis
Smoking
Obstructive lung disease
Neuromuscular weakness
Cytotoxic drugs
Acute respiratory distress syndrome
Viral infections

overwhelming predominance of neutrophils, intracellular organisms, and the predominance of a single morphologic bacterial form further strengthens the case. Finally, the diagnosis is established unequivocally by recovering the same organism from blood and sputum or pleural fluid cultures. The presentation is not always so classic, even with community-acquired pneumonia: fever may be mild, infiltrates may be subtle, and self-medication with antibiotics often obscures a bacteriologic diagnosis.

In the ICU, making a correct clinical diagnosis of pneumonia can be difficult for several reasons. Fever and leukocytosis are nonspecific, and patients often have several potential nonpulmonary sites to explain these findings. In addition, the radiographic infiltrates that suggest pneumonia are mimicked by atelectasis, aspiration pneumonitis, pulmonary embolism and infarction, pleural effusion, and pulmonary edema. Computed tomography (CT) sharpens discrimination but may not settle the issue. Finally, widespread use of antibiotics inhibits the ability to recover a single pathogenic organism, and even when sputum cultures are positive, small numbers of colonizing bacteria are usually recovered.

Causative Organism

The organisms causing pneumonia differ dramatically, depending on site of acquisition—community versus hospital. Common causes of community-acquired pneumonia and their clinical associations are shown in Table 26-3. In the community, streptococci, especially *Pneumococcus* and, *Haemophilus influenzae, Mycoplasma,* and viruses are the most common pathogens in otherwise "healthy" adults. Many underlying conditions vary this spectrum, however. In addition to the organisms listed, patients with alcoholism, diabetes, or heart failure are predisposed to infection with *Klebsiella, Legionella,* enteric Gram-negative rods, and *Staphylococcus.* When aspiration is likely (e.g., alcoholism, drug abuse, esophageal disorders), *Bacteroides* and other anaerobes are more prevalent. *S. aureus* frequently is recovered from patients with "postinfluenza" pneumonia, and *Pseudomonas* species and *Staphylococcus* are common etiologic organisms among patients with cystic fibrosis. In fact, staphylococcal disease including MRSA is now frequently encountered in patients with severe community-acquired pneumonia. Pneumonia acquired in chronic nursing care facilities or within 3 weeks of hospital discharge is likely to be caused by organisms usually recovered in hospital-acquired infections.

For pneumonias that develop after the first few days in the ICU, a different, hospital-specific spectrum predominates. Such infections are frequently polymicrobial. Gram-negative rods (*Pseudomonas aeruginosa, Klebsiella* species, *Enterobacter* species, *Actinetobacter* species, *E. coli, Proteus,* and *Serratia*) cause approximately 50% of all ICU pneumonias. Which Gram-negative organism predominates at a given hospital has a great deal to do with antibiotic pressure placed on the environment. *Acinetobacter,* for example, represents a significant threat in some hospitals, but by no means all. Interestingly, *Acinetobacter* species infections have been exceedingly common among servicemen injured in Iraq. *S. aureus* causes another 10% to 20% of infections and its incidence appears to be rising. The predominance of Gram-negative rods and *Staphylococcus* seen in the hospitalized patient is explained partially by the rapid rate at which the oropharynx of the critically ill patient becomes colonized. Almost all critically ill patients are colonized with

nonnative Gram-negative bacteria (many of which are antibiotic resistant) by the third hospital day.

All too often, a specific pathogen cannot be identified, despite good sampling methods and symptoms compatible with acute pneumonia. Polymicrobial causation mixed aerobic/anaerobic infection, *Mycoplasma, Chlamydia, Legionella,* and viral agents become more likely candidates under these conditions. Fungal pneumonia (*Candida/Torulopsis* species, *Aspergillus,* or *Mucor*) must be considered in the neutropenic or severely debilitated patient (<500 neutrophils/mm^3) but it occurs only rarely in the immunocompetent patient. When lung involvement occurs in the immunocompetent patient, it usually is the result of hematogenous seeding with *Candida* in a predisposed host. For some patients with chronic destructive lung diseases (e.g., chronic obstructive pulmonary disease [COPD], healed cavitary tuberculosis), *Aspergillus* can produce a primary invasive pneumonia.

Patients infected with HIV present a unique set of problems. When the CD4 T cell counts are normal, patients infected with HIV are susceptible to the same organisms as any other adult in the risk categories outlined in Table 26-3. As the CD4

TABLE 26-3 CLINICAL ASSOCIATIONS IN COMMUNITY-ACQUIRED PNEUMONIA

PATIENT CHARACTERISTICS	LIKELY ORGANISMS
Healthy young adult	*S. pneumoniae, Mycoplasma,* viruses, *Chlamydia*
Healthy adult	*S. pneumoniae, H. influenzae, Mycoplasma*

Prone to aspiration
  Stroke
  Esophageal disease
  Alcoholism
  Seizures
  Alcohol abuse
  Recent dental work
	S. pneumoniae, Bacteroides, oral anaerobes

Chronically ill
  Diabetes
  COPD
  Alcoholism
  Heart failure
  Low-dose corticosteroids
	All organisms listed for healthy adult plus *Klebsiella* spp., enteric Gram-negatives, *Legionella, S. aureus, Branhamella* spp.

Postinfluenza	*S. pneumoniae, S. aureus, H. influenzae*
Cystic fibrosis	*S. aureus, Pseudomonas* spp.
AIDS or HIV with CD4 < 200	*P. carinii, S. pneumoniae, H. influenzae, M. tuberculosis,* fungal infection (geographic predilection)
Neutropenia	All organisms listed for chronically ill plus *Aspergillus, Mucor,* and *Candida*

count declines, and especially as it falls below 200 cells/mm^3, the spectrum of infecting organisms broadens. Although routine bacterial pathogens still predominate, *Pneumocystis carinii (jiroveci)*, *Mycobacterium tuberculosis*, atypical mycobacteria, and fungal infections become more likely. There is a rough correlation between the CD4 count and the infecting organism, but the linkage is not sufficiently strong to forgo detailed evaluation for presumptive diagnosis. Potential pathogens also are influenced by the prior use of prophylactic therapy. Oral trimethoprim-sulfamethoxazole prophylaxis, for example, has dramatically reduced the incidence of *Pneumocystis* and *Toxoplasmosis* infections.

Regardless of the patient substrate, the choice of initial therapy for a bacterial pneumonia is always accompanied by some uncertainty, even in the presence of a Gram stain "typical" of a specific organism. Historical features can help immensely in sorting through the diagnostic possibilities. For example, the sudden onset of chills, pleurisy, rigors, and high temperature are characteristic features for community-acquired *Pneumococcus* in a young adult. On the other hand, these findings may be inconspicuous in an older person, in whom confusion or stupor often predominate. A history of seizures, drug abuse, alcoholism, or swallowing disorder focuses attention on aspiration. Recent travel history, occupational or recreational exposure, and concurrent family illnesses can help diagnose an unusual organism (Table 26-4). In the absence of intrinsic cardiac conduction abnormality or intense β-blockade, a pulse rate that fails to rise in proportion to fever (pulse–temperature dissociation) suggests an "intracellular pathogen" such as *Legionella, Rickettsia, Mycoplasma,* Q fever, psittacosis, virus, or tularemia. *Mycoplasma* often has accompanying pharyngitis, myringitis, or conjunctivitis. Contrary to popular teaching, extrapulmonary symptoms (diarrhea, central nervous system disease) are no more common in Legionnaires disease than in other bacterial pneumonia.

Unlike community-acquired pneumonia, nosocomial pneumonia offers few historical clues to diagnosis. Occasionally, however, a skin rash, gingival disease, or purulent sinus drainage helps narrow the possibilities. Numerous classic radiographic features have been described, including lobar consolidation without air bronchograms (central obstruction), bulging fissures (*Klebsiella*), infiltrate with ipsilateral hilar adenopathy (histoplasmosis,

TABLE 26-4 CLUES TO UNUSUAL CAUSES OF PNEUMONIA

DIAGNOSIS	HISTORICAL CLUE
Histoplasmosis	Excavation, bird exposure, Ohio Valley travel
Coccidiomycosis	Travel to southwestern United States, California
Tularemia	Tick bite or exposure to skinned animals
Brucellosis	Slaughterhouse work
Psittacosis	Exposure to pet birds
Q fever	Sheep contact
Varicella	Family exposure
Measles	Family exposure
Respiratory syncytial virus	Family exposure
Blastomycosis	Hunting, deep woods exposure
Ehrlichiosis	Tick bite

tularemia, tuberculosis), widespread cavitation (*Staphylococcus, Aspergillus*), and sequential progression to multilobar involvement (*Legionella*). These findings are not sufficiently consistent, however, to be of real value in confirming the diagnosis.

Diagnostic techniques

Although the history provides clues to the etiologic organism, laboratory studies are the cornerstone of the workup. Leukopenia often results from overwhelming infections, particularly those that are due to *Staphylococcus, Pneumococcus,* or Gram-negative organisms. A differential count that is not significantly left-shifted suggests the possibility of virus, *Mycoplasma,* or *Legionella.* Cultures of blood and pleural fluid (when present) must be obtained, and if positive, they are the most convincing evidence of a causative organism. Unfortunately, such specimens are usually nondiagnostic, even in seriously ill patients, and sampling of pulmonary secretions becomes the primary diagnostic modality.

The aggressiveness of the diagnostic evaluation should parallel the severity of the illness. In an otherwise healthy young person with a lobar pneumonia and good oxygenation, empiric therapy or treatment based on Gram stain alone is acceptable. For the septic, profoundly hypoxemic or immunocompromised patient, however, a more systematic evaluation is often prudent. When performed correctly, stain and culture of pulmonary secretions or alveolar lavage fluid remain the most likely techniques to yield a diagnosis. For patients with severe community-acquired pneumonia, high-quality sputum often is obtained immediately after endotracheal intubation because forceful coughing and suctioning at this time often yield copious lung secretions not yet contaminated by ICU colonization. Expectorated sputum is appropriate for analysis and culture only if there is a high ratio of inflammatory to epithelial cells. Apart from the Gram stain, direct immunofluorescent antibody staining for *Legionella* and tuberculosis are other useful methods for processing the expectorated sample that can yield an immediate, but presumptive, diagnosis. Inhalation of a hypertonic aerosol, particularly if given via an ultrasonic nebulizer, can stimulate a productive cough in patients otherwise unable to expectorate. When adequate sputum is not expectorated, nasotracheal suctioning can be helpful. Transtracheal aspiration has been all but abandoned with wide availability of fiberoptic bronchoscopy.

Properly performed on well-selected patients, fiberoptic bronchoscopy is a valuable technique for evaluation of pneumonic infection. In general, bronchoscopic procedures should be reserved for those who are seriously ill, immunocompromised, or unresponsive to conventional therapy. The safety and ease of bronchoscopy are facilitated by the presence of an endotracheal tube. When a decision is made to perform bronchoscopy, bronchoalveolar lavage and protected brush sampling from the involved region are both reasonable alternatives. Of these, lavage methodology is perhaps more popular, as it is relatively easier, and the protected brush seldom conflicts with or adds to its accuracy. If the lavage specimen yields a predominance of polymorphonuclear leukocytes and more than 10^3 to 10^4 organisms/mL are isolated, infection with the recovered organism is likely. Fewer bacteria suggest an active infection but also may be seen with a partially treated bacterial pneumonia. Blind suctioning, conducted with or without lavage through a wedged catheter ("mini-BAL"), can be performed proficiently by respiratory therapists or trained nurses. In the setting of diffuse pneumonia, this is a low-cost and generally effective sampling option. Only bronchoscopy, however, offers the directed sampling so often necessary.

Performing transbronchial biopsies to obtain tissue for histologic examination and/or culture is more hazardous in mechanically ventilated patients. Moreover, empirically chosen antibiotics are usually effective in addressing potential pathogens in patients who are immune competent. Although not performed commonly because of the risk of pneumothorax, transbronchial biopsy may be attempted when tissue recovery is essential, oxygenation can be well maintained, and coagulopathy is not present. In this setting, the only diagnostic alternatives are open or thoracoscopic lung biopsy. (The latter may not be feasible because of altered anatomy, high ventilation requirements, or refractory hypoxemia.) The risk of developing a pneumothorax while on the mechanical ventilator must be balanced against the potential yield and the clinician's ability to promptly recognize and evacuate the air leak. (Note that the incidence of pneumothorax is 100% after open lung biopsy.) In addition, there are situations in which a diagnosis can be made only by tissue biopsy. Open lung biopsy is rarely necessary for patients with intact host defenses, and the value in even compromised hosts is arguable. Transthoracic needle aspiration often yields an adequate specimen but exposes the patient to attendant risks of pneumothorax and bleeding.

The optimal diagnostic evaluation of a pneumonic process for patients infected with HIV continues to evolve. For patients with normal or minimally reduced CD4 counts, mild to moderate illness, and a history and examination compatible with acute bacterial pneumonia, empiric antibacterial therapy after obtaining cultures is reasonable. For patients with reduced CD4 counts, progressive dyspnea, nonproductive cough, elevated lactic dehydrogenase (LDH), and a radiograph with an interstitial or ground glass pattern, empiric therapy for *Pneumocystis* and close observation may be reasonable. (This is especially true in the absence of *Pneumocystis* prophylaxis.) For patients with low CD4 counts, severe hypoxemia, uncharacteristic chest X-ray infiltrates, or an unusual exposure history, early bronchoscopy is the most prudent option. When bronchoscopy is performed, bronchoalveolar lavage alone is often not sufficient; fungal infections, tuberculosis, and even *Pneumocystis* are missed at an unacceptable rate without transbronchial biopsy. Because of the wide variety of potential radiographic presentations of tuberculosis, it probably is wise for all patients with HIV and abnormal chest radiographs to be placed in respiratory isolation until a diagnosis of tuberculosis can be excluded reasonably.

Treatment

Nutritional, fluid, electrolyte, and oxygen support of the patient with bacterial pneumonia are not controversial and are applied universally. The initial choice of antibiotic(s) must be guided not only by the nature of the suspected organism but also by the severity of the illness and underlying patient factors. Thus, although treatment should be directed as specifically as possible for patients who are only moderately ill, the initial therapy of a fragile patient with serious illness should include "broad-spectrum" coverage. It also makes sense to administer the chosen antibiotics as quickly as is feasible. There is little margin for error for critically ill patients with pneumonia; however, one can never treat all potential pathogens. Holes in coverage always exist, and there is almost always more than one acceptable antibiotic combination. The selection of antibiotic therapy represents a calculated bet against the most likely organisms.

Recognizing the imprecision of the following descriptions, otherwise healthy patients with community-acquired pneumonia caused by an unknown organism who exhibit little systemic toxicity can be treated initially with either ampicillin or a macrolide antibiotic, such as azithromycin or clarithromycin. Macrolides, fluoroquinolones, and doxycycline are good options when atypical organisms are suspected. If the same patient appears toxic, reasonable initial treatments include ceftriaxone with or without azithromycin, levofloxacin, or moxifloxacin with ceftriaxone, or an extended-spectrum penicillin. The following caveats apply: If postinfluenza pneumonia (*Staphylococcus*) is suspected or if the patient is from a geographic region with a high prevalence of penicillin-resistant pneumococci, the addition or substitution of vancomycin should be considered. For patients with a high likelihood of aspiration, clindamycin alone or amoxicillin–clavulanate with metronidazole represent good initial choices. Community-acquired pneumonia in a patient with HIV was discussed earlier.

Because a second chance to institute the correct therapy cannot be guaranteed, broad empiric coverage is necessary for the toxic patient with nosocomial pneumonia. Recognizing that many toxic-appearing patients will not have pneumonia documented, nonetheless, coverage in this situation must include enteric Gram-negative rods (including multiply resistant organisms), *Streptococcus* (including penicillin-resistant organisms), and *Staphylococcus* (including MRSA). Important clues to etiology can be gleaned from knowledge of the patient's recent antibiotic treatment, the resident flora of the ICU, the patient's underlying illnesses, and available culture data. Yet, in the majority of instances, therapy must be initiated empirically. Regardless of the appearance of the Gram stain, initial therapy for critically ill patients should include a coverage for multiresistant Gram-negative bacilli, such as an extended-spectrum penicillin plus an aminoglycoside or appropriate fluoroquinolone (e.g., ciprofloxacin), or a third-generation cephalosporin (e.g., ceftazidime) plus an aminoglycoside or fluoroquinolone. For patients predisposed to staphylococcal infection (e.g., recent influenza, neutropenia, institutional prevalence or a suggestive sputum Gram stain), vancomycin represents first-line coverage. A fluroquinolone, macrolide, or doxycycline should be added if there is an "atypical" clinical or radiographic presentation or if fever persists despite usual therapy.

Highly resistant bacteria can be transferred between patients in the ICU, necessitating measures to decrease cross-contamination. Careful hand washing or use of a bactericidal lotion between patient contacts dramatically decreases the risk of nosocomial infection. Use of gloves does not diminish the need for hand washing and it is essential that gloves be changed between patient contacts. Whenever suctioning intubated patients, gloves should be worn on both hands to prevent staff acquisition and transfer of pathogens including herpes viruses.

One pneumonic infection that deserves special discussion is pulmonary tuberculosis. Although patients may be admitted to the ICU with signs and symptoms typical of pulmonary tuberculosis (cavitary apical infiltrates, cachexia, fever), the presentation often is subtler. Tuberculosis in the ICU can take on almost any clinical or radiographic presentation. Cavitary lung disease is only marginally more common than other frequently encountered variants: punctate interstitial infiltrates ("miliary pattern"), lobar pneumonia, "empyema," lung nodule, or diffuse bilateral infiltrates compatible with acute respiratory distress syndrome (ARDS). When the suspicion of tuberculosis is high, respiratory isolation should be instituted as quickly as possible and maintained until firm evidence suggests that the likelihood of contagion is low. (This is accomplished simply by examining two or more good-quality sputum smears for acid-fast organisms.) The implications of missing a case of tuberculosis are enormous: potential death or disability of the infected patient and transmission of infection to the staff and other nearby immunocompromised patients.

Viral Pneumonia

Certain forms of viral pneumonia occur with distressing frequency in severely immunocompromised patients (e.g., CMV in transplant recipients). Although rhinitis, sinusitis, laryngitis, and other familiar manifestations of the "common cold" afflict most persons one or more times per year, viral disease rarely extends to the alveolar level in immunocompetent adults. Yet, certain classes of organism—notably adenovirus, influenza, varicella-zoster, and most recently the coronavirus responsible for severe acute respiratory syndrome (SARS)—can cause devastating illness in exposed individuals who are vulnerable. These diseases generally present with a diffuse bronchopneumonia or ARDS. In addition to general supportive measures applied to patients in respiratory failure, isolation is required and viral antimicrobials should be considered. For example, acyclovir (varicella), rimantadine (influenza), and ribavirin (adenovirus) each offer modest benefit when used in timely fashion in well-selected cases. Perhaps the most important aspect in the management of these pneumonias is to take appropriate measures to prevent the spread of these contagious diseases to health care workers and to the patients they treat. The importance of such precautions was dramatically emphasized in the high incidence of illness among physicians during the SARS outbreak of 2003. When an appropriate vaccine is available for a contagious disease (e.g., influenza), immunization of exposed individuals is prudent.

■ EMPYEMA AND PARAPNEUMONIC EFFUSIONS

Definition

Small amounts of pleural fluid routinely accumulate adjacent to pneumonias and such collections are termed "parapneumonic effusions." Most parapneumonic effusions are intermediate or even transudative in nature (protein <3.5 gm/dL or 50% of the serum level; LDH < 200 U/dL or 60% of the serum level), freely flowing, and self-limited. The term "complicated parapneumonic effusion" has been applied to effusion with loculations, the characteristics of which fall somewhere between an uncomplicated, self-resolving parapneumonic effusion and an empyema. Usually exudative by protein and LDH criteria, leukocyte counts usually are less than 20,000/mm^3, and glucose levels fall between the serum value and 20 mg/dL. The pH of such effusions is commonly regarded as a discriminator of the need for drainage, but its value is often limited. Although it is true that the lower the pH, the more likely a pleural effusion is to have characteristics of an empyema (see following), the pH alone neither makes the diagnosis of an empyema nor dictates a particular course of action. Effusions with a pH less than 7.0 (with a normal arterial pH) are likely to be empyemas and are likely to require tube thoracostomy but such associations are not always valid. An acidic, thin, clear, or slightly cloudy sterile fluid does not necessarily require tube thoracostomy, whereas a thick, viscous, protein- and leukocyte-rich effusion would require thoracostomy, regardless of fluid pH. As a general rule, freely flowing effusions that separate the lung from the chest wall by more than 1 cm on a lateral decubitus film, those that are loculated, and those that do not flow freely, should be sampled and/or drained. The existence of parietal pleural thickening documented on a contrast-enhanced CT scan suggests an intense inflammatory response and probable empyema. The ease and safety of thoracentesis in the ICU may be enhanced by using ultrasound localization.

Empyema is defined as an effusion with organisms detected by Gram stain or as "pus" in the pleural space. Unfortunately, observers vary widely in their definition of "pus." The diagnosis of empyema is not made by laboratory testing, and there are no specific laboratory cutoffs for what constitutes an empyema. Not all empyemas grow bacteria in culture, perhaps because antibiotic therapy has already been administered or the responsible organism is inherently difficult to isolate (e.g., anaerobes). Many empyemas do not have microorganisms visible on Gram stain examination. If infected with bacteria, especially anaerobic bacteria, the odor of an empyema is memorable. Generally accepted characteristics of an empyema are grossly cloudy or opaque appearance and thick, viscous character because of high levels of protein and leukocytes. Certainly, not all infected pleural fluids are thick. Yet, it is the physical characteristics of the fluid that make empyema important to diagnose and treat appropriately. Intrapleural streptokinase can reduce the need for pleural decortication if used early in the clinical course and is often helpful later when tube drainage slows and pockets remain. Intrapleural streptokinase is associated with a low risk of either allergic reaction or systemic coagulopathy. Several types of pleural effusions can mimic an empyema: chylothorax, rheumatoid effusion, tuberculous effusion, and resolving hemothorax all can have the thick, turbid appearance characteristic of empyema.

The clinical presentation of empyema can be subtle. It is not uncommon for elderly or debilitated patients to have empyema as the primary cause of or co-contributor to chronic wasting illness. The diagnosis should be suspected in patients with unresolving or hectic fever and pleural effusions that do not improve with antibiotic therapy. Empyema becomes more likely if the suspect fluid collection is adjacent to pneumonia. Because ICU chest films are often taken supine or semi-upright, the classic "layering" of an effusion can be missed. Although decubitus views and ultrasound enhance the likelihood of finding an effusion, CT currently is the definitive way to confirm a free or loculated fluid collection, especially if small or loculated. For febrile or frankly septic patients, especially those with an underlying pneumonia, the search for an empyema is reasonable.

Therapy

Three basic principles apply to treating empyema: early diagnosis, appropriate antibiotic therapy, and thorough drainage. Of these, drainage is most important. Because there are no radiographic or physical examination features to distinguish an empyema from a routine pleural effusion, thoracentesis is required. Early diagnosis minimizes both early (sepsis and respiratory failure) and late complications (fibrothorax and debilitation). When turbid, viscous, pleural fluid (especially if foul smelling) is obtained at thoracentesis, cultures for aerobic and anaerobic bacteria, tuberculosis, and fungi should be sent. In addition to routine cell counts and chemistry analysis, it is prudent to obtain triglyceride and cholesterol levels to exclude a diagnosis of chylothorax, which can have an empyema-like (turbid) appearance.

(Effusions because of rheumatoid disease also can have a similar appearance.) The pleural fluid should be Gram stained and sputum and blood cultures obtained. Antibiotic coverage should be chosen initially on the basis of the Gram stain and then fine-tuned by culture results. The usual etiologic suspects for pneumonia also cause empyema (*Streptococcus pneumoniae, H. influenzae,* anaerobic mouth flora); however, staphylococci also should be covered.

Prompt insertion of a thoracostomy tube(s) of sufficient caliber to completely drain the pleural space usually is indicated. Several tubes often are necessary when the fluid is multiloculated. Chest CT guidance can be invaluable in guiding placement. Effusions that do not resolve with antibiotics and tube thoracostomy may require exploration and drainage by thoracotomy or video-assisted thorascopy (VATS). Failure to resolve the acute process satisfactorily can require later pleural stripping or decortication. Relatively large collections of fluid that form after appropriate antibiotic therapy is initiated can usually be managed by serial thoracentesis, rather than by indwelling chest tube. The latter becomes necessary, however, if the patient unexpectedly remains toxic appearing or the fluid loculates.

■ INTRAVASCULAR CATHETER-RELATED INFECTIONS

Intravascular catheter-related infections remain one of the top three causes of nosocomial sepsis, however, in ICUs with organized prevention plans, the incidence can be reduced to a very low level. Despite better antibiotics and improved understanding of the mechanisms of catheter-related infections, the case fatality rate for catheter-associated bacteremia remains between 10% and 20%.

Mechanisms

Three basic mechanisms can produce catheter-related infections. (a) Most commonly, catheters are colonized at the skin–air interface, after which bacteria migrate along their outer surfaces. Subcutaneous and eventual intravascular migration results in local infection, or bacteremia if bacterial growth is uncontrolled by host defense or antibiotic therapy. (b) Catheters also can become colonized by exposure to circulating microorganisms introduced into the circulation at a distant site. As foreign bodies, catheters routinely form a "fibrin sheath" around the catheter in the vessel lumen. This microenvironment is a stagnant, fertile environment for pathogen growth. Sources of bacteria or fungi far distant from the catheter can seed these indwelling lines. (c) Only rarely, catheter-related infections are due to the infusion of a contaminated intravenous fluid or drug. Although, in theory, such infusate contamination can occur with any drug, the problem has been reported most often with parenteral nutrition solutions and a first-generation formulation of propofol, an intravenous sedative/anesthetic with a lipid vehicle.

Risk Factors

Characteristics of patients at particular risk for catheter-related infection include diabetes mellitus, immunosuppressive therapy (especially neutropenia), immune deficiency diseases, skin diseases at the insertion site, and presence of sepsis from a distinct source. Physician and environmental factors increasing the risk of intravascular catheter infections include (a) catheter placement under emergency or nonsterile conditions, (b) insertion of multilumen catheters, (c) catheterization of a central vein, (d) prolonged catheterization at a single site, (e) placement by surgical cutdown, and (f) inexperience of the operator. Most catheter infections can be prevented by using sterile technique when inserting, dressing, changing, and reconnecting catheters and by minimizing the frequency of catheter entry. Rigorous sterility during insertion is essential; apart from sterile gloves, wide sterile barriers, surgical gowns, caps, and masks should be used for elective insertions. Chlorhexidine is superior to provodine-iodine solutions for skin preparation. Inexperience with catheter insertion is a powerful risk for infection. (It is not clear whether catheters become contaminated during insertion or if less-experienced operators are prone to produce more tissue trauma during the insertion process.) Multilumen catheters or catheters entered repeatedly (even for antibiotic administration) seem to have a higher infection rate. Neither antibiotic ointment applied at the catheter entry site nor systemic antibiotics convincingly decrease the risk of bacteremia.

There is no clear evidence regarding the relative infective risk of internal jugular and subclavian sites when the duration of catheterization is controlled. Although the risk of pneumothorax is averted, the femoral approach limits leg movement, predisposes to deep venous thrombosis, and places the catheter in a region at risk for contamination by urine and stool, probably explaining the higher infection risk compared to sites above the waist. Central venous catheters are more likely to become infected than peripheral catheters (in part because of duration of catheterization). Peripherally inserted central catheters (PICC), which are usually inserted via a brachial vein, provide intermediate to long-term central access with a somewhat lower risk of infection. Pulmonary artery monitoring catheters and multilumen catheters (risk, 10% to 20%) are more likely to become infected than are single-lumen catheters (risk, approx. 5%). Interestingly, venous catheters are more likely to be infected than arterial catheters. Whether this differential risk is related to the shorter duration of arterial catheterization, the greater flow of blood in the artery, the shorter length of the arterial cannula, or the site of placement (usually in the radial artery), is unclear. Hypertonic fluids (peripheral total parenteral nutrition [TPN]) or highly caustic drugs (e.g., amphotericin, diazepam, phenytoin, erythromycin) may induce a chemical phlebitis, facilitating bacterial superinfection.

To minimize the risk of infection, intravenous sites should be closely monitored and connecting tubing should be changed every 24 to 48 h. Blood withdrawal increases the risk of infection, as does the filling of tubing systems in advance of their use. Even minute quantities of blood or fat provide nutrients adequate to support the growth of most bacteria; therefore, changing tubing after infusing blood or lipids reduces infection risk. Continuous flush solutions and pressure-monitoring devices attached to arterial catheters pose special hazards. Reducing the number of catheter entries for blood sampling will reduce infection risk. It is especially important to avoid contamination of pressure measuring catheters during calibration. Contamination of Swan–Ganz catheters may be reduced by minimizing the number of cardiac output determinations and by using sterile precautions during preparation and introduction of the injectate. Because of the escalating risk of infection, central venous and arterial catheters should be removed within 3 to 5 days of placement whenever possible. Obviously, there are situations in which all potential access sites have been exhausted or the risk of catheter reinsertion outweighs the risk of infection posed by leaving an existing catheter in place. Therefore, the need for and timing of catheter replacement must be individualized. There are no credible data to support a practice of routine changing of catheters over a flexible guidewire, and doing so in patients with established severe sepsis makes little sense unless all other sites and options for catheter insertion have been exhausted. When receiving a patient from another health care facility, as a general rule it is reasonable to treat indwelling catheters as contaminated, regardless of their duration of insertion.

Diagnosis

Although redness, pain, and swelling around the insertion site strongly suggest infection, these signs are often absent in patients with catheter-related infection. Local (soft-tissue) catheter infections may be confirmed by Gram staining and culturing the catheter and by "milking the wound" to provide material for examination. Because intravascular infections usually produce recurrent and sometimes continuous low-level bacteremia, collecting several sets of cultures obtained over hours to days is sensible. A positive blood culture withdrawn through a potentially contaminated intravenous line does not necessarily establish a diagnosis of catheter sepsis; it is possible that the patient has systemic bacteremia from another source. That supposition is bolstered if the same organism is simultaneously recovered from a clean distant venipuncture site. However, if cultures from the catheter are positive but cultures from a peripheral stick negative, the catheter is suspect, especially if the catheter-obtained cultures grow rapidly. In patients with suspected "line" sepsis, the catheter, tubing, and fluids should be replaced with fresh components. Before catheter removal, the skin should be cleansed with chlorhexidine. The distal centimeter of the catheter tip should then be sent in a sterile container for culture and Gram stain. Semiquantitative culturing is performed by rolling the tip of the catheter across a culture plate. If more than 15 colonies of a single organism are isolated, infection is more likely than colonization. The catheter tip should not be placed into any solution for transport—doing so renders quantitative culturing impossible. Routine catheter changes over a guidewire are not rational in patients with sepsis or inflamed entry sites and are not necessary for asymptomatic patients. Guidewire changes might make sense for patients in whom alternate sites for catheter insertion have been exhausted or who are deemed to be at high risk for insertion of a catheter at a fresh site (e.g., coagulopathy, tenuous respiratory status, bilateral femoral vein thrombosis).

Common Organisms

S. aureus, S. epidermidis, and *Candida* cause most catheter-related infections, although enteric Gram-negative rods also are recovered occasionally. Although rare, blood cultures growing *Enterobacter agglomerans, Pseudomonas cepacia, E. cloacae, Serratia marcescens, Citrobacter freundii,* or *Corynebacterium* species should suggest a contaminated intravenous solution.

Treatment

In almost all cases, contaminated catheters should be removed and cultured as outlined earlier (this includes PICC lines, temporary dialysis catheters, Portacath and Hickman devices). Blood cultures should be obtained from a site separate from the catheter insertion site. Considering the high incidence of MRSA in many ICUs, initial empiric antibiotic therapy for the patient with sepsis from a suspected intravenous line source should include vancomycin in doses adjusted for renal function. In units in which MRSA is rare, an antistaphylococcal penicillin is a reasonable initial choice in nonallergic patients. In either case, additional coverage for Gram-negative organisms should be included. Recovery of *Candida* from the catheter tip and blood culture usually requires parenteral caspofungin, fluconazole, or amphotericin B therapy. Vancomycin-resistant staphylococci may respond to linezolid or quinupristin/dalfopristin.

Persistent Bacteremia

For patients with persistent bacteremia or fungemia, catheter infection and septic thrombophlebitis must be distinguished from bacterial endocarditis. The diagnosis of endocarditis usually obligates treatment with parenteral antibiotics for 4 to 6 weeks, whereas shorter courses of therapy are reasonable for line infections after the catheter is removed. The following factors all favor a diagnosis of endocarditis: (a) a new or changing (especially regurgitant) heart murmur; (b) valvular vegetations on echocardiogram; (c) physical stigmata of endocarditis; and (d) persistent bacteremia or fungemia after removal of the suspect catheter. Negative blood cultures should not dissuade the clinician from a diagnosis of endocarditis for patients with other signs: a small fraction of patients remain culture-negative off antibiotics, and an even larger group is difficult to be diagnosed because antibiotics suppress bacterial recovery. The transesophageal echocardiogram

(TEE) has greatly enhanced the sensitivity of echocardiography to detect and stage heart valve lesions. Vegetations on the right-sided valves do not firmly establish a diagnosis of bacterial endocarditis with certainty; central venous and pulmonary artery catheters crossing these valves can induce sterile vegetations.

It is difficult to make generalizations about endocarditis in critically ill patients because the condition may have been acquired in the community or may be a nosocomial problem, situations associated with vastly different etiologic organisms, locations, and treatments. For patients with prosthetic valves who do not inject illicit substances, the left-sided heart valves (mitral and aortic) are those most often affected, and in such cases, the disease is either a subacute or acute problem caused by streptococci (40%), *S. aureus* (20% to 30%), or *Enterococcus* (10% to 20%). The *viridans* group of *Streptococcus* is a common cause of the subacute form, whereas the acute variety is more commonly *Staphylococcus*. For patients with prosthetic valves who inject intravenous drugs and for hospitalized patients subject to nosocomial bacteremia, the disease differs. There endocarditis is much more likely to be acute in nature and is most commonly caused by staphylococcal or streptococcal species. For these patient groups, Gram-negative rods and *Candida* also are

recovered with a much greater frequency. Infections developing while in an ICU and those associated with intravenous drug abuse are much more likely to occur on right-sided heart valves.

For patients with suspected endocarditis, several blood cultures should be obtained (preferably from different sites and before initiating antibiotic therapy). Recovery of organisms relates partially to the volume of blood cultured. A 12-lead electrocardiogram also should be obtained to look for evidence of conduction defects or arrhythmias, which suggest valve ring abscess. When a clinical diagnosis of endocarditis is confirmed, in most cases an echocardiogram should be performed to look for vegetations, valve ring abscess, and rupture of valve leaflets. Each of these conditions is associated with increased morbidity (peripheral emboli), the need for surgical intervention, and mortality (possibly 50% higher than in the absence of these findings). The sensitivity of echocardiography has improved since the introduction of the TEE, which is capable of detecting small vegetations and those in positions previously not visible by surface echocardiography.

Intravascular foreign bodies (venous and arterial catheters, pacing wires) should be removed, if possible. Empiric antibiotic therapy should be initiated against the most likely organisms based on history or clinical situation (Table 26-5). If valvular

TABLE 26-5 CAUSES AND THERAPY OF ENDOCARDITIS

PATIENT CHARACTERISTIC	LIKELY ORGANISMS	INITIAL THERAPY
"Normal" host, community-acquired infection	Streptococcus (especially viridans) *S. aureus* Enterococcus	Nafcillin or oxacillin plus penicillin and gentamicin Substitute vancomycin in penicillin allergic patients or if resistant Staphylococcus or Enterococcus recovered
Prosthetic valve disease	Early postoperative S. epidermidis Gram-negative rods Diphtheroids Late postoperative (as above for "normals")	Vancomycin plus aminoglycoside As above for "normals"
Intravenous drug users	*S. epidermidis* S. aureus including MRSA, Gram-negative rods Candida	Vancomycin plus aminoglycoside Amphotericin B, consider 5-flucytocisine and surgery
ICU acquired	Same organisms and therapy as for IV drug users	

insufficiency, valve ring abscess, or fungal endocarditis is suspected or found, consultation with a cardiothoracic surgeon is indicated. Although most cases of subacute bacterial endocarditis on native valves can be managed successfully with antibiotics alone, Gram-negative or fungal infections, valvular incompetence, valve ring abscess, and disease on a prosthetic valve often require surgical intervention.

Persistent unexplained bacteremia (or, more rarely, fungemia), particularly when accompanied by pain, swelling, or redness at an intravenous site and recovery of a catheter-related organism, may signal suppurative thrombophlebitis, a condition often confused with endocarditis. A low threshold for surgical exploration should be maintained because this often subtle and highly lethal disease seldom will be cured unless the suppurated vessel is excised, despite the use of appropriate antibiotics.

■ INFECTIOUS DIARRHEA

Diarrhea developing in the ICU is an extremely common problem. Its etiology often is multifactorial and rarely caused by bacteria associated with usual outpatient infectious diarrhea (e.g., *Salmonella*, *Shigella*, *Campylobacter*, and *Yersinia*). When "infectious," a much more common condition is antibiotic associated or "pseudomembranous colitis," more commonly known as "*C. difficile*" colitis. Although it is entirely reasonable to perform stool cultures and to examine the stool for inflammatory cells, ova, and parasites, repeated culturing of patients with loose stools is cumbersome, expensive, and of very low yield.

Pathophysiology

Pseudomembranous colitis is caused by toxins produced by *Clostridium difficile*. This clostridial toxin directly attacks colonic cells, in some cases producing the areas of mucosal damage that form the characteristic "pseudomembrane." Although classically described after intravenous clindamycin therapy, *C. difficile* may overgrow the normal flora of patients receiving essentially any parenteral or oral antibiotic. Less commonly, colonic overgrowth in response to antibiotic therapy by other microorganisms (e.g., *Staphylococcus*, *Candida*) can give rise to a similar picture. Although years ago *C. difficile* colitis was an uncommon nuisance, now mutations in the bacteria have made the disease potentially lethal.

Signs and Symptoms

C. difficile colitis typically presents with watery diarrhea on the fourth to ninth day of antibiotic therapy. Although usually guaiac-positive, the stool is rarely bloody. However, bloody stools may result from one form of the disease localized to the hepatic flexure. Classically, crampy periumbilical and hypogastric pain and low-grade fever were common, and an "acute abdomen" was rare (see Chapter 37). Now high fever, profound leukocytosis, and a presentation suggestive of bowel ischemia or infarction (elevated lactate) are often seen.

Diagnosis

No routine laboratory test is diagnostic, but leukocytosis occurs in almost 80% of cases. As with other forms of inflammatory colitis, red blood cells and leukocytes usually are detectable in the stool specimen. Diagnosis is confirmed by culturing *C. difficile* in profusion from the stool or by detecting bacterial toxin in a fecal specimen. The toxin assay is, readily available, and less sensitive but more specific than stool culture. Some patients without *C. difficile* colitis have small numbers of the bacteria isolated from stool. If a diagnosis of staphylococcal- or candidal-antibiotic-associated diarrhea is being entertained, the microbiology laboratory should be notified when the stool specimen is submitted. Growth of *Staphylococcus* or *Candida* may not be reported as pathogenic unless near-pure cultures result or unless the laboratory is alerted in advance. If done, sigmoidoscopy usually visualizes the colonic pseudomembrane, but in a small fraction of patients (about 10%), only the right colon is involved. In such cases, full colonoscopy is required to find the characteristic lesions. In clinical practice, empirical therapy is usually initiated without endoscopy once the diagnosis is entertained.

Treatment

Systemic antibiotics should be minimized, and fluid and electrolyte support should be administered. Antidiarrheal agents should be avoided, because they may prolong colonic dwell time, thereby increasing the severity of the colitis. There is no evidence that using corticosteroids or that giving lactobacilli to change the fecal flora is beneficial. Because the toxin as well as the organism may be transmitted nosocomially, all patients with this disease should be placed on contact isolation. Because it is effective, inexpensive, and not associated with the induction of bacterial resistance seen with vancomycin, metronidazole in doses of 500 mg *enterally* every 8 h for 10 days is the therapy of choice. Vancomycin (125 to 250 mg *enterally* every 6 h) for 10 days is appropriate in documented metronidazole failures. Intravenous metronidazole and vancomycin are less effective. Bacitracin also has been used in doses of 25,000 units orally, four times daily, but is of uncertain benefit. Treatment may fail because of reinfection, emergence of a vancomycin-resistant strain (rare), or bacterial transformation into a dormant spore phase. When therapy fails, relapses usually occur within 2 weeks of stopping treatment and will respond to a second long course of metronidazole. It should be kept in mind that most episodes of recurrent or persistent diarrhea are not due to colitis associated with *C. difficile* but with one of the more benign noninfectious causes outlined earlier. Alcohol-based hand washing products commonly used in ICUs do kill the *C. difficile* bacteria, but do not kill the organism's spores. Therefore, it is important to decontaminate one's hands regularly with a prolonged soap and water wash.

■ SINUSITIS

Although radiographic evidence of sinusitis can be demonstrated in many supine patients with nasogastric tubes, nasal packing, or nasotracheal tubes, sinusitis often is overlooked as a source of occult fever in critically ill patients. Nosocomial sinusitis usually is polymicrobial with Gram-negative rods and staphylococci predominating. Frequently, cryptic fever is the only clinical feature. Headache and facial pain may be impossible to detect in comatose or intubated patients. Nasal discharge usually is absent. The paucity of overt clinical signs may allow purulent sinusitis to advance to a life-threatening infection of the central nervous system. Its remote position and contiguity to vital structures renders sphenoid sinusitis an unusually insidious process. Because bedside sinus radiographs are worthless (particularly for visualizing the sphenoid sinus), CT of the head with attention directed to the sinuses is the preferred method of diagnosis.

The best treatment for nosocomial sinusitis is prevention. Raising the head of the bed to a more physiological position may promote sinus drainage. Whenever possible, insertion of ostia-obstructing tubes into the nose should be avoided. For orally intubated patients, a standard orogastric tube can be placed easily for aspiration of the stomach, medication delivery, or feeding. Orogastric passage

does not increase the level of patient discomfort and completely avoids the problems of ostial obstruction. When feeding tubes must be inserted through the nose, small-bore, flexible tubes are preferable. Most cases of sinusitis respond to tube removal, decongestants, and antibiotics. Empiric antibiotic selection should include an antistaphylococcal penicillin and an aminoglycoside. More specific therapy can be guided by Gram stain and culture of sinus cavity aspirates. For community-acquired sinusitis, *H. influenzae* is a common etiologic organism that often requires therapy with a β-lactamase-resistant drug, such as a third-generation cephalosporin. Surgical intervention may be necessary for patients with suppurative complications of sinusitis (e.g., retroorbital cellulitis, osteomyelitis, and brain abscess).

■ MENINGITIS

Diagnosis

Bacterial meningitis should be suspected in all patients with mental status changes, fever, and signs of meningeal irritation. Suspected bacterial meningitis is a genuine medical emergency that demands a precipitous workup and immediate broad-spectrum coverage. When neurologic symptoms begin, they often progress rapidly, but most patients with bacterial meningitis are ill for days beforehand. The presentation often is subtle in the ICU, where intubation and sedation, limit communication. Fever, leukocytosis, and an otherwise unexplained change in mental status may be the only clues. When meningitis results from malignancy, tuberculosis, or fungal infection, the clinical picture is even subtler and more likely to include focal neurologic deficits, and perhaps seizures. Although focal deficits are possible with uncomplicated meningitis, the presence of focal *lesions* should raise the possibility of an underlying or complicating brain abscess, subdural empyema, or epidural abscess. Bacterial meningitis may be mimicked by several noninfectious conditions, including drug reactions to trimethoprim-sulfamethoxazole, ibuprofen, and OKT3; carcinomatous meningitis; subarachnoid hemorrhage; systemic lupus; and sarcoidosis.

Organisms

The microbiologic etiology varies with the site of acquisition (community versus hospital) and patient age. The *Pneumococcus* remains the most common organism in community-acquired adult meningitis. Sinusitis, otitis, pneumonia, and endocarditis coexist frequently. *Neisseria meningitidis* is the second most frequent cause of sporadic meningitis. Nontypeable strains of *H. influenzae* represent the third. Although unusual in any setting, *Listeria* and enteric Gram-negative rods are especially rare when meningitis is acquired outside the hospital. In hospital-acquired meningitis, *S. aureus* or *S. epidermidis* and enteric Gram-negative rods are the leading etiologies, particularly following brain surgery.

Diagnostic techniques

Examination and culture of spinal fluid offer the only conclusive method of diagnosing meningitis. In the absence of papilledema or focal neurologic deficits suggestive of a mass lesion, lumbar puncture (LP) may be performed safely without CT scanning. (Full dose anticoagulation, uncontrolled coagulopathy, and significant thrombocytopenia constitute other relative contraindications to LP.) An LP may be impossible technically because of poor patient cooperation or lumbar disease. In such patients, LP under fluoroscopy or cisternal puncture may secure a specimen of spinal fluid.

Spinal fluid pleocytosis with a granulocytic predominance usually is documented in patients infected with bacteria. (Lymphocytic predominance suggests aseptic meningitis, herpes simplex encephalitis, lyme disease, listeriosis, tuberculosis, partially treated bacterial meningitis, or other nonbacterial cause. In the absence of a traumatic tap, large numbers of erythrocytes are rarely seen in the cerebrospinal fluid (CSF) of bacterial meningitis and suggest such alternatives as herpes encephalitis, head trauma, and subarachnoid hemorrhage. Eosinophils suggest a parasitic, cryptococcal, or coccidioidomycotic origin, or a drug-related cause, such as those because of nonsteroidals, ciprofloxacin, vancomycin, and trimethoprim-sulfamethoxazole. With bacterial meningitis, the spinal fluid glucose level usually is less than 50% of the peripheral blood glucose value and CSF protein concentration often exceeds 100 mg/dL. Gram stain of spun spinal fluid demonstrates the organism in three of four cases of bacterial meningitis. It should be noted that seizures, tumors, trauma, and intracranial hemorrhage can mimic the CSF picture of meningitis. In particular, subarachnoid hemorrhage can present remarkably like bacterial meningitis.

If the diagnosis of subarachnoid hemorrhage is not clear from head CT scan, it is useful to centrifuge a sample of freshly obtained spinal fluid and then examine the fluid for xanthochromia characteristic of subarachnoid hemorrhage.

Culture establishes a definitive diagnosis of meningitis. Although cultures of spinal fluid are positive in more than 90% of untreated cases of bacterial meningitis, the specimen may be rendered sterile by even a single dose of oral antibiotic. However, antibiotics rarely change the pattern of cells, glucose, or protein measurements in CSF for 12 to 24 h. Leukocyte counts of 100/mm^3, protein levels higher than 100 mg/dL, and glucose values lower than 30 mg/dL are typical in bacterial meningitis. If spinal fluid cultures are sterile, antigen agglutination tests may reveal the etiology, especially when *Pneumococcus* or *H. influenzae* is causative. Because of wide cross-reactivity, these agglutination tests are least helpful in establishing or ruling out *Neisseria* infections. Blood cultures, positive in one third of patients with bacterial meningitis, should be obtained before instituting antibiotics. After the diagnosis of bacterial meningitis has been established, the clinician should be careful to exclude underlying pneumonia, abscess, or endocarditis before deciding on the dosing and duration of treatment. Viral, neoplastic, fungal, and tuberculous organisms all cause meningitis but generally present less urgently than acute bacterial meningitis.

Treatment

Although not nearly as contagious as widely feared, patients with suspected bacterial meningitis probably should be isolated until the organism is identified and 24 to 48 h of antibiotic therapy have been administered. Even if spinal fluid cannot be obtained because of technical problems or concern over safety of the procedure, antibiotics should be administered as rapidly as feasible. If LP is contraindicated, unavoidably delayed, or technically impossible, empiric therapy should be initiated as efforts are undertaken to establish a delayed diagnosis by blood culture or antigen testing. Ideally, antibiotic therapy and its route of administration (intravenous, intrathecal) should be guided by Gram stain of centrifuged spinal fluid and modified in accordance with its culture. Although meningeal inflammation improves the penetration of most antibiotics into the CSF, certain drugs cross much more efficiently than others. For example, penicillin, chloramphenicol, and selected third-generation cephalosporins (e.g., ceftriaxone) cross the blood–brain barrier easily, whereas aminoglycosides and other cephalosporins may fail to achieve effective concentrations. Penicillin has long been the drug of choice for community-acquired meningitis when lancet-shaped Gram-positive cocci are present unequivocally. Yet, because the risk of penicillin-resistant *Pneumococcus* is significant, a good empirical regimen for initial coverage is a third-generation cephalosporin (or meropenem) and vancomycin. Small Gram-negative rods suggest *H. influenzae,* making a third-generation cephalosporin (e.g., cefotaxime, ceftriaxone) the drug of choice. If Gram stain suggests an enteric (large) Gram-negative rod or if there is evidence of a parameningeal focus (sinusitis, spinal osteomyelitis), an aminoglycoside should be added to a third-generation cephalosporin. (Aminoglycosides are never sufficient therapy alone, and even when clearly indicated for Gram-negative infections, consideration should be given to intrathecal administration.) For cases in which spinal fluid cannot be obtained or is nondiagnostic, a third-generation cephalosporin and vancomycin with or without ampicillin (if *Listeria* is considered) is the safest alternative. Because the spectrum of causative organisms in the hospitalized patient is so broad, initial therapy should include vancomycin, and a third-generation cephalosporin, or meropenem. Because acid-fast smears and cultures are negative in most patients with tuberculous meningitis, empiric antituberculous therapy should be considered for patients with chronic meningitis syndromes, especially if the CSF glucose concentration is low.

Although still somewhat controversial, preadministration or coadministration of dexamethasone with antibiotics may decrease the risk of long-term neurological deficits in patients with meningitis. This effect has been shown most convincingly for pneumococcal disease. If dexamethasone is given, typical doses are 10 mg IV every 6 h for 2 to 4 days. Benefits of corticosteroid therapy are unproven if begun hours or days after beginning antimicrobial therapy.

Patients with acquired immunodeficiency syndrome (AIDS) certainly can acquire any form of bacterial meningitis, but a diagnosis of *Cryptococcus neoformans*, the most common cause of meningitis in AIDS, must be pursued. The CSF inflammatory response in patients with AIDS is often minimal; therefore, absence of an impressive pleocytosis should not dissuade one from the diagnosis of meningitis, especially if the glucose is low. Although an India ink examination of CSF reveals organisms in only 50% of cases, the CSF cryptococcal antigen is positive in almost 90%. Combining these two tests promptly identifies the disease in most patients. The remainder are diagnosed when cultures return positive. Because cryptococcal infection is so frequently a cause of meningitis in patients with AIDS, empiric amphotericin B probably is indicated unless CSF examination clearly indicates a bacterial cause. Tuberculous meningitis should also be considered when the patient infected with HIV presents with a syndrome of meningitis but has minimal CSF abnormalities. The higher frequency of brain abscess, toxoplasmosis, and central nervous system lymphoma in HIV-infected individuals necessitates a low threshold for head CT or MRI scanning, especially if focal defects are apparent on examination.

Complications

Four important complications of acute bacterial meningitis are (a) cerebral edema, (b) inappropriate antidiuretic hormone (ADH) syndrome, (c) obstructive hydrocephalus, and (d) seizures. Because one in three adults with meningitis experiences seizures, prophylactic anticonvulsant therapy is rational. Signs of increased intracranial pressure (e.g., lethargy, papilledema, cranial nerve palsies, hemiparesis) should prompt emergent evaluation for cerebral edema or hydrocephalus by CT scanning. Unexplained hyponatremia (usually in conjunction with concentrated urine) should raise concern for syndrome of inappropriate antidiuretic hormone secretion (SIADH). Although rare, high volume urine output with a rising serum sodium level should prompt consideration of pituitary injury with diabetes insipidus.

Craniotomy patients are at particular risk of meningitis caused by *Staphylococcus* and Gram-negative rods in the early postoperative period. Conversely, the *Pneumococcus* is responsible for more than 90% of late meningeal infections in patients with persistent posttraumatic CSF leakage. Septic cerebral embolism (e.g., from subacute bacterial endocarditis) and parameningeal infections (epidural abscess, brain abscess, sinusitis, and otitis media) are often confused with meningitis because they produce similar symptomatology and CSF pleocytosis. Paraspinal tenderness accompanied by radicular pain or weakness should be a clue to epidural abscess. *S. aureus* is the causative organism in more than one half of such cases. Brain abscess most often is a polymicrobial infection because of *Staphylococcus, Streptococcus,* and anaerobes. Abscess may develop by extension from the sinuses or ears or by hematogenous seeding (infected dialysis shunts, heart valves) or long-standing purulent lung disease (abscess, bronchiectasis). Brain abscess rarely is confused with uncomplicated bacterial meningitis because it usually presents with a less-toxic picture and with focal neurologic signs. Unless otherwise guided by results of culture, penicillin together with chloramphenicol or metronidazole should comprise the treatment. In selected cases, a third-generation cephalosporin or antistaphylococcal agent may be indicated. Surgical intervention generally is reserved for lesions that compress vital structures, those unresponsive to medical management, and those for which malignancy is a strong alternative possibility.

■ SOFT TISSUE INFECTIONS

Most skin infections seen in the ICU are polymicrobial because they result from wounds incurred in surgical or accidental trauma, decubitus ulcers, and therapeutic or illicit vascular punctures or because they occur in patients with compromised defenses and vascular insufficiency (especially diabetes). Necrotizing infections of the soft tissues are characterized by fulminant destruction of tissue, often (but not invariably) accompanied by impressive systemic toxicity and always by a substantial risk of mortality. Microthrombosis, a tendency to spread along facial planes and relatively little inflammatory cellular infiltrate characterize their pathology. Eponyms such as Fournier's gangrene (pelvicoperineal necrotizing cellulitis), Ludwig's angina (cervicofacial necrotizing fasciitis), and Lemierre syndrome (pharyngeal-jugular thrombophlebitis) have been applied to recognized variants of necrotizing cellulitis and necrotizing fasciitis.

Among the most impressive of these are gas-producing infections, which usually develop in the setting of tissue ischemia or gross contamination. Risk factors for gas-forming infection include diabetes, penetrating foot lesions, peripheral vascular disease, and open trauma. Gas-producing infections may be classic gas gangrene with myonecrosis or a mixed organism (synergistic) necrotizing fasciitis. Both may spread with alarming speed. A mixture of aerobic and anaerobic organisms (Gram-positive cocci and Gram-negative rods)

causes most gas-producing soft tissue infections. Classic clostridial gangrene occurs less commonly.

Necrotizing fasciitis is a pernicious infection that may easily elude detection until it is far advanced. Diabetic patients usually have an obvious portal of entry in the foot or lower extremity, but have relatively few signs of toxicity and relatively little local pain. Because such infections are usually due to gas-forming organisms, imaging of the lower extremity may be diagnostic. A different picture—"Type 2" necrotizing fasciitis—is usually presented by non-diabetic patients who have high fever, often an inconspicuous portal of entry, and intense local pain out of proportion to the physical findings. Although infection may be polymicrobial, group A *Streptococcus* (or "GAS") is the primary pathogen in most such cases. To achieve a successful outcome, a combined medical/surgical treatment approach must be executed rapidly. Cultures of blood should be obtained, in conjunction with biopsy or aspiration culture of the affected tissue. The primary indication for surgical intervention is severe pain in conjunction with a compatible clinical setting, toxic signs, and elevated creatine kinase. Physical examination may be seriously misleading. Disease-consistent imaging studies may be supportive but are not required. If not up to date, tetanus immunization and toxoid should be administered. Although the choice of antibiotics should be guided by Gram stain and culture, empiric regimens usually include an antistaphylococcal penicillin and clindamycin or metronidazole. Wider Gram-negative coverage may be advisable in patients who have been recently exposed to antibiotics or who have been hospitalized for longer periods. Extensive debridement (or amputation) frequently is required for control. Reexploration of the wound is usually indicated after 24h to ensure effective debridement of necrotic debris.

A particularly virulent form of lower extremity tissue necrosis follows systemic or local infection with the bacteria *Vibrio vulnificus.* More common in the immunocompromised, especially patients with cirrhosis, the infection causes a rapidly progressive syndrome beginning with abdominal pain and blistering dermatitis. Within hours, microvascular thrombosis infarcts huge masses of tissue, sometimes whole limbs. Not surprising because of the ferocity of the illness, it is often fatal despite prompt treatment with ceftriaxone and doxycycline—the recommended antibiotics.

Most soft tissue infections at intravenous sites are the result of *Streptococcus* and *Staphylococcus* inoculated from the skin. In the colonized ICU patient, Gram-negative rods may be causative. Removal of the catheter, application of warm compresses, and administration of analgesics and antibiotics usually resolve such infections rapidly. Treatment with a penicillinase-resistant penicillin usually will suffice. In less-serious cases, oral therapy is acceptable. If methicillin-resistant staphylococci are likely, vancomycin represents appropriate initial therapy.

Toxigenic infections present a unique set of characteristics. "Toxic shock" syndrome, an uncommon but lethal disease often mediated by the *Staphylococcus* toxin TSST-1, was first reported in menstruating women using high-absorbency tampons. It is now recognized, however, that this syndrome occurs in many settings and can result from streptococci as well. Traumatic or postoperative wound infections may serve as the source for the toxin, even when the surgical wound itself appears uninfected. Toxic shock syndrome should be suspected in any patient with the triad of fever, erythematous (eventually exfoliative) rash, and shock. Therefore, toxic shock can be confused with Rocky Mountain spotted fever, Stevens–Johnson syndrome, leptospirosis, measles, or drug eruption. Because toxic shock syndrome is a toxin-mediated disease, local cultures are often positive for *Staphylococcus,* but blood cultures usually are negative. Therapy includes appropriate drainage (surgical drainage of wounds, removal of tampons), antistaphylococcal antibiotics (vancomycin is a good initial choice), and general supportive therapy with fluids, oxygen, and vasopressors.

■ INFECTION IN THE IMMUNOCOMPROMISED HOST

General Considerations

Few clinical problems present a greater diagnostic challenge than fever in the immunocompromised host. Because such patients often have impaired function of multiple organ systems and undergo treatment with toxic chemotherapeutic agents, possible etiologies span a wide range of noninfectious and infectious agents. Multiple causes frequently coexist. Patients in this category have primary deficits of T-lymphocyte (cell-mediated), B-cell (antibody), or granulocyte (phagocytic) function. Knowledge of the type of immune deficit can help narrow the differential diagnosis. For example, T-cell disorders predispose patients to viruses and fungi, whereas B-cell disorders and granulocytopenia

predispose patients to bacterial pathogens. Although loss of humoral immunity and T-cell function predispose patients to infection, profound neutropenia (<1,000 granulocytes/mm^3) is the defect that represents the greatest risk to life. Infections constitute a true medical emergency. In this setting, the speed with which appropriate therapy is begun largely determines outcome. Unfortunately, establishing a specific diagnosis often proves difficult. Such patients frequently fail to produce suppuration or other localizing signs of inflammation. Regardless of the type of immune defect or site of inflammation, the etiologic organism usually is one that normally resides as a commensal in the host. Although any site may be the target of infection, a few problems are characteristic in the neutropenic patient. These include mucosal infections (e.g., mucositis, gingivitis), "primary bacteremia," soft tissue phlegmons (e.g., perirectal abscess), and atypical pulmonary infiltration.

Pulmonary Infiltrates

The problem of diagnosing pulmonary infiltrates in the immunocompromised patient is complex, and only a few salient features can be covered here. For febrile neutropenic patients, infection must always be the leading diagnostic consideration; however, progression of the primary neoplastic process, hemorrhage, pulmonary edema, graft-versus-host disease, radiation, and drug reaction are frequent causes of pulmonary infiltrates. Although virtually any organism can cause pulmonary infiltration in the compromised host, the clinician often can integrate knowledge of the immune defect, epidemiology, and clinical and laboratory data to narrow the spectrum of likely possibilities and formulate a logical approach. As a first consideration, the underlying disease may give some clue to the nature of the pathogen. For example, AIDS, a problem predominantly of helper T lymphocytes, so predisposes a patient to *Pneumocystis,* mycobacteria, fungal, and cytomegalovirus (CMV) infections that a presumptive diagnosis often is suggested by the radiographic and clinical pictures alone. Nonetheless, the spectrum of possibilities remains wide until the cause is confirmed by biopsy or fluid examination. Epidemiologic factors also are important to consider. The duration of hospitalization before the development of pneumonitis influences the microbiology. For example, *Pseudomonas, Candida,* and *Aspergillus* infections are most likely to develop after many days in the hospital, whereas the likelihood of routine (community prevalent) pathogens wanes after the first few days of hospital confinement. Renal transplant recipients are unusually prone to CMV, herpes simplex, *Cryptococcus, Aspergillus,* and *P. carinii* infections during the period of maximal T cell suppression, 1 to 6 months after operation. Neutropenic patients are highly susceptible to Gram-negative bacteria and fungal infections. (*Aspergillus* and *Mucor* become common infecting organisms if neutropenia is sustained longer than 3 weeks.) Concurrent infection with two or more organisms occurs commonly in patients with AIDS and in those undergoing renal or marrow transplantation. CMV, *Cryptococcus,* and *Nocardia* frequently are recovered in conjunction with other pathogens. (CMV and *Pneumocystis* are commonly associated.) Superinfections also occur frequently in immunosuppressed patients, particularly during sustained neutropenia and prolonged high-dose immunosuppressive therapy.

Certain clinical findings are especially noteworthy. *Legionella, Strongyloides,* and *Cryptosporidium* may cause diarrhea and pulmonary infiltration. Concurrent infiltration of lungs and skin may result from *Pseudomonas, Aspergillus, Candida,* and varicella–zoster. Hepatic and pulmonary diseases tend to coexist during infections with CMV, *Nocardia,* mycobacteria, and necrotizing bacteria (*Pseudomonas, Staphylococcus*).

Evaluation and Therapeutic Approach to Pulmonary Infiltrates

Unfortunately, these problems often defy easy diagnosis and a tissue biopsy frequently is needed. The pace of the disease may be very rapid, so that the objective is to cover broadly while attempting to establish a specific etiologic diagnosis expediently and safely. Two important questions must be answered to deal effectively with a life-threatening pulmonary process in a compromised host. First, considering that the process seems to be infectious and that the course cannot be determined easily, does a precise diagnosis need to be established or is empirical therapy sufficient? Second, if a precise diagnosis is required, what is the most efficacious technique for a fragile, critically ill patient? These questions are not straightforward and remain the subject of intense controversy. In general, the approach should vary with the severity of illness, the pace of advancement, the coagulation and ventilation status, the strength

of ancillary information, and the experience of available personnel with specific invasive procedures. If diffuse infiltrates cannot be distinguished confidently from pulmonary edema despite CT imaging, a brief trial of diuresis may be prudent before proceeding to invasive diagnostic measures. Even when pneumonitis is certain, the astute clinician considers the potential contributions of hypoproteinemia and hydrostatic forces to the density of the infiltrates.

Ancillary Data

Both the characteristics of the chest radiograph at any single point in time and its rate of progression can provide helpful diagnostic clues. Localized infiltrates, either consolidated or nodular, are most consistent with bacterial or fungal infection, hemorrhage, or thromboembolic disease. Bilateral "interstitial" infiltrates, on the other hand, suggest volume overload, *Pneumocystis,* mycobacteria, or virus. However, serious lung infections may develop without causing pulmonary infiltrates, particularly in neutropenic patients. A fulminant evolution suggests a bacterial process or a noninfectious etiology (fluid overload, embolism, ARDS). Conversely, a process requiring 1 to 2 weeks for full expression calls to mind mycobacterial, parasitic, or systemic fungal diseases. The severity of hypoxemia is another key observation. Explosive life-threatening depressions of blood oxygen tension are typical for bacterial, viral, and *Pneumocystis* infections but are less common with more indolent fungal and mycobacterial processes. Examination of body fluids from extrapulmonary sources can suggest a presumptive diagnosis for the chest infiltrate. Spinal fluid may demonstrate *Cryptococcus* but does not prove that the roentgenographic infiltrates are related. Nonetheless, in the appropriate setting, pleural and joint fluids should be tapped, examined, and cultured, and a stool specimen should be sent for parasite detection. Although blood cultures are unquestionably important, serologic testing rarely provides definitive information in an appropriate time frame.

Pulmonary Secretions and Tissue

Sputum is produced less frequently by the compromised host than by immunocompetent patients, especially when neutropenia is present. Nonetheless, when sputum can be obtained, its careful examination may reveal the responsible pathogen. In addition to the routine Gram stain, a direct fluorescent antibody test for *Legionella,* a phase contrast or cytologic preparation for *Blastomycosis,* an acid-fast stain for mycobacteria and *Nocardia,* and a silver stain for *Pneumocystis* and fungal elements are highly worthwhile. Concentrated sputum specimens may reveal *Strongyloides.* In patients with AIDS, such a profusion of *Pneumocystis* organisms is harbored that expectorated specimens often reveal them. Unfortunately, cultures of many pathogens require days to weeks for growth, and the nearly universal practice of early, multiple broad-spectrum antibiotic use routinely obscures the diagnosis.

The Need for Biopsy

If a specific diagnosis is not in hand after review of clinical data and laboratory results, the next step should be guided by the strength of clinical suspicion and the urgency of making the correct diagnosis. In most instances, bronchoscopy should be the first invasive procedure. Although coagulopathy and the need for mechanical ventilation are moderate contraindications to forceps biopsy, lavage is virtually always feasible, and gentle, protected specimen brushings can be obtained safely when care is taken to administer platelets and/or deficient clotting factors beforehand. Bronchoscopic yield varies greatly with the disease process and with the timing and method of conducting this procedure. For example, when all specimen-gathering techniques (biopsy, brushings, and lavage) are used, a specific diagnosis can be established about 50% of the time. In special instances, such as patients with AIDS, the yield is considerably higher.

Open lung biopsy often is delayed because of its perceived morbidity and expense. In fact, open biopsy, a 20- to 40-min procedure, is usually well tolerated and often helpful if conducted early in the course of the illness. It is the most reliable means of securing tissue for histologic diagnosis while establishing effective hemostasis in patients at high risk for bleeding. VATS is another approach of merit in patients with good hemostasis. The expense of open biopsy should be considered along with the high cost of empiric antibiotic therapy. Not only are multidrug combinations expensive, but also some of the commonly used agents carry substantial risk of toxicity for kidneys and bone marrow. Whatever the value of open lung biopsy may be when undertaken early in the course of disease, it is clearly less valuable after broad-spectrum antibiotics have been given for a prolonged period. In such instances, it is

unusual for open biopsy to add sufficient new information to warrant its attendant drawbacks. Failure to define a specific etiology should not mandate continuation of empiric antibiotics indefinitely. Not only can antibiotic management be streamlined when a specific diagnosis has been made, but also rational reductions in therapy can be made in the patient improving on multiple drugs. Usually, this takes the form of removing the next least likely beneficial or most toxic antibiotic from the combination every 1 to 2 days. The process of trimming antibiotic coverage often is delayed until patients are no longer granulocytopenic. Even while patients remain on multiple antibiotics, the clinician must remain alert to "superinfection" with a new or resistant organism. Furthermore, if a patient fails to improve with specific therapy directed against a known pathogen, a second organism commonly is present. For example, patients with AIDS and confirmed *Pneumocystis* pneumonia who fail to respond to trimethoprim-sulfamethoxazole often have coexistent CMV infection. When no specific diagnosis has been made and the clinician is forced to choose a regimen, it should be remembered that *Legionella* and *Pneumocystis* are among the most lethal and common pathogens. For the immunocompromised patient without a diagnosis, a third-generation cephalosporin and an aminoglycoside or quinolone, plus erythromycin or doxycycline and trimethoprim-sulfamethoxazole, are often chosen as initial therapy. When methicillin-resistant staphylococci are prevalent, vancomycin often is added or substituted. In centers in which fungi present a major problem, potent antifungals (e.g., amphotericin) are often begun very early in the course. The use of ultra–broad-spectrum antibiotics (such as imipenem) may help to greatly simplify initial coverage, but such drugs present their own set of problems in terms of expense and the induction of multiply resistant bacteria.

Nonpulmonary Sites of Infection

Neutropenia most frequently is an iatrogenic complication of antineoplastic chemotherapy. These same drugs profoundly impair host ability to maintain the integrity of tissues having rapid cellular turnover (e.g., bowel wall and the mucosa of gingiva and rectum). Therefore, it is not surprising that diffuse necrotizing colitis, anorectal cellulitis, and typhlitis (a severe bacterial infection of the cecum mimicking appendicitis) occur relatively frequently. Violation of the normally intact integument by intravenous catheters, surgical incisions, or decubitus ulcers also opens a portal for bacterial entry. Therefore, for febrile neutropenic patients, physical examination should routinely include catheter entry sites and the gingival and perirectal regions. Lack of tenderness with gentle palpation of the anal verge usually suffices to exclude this as a site of infection. All too often, no site is found for bacteremia or the sepsis syndrome.

General Principles

Survival of the neutropenic patient depends on early empiric therapy with more than one antibiotic effective against the infecting organism. The most common organisms include Gram-negative rods (particularly *Pseudomonas*), *Staphylococcus,* and fungi (e.g., *Aspergillus* and *Candida*). Patients with impaired cell-mediated immunity are more likely to be infected with *Pneumocystis* or *Candida.* When a site of infection is clearly definable, antibiotics should be chosen against the likely organisms. However, neutropenic patients frequently lack localizing signs of inflammation and no likely source is found in most cases (even with careful examination). In such cases, cultures of blood, urine, sputum, and skin lesions should be obtained. Even though pyuria may be absent, microscopic examination of the urine may reveal large numbers of organisms. Broad-spectrum antibiotics, including extended-spectrum penicillin or third-generation cephalosporin plus an aminoglycoside, should be initiated. The empiric use of vancomycin is unwarranted unless the patient is allergic to penicillin or there is a reason to suspect a methicillin-resistant *Staphylococcus* infection. In many centers, amphotericin or other antifungal agent is begun if the patient remains febrile for more than 72 h after institution of broad-spectrum antibiotics.

■ POSTSPLENECTOMY INFECTIONS

Serious infections after splenectomy usually are due to encapsulated bacteria (e.g., pneumococci, *Salmonella, Haemophilus*). Loss of the spleen's phagocytic function allows unchecked bacterial proliferation. Similarly, loss of hepatic phagocytic function in patients with cirrhosis makes them subject to overwhelming infection. *Salmonella* and *Vibrio* species are two unusual pathogens seen in such patients. Therefore, in patients without a functional spleen (e.g., sickle cell disease), the prevention of infections and the early institution of antibiotics are essential.

■ SUGGESTED READINGS

Berenholtz SM, Pronovost PJ, Lipsett PA, et al. Eliminating catheter related bloodstream infections in the intensive care unit. *Crit Care Med.* 2004;32:2014–2020.

Bonten MJ. Prevention of infection in the intensive care unit. *Curr Opin Crit Care.* 2004;10(5):364–368.

Casburn-Jones AC, Farthing MJ. Management of infectious diarrhoea. *Gut.* 2004;53(2):296–305.

Craven DE. Preventing ventilator associated pneumonia in adults. *Chest.* 2006;130:251–260.

Hollm-Delgado MG, Allard R, Pilon PA. Invasive group A streptococcal infections, clinical manifestations and their predictors, Montreal, 1995–2001. *Emerg Infect Dis.* 2005;11(1):77–82.

Kollef MH. Prevention of hospital associated pneumonia and ventilator associated pneumonia. *Crit Care Med.* 2004;32:1396–1405.

O'Grady NP, Barie PS, Bartlett JG. Guidelines for reevaluation of new fever in critically ill adult patient: 2008 updates form the American College of Critical Care Medicine and the Infectious Diseases Society of America. *Crit Care Med.* 2008;36:1330–1349.

Porzecanski I, Bowton DL. Diagnosis and treatment of ventilator associated pneumonia. *Chest.* 2006;130:597–604.

Poutanen SM, Simor AE. *Clostridium difficile*-associated diarrhea in adults. *CMAJ.* 2004;171(1):51–58.

Quagliarello VJ, Scheld WM. Treatment of bacterial meningitis. *N Eng J Med.* 1997;336(10):708–716.

Safdar N, Kluger DM, Maki DG. A review of risk factors for catheter-related bloodstream infection caused by percutaneously inserted noncuffed central venous catheters: Implications for preventive strategies. *Medicine.* 2002;81(6):466–479.

Seal DV. Necrotizing fasciitis. *Curr Opin Infect Dis.* 2001;14(2):127–132.

Shorr AF, Susla GM, O'Grady NP. Pulmonary infiltrates in the non-HIV-infected immunocompromised patient: Etiologies, diagnostic strategies, and outcomes. *Chest.* 2004;125(1):260–271.

Severe Sepsis

KEY POINTS

1 Severe sepsis is a syndrome caused by infection and defined by the presence of vital sign abnormalities and new organ system failure caused by the ensuing inflammation and coagulation. It differs from severe systemic inflammatory response syndrome only by the fact that infection is present.

2 Severe sepsis is common and carries a 30% to 40% risk of death. Outcome is influenced strongly by the number and severity of organ system failures that occur. Average mortality risk increases approximately 15% to 20% for each organ system failure.

3 The lung and circulatory system are the two most commonly failing organ systems. Both manifest dysfunction early in the septic process. Circulatory failure usually reverses within days or is fatal, whereas respiratory failure often requires 1 to 2 weeks of ventilatory support. Transient oliguria is very common, but frank renal failure requiring dialysis is rare. Cognitive function may remain abnormal for months.

4 Infection source control, directed cultures, and targeted antimicrobial therapy are essential but not sufficient to cure severe sepsis.

5 Early fluid replacement and vasopressor therapy are keystones of circulatory support. Glucocorticoid and mineralocorticoid therapy is indicated for patients with frank adrenal insufficiency and may constitute a reasonable therapeutic trial for patients with shock refractory to vasopressor support.

6 Human recombinant activated protein C reduces the morbidity and mortality in severe sepsis and is indicated for patients without a high risk of bleeding complications who are likely to die.

■ TERMINOLOGY

Standardized definitions of three important clinical conditions—systemic inflammatory response syndrome (SIRS), sepsis, and severe sepsis are well accepted. The constellation of fever or hypothermia, tachycardia, tachypnea, and leukocytosis or leukopenia defines SIRS. SIRS represents a body's response to inflammation that may or may not be due to infection. When a major organ system malfunction results from this process, the syndrome is termed "severe SIRS." Common parameters for vital sign abnormalities of SIRS are a temperature lower than 96°F (36°C) or higher than 100.4°F (38°C), a pulse greater than 90 to 100 beats/min in the absence of intrinsic heart disease or pharmacotherapy limiting heart rate response, and tachypnea with a respiratory rate higher than 20 breaths/min. In mechanically ventilated patients, a minute volume criterion of 10 L/min is customarily applied. Abnormalities in the circulating leukocyte (WBC) count (>10,000/mm^3 or <4,000/mm^3) are frequent enough in SIRS to constitute a diagnostic hallmark.

When SIRS is caused by infection, the condition is termed "sepsis." Correspondingly, when an acute organ system dysfunction occurs in a patient with infection-induced SIRS, the resulting syndrome is called severe sepsis. Hypotensive cardiovascular system failure and those who are normotensive with evidence of systemic hypoperfusion (i.e., lactic acidosis) are said to have "septic shock." Although strict criteria are lacking, the multiple organ failure syndrome is highly lethal, progressive cumulative failure of organs. The relationship of infection, SIRS, severe SIRS, sepsis, and severe sepsis are illustrated **1** in Figure 27-1. An operational definition of severe sepsis is outlined in Table 27-1.

■ EPIDEMIOLOGY

The millions of cases of severe sepsis that occur each year in the world present huge medical, social, and economic problems. Patients average 55 to 60 years of age, and for unclear reasons, there is a male predominance; however, severe sepsis has no age or gender boundaries. With the exception of a spike in frequency in the first year of life, severe

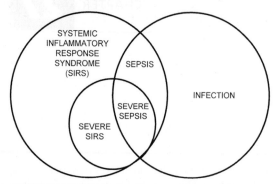

■ **FIGURE 27-1** SIRS is defined by a specific pattern of vital sign abnormalities. Infection is the presence of a microbe within the host at a normally sterile site. When infection causes SIRS, the resulting syndrome is called sepsis (central overlap). If an organ failure results from sepsis, the syndrome is called severe sepsis.

sepsis has a low incidence throughout early adulthood, then an exponentially rising incidence, mortality rate, and cost, after the age of 50. Although sepsis can develop in perfectly healthy persons in the community, most patients have been hospitalized for several days before recognition of the condition. Victims of trauma, immunosuppressed patients, and patients with chronic debilitating medical conditions (e.g., diabetes, chronic obstructive lung disease) or undergoing complicated surgical procedures are most at risk.

Overall, 30% to 40% of patients with severe sepsis die despite receiving "standard therapy" consisting of antimicrobial therapy and organ system support with fluids, vasoactive drugs, mechanical ventilation, dialysis, and nutrition therapy. Elderly and hypothermic patients have a substantially worse prognosis than those without these factors; however,

the best practical clinical predictor of outcome is the number of dysfunctional organ systems. Among the possible organ failures, circulatory failure (shock) has a disproportionate negative prognostic value. The morbidity and mortality of severe sepsis remain unacceptably high, and billions of dollars are spent caring for this desperately ill group of patients. Fortunately, survivors usually eventually regain premorbid levels of function in most organs; however, there is a growing awareness that a significant proportion of patients are left with long-lasting cognitive and neuromuscular impairment.

The average survivor requires 7 to 14 days of intensive care support, with much of this time spent on a ventilator. After intensive care unit (ICU) discharge, an additional 10- to 14-day hospital stay is typical. Thus, the hospital length of stay for survivors averages 3 to 5 weeks. After hospital discharge, long-term skilled inpatient care or challenging home care is often required. Most survivors are discharged on numerous medications; see physicians frequently during the year after discharge and are readmitted one or more times for treatment of complications. Many are shocked to learn that severe sepsis victims typically generate a hospital bill of $150,000 to $200,000 and million dollar bills are not unheard of.

■ RELATIONSHIP OF INFECTION TO SEPSIS

Recovery of a pure growth of a pathogen from a normally sterile site (e.g., blood or joint or cerebrospinal fluid [CSF]) diagnoses *infection*; however, most infected patients do not develop severe sepsis.

TABLE 27-1 SEPSIS SYNDROME CRITERIA

I. Clinical evidence of infection (required)

II. Major criteria (two of four required)
Fever or hypothermia (temperature >100.4°F or <96°F)
Tachypnea or high minute ventilation (respiratory rate >20 or minute ventilation >10 L)
Tachycardia (pulse >90 in absence of intrinsic heart disease or drug therapy inhibiting tachycardia)
Leukocytosis or leukopenia (WBC >10,000/mm³ or <4,000/mm³) or >10% band forms on differential

III. Acute impairment of organ system function (one required)
Altered mental status (reduction in Glasgow coma score >2 points)
Hypotension (SBP <90 mm Hg or fall in BP >40 mm Hg refractory to fluid challenge)
Impaired gas exchange or acute respiratory distress syndrome (PaO_2/FiO_2 ratio <300)
Metabolic acidosis/lactic acidosis
Oliguria or renal failure (urine output <0.5 mL/kg/h)
Hyperbilirubinemia
Coagulopathy (platelet count <80,000/mm³ or a 50% decline within 48 h; INR >2.0; PTT >1.5 × control with elevated fibrin degradation products)

This fact suggests that it is not infection per se that is etiologic but rather the combination of infection and host response that determines if an individual will develop severe sepsis. Interestingly, a clear microbiologic explanation is absent in many patients even though cultures grow some organism 60% to 80% of the time. Many of these "positive" cultures are obtained long after severe sepsis is established and represent insignificant colonization, contamination, or superinfection. Common examples include growth of skin flora in one of several blood culture bottles, the recovery of a light growth of *Staphylococcus aureus* from sputum of a ventilated patient, or demonstration of a few colonies of *Candida albicans* in the urine of a patient with an indwelling urinary catheter. Perhaps the most convincing evidence of infection comes when several blood cultures obtained at the onset of the episode grow an identical pathogen consistent with the patient's clinical situation, for example, recovery of *Escherichia coli* in multiple blood cultures from an elderly man with bladder outlet obstruction and pyuria. Unfortunately, positive blood cultures are seen in no more than 20% to 30% of severe sepsis patients, and blood cultures are very rarely (perhaps as low as 1%) positive if obtained after antimicrobial therapy is started. Despite historical teaching, there is little prognostic import of having positive blood cultures, unless bacteremia cannot be eradicated. Inability to clear the circulation of organisms is often associated with an unresolved focus of infection (e.g., endocarditis or an infected foreign object) and portends a worse prognosis.

Remarkably, the severity of the host response depends little on the presence of infection. In fact, noninfected patients with severe SIRS caused by pancreatitis, trauma, or burns have similar biochemical changes and identical physiology, clinical presentation, and outcome as infected patients with severe sepsis. Again, this observation suggests that infection is not essential but rather that microbiologic stimulation acts merely as one disease trigger.

Consistently, the lung is the most common site of infection leading to severe sepsis accounting for roughly half of all the cases. Intra-abdominal infections (20% to 25%) and urinary tract infections (approx. 10%) are the next most common, with all other sites comprising the remaining 15% of infections. Despite these statistics, in an individual, any site of infection may occur, thus a thoughtful assessment must be conducted every time severe sepsis develops.

■ MICROBIOLOGY

Bacteria, fungi, parasites, and viruses all can incite severe sepsis. Probably, because of the relatively high incidence of bacterial infections and relative ease in recovery of the organisms, bacteria are most commonly implicated. Limitations of diagnostic techniques make viruses least commonly identified. Historically, fungal infections were rarely etiologic in immunocompetent hosts but with improved antibacterial agents and support techniques, more and more immunocompetent patients are surviving long enough to acquire a fungal infection. Distressingly, the frequency of fungal, particularly *Candidal*, infection is rising dramatically and now accounts for almost 10% of all episodes of severe sepsis.

When a bacterial pathogen is identified, the frequency of Gram-positive versus Gram-negative bacteria is roughly 50:50. Discussions of the likelihood of Gram-positive versus Gram-negative infection are of limited value; the prevalence of organisms varies by location and over time, "cycling" under antibiotic pressure. Furthermore, knowing the frequency of each type of bacteria in a population is not particularly helpful in designing therapy for one patient except that it can highlight unusual local resistance patterns. For example, in some parts of the south-eastern United States half of all *Pneumococcus* isolates are at least of intermediate resistance to penicillin. In addition, now in some ICUs the single most common organism causing severe sepsis is a highly resistant nosocomial pathogen, typically methicillin-resistant *S. aureus* (MRSA) or vancomycin-resistant *Enterococcus*. Regardless, in most circumstances, critically ill patients require prompt empiric therapy for all reasonably likely organisms until culture data are available.

■ PATHOPHYSIOLOGY

The severity of severe sepsis is determined more by the specificity and ferocity of the host response than by the inciting organism. Ironically, the same inflammatory and coagulopathic mechanisms that are detrimental when undirected in the septic patient are probably beneficial on the average day. Certainly, both confined inflammation and accelerated coagulation are beneficial when they limit spread of local infection or injury. It is only when rogue, diffuse, unbridled inflammation or coagulation occurs that they are detrimental.

Historically, excessive inflammation was considered the major, if not sole, pathogenetic factor in

TABLE 27-2 COMMON MEDIATORS OF SEPSIS AND THEIR ACTIONS

AGENT	ACTION
Cellular elements	
Monocytes and macrophages	Cytokine production, tissue factor expression
Neutrophils	Tissue destruction via oxidant and protease mechanisms
Eicosanoids	
Prostaglandins	
Prostacyclin	Vasodilation, inhibition of platelet aggregation
Thromboxane	Vasoconstriction, platelet aggregation
E series prostaglandins	Renal vasodilation, inhibition of cytokine generation
Leukotrienes	Vasodilation, increased vascular permeability, leukocyte chemotaxis
Cytokines	
Tumor necrosis factor	Activates neutrophils, causes IL-1, IL-6, and IL-8 production, promotes leukocyte/vessel wall adhesion
Interleukin-1	
Interleukin-6	
Interleukin-8	Neutrophil chemoattractant
Oxidants	
H_2O_2, $HOCl_2^-$, O_2^-	Direct injury of lipids, nucleotides, and proteins
Proteases	Destruction of vital cellular proteins, including antioxidants
Clotting proteins	
Thrombin	Microvascular thrombosis, leukocyte activation, inhibition of fibrinolysis

severe sepsis. This paradigm envisioned a multistage inflammatory "cascade" in which an initial trigger caused production of a few "early" mediators, followed over hours by a larger number of secondary mediators (Table 27-2). It is now clear that inflammation is but one of at least three important pathophysiologic pathways that also includes enhanced coagulation and impaired thrombolysis.

The trigger for severe sepsis is often a protein, lipid, or carbohydrate toxin shed from a microbe but may be activated complement, a clotting cascade component, or dead host tissue. The most notorious inciting toxin is endotoxin, the integral cell wall lipopolysaccharide component of Gram-negative bacteria. However, it is far from being the only important toxin; staphylococcal toxic shock syndrome toxin (TSST-1) and group B streptococcal (GBS) toxin are other well-recognized triggers. The triggering compound usually is only present transiently in the circulation and commonly escapes detection, even when sophisticated monitoring is performed. For example, less than one half of patients exhibiting septic shock ever have detectable endotoxin in plasma. This fact may help to explain the failure of antidotes developed to bind and neutralize circulating toxins. Development of sepsis does not require bacteremia or endovascular infection; toxic products may be released into the bloodstream from localized sites (e.g., abscesses) or

directly from the colon (gut translocation), even when viable organisms do not circulate.

Tumor necrosis factor (TNF) and interleukin 1 (IL-1) have received the most attention as targets for modifying the septic response because they are potent, rapidly produced inflammatory compounds found in the tissues and circulation of many septic patients (Table 27-3). However, controversy exists regarding the significance of circulating cytokines, and clinical trials designed to lessen levels of these compounds have not reduced mortality. That controversy not withstanding, these cytokines are major stimulants of other mediators, including IL-6, IL-8, enzymes, prostaglandins, leukotrienes, oxidant radicals, platelet-activating factor, and nitric oxide and activate coagulation.

There is growing appreciation that abnormal coagulation is nearly universal in severe sepsis and that a complex interplay exists between clotting and inflammation. At the outset of the syndrome, tissue factor expressed by leukocytes and endothelium and cytokines lead to the production of thrombin by stimulating clotting factors V and VIII. Initially, the natural anticlotting systems (e.g., protein C, protein S, antithrombin) counteract the accelerated clotting. In this process, clotting proteins are consumed forming thrombi, and anticlotting proteins are depleted trying to inhibit clot formation. Because sepsis also impairs the host's

TABLE 27-3 EXPERIMENTAL THERAPIES FOR SEPSIS

CATEGORY	PROPOSED ACTION	RESULT
Corticosteroids	Nonspecific anti-inflammatory	Multiple failed human trials, possibly increases infection risk
	Replacement of relative adrenal insufficiency	One positive human trial not confirmed in larger subsequent study
Naloxone	Opioid receptor antagonist	May transiently raise blood pressure, no effect on survival
Cyclooxygenase inhibitors	Reduce thromboxane and prostacyclin	Improved vital signs, no effect on survival, overall safe
Antiendotoxins	Inactivate Gram-negative toxins	Several failed trials, possible harm suspected from one agent; trials ongoing
IL-1 receptor antagonist	Block IL-1 action	No improvement in physiology or survival
TNF antibodies	Inactivate TNF	No certain benefit; no evidence of harm; trials ongoing
TNF receptor antagonists	Block TNF action	Dose-dependent increase in mortality
Antioxidants	Prevent oxidant-mediated cellular injury	Trials ongoing
Toll-like receptor antagonists	Block inflammatory signal transduction	Positive Phase II human trails, studies ongoing
Tissue factor pathway inhibitor	Inhibit tissue factor activation of coagulation	Studies ongoing

ability to convert inactive anticlotting precursors to functioning proteins, clotting proceeds unopposed. As a second line of defense, endogenous fibrinolytic systems (e.g., plasminogen) are activated to dissolve the microvessel clogging thrombi, increasing plasma levels of clot degradation products. Although routine clotting assays (e.g., prothrombin and activated partial thromboplastin times) may be near normal, abnormalities of clotting and anticlotting systems can be detected using more sensitive laboratory tests. For example, essentially all patients have elevated fibrin degradation products (e.g., d-dimers) and the vast majority have depleted levels of specific clotting and anticlotting proteins. Unfortunately, thrombin also augments levels of plasminogen activator inhibitor 1 (PAI-1) and thrombin-activatable fibrinolysis inhibitor (TAFI), both antagonists of endogenous thrombolysis. Together, the net effect of PAI-1 and TAFI is to stabilize whatever thrombi form impairing tissue perfusion. Finally, thrombin independently promotes adherence of leukocytes to endothelial cells leading to vessel wall damage. The complex interrelationship of the three major pathways (inflammation, coagulation, and fibrinolysis) is illustrated in Figure 27-2.

■ CLINICAL DIAGNOSIS

Sepsis has many classic presentations: group B streptococcal sepsis in newborns, meningococcemia in young children, and staphylococcal toxic shock syndrome of adults. Unfortunately, such "classic presentations," which include recovery of a specific organism, are exceptional. Sepsis is a clinical diagnosis, not one made by noting a single specific laboratory value or positive culture.

Although fever is present in more than 90% of diagnosed cases, it may be minimal or absent in elderly patients, patients with chronic renal failure, or patients receiving steroids or other anti-inflammatory drugs. Hypothermia occurs in approximately 10% of cases of sepsis and is a particularly poor prognostic sign, with mortality rates in hypothermic patients approaching 80%. This high mortality rate is not due to the reduced temperature itself but rather the close linkage of hypothermia with chronic underlying disease, shock, and Gram-negative bacteremia, and a more ferocious host inflammatory response.

Respiratory rate is a key vital sign, because tachypnea is an early harbinger of severe sepsis. Although it is possible to have near-normal lung function, the diagnosis of severe sepsis should

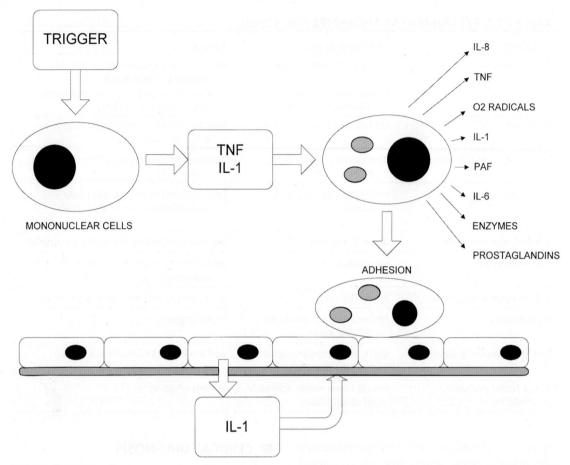

■ **FIGURE 27-2** Simplified representation of the early biochemical events in sepsis syndrome. In most cases, an inflammatory stimulus (*upper left*) activates tissue-based and circulating mononuclear cells. The resulting production of tumor necrosis factor (TNF) and interleukin 1 (IL-1) can activate every nucleated cell. In response to TNF, other cells, especially neutrophils (*upper right*), release additional interleukins, more TNF, oxidant radicals, prostaglandins, leukotrienes, and proteases. TNF and IL-1 also activate adhesion molecules on neutrophils and vascular endothelium, resulting in cellular binding and vessel injury (*bottom*). Simultaneously, activation of tissue factor on white blood cells and endothelial cells results in accelerated clotting and inhibition of fibrinolysis.

be questioned in patients without tachypnea or abnormalities of gas exchange; more than 90% of patients develop hypoxemia sufficient to require oxygen (usually a PaO_2/FiO_2 ratio below 300), and nearly 75% of severe sepsis victims require mechanical ventilation. Likewise, unless patients have intrinsic cardiac conduction system disease or are receiving medications to prevent tachycardia (e.g., β-blockers, calcium channel blockers), tachycardia is almost guaranteed. Abnormalities in circulating leukocyte (WBC) count (>10,000 cells/mm³ or <4,000 cells/mm³) are frequent enough to be considered an important diagnostic criterion.

Although there will always be some diagnostic uncertainty, bedside recognition of severe sepsis is usually not difficult. Among ICU patients, the vital signs and leukocyte abnormalities noted above are nearly universal, giving essentially all ICU residents a diagnosis of SIRS. In that setting, the simultaneous use of one or more antibiotics, a vasoactive drug, and a mechanical ventilator almost always identifies a patient with severe sepsis most likely with two or three failing organ systems.

■ ORGAN SYSTEM FAILURES

In fatal cases of severe sepsis, it is the cumulative effects of organ system failures that cause patients to succumb. Therefore, understanding the usual onset, duration, and resolution of organ failure and methods of support assume paramount importance. A clear relationship between the number of organ

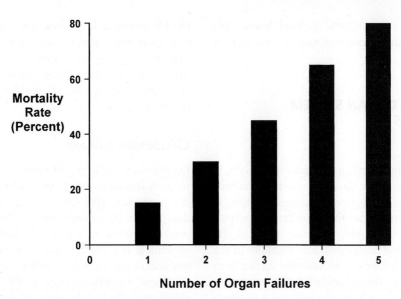

■ **FIGURE 27-3** Relationship between mortality and the number of organ systems failing because of sepsis. Each additional failing organ system raises the overall mortality rate by 15% to 20%.

failures and mortality exists. Each new organ system failure adds roughly 15% to 20% to the baseline risk of death of 10% to 15% for ICU residents (Fig. 27-3). Patients typically average two to three failing organ systems at the time of diagnosis. The frequency of various organ failures noted at the time of diagnosis is shown in Figure 27-4. The most common constellation is the development of pulmonary dysfunction and shock. (Most patients developing shock also will be oliguric at least transiently.) Despite the multiplicity of causes, the pattern of organ failures in severe sepsis is remarkably similar among patients, with lung and circulatory failure developing rapidly (usually within 72 h). Central nervous system (CNS) dysfunction tends to develop later although confusion can be the

predominant manifestation of severe sepsis in the elderly. Even though coagulation abnormalities exist in almost all severe sepsis victims, overt disseminated intravascular coagulation (DIC) occurs in only 10% to 15%, and the timing and its clinical recognition are less predictable.

Not only does the number of organ system failures correlate with outcome, but also the severity of each is important. For example, patients requiring high dose vasopressors (>15 μg/kg of dopamine or >7 μg of norepinephrine) have mortality rates approaching 60% compared to 40% for patients requiring lower vasopressor doses. Likewise, the mortality associated with a creatinine higher than 3.5 mg/dL as the result of sepsis may reach 80%, whereas a creatinine level of 2 to 3.5 carries a

■ **FIGURE 27-4** Prevalence of organ system failures at the time of diagnosis of severe sepsis. ARDS, acute respiratory distress syndrome; CNS, central nervous system.

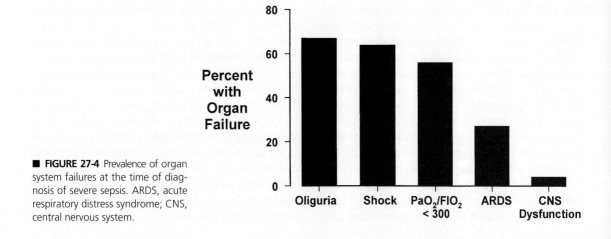

mortality risk of near 50%. A level lower than 2.0 mg/dL predicts approximately a 30% risk of death.

■ SPECIFIC ORGAN SYSTEM FAILURES

Pulmonary

3 Pulmonary failure rarely is absent and usually is the first organ failure to be recognized. Perhaps respiratory failure is common because the lung is the only organ to receive the entire cardiac output, promptly and thoroughly exposing it to all the inflammatory and coagulation abnormalities of the circulation. The lung's huge vascular surface area and delicate endothelial–epithelial capillary structure also may play a role. Or, perhaps it is much simpler, in that patients complain of dyspnea when they become hypoxemic or lung compliance declines and techniques for detecting pulmonary dysfunction (oximetry, arterial blood gases, and chest radiography) are applied promptly to ill-appearing patients.

Sepsis puts many demands on the respiratory system, requiring an increased minute ventilation to maintain oxygenation and compensate for metabolic (lactic) acidosis. Airflow resistance is increased, and lung compliance is reduced, resulting in an overall increase in the work of breathing. These increased demands occur at a time when ventilatory power is compromised by diaphragmatic dysfunction and reduced respiratory muscle perfusion. The shortfall in muscle oxygen supply often leads to combined hypoxic and hypercapnic respiratory failure.

Most patients with severe sepsis require mechanical ventilation. The average duration of mechanical ventilation for survivors is 7 to 10 days. Fortunately, fewer than 5% of patients require chronic ventilation and less than 1 in 10 patients requires long-term oxygen therapy. Overall, almost half of patients develop acute respiratory distress syndrome (ARDS), defined as a PaO_2/FiO_2 ratio less than 200 with diffuse bilateral infiltrates resembling pulmonary edema on chest radiograph (not the result of left atrial hypertension). If ARDS develops, it happens rapidly, with most afflicted patients manifesting the syndrome within 48 h of onset. Interestingly, there is only a rough correlation of PaO_2/FiO_2 ratio (*P/F* ratio) with mortality until the ratio falls below 100, at which time the *P/F* ratio becomes a powerful predictor of death. Paradoxically, the chest radiograph adds little prognostic information after the P/F ratio and lung compliance are considered. The good news about pulmonary dysfunction is that in essentially all survivors, the most severe manifestations of lung injury reverse within 30 days, although a year may be required for near-complete recovery.

Circulatory Failure

Hypotension sufficient to meet criteria for shock (a mean arterial pressure <60 to 65 mm Hg, systolic blood pressure [BP] <90, or a fall in BP of more than 40 mm Hg unresponsive to fluid administration) is present in about one half of all septic patients at the time of diagnosis and develops in one half of the remainder within the first few days of illness. Understandably, of all organ failures, shock typically has the shortest duration, averaging only 2 to 3 days. "Chronic" shock is rare: patients not reversing the shock state usually die quickly. Surprisingly, blood pressure alone is a poor indicator of prognosis—pharmacologic elevation of blood pressure usually can be achieved; therefore, the blood pressure of treated patients with "shock" does not differ from that of patients without shock. Hence, clinicians can be lulled into a false sense of security if vasopressor requirements are not considered when evaluating blood pressure. Patients who require even low doses of a vasopressor after adequate volume replacement have a mortality rate of nearly 40%, and the need for high doses of a vasoactive drug is associated with nearly a 60% mortality rate.

For most hypotensive patients with severe sepsis, invasive monitoring will initially reveal a low central venous pressure (CVP) or pulmonary artery occlusion pressure (PAOP) and a normal or elevated cardiac output with a low systemic vascular resistance (SVR). For the vast majority of patients, pulmonary artery catheter placement increases the risk of arrhythmias but adds little or no useful information and is usually not necessary. Intravascular pressures usually are low because of a combination of reduced intake (anorexia), increased measurable losses (vomiting or diarrhea), increased insensible losses (sweating and tachypnea), and increased vascular permeability. Therefore, initial fluid requirements for resuscitation are substantial. It is common to infuse 4 to 6 L of crystalloid within the first 6 h to raise the intravascular filling pressures into a range optimizing blood pressure and cardiac performance. Fluid deficits typically average 10 L or more in the first 24 h.

Severe sepsis can also cause ventricular dilation and blunt myocardial contractility sufficiently to reduce cardiac output. Therefore, it is easy to see how septic shock with an elevated cardiac filling pressure and a low or low normal cardiac output may be mistakenly labeled "cardiogenic shock." The key to differentiation when there is diagnostic uncertainty is calculation of the SVR, which is reduced in septic shock but elevated in cardiogenic shock. Unfortunately, the hemodynamic situation can be confusing when septic (vasodilatory) shock occurs in a patient with chronic congestive heart failure, the net result being a hypotensive patient with elevated intravascular filling pressures, a low-cardiac output, and a near-normal SVR.

When volume challenged, septic shock survivors demonstrate a rise in cardiac output, but the slope of the cardiac performance curve is flatter than that of normal subjects. Failure to raise the cardiac output when intravascular pressures are boosted is a poor prognostic sign that may reflect impaired cardiovascular reserve or presence of myocardial depressant factors.

Renal Failure

Oliguria (urine output < 0.5 mL/kg/h) is very common early in severe sepsis and tracks closely with shock. Up to 80% of patients develop at least transient oliguria, but it rarely persists beyond several days. Although the creatinine often rises modestly (range, 2 to 3 mg/dL) it is uncommon to develop frank renal failure. Overall, typically only 10% to 15% of patients with sepsis require renal replacement therapy, and in more than 90% of survivors, dialytic support is brief (7 to 10 days). It is rare to develop permanent dialysis-dependent renal insufficiency from sepsis unless baseline kidney function is significantly impaired; the elderly and patients with diabetes are at greatest risk for this complication. Interventions that can reduce the incidence of renal failure are to promptly treat hypovolemia and shock and to avoid use of nephrotoxic drugs (e.g., IV radiographic contrast, aminoglycosides) whenever possible. Use of agents like *N*-acetyl-cysteine which are renal-protective in other settings have not yet been shown to be beneficial in severe sepsis.

Metabolic Acidosis

The pathogenesis of lactic acidosis in severe sepsis is controversial. Clearly, in some patients with low oxygen delivery (DO_2) resulting from hypoxemia, anemia, or low cardiac output, impaired DO_2 alone can cause anaerobic metabolism. In other patients, lactic acidosis results from either maldistribution of cardiac output or from cellular malfunction, probably at the mitochondrial level. In a sense, the mitochondrial failure can be viewed as "organelle" failure much like other organ failures. Boosting DO_2 to prevent or reverse anaerobic metabolism and lactic acidosis has been extensively studied. It is clear that increasing DO_2 to some arbitrary supranormal value in established sepsis does not reverse anaerobic metabolism and may be harmful. By contrast, early vigorous resuscitation sufficient to correct insufficient oxygen delivery and eliminate circulating lactate in the first few hours of the disease is likely beneficial. The finding that elevated lactate levels can occur in the absence of hypotension has been an important discovery because it can be used to identify a cohort of patients who may benefit from prompt, vigorous, protocolized resuscitative efforts.

Coagulation Disorders

The cause of coagulation disorders in patients with severe sepsis is usually multifactorial. The two most important mechanisms are tissue factor expression on endothelial cells and leukocytes and cytokine generation. The incidence of coagulation disorders varies depending on the defining criteria. For example, essentially all patients have reduced levels of specific clotting and anticlotting proteins and elevated clot degradation products. (Nearly, 100% of victims have elevated d-dimer levels, and 90% have reduced protein C levels.) Likewise, modest thrombocytopenia (platelet counts 75,000 to 100,000/mm³), minimal reductions in fibrinogen, and small prolongations of the prothrombin and partial thromboplastin times are very common. However, full-blown DIC occurs in only 10% to 20%. Although uncommon, when DIC occurs, it carries an extremely poor prognosis, with mortality rates in excess of 50%.

Central Nervous System Failure

A slight decline in CNS function, often measured as deterioration in the Glasgow coma score, is usually a later manifestation of sepsis. Surprisingly, even a modest deterioration in cerebral function on this scale portends a dismal prognosis. It is interesting that any clinical scale of CNS function that relies so heavily on volitional actions can predict outcome, considering the frequency of use of sedative and paralytic agents. As the mortality rate of severe sepsis has declined, it has become apparent that long-term cognitive problems are very common among survivors. Persistent difficulty with memory, concentration, and executive functioning can dramatically disrupt the lives of survivors.

Gastrointestinal Failure

The gut is an early victim of the septic response, in that perfusion is diverted to more "essential" organs. Therefore, peristaltic function often temporarily ceases, producing ileus. For this reason, few physicians attempt full enteral nutrition until hemodynamic stability is achieved, even though no credible data suggest early feeding is impractical or unsafe. Because gut motility resumes shortly after BP and oxygenation are stabilized, enteral feeding usually is feasible 1 to 2 days after the onset of sepsis.

In the distant past, significant upper GI bleeding resulting from gut ischemia occurred with substantial frequency (near 30%) unless pharmacologic prophylaxis was undertaken or early feeding begun. Now the combination of early resuscitation, earlier feeding, and nearly routine use of gastric acid suppression has all but eliminated life-threatening GI bleeding. Although controversial, the hypoperfusion of colonic mucosa also has been associated with leakage or "translocation" of bacteria and their toxins to the lymphatic and portal circulations.

Profound hypotension, especially when prolonged, also can lead to hepatocellular injury—the so-called shock liver syndrome. Shock liver is characterized by significant increases in hepatic transaminases and bilirubin, whereas alkaline phosphatase tends to remain in the normal range or rise minimally and impairment of hepatic synthetic function is rare.

■ SEPSIS THERAPY

Over the last few years, the treatment of severe sepsis has changed perhaps more than any other condition discussed in this book. Even though the foundation of severe sepsis treatment still contains infection source control, cultures, appropriate antibiotics, and prompt circulatory and ventilatory support, clinical trials have given us information about how to best perform these treatments. A specific lifesaving therapy directed against inflammation and coagulopathy, human recombinant activated protein C (rhAPC), has been added to the therapeutic armamentarium but remains underused. Perhaps

the most important development in the care of the severe sepsis patient has been the recognition that outcomes can be optimized and money can be saved by applying a protocol-based approach to care delivered by experts.

Antimicrobial Therapy

Drainage of closed-space infection and removal of infected foreign bodies or devitalized tissue are time tested and essential but not sufficient for cure of severe sepsis. Initially, a low threshold for obtaining cultures of blood, urine, and sputum should be held. Cultures of wound discharge, ascitic fluid, pleural fluid, and CSF should be performed as indicated by the history and examination. The likelihood of making a culture diagnosis is maximized by obtaining specimens before antibiotics are initiated, but in some circumstances, this is not practical. For example, in a septic patient with suspected meningitis and a focal neurological defect, it is prudent to obtain a head CT before lumbar puncture; however, it probably is not wise to delay antibiotic therapy while awaiting a scan. In this situation, it is better to begin empiric therapy, even if it may delay or obscure a specific bacteriologic diagnosis. In this scenario, blood cultures could be obtained before antibiotics and might yield a diagnosis.

The most antimicrobial agents can do is kill the offending organism; they do not reverse the inflammatory–coagulopathic process. This fact notwithstanding, it makes sense to initiate antibiotics in a timely fashion. Until recently, there has been little evidence to suggest that minutes or perhaps even hours in the time to administer antibiotics made a difference in outcomes. However, data now indicate that for patients with septic shock, perhaps only half of all victims receive antibiotics in the first 6 h of their illness, with the remainder taking up to 36 h to get antimicrobial treatment. Longer time to antibiotic administration is associated with higher mortality. For patients without shock the urgency with which antibiotics must be given is less certain. For example, the national effort to rapidly administer antibiotics to patients with community-acquired pneumonia is associated with tiny improvements in survival.

Ultimately, establishing appropriate antibiotic coverage is important; patients with sepsis who do not have the offending organisms properly treated have a higher mortality rate than those given adequate coverage. This observation should be interpreted cautiously, however. The reason for "inadequate" antibiotic coverage is often that patients are infected with highly resistant or unusual organisms as the result of chronic illness, long hospital stays, previous antibiotic exposure, or an immunocompromised state. Failure to respond to seemingly appropriate antimicrobial therapy may be the result of an undrained closed-space infection (e.g., empyema, intraabdominal abscess), presence of a resistant organism(s), insufficient drug levels, or most commonly simply insufficient time for response after starting therapy.

Antibiotics should be chosen based on individual patient factors (e.g., immunosuppression, allergies, and underlying chronic illnesses), the presumptive site of infection, pattern of local antibiotic resistance, and examination of body fluids/specimens. For the severe sepsis patient, unless the etiologic agent is known with a very high degree of certainty, broad-spectrum antibiotic coverage is indicated until culture and sensitivity data return. Unfortunately, changes in resistance patterns induced by injudicious past use of antibiotics now frequently necessitate three or sometimes even four antibiotics to provide empiric coverage. The stark reality is that we are unable to anticipate or provide empiric therapy for all possible organisms.

In the absence of diagnostic clinical specimens, the presumed site of infection probably is the most helpful information on which to select antibiotics. An in-depth discussion of appropriate empiric coverage based on the presumptive site of infection is covered in Chapter 26. Because lung and abdominal infections are most common, when no clear site of infection can be found, therapy with a third-generation cephalosporin or extended-spectrum penicillin and a quinolone or aminoglycoside is a reasonable first combination. In many cases, vancomycin also should be added to primary coverage if penicillin-resistant *Pneumococci* or methicillin-resistant *Staphylococci* are prevalent regional pathogens. When an "atypical" organism is suspected as the cause of pneumonia, a quinolone, doxycycline, or macrolide should be included in coverage. Because most antibiotics are concentrated in urine, bacterial urinary tract infections are usually easily treated with almost any antibiotic, unless drainage is obstructed. In suspected meningitis, initial therapy should always include at least vancomycin and a third-generation cephalosporin. Finally, high suspicion of an anaerobic infection should usually prompt addition of metronidazole or clindamycin. Within reason, it is best to begin therapy in the critically ill patients with "too broad" a spectrum and then narrow coverage as more clinical data become available. With that caveat, antibiotic coverage should be reassessed on a daily basis and unnecessary drugs should be stopped promptly. Contrary to popular belief, antibiotic therapy is not benign. Use of excessive or unnecessary antibiotics is costly, risks allergic reactions and toxicity, and perhaps most importantly, breeds the emergence of highly resistant bacteria that can harm future patients. Obviously, even when appropriate initial antibiotic choices are made, the doses must be adjusted to ever-changing levels of renal and hepatic function.

Respiratory Support

Because of the high frequency of hypoxemic respiratory failure, airway intubation, supplemental oxygen, and mechanical ventilation usually are necessary. The specifics of airway control and the principles and problems of mechanical ventilation are presented in detail in Chapters 6 to 9; however, some unique features of sepsis-induced lung injury deserve mention. More than 80% of sepsis victims eventually develop respiratory failure sufficient to require mechanical ventilation, and nearly all require supplemental oxygen. Therefore, for patients with severe sepsis, tachypnea (respiratory rate higher than 30), and marginal oxygenation, it is prudent to plan for elective intubation. It is counterproductive to pretend that rapidly evolving tachypnea and desaturation will resolve spontaneously. Doing so often results in emergent intubation of an apneic patient, and only rarely can patients sustain a respiratory rate greater than 30 breaths per minute. Similarly, the prolonged duration of respiratory failure and the high levels of support required usually portend failure of noninvasive ventilation strategies.

There is no clear best mode of ventilation for all septic patients; however, it makes sense to provide full support (assist control, pressure control, or intermittent mandatory ventilation [IMV] at a rate sufficient to provide more than 75% of the minute ventilation requirement). Full support, especially for patients in shock, permits redistribution of cardiac output from the respiratory muscles to other parts of the body. The effect of ventilatory support can be substantial, in many cases amounting to an effective 20% boost in systemic oxygen delivery.

Often, the drive to breathe is so high that sedation is needed to match the respiratory efforts of man and machine. Fortunately, paralysis is rarely necessary if appropriate sedation is provided and the ventilator is adjusted carefully. To maximize patient matching and comfort, special consideration should be given to altering the gas flow delivery pattern and flow rate.

For patients with sepsis-induced acute lung injury, initial tidal volume selection should approximate that of a normal spontaneous breath (5 to 7 mL/kg of ideal body weight), provided the resulting plateau pressures are below 30 cm H_2O. Higher plateau pressures mandate additional tidal volume reductions. Despite this recommendation, there is no known "safe" plateau pressure, and values less than 30 cm H_2O should not encourage use of a higher tidal volume. Limiting plateau pressure reduces alveolar stretch, hence the risk of classical barotrauma and "biotrauma," the name given to the local and systemic inflammatory response generated by imprudent ventilation. Use of a normal-size tidal breath almost always results in patients increasing their respiratory rate to near 30 breaths per minute to maintain constant minute ventilation. The tachypnea and mild hypercapnia ($PaCO_2$ 45 to 50 mm Hg) that result distress some health care professionals; however, tachypnea is not harmful and is usually easily managed by adjusting inspiratory flow rates and providing modest sedation. The rare patient ventilated with lower tidal volumes will have such drive, so as to "double stack" breaths. When flow rate adjustments and sedation fail to control this dyssynchrony, tidal volumes may be increased cautiously.

Supplemental oxygen should be administered to maintain an acceptable saturation (in most cases, SaO_2 higher than 88%). The real and immediate risk of hypoxemia should not be traded for the theoretical future risk of oxygen toxicity. These lower saturation limits are acceptable for young, otherwise healthy patients, whereas higher targets may be appropriate for patients with myocardial ischemia or recent stroke. Uncertainties surround the potential for oxygen toxicity; however, common practice is to attempt to reduce FiO_2 to a level of 0.6 or less, provided saturation is acceptable. If higher FiO_2 is required, sequential upward titration of PEEP usually is undertaken. The "best PEEP" is the lowest PEEP that provides acceptable O_2 delivery with an FiO_2 at or below 0.6. Some minimal level of PEEP (5 to 10 cm H_2O) is probably beneficial for all mechanically ventilated patients to raise functional residual capacity and minimize injury induced by the repeated phasic opening and clos-

ing of alveoli. Randomized trials in acute lung injury have failed to show a benefit of higher levels of PEEP (12 to 15 cm H_2O) compared to lesser amounts (see Chapters 8 and 9). Despite the emotion sometimes surrounding the selection of PEEP and FiO_2 and use of other measures to improve oxygenation, most patients with sepsis-induced ARDS end up receiving an FiO_2 between 40% and 60% and PEEP of 8 to 10 cm H_2O pressure and require no extraordinary interventions.

Contrary to long-standing belief that fluid administration will increase the likelihood of positive pressure ventilation, data from hospitals undertaking a protocolized approach to the resuscitation of patients with septic shock suggest that prompt fluid resuscitation reduces the need for mechanical ventilation. Another important development in the care of the patient with sepsis-induced lung injury has to do with fluid management after shock has resolved. Minimizing nonessential fluid intake and using diuretics to target a CVP less than 4 mm Hg can shorten the period of mechanical ventilation by 2 to 3 days, without increasing the incidence of recurrent shock or renal failure.

Cardiovascular Support

Septic shock usually is defined as a mean arterial pressure less than 60 to 65 mm Hg, or systolic BP lower than 90 mm Hg or a decrease in normal systolic BP of more than 40 mm Hg unresponsive to fluid administration. The definition has been **5** expanded to include patients who have reduced central venous hemoglobin saturations or elevated arterial lactate concentrations regardless of blood pressure.

At the onset of the syndrome, most patients with sepsis-induced shock have substantial volume depletion with variable degrees of systemic vascular dilation and myocardial dysfunction. Ventricular filling pressures are usually low because patients have been deprived of oral intake, have increased fluid losses (from sweating, panting, vomiting, or diarrhea), and have dilated capacitance vessels and increased endothelial permeability. The average septic patient requires 4 to 6 L of crystalloid fluid replacement or a comparable volume-expanding amount of colloid within the first few hours to optimize ventricular performance and perhaps double that amount of fluid in the first 24 h.

There is no proven difference in efficacy of crystalloid and colloid, although recent metaanalyses suggest crystalloid may be the better choice. Obviously, a smaller volume of colloid will be required to achieve any given increase in intravascular pressure; however, neither colloid nor crystalloid is confined entirely to the vascular compartment in sepsis. Although less colloid is required, volume expansion is achieved at substantial cost—colloid risks allergic reactions, and its price is often many times that of an equivalent dose of crystalloid. Results of one randomized controlled trial are concerning because they indicate one colloid, pentastarch, causes more renal insufficiency compared to crystalloid therapy. Because hemodilution accompanies resuscitation with colloid or crystalloid, administration of packed red blood cells is often used to maintain hemoglobin concentrations in an acceptable range.

Despite informative clinical trials highlighting the benefits of prompt significant fluid administration, there remains controversy with regard to the optimal fluid volume infused, rate of administration, or method of monitoring the adequacy of therapy. Each physician seems to have a different level of comfort with regard to the amount of fluid infused before instituting invasive monitoring or starting a vasoactive drug. The widely proffered recommendation to "replace circulating volume" before instituting a vasoactive drug is sensible but nebulous, because there are no certain guidelines for intravascular filling pressure goals or even which pressure to target (CVP or PAOP). One resuscitation strategy shown to reduce mortality in septic shock used a target central venous pressure of 8 to 12 mm Hg.

Treatment strategies range from giving fluid boluses guided only by the clinical exam (i.e., blood pressure, pulse rate, skin color and temperature, and urine output) to the addition of central venous pressure measurement, all the way to pulmonary artery catheterization with mixed venous oxygen saturation monitoring. Although the best measure of left ventricular filling is probably the PAOP, even when PAOP is known, left ventricle preload remains uncertain because of the difficulty measuring ventricular compliance and juxtacardiac (pleural) pressure. Thus, when using an invasive monitoring strategy, the optimal ventricular filling pressure must be derived empirically and should be reevaluated frequently. Typically, this is accomplished by measuring hemodynamics (CVP or PAOP) in response to frequent serial fluid challenges.

When a fluid challenge is used, it is important to use a bolus of sufficient volume to cause a detectable change. A commonly selected "bolus" size, 500 mL, has been shown to produce no measurable change in blood pressure, intravascular filling pressures, or cardiac output. Thus, it makes sense to use larger fluid challenges ($\geq$15 mL/kg) unless there is a strong suspicion that cardiac performance is profoundly impaired. Likewise, it is logical to administer the bolus as rapidly as possible to maximize the chance of achieving and seeing a hemodynamic effect.

Although confirmatory trials are underway, data suggest that a treatment strategy of early "goal-directed" therapy (EGDT) dramatically improves survival in severe sepsis. This strategy uses fluids to achieve a target CVP (8 to 12 mm Hg) followed by vasopressors to attain a target mean arterial pressure of 65 to 95 mm Hg. Then, patients with persistently low superior vena cava oxygen saturations (<70%) are given red blood cells if anemic, or dobutamine if not anemic to reach a specific superior vena caval saturation target. In contrast to previous potentially harmful strategies targeting an arbitrary level of oxygen delivery in established sepsis, this strategy focuses on *early* (first 6 h) correction of circulatory abnormalities.

A detailed discussion of vasopressor therapy is provided in Chapter 3; however, a few points deserve highlighting. Vasopressors are of limited effectiveness in volume-depleted patients and can be detrimental if given in doses that compromise tissue perfusion. In septic shock, hypotension is predominately the result of reduced systemic vascular resistance, with a lesser contribution from impaired cardiac contractility. Thus, drugs with both β-adrenergic (cardiac stimulatory) and α-adrenergic (vasoconstrictive) properties make sense. As a practical matter, in the fluid unresponsive patient, physicians usually initiate circulatory support with dopamine (5 μg/kg/min) or norepinephrine (2 μg/min) and then titrate the infusion upward as needed. Historically, dopamine has been favored because of its alleged "renal protective" effects; however, it is rapidly being supplanted by norepinephrine because it is clear that dopamine does not protect the kidney, is less effective at raising blood pressure, and is more likely to cause tachycardia. When profound reductions in SVR are responsible for hypotension, it is also common to add a pure α-adrenergic agent (e.g., neosynephrine) to the pharmacologic regimen. Although empiric, some clinicians add dobutamine to an existing vasopressor regimen if cardiac index appears inappropriately low (<2.5 L/min/m^2).

Recognition that many patients with septic shock have low plasma vasopressin levels and administration of low doses of vasopressin (0.01 to 0.04 U/min) raise blood pressure has lead many clinicians to use vasopressin routinely or in patients with hypotension resistant to moderate doses of catecholamines. Results of a large randomized trial of vasopressin in septic shock indicate that low doses of vasopressin are safe and effective at raising blood pressure, but do not afford significant benefits with regard to survival compared to catecholamines alone.

One widely held misconception is that the use of potent vasoconstrictive agents (e.g., norepinephrine, phenylephrine, vasopressin) "guarantees" a poor outcome. To the contrary, sometimes it is only after norepinephrine is begun that SVR increases, in turn raising the mean arterial pressure and organ perfusion. In certain settings (e.g., cor pulmonale), failure to raise systemic blood pressure will deprive the heart of the coronary perfusion gradient it needs to pump effectively.

Physicians and nurses often become anxious when the required dose of any vasoactive drug is higher than that used in their past experience. However, it should be kept in mind that individual patient responsiveness to vasopressors can differ widely (perhaps a log variation in dose). Therefore, there are no absolute limits for vasopressor doses in shock and no evidence that using "modest" doses of two or three vasopressors is superior to "high" doses of a single agent. When very high doses of vasoactive agents are required, consideration should be given to several specific causes of refractory hypotension, including intravascular volume depletion, adrenal insufficiency, profound acidosis, pericardial constriction or tamponade, and tension pneumothorax.

Brief high-dose corticosteroid therapy has consistently failed to improve outcomes in septic shock. Based upon results of one widely debated study, the use of longer courses of lower-dose steroid therapy became common place. This study popularized the concept of "relative adrenal insufficiency" defined by failure to increase serum cortisol levels by at least $9\,\mu g/dL$ after a $250\,\mu g$ dose of intravenous adrenocorticotropic hormone (ACTH). Mortality rates were reportedly reduced when ACTH "nonresponders" are treated for 7 days with a combination of hydrocortisone 50 mg q6h and fludrocortisone 50 mg per day. The results of this trial suggested that caution is indicated; "responders" given this steroid combination had nominally higher mortality rates than those not treated. The controversy over corticosteroid use has been fueled by a larger, randomized, blinded international multicenter trial that failed to confirm the benefits of corticosteroid in any group studied. While each clinician will have a different interpretation of these results, the following strategy is defensible. For patients with septic shock who respond to administration of fluid and low or modest doses of vasopressors, neither provocative adrenal testing nor corticosteroid administration is indicated. For patients refractory to aggressive fluid replacement and moderate or high dose vasopressors, measurement of random plasma cortisol may be informative; if low, i.e., true adrenal insufficiency, administration of glucocorticosteroid is indicated. If the baseline cortisol is in or above the normal range, ACTH stimulation testing to identify a "nonresponder" is probably unnecessary.

After initial resuscitation, a functioning brain, adequate (>0.5 mL/kg/h) urine output, evidence of adequate peripheral skin and digit perfusion, and a reasonable level of oxygenation and blood pressure are appropriate goals. These clinical perfusion goals usually are met when cardiac output is in the 7- to 10-L range, arterial lactate concentrations are declining, and oxygen delivery measurements are slightly above those for a resting healthy patient.

Human Recombinant Activated Protein C

rhAPC reduces inflammation, downregulates coagulation, and inhibits the antithrombolytic actions of PAI-1 and TAFI. rhAPC is given by continuous infusion in a dose of $24\,\mu g/kg/h$ for 96 h. Among severe sepsis patients treated within the first 2 days of illness, relative reductions in mortality of 20% to 30% have been observed. Mortality benefits persist at least through two and one-half years of follow-up. The largest decrease in mortality is seen when patients with shock, two or more failing organ systems, or high severity of illness scores are treated within the first day. Patients with overt DIC also appear to have large reductions in mortality. In addition to the survival benefit, early treatment is associated with fewer days on a vasopressor, on a ventilator, in the ICU, and in the hospital, compared to delayed or no rhAPC therapy.

The sole toxicity of rhAPC is bleeding, seen in 1.5% to 2.5% more patients than those not treated (a risk comparable in magnitude to anticoagulation with heparin). The risk of serious bleeding can be minimized by not treating patients with less than 30,000 platelets/mm^3, overt hemorrhage, recent stroke, or intracranial or spinal surgery or injury. Avoiding treatment within 12 h of surgery or trauma and stopping the drug for 2 h before performing invasive vascular procedures also act to minimize bleeding risk. Although the costs are recouped by 1 to 2 fewer days in the ICU on a ventilator, the major impediment to widespread use has been the drug's substantial cost (approx. $7,000 per course of therapy).

Glucose Control

For critically ill patients with stroke, myocardial infarction, and cardiac arrest, the development of hyperglycemia is associated with worse outcomes than normoglycemia. In addition, high serum glucose concentrations impair neutrophil function and exert a procoagulant effect in patients with severe sepsis. Hence, it was reasonable to investigate the benefits of "tight" glucose control in the ICU. Among postoperative patients, stringent control of glucose (80 to 110 mg/dL) reduces the risk of developing severe sepsis and of dying compared to a more traditional glycemic range. This observation prompted numerous studies of strict glucose control that have failed to confirm the survival benefit initially observed. Furthermore, several of these investigations have found a substantial incidence of hypoglycemia. Furthermore, glycemic control is not a trivial undertaking; it usually requires a continuous insulin infusion with hourly monitoring of blood glucose entailing substantial labor expenditure.

Despite the conflicting data regarding benefits and risks, clinicians must make a practical decision: Do I attempt to manage glucose levels, and if so, how? At present, a prudent course of action is to maintain glucose levels near normal, probably in the 100 to 150 mg/dL range. To prevent hypoglycemia, frequent monitoring and measured changes in insulin doses are indicated. Careful attention should be given to patients who develop renal failure and those who have nutrition support discontinued because both populations are at particular risk for hypoglycemia.

Therapy of Metabolic Acidosis

Lactic acidosis is common in severe sepsis patients. Fortunately, it is usually a mild and self-limited problem that resolves when intravascular volume deficits are corrected. When lactic acidosis results from low cardiac output and hypotension, it is likely to be improved by increasing arterial pressure. The benefits of fluids, vasoactive drugs, or red blood cells appear to be confined to resuscitation shortly after the onset of shock. Conversely, when cardiac output and arterial pressure are normal or high, no data convincingly demonstrate a benefit of further increasing output or oxygen delivery, especially in patients with established organ failures. Survival correlates best with lactate levels and not serum pH; therefore, buffering an abnormal pH with sodium bicarbonate or dichloroacetate does not improve outcome, unless the underlying reason for lactate generation is corrected simultaneously. Even though experimental data do not support the practice, as a practical matter, many physicians feel compelled to intervene when pH declines below 7.10.

Support of the Kidney

The kidney commonly experiences transient dysfunction early in the septic process; more than 40% of patients develop transient oliguria, which is usually reversed by simple fluid administration to correct underlying volume depletion. For patients with shock, a combination of volume repletion and vasoactive drug administration may be required to raise cardiac output or SVR sufficiently to perfuse the kidney. There is no credible clinical evidence indicating that the use of dopamine (in any dose range) serves to protect the kidney from injury or improve outcome. Likewise, diuretic therapy has not been shown to improve outcome in oliguric patients. Perhaps the most important interventions to protect the kidneys of patients with sepsis are early circulatory resuscitation and avoidance of potentially nephrotoxic medications whenever possible. As renal function declines early in the septic process, any number of toxic drugs may accumulate to the point that they cause systemic toxicity or accentuate the injury to the kidney. Probably, the most important class of compounds in this regard are antibiotics. Intermittent high-flow hemodialysis has been the traditional method for renal replacement therapy; however, continuous hemofiltration/hemodiafiltration is growing in popularity. Because continuous filtration avoids rapid fluid shifts and can be performed in the ICU by bedside nurses, it has become the preferred method by many nephrologists and intensivists, especially for the patient with septic shock. It should not be overlooked that the kidneys also may be the source of sepsis, making it important to exclude urinary tract infection—especially that associated with obstruction.

Nutritional Support

A thorough discussion of nutritional assessment and support is provided in Chapter 16. As with all other critically ill patients, there are two basic "truths" about nutrition. First, prolonged starvation (weeks to months) is fatal, and second, any patient can tolerate days without feeding. Almost every other aspect of nutritional support is argued. Even with the disagreements about nutrition, there are some common practices. For better or worse, nutritional support usually is withheld until hemodynamic stability is achieved (1 to 2 days). Most practitioners now favor the enteral route of support because it provides more complete nutrition, preserves gut mucosa, and favorably impacts immune function. In addition, enteral nutrition is substantially less expensive than intravenous supplementation and avoids the complications associated with central venous catheters and hypertonic glucose solutions required for effective parenteral nutrition. At this time, there is no compelling evidence to suggest that any particular enteral feeding formula or particular balance of components is superior to another for the patient with sepsis, although there is a growing body of evidence to suggest that diets rich in omega 3 fatty acids may be beneficial.

Simply stated, the current level of knowledge supports giving a balanced mixture of carbohydrate, protein, and lipid (based on the patient's estimated needs) via an enteral route after hemodynamic stability is achieved. For patients with prolonged (>5 days) gut dysfunction, parenteral nutrition may be indicated.

■ SUGGESTED READINGS

Bernard GR, Vincent JL, Laterre PF, et al. Efficacy and safety of recombinant human activated protein C for severe sepsis. *N Engl J Med*. 2001;344(10):699–709.

Dellinger RP, Levy MM, Carlet JM, et al. Surviving sepsis campaign: International guidelines for management of severe sepsis and septic shock 2008. *Crit Care Med*. 2008;36:296–327.

Rivers E, Nguyen B, Havstad S, et al. Early goal-directed therapy in the treatment of severe sepsis and septic shock. *N Engl J Med*. 2001;345(19):1368–1377.

Russell JA, Walley KR, Singer J, et al. Vasopressin versus norepinephrine infusion in patients with septic shock. *N Engl J Med*. 2008;358: 877–887.

Sprung C, Annane D, Keh D, et al. Hydrocortisone therapy for patients with septic shock. *N Engl J Med*. 2008;358:111–124.

Thompson BT. Glucose control in sepsis. *Clin Chest Med*. 2008;29: 713–720.

Wheeler AP. Recent developments in the diagnosis and management of severe sepsis. *Chest*. 2007;132:1967–1976.

Wheeler AP, Bernard GR. Acute lung injury and acute respiratory distress syndrome: A clinical review. *Lancet*. 2007;369:1553–1564.

Wheeler AP, Steingrub J, Schmidt GA, et al. A retrospective observational study of drotrecogin alfa (activated) in adults with severe sepsis: A comparison with a controlled clinical trial. *Crit Care Med*. 2008;36:14–23.

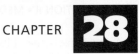
Thermal Disorders

■ NORMAL TEMPERATURE REGULATION

Body temperature is normally tightly regulated **1** between 36°C and 37.5°C. The net temperature is the result of the balance between heat generated and that lost. Heat dissipation occurs primarily by radiation and evaporation at the skin surface with a lesser contribution from exhaled gas. When heat production rises (e.g., exercise) or heat loss declines (e.g., environmental exposure), sweating, cutaneous vasodilation, and hyperventilation attempt to return temperature toward normal. Behavioral responses (shedding clothing, drinking cool liquids, cessation of exercise, etc.) also serve to lower the temperature. If compensatory mechanisms fail to keep pace with heat generation, body temperature rises. Significant reductions in body temperature are usually the result of exposure to low ambient temperatures. Vasoconstriction and behavioral responses (donning extra clothing, seeking a warm environment, etc.) attempt to counteract excessive heat loss, but exercise and shivering are the only effective compensatory methods for raising heat production. In general, the body is much better adapted to losing excess heat than it is to rapid heat production.

Aging impairs the ability to sense temperature extremes and blunts thermoregulation, thus the elderly are at highest risk for most temperature disorders. When cold, older patients are less able to generate heat because of decreased body weight and fat stores, decreased exercise and shivering capacity, and a reduced ability to vasoconstrict peripheral vessels. When hot, the elderly have impaired vasodilation. Older patients are also more likely to develop diseases that can either induce temperature changes (e.g., sepsis, hypothyroidism, renal failure) or impair their ability to respond to thermal challenges (e.g., peripheral vascular disease, depression, heart failure, and stroke). These very same conditions are likely to be treated with medications that further impair temperature sensing, regulation, and compensation. Finally, the elderly are most prone to financial barriers preventing environmental heating or cooling.

■ TEMPERATURE MEASUREMENT

Types of Measuring Devices

2 The technique used to measure temperature is critical in detecting fever or hypothermia. Mercury thermometers are usually unable to detect temperatures less than 34.4°C (94°F) or greater than 40.6°C (105°F) and fail to record values below the initial "shaken" level. Mercury thermometers respond slowly to temperature changes, making use of an electronic device or thermocouple (e.g., on a pulmonary artery catheter or indwelling urinary catheter) preferable when recording temperature extremes and rapid fluctuations. Infrared-sensing ear canal probes capable of accurate estimation of core temperature within seconds are now quite accurate. Plastic-strip thermometers have limited accuracy and recording range.

Sites of Measurement

Regardless of which site is chosen, it is important to be consistent in location and units. If throughout the day the temperature is sometimes measured orally, other times in the axilla, and occasionally using an indwelling pulmonary artery catheter and is sporadically recorded in Fahrenheit and other times Centigrade degrees, confusion about temperature trends is sure to ensue.

Measured oral temperatures are routinely less than their true value when respiratory rates exceed 18 breaths/min. Rectal temperatures avoid the artifacts of oral recordings because of varying respiratory rates, poor thermometer–patient contact, and aberrations caused by smoking or drinking hot or cold liquids. Although usually accurate, rectal temperatures may be spuriously low in patients with colonic impaction and may be slow to respond when rewarming the hypothermic patient if the temperature probe is lodged in cold stool. Axillary temperatures often underestimate core temperature because of poor thermometer–skin contact and wide differences between skin and core temperature. Obviously, a significantly elevated axillary temperature indicates fever. Esophageal measurement is an accurate "noninvasive" way to measure core temperature not commonly used because it requires specialized equipment. Infrared sensing of external ear canal temperature closely parallels core temperature and is not subject to influence by eating, drinking, or smoking as is oral temperature. The temperature of pulmonary artery blood may be continuously monitored using a thermistor-tipped pulmonary artery catheter and that of urine can be measured in the bladder using a thermistor-equipped indwelling catheter.

■ HYPOTHERMIA

Definition and Problems in Detection

Patients with uremia, hypothyroidism, malnutrition, and congestive heart failure often have mildly reduced (1°C to 2°C) basal temperatures. In these patients, a "normal" or slightly increased temperature may represent fever. Clinical hypothermia, a core temperature below 35°C, frequently escapes detection because symptoms are nonspecific and because most thermometers fail to record in the appropriate range.

Etiology

Hypothermia can occur at any time of the year and is usually multifactorial in origin. Outdoor adventurers and the destitute are at highest risk. Among the latter group, environmental exposure following **3** intoxication or a neurological event is a common sequence of events. It is important to know that extreme ambient cold is not necessary to cause hypothermia, and a substantial number of cases occur at mild temperatures. Hypothermia may also be caused by medications that (a) alter the perception of cold, (b) increase heat loss through vasodilation, or (c) inhibit heat generation. (Phenothiazines and barbiturates are frequent offenders.) Common contributing metabolic conditions include adrenal insufficiency, hypoglycemia, and myxedema. Because hypothyroidism decreases heat production, blunts the shivering response, and impairs temperature perception, it is an etiologic factor in up to 10% of cases of hypothermia. Hypopituitarism, severe sepsis, diabetic ketoacidosis, malnutrition, and mass lesions of the central nervous system (CNS) may also induce hypothermia. (The topic of hypothermic sepsis is discussed in Chapter 27.) An intact skin covering and the ability to vasoconstrict are essential to the regulation of core temperature. Hence, both burns and spinal cord injuries impair the ability to conserve heat. Hypothermia is commonly observed during and immediately after general anesthesia because of the exposure of the body to low ambient temperatures and the use of drugs that blunt the vasoconstrictor response (e.g., neuromuscular blockers).

Clinical Manifestations

Because physiologic changes are not precisely linked to specific temperature landmarks, it is best to classify hypothermia in broad categories: mild (32°C to 35°C), moderate (28°C to 32°C), and severe (<28°C). Vasoconstriction to conserve heat and shivering to generate heat are important initial compensatory mechanisms to prevent hypothermia. Unfortunately, both responses are blunted by a variety of underlying diseases or drugs and by profound hypothermia. Progressive hypothermia depresses metabolism of essentially all organ systems. Common physiologic events occurring during hypothermia are illustrated in Figure 28-1.

Cardiovascular

Mild hypothermia initially increases heart rate, blood pressure, and cardiac output through sympathetic stimulation. As temperature falls, heart rate and cardiac output decline as vasoconstriction maintains blood pressure. Moderate hypothermia decreases cardiac conduction and slows repolarization prolonging all measured electrocardiographic (ECG) intervals, eventually causing atrioventricular (AV) nodal blockade. Characteristic deformations of the J point (Osbourn waves) may be seen on the ECG but are neither sensitive nor specific indicators of core temperature. In advanced hypothermia, disproportionate reductions of cardiac output and blood pressure often result in metabolic acidosis. Myocardial irritability, manifest by any number of arrhythmias, increases at temperatures less than 28°C, but eventually asystole supervenes as temperatures fall below 20°C.

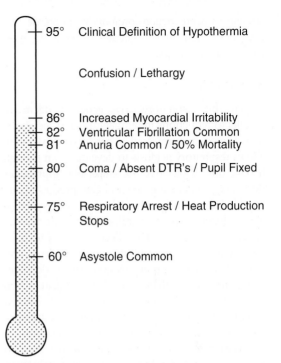

95°	Clinical Definition of Hypothermia
	Confusion / Lethargy
86°	Increased Myocardial Irritability
82°	Ventricular Fibrillation Common
81°	Anuria Common / 50% Mortality
80°	Coma / Absent DTR's / Pupil Fixed
75°	Respiratory Arrest / Heat Production Stops
60°	Asystole Common

■ **FIGURE 28-1** Benchmarks in hypothermia.

Neurological

Cerebral oxygen consumption is roughly halved for each 10°C (18°F) decline in temperature, greatly increasing the CNS's tolerance of reduced perfusion. Initial CNS responses to hypothermia include decreased respiratory drive, lethargy, confusion, and fatigue. As temperatures fall below 32°C, hallucinations and a reduced level of consciousness are seen. Coma usually develops when core temperatures fall below 28°C, and at slightly lower temperatures, the EEG may even become electrically silent. Concurrent with the loss of consciousness, deep tendon reflexes disappear and the pupils become fixed. Asymmetric neurological deficits rarely result from hypothermia, unless an independent CNS event (trauma or stroke) is the precipitant. Complete neurological recovery is possible following an hour or more of asystolic cardiac resuscitation of patients with hypothermia.

Renal

Early in hypothermia, the combination of increased cardiac output, vasoconstriction, and renal tubular unresponsiveness to antidiuretic hormone produces a "cold diuresis." The resulting large-volume dilute urine output (often with an osmolarity < 60 mOsm/L) leads to intravascular volume depletion. Later in the course of hypothermia, volume contraction, a low cardiac output, and arterial vasoconstriction profoundly decrease the renal blood flow. At temperatures below 27°C, most patients become anuric.

Respiratory

Hypercarbic respiratory drive generally decreases parallel to reductions in temperature and metabolic rate. Hence, a suppressed hypercarbic drive often allows respiratory acidosis to develop, even though hypoxic drive is preserved. As temperature approaches 30°C, oxygen consumption and CO_2 production are roughly halved. Early in hypothermia, the oxyhemoglobin dissociation curve shifts leftward, decreasing tissue oxygen delivery. This effect is offset by increasing lactic acidosis resulting from hypoxia and reduced cardiac output. Despite these derangements, net oxygen delivery is often adequate, given the profound reductions in consumption. Altered consciousness and an increased volume of respiratory secretions warrant a low threshold for intubation.

Unnecessary controversy exists with regard to interpreting arterial blood gas (ABG) values in hypothermia. Standard practice is to warm ABG samples to 37°C for analysis. When this is done, higher partial pressures of oxygen (PaO_2) and carbon dioxide ($PaCO_2$) and lower pH are observed than those that exist in vivo. ($PaCO_2$ and PaO_2 tensions are elevated by 4% to 7% per 1°C, and the pH is reduced by approx. 0.02 units per 1°C fall in temperature.) To the naïve physician, the reported ABG values may prompt poor clinical decisions: (a) the use of sodium bicarbonate to treat an artifactual acidosis, (b) overventilation in response to artifactual hypercarbia, and (c) withholding supplemental oxygen because reported PaO_2 values appear adequate. Hence, even though there is no need to "correct" the blood gas values for temperature, making sure that adequate oxygen is administered is important.

Hematologic

Hypothermia-induced diuresis decreases plasma volume, causing hemoconcentration (approx. 2% rise in hematocrit per °C) and increased serum viscosity. The resulting sluggish blood flow predisposes to deep venous thrombosis. Total leukocyte counts are usually normal or slightly increased, but isolated granulocytopenia may be seen. Thrombocytopenia, a common finding, is believed to result from platelet sequestration. Hypothermia impairs coagulation enzyme activities leading to impaired intrinsic and extrinsic clotting function.

Other Complications

Hyperglycemia is common as cold impairs pancreatic insulin release and increases counterregulatory hormone levels, including those of cortisol, epinephrine, glucagon, and growth hormone. Because it is relatively frequent and easily diagnosed and treated, hypothyroidism should be sought. Skeletal and cardiac muscle enzymes may increase in response to membrane dysfunction or rhabdomyolysis. Because hypothermia increases gastric acid production, it is sound to prescribe an acid-suppressing medication. Pancreatitis, ileus, and venous thrombosis are common. Although venous thrombosis often complicates hypothermia, subcutaneous heparin is poorly absorbed. Thus initially, pneumatic compression devices may be the best option for prophylaxis. Coexisting or precipitating infections (particularly pneumonia and meningitis) complicate as many as 40% of hypothermia cases. Cold-induced stiffness of the abdominal wall or neck often confounds clinical interpretation by simulating acute abdomen or meningitis.

Treatment

General Principles

Many hypothermia deaths are iatrogenic. Overly aggressive treatment, including excessive catecholamines, and prophylactic pacemaker insertion should be avoided; rewarming, close observation, gentle patient handling, and a search for underlying causes are key factors in successful therapy. Because patients with mild-to-moderate hypothermia already have maximal vasoconstriction, exogenous vasoconstrictor drugs often only serve to induce arrhythmias. With profound hypothermia (<28°C), vasoconstrictors may be useful to restore vascular tone. Fluids should be replaced as necessary to maintain blood pressure and vital organ perfusion. Central venous catheters are preferred for fluid and drug administration because peripheral intravenous lines are difficult to place (because of vasoconstriction) and allow only sluggish infusion. Catheters should not be advanced into the right atrium or ventricle, where they may stimulate life-threatening arrhythmias. (In most situations, it is probably best to avoid pulmonary artery catheterization.)

Serum amylase should be measured to detect pancreatitis—a complication seen in 20% to 30% of severe cases. Hypothyroidism, a common precipitant of hypothermia, should also be sought. Because many patients either have infection as a precipitating cause or develop an infection as a result of the hypothermia, it is prudent to obtain cultures of blood, urine, sputum, and spinal fluid if clinically indicated and then begin empiric antibiotics. Empiric coverage should probably include that for pneumonia and bacterial meningitis if suspected. (Fortunately, such regimens will treat essentially all skin and urinary tract infections.) A gently inserted nasogastric tube is useful in management to counter gut hypomotility and can be used for rewarming gastric lavage. Because many medications have prolonged actions in hypothermia, all drugs must be given cautiously, particularly those that are hepatically degraded. Finally, it should be emphasized that prolonged resuscitative efforts (hours) can prove successful in hypothermia. Therefore, patients with hypothermia must be rewarmed to temperatures exceeding 29°C (85°F) before death is declared.

Rewarming

The aggressiveness with which hypothermia is reversed depends not only on the depth of temperature depression but also on the physiologic manifestations. Caution must be exercised in reversing well-tolerated hypothermia. Because wet clothing can increase evaporative heat loss, it should be removed. Passive external rewarming with ordinary blankets is usually adequate if the temperature is higher than 33°C and typically results in temperature increases of 0.5°C to 2°C/h. Covering the head and neck is especially important, as these sites account for substantial heat loss. Historically, active external rewarming was controversial because it was believed to divert warm blood from the vital organs to the body surface and return very cold blood from the limbs to the central core. This phenomenon, known as "afterdrop," is likely to be unimportant provided external heating is continued until the core temperature normalizes. Active external rewarming can increase core temperature by as much as 1.5°C to 2.5°C/h. Advantages of this noninvasive method include wide availability of forced heated air devices. A risk of improperly conducted active external rewarming includes skin burns. Warm water immersion is largely impractical and makes access to the patient difficult in the event of an emergency.

Internal rewarming may be performed by several methods. The simplest, universally available techniques are the administration of heated IV fluids and, for the intubated patient, inhalation of warmed humidified air. It makes sense to use only warmed fluids; administration of room temperature or colder solutions will lower the temperature

further. The specific heat of water (1 kcal/kg/°C) is slightly higher than that of the human body (0.83 kcal/kg/°C), thus administration of heated IV saline is a relatively efficient warming method. Obviously this technique is limited by the maximum volume and temperature of fluid that can be administered. Because fluids can only be safely heated to 40°C to 42°C, each liter infused raises the patient's temperatures less than 1°C. Because it contains less water, warmed, fully humidified oxygen delivers heat more slowly, raising core temperature well less than 1°C/h. Although safe to deliver gas at temperatures up to 45°C, most commercial heaters limit gas temperatures at 41°C to 42°C.

Lavages of the stomach, bladder, colon, and pleural spaces have all been reported as potential methods of internal rewarming, but their effectiveness and safety are unknown. Peritoneal lavage with warmed fluid is an attractive option because it may raise core temperature as quickly as 4°C/h and can be instituted rapidly. Internal rewarming using dialysis or hemofiltration machines is a safe, effective, widely available method that can be rapidly instituted. Typically, temperature increases of 2°C to 3°C/h can be achieved. Cardiopulmonary bypass and mediastinal lavage are the most rapid rewarming methods (7°C to 10°C/h), but for obvious logistical and safety reasons, they are not the techniques of choice for most patients.

Patients with Cardiovascular Instability

The primary therapeutic goal in patients with life-threatening arrhythmias should be rewarming the core quickly to temperatures greater than 29°C, a threshold below which defibrillation and antiarrhythmic therapy are often ineffective. There are no controlled trials demonstrating superiority or even effectiveness of one antiarrhythmic over others. Transvenous pacemakers increase myocardial irritability and the risk of ventricular fibrillation. Therefore, they should not be used in the absence of a clear indication and only after transthoracic pacing has failed. For the profoundly cold patient suffering cardiac arrest, cardiopulmonary bypass represents an attractive option in which perfusion and rewarming occur simultaneously.

Diagnosis of Death

Resuscitative efforts lasting even hours can prove successful in hypothermia and survival after core temperatures as low as 14°C have been reported.

Therefore, unless there are obvious other lethal injuries or the victim is frozen solid, patients with hypothermia should be rewarmed to temperatures greater than 29°C before death is declared.

■ HYPERTHERMIA

Causes of Temperature Elevation

In the intensive care unit (ICU), sudden temperature elevations usually signal infection, making it prudent to perform a directed physical examination and, if indicated, obtain appropriate cultures and institute empirical antibiotics. Although infection is the most common explanation, several life-threatening noninfectious causes of fever are frequently overlooked (Table 28-1). Interestingly, fever in ICU patients rarely responds well to acetaminophen; nonsteroidal anti-inflammatory drugs (e.g., ibuprofen) are much more effective.

■ SYNDROMES OF EXTREME HYPERTHERMIA

Regardless of etiology, high temperatures injure cells. In humans, as little as an hour of core temperatures greater than 40°C (105°F) *may* damage the CNS, and temperatures higher than 50°C (120°F) can cause injury within minutes. Hence, high fevers should be reduced to safer levels as quickly as possible. On the other hand, there are little, if any, data to suggest that reducing temperatures below 40°C is routinely necessary and could even be detrimental depending on the method used to lower the temperature.

Four noninfectious conditions producing high fever in the ICU include (a) classic or nonexertional heatstroke, (b) exertional heatstroke, (c) malignant hyperthermia, and (d) neuroleptic malignant syndrome (NMS). All are associated with dramatic elevations in core temperature and demand rapid recognition and therapy. Clinical features, etiology,

and treatment of these diseases are contrasted in Table 28-2. The related problems of anticholinergic and stimulant toxicity and serotonin syndrome are discussed in Chapter 33 and that of thyroid storm in Chapter 32.

Nonexertional (Classic) Heatstroke

Definition and Clinical Presentation

Classic heatstroke is a potentially lethal disorder that should be suspected in patients exposed to **4** high ambient temperatures who exhibit the triad of (a) fever higher than 40°C (105°F), (b) hot dry skin, and (c) CNS dysfunction. The cognitive abnormalities may include lethargy, delirium, seizures, cerebellar dysfunction, and coma. An antecedent history of physical activity is usually absent. Tragic cases of children locked in automobiles for just minutes illustrate how rapidly heatstroke can occur when ambient temperatures reach 43°C to 54°C. Tachycardia and tachypnea are nearly universal, and hypotension is seen in about a quarter of victims. Other organ systems (renal, hematologic) are frequently affected, but their involvement is not necessary for diagnosis.

Mechanisms

Usually, when temperature rises, cardiac output increases, cutaneous vasodilation occurs, blood flow is redirected from the core to the surface, and sweating begins. Evaporation of sweat normally is responsible for more than 50% of heat dissipation, but high humidity and poor air circulation impair the efficiency of this process. The huge capacity for heat dissipation is evidenced by the facts that evaporation of less than 2 mL of sweat results in more than a kilocalorie of heat loss and humans are capable of up to 2 L of sweat production per hour. When compensatory mechanisms cannot shed sufficient heat, temperature rises.

TABLE 28-1 NONINFECTIOUS CAUSES OF FEVER

Heatstroke	Pheochromocytoma
Neuroleptic malignant syndrome	Status epilepticus
Malignant hyperthermia	Vasculitis
Drug allergy	Crystalline arthritis (gout and pseudogout)
Transfusion reaction	α-Agonist drugs
Autonomic insufficiency	Anticholinergic toxicity
Malignancy	Salicylate intoxication
Stroke or CNS hemorrhage	Lithium intoxication
Alcohol withdrawal/delirium tremens	Serotonin syndrome
Hyperthyroidism	Stimulant (cocaine, amphetamine) ingestion

CNS, central nervous system.

TABLE 28-2 FEATURES OF HEATSTROKE, NMS, AND MALIGNANT HYPERTHERMIA

FEATURE	MALIGNANT HYPERTHERMIA	NEUROLEPTIC MALIGNANT SYNDROME	CLASSIC HEATSTROKE	EXERTIONAL HEATSTROKE
Usual age	Children and young adults	Young adults	Elderly	Any age
Common precipitants	Succinylcholine, halogenated anesthetics	Neuroleptics	Diuretics, tricyclics, anticholinergics	Hot environment Confining garb
Mechanism	Abnormal muscle calcium metabolism	Reduced brain dopamine levels	Impaired heat loss	Impaired heat loss
Therapy	Remove offending drug Dantrolene	Remove offending drug Dantrolene Bromocriptine	External cooling	External cooling Fluid replacement

In the past, heatstroke was believed to be a simple process of direct cellular damage from high temperatures, but in recent years, it has become clear that mechanistically the disease is much more complex. In fact, heatstroke shares the three cardinal pathophysiologic features of severe sepsis: activation of clotting by expression of tissue factor, inhibition of endogenous fibrinolysis, and generation of proinflammatory cytokines like tumor necrosis factor and interleukin-1. Collectively, these processes lead to endothelial cell damage and microvascular thrombosis resulting in organ failures.

Causes

Nonexertional heatstroke can occur in anyone but is most common among the elderly because of five factors that impair ability to dissipate heat, including (a) decreased sweat production, (b) decreased skin blood flow, (c) limited cardiac compensation, (d) impaired hypothalamic regulation, and (e) use of drugs impairing heat loss. Old, poor, and urban residents are at the highest risk by virtue of the fact that they may not be able to afford to cool their homes and do not feel safe enough to leave doors and windows ajar.

Among younger people, prescription or illicit drug use is a common contributing factor. CNS tumors, stroke, and certain drugs (e.g., cocaine, ecstasy [MDMA], lysergic acid diethylamide [LSD], amphetamines) may disrupt hypothalamic heat regulation. Other drugs may produce heatstroke through increased heat production (e.g., cocaine, tricyclics, lithium, or alcohol withdrawal), by

impairing heat loss (e.g., anticholinergics, phenothiazines, diphenhydramine, diuretics, and tricyclic antidepressants) or by a combination of these two mechanisms. Impaired heat loss may also be seen with extensive burns or skin diseases (e.g., scleroderma) and with the use of occlusive dressings or ointments that cover large skin areas.

Laboratory Studies

ABGs typically reveal a pure respiratory alkalosis. Occasionally, lactic acidosis is superimposed, but it is much more common among patients with *exertional* heatstroke. Hypophosphatemia and hypokalemia are frequent. Although rhabdomyolysis may occur and result in hyperphosphatemia, hypocalcemia, hyperkalemia, and elevations in creatinine phosphokinase (CPK) and serum aspartate aminotransferase (AST), rhabdomyolysis is much more likely with exertional heatstroke. Although most patients have subclinical coagulation changes (e.g., elevated d-dimers, reduced protein C levels), overt disseminated intravascular coagulation is seen in only about 10% of patients.

Complications and Prognosis

Heatstroke can result in the failure of any organ system and unfortunately, up to 20% of heatstroke victims sustain permanent brain injury. Acute respiratory distress syndrome, pancreatitis, hepatic failure, and bowel ischemia are all well described. Of all organs, the kidney is at highest risk of injury from ensuing dehydration, hyperuricemia, and rhabdomyolysis. However, renal injury is much more common in exertional heatstroke because of the higher incidence of volume depletion and rhabdomyolysis.

Treatment

With the exception of therapy to rapidly lower temperature, the treatment of heatstroke is supportive. Core temperature should be lowered to below 39°C as quickly as possible. The most effective method of cooling is combining convection and evaporation, not conduction. Spraying unclothed victims with tepid water (15°C to 20°C) and using a fan to promote evaporation cools most patients to less than 40°C within 60 min. Ice packing or cold water immersion produces conductive heat loss rapidly but has major limitations apart from the difficulty of implementation. Attempts at conductive cooling result in intense peripheral vasoconstriction and shivering, which serve to sustain core temperature. Now, a variety of commercially available intravascular and surface cooling devices are used that reliably lower the body temperature, but often at substantial cost. In addition, there is no evidence that such devices are safer or yield superior clinical outcomes to lower technology approaches. Regardless of the cooling method, patients should be monitored closely for temperature rebound after initial control.

Fluid deficits in adults with classic heatstroke average just 2 L, but the extent of volume depletion is highly variable. If hypotension is present, more aggressive fluid replacement, perhaps guided by central venous pressure monitoring, should be undertaken. Cooling the infused fluids below room temperature, perhaps as low as 4°C, is a simple adjunctive method of temperature reduction. α-agonists and atropine should be avoided if possible because drug-induced peripheral vasoconstriction further impairs heat loss. Dantrolene has been shown to be ineffective.

Exertional Heatstroke

Definition and Clinical Presentation

In distinction to its nonexertional counterpart, exertional heatstroke is diagnosed when the triad of (a) fever higher than 40°C (105°F), (b) hot dry skin, and (c) CNS dysfunction occur in the setting of strenuous physical exertion.

Causes

Exertional heatstroke is usually the result of vigorous physical exercise by an otherwise healthy person in a hot humid environment; however, exercise alone can initiate the syndrome. Victims

of exertional heatstroke are commonly involved in activities they continue long after perceiving the sensation of extreme heat (e.g., military training, firefighting, law enforcement, athletic activity). Furthermore, these patients often are wearing heavy or restrictive equipment that impairs heat loss. In addition to environmental stress, predisposing factors include dehydration and lack of training and acclimatization. In recent years, several high-profile deaths have been linked to the concurrent use of stimulants (e.g., cocaine, amphetamines) or over-the-counter weight-loss drugs (e.g., ephedra) during athletic training. Rarely, occult sickle cell trait and sickle C disease have been discovered in apparently healthy, African American military recruits after they suffered exertional heatstroke.

Clinical Features

Clinical features include fever, altered mental status, hypotension, tachycardia, and tachypnea. Laboratory data frequently suggest a diagnosis of rhabdomyolysis with elevated AST, CPK, and myoglobinuria. Renal function tests are often abnormal as a result of dehydration and rhabdomyolysis. Hemoconcentration can be profound and tends to be more frequent and severe in exertional than classic heatstroke because of the greater fluid losses. Thus, fluid replacement using cooled isotonic crystalloid is indicated. When intravascular volume status is uncertain, monitoring the central venous pressure can be helpful.

Treatment

The best treatment of exertional heatstroke is its prevention through acclimatization, appropriate dress, modification of work or exercise schedules, and adequate hydration. An established disease therapy includes discontinuing activity, moving the patients to a cooler location, rehydration, and external cooling. As with nonexertional heatstroke, removal of clothing and spraying the patients with tepid water appears to be the most effective method to rapidly lower the temperature. Blowing a fan across the disrobed victim accelerates evaporative heat loss. Even with rapid lowering of body temperature, mortality rates as high as 10% have been reported. Dantrolene is not effective.

Malignant Hyperthermia

Causes

Malignant hyperthermia is a rare but dramatic heritable disorder caused by excessive heat generation resulting from dysfunctional calcium channels in skeletal muscle. The genetic predisposition is expressed following exposure to halogenated inhalational anesthetics and/or depolarizing neuromuscular blocking drugs. Halothane and succinylcholine cause more than 80% of all cases, although other inhaled anesthetics, neuromuscular blockers, ketamine, and phencyclidine (PCP) have been implicated. Malignant hyperthermia is distinctly more common among young people, especially those with a history of congenital myotonia or a muscular dystrophy. (More than half of all cases occur in children <15 years old.)

Clinical Diagnosis

The diagnosis is a clinical one triggered by the occurrence of (a) muscular rigidity, (b) high (commonly 41°C to 45°C) and rapidly rising fever (often 2°C/min), and (c) acidosis, occurring in an appropriate clinical setting. Temperature may begin rising within minutes of drug exposure, although hyperthermia can be delayed up to 12 h. Therefore, the condition should be considered in the differential diagnosis of early, severe postoperative fever. Extreme muscle activity massively increases oxygen consumption and CO_2 production; the resulting tissue hypoxia eventually leads to lactate formation. Hence, a combined metabolic and respiratory acidosis is frequently seen. Tachycardia, tachypnea, ventricular arrhythmias, and skin mottling are common clinical signs. Phosphate, potassium, uric acid, and muscle enzymes (CPK, lactic dehydrogenase [LDH], and aldolase) are routinely elevated as a result of rhabdomyolysis.

Complications

Massive increases in metabolic rate cause hypercapnia, hypoxemia, and hypoglycemia in a large percentage of cases. When not promptly treated, malignant hyperthermia can produce severe muscle damage with necrosis and soft tissue calcification. Renal injury resulting from circulating myoglobin may be attenuated or even averted by alkalinizing the urine and by maintaining blood pressure and renal tubular flow. High cardiac output with low systemic vascular resistance may result in hypotension, but dopamine or α-agonists should be used cautiously because vasoconstriction may retard heat loss. Tissue hypoxia is more intense in malignant hyperthermia than in heatstroke or NMS, accounting for a higher incidence of cardiac arrhythmias and muscular damage.

Direct thermal toxicity may cause neuronal death. The hippocampus and the Purkinje cell layer of the cerebellum are particularly vulnerable, accounting for a high incidence of movement disorders after recovery. Prophylactic anticonvulsants may prevent the seizures that occur in many cases. Likewise, histamine blockers or proton pump inhibitors are indicated to counteract the tendency for GI hemorrhage. Although transaminase elevations are common, hepatic necrosis is infrequent. Late hematologic effects include increased leukocyte and platelet counts, coagulopathy resulting from impaired liver function, and direct thermal activation of platelets and clotting factors.

Treatment

Malignant hyperthermia is a true emergency with mortality proportional to the magnitude and duration of peak temperature. Even brief delays in therapy may prove fatal. Temperature should be continuously monitored until it stabilizes below 39°C. Exposure to potentially offending volatile anesthetics and paralytics must be stopped as soon as feasible, and it is wise to terminate any operative procedure if possible. In the exceptional case where a surgical procedure cannot be aborted, drugs believed to be safe include nitrous oxide, barbiturates, benzodiazepines, pancuronium, and opiates. Ventilation with 100% oxygen should be started immediately. Direct external cooling with a fanned water mist dissipates heat while awaiting definitive therapy with dantrolene. Shivering caused by external cooling can be controlled with benzodiazepines and nondepolarizing neuromuscular blockers.

Dantrolene stops the runaway heat generation by inhibiting calcium release from sarcoplasmic reticulum. Doses of 2.5 mg/kg should be initiated swiftly and can be repeated at 5-min intervals as long as hyperthermia persists. If available, a central venous catheter should be used for administration to avoid phlebitis induced by the strongly alkaline solution. As a rule, improvement occurs quickly if recognition and treatment are prompt. (Failure to improve with doses of 10 mg/kg should raise questions about the diagnosis.) An additional infusion of 10 mg/kg given over a 24-h period has been advocated after initial temperature control is achieved. By inhibiting calcium release, dantrolene can cause muscle weakness, perhaps even sufficient to impair spontaneous ventilation. Thus, an extra measure of caution should be exercised in extubating patients treated with dantrolene. Corticosteroids and traditional antipyretics are ineffective.

Because patients with malignant hyperthermia usually have normal intravascular volume, fluid requirements are minimal. Although debated, fluid loading to promote urine flow and serum alkalinization with sodium bicarbonate may be useful to prevent myoglobinuric renal tubular injury. Hyperkalemia can be treated initially in a conventional manner using sodium bicarbonate for pH correction, insulin and glucose to transfer potassium into cells, and calcium to stabilize membranes (see Chapter 13). Nonhyperkalemia-related arrhythmias are best treated by controlling the underlying disorder, although lidocaine and β-blockers may be useful. Because this disorder involves calcium metabolism abnormalities, it is commonly recommended to avoid calcium channel blockers.

6 Neuroleptic Malignant Syndrome (Drug-induced Central Hyperthermia)

Definition

Like malignant hyperthermia, NMS is a rare drug-associated hyperthermic syndrome characterized by fever, muscle rigidity, and altered mentation and frequently accompanied by pulmonary dysfunction and autonomic instability. It differs, however, regarding precipitating factors, underlying mechanism, time course, prognosis, and patient substrate. The differential diagnosis of neuroleptic NMS includes heatstroke, thyroid storm, tetanus, pheochromocytoma, anticholinergic or lithium toxicity, delirium tremens, monoamine oxidase (MAO) inhibitor crisis, and the serotonin syndrome.

Causes

The precise mechanism of NMS is unknown, but its genesis involves some combination of drug-induced changes in dopamine levels in the brain and skeletal muscle of susceptible individuals. Two lines of clinically relevant evidence support this conclusion. The first is that antipsychotic drugs that decrease dopamine's inhibitory effects on serotonin-mediated heat generation or that directly alter brain serotonin levels have been associated with the condition. The second line of evidence is that abrupt withdrawal of anti-Parkinsonian agents (dopaminergic agents), such as levodopa–carbidopa and amantadine, may precipitate the disease. The association of NMS with discontinuation of dopaminergic drugs is mechanistically interesting because dopaminergic drugs not only act in the brain but also have direct muscle-relaxing properties. Oddly, there are no reports of NMS following abrupt cessation of prolonged dopamine infusions. For reasons that are unclear, dehydration and extreme muscular activity predispose to NMS.

The association of NMS with neuroleptics is unarguable and the typical antipsychotics (e.g., haloperidol, chlorpromazine, fluphenazine) are thought to be more likely to cause the syndrome than are the atypical antipsychotics (e.g., clozapine, olanzapine, risperidone). Without a doubt, NMS is a very odd disease; it occurs in only a tiny minority of those exposed to neuroleptics. Patients developing the disease when treated with one antipsychotic are unlikely to manifest the syndrome when treated with another, despite an ostensibly identical mechanism of action, and there does not appear to be a clear dose–risk relationship. Furthermore, NMS can occur at any time a patient is receiving a neuroleptic and has even been reported up to 3 weeks after discontinuing therapy. Moreover, although many cases have been identified following an increased neuroleptic dosing, there are numerous reports linking NMS to antipsychotic withdrawal. Interestingly, even though abrupt changes in neuroleptic doses are routine in the ICU, NMS has rarely been reported. Mysteriously, NMS even shares some features with malignant hyperthermia. Many NMS victims have been found to have abnormalities in skeletal muscle calcium release, and most respond to the calcium modulator dantrolene. Although the degree of crossover between malignant hyperthermia and NMS is unknown, some patients who have had malignant hyperthermia undergo uneventful therapy with neuroleptic drugs.

Clinical Features

There are no rigid criteria for the diagnosis of NMS. Rapid onset of fever higher than 38°C, muscle rigidity, delirium, tachycardia, hypertension, diaphoresis, and extrapyramidal movements characterize the syndrome. In most cases, extrapyramidal symptoms antedate the fever and autonomic abnormalities. As is evident, clinical features alone may not distinguish this syndrome from malignant hyperthermia (especially in a postoperative patient treated with haloperidol). Symptoms develop over 24 to 72 h and usually last about 10 days, although they can persist up to 6 weeks. Even with optimal treatment, NMS is fatal in 20% to 30% of cases and is frequently complicated by rhabdomyolysis, acute myocardial infarction, and persistent movement disorders.

Laboratory

Laboratory abnormalities are all nonspecific and include leukocytosis and elevated values for CPK, creatinine, and liver transaminases. Lumbar puncture and head computed tomography are not diagnostic but may be necessary to exclude mass lesions and infections from the differential diagnosis.

Treatment

The initial treatment of NMS requires stopping the suspected offending drug and beginning external cooling. All neuroleptics and dopamine antagonists, such as metoclopramide, should be withheld at least until the disease abates. Intravascular fluids should be administered based on estimated deficits, blood pressure, pulse and urine output values, or central venous pressure measurements. The effectiveness of pharmacologic therapy for NMS is far less certain than for malignant hyperthermia, and there are no comparative trials of the advocated treatments. Dantrolene (2.5 mg/kg IV every 5 min up to approx. 10 mg/kg) has been recommended until hyperthermia and excessive muscular activity are corrected. After initial symptom control, a daily infusion of 10 mg/kg has been suggested. Unfortunately, there are little, if any, data about the optimal duration of therapy, and high doses or prolonged courses of dantrolene can cause hepatotoxicity. Dantrolene given by peripheral IV is almost certain to cause chemical phlebitis because of its profound alkaline pH. Bromocriptine, a dopamine agonist, in doses of 2.5 to 10 mg given at 6-h intervals, has been reported as an effective alternative to dantrolene. Bromocriptine controls rigidity and fever within hours, but dosing may be limited by its most common side effects, hypotension and delirium. Success has also been reported using combinations of the anti-Parkinson's drugs levodopa–carbidopa and amantadine in typical doses.

■ SUGGESTED READINGS

Halloran LL, Bernard DW. Management of drug-induced hyperthermia. *Curr Opin Pediatr.* 2004;16:211–215.

Kempainen RR, Brunette DD. The evaluation and management of accidental hypothermia. *Respir Care.* 2004;49:192–205.

Krause T, Gerberhagen MU, Fiege M, et al. Dantrolene: A review of its pharmacology, therapeutic use and new developments. *Anaesthesia.* 2004;59:364–373.

Mallet ML. Pathophysiology of accidental hypothermia. *Q J Med.* 2002;95:775–785.

Stowell KM. Malignant hyperthermia: A pharmacogenetic disorder *Pharmacogenomics.* 2008;9:1657–1672.

Strawn JR, Keck PE, Caroff SN. Neuroleptic malignant syndrome. *Am J Psychiatry.* 2007;164:870–876.

Sucholeiki R. Heatstroke. *Semin Neurol.* 2005;25:307–314.

Acute Kidney Injury and Renal Replacement Therapy

The kidney's excretory function can be replaced mechanically and its metabolic functions can be compensated by the actions of the lung or liver or replaced by drugs. Therefore, the kidney is the only major organ whose total failure is not necessarily fatal. Yet the development of acute kidney injury (AKI) in a critically ill patient is associated with significantly higher morbidity and mortality. A greater appreciation of the importance of maintaining adequate perfusion and avoiding nephrotoxic compounds might have reduced the incidence and severity of AKI, but for an aging population with an increasing incidence of diabetes and hypertension. Fortunately, the safety and efficiency of renal replacement therapy (RRT) has improved permitting treatment of patients who previously would have not been candidates.

■ INDICES OF RENAL FUNCTION AND INJURY

Urine Volume

Urine volume usually tracks kidney perfusion, whereas urine specific gravity and osmolality parallel concentrating ability (tubular function). Therefore, renal blood flow is probably adequate in nonoliguric patients and patients producing concentrated urine are unlikely to have significant tubular damage. However, it is important to note that concentrated urine does not imply normal perfusion; the standard response of the kidney to inadequate perfusion is to concentrate the urine. Certain calculated indices have long been used to distinguish problems of perfusion from those of tubular dysfunction but all of these measures have a much lower specificity than commonly believed (Table 29-1).

Blood Urea Nitrogen

Because the kidney is the primary filter of nitrogenous waste, blood urea nitrogen (BUN) and creatinine track renal function, but do so imperfectly. The extreme variation of urea load and the ability of the proximal tubule to absorb filtered urea render BUN less reliable than creatinine for this purpose. For example, rhabdomyolysis, increased protein ingestion, gastrointestinal (GI) bleeding, and corticosteroid use may all increase the BUN, whereas liver disease, low protein diets, or low

1

TABLE 29-1   LABORATORY INDICES IN ACUTE RENAL FAILURE

	PRERENAL	INTRARENAL
BUN/creatinine	>10:1	Approx. 10:1
Urinary Na⁺ concentration	<20 mEq/L	>40 mEq/L
Urine specific gravity	>1.020	1.010–1.020
Urine osmolality	>500 mOsm/L	<300–400 mOsm/L
Urine creatinine/plasma creatinine	>40	<20
Urine Na⁺/creatinine clearance	<1	>2
Na⁺ clearance/creatinine clearance (FeNa)	<1	>1
Urine sediment	Normal or hyaline casts	Active with granular casts

muscle mass decrease BUN. In addition, when urine flow declines because of volume depletion, the BUN rises disproportionately, as it is reabsorbed along with sodium and water. Conversely, when glomerular filtration rate (GFR) is increased such as in pregnancy and during aggressive volume resuscitation, the BUN declines. As general guidelines, the BUN increases by 10 to 15 mg/dL/day and creatinine by 1 to 2.5 mg/dL/day after abrupt renal shutdown. The serum potassium (K^+) usually rises less than 0.5 mEq mg/dL/day, and bicarbonate (HCO_3^-) falls by about 1 mEq/L day. Under the catabolic stress of burns, trauma, rhabdomyolysis, steroids, severe sepsis, or starvation, the rates of change of these parameters may be doubled.

Creatinine

In contrast to BUN, daily creatinine production is more consistent. Patients with low muscle mass from starvation, limb amputation, or neuromuscular disease and those with a protein-restricted diet, have on average lower creatinine values than patients with conventional diets and body composition. A rising creatinine indicates that the rate of production exceeds its combined clearance by filtration and proximal tubular secretion because the kidney does not reabsorb or metabolize creatinine. For these reasons, a stable elevation of creatinine implies that a new steady state has been achieved at a decreased GFR. The best method to determine GFR is a 24-h urine collection but logistical problems, the inherent delay imposed, and the high incidence of severe oliguria usually make this impractical. Consequently, GFR is typically estimated using the Cockcroft–Gault equation: GFR (mL/min) = [(140 − age in years) × weight in

kilograms]/(Serum creatinine × 72) or the more complex modification of diet in renal disease (MDRD) equation: GFR (mL/min/1.73 m²) = 170 × (Serum creatinine)$^{-0.999}$ × age (years)$^{-0.176}$ × 0.762 (if female) × 1.8 (if African American) × BUN (mg/dL)$^{-0.170}$ × albumin (g/dL)$^{0.318}$. Fortunately, both of these equations are widely available in online calculator sites.

It is important to understand that because serum creatinine increases lag behind the deterioration in actual GFR, kidney function cannot be reliably assessed until creatinine stabilizes. For this reason, drug doses are usually overestimated by the calculated GFR during the evolution of AKI. Thus, if a patient becomes anuric or severely oliguric, it is probably best to estimate drug dosing based on a GFR of zero. Without intervention, creatinine usually plateaus at 12 to 15 mg/dL, depending on catabolic state. (Rhabdomyolysis can cause creatinine to exceed this value.)

Normally, about 15% of urinary creatinine is secreted by the proximal tubule (a higher fraction in renal failure). As a result, drugs that compete with creatinine for tubular secretion like trimethoprim and cimetidine may increase serum creatinine despite a preserved GFR. One creatinine assay method (alkaline picrate) is subject to interference by acetoacetate, flucytosine, and cefoxitin, causing artifactual elevations in measured serum creatinine.

Cystatin C

Because creatinine and BUN are flawed, better measures of function have been sought. Cystatin C, a proteinase inhibitor synthesized and released at a nearly constant rate by all nucleated cells, is an

TABLE 29-2 RIFLE CRITERIA FOR ACUTE KIDNEY INJURY

STAGE	GFR CRITERIA	URINE OUTPUT CRITERIA	ASSOCIATED MORTALITY RATE
Risk	1.5-Fold creatinine increase or GFR decrease >25%	<0.5 mL/kg/h for 6 h	20%–40%
Injury	2-Fold creatinine increase or GFR decrease >50%	<0.5 mL/kg/h for 12 h	40%–50%
Failure	3-Fold creatinine increase or GFR decrease >75% or Creatinine ≥4 mg/dL (with acute rise >0.5 mg/dL)	<0.3 mL/kg/h for 24 h or Anuria for 12 h	55%–75%
Loss	Persistent failure for >4 weeks		
ESRD	End-stage renal disease		

attractive option. This compound is filtered by the glomerulus and is completely metabolized by the proximal renal tubule without secretion or reabsorption. Hence, increases in serum levels correlate well with declines in GFR. In addition, the rise in serum cystatin C after kidney injury may precede increases in serum creatinine by 1 to 2 days providing an early marker of injury. The major drawback of cystatin C currently is limited assay availability.

New Markers of Kidney Injury

In an attempt to identify very early AKI and better localize the site of injury within the kidney, several new biomarkers have been investigated. Three of these compounds, Interleukin 18 (IL-18), kidney injury molecule 1 (KIM-1), and neutrophil gelatinase-associated lipocalin (NGAL) demonstrate promise. After renal insult, all three compounds have been identified in serum well before creatinine or BUN become abnormal.

■ DEFINITIONS OF ACUTE KIDNEY INJURY

Innumerable definitions of "renal failure" have been used causing difficulty interpreting the literature in this field. Traditionally, a rise in creatinine of 0.5 mg/dL or a doubling of creatinine or (halving of calculated GFR) has been considered clinically significant. Oliguria has been defined variably as urine production less than 400 mL/day or less than 0.5 mL/kg/h. The mortality of oliguric renal failure is at least twofold greater than nonoliguric failure, and for survivors time to recover function is shorter among nonoliguric patients. Reasons for these observations are uncertain but probably

reflect differences in severity of AKI and perhaps etiology. Unfortunately, little data suggest that "converting" oliguric to nonoliguric renal failure using diuretics alters outcome.

In the last few years, the development of a standardized staging system, RIFLE, has been useful. The RIFLE system (Table 29-2) uses calculated GFR and urine output to classify patients along a continuum of risk, injury, or failure, and then fine-tunes the duration of failure as either persistent loss (>4 weeks) or end-stage disease (>3 months). The system has been validated in a variety of critically ill populations. Recent data suggest that perhaps even smaller changes in creatinine (0.3 mg/dL) than those of the RIFLE risk group are associated with an increased length of stay needed for RRT and risk of death.

■ ETIOLOGY OF ACUTE KIDNEY INJURY

Approximately, 20% of critically ill patients develop AKI—an incidence five times that of the general hospital population. The risk of developing AKI is highest among patients who have underlying renal impairment. Roughly, 25% of these patients or 5% of all ICU residents will receive RRT. The etiology of AKI differs drastically, depending on whether the condition develops in or outside the hospital and varies with the chronicity of the process. For example, poorly controlled hypertension and diabetes mellitus are the most common etiologies of slowly developing renal failure outside the hospital. When *AKI* develops outside the hospital, glomerulonephritis (GN), vasculitis, and obstructive uropathy are common causes. By contrast, AKI developing in the hospital is much more likely to

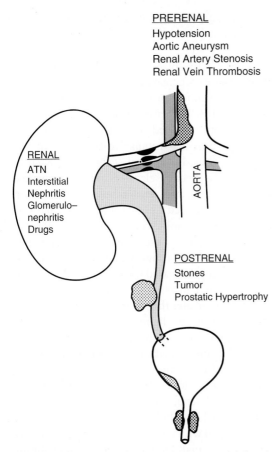

PRERENAL
Hypotension
Aortic Aneurysm
Renal Artery Stenosis
Renal Vein Thrombosis

RENAL
ATN
Interstitial
Nephritis
Glomerulo–
nephritis
Drugs

AORTA

POSTRENAL
Stones
Tumor
Prostatic Hypertrophy

■ **FIGURE 29-1** Common causes of acute renal failure in the intensive care unit.

be the result of hypoperfusion or drug toxicity—often now on a background of mild chronic renal dysfunction.

AKI may result from a variety of causes acting through one of three common mechanisms: (a) hypoperfusion (prerenal), (b) outlet obstruction (postrenal), or (c) parenchymal disease (intrarenal) (Fig. 29-1).

Prerenal Failure

2 Hypoperfusion accounts for half of all cases of AKI; hence, prevention of hypotension or its rapid reversal is probably the most effective therapy. Although prolonged ischemia alone may lead to AKI, in most cases the etiology is multifactorial (i.e., severe sepsis, drugs, and hypotension). In general, mean arterial pressures less than 60 to 70 mm Hg for longer than 30 min risk injury, particularly if there is accompanying hypoxia. Hypoperfusion results from circulatory failure, hypotension, vascular obstruction (e.g., renal artery stenosis, vasculitis, embolization

of bland clot or cholesterol or maldistribution of cardiac output (CO), as in severe sepsis. The hepatorenal syndrome (see Chapter 31) and the renal response to positive end-expiratory pressure (PEEP) mimic prerenal physiology by redistributing blood flow away from the filtering glomerulus.

Marked increases in intra-abdominal pressure (abdominal compartment syndrome), usually greater than 25 mm Hg, resulting from the accumulation of ascitic fluid or blood, can also produce a prerenal state. It is uncertain if elevated abdominal pressures lessen urine flow by reducing CO through impaired venous return; by obstructing kidney arterial supply or venous outflow; or by compressing the kidney parenchyma directly. It appears unlikely that ureteral obstruction is etiologic because placement of ureteral stents does not improve flow. Regardless of mechanism, when elevated pressures are responsible for oliguria, decompressive laparotomy or paracentesis is associated with a near immediate restoration of urine flow.

Indicators of Intravascular Volume Status

Orthostatic blood pressure is a helpful clinical measure of intravascular volume status in healthy persons. However, few critically ill patients can be tested in this fashion, and autonomic insufficiency renders such changes less reliable in patients who are diabetic, elderly, or bedridden. Dry mucous membranes, skin laxity, and absence of axillary moisture may also be clues to hypovolemia. Unfortunately, these signs, too, prove unreliable in patients with hyperpnea or advanced age. For the hospitalized patient, a persistently negative fluid balance supports a prerenal diagnosis.

Response to fluid challenge is the diagnostic hallmark of prerenal disease. The rate and volume of fluid administered must be customized taking into account the estimated magnitude of the deficit, and cardiopulmonary reserves. Repeated boluses of 15 to 20 mL/kg are typically administered until deemed futile or function improves. Because noninvasive methods to assess fluid status (chest radiograph and echocardiogram) are insensitive tests of intravascular depletion, invasive monitoring is often undertaken (see Chapter 2). The need for invasive monitoring is controversial, however, because no particular values for central venous pressure (CVP), pulmonary artery occlusion pressure (PAOP), CO, or systemic vascular resistance (SVR) guarantee sufficient or inadequate renal blood flow. That is, glomerular pressure and flow are poorly gauged by these hemodynamic measures. Nevertheless, a low intravascular pressure (i.e., CVP ≤2 or PAOP ≤5 mm Hg) can be diagnostically helpful, especially if CO is reduced concomitantly.

In prerenal failure initially the urinalysis is normal or minimally abnormal with hyaline casts and other nonspecific sediment; however, if the injury is sufficient to induce tubular damage, typical ATN sediment will be present. A prerenal state prompts the tubule to reabsorb Na^+ and water, yielding concentrated urine with low Na^+. A urine Na^+ less than 20 mEq/L, urine osmolality greater than 500 mOsm/L, and the urine specific gravity greater than 1.015 are typical. The fractional excretion of sodium (FeNa) is another commonly used index to identify the prerenal state that measures the percentage of filtered sodium that is excreted. FeNa is calculated as the ratio of the urine Na^+ concentration times the plasma creatinine concentration to the product of the plasma Na^+ concentration times the urine creatinine concentration. FeNa = ([Urine Na^+] × [Plasma creatinine])/([Plasma Na^+] × [Urine creatinine]) × 100. FeNa values less than 1% are generally indicative of prerenal disease, whereas values greater than 3% usually represent acute tubular necrosis (ATN). Intermediate values are not helpful and there are exceptions to this rule. For example, up to 10% of cases of ATN have a low FeNa. For urine Na^+ or FeNa measurements to be valid, the underlying Na^+ reabsorbing capacity of the renal tubule must be intact. For this reason, chronic renal failure, hypoaldosteronism, and metabolic alkalosis may all render tests of urine Na^+ invalid. Likewise, diuretic therapy invalidates urine Na^+ determinations for at least 24 h. Osmotic agents

(glucose, mannitol, radiographic contrast) also confuse interpretation of urine chemistry values by diluting the urine.

Although the BUN may be disproportionately high because of increased urea production resulting from tetracycline, corticosteroids, or GI bleeding, an elevated BUN/creatinine ratio more commonly results from reduced tubular urine flow and increased proximal tubular reabsorption of urea nitrogen. Thus, in prerenal states the BUN/creatinine ratio is usually elevated (>10:1; sometimes >20:1). Because the renal tubules cannot absorb creatinine, reduced tubular flow rates have no effect on the creatinine concentration if GFR is preserved. Comparing urea clearance to creatinine clearance will determine whether increased urea production or decreased urea excretion is the cause of an elevated BUN. If the urea/creatinine clearance ratio is greater than 1, increased production is the likely etiology. The most common clinical task is to differentiate prerenal disease from ATN. Table 29-1 compares the more common renal function indicators in these two conditions. Imaging studies of the kidneys may also provide clues to the cause of renal failure (Table 29-3). In most forms of AKI, the kidneys will be of normal size when imaged with ultrasound or computed tomography (CT). Small kidneys suggest a more chronic process (e.g., diabetes or hypertension) with a superimposed insult.

Postrenal Failure

Once prerenal causes have been excluded, obstructive or postrenal causes (e.g., urinary calculi or clots, tumor, prostatic hypertrophy, retroperitoneal

---

TABLE 29-3   KIDNEY SIZE AS A CLUE TO THE ETIOLOGY OF RENAL FAILURE

NORMAL	ENLARGED	SMALL
Acute glomerulonephritis	Amyloidosis	Chronic renal failure
Acute tubular necrosis	Acute glomerulonephritis	Chronic hypertension
Acute cortical necrosis	Acute interstitial nephritis	
Acute interstitial nephritis	Obstructive uropathy	
Hepatorenal syndrome	Renal vein thrombosis	
Malignant hypertension	Acute transplant rejection	
Renal artery obstruction		
Scleroderma		

hemorrhage) should be considered. Even though obstructive disease accounts for less than 10% of cases of AKI, this reversible problem cannot be overlooked. Because of the low risk and cost, practically every patient developing AKI should have an imaging study to exclude obstruction. The pattern of decline in urine flow can provide a valuable clue to the presence of obstructive disease. In both prerenal and intrarenal failure, the development of oliguria or anuria is usually gradual over hours to days, whereas an abrupt cessation of flow often occurs with obstructive uropathy. (Urethral obstruction by prostatic enlargement, trauma, or blood clot is the most common cause of anuria.) In catheterized patients, a clogged or dysfunctional catheter is a common cause for sudden "anuria" in which case flushing the catheter is diagnostic and theraputic. Upper tract obstruction produces anuria only if bilateral or if it occurs in a patient with a single kidney or drainage pathway. In this setting, tumor (e.g., bladder, kidney, prostatic, or ovarian), stone, and clot are the most common etiologies. Urethral obstruction may be immediately excluded or confirmed by the attempt to place a catheter into the bladder. Because of the high incidence of urinary collecting system abnormalities, however, urinary bladder catheterization alone never excludes the possibility of more proximal obstructive uropathy. Renal ultrasonography and CT scan can detect hydronephrosis and urinary obstruction within or proximal to the bladder and have supplanted the outmoded intravenous pyelogram (IVP).

In obstructive uropathy, the urinalysis is usually normal, at least initially, and urine studies are seldom enlightening. A notable exception would be discovery of hematuria suggesting papillary necrosis or obstruction by stone, clot, or tumor.

Intrarenal Failure

The history, urinalysis, and urinary chemistry profile provide clues to distinguish prerenal from intrarenal causes of AKI (Tables 29-1 and 29-4). However, no single index of renal function yields a **3** specific diagnosis in AKI. For example, although the FeNa is usually greater than 1 when "intrarenal" failure occurs, diuretic use, glycosuria, mannitol, and prolonged urinary obstruction can produce identical findings. Similarly, the urinalysis can be very informative if it reveals red cell casts (vasculitis or GN), eosinophils (acute interstitial nephritis [AIN]), or crystals (ethylene glycol, uric acid nephropathy), but is rarely unequivocal. The size of the

TABLE 29-4 URINE SEDIMENT IN ACUTE KIDNEY INJURY

URINE SEDIMENT	ASSOCIATED ETIOLOGY
Red cell casts	Glomerulonephritis, vasculitis, trauma
Heme pigmented casts	Hemoglobinuria, myoglobinuria
Leukocyte casts	Pyelonephritis, papillary necrosis
Renal tubular casts	Acute tubular necrosis
"Muddy" granular casts	Acute tubular necrosis
Leukocytes	Urinary infection; interstitial nephritis
Eosinophils	Interstitial nephritis
Crystals	Urate, oxalate (ethylene glycol)

kidneys may also provide a useful clue to the etiology of renal failure. If the kidneys are small, then renal failure is at least in part chronic. By contrast, normal-size or large kidneys are much more common in acute renal failure. Renal enlargement is indicative of a limited number of acute etiologies, including obstruction, renal vein thrombosis, and transplant rejection (see Table 29-3).

There are three major categories of acute intrarenal failure: (a) tubular disorders, (b) interstitial nephritis, and (c) GN and small vessel vasculitis.

Tubular Disorders

The most common form of AKI results from tubular injury commonly called acute tubular necrosis (ATN). ATN is not a unique entity and should be considered the severe extreme of the continuum of AKI induced by ischemia and drugs. ATN manifests clinically as an abnormal urinalysis featuring muddy brown and epithelial cell casts, a high urinary Na^+ greater than 40 mEq/L, a FeNa greater than 2%, and a urine osmolality less than 400 mOsm/L reflecting the loss of tubular concentrating ability.

ATN is usually multifactorial in etiology, but drugs often play a role. Aminoglycosides, amphotericin, contrast media, cyclosporine, platinum-based chemotherapeutic agents, angiotensin-converting enzyme (ACE) inhibitors, and nonsteroidal anti-inflammatory drugs (NSAIDs) are most commonly implicated. Elderly, dehydrated, hypertensive, and diabetic patients and those with mild underlying renal dysfunction and myeloma are at particular risk of drug-induced AKI. Aminoglycosides cause renal insufficiency in 10% to 20% of patients who receive them by binding and injuring cellular proteins in the proximal tubule. Damage is most likely with sustained elevated trough drug levels. (Peak levels correlate with bacterial killing, whereas trough levels predict toxicity.) Toxicity is potentiated by preexisting renal disease, volume depletion, and concomitant use of other nephrotoxins. Because prolonged exposure of the renal tubule to drug and not peak levels appears to be the critical determinant of damage, dosing once daily (e.g., gentamicin 5 mg/kg) lowers the risk of nephrotoxicity. Such a dosing schedule is also more convenient and less costly. Because the *duration* of exposure is also a risk factor, limiting the length of therapy reduces risk. When using aminoglycosides, frequent mistakes are to administer multiple daily doses and to empirically treat for prolonged periods without a clear indication. Although aminoglycoside loading doses need no modification, maintenance doses should be reduced in proportion to GFR. (For example, a patient with 50% of predicted GFR should receive approx. 50% of the standard maintenance dose.) Serum trough levels should not be determined until after five half-lives when steady-state concentrations are achieved. Fortunately, aminoglycoside use has declined dramatically with the development of less-toxic alternatives, and almost all patients with aminoglycoside-induced AKI recover sufficient function to obviate long-term dialysis.

Radiographic contrast-induced nephropathy (CIN) is a rare cause of AKI in patients with normal baseline renal function but frequently produces AKI in patients with underlying volume depletion, renal disease, diabetes mellitus, or paraproteinemia. Fortunately, an isolated rise in creatinine is much more common than full-blown AKI requiring dialysis. Risk is higher among patients receiving hypertonic and ionic contrast agents, and is proportional to the number of exposures and volume of contrast (highest with doses > 2 mL/kg). Consequently, it makes sense to bundle together imaging studies requiring intravenous contrast to minimize exposure and select the contrast agent carefully in at-risk patients. Although not studied in large randomized trials, volume loading appears to be beneficial for prevention of CIN. For this purpose current evidence suggests that isotonic fluids are superior to hypotonic fluids

and that perhaps $NaHCO_3$ may be superior to NaCl. A $NaHCO_3$ solution (154 mEq Na/L) is given as a 3 mL/kg infusion in the hour before contrast exposure and is followed by doses of 1 mg/kg/h for 6 h. The mechanism of protection is unknown but probably involves a combination of volume expansion (enhanced tubular flow) and an antioxidant effect. When time for pretreatment is available, two to four doses of oral *n*-acetylcysteine (NAC) (600 mg q12h) significantly reduces the risk of CIN and is safe and inexpensive. Most oral NAC regimens begin 24 to 48 h before contrast exposure, limiting their usefulness in the emergent setting. Although safe, the effectiveness of immediate pretreatment with intravenous NAC is unknown. Although logical, the value of "prophylactic dialysis" to remove contrast is controversial and has obvious risks and costs not incurred with other options.

NSAIDs may impair renal function in patients with prerenal azotemia, shock, heart failure, cirrhosis, and nephrotic syndrome, but their risks to the average intensive care unit (ICU) patient have probably been exaggerated. Prostaglandin E_2 (PGE_2), an endogenous vasodilator, is pivotal in maintaining renal blood flow in patients with high renin/angiotensin states. In such patients, NSAIDs can block PGE_2 formation, decreasing renal blood flow. Furthermore, NSAIDs encourage sodium, potassium, and fluid retention and inhibit diuretic action. If NSAIDs are used, aspirin, sulindac, and ibuprofen are perhaps the best options. Despite concerns regarding chronic use, there is no evidence that short-term use of NSAIDs (COX2 or nonselective) blockers in usual doses increases risk of cardiovascular death.

ACE inhibitors block formation of angiotensin II thereby reducing systemic blood pressure and dilating postglomerular arterioles. Both effects reduce glomerular perfusion pressure and may precipitate AKI when perfusion is marginal, especially among patients with bilateral renal artery stenosis or a single kidney. Beginning an ACE inhibitor in a critically ill patient with congestive heart failure and a concomitant creatinine elevation is often a difficult decision, especially if renal artery anatomy is not known. Fortunately, for most patients, the increased CO stemming from reduced afterload provides more benefit than any direct negative effect of the ACE inhibitor on renal blood flow. If renal function deteriorates, prompt discontinuation of the ACE inhibitor usually results in rapid return of renal function to baseline. The combination of ACE inhibitors and NSAIDs is especially detrimental to renal function because of the synergistic effects on perfusion.

The cellular pigments, myoglobin, and hemoglobin may induce AKI when released into serum during hemolysis or rhabdomyolysis. Both myoglobin and hemoglobin precipitate in the renal tubules, obstructing them by forming pigmented tubular casts. Trauma, severe sepsis, seizures, statin toxicity, prolonged immobilization, and hyperthermic illnesses like neuroleptic malignant syndrome and heatstroke can all be etiologic. Half of all patients have no complaints of muscle pain, tenderness, or weakness. Clues to rhabdomyolysis include rapidly increasing creatinine with disproportionate rises in K^+, PO_4^-, and uric acid. Volume loading with isotonic saline or bicarbonate, osmotic diuretics, and alkalinizing agents may help to keep these pigments in solution, thus encouraging their elimination and preventing AKI.

Among patients with lymphoid malignancies who have a high tumor burden, spontaneous tumor death or that from chemotherapy and/or radiation releases large quantities of uric acid which can rapidly produce AKI. Patients with tumor lysis syndrome have rapidly increasing levels of released intracellular components K^+, PO_4^-, and a resulting fall in serum Ca^{2+}. Use of the xanthine oxidase inhibitor, allopurinol, to stop uric acid formation, or rasburicase, a synthetic urate oxidase enzyme to degrade uric acid is beneficial. Adequate hydration is a key prophylactic step but urinary alkalanization is probably not helpful.

Interstitial Nephritis

AIN is a common but frequently unrecognized drug-induced allergic event in the renal interstitium. Penicillins, cephalosporins, sulfonamides, quinolones, rifampin, thiazides, furosemide, NSAIDs, allopurinol, and cimetidine are reported causes. AIN may present with fever, eosinophilia, and rash; however, oliguria and a rising creatinine are often the only indications. Laboratory clues to diagnosis include eosinophilia in about 1/4 of cases and eosinophiluria in about 2/3 of patients. Hansel's stain is necessary to document urinary eosinophilia. (Wright's stain is pH dependent and often fails to demonstrate eosinophils in the urine.) Removal of the suspect offending drug is indicated, and although controversial, corticosteroids are often tried.

Glomerulonephritis and Vasculitis

Although GN and vasculitis represent a relatively common etiology for AKI developing outside the hospital, they are uncommon causes of abrupt renal failure in the ICU. The diverse spectrum of these disorders includes poststreptococcal GN, rickettsial infection, subacute bacterial endocarditis, systemic lupus erythematous (SLE), malignant hypertension, and drug-related vasculitis. Urinalysis reveals an active sediment containing leukocytes, protein, and the hallmark of GN, red blood cell (RBC) casts. Specific diagnosis may be aided by measurement of serum complement, antinuclear cytoplasmic antibodies (ANCA) and antinuclear antibody (ANA) studies, rheumatoid factor, hepatitis B surface antigen, and blood culture. Therapy is directed at the underlying condition (e.g., antibiotics for infection including endocarditis, steroids for SLE, and cytotoxic therapy for Wegener's and polyarteritis).

■ COMPLICATIONS AND TREATMENT OF ACUTE RENAL FAILURE

Prevention

Because the only therapy after AKI is established is supportive, it is clear that the best treatment is prevention. Avoiding hypotension and hypoxia and recognizing urinary obstruction can prevent the majority of cases of AKI. Parsimonious use of nephrotoxic drugs in appropriate doses is the next most important preventative measure. Volume expansion with isotonic saline or sodium bicarbonate is effective prophylaxis against AKI induced by contrast agents, rhabdomyolysis, cisplatinum, methotrexate, or cyclophosphamide. NAC and perhaps aminophylline can also limit the extent of contrast-related damage.

Established Oliguric Renal Failure

Prolonged illness before admission and delays in transferring patients from the general care floor or another hospital often postpone the diagnosis of oliguric AKI until 12 to 48 h after its onset. Even if evaluation is delayed, it is prudent to exclude obstructive uropathy. When presented with a patient with *established* oliguric AKI, several measures should be undertaken to prevent additional injury and perhaps forestall or avert the need for dialysis or hemofiltration (HF). First, all nonessential nephrotoxins should be discontinued and any necessary drug cleared by the kidney should have its dose modified based on the assumption of a zero GFR. Second, limit fluid intake by discontinuing "maintenance fluids" and unnecessary drugs, and concentrating the required drugs makes common sense. Next, because K^+ and PO_4^- levels rise as the result of normal metabolism, intake of K^+ and PO_4^{-3} should be minimized unless the patient exhibits significant symptomatic hypokalemia or hypophosphatemia. (Do not forget to modify the diet.) If PO_4^{-3} levels are already elevated, it makes sense to begin oral PO_4^{-3} binders. Likewise, if the patient is hyperkalemic, oral or rectal K binding resin should be initiated. Potassium binding resins exchange Na^+ for K^+ and can contribute to volume overload. Mg supplements should be discontinued to avoid exceeding the limited excretory capacity. Providing HCO_3^- enterally can blunt the development of academia. Finally, it is wise to involve a nephrologist *early* in the care of the patient. Not only may they provide valuable advice, but it is also simple courtesy to inform them about potential dialysis candidates so that they may best schedule any required intervention.

Early Oliguric Renal Failure

For patients seen shortly after developing oliguria, the initial approach should be to eliminate prerenal factors, exclude obstructive uropathy, and when possible, reverse oliguria. After prerenal and postrenal causes have been excluded, careful review of the history, physical examination, and laboratory and medication records may give clues to the cause. Unfortunately, AKI often occurs in the setting of multiorgan failure where potential etiologies are numerous. In this situation, combined renal and respiratory insufficiency is particularly ominous, with mortality exceeding 90% in several published series. Interestingly, even with appropriate dialysis, morbidity and mortality remain high as a result of nonuremic causes (Table 29-5). In patients with acute renal failure, supportive care must be meticulous to maximize chances for survival. It is most important to avoid such iatrogenic complications as infection related to monitoring devices, fluid and electrolyte imbalances, drug toxicity, and inappropriate nutritional support.

Hemodynamic Management

Nonoliguric AKI is associated with lower mortality than the oliguric variety. Unfortunately, this fact is often misinterpreted. A response to measures designed to restore urine flow is not necessarily an indication of improved renal function, but may simply serve as an indicator of a patient's overall physiologic condition and the severity of the underlying injury. Perhaps responders have better baseline renal function or more cardiovascular reserve than nonresponders. Although it is not proved that restoring urine flow reduces mortality, attempting to restore flow is still probably worthwhile because it vastly simplifies fluid management.

When attempting to reverse oliguria, a fluid challenge of 15 to 30 mL/kg of isotonic crystalloid should be performed first unless there are obvious signs of intravascular congestion. Invasive monitoring can be considered in patients with tenuous cardiopulmonary reserve and when volume status is particularly difficult to assess (e.g., edema, hypoproteinemia). The limitations of invasive monitoring catheter must be recognized; no combination of measurements guarantees adequate glomerular flow. (Nevertheless, a low CVP, PAOP, and CO with

TABLE 29-5 COMPLICATIONS OF ACUTE KIDNEY INJURY

METABOLIC	CARDIOVASCULAR	NEUROLOGICAL
Metabolic acidosis	Fluid overload	Neuropathy
Hyperkalemia	Hypertension	Dementia
Hypocalcemia	Arrhythmias	Seizures
Hyperphosphatemia	Pericarditis	
Hyperuricemia		
HEMATOLOGIC	**GASTROINTESTINAL**	**INFECTIOUS**
Anemia	Nausea and vomiting	Urinary tract
Coagulopathy	GI bleeding	IV-catheter Sepsis
		Pneumonia

GI, gastrointestinal.

increased SVR suggest that more fluid may be beneficial.) Next a single sizeable dose of loop diuretic (e.g., furosemide, 1 mg/kg) can be tried but it makes little sense to continue diuretics in established oliguria, and observational studies suggest possible harm from continued use. Although single doses of osmotic diuretic (mannitol, 25 to 50 gm) may also be effective, any potential benefit needs to be balanced against the risk of volume overload and hyperosmolarity. Measures to reverse the oliguric state are most likely to be successful when undertaken shortly after the reduction in urine flow. When 8 or more hours have elapsed, efforts to restore urine flow by volume loading routinely fail.

Once assured that intravascular volume is adequate, vasoactive drug therapy may be helpful in the hypotensive acutely oliguric patient. Any drug that raises mean arterial pressure of 60 to 65 mm Hg is likely to boost urine output. There are no data to indicate superiority of one vasopressor over another, although currently norepinephrine is used most commonly. Historically, "low dose" dopamine was often chosen as a first-line agent because of its ability to increase CO through β-adrenergic receptor stimulation and increase renal blood flow via dopaminergic receptor stimulation. It is now clear that low-dose dopamine does not prevent the development, alter progression, or hasten recovery of AKI. Although it is perfectly fine to use dopamine as a vasopressor, there is no beneficial effect associated with doses that do not boost perfusion pressure.

Electrolyte Disorders

Hyperkalemia, hyponatremia, hypermagnesemia, and hyperphosphatemia are the major electrolyte disturbances of AKI. The primary approach to each disorder is to modify input and/or enhance removal of solute or fluid, as detailed in Fluids and Electrolyte Disorders, Chapter 13. It is worth noting here that oral PO_4^{-3} binders (aluminum-containing antacids) are usually capable of suppressing the serum PO_4^{-3} sufficiently to prevent hypocalcemia. Because Mg^{2+} excretion is impaired in patients with AKI, Mg^{2+} containing products (antacids and cathartics) should be avoided.

Water, Na^+, and K^+ intake should be adjusted to match measured urinary output and normalize serum values. In the resolution phase of ATN (3 to 4 weeks after onset), patients frequently undergo a polyuric period during which fluid losses may be life-threatening unless appropriately replaced. The cause of the polyuric phase is not known with certainty, but probably results from tubular dysfunction in the face of recovering GFR and excess total body water.

Infection

Infection-induced multiple organ failure is arguably the most common cause of death in acute renal failure. With the possible exception of pyocystis, a pus-filled nondraining bladder, the infections acquired by patients with AKI do not differ from those of other ICU patients. In decreasing frequency, nosocomial pneumonia and IV catheter–related infections lead the list. Among patients dying with renal failure, however, there may be a disproportionate occurrence of intra-abdominal sepsis. The clues to suspect infection and the techniques to diagnose and treat various infections are outlined in Chapter 26.

Bleeding Disorders

Hemorrhage (primarily GI) accounts for a substantial number of deaths among patients with AKI. Bleeding is common because of the inhibitory actions of uremic toxins on platelets and factor VIII. The key to reversing coagulation disorders is to improve the environment in which the platelets and clotting factors function. Most commonly this is accomplished through adequate dialysis. Replacement of factor VIII with purified concentrates, cryoprecipitate, or fresh frozen plasma (FFP) may transiently help to correct bleeding defects (see Chapters 14 and 30). Likewise, arginine vasopressin (DDAVP) will temporarily improve hemostasis in uremic patients by increasing levels of factor VIII complex. (Unfortunately, tachyphylaxis is seen within just one or two doses.) Platelet transfusions may also briefly improve hemostasis before invasive procedures.

Nutrition

The production of uremic toxins can be reduced by minimizing catabolism and providing sufficient calories to prevent protein wasting. Except in AIN and some forms of renal vasculitis, corticosteroids should be avoided because of their catabolic effects and impact on immune function. For most AKI victims, caloric requirements generally range from 2,500 to 3,000 calories per day. Sufficient carbohydrate (>100 gm/day) and fat calories should be provided to prevent the catabolism of protein for energy production. In patients who do not undergo dialysis, protein intake should be limited to less than 50 gm/day, the majority of which should be of high biological value. In dialyzed patients, protein intake may be liberalized (80 to 100 gm/day); however, it should be recognized that higher protein intake may necessitate more frequent dialysis. Folate and pyridoxine must be supplemented because they are lost through hemodialysis (HD). If total parenteral nutrition (TPN) is used, a formulation low in Na^+, Mg^{2+}, PO_4^{-3}, and K^+ is mandatory. Enteral feeding is preferred because of the lower fluid volume, infection risk, and costs.

Drug Therapy

4 The need for every medication should be questioned in AKI. Any drug that may impair renal function should be discontinued or its dosage appropriately modified. Renally metabolized or excreted drugs require dose modification. As a general guideline, the dosage needs revision in proportion to its percentage of elimination by the kidney and the degree of renal impairment. Dosing of each drug susceptible to renal excretion should be guided by published nomograms. Even when dosage is precisely calculated, it is probably prudent to follow levels of drugs with a low therapeutic index.

Renal Replacement Therapy

Indications

Indications for HD or HF are (a) fluid overload, (b) refractory hyperkalemia or hypermagnesemia, (c) life-threatening metabolic acidosis, (d) symptomatic uremia (e.g., pericarditis, seizures, encephalopathy), and (e) presence of a dialyzable toxin (salicylate, methanol, ethylene glycol).

Overview of Methods

5 The terminology surrounding RRT is confusing, but each technique's name is derived from three basic characteristics: (a) the method used to remove the solutes (diffusion, convection, or a combination), (b) whether the process is intermittent or continuous, and (c) the access site (arteriovenous, venovenous, or peritoneal). Two basic methods of fluid and solute removal can be used: *HF*, a process in which fluid and the solutes it contains are removed from blood by convection; or hemodialysis or peritoneal *dialysis*, in which solutes diffuse down a concentration gradient. These techniques

are usually combined as *hemodiafiltration*, a system combining diffusion and convection to remove fluid and solute from blood.

Access to the circulation is achieved by inserting either a multilumen venous catheter or one arterial catheter for supply and one venous catheter for blood return. Jugular, subclavian, and femoral venous sites are all acceptable. When an artery is used, it is almost always a femoral vessel, necessitating that the patient remains supine. Venovenous access is usually preferred because only one catheter is needed and it avoids risks of limb ischemia from artery occlusion by the catheter itself, clot, or cholesterol embolism. Avoiding arterial access also precludes arterial air embolism and permits less-intense anticoagulation. Because arteriovenous methods usually use the patient's blood pressure to power flow through the circuit, problems of low flow in patients with hypotension or peripheral arterial disease are common. The more commonly used venovenous filtration overcomes this problem by introducing an extracorporeal pump. The higher blood flows (≥ 200 mL/min) through this apparatus easily compensate for the "recirculation" that occurs through the adjacent ports. Because of their comparatively rigid construction and large diameter, dialysis catheters are more prone to perforate vascular structures during insertion and erode through vessel walls over time than conventional venous access catheters. Particular care should be used during insertion, making sure that the catheter advances easily over the guidewire. If inserted in the neck or thorax, a radiograph should be obtained to confirm that the catheter tip is aligned with the luminal axis and does not terminate in the heart.

Because flow rates and solute clearance achieved with HF alone are lower, the process is typically done continuously. By contrast, the higher flow rates and solute clearance of HD permit intermittent sessions. A summary of the characteristics of each of the blood purification methods is provided in Table 29-6 and is discussed in detail below.

Hemofiltration

HF is the removal of solute containing fluid by convection across a semipermeable membrane. HF can be accomplished using an extracorporeal pump to power the flow of venous blood or by using the patient's arteriovenous pressure gradient to drive flow through a hollow fiber cartridge (often called a

TABLE 29-6   CHARACTERISTICS OF RENAL REPLACEMENT METHODS

| | EFFICIENCY OF SOLUTE REMOVAL | | DYSEQUILIBRIUM SYNDROME | HEMODYNAMIC INSTABILITY | HYPOXEMIA | PROTEIN LOSSES | WORKLOAD | COST |
	SMALL	LARGE						
Peritoneal dialysis	Low	Medium	Rare	Rare	High volume	Present	High	Low
Continuous venovenous hemodiafiltration	High	Low	None	None	None	Absent	High	Highest
Intermittent hemodialysis	Very high	Low	Frequent	Frequent	Technique dependent (acetate/cuprophane)	Absent	Lower	Intermediate

"kidney"). Typically, non–pump-aided filtration becomes ineffective when mean arterial pressure is less than 60 mm Hg. The filtration rate can be increased by restricting cartridge outflow (raising downstream venous pressure), by increasing the cartridge inflow pressure (either arterial pressure or pump pressure), or by increasing blood flow rate or the transmembrane filtration pressure by applying suction to the shell surrounding the permeable fibers (Fig. 29-2). (Obviously, increasing the cartridge surface area will also boost filtration rate.) Conversely, filtration may be decreased by restricting blood inflow or pump supply pressure.

In it simplest form, HF removes solutes in exactly the concentrations in which they are present in blood, as they are passively carried across the cartridge's semipermeable membrane in the plasma extract. Decreases in *plasma* urea or creatinine concentrations result by replacing the extracted ultrafiltrate with a nonurea/creatinine containing electrolyte solution, in essence diluting the plasma. As a result, changes in solute concentrations are slow. Although not at first obvious, infusing the replacement fluid upstream of the cartridge can increase urea clearance by diluting plasma concentrations, which encourages movement of urea from the freely permeable red cells into plasma.

When HF is applied continuously, the process is termed continuous venovenous HF (CVVH) or continuous arteriovenous HF (CAVH), depending on the route of circulatory access. The term "slow continuous ultrafiltration" (SCUF) has been used to describe ths same processes when conducted at low flow rates. The term high volume HF (HVHF) is used when clearance rates exceed 35 mL/kg/h.

HF has several advantages over HD; one among them is its ability to be safely conducted by ICU nurses. Undoubtedly, the major benefit of HF is that it is much less likely to result in hypotension or cerebral edema than HD in part because of slower changes in plasma osmolality. The continuous nature of the filtration also tends to reduce body temperature which may raise blood pressure by increasing SVR. For these reasons, HF has become a favored technique to treat the hemodynamically unstable patient. The relative inefficiency of solute clearance is offset by its continuous application. Even though solute clearance rates are usually low, prodigious fluid removal rates (1 to 3 L/h) are possible.

The major disadvantages to HF are that it requires anticoagulation, is costly and labor intensive. CVVH usually requires a one-to-one nurse to patient assignment because each day 10 to 20 L of ultrafiltrate must be discarded and replaced using an appropriate volume of an expensive, proprietary electrolyte solution. Without careful monitoring of output, patients are prone to volume depletion. Unless blood flow rates are high, anticoagulation (usually with heparin at 300 to 400 U/h) is required, and unfortunately, the anticoagulant effect often becomes systemic. Regional citrate anticoagulation reversed using a Ca^{2+}/Mg^{2+} mixture is a more cum-

HEMOFILTRATION

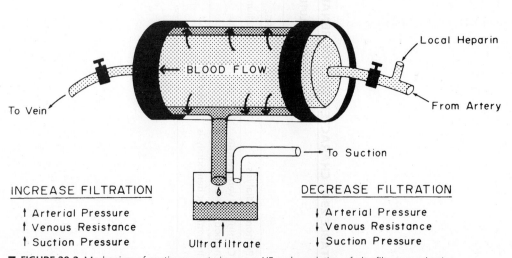

■ FIGURE 29-2 Mechanism of continuous arteriovenous HF and regulation of ultrafiltrate production.

bersome alternative. Cartridge clotting is common despite anticoagulation. Despite physician preferences, no compelling data indicate a survival advantage of continuous HF over intermittent HD.

Hemodialysis

HD differs from HF in that a dialytic fluid replaces air on the opposite side of the semipermeable membrane from the blood. As a result, solutes not only filter from blood across the membrane governed by pore size, but also diffuse down a concentration gradient as the dialysate is continuously exchanged using countercurrent flow. It is by combining convection and diffusion that HD achieves high solute clearance rates. Because the membrane is permeable in both directions, electrolytes in the dialysate equilibrate with those in plasma. Hence, the electrolytic composition of the dialysis fluid should roughly approximate desired plasma electrolyte concentrations. Back-filtration of dialysate into the patient necessitates sterility. By altering the pressure of blood on one side of the dialysis membrane and the pressure of the dialysate on the other, the amount of fluid filtered during HD can be precisely controlled. (Increasing the transmembrane gradient results in greater fluid losses.) HD machines can be used for HF by simply plugging the dialysate infusion port and using the outflow port to drain the plasma ultrafiltrate.

Although more efficient than HF or peritoneal dialysis (PD), HD requires cardiovascular stability; rapid shifts of fluid between intracellular and extracellular compartments induced by changes in osmolality are not well tolerated by hemodynamically unstable patients. Hypotension during HD is the most common significant problem. Fluid and electrolyte shifts, reactions to the dialysis membrane or dialysate, and impaired cardiac performance all play a part. Many hypotensive episodes result from the rapid reduction in plasma osmolality as urea is cleared. When this happens, water moves from the now hypotonic plasma into cells, resulting in intravascular volume contraction and cellular edema. (Interestingly, HF has the opposite effect on cellular hydration; as water is filtered, plasma protein concentrations rise, leading to a net flux of water from cells into the plasma.) Another mechanism of hypotension is excessively rapid filtration reducing preload. Intravascular volume deficits respond quickly to crystalloid or colloid replacement and low-dose vasopressor support. If transfusion is planned, administration of blood during HD helps to minimize hypotension. If hypotension recurs with each dialysis session or occurs after only small volumes of fluid have been removed, a reaction to the dialysis membrane or to acetate in the dialysis bath should be suspected. Fortunately, improvements in material technology have made this problem rare. Intolerance to HD is particularly common early in the treatment course.

During HD, intraneuronal tonicity may not track the abrupt shifts in fluid/solute composition that occur in the extracellular compartment, producing the "dialysis disequilibrium" syndrome. Nausea, vomiting, confusion, seizures, and coma may all be manifestations of the syndrome most common in patients with high BUN concentrations undergoing initial dialysis. Disequilibrium can be minimized by using brief dialysis sessions, lower flow rates, and a small surface area cartridge. Administration of osmotically active compounds (NaCl, mannitol, or dextrose) can also reduce the frequency and severity of the syndrome.

Depending on choice of membrane and dialysate, hypoxemia during HD may result from leukostasis within the pulmonary capillaries (cuprophane membrane) or from hypoventilation (acetate buffer). Hypoventilation occurs as CO_2 diffuses into the dialysate, reducing the stimulation of ventilatory chemoreceptors.

Using a naming convention identical to HF, HD is termed intermittent or continuous, and venovenous or arteriovenous, depending on circulatory access. The term SLED, slow low efficiency dialysis, is associated with long or continuous dialysis using lower blood flow and dialysate rates. The term *hemodiafiltration* is used to describe the process of HD with net filtration of fluid.

Peritoneal Dialysis

PD can be undertaken in most patients who have a freely communicating and uninflamed peritoneal cavity, but it is considerably less efficient than HD in removing toxins or correcting electrolyte imbalances. The major advantages of PD are the absence of significant hemodynamic effect and lack of need for vascular access. The process requires insertion of a peritoneal catheter, which incurs minimal risk. After catheter insertion, 1 to 3 L of dialysis solution is slowly introduced into the peritoneal cavity and allowed to "dwell" for 30 to 40 min before 20 to 30 min of drainage. This 1-h dialysis cycle can be continuously repeated or can be automated using a "cycler." An osmotic gradient for fluid removal is created by using hyperosmolar (350 to 490 mOsm/L) glucose concentrations (1.5 to 4.25 gm/dL) in the dialysate. Standard concentrations of Na^+ and Cl^- are slightly hypotonic compared to plasma. Concentrations of K^+ and Ca^{2+} can be varied from patient to patient. Although hemodynamically well tolerated, PD is not always feasible or risk free. The technique cannot be performed in patients with recent laparotomy, abdominal drains, or active intra-abdominal infection. In addition, abdominal distention during high-volume PD may drive the diaphragm cephalad, causing atelectasis, hypoxemia, and increased work of breathing. Instilled dialysate may also leak into the chest, resulting in pleural effusion further impairing lung function. Electrolyte imbalance, significant hyperglycemia, and peritonitis are commonly encountered. There are no clear data to indicate that PD is better or worse than HD with regard to survival.

Timing and Intensity of RRT

Strong opinion exists with regard to optimal intensity and timing for initiation of RRT. Because uremia exerts global negative metabolic effects, it makes sense to begin RRT as soon as it is clear that intervention will be needed and to provide sufficient support to normalize blood chemistry values. Retrospective and nonrandomized studies support earlier and more intense treatment by demonstrating improved survival and functional recovery, but these findings have not been corroborated by prospective randomized studies. In what may be the definitive study of dialysis intensity in which patients could cross over between intermittent and continuous methods of support, no difference between an intense or conventional RRT strategy was found. Hence, current information suggests that for most patients with AKI the outcomes of thrice weekly intermittent HD sessions are equal to daily intermittent HD or continuous RRT support. One exception to this rule includes hemodynamically unstable patients where CVVH may be safer. Another exception would be where toxin removal (ethylene glycol, methanol, lithium) is the goal in which case intense continuous RRT is often continued until the toxin is undetectable.

■ PROGNOSIS

The survival of patients with AKI is more determined by the underlying conditions precipitating renal failure than by renal dysfunction itself. Rarely do patients die from renal failure if dialysis is instituted. Recent data indicate that among patients who do not succumb to their underlying illness, recovery of function is the rule rather than the exception with one caveat: functional recovery is much less likely for patients with chronic renal dysfunction before superimposed acute injury.

■ SUGGESTED READINGS

Bellomo R, Ronco C, D'Amico G, et al. Acute renal failure: Definition, outcome measures, animal models, fluid therapy and information technology needs; the second international consensus conference of the acute dialysis quality initiative (ADQI) group. *Crit Care.* 2004;8:R204–R212.

Friedrich JO, Adhikari N, Herridge MS, et al. Meta-analysis: Low-dose dopamine increases urine output but does not prevent renal dysfunction or death. *Ann Intern Med.* 2005;142(7):510–524.

John S, Eckardt K-U. Renal replacement strategies in the ICU. *Chest.* 2007;132:1379–1388.

Moreau R, Lebrec D, Acute kidney injury: New concepts: Hepatorenal syndrome the role of vasopressors. *Nephron Physiol.* 2008;109:73–79.

Ronco C, Ricci Z. Renal replacement therapies: Physiological review. *Intensive Care Med.* 2008;34:2139–2146.

The VA/NIH Acute Renal Failure Trial Network. Intensity of renal support in critically ill patients with acute kidney injury. *N Engl J Med.* 2008;359:7–20.

Uchino S, Kellum JA, Bellomo R, et al. Acute renal failure in critically ill patients: A multinational, multicenter study. *JAMA.* 2005;294:813–818.

Weisbord SD, Palevsky PM. Radiocontrast-induced acute renal failure. *J Intensive Care Med.* 2005;20(2):63–75.

Clotting and Bleeding Disorders and Anticoagulation Therapy

KEY POINTS

1 A prothrombin time, an activated partial thromboplastin time, and a platelet count done after a careful detailed history, which includes a review of current medications, can detect essentially all significant acquired bleeding disorders seen in the ICU.

2 Coagulation tests are often indiscriminately performed. The activated partial thromboplastin time is rarely necessary unless a patient is receiving heparin, and the prothrombin time is of essentially no use to monitor heparin's effects. Neither is informative during low molecular weight heparin treatment.

3 Platelet numbers correlate roughly with the tendency to bleed. At platelet counts greater than 50,000 mm³, the risk of spontaneous bleeding is low, platelet transfusions are rarely necessary, and most procedures can be safely performed provided platelets function normally. By contrast, platelets counts less than 20,000 mm³ are associated with spontaneous hemorrhage and are often treated with platelet transfusions. Platelet counts do not provide information about platelet function.

4 Most bleeding disorders seen in the ICU are the result of acquired deficiencies of multiple clotting factors, whereas most hereditary disorders are rare and stem from a single soluble factor deficiency. Hemophilia A (factor VIII deficiency) and Hemophilia B (factor IX) deficiency constitute 90% or more of clinically significant hereditary bleeding disorders. Because these two conditions can be detected by an activated partial thromboplastin time and are rarely the result of a spontaneous mutation, they can be easily excluded from consideration by family history and a simple blood test.

5 Liver disease, vitamin K deficiency, dilutional coagulopathy, and disseminated intravascular coagulation are the most common soluble factor problems encountered in the ICU. All

can produce elevations of the prothrombin time and activated partial thromboplastin time. The presence of high levels of FDPs and a lower platelet count favors disseminated intravascular coagulation. Vitamin K deficiency and liver disease can often be distinguished by searching for additional historical or chemical evidence of a liver disease, especially a problem of synthetic function. Although dilution and disseminated intravascular coagulation can appear similar, dilutional coagulopathy is less likely to exhibit fibrin degradation products.

6 When using unfractionated heparin for thromboembolism, a loading dose followed by a continuous infusion is almost always necessary to achieve the usual target level of anticoagulation of an activated partial thromboplastin time 1.5 to 2 times baseline. Subtherapeutic activated partial thromboplastin times usually require an additional bolus and increases in infusion rate of 20% to 25% for correction. For most patients, low molecular weight heparin are safer, more effective alternatives that do not require in vitro monitoring.

7 Identifying thrombophilia is uncommon. Clues that could trigger a laboratory search for a thrombotic condition are unprovoked clotting, clotting at an early age, repeated episodes of thrombosis, a positive family history of clotting, and a history of repeated spontaneous abortions.

In the intensive care unit (ICU), bleeding disorders are diagnosed substantially more commonly than clotting disorders even though thrombotic diseases (e.g., stroke, myocardial infarction, thromboembolism) are substantially more common and lethal. The disparity in diagnostic rates occurs in part because bleeding is visible, whereas thrombotic conditions have more protean manifestations. This variation is also partly explained by the fact that the most commonly available in vitro laboratory tests reflect defective clotting, not a thrombotic tendency, and less is known about disorders producing excessive thrombosis. Although no single routine laboratory test is indicative of overall clotting function, nearly all clinically significant bleeding disorders can be screened for by adding an activated partial thromboplastin time (aPTT) and platelet count to the prothrombin time (PT). Unfortunately, no abnormal in vitro clotting test value accurately predicts that bleeding will occur, nor do normal values preclude bleeding.

■ BLEEDING DISORDERS

Vascular endothelium, clotting proteins, and platelets are the components of hemostasis. Only when two or more of these hemostatic pathways are defective, spontaneous or uncontrollable hemorrhage is likely; impairment of any single factor seldom provokes clinical bleeding. However, since many patients are in the ICU because they have conditions that breach vascular integrity (e.g., surgery, trauma, and sepsis), it only requires the addition of a platelet or soluble factor disorder to induce bleeding.

Approach to the Bleeding Patient

History

The history provides important clues to the etiology of bleeding. With few exceptions, the rare hereditary disorders produce deficiency or dysfunction of a single clotting factor, whereas the much more common acquired disorders cause multiple factor abnormalities. All congenital bleeding disorders are inherited in an autosomal fashion, except for the sex-linked recessive hemophilias and the very rare Wiskott–Aldrich syndrome. The most common inherited bleeding disorder is von Willebrand disease (vWD), an autosomal dominant condition that produces combined platelet-vessel wall dysfunction in up to 1% of the population. Fortunately, despite its prevalence, vWD is usually so mild that it remains undiagnosed. Although much less common, the hemophilias are the most likely genetic disorders to result in clinically significant bleeding. Deficiency of factor VIII (hemophilia A) may be up to ten times more common than the milder factor IX deficiency (hemophilia B). Unlike vWD, which affects men and women with equal frequency, the X-linked recessive inheritance pattern of the hemophilias dictates an almost exclusively male occurrence. (Some female carriers have factor levels as low as 50% and can exhibit mild increased bleeding tendencies.) All other inherited factor deficiencies are very rare autosomal recessive conditions; for these reasons, a thorough negative family history virtually excludes a diagnosis of hereditary coagulopathy. Furthermore, almost all inherited coagulation disorders manifest in childhood, making a new diagnosis in an adult a distinct rarity.

In taking the history, patient reports of "easy bleeding," excessive bruising, or heavy menses are so common and nonspecific that they are all but useless. Detailed answers to the following questions should be sought: (a) Has there been excessive bleeding during or after surgery (especially oral surgery) or following significant trauma? (b) Has bleeding required transfusion or reoperation? The answers to these two questions can be very telling; an adult who has never experienced significant bleeding spontaneously or following surgery or trauma is extremely unlikely to have a hereditary disorder (at least one of clinical significance). If there is a suggestive history, the following questions help confirm the problem and point to the cause: (a) When did hemorrhage occur in relation to trauma or surgery? (Intraoperative bleeding suggests a platelet or vessel disorder, whereas delayed bleeding is more indicative of a soluble factor problem.) (b) What drugs have been taken? Particular attention should be paid to drugs affecting platelet numbers (e.g., immunosuppressive chemotherapy and alcohol) or function (e.g., aspirin, clopidogrel, glycoprotein IIb/IIIa inhibitors, and nonsteroidal anti-inflammatory agents) or those impairing synthesis of vitamin K–dependent clotting proteins (e.g., warfarin and antibiotics).

Physical Examination

Petechiae (especially in dependent, high venous pressure areas), purpura, and persistent oozing from skin punctures or mucosal sites are most characteristic of platelet disorders. Palpable purpura is a sign of small artery occlusion usually associated with vasculitis of collagen–vascular disease (i.e., polyarteritis, systemic lupus erythematosus [SLE]), endocarditis, or severe sepsis. Larger vessel occlusions from disseminated intravascular coagulation (DIC) may cause the extensive ecchymoses of purpura fulminans. By contrast, factor deficiencies (especially the hemophilias) usually cause deep muscle and joint bleeding resulting in ecchymoses, hematomas, and the most characteristic feature, hemarthroses.

Laboratory Tests

Basic screening tests of clotting function are indicated for patients undergoing surgery or invasive procedures and for those with a history that suggests a bleeding disorder. Clotting tests are also useful in patients undergoing massive transfusion, anticoagulation, or thrombolytic therapy. When indicated, a platelet count, PT, and aPTT usually suffice to exclude clinically important bleeding disorders. (Neither the PT nor aPTT will detect factor XIII deficiency, fortunately a rare cause of hemorrhage.) Not all prolongations of the PT and/or aPTT signify an increased risk of hemorrhage. For example, deficiencies of factor XII, high-molecular-weight kininogen or prekallikrein or the presence of anticardiolipin antibody, also known as lupus anticoagulant, may prolong in vitro clotting tests without increasing bleeding risk. (In fact, anticardiolipin antibodies are more likely to result in clotting than bleeding.)

It has long been routine to measure PT, aPTT, and platelet count at the time of admission in almost all hospitalized patients. However, in the absence of a history suggesting hemophilia, vWD,

2 or heparin use, measurement of the aPTT is extremely unlikely to yield a true positive abnormality and thus is wasteful of money and blood. Likewise, the common practice of measuring both the PT and aPTT in all patients receiving warfarin or heparin is also uneconomical; aPTT determinations are unnecessary during therapy with only warfarin, and PT measurements rarely add to the care of patients receiving only heparin. PT and aPTT ordering should be unlinked and tailored to the clinical situation.

■ PLATELET DISORDERS

Thrombocytopenia

Thrombocytopenia, the most common coagulation disorder among ICU patients, is not only associated with an increased risk of bleeding but serves as an independent predictor of outcome. Normally, platelet counts average 250,000/mm^3 and display little day-to-day variability in individuals; therefore, a 50% decline in platelet levels usually represents a

3 significant change. In the absence of bleeding, most physicians do not display concerns until levels dip to 100,000/mm^3 (<10 platelets per high-power field on peripheral blood smear). As platelet counts fall below this threshold, bleeding risk increases progressively and even more so if functional platelet

abnormalities coexist. A search for the cause of thrombocytopenia and periodic rechecking of platelet counts is prudent when levels decrease by 50% and certainly when they reach 100,000/mm^3. Although counts greater than 50,000/mm^3 are acceptable for most types of surgery, levels greater than 100,000/mm^3 are preferred for cardiac procedures or neurosurgery. Spontaneous bleeding is rare with greater than 20,000/mm^3 normally functioning platelets, but at this level bleeding may occur even with minor trauma. When counts fall below 20,000/mm^3, spontaneous bleeding is possible. Normally, about 10% of platelets appear "large" on the peripheral smear, reflecting recent production. These young platelets produced by an active marrow are more hemostatically effective. Therefore, at any given count, bleeding is more likely to occur if thrombocytopenia results from impaired platelet production (rather than increased destruction). Common causes of thrombocytopenia are outlined in Table 30-1. Among all causes, idiopathic thrombocytopenia (ITP), acute leukemia, and aplastic crisis are the most likely causes of *severe* thrombocytopenia (<10,000/mm^3).

Mechanistically, thrombocytopenia is usually classified as a problem of production or destruction, but low counts can also result from dilution, splenic sequestration, or artifact. Spurious thrombocytopenia can occur when platelets form large clumps after being exposed to the anticoagulant EDTA. Spurious thrombocytopenia can be detected by automated testing of a heparinized sample or directly examining a bedside peripheral smear. Although there are no reliable rules of thumb, replacement of the entire blood volume within a day, or half within 3 to 4 h is typically required to precipitate a dilutional coagulopathy. The occurrence of dilutional coagulopathy is so variable that a strategy that advocates a fixed recipe of blood product replacement does not make sense. Although one might suspect that mild thrombocytopenia would result from dilution, surprisingly in cases where 20 or more units of blood products are transfused, platelet counts less than 50,000/mm^3 are common. Dilutional coagulopathy is also frequently compounded by hypothermia resulting from ambient exposure, infusion of large volumes of cool fluids, and by acidosis resulting from underperfusion and infusion of acidic fluids.

Because up to one third of all platelets are in the spleen at any given time, splenic enlargement, typically from the portal hypertension of cirrhosis, and ITP can lower circulating counts.

TABLE 30-1 CAUSES OF THROMBOCYTOPENIA

PRODUCTION DEFECTS	CONSUMPTION DEFECTS
IMPAIRED PRODUCTION	IMMUNE-MEDIATED DESTRUCTION

Drugs (alcohol, chemotherapy)
Infection (measles, mumps, EBV,
   TB, HIV, parvovirus, hepatitis C)
Myelodysplasia
Radiation
Liver disease
	ITP
	Drugs (heparin, quinine, valproic
	   acid, sulfonamide, phenytoin)
	Lymphoma
	Systemic lupus
	Alloimmunization/posttransfusion

INEFFECTIVE PRODUCTION	NONIMMUNE-MEDIATED DESTRUCTION
B_{12}/folate deficiency Myeloproliferative disease	DIC Postbypass pump Splenomegaly Prosthetic cardiac valves Thrombotic thrombocytopenic purpura Hemolytic uremic syndrome Preeclampsia and HELLP syndrome

Anemia, leukopenia, and a normal or hyperplastic marrow usually accompany thrombocytopenia from hypersplenism.

Impaired Production

In the ICU, isolated platelet production defects are uncommon; when inadequate production accounts for thrombocytopenia, anemia and leukopenia usually coexist (i.e., complete marrow failure). In such cases, platelets are small and bone marrow examination shows a decreased number of megakaryocytes. Marrow failure may result from alcohol or radiation; a deficiency of vitamin B_{12} or folate; infection with hepatitis B, Epstein-Barr virus, parvovirus, or cytomegalovirus; cytotoxic chemotherapy; or marrow infiltration with tumor, fibrosis, or granuloma. Selective failure of platelet production may occur with the use of gold, sulfas, and thiazides.

Increased Consumption

Excessive platelet consumption is the most common cause of thrombocytopenia and may be due to immunologic or nonimmunologic mechanisms. Laboratory clues to excessive platelet consumption include disproportionate numbers of large (young) platelets on peripheral smear and an increased number of marrow megakaryocytes. Nonimmunologic platelet consumption occurs in DIC, severe sepsis, some malignancies, microangiopathic hemolysis, and following cardiopulmonary bypass

and splenic sequestration. Thrombotic thrombocytopenic purpura (TTP) and hemolytic uremic syndrome (HUS) are other nonimmunologic cause of thrombocytopenia in which platelets aggregate with abnormally large von Willebrand factor (vWF) multimers that result from a deficiency in a vWF-cleaving protease. The often profound thrombocytopenia is accompanied by elevated serum lactate dehydrogenase (LDH) levels and the presence of schistocytes on the peripheral smear representing mechanical erythrocyte destruction. Only microangiopathic hemolytic anemia and thrombocytopenia are required for the diagnosis, despite the description of a classic "pentad," which also includes renal dysfunction, neurologic abnormalities, and low grade fever. Numerous conditions, including cancer, pregnancy, antiphospholipid antibody syndrome, and pneumococcal infection can be associated with "TTP-like" syndromes as can medications, such as cyclosporine, clopidogrel, and some chemotherapeutic agents. The absence of significant fever and normal aPTT and PT seen with TTP-HUS can sometimes help differentiate it from DIC, which also can exhibit schistocytes on the peripheral smear. Unfortunately, increased coagulation parameters are not universally present in DIC, making the distinction difficult at times. HELLP syndrome (hemolysis, elevated liver enzymes, and low platelets) of pregnancy represents another condition with hemolysis and thrombocytopenia that may be difficult to discriminate from TTP-HUS. Elevated liver enzymes may be helpful in differentiating the two, but pregnancy itself is not distinguishing since it is also a risk factor for TTP. Since HELLP syndrome usually resolves within 72 h of delivery, continued worsening of thrombocytopenia beyond this time should prompt strong consideration of TTP-HUS.

Immune-mediated thrombocytopenia occurs via production of platelet antibodies with subsequent destruction. The antibodies can be idiopathic, or induced by drugs, infections (e.g., cytomegalovirus, human immunodeficiency virus, Epstein-Barr virus, parvovirus), or alloimmune following transfusion or transplantation. Many drugs have been implicated as causes of thrombocytopenia. An extensive current list can be found at http://moon.ouhsc.edu/jgeorge/DITP.html. Drug-induced destruction of platelets usually occurs via the formation of antiplatelet antibodies, which bind normal platelets in the presence of the sensitizing drug but a few drugs, such as procainamide, induce autoantibodies that react with platelets even in the absence of the drug. A third mechanism of drug-induced thrombocytopenia involves a direct interaction between drug and platelets resulting in immune destruction. Tirofiban, for example, interacts with the glycoprotein IIb/IIIa receptor on platelets, changing their shape and thereby facilitating antibody recognition. Heparin, one of the most common drugs associated with thrombocytopenia, similarly binds platelet factor 4 (PF4) forming an immune complex which is recognized and destroyed.

Drug-induced thrombocytopenia can be overlooked because its onset is often a week or more after beginning the medication and there are no distinguishing clinical features. Nonetheless, recognition is important because the problem may sometimes be reversed by simply discontinuing the offending agent. After drug discontinuation, platelet counts often rise substantially within 5 days but full recovery may take 3 to 4 weeks. Platelet transfusions and corticosteroids may help restore platelet counts rapidly once the inciting drug is removed.

In acute ITP, immunologic platelet destruction usually follows a childhood viral illness. Steroids are frequently helpful if thrombocytopenia persists more than several weeks. In adults, ITP usually presents as a chronic disease, with counts ranging from 20,000 to 80,000/mm³. The spleen is the major site of platelet destruction of the IgG coated platelets. Splenectomy is indicated in the 10% to 20% of patients who fail to respond to steroids,

or immune globulin. Anemia in ITP is secondary to blood loss, not immune hemolysis. Interestingly, despite sometimes profound reductions in platelet count, life-threatening bleeding is rare.

Platelet Dysfunction

By impairing platelet function, drug effects, uremia, DIC, leukemia, vWD, and paraproteinemia can cause bleeding despite normal platelet counts. If performed, the bleeding time is abnormal. The most common drugs to impair platelet function are listed in Table 30-2. Function may be impaired by drug combinations even when any single drug acting alone would be well tolerated. (The most common combinations causing platelet dysfunction are aspirin and alcohol and aspirin and clopidogrel.) Aspirin impairs platelet function irreversibly, so hemostasis is restored only by transfusion or formation of new platelets over a period of days. (Platelets can be generated at a rate sufficient to restore functioning levels by 10% to 30% each day.) The glycoprotein IIb/IIIa inhibitors alone or in combination with aspirin are commonly used to deter thrombosis after coronary interventions, and while all of these agents impair platelet function, the effects of abciximab persist until new platelets are produced. Similarly, clopidogrel impairs coagulation for days by inhibiting adenosine diphosphate induced-platelet aggregation preventing activation of the IIb/IIIa mechanism. In bleeding patients exposed to these medications, discontinuation of the drug may not be sufficient to return platelet function to normal and platelet transfusion may be needed. Alcohol inhibits platelet production and action in several ways. Heavy alcohol usage predisposes to trauma, encourages nutritional deficiencies, and directly injures the marrow. Given in high doses, most penicillins bind to the platelet surface, preventing interaction with vWF. (This does not occur with methicillin or cephalosporins.)

TABLE 30-2 DRUGS INHIBITING PLATELET FUNCTION
Aspirin
Nonsteroidal anti-inflammatory drugs (NSAIDs)
Alcohol
High-dose penicillins
Moxalactam
Heparin
Glycoprotein IIb/IIIa inhibitors

Although patients with end-stage renal disease may have mild thrombocytopenia, more often they have a normal number of, but dysfunctional, platelets. The pathophysiology of "uremic coagulopathy" is uncertain but likely multifactorial. One factor is anemia causing platelets to travel in a more midstream position within vessels, rendering them further away and less likely to react to endothelial damage. In addition, uremic toxins result in dysfunctional vWF and vWF–factor VIII complex and impaired platelet aggregation.

Therapy of Platelet Dysfunction

Bleeding rarely occurs in patients with platelet dysfunction alone. As a first step, potentially offending medications should be discontinued. Unless sequestered or destroyed, transfused platelets quickly restore coagulation competency. Platelet transfusions will effectively correct dysfunction induced by aspirin, clopidogrel, or the cardiac bypass pump. Platelet transfusion is also transiently useful when the platelet environment is abnormal, as in uremia, paraproteinemia, or after treatment with high-dose penicillin or dextran. However, it is better to correct the underlying defect using dialysis, plasmapheresis, or by discontinuing the offending drug.

Treatment of chronic dialysis in patients who are bleeding requires a multifaceted approach, including adequate dialysis to remove uremic toxins. Functional defects caused by uremia and vWD may at least temporarily be corrected with fresh frozen plasma (FFP), arginine vasopressin also known as desmopressin (DDAVP), or cryoprecipitate. By releasing factor VIII/vWF multimers, DDAVP in doses of $0.3\,\mu g/kg$ IV or $3\,\mu g/kg$ intranasally correct clotting abnormalities in at least half of all patients within 1 h. Unfortunately, effectiveness is limited by tachyphylaxis, which occurs usually by the second dose. By increasing the levels of functional factor VIII, vWF, and fibrinogen, cryoprecipitate is also useful in uremic coagulopathy. For long-term therapy, estrogens may be helpful. Although their mechanism of action is not entirely understood, estradiol working through estrogen receptors can increase clotting within a day of starting therapy.

■ INTERPRETATION OF ABNORMAL CLOTTING TESTS

Surprisingly, the most common cause of an abnormal clotting assay is not a physiological problem or even laboratory error but rather an improperly obtained sample. There are several common causes of this so-called preanalytical error. Accurate results from aPTT and PT testing require a specific ratio (9:1) of plasma to anticoagulant (typically sodium citrate in a "blue top" tube). If the tube is underfilled both values will be prolonged. Conversely, if the tube is forcefully overfilled, clotting times will be shortened. Another potential source of error occurs if blood is contaminated with a second anticoagulant. This error typically occurs in one of two ways: blood is drawn from a heparin-containing catheter; or blood is placed into the wrong tube then transferred to the correct tube. For example, blood initially drawn into an EDTA or heparin containing tube which is then transferred to a citrate tube will yield prolonged PT and aPTT values. Another problem results when blood is not promptly and gently mixed with anticoagulant. For example, initial collection of blood into a tube not containing anticoagulant; delay in transferring blood from a syringe to an anticoagulant containing tube; and failure to mix blood in with the anticoagulant—all can artificially prolong the PT and aPTT. Conversely, hemolysis or excessively vigorous agitation of blood with citrate will artificially shorten the PT and aPTT. Excessive tourniquet time elevates vWF and factor VIII levels also resulting in falsely shortened PT and aPTT. Since both the aPTT and PT are performed on platelet-depleted plasma, thrombocytopenia does not alter their in vitro value.

In general, an isolated PT prolongation of 2 or 3 s or an aPTT prolonged by as much as 5 s should not raise concern in the absence of bleeding. In fact, aPTT abnormalities of such a magnitude usually do not warrant further investigation because very few disorders occurring in the ICU cause an isolated progressive prolongation of the aPTT (exception: unfractionated heparin [UFH] therapy), and the history will dictate further evaluation for hemophilia or vWD. On the other hand, it is often prudent to recheck a prolonged PT of even a few seconds because many diseases or interventions occurring in the ICU can progressively extend the PT (e.g., antibiotic therapy, starvation, progressive hepatic failure).

The PT or aPTT may be prolonged individually or together. Each potential combination of abnormalities suggests a limited specific set of diagnostic possibilities and an optimal plan for evaluation. Potential diagnoses and their evaluation are summarized in Table 30-3 and discussed below.

TABLE 30-3 CAUSES OF A PROLONGED PT

Liver disease
Vitamin K deficiency/malnutrition
Warfarin therapy
Broad-spectrum antibiotic therapy
Disseminated intravascular coagulation
Dilutional coagulopathy
Circulating anticoagulants (i.e., antiphospholipid
  antibodies)
Salicylate poisoning
Massive heparin overdose

Prothrombin Time

The PT is a test of the tissue factor (formerly extrinsic) clotting pathway in which factor VII is activated by adding complete tissue thromboplastin and calcium to a platelet-depleted citrated sample. This process sequentially triggers factors X, V, II, and then fibrinogen. Because the endpoint of the test is clot formation, deficiencies of factor VII (or any factor at or distal to factor X) can prolong the PT (Fig. 30-1). The PT is relatively resistant to change, typically requiring factor levels to fall to 10% of normal or less before becoming prolonged. An acquired inhibitor to one of these same factors will also prolong the PT. (Inhibitors can be detected by mixing the suspect plasma in a 1:1 ratio with normal plasma; a persistently abnormal PT indicates presence of an inhibitor.) Common causes of a prolonged PT are listed in Table 30-3. Even though heparin inhibits some factors in this test of the tissue factor pathway, it is a rare cause of significant PT prolongation because there are fewer factors sensitive to heparin in the tissue factor pathway and a greater degree of inhibition is required for PT prolongation. In addition, some PT assay systems contain heparin-neutralizing compounds. (Massive heparin levels can overcome these inhibitors.)

The very uncommon combination of a normal aPTT with a prolonged PT is uniquely explained by a deficiency of factor VII. This combination is rarely seen on a chronic basis (i.e., genetic deficiency of factor VII or acquired inhibitor), but because factor VII has the shortest half-life of all vitamin K–dependent clotting proteins (approx. 6 h), transient, isolated prolongation of PT can occur in early vitamin K deficiency, hepatic failure, DIC, or warfarin therapy.

Activated Partial Thromboplastin Time

The aPTT tests the contact activation (formerly intrinsic) pathway by adding kaolin, silica or other particulate, and phospholipid (in lieu of complete thromboplastin) to activate coagulation, hence the name *activated partial* thromboplastin time. In sequence, factor XII activates factor XI, then IX, and VIII which then triggers the common sequence of factor X–V through fibrin formation. Hence, the

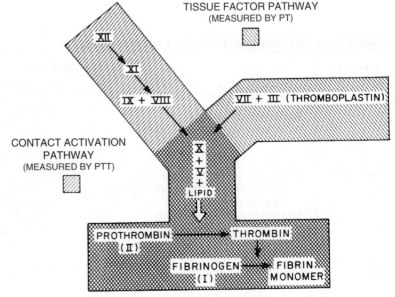

■ **FIGURE 30-1** Relationship of PT and aPTT to the clotting cascade. Deficiencies of factors in the doubly cross-hatched region (the intersection of contact and tissue factor pathways) produce abnormalities of both tests. The thrombin time tests only the final conversion of fibrinogen to fibrin monomer. Factor XIII (*not shown*) stabilizes the linkup of fibrin monomers into organized clot.

TABLE 30-4 CAUSES OF A PROLONGED PARTIAL THROMBOPLASTIN TIME

Spurious results (underfilled tube)
Polycythemia
Delay in performing assay
Heparin
Antiphospholipid antibodies
Hemophilia A and B
von Willebrand disease

aPTT tests all factors except for VII and XIII, making it a sensitive overall test of clotting abnormalities but less specific than the PT for the same reason (see Fig. 30-1). Single factors unique to the contact activation pathway must decline to only 15% to 30% of normal before the aPTT is prolonged. Milder deficiencies of multiple factors can also prolong the aPTT. In the absence of heparin, the discovery of a normal PT with a prolonged aPTT usually indicates an inherited deficiency or dysfunction of factors VIII, IX, XI, or XII (most often hemophilia A or B or vWD). Common causes of a prolonged aPTT are listed in Table 30-4. Inherited disorders of the common pathway (factors II, V, X, and fibrinogen) are rarely to blame. Among these, fibrinogen deficiency can be quickly excluded by direct measurement. Prekallikrein, high-molecular-weight kininogen (HMWK), and factor XII deficiencies will also prolong the aPTT, but the former two are rare, and none of the three increases the risk of bleeding despite altering the aPTT.

Combined PT and aPTT Abnormalities

Because the contact and tissue factor pathways share multiple factors (X through II), diseases or therapies altering one pathway often affect the other. When both the PT and aPTT are abnormal, simultaneous treatment with heparin and warfarin or an acquired bleeding disorder affecting multiple factors (e.g., liver disease, DIC, fibrinolytic therapy) is almost always responsible. Table 30-5 provides an overview of the diseases and defects in which isolated or combined abnormalities of the PT and aPTT are seen.

Anti-Xa Activity Assay

One test being used with increasing frequency because of the popularity of low-molecular-weight heparins (LMWHs) is the anti-Xa activity assay. Methodology is straight forward: an excess of factor Xa and antithrombin (AT) are added to platelet-poor, citrated patient plasma. Any heparinoid in the test sample binds to the exogenous AT impairing the activity of the added Xa which is detected as a decrease in the cleavage of an added chromogenic substrate, relative to control. LMWHs and direct Xa inhibitors such as fondaparinux bind to AT through a 5-oligosaccharide sequence, but unlike the longer UFH, do not have sufficient length to bind to thrombin (factor IIa). As a result, the PT and aPTT demonstrate minimal changes (on average 1 to 4 s) despite effective anticoagulation.

TABLE 30-5 INTERPRETATION OF PT AND APTT TESTS

ACTIVATED APTT	PROTHROMBIN TIME	
	NORMAL	**PROLONGED**

Normal	Defect: Factor XIII
	Frequency: very rare
	    Dx test: Urea solubility assay
		Defect: Isolated to tissue factor pathway
		    (e.g., early: starvation, warfarin, liver
		    disease, DIC, or dilution)
		Frequency: relatively common but transient
		    Dx test: Factor VII assay

Prolonged	Defect: contact pathway (e.g., heparin,
	    hemophilia A and B, von Willebrand's)
	    Frequency: uncommon
	Dx test (exclude heparin) then:
	    If bleeding, check: VIII, IX, XI levels
	    No bleeding, check: prekallikrein, XII,
	    high-molecular-weight kininogen
		Defect: Combined contact/tissue factor
		    defect (e.g., DIC, liver failure, warfarin,
		    starvation, thrombolytic R$_x$)
		Frequency: most common
		    Dx test: DIC panel; fibrinogen; factors II,
		    V, X; liver function assessment

Activated Clotting Time

In locations like the cardiac catheterization lab, where a real time *estimate* of clotting is necessary, the activated clotting time (ACT) is often used, especially to monitor UFH or bivalirudin activity. The ACT is a nonspecific test which reports the time for an activating agent (e.g., celite, kaolin, glass particles) to produce clot in whole blood, thereby evaluating soluble factor and platelet function in toto. Because neither the reagents nor clot detection method (e.g., resistance to mechanical deformation of clot or changes in the electrical or mechanical properties of the blood) is standardized, results of different assay systems are not equivalent and the ACT correlates poorly with aPTT, PT, and anti-Xa assays.

Thrombin Time

The thrombin time is a test of the final step in the coagulation cascade, performed by adding thrombin to an anticoagulated sample, thereby converting fibrinogen to fibrin (see Fig. 30-1). Because only the terminal step in a complex clotting array is evaluated by this test, it detects a limited number of clotting abnormalities. Fibrinogen levels less than 100 mg/dL, most commonly from DIC, thrombolytic therapy, or dysfunctional fibrinogen, may prolong the thrombin time. UFH, fibrin degradation products (FDPs), and abnormal immunoglobulins also prolong the thrombin time by interfering with thrombin-induced fibrinogen conversion. (If heparin is the etiology, the reptilase time will be normal.) Direct thrombin inhibitors (e.g., hirudin, argatroban) will not only prolong the PT, aPTT, and thrombin time but the reptilase time as well.

Bleeding Time

Together, a platelet count and bleeding time effectively screen for platelet problems by testing the platelet number, adhesion, and aggregation. The bleeding time is primarily a test of platelet function but is also influenced by platelet number and tissue fragility and edema. Accuracy is highly subject to technician expertise. As a general rule, the bleeding time becomes a less reliable index of platelet function when counts fall below 100,000/mm³, will often be prolonged if platelets number is less than 80,000/mm³, and will almost always be prolonged if counts dip below 50,000/mm³. Unfortunately, a normal or high platelet count does not ensure a normal bleeding time, as function may be selectively impaired. The bleeding time is often abnormal in patients with uremia and in those receiving drugs that impair platelet function (e.g., aspirin and other nonsteroidal anti-inflammatory drugs, β-lactam antibiotics, and direct thrombin or IIb/IIIa inhibitors). Bleeding time is also prolonged by rare, inherited platelet disorders (Bernard–Soulier, Glanzmann syndrome, and Wiskott–Aldrich syndrome), by vWD, and by severe hypofibrinogenemia. One common and important artifact that can prolong bleeding time is anemia. By altering blood rheology and diluting platelets in a larger volume of plasma, anemia prolongs bleeding time. The degree of bleeding time prolongation correlates poorly with the tendency to bleed. Because of both the technical difficulty and limited predictive value of bleeding times, they are rarely performed in critically ill patients.

Inhibitor Testing

Roughly, only 30% activity of each clotting factor is needed to result in normal clotting assays, hence, combining equal portions of normal plasma (or a standardized reagent) and plasma from a patient with a factor deficiency will yield normal PT and aPTT results, unless a factor inhibitor (e.g., anticardiolipin antibody, factor VIII inhibitor) is present.

Fibrinogen Levels and Fibrin Degradation Products

Fibrinogen levels may be reduced as a result of impaired production or increased consumption. Because fibrinogen is an acute phase reactant released from the liver, it may be elevated in hepatitis or other conditions that cause liver inflammation (e.g., severe sepsis). Therefore, even if consumption is increased, fibrinogen levels may remain in the normal range.

The term FDP is general one that describes the breakdown products of fibrin *and* fibrinogen generated by the enzymatic action of plasmin. The d-dimer is a specific subtype of FDP produced only by degradation of fibrin from intact clot. Unfortunately, both assays lack specificity and are positive in patients with thrombotic diseases (e.g., venous thromboembolism, myocardial infarction, and in DIC). In fact, both can be elevated in patients with cancer and pregnancy and because of impaired hepatic clearance, chronic liver disease can also result in elevated levels. Commercially available assay methods differ significantly (i.e., Latex or red blood cell agglutination or ELISA) resulting in widely divergent sensitivities. If using a d-dimer assay as an adjunctive test for thromboembolic disease diagnosis, it is imperative to use an ultrasensitive assay to avoid false negative results. In general, assays using latex agglutination methods are least sensitive. Even in the very unlikely event an inpatient's d-dimer assay is negative; it is imprudent to use this test alone as definitive evidence of absence of clot (also see Chapter 23). By contrast, a negative *sensitive* d-dimer assay performed in an outpatient at low risk for thromboembolism all but excludes the disease.

■ SPECIFIC CLOTTING DISORDERS

Heparin-Induced Thrombocytopenia

Two forms of heparin-induced thrombocytopenia (HIT) are described. Type I is a common, mild, transient, self-limited, nonimmunologic variety that appears quickly (<5 days) after initiating heparin. Type I HIT occurs in up to 20% of heparin-exposed patients but is not associated with bleeding or clotting complications and does not necessitate discontinuing heparin therapy. The second more serious type of HIT (Type II) is the result of IgG antibodies that cross-react with heparin and PF4 antigens. Onset is usually about 1 week after initiation of heparin but may occur as rapidly as 24 h in a presensitized patient. Although both forms of HIT are more common among patients receiving high-dose UFH, even the modest amounts used for subcutaneous deep venous thrombosis (DVT) prophylaxis or intravenous catheter flushing can cause disease. An estimated 1% to 5% of UFH recipients will develop Type II HIT but the syndrome is significantly (perhaps 10-fold) less common among patients receiving LMWHs. With Type II HIT typically, platelets decline to the 50,000/mm^3 range, but 10% to 15% of victims will maintain counts near 150,000/mm^3. The diagnosis of HIT is confirmed by finding heparin cross-reacting antibodies that activate platelets resulting in serotonin release. (Unfortunately, the serotonin release assay is not widely available and rarely in a timely fashion, hence many diagnoses are false positive made on the basis of tests for cross-reacting IgG antibodies alone.) Type II HIT is a serious problem with 50% of patients or more

developing venous or arterial thrombosis. Ironically, despite thrombocytopenia, clotting (e.g., DVT, PE, stroke, myocardial infarction, limb arterial occlusion) is much more common than hemorrhage. Withdrawal of heparin is mandatory but not sufficient treatment, and thromboses have been reported up to a month after stopping heparin. In addition to the immediate discontinuation of heparin, anticoagulation with a direct thrombin inhibitor (e.g., lepirudin) or heparinoid (e.g., danaparoid) is required. Although some clinicians have used fondaparinux in this setting, emerging reports of HIT associated with fondaparinux use should discourage this practice. Warfarin should be withheld until platelet counts rise above 100,000/mm^3 to avoid potentially worsening the situation by lowering protein C levels at a time the patient is prone to thrombosis. Platelet transfusions should be avoided if possible. Reexposure of patients with confirmed Type II HIT to heparin is controversial but is sometimes inescapable. If unavoidable, it is probably safest to use a LMWH and to delay exposure for at least 3 months and until PF4 antibodies have disappeared from the circulation.

Hemophilia

The hemophilias are sex-linked recessive diseases producing clinical bleeding in affected males. Spontaneous hemorrhage in hemophilia A (factor VIII deficiency) or hemophilia B (factor IX deficiency) usually occurs only when factor levels dip below 5% of normal (most commonly <1%). Therefore, heterozygous female carriers possessing 50% of normal factor VIII or IX levels are spared bleeding complications. Despite these guidelines, a less-than-ideal correlation exists between factor levels and bleeding tendency. Laboratory examination in both diseases most commonly reveals a prolonged aPTT, with normal PT, platelet count, bleeding time, and thrombin time. Specific levels of factors VIII and IX are required to distinguish hemophilia A from B.

The urgency of therapy must be guided by the amount and location of bleeding; massive hemorrhage or bleeding into the brain or upper airway is most urgent. Surgery and invasive procedures in hemophiliacs require maintenance of factor levels greater than 50% for 14 days following the procedure. In critical operative sites (e.g., brain, spinal cord), activities approaching 100% are desirable. Topical aminocaproic acid may be effective at controlling localized mucosal or venipuncture bleeding. Although factor VIII is present in FFP cryoprecipitate and factor VIII concentrates, recombinant factor VIII is the most practical replacement product because of safety and fluid volume considerations. The 8- to 12-h half-life of transfused factor VIII typically mandates twice daily dosing. Replacement of factor IX can be accomplished using FFP, purified factor IX concentrates (also known as prothrombin complex concentrates [PCCs]), or recombinant factor IX. PCCs contain factors VII, IX, and X as well as trace amounts of factors VIII, VIIa, and IXa, the concentrations of each varying by manufacturer. Care must be exercised in administration of PCCs, which may excessively activate clotting. The biological half-life of factor IX is longer than factor VIII, permitting once daily dosing for most patients. (For detailed recommendations on the replacement of factors VIII and IX, see Chapter 14.)

Liver Disease

5 Apart from its role in clearing FDPs, the liver produces albumin and all clotting factors except the factor VIII–vWF complex. Therefore, a low serum albumin concentration supports hepatic insufficiency as the etiology of the coagulation disorder. When the liver is responsible for a coagulopathy, laboratory examination typically reveals decreased fibrinogen, increased circulating levels of FDPs, prolonged PT and aPTT, and an increased thrombin time (because of FDPs). Such a laboratory pattern is identical to that seen with DIC; however, detecting d-dimers and fibrin monomers favors a diagnosis of DIC.

Liver disease and vitamin K deficiency decrease levels of factor VII, the vitamin K–dependent factor with the shortest half-life (6h). This reduction leads to early increases in the PT. Because multiple factors (II, VII, IX, and X) are deficient in liver disease, FFP is the replacement product of choice if immediate correction is necessary. In less-urgent situations, vitamin K will usually suffice if there is a vestige of hepatic synthetic function. Vitamin K should also be given empirically to virtually all patients with liver-related coagulopathy because it is difficult to distinguish liver disease from pure vitamin K deficiency. In urgent situations, vitamin K can be given intravenously; in less-urgent situations, oral dosing is sufficient. Platelet counts are usually normal in liver disease unless there is coexisting hypersplenism or DIC. When platelet counts

are significantly decreased ($<50,000/mm^3$), platelet concentrates may be administered but unfortunately are often ineffective.

Vitamin K Deficiency—Warfarin Excess

Vitamin K deficiency may develop in any patient deprived of a balanced diet for 7 to 14 days. Because antibiotics may eliminate the enteric bacteria required for the production of vitamin K when intake is insufficient, malnourished patients and those receiving broad-spectrum antibiotic therapy are at particular risk. Fat-soluble vitamin K is incompatible with many total parenteral nutrition preparations and, if omitted, must be given separately. Warfarin compounds induce vitamin K deficiency by preventing carboxylation to the active form. Malabsorption (from pancreatic insufficiency) and bile salt deficiency (from ductal obstruction) may also prevent vitamin K absorption.

Vitamin K is required for the formation of factors II, VII, IX, and X. Although depletion of vitamin K eventually extends both the PT and aPTT, prolongation of the PT is more marked and occurs earlier because factor VII (tissue factor pathway) has the shortest half-life of all clotting proteins. (Very rarely vitamin K deficiency leads to seemingly paradoxical thrombosis by reducing the production of the anticlotting proteins C, S, and AT.) FFP corrects the clotting disorder of vitamin K deficiency very rapidly (two to four bags usually suffice). Vitamin K alone usually corrects the deficiency within 24h if liver function is normal. However, when hepatic disease is far advanced, vitamin K is ineffective and is analogous to bringing raw materials to a factory that is closed.

When vitamin K is used to reverse warfarin effect, its dose and route of administration should be guided by the urgency of the situation and the anticipated need for resuming warfarin anticoagulation. For example, during life-threatening hemorrhage, FFP and a large dose of vitamin K (10 mg) can be given intravenously to a patient who will not have warfarin restarted. By contrast, for a patient with only an excessively prolonged PT who must continue on long-term anticoagulation (e.g., mechanical mitral valve), a small dose (1 to 2 mg) of vitamin K orally is the most appropriate course of therapy. (Using large doses of vitamin K will prevent reestablishing warfarin anticoagulation for days to weeks.)

Disseminated Intravascular Coagulation

DIC should be strongly considered in any patient with the combination of diffuse bleeding or clotting, elevations in PT and aPTT, and a decreased platelet count. DIC is not self-perpetuating but requires continuous activation of the clotting mechanism. Such stimulation most frequently results from vascular damage or sepsis. In DIC, thrombin activation stimulates plasmin-mediated thrombolysis. FDPs are formed in this process. With concurrent clotting and fibrinolysis, factors V, VII, fibrinogen, and platelets are rapidly consumed. Bleeding results if consumption outstrips production. The causes of DIC are numerous but usually relate to tissue inflammation from infection, trauma, tumor, or release of the products of conception into the circulation. Cytotoxic drugs, heat stroke, envenomations, and shock, as well as vascular disruption (e.g., aortic aneurysm) may also cause DIC.

Diagnosis of DIC is usually straightforward. Early in the course, the aPTT may be shortened as thromboplastin is released into the circulation. Later, the PT and aPTT are prolonged because of depletion of fibrinogen, factors V and VII, and the anticoagulant action of FDPs. The platelet count is usually less than 150,000/mm^3 and fibrinogen usually less than 150 mg%. (Fibrinogen concentration may be in the normal range if levels were initially elevated, as with hepatitis or pregnancy.) The hallmark of DIC is an increase in the levels of FDPs to titers greater than 1:40. Large platelets are usually seen on peripheral smear along with fragmented red blood cells (RBCs) suggestive of microangiopathic hemolysis. A laboratory picture similar to DIC may be seen in dilutional coagulopathy or in hepatic failure if complicated by thrombocytopenia from splenic sequestration or platelet destruction.

The treatment of DIC associated with bleeding is to reverse the underlying cause and to supplement consumed clotting factors. Thus, typically, treatment involves removal of dead or infected tissue and giving antibiotics if infection is suspected. Platelets should be administered for severe thrombocytopenia. FFP may be used to replace most soluble factors. Cryoprecipitate may be used to replace fibrinogen if levels are markedly depressed. When severe sepsis is the cause, human recombinant activated protein C (rhAPC) should be strongly considered as part of the treatment regimen. When administered to septic DIC victims, rhAPC is associated with a nearly 50% decrease in the risk of death. There is no clear evidence that heparin is beneficial for DIC, except possibly when secondary to acute promyelocytic leukemia (APL). All transretinoic acid can be very beneficial in patients with APL by inducing differentiation of immature cells, hence reducing coagulopathy.

Dilutional Coagulopathy

Dilutional coagulopathy occurs during massive hemorrhage, when replacement of a substantial fraction of the circulating volume leads to washout of platelets and clotting factors. After 10 units of packed RBCs are transfused, it is prudent to begin regular monitoring of the PT and platelet count, although dilutional effects are rarely seen before 15 units are transfused. If platelet counts fall below 50,000/mm^3, random donor platelets are recommended. PT increases can be corrected with FFP. In addition to replacing deficient clotting proteins, preventing hypothermia is essential to optimize clotting enzyme function. The major diagnostic dilemma is to separate dilutional coagulopathy (increased PT and aPTT, decreased platelet count) from DIC, a distinction that is most reliably made by FDP assay. While awaiting laboratory confirmation, the best strategy is to administer 2 to 4 units of FFP; if the clotting disorder is dilutional, FFP will usually correct the defect.

Acquired Inhibitors of Coagulation

Circulating anticoagulants are immunoglobulins that inhibit the action of clotting proteins. Circulating inhibitors are most commonly seen in patients with pregnancy, hemophilia, rheumatoid arthritis, cancer, systemic lupus, advanced age, and with certain drugs (e.g., penicillin and chlorpromazine). The most notable inhibitor occurs in systemic lupus in which the action of factors II, V, IX, and X is impaired. Although termed the "lupus anticoagulant," also known as antiphospholipid and anticardiolipin antibody, such proteins are much more commonly associated with thrombosis than hemorrhage. Screening for a circulating anticoagulant is done by performing a PT and aPTT on a mixture of equal parts of normal and patient plasma. If a simple factor deficiency is the cause of abnormal clotting, the addition of normal plasma will provide 50% activity and will normalize clotting tests. However, if an inhibitor is present, clotting tests remain abnormal. Circulating anticoagulants often increase only the more sensitive aPTT mimicking the laboratory findings of hemophilia. (Antiphospholipid antibodies are also commonly associated with mild thrombocytopenia.) In urgent circumstances, therapy may include massive replacement of the affected factors or the use of activated factor X. In the long term, immunosuppressive therapy with cyclophosphamide, prednisone, or intravenous immune globulin may be helpful.

von Willebrand Disease

vWD, an autosomal dominant trait, decreases the activity of the factor VIII–vWF complex, thereby reducing the adherence of platelets to sites of vascular injury. vWD is usually subclinical but when overt, presents with hemorrhage after trauma, mucosal bleeding, or menorrhagia. Laboratory findings include an increased bleeding time with a normal platelet count and a prolonged aPTT. Because factor VIII-vWF is an acute phase reactant, the physiological stress of illness or even hemorrhage may increase plasma factor levels, thereby obscuring the diagnosis. Several subtypes of vWD exist, each requiring a slightly different diagnostic approach and treatment. Because of the complexities of diagnosing and treating vWD, hematological consultation is strongly recommended. Intermediate purity factor VIII concentrates contain vWF multimers useful in treating the condition and now present a very low risk of viral infection. Cryoprecipitate may be used to replace vWF, but as a pooled blood product, cryoprecipitate risks viral contamination avoided by use of factor VIII concentrates. Target vWF levels in bleeding patients or those undergoing surgery are 80 to 100 units/dL in the immediate perioperative period. The vasopressin analog desmopressin (DDAVP) may be used to transiently increase the endogenous release of factor VIII in most forms of vWF. Use of DDAVP may avoid transfusion in patients requiring only temporary normalization of hemostasis (e.g., patients undergoing brief invasive procedures). Tachyphylaxis rapidly occurs to DDAVP limiting its usefulness to just one to two doses.

Paraproteinemia

When present in large amounts, serum proteins of the IgG, IgM, and IgA classes may impair clotting. Such problems usually occur in patients with myeloma or Waldenström's macroglobulinemia. Plasmapheresis reduces the serum protein level and reverses the coagulopathy.

Thrombolytic Therapy

Almost any in vitro clotting test will confirm the presence of a "lytic state" during the administration of thrombolytic agents (e.g., streptokinase, urokinase, or tissue plasminogen activator [tPA]). The thrombin time, however, most directly monitors the effect of thrombolytic drugs by examining the final step in the clotting cascade (the conversion of fibrinogen to fibrin). As an index of the effectiveness of thrombolytic activity, the thrombin time should be maintained two to five times the baseline value when assessed 4 h after the initiation of therapy. If bleeding occurs during thrombolytic therapy, cryoprecipitate and FFP can rapidly correct the clotting abnormalities. Because hemorrhage during thrombolytic therapy is usually a consequence of poor patient selection (e.g., elderly, traumatized) or the result of invasive procedures during the lytic period, most bleeding episodes can be avoided. Because of issues of product availability and safety, tPA is now used almost exclusively.

Anticoagulant Therapy

Heparins

Anticoagulation therapy is difficult because there are risks of thrombosis from underdosing, risks of bleeding from excessive dosing, and current monitoring tests are only crude indirect measures of the risk of clotting or bleeding. Fortunately, serious bleeding during anticoagulation is uncommon and usually indicates a coexisting disturbance of vascular integrity or platelet function. As a corollary, gastrointestinal or genitourinary tract hemorrhage occurring at therapeutic levels of anticoagulation usually indicates an underlying structural lesion. Recognized risk factors for anticoagulant-induced bleeding include advanced age, alcohol and antiplatelet agent use, and female gender.

UFH, a heterogeneous drug with a half-life of 60 to 90 min, has been the traditional choice for acute anticoagulation. Used subcutaneously in fixed doses for thromboembolism prophylaxis (5,000 to 8,000 units), the aPTT usually remains unaffected and bleeding is very rare unless HIT occurs. There are little if any data to support the use of twice daily UFH for prophylaxis. By contrast, dosing every 8 h is of proven effectiveness.

When UFH is used for full "therapeutic" anticoagulation, the goal is to promptly prolong the aPTT to 1.5 to 2 times the control value. (Either the patient's baseline aPTT or the midpoint of the laboratory normal range may be targeted.) Failure to achieve this goal within the first day is associated with an increased risk of clot extension and recurrent embolism. The best method of rapidly achieving and maintaining the therapeutic goal is to use one of several validated heparin dosing protocols. To achieve prompt success, UFH demands starting treatment with a bolus of heparin (≥80 units/kg) and an initial hourly infusion of ≥18 units/kg. However, even when using a dosing protocol, underanticoagulation and overanticoagulation are all too frequent.

Despite little evidence to suggest anything more than weak correlation between aPTT values between 1.5 and 3 times control and bleeding tendency, physicians have strong fears of anticoagulation-induced bleeding. However, if the PT or aPTT are "infinitely" prolonged (>100 s), the tendency for unprovoked bleeding may be increased. Because UFH inhibits the action of thrombin and factor Xa, in high doses it can prolong the PT as well as the aPTT. The therapy of UFH overdose includes discontinuation of the drug, and in the hemorrhaging patient, administration of protamine sulfate (1 mg/100 units of circulating heparin). Except following cardiopulmonary bypass, protamine is rarely given in practice because of safety concerns and the difficulty in knowing how much should be administered.

Much more common than UFH excess is underdosing. In patients with active thrombosis, larger doses than those commonly used may be required to interrupt clotting. Unfortunately, there is no way to standardize the "clot burden" to guide therapy. The most common error in UFH dosing is failure to administer a heparin bolus and increase the rate of infusion for patients with subtherapeutic aPTTs. Failure to rebolus and increase infusion rates results in an aPTT in the therapeutic range only 50% to 60% of the time. When a "high" aPTT is encountered, physicians often discontinue UFH infusions for extended periods of time, the result being subtherapeutic anticoagulation when next measured. In most cases, prolongation of the aPTT to more than two times control does not require interruption of UFH infusion, but merely reducing the infusion rate by 20% to 25%. Interruption of a continuous infusion of UFH for more than 2 to 3 h will almost always result in a subtherapeutic aPTT, except in the setting of massive overdosage. (It obviously makes sense to interrupt administration in a bleeding patient.)

Overall, HIT develops in up to 20% of hospitalized patients given heparin, but most cases are the clinically insignificant nonimmune "Type I." The much more serious Type II HIT is induced by the formation of antibodies to heparin that cross-react with platelet surface antigens. Type II HIT rarely manifests before 7 days of heparin therapy in unsensitized patients and is most common in patients receiving higher doses. However, the syndrome may occur at any time during heparin therapy and has been reported in patients only receiving subcutaneous dosing or the tiny amounts infused in the maintenance of continuously flushing vascular-access catheters. The incidence of both varieties of HIT is reduced by using LMWH. The most serious complication of HIT is not bleeding but thrombosis. Up to 50% of patients developing Type II HIT experience thrombosis, the "white clot syndrome" of diffuse venous and arterial thrombosis induced by platelet aggregation. The development of thrombosis is associated with a mortality rate as high as 25%. Treatment of HIT should include discontinuing heparin and starting an alternate method of anticoagulation (e.g., direct thrombin inhibitor). Platelet transfusions should be avoided. Among patients developing HIT, future heparin exposure should be avoided if at all possible; however, if unavoidable, waiting until PF4 antibody levels are undetectable and minimizing the duration of exposure may be the safest course of action.

LMWHs are AT activators purified from UFH. Low endothelial uptake and serum protein binding provide for high bioavailability and slower clearance. The result is that appropriate doses of intermittent subcutaneous LMWH can be used for thromboembolism prophylaxis or treatment. Minor interactions of LMWH with vWF produce fewer platelet inhibitory actions than UFH and may account for the lower incidence of hemorrhage observed when using LMWH. LMWHs also have a lower incidence of HIT than UFH. The safety and efficacy of LMWH for treatment of thromboembolism in and out of the hospital have been clearly demonstrated. Outpatient therapy is also associated with significant reductions in cost. Given the lower incidence of HIT, and bleeding; predictability of anticoagulation with LMWH compared to UFH; and issues of patient satisfaction, it is hard to understand why the marginally higher acquisition costs deter the use of LMWH.

All forms of heparin are cleared at least in part by the kidney. Hence, significant reductions in glomerular filtration rate (i.e., GFR < 30 mL/min) necessitate reducing doses for both prophylaxis and treatment. Unfortunately, there are no good guidelines on how to modify prophylactic doses of UFH, but with regard to one LMWH, enoxaparin, study indicates dose reduction from 40 to 30 mg per day is probably appropriate for most average-sized patients. With regard to therapeutic dosing in renal insufficiency, three choices exist: (a) use of UFH and monitoring of aPTTs, (b) use of reduced doses (1 mg/kg daily) of enoxaparin (the sole LMWH with published guidelines), or (c) empiric use of a LMWH and monitoring anti-Xa activity levels. Uncertainty continues regarding how to treat morbidly obese patients with heparins. There are few data to guide dosing of UFH but as a practical matter, obese patients are rarely given doses derived from accepted nomograms. For example, a 200-kg patient is very unlikely to receive an UFH bolus of 16,000 units and an infusion of 3,600 units/h. Although not proven to be safer, instead it is more likely, that a "conventional" dose of heparin is started and the therapeutic aPTT approached slowly from below. Current data suggest that if a LMWH is to be used in the morbidly obese patent, dosing should be based on *actual* body weight. In this setting, checking anti-Xa activity levels is probably prudent to avoid under- or overanticoagulation.

Fondapariunux

Fondapariunux is a synthetic pentasaccharide inhibitor of factor Xa. Weight-based dosing is used for prevention and treatment of thromboembolic disease. The purported advantage of fondaparinux, avoidance of HIT, is now in question with reports of an association between the drug and PF4 antibody formation. Three significant limitations to use of fondaparinux are: uncertainty of dosing for patients less than 100 lb lack of a reversing agent; and exclusive renal clearance. Because fondaparinux is cleared by the kidney and has a half-life near 17 h in patients with normal renal function, it should not be used in patients with renal insufficiency.

Warfarin

Warfarin inhibits production of vitamin K–dependent proteins (II, VII, IX, X) prolonging the PT to a greater degree than the aPTT. The intensity and duration of warfarin anticoagulation should be guided by the severity of the thrombotic consequences. Because of interlaboratory variation in testing procedures, most hospitals now report the PT and an "international normalized ratio" (INR). INR reporting permits comparison of the intensity of warfarin anticoagulation among hospitals. The goal of warfarin therapy in thromboembolism has traditionally been to maintain PT 1.5 to 2.5 times the patient's baseline or laboratory control (INR 3 to 4.5). More intense anticoagulation has been advocated for patients with mural cardiac thrombi and mechanical prosthetic heart valves. However, evidence suggests that PT values 1.25 to 1.5 times control (INR 2 to 3) are adequate for most conditions and less-intense anticoagulation may lower hemorrhage risk.

Changes in previously stable INRs are often due to fluctuations in warfarin metabolism or protein binding induced by the addition or discontinuation of other drugs (e.g., erythromycin, phenobarbital, and phenytoin). Anticoagulation intensity is also increased by drugs that compete with warfarin for albumin binding (sulfas, sulfonureas, indomethacin, and phenylbutazone). In patients with warfarin-induced bleeding and firm indications for chronic anticoagulation (i.e., prosthetic heart valves, recurrent embolism), interruption of warfarin for 2 to 4 days is usually uneventful. If more precise control of anticoagulation is needed, UFH or LMWH may be temporarily substituted. Vitamin K is usually sufficient to reverse the anticoagulant effect of warfarin in patients with an excessively prolonged PT without bleeding. However, vitamin K does not provide ideal reversal because its effect may be delayed 6 to 24 h, and re-anticoagulation may be difficult if more than 1 mg of vitamin K is given. In more urgent cases, (e.g., an invasive procedure) FFP will promptly (but temporarily) reverse anticoagulation. Off label use of activated factor VIIa to treat warfarin overdose should be discouraged because of uncertain safety and efficacy.

Skin necrosis is a rare complication of warfarin anticoagulation traditionally associated with use of "loading doses," especially when given to patients not receiving concurrent AT therapy (i.e., UFH, LMWH). Warfarin-induced necrosis is most likely to occur in patients with hereditary or acquired protein C–deficiency, (especially those with HIT). Pathologically, the mechanism of necrosis is the formation of microvascular thrombi, leading to the hypothesis that necrosis is the result of inhibiting production of the anticlotting vitamin K–dependent proteins C and S.

TABLE 30-6 IDENTIFIED HYPERCOAGULABLE DISORDERS

Activated protein C resistance (factor V Leiden)
Prothrombin 20210 mutation
Protein C deficiency
Protein S deficiency
Antithrombin deficiency
Anticardiolipin antibody
Dysfibrinogenemias

■ HYPERCOAGULABLE DISORDERS

Knowledge regarding hypercoagulable disorders, also called thrombophilias, is much less complete than that for bleeding disorders. Routinely available laboratory tests cannot reliably predict a thrombotic tendency, and the assays possibly useful to predict thrombotic tendency are expensive, prone to artifact, and not widely available. Even though 20% to 40% of patients with thrombotic episodes are at least heterozygous for the factor V Leiden (activated protein C [APC] resistance) or prothrombin 20210 mutations, most episodes of arterial and venous thromboses cannot be attributed to any inherited or acquired prothrombotic blood disorder. Most patients with a thrombotic event do, however, have the risk factors of stasis and vascular intimal damage or inflammation. The most common identifiable hypercoagulable disorders are outlined in Table 30-6. Useful clinical clues to raise suspicion of an inherited or acquired thrombotic tendency are outlined in Table 30-7.

Inherited Thrombotic Disorders

Deficient quantities or activity of three specific plasma proteins, AT, protein C, and protein S, have been linked to a thrombotic tendency. Even though these conditions have long been appreciated, they are dwarfed in frequency and probably importance

TABLE 30-7 CLINICAL CLUES TO HYPERCOAGULABLE DISORDERS

Family history of thrombotic events (usually venous)
Thrombotic event at an early age
Thrombosis without identifiable risk factor
Recurrent clotting episodes
Thrombosis at unusual site (upper extremity)
Recurrent spontaneous abortions

by the factor V Leiden (APC resistance) and prothrombin 20210 mutations. Quantitative, genetic, and functional assays now exist for numerous mutations; however, testing is expensive and interpretation complicated. For example, levels of all these clotting proteins can be altered by liver disease, DIC, pregnancy, anticoagulation, or the occurrence of a thrombotic event not precipitated by the protein deficiency. Hence, the involvement of an expert hematologist in the evaluation of patients with a suspected prothrombotic disorder is prudent.

Unfortunately, there are no reliable clinical features to distinguish patients with thrombophilia from patients without heritable clotting disorders except perhaps a strong family history of thrombosis. (When clotting occurs, DVT of the leg appears to be the most likely event. Arterial thrombosis or visceral, cerebral, or upper extremity thromboses occur rarely.)

Substantial controversy exists about the wisdom of testing for thrombophilias. Because the factor V and prothrombin mutations are very prevalent, but the risk of thrombosis in the absence of additional risk factors is quite low, it does not make sense to test a broad population of asymptomatic patients. An impassioned argument is often made to test patients developing thrombosis who have few or no recognized risk factors for thromboembolism or those having a second or third clotting episode. Reasons for such an approach usually include "knowing" about future risk to the patient and relatives but unfortunately, there is no consensus about what should be done for patients with thrombosis and a concurrent mutation versus those lacking the mutation. That is, it is unclear if the duration of anticoagulation should be extended and if so, for how long. In addition, it is already recommended that patients with a second or third clotting episode receive lifelong anticoagulation, mitigating the need for diagnosis. The idea that asymptomatic family members should be tested at first blush makes sense but is complicated. First, most affected individuals do not experience thrombotic episodes unless additional risk factors are superimposed. Thus, lifelong prophylactic anticoagulation for asymptomatic carriers is not indicated and may confer substantial bleeding risk. Second, knowing that a relative has a mutation is not required to administer prophylaxis when additional risk factors develop (e.g., trauma, surgery, immobilization). Finally, diagnosing thrombophilia in an asymptomatic individual can have devastating unintended consequences for insurability, employment and reproductive choices. Hence, consultation with a genetic counselor before testing is wise. If after careful consideration testing is believe to be indicted, first steps in the evaluation of patients with a suspected clotting disorder include testing for factor V Leiden, prothrombin 20210, AT, and proteins C and S.

Factor V Leiden

Factor V Leiden is the most prevalent thrombophilia. Although as much as 6% of the white population may be heterozygous for the disorder, the condition is substantially less prevalent among peoples of Native American, Hispanic, African, or Asian ancestry. The most common defect, a single amino acid substitution renders factor V resistant to the neutralizing effects of APC. The genetic assay offers the advantage that it can be performed in patients with active thrombosis or those receiving anticoagulant therapy, but will not detect APC resistance caused by any other defect except the arginine–glycine substitution. Despite its frequency, the risk of thrombosis associated with the factor V mutation is substantially less than that for a person with protein C, S, or AT deficiency. It should be noted that some functional assays for protein S are sensitive to APC resistance and can yield a false diagnosis of protein S deficiency. Homozygotes are rare, and most thromboses occur among heterozygotes with multiple conventional risk factors.

Prothrombin Gene Mutation

A mutation at nucleotide pair 20210 in the gene coding for prothrombin is the second most common thrombophilia. The transformation is associated with an increase in circulating protein levels of about 30%. Like factor V Leiden, this mutation is very rare in patients of Asian or African descent, but can be found in up to 7% of whites. Alone, the prothrombin mutation is believed to increase the risk of clotting three- to fourfold but when it coexists with the factor V mutation, thromboembolism risk may be 20-fold higher than in individuals without either defect. Patients with the mutation cannot be detected merely by measuring the plasma prothrombin levels because substantial overlap exists with normals; genotyping is necessary for diagnosis.

Antithrombin

AT, formerly known as antithrombin III, is a naturally occurring serine protease plasma anticoagulant that acts to inhibit the action of activated factors IX, X, XI, and most importantly thrombin. The rate at which AT inactivates thrombin is dramatically increased (up to 10,000-fold) by the addition of heparin. AT deficiency is usually inherited as an autosomal dominant trait, with somewhere between 1 in 2,000 and 1 in 5,000 heterozygous for the protein. Heterozygotes are at increased risk for thromboses. Deficient homozygotes have not been identified, suggesting that such a severe deficiency is lethal. Spontaneous mutations (acquired disease) have rarely been described, and pregnancy, liver disease, DIC, nephrotic syndrome, and acute thromboses have been reported to reduce AT levels in genetically normal persons. Clinically, the disorder is usually suspected when the deficient protein renders patients clot resistant to the effects of heparin. Two general types of AT deficiency have been identified: reductions in plasma protein level or activity. The most common form of the disorder is a combined reduction in plasma protein level and functional activity. Normal AT levels but decreased functional activity represents the next most common form of the disorder. Immunological assays can measure the protein level, but functional assays are usually required to quantitate protein anticoagulant activity in the absence of heparin (progressive assay) or in the presence of heparin (heparin cofactor assay). An AT concentrate is now available for treatment of deficient patients; however, the mainstay of therapy remains lifelong anticoagulation for patients with demonstrated thrombotic events and AT deficiency.

Protein C Deficiency

The clinical presentation of protein C deficiency, a thrombin-activated vitamin K–dependent serine protease, is similar to that of AT deficiency. APC inhibits the activity of factors VIIIa and Va and increases fibrinolytic activity. As many as 1 in 200 persons in the general population is heterozygous for the autosomally dominant inherited condition and exhibits partial deficiency. Protein C levels can also be reduced by liver disease, DIC, use of chemotherapy, or the occurrence of acute thromboses. Warfarin reduces protein C and S levels, making laboratory determinations during therapy unreliable. Submaximal function of the enzyme may also result even when levels are normal. The importance of protein C deficiency is less certain than that for AT; most patients with reduced protein C levels are asymptomatic. Therapy for protein C deficiency includes chronic warfarin initiated during antithrombin coverage. Purified protein C and APC infusions are investigational. Although rare, skin necrosis has been associated with the institution of warfarin without concomitant heparin and when loading doses are used.

Protein S Deficiency

Protein S, another vitamin K–dependent protein, complexes with APC, potentiating its anticoagulant effect. Although protein assays for protein S exist, the free protein fraction is difficult to measure reliably. The most common form of protein S deficiency is a decrease in total level, though disorders in which the functional activity is decreased with normal total activity have also been described. Therapy for protein S deficiency is warfarin anticoagulation begun during heparin.

Lupus Anticoagulant/Antiphospholipid (Anticardiolipin) Antibody

Antiphospholipid antibody (APLA) is an IgG antibody directed against cardiolipin phospholipid, which constitutes a substantial risk for thrombosis and spontaneous abortions. Antibody titer correlates with the risk for thrombosis. APLA should be suspected in an appropriate clinical setting when the baseline aPTT is prolonged, especially if the platelet count is low. APLA can be confirmed using and factor Xa assay, a kaolin-activated aPTT, a dilute Russell viper venom time or a dilute one-stage PT. Alternatively, direct measurement of antibody titer can be performed. Therapy for patients with APLA syndrome includes increased intensity warfarin anticoagulation.

■ **SUGGESTED READINGS**

Gando S, Iba T, Eguchi Y, et al. A multicenter, prospective validation of disseminated intravascular coagulation diagnostic criteria for critically ill patients: Comparing current criteria. *Crit Care Med.* 2006;34(3):625–631.

Mercer KW, Macik B, Williams ME. Hematologic disorders in critically ill patients. *Semin Respir Crit Care Med.* 2006;27:286–296.

Rice TW, Wheeler AP. Coagulopathy in critically ill patients: Part 1—Platelet disorders. *Chest.* 2009;136: in press.

Visentin GP, Liu CY. Drug-induced thrombocytopenia. *Hematol Oncol Clin North Am.* 2007;21:685–696.

Warkentin TE, Greinacher A, Koster A, et al. Treatment and prevention of heparin induced thrombocytopenia. *Chest.* 2008;133:340–380.

Wheeler AP, Rice TW. Coagulopathy in critically ill patients: Part 2—Soluble clotting factors and hemostatic testing. *Chest.* 2009;136: in press.

Whitlatch NL, Ortel TL. Thrombophilias: When should we test and how does it help? *Semin Respir Crit Care Med.* 2008;29:25–39.

Hepatic Failure

■ CLASSIFICATION

Hepatic failure can arise as a primary process in a previously healthy person (e.g., acetaminophen overdose, acute viral hepatitis), through the progression of a chronic liver disease (e.g., cirrhosis, chronic viral hepatitis), or as part of the multiorgan failure syndrome. Whatever the cause, key manifestations are shared as one or more of the five major functions of the liver are disrupted: (a) maintenance of acid–base balance through lactate metabolism, (b) detoxification, (c) glucose and lipid metabolism, (d) protein synthesis (including clotting factors and albumin), and (e) phagocytic clearance of organisms and circulating debris.

The classification of hepatic failure can be confusing. Recently, a three-tiered categorization of acute hepatic failure (AHF) has been proposed based upon the pace of progression: *hyperacute* developing in less than a week, *acute* evolving over 1 to 4 weeks and, subacute occurring over 5 to 26 weeks. This system has some utility for predicting etiology and outcomes but is not clearly superior to the traditional designation *fulminant hepatic failure* defined as the development of encephalopathy within 8 weeks of onset of symptoms. For simplicity, the general term AHF will be used in this chapter. Chronic liver disease present for more than 6 months will be discussed separately because of the vastly different spectrum of complications.

■ ACUTE HEPATIC FAILURE

Clinical Features

The diagnosis of AHF cannot be made until coagulopathy and central nervous system (CNS) dysfunction (encephalopathy) are present. Irritability, confusion, and vomiting are all early signs of CNS involvement. The rate of progression of encephalopathy can be astonishing, with patients evolving from normal mental status to obtundation in hours. Fever is common early in the course, whereas hypothermia is more frequent later. The patient with AHF is typically tremulous and hyperventilating; "liver flap" (asterixis) and sustained clonus often can be elicited. Hypoxemia is present in most patients, and acute lung injury (ALI) complicates about one third of all cases. Although ascites and peripheral edema may occur in AHF, these signs result from portal hypertension and hypoalbuminemia making them much more common among patients with chronic liver disease.

Laboratory Features

Leukocytosis with neutrophilia and transaminase elevations usually are present in AHF. Marked hyperbilirubinemia commonly precedes a fall in albumin and prolongation of the prothrombin time (PT). Extensive hepatocyte destruction may impair glycogen storage and gluconeogenesis, giving rise to hypoglycemia. Low-grade disseminated intravascular coagulation (DIC) commonly results from decreased synthesis of clotting factors, together with failure of the liver to clear fibrin degradation products. Deficient hepatic production of antithrombin proteins predisposes to thrombosis. In AHF with hepatic encephalopathy, ammonia concentrations usually are elevated; a normal value may help to exclude the diagnosis. However, ammonia levels may be surprisingly low in patients with severe protein malnutrition. Furthermore, the degree of elevation correlates so poorly with changes in clinical status as to limit its utility for following a patient's progress.

Etiology

AHF has a wide variety of causes (Table 31-1). However, approximately 50% of cases are proven to result from acetaminophen toxicity (see Chapter 33), and

TABLE 31-1 CAUSES OF AHF

INFECTIONS	
Viral	**Chemical hepatotoxins**
Hepatitis A, B, C, D, E	Carbon tetrachloride
Adenovirus	Benzene
Varicella–Zoster	Ethylene glycol
Cytomegalovirus	Ethanol
Epstein–Barr	Phosphorus
Human immunodeficiency virus	**Cardiovascular**
	Portal vein thrombosis
Drug/Toxins	Budd–Chiari syndrome
Acetaminophen	Shock
Tetracycline	**Miscellaneous**
Isoniazid	Sickle cell disease
Rifampin	Reye syndrome
Phenytoin	Fatty liver of pregnancy
Methyldopa	Autoimmune hepatitis
Ketoconazole	Wilson disease
Valproic acid	Heatstroke
Anabolic steroids	
Sulfonamides	
Halogenated anesthetics	
Amanita phalloides mushrooms	
Vitamin A	
Herbal remedies	

sophisticated testing reveals that a substantial proportion of cases previously classified as "indeterminate" (the second most common etiologic category) are likely acetaminophen related. The third most common cause is viral infection.

Acetaminophen

Acetaminophen is safe when taken in recommended doses, but ingestion of as little as 6 gm may be fatal. (Usually, a fatal dose exceeds 140 mg/kg.) Toxicity is most likely among patients with chronic liver disease and those abusing alcohol. Because acetaminophen is rapidly absorbed and usually quickly metabolized, most AHF patients will have low or undetectable acetaminophen levels at presentation. After ingestion of a toxic dose, symptoms are minimal for the first day, with the exception of nausea and vomiting. One to two days later, deteriorating liver function tests, right upper quadrant pain, and oliguria (because of antidiuretic hormonelike effects) become evident. At this time, transaminases may peak in the tens of thousands of units. Within 3 to 5 days, a rising bilirubin and PT are seen as hepatic transaminases and albumin decline. In this most advanced stage, mental status may decline and renal failure develop. If the patient is to spontaneously recover, improvement is typically noted between days 5 and 7. Of all causes acetaminophen-induced AHF has the highest rate of spontaneous recovery, but predicting who will recover and who will die without transplantation is difficult. Poor prognostic factors are late presentation, the presence of coagulopathy, metabolic acidosis, renal failure, and cerebral edema.

When the time of ingestion is known, the risk of toxicity from an isolated acute acetaminophen ingestion may be predicted from the Rumack–Matthew nomogram. (Concentrations > 140 mg/dL ≥ 4 h are predictive of toxicity.) Unfortunately, the time of ingestion is rarely certain and patients with chronic exposure, preexisting liver disease, or significant alcohol use may develop toxicity at much lower concentrations than the nomogram predicts. For these reasons, it makes sense to administer N-acetylcysteine (NAC) as quickly as possible to AHF victims unless certain acetaminophen is not the cause. NAC protects by directly binding the toxic acetaminophen metabolites and repleting intracellular glutathione. Historically, an oral loading dose of 140 mg/kg followed by 17 additional doses of 70 mg/kg at 4-h intervals has been used. Vomiting is so common with oral NAC that "prophylactic" antiemetics are usually needed. Intravenous NAC, free of emetogenic effects, is available, safe, affordable, and at least as effective as the older, less-convenient oral regimen.

Viral Hepatitis

The risk of developing AHF from viral hepatitis is small (<1%), but because viral infection is common, collectively viral infections represent the third most cause of AHF. Numerous agents including hepatitis A to E, Epstein–Barr virus, and cytomegalovirus can cause severe hepatitis. Hepatitis B and C account for more than 90% of cases; with hepatitis A contributing another 5%. Hepatitis B and C are transmitted predominantly through the exchange of body fluids (e.g., transfusion, needle stick, or sexual intercourse). Although blood transfer represents the highest relative risk, saliva and semen are also vehicles. Hepatitis B immunization, testing the donated blood supply and evaluating the liver function tests of donors, has dramatically reduced the risk of transfusion-induced disease. After exposure to the hepatitis B virus, a 2- to 3-month incubation period passes as the virus proliferates. During this time, viral surface antigen (HbsAg) can be detected in the serum of infected patients. Nonspecific, gastrointestinal (GI), systemic, and rheumatologic symptoms precede the onset of jaundice and elevations in liver transaminases and, in most patients, by the disappearance of HbsAg. In a small minority of patients, HbsAg persists in the circulation signifying the presence of chronic disease and high infectivity. Antibodies to the core antigen appear in the serum during the incubation period and are typically present for several months after the illness resolves. Antibodies to HbsAg develop during the period of convalescence and may persist for years. Most patients do not require treatment for acute hepatitis B infection, and the value of antivirals or interferon therapy for patients with hepatitis B induced AHF is debated. The delta agent, or hepatitis D, creates disease by coinfecting or superinfecting patients with hepatitis B, producing a highly lethal combination.

In contrast to hepatitis B, hepatitis C is more likely to be clinically subtle in its initial stages and is a rare cause of AHF. Jaundice is uncommon with the acute illness, and when it does occur, is mild. Despite mild initial illness, hepatitis C is a major cause of chronic liver disease and cirrhosis. Even though 40% of infected individuals clear the virus spontaneously, if persistent infection is discovered,

treatment with interferon alpha and antivirals accelerate viral clearance. Because different genotypes of the virus have differential response rates and treatment is complex, expensive, and side effect laden, consultation with a hepatologist is prudent. Because coinfection is common, patients diagnosed with hepatitis C should be tested for HIV and vice versa.

Hepatitis A and E differ in many respects from hepatitis B or C. Both A and E are acquired by the fecal–oral route and often produce asymptomatic infection, especially in children. (Adults often are more symptomatic). After ingestion, an average incubation period of a month precedes the onset of nonspecific constitutional and GI symptoms. In some patients, an icteric phase follows, which is associated with abnormalities of transaminases and coincides with the appearance of IgM antibodies. Fortunately, hepatitis A and E uncommonly are associated with either AHF or chronic infection. The exception to this rule may be pregnant women who appear to be more severely affected by hepatitis E. Cytomegalovirus and Epstein–Barr virus are much less common causes of clinically important hepatitis and only rarely are associated with AHF.

Ischemia

Although ischemic AHF occurs only rarely as a primary process (e.g., Budd–Chiari, sickle cell crisis), life-threatening hepatic dysfunction often develops in patients with limited reserves, when another even relatively minor insult tips the balance. This injury can occur when nutritive flow is compromised by congestive heart failure or shock or when hepatocytes are damaged by circulating inflammatory mediators (e.g., severe sepsis) or severe hypoxemia.

Treatment

Initial Evaluation

Most patients with AHF should be cared for in an ICU because of their numerous physiologic problems and need for close monitoring. Because AHF patients are complex and encouraging survival rates have been achieved with transplantation, potential candidates should be transferred early in their course to a facility with transplant capability and resources necessary to manage complications. Unfortunately, transplantation carries its own set of risks, and at least half of all good candidates die while waiting for a liver. Transplantation is best reserved for the otherwise healthy patient with isolated liver failure. For example, it clearly cannot benefit patients with metastatic carcinoma or those who have sustained irreversible brain damage from hypoxia, intracranial bleeding, or intracranial hypertension.

The first step after confirming respiratory and hemodynamic adequacy is to try to determine the etiology of AHF. An in-depth history should be obtained that includes medications (e.g., herbal remedies, vitamins, estrogens); a dietary history targeting potential sources of hepatitis (e.g., travel, raw seafood consumption, and sick contacts) and; hepatotoxin exposure (e.g., alcohol, carbon tetrachloride, mushrooms). Obviously, a detailed history of transfusion, needle sharing, and sexual activity is essential. A toxicological survey should be obtained that includes acetaminophen levels. A panel of serologic tests should be sent to search for viral causes listed in Table 31-1. Although rare in patients under 40, ceruloplasmin, serum copper, and a 24-h urine for copper should be sent to look for Wilson disease. Autoimmune hepatitis can be excluded by laboratory testing for antinuclear antibody, antimitochondrial antibody, and anti–smooth-muscle antibody. A pregnancy test should be obtained for all women with childbearing potential. Basic laboratory studies including blood counts, bilirubin, transaminases, platelets, electrolytes, creatinine, an arterial blood gas, and tests of hepatic synthetic function (albumin and PTs) should be obtained. It is also reasonable to perform an ultrasound examination of the liver to evaluate its size, echogenicity, bile duct anatomy, portal and hepatic vein patency, and to look for ascites. In many cases, and essentially all cases where transplantation is a consideration, a contrasted abdominal computed tomographic (CT) scan will be performed to evaluate liver and spleen size and texture and vascular anatomy. Obviously, the decision to administer contrast media should be well reasoned given the risks of contrast-induced nephropathy. As initial data are being gathered, potential consultants, (e.g., hepatologist, transplant surgeons, and neurosurgeons) should be contacted.

Supportive Care

Patients should be positioned with the head of the bed elevated to decrease the risks of aspiration and cerebral edema. Neurological status should be monitored frequently, typically every 1 to 2 h. Prophylactic therapy for gastric ulceration should be undertaken. Special vigilance for hypoglycemia should be maintained because it is a common, potentially lethal, and easily treated cause of altered mental status. Supportive care includes maintenance of adequate nutrition and hemodynamic support as well as monitoring for the most frequent complications: (a) encephalopathy and cerebral edema, (b) infection, (c) coagulopathy and bleeding, and (d) renal failure.

N-acetylcysteine

NAC is indicated for treatment of proven or suspected acetaminophen toxicity as described above. In addition, a randomized trial of NAC versus placebo for nonacetaminophen-induced AHF suggests a substantial survival benefit (52% vs. 30%) for patients with Grade I or II encephalopathy at the time treatment was started. Given the safety profile, cost, and ease of administration, a strong case can be made to administer NAC to Grade I and II AHF patients, regardless of etiology, while awaiting confirmatory trials.

Complications

Encephalopathy

The causes of encephalopathy in liver failure are poorly understood, but almost certainly differ **2** between patients with acute and chronic disease. Intracranial hypertension induced by cerebral edema is the most common cause of encephalopathy in AHF but seldom complicates chronic liver disease. A standardized grading system for encephalopathy is presented in Table 31-2. Even though cerebral edema is usually the cause of altered mental status, hypoglycemia, infection, electrolyte imbalance, drug toxicity, and hypoxemia cannot be overlooked. The risk of cerebral edema is proportional to the speed of encephalopathy development

---

TABLE 31-2   CLASSIFICATION OF HEPATIC ENCEPHALOPATHY

Grade 0: Normal
Grade I: Behavioral alteration without change in level of consciousness
Grade II: Disorientation, hallucinations, drowsiness, asterixis
Grade III: Somnolent but arousable, confusion, incoherent speech
Grade IVA: Unconscious but arousable
Grade IVB: Unresponsive to pain

and is a serious problem; up to 25% of AHF deaths are attributable to cerebral edema. The mechanism of edema formation is not fully understood but likely involves ammonia uptake by astrocytes which is then converted to osmotically active glutamine which attracts water causing edema. Patients with chronic liver disease appear to be able to export other organic osmolar substances at a rate capable of offsetting this effect (probably because of lower rates of ammonia formation). Physical examination is rarely helpful in detecting cerebral edema, and even the head CT scan is relatively insensitive to this diagnosis. (The CT is helpful to rule out other causes of altered mental status like intracranial hemorrhage or metastatic disease.) To monitor intracranial pressure (ICP) accurately, an invasive monitor must be inserted. (See Chapter 34, Neurological Emergencies.) The decision to insert an ICP monitor is usually controversial because it necessitates sedation and intubation and by the time the procedure is considered, essentially all patients have significant coagulopathy. Even though supportive data are lacking, understandably most neurosurgeons require a platelet count greater than 50,000/mm^3 and a PT ≤1.5 times normal before monitor placement. (Normalizing the PT often requires 8 to 12 units of fresh frozen plasma [FFP]) The controversy over invasive monitoring is enhanced by absence of data of improved outcomes. Because the risk of procedural bleeding is associated with the "depth" of device placement, epidural monitors are favored over subdural or intraventricular devices. If employed, the ICP monitor is typically inserted as patients enter stage III encephalopathy.

When invasive monitoring is used, maintaining the cerebral perfusion pressure (CPP), defined as the difference between the mean arterial pressure and ICP, greater than 50 to 60 mm Hg appears to be an important goal. Poor neurological outcomes are associated with CPP values less than 40, especially if they persist for ≥2 h. CPP can be increased by raising mean arterial pressure with vasopressor and/or lowering ICP. Simple measures including elevation of the head of the bed to 30 degree and avoiding excessive fluid administration, coughing, and Valsalva maneuvers can reduce ICP. Keeping the head midline and avoiding neck flexion prevents compromise of jugular vein outflow. Unfortunately, even when diagnosed, the elevated ICP of AHF often fails to respond to treatments effective for edema from other causes. Surgical decompression and dexamethasone are of no benefit. Hyperventilation (PaCO$_2$

30 to 35 mm Hg) is only transiently helpful, and although mannitol (0.5 to 1 mg/kg every 6 h) may temporarily reduce edema, there is little evidence that survival is increased. When mannitol is used, serum osmolarity should not exceed 310 to 320 mOsm. (Mannitol is not useful in patients who have developed oliguria because it cannot be excreted). Hypertonic saline targeting a serum sodium of 145 to 155 has not been tested as a treatment for AHF induced cerebral edema, but may have prophylactic value. In desperate situations, deep sedation with propofol or barbiturates with or without paralysis can reduce cerebral oxygen consumption and ICP. A small human study suggests there may be a role for therapeutic hypothermia (core temperature 32°C to 33°C) in reducing ICP. In distinction to portosystemic encephalopathy (PSE) of chronic liver disease, lactulose offers little benefit for the encephalopathy of AHF.

Infection

Acute and chronic liver failure predisposes to infection by decreasing opsonins, complement levels, and phagocytosis. Up to 80% of AHF victims develop serious infections, 25% of which are bacteremic. Ten to twenty percent of patients with AHF die of bacterial infection. Interestingly, fever and leukocytosis occur in a minority of cases and there is a surprisingly high rate of positive blood cultures despite few signs of infection. Pneumonia, urinary tract and catheter-related sepsis are common, largely preventable infections, with good supportive care. Spontaneous bacterial peritonitis (SBP) which is common among patients with ascites from portal hypertension of chronic liver failure is relatively uncommon in AHF. Avoiding serious infection is critical because it is life threatening in and of itself and development of infection almost always disqualifies the patient for transplantation. *Staphylococcus* and *Streptococcus*, followed by Gram-negative rods, are the predominant organisms. Randomized trials have shown prophylactic antibiotics decrease the incidence of infection without altering mortality; nevertheless, antibiotics are usually administered. As antibacterial coverage has been escalated, more fungal infections (especially *Candida*) have been observed.

Coagulation Disorders and Bleeding

Coagulopathy is frequent in AHF because all clotting factors are produced by the liver, with the exception of factor VIII/von Willebrand's factor (see

Chapter 30). Failure to produce clotting factors results in elevation of the PT and activated partial thromboplastin time (aPTT). In addition, function of Kupffer cells which normally clear clot degradation products from the circulation is lost increasing the risk of DIC. When thrombocytopenia occurs, it is usually due to DIC, often from infection. Interestingly, despite the high frequency of abnormal clotting studies spontaneous bleeding is uncommon. (When it occurs, gastritis and esophagitis are the most common sources.) This rarity of bleeding may be explained by the fact that the liver also produces anticlotting factors (antithrombin and proteins C and S) which decline concurrently. Second, patients with AHF rarely have significant portal hypertension making variceal bleeding very rare.

Because there is a poor correlation between laboratory studies and spontaneous bleeding risk, routine correction of clotting tests is not warranted. Despite absence of data to support correction of clotting studies before performing invasive procedures, it is almost always attempted, especially before intracranial pressure monitor insertion. Importantly, up to 25% of patients are vitamin K deficient and doses of 10 mg/day safely augment production of factors II, VII, IX, X when there is residual synthetic function. Hence, vitamin K should be tried in most patients. When synthetic function is inadequate, FFP can be used to correct the PT before an invasive procedure or to treat active bleeding. FFP is not routinely indicated for correction of abnormal clotting parameters because it presents a volume challenge that may increase intracranial pressure, risks infection and immunologic reaction, and obscures the ability to gauge the liver's endogenous clotting factor production. Furthermore, prophylactic administration of FFP has been shown to not decrease bleeding risk. In the bleeding patient who cannot tolerate the FFP volume required to correct the PT, isovolemic plasmaphresis can be performed. Obviously, plasmaphresis requires large-bore venous access and incurs significant costs.

Since fibrinogen is an acute phase reactant produced by the liver, levels are unpredictable in AHF. In patients who are bleeding, measurement of fibrinogen is warranted if coagulation parameters are not normalized by FFP. When levels fall below 100 mg/dL, cryoprecipitate is the most effective fibrinogen replacement. There are no reliable data to guide platelet transfusions but consensus suggests a transfusion threshold of 50,000/mm^3. Recently, there has been interest in use of human recombinant activated factor VII (rhVIIa) for hemorrhage in a variety of settings. Uncontrolled reports of rhVIIa use in liver transplant surgery and observations that the drug rapidly corrects the PT have fuelled interest. Unfortunately, controlled trials have shown little clinical benefit (1 to 3 unit reductions in packed red cell use) and an increase in thrombotic complications. Given that data, it seems reasonable to reserve use of rhVIIa for hemorrhage that persists after restoration of platelet and soluble factor levels using conventional blood products.

Acute Kidney Injury

Acute kidney injury (AKI) develops in up to 75% of all patients with AHF most commonly from the direct toxicity of acetaminophen. When AKI occurs **4** in patients with non–acetaminophen-induced AHF, hypotension from volume depletion and severe sepsis are the most common causes. Blood urea nitrogen (BUN) levels are not a reliable indicator of renal function in AHF because production of urea nitrogen by the liver is impaired. The diagnosis and therapy of AKI is outlined elsewhere (see Chapter 29).

Nutrition

Although sufficient calories and protein of high biologic value must be provided, high-protein loads should be avoided in AHF. Vitamin K, thiamine, and folate are required by most patients. Sufficient glucose should be given to prevent hypoglycemia and to provide protein-sparing effects (see Chapter 16). It may be advantageous to use branched-chain (rather than aromatic) amino acids to minimize encephalopathy. Restoring a positive nitrogen balance is a major goal of nutritional repletion and may be assessed by standard tests of urine urea nitrogen. Lipid infusions are of limited usefulness because the failing liver cannot process fats readily.

Pulmonary Complications

Aspiration, pneumonia, atelectasis, and abnormal ventilation–perfusion (*V/Q*) matching all contribute to the frequent development of hypoxemia in patients with AHF. Acute *V/Q* mismatching probably is due to failure of the damaged liver to clear vasodilating humoral substances. A reduced level of consciousness, abdominal distention, and splinting from pain caused by a swollen liver all can produce hypoxemia by causing atelectasis. Pulmonary edema because of fluid overload, hypoalbuminemia, impaired cardiac contractility, and increased vascular permeability all may occur. As patients enter Stage III encephalopathy, most will require intubation and mechanical ventilation.

Miscellaneous Complications

Many hepatically metabolized drugs are potentially lethal in AHF. Because narcotics, sedatives, and anesthetics severely depress mental status and glottic reflexes in these sensitive patients, indiscriminate use may be fatal; careful dosing and monitoring are mandatory. Long-acting sedatives given frequently or in large doses should be avoided because of cumulative drug effects. If sedation is necessary, small doses of short-acting drugs without active metabolites (e.g., oxazepam) should be used. If neuromuscular paralytic agents are used, those not requiring hepatic metabolism are favored (e.g., succinylcholine, pancuronium, and atracurium).

Prognosis

Outcome is determined largely by patient characteristics and the cause and severity of hepatic failure and is best for patients between the ages of 10 and 40 years. AHF caused by non-A or non-B hepatitis or drugs (exclusive of acetaminophen) is associated with poor prognosis. Similarly, development of coma, a bilirubin greater than 18 mg/dL, an arterial pH less than 7.30, an international normalized ratio (INR) greater than 3.5, and less than 10% activity of any specific clotting factor are poor prognostic indicators. The occurrence of any other associated organ failure (e.g., ALI or AKI) also dramatically reduces the chances for survival. These factors have been amalgamated into a single index: the model for end-stage liver disease (MELD) score calculated as = 10 [0.957 × ln(serum creatinine) + 0.378 × ln(serum bilirubin) + 1.120 × ln(INR) + 0.643)]. In addition to becoming a useful prognosticator, the MELD score has become the standard for ranking transplant candidates.

■ CHRONIC LIVER FAILURE

Etiology and Pathophysiology

Alcoholism, chronic viral hepatitis (hepatitis B and C) and nonalcoholic steatohepatitis (NASH) are the most common causes of chronic liver failure and cirrhosis. In addition to loss of hepatic functions including drug, toxin, glucose and lipid metabolism, and synthesis of clotting factors and albumin, cirrhosis presents a unique mechanical problem—portal hypertension. As the cirrhotic liver shrinks from scarring, cephalad flow of blood from the portal to hepatic veins is blocked. As portal pressure rises, blood shunts around the liver to the lower pressure vessels of the stomach, esophagus, abdominal wall, and rectum dilating these fragile vessels into varices. The same portal pressure increase transudes ascitic fluid and causes splenomegaly by increasing back pressure in the splenic vein.

Clinical and Laboratory Features

Portal hypertension leads to splenomegaly and causes formation of ascites, occasionally severe enough to produce umbilical herniation. Thrombocytopenia is common as splenic dilation sequesters platelets and hepatically produced thrombopoesis factors decline. The tendency for ascites formation is enhanced by hypoalbuminemia due to loss of normal albumin synthesis. Shunting of blood around the liver leads to findings of *caput medusae* as veins on the anterior abdominal wall dilate and to the frequent occurrence of hemorrhoids. The internal manifestations of vascular shunting are esophageal and gastric varices. Gynecomastia, spider telangestasia, and palmar erythema are probably related to failure of the damaged liver to clear estrogenic and vasodilating humoral substances. Impaired metabolic function from loss of hepatocytes typically results in a low BUN. Jaundice results from impaired bilirubin metabolism and the frequent findings of echymoses stem from impaired coagulation factor synthesis, often manifest as a prolongation of the PT. Although the MELD score described above is now commonly used to describe severity of illness among patients with acutely decompensated liver failure, the Child-Pugh criteria (Table 31-3) are often used to categorize patients with chronic liver disease.

Treatment and Complications

Encephalopathy

Hepatic encephalopathy, also known as PSE, is the most common cause of altered mental status in chronic liver disease but it is important to exclude other more readily reversible causes of altered consciousness including (a) hypoglycemia, (b) infection (especially spontaneous bacterial peritonitis),

TABLE 31-3 CHILD-PUGH CLASSIFICATION OF CHRONIC LIVER DISEASE

PARAMETER	SCORE		
	1 POINT	2 POINTS	3 POINTS
Bilirubin	<2	2–3	>3
Albumin	>3.5	3.5–2.8	<2.8
International normalized ratio (INR)	<1.7	1.7–2.3	>2.3
Ascites	Absent	Mild to moderate	Severe/refractory
Encephalopathy grade	0	I–II	III–IV

(c) electrolyte imbalance (e.g., hyponatremia), (d) drugs (particularly sedatives), (e) hypoxemia, and (f) thiamine deficiency. Hypoglycemia is important because it develops in as many as 40% of all patients, can cause permanent damage, and is easily reversible. Likewise, thiamine deficiency is perilous but easily corrected.

PSE arises when cirrhosis causes shunting of toxin-laden portal blood around the liver into the systemic circulation. Ammonia, fatty acids, mercaptans, and other false neurotransmitters have been implicated as causative, but there is no clear consensus on etiology. Encephalopathy may produce focal neurological deficits as well as alterations in consciousness, and cognition. In salvageable patients, mental status responds to appropriate therapy within several days. The standard grading system for encephalopathy is presented in Table 31-2.

Regardless of the specific mechanism, a number of precipitating factors worsen PSE. High protein intake or GI hemorrhage increases the protein load and toxin production. Intravascular volume depletion from bleeding or diuretic use worsens mental status by reducing hepatic and renal perfusion and predisposing patients to contraction alkalosis. In turn, alkalosis and hypokalemia increase ammonia production and impair its renal excretion, further worsening mental status. Excessive withdrawal of ascitic fluid may redistribute fluid from the vascular space to the peritoneal cavity, further decreasing hepatic perfusion. Because of the complications of hypovolemia, weight lost through the use of diuretics or fluid restriction usually should not exceed 1 to 2 lb per day. Failing renal function accentuates the accumulation of toxins. Almost any systemic infection may alter mental status, but the most common infection precipitating PSE is spontaneous bacterial peritonitis. All drugs (but particularly sedatives and narcotics) must be used with extreme caution when hepatic metabolism is impaired.

The diagnosis of PSE is made on clinical grounds and can be supported by elevated blood ammonia levels or specific electroencephalogram (EEG) findings. Although an EEG occasionally demonstrates characteristic abnormalities (high-amplitude δ and triphasic waves), unfortunately, the EEG usually shows only nonspecific, diffuse slowing. CT scanning of the brain can reveal intracranial hemorrhage or nonspecific cerebral edema but cannot confirm a diagnosis of hepatic encephalopathy. When there is concern for the possibility of meningitis, lumbar puncture should be performed. For patients with subtle encephalopathy or in cases where the diagnosis is in doubt, a therapeutic trial should be undertaken after other causes of reversible encephalopathy are excluded. Response usually occurs within 3 to 4 days if the diagnosis is correct. Correction of precipitating causes (bleeding, drugs, infection, alkalosis, hypovolemia) is key to improvement. However, when PSE is established, restricting protein intake (0.25 to 0.5 gm/kg/day) and preventing GI bleeding reduce the substrate available for the production of cerebral toxins. Aromatic amino acids (e.g., phenylalanine, tyrosine) have been implicated in the encephalopathy of liver failure; therefore, diets high in branched-chain amino acids (e.g., valine, leucine, and isoleucine) have been advocated.

Laxatives and enemas decrease fecal generation of nitrogenous toxins, but profuse or protracted diarrhea sufficient to cause fluid depletion and electrolyte abnormalities must be avoided.

Lactulose, a synthetic nonabsorbable and disaccharide, usually is used to reduce the intestinal burden of toxins. Lactulose is broken down by colonic bacteria to lactic and acetic acids, compounds that promote bowel transit. Initially, 15 to 30 mL is given every 6 h and then the dose is modified to produce three loose stools per day. As with other laxatives, excessive diarrhea may deplete intravascular volume, worsening hepatic encephalopathy and sometimes precipitating the hepatorenal syndrome (HRS). Neomycin is a poorly absorbed broad-spectrum antibiotic sometimes used as an alternative. When given in 2- to 4-gm oral doses or administered as an enema once or twice daily, neomycin reduces the number of intestinal bacteria forming these toxic compounds. Because as much as 5% of the drug may be absorbed systemically, renal insufficiency may occur when large doses are given to patients with preexisting renal dysfunction. Ototoxicity is another risk. Occasionally, patients respond to neomycin but not to lactulose, or vice versa.

Ascites and Hepatic Hydrothorax

Ascites frequently is present in chronic liver disease, and on occasion, a pleuroperitoneal communication may allow ascitic fluid to enter the chest, producing a symptomatic pleural effusion (hepatic hydrothorax). Although the natural tendency is to drain such pleural effusions, the positive pressure inside the ascites-filled abdomen and the average negative pleural pressure typically refill the pleural space in hours to days. In this setting, it is important to avoid tube thoracostomy. Insertion of a chest tube often results in a never-ending flow of pleural fluid, which leads to protein and lymphocyte depletion. The development of ascites with or without pleural fluid may impair ventilation and increase the work of breathing. Usually, sodium and water restriction and diuretic therapy are sufficient to limit ascites to manageable levels. Spironolactone, a potassium-sparing diuretic, alone or in combination with a loop diuretic, usually is effective. When diuretics fail, large-volume paracentesis may temporarily improve gas exchange and patient comfort. Rarely, ascites can become so tense that venous return is impaired and urine flow declines, in essence, "abdominal tamponade," also known as the abdominal compartment syndrome. The mechanism of reductions in urine flow is uncertain but might be the result of decreased venous return, or compression of renal veins or arteries. Ureteral obstruction appears unlikely.

Regardless of mechanism, decompression of the abdomen by paracentesis rapidly restores urine output. Removal of large volumes of ascites can, on occasion, precipitate hypotension, which responds to intravenous volume replacement. Controversy persists about the relative benefits of colloid and crystalloid in this situation.

Spontaneous Bacterial Peritonitis

SBP is a common complication of chronic liver disease in which bacteria seed the peritoneal cavity. Hypoperfusion often precipitates SBP, presumably by impairing bowel wall integrity. For this reason, many clinicians routinely administer antibiotics to patients with cirrhosis and ascites who develop significant GI bleeding. In patients with ascites, sudden deterioration of renal function or mental status, rapid weight gain, and ascites that becomes resistant to diuretic therapy all should prompt consideration of SBP. Classically, SBP may be recognized by the triad of fever, abdominal pain, and encephalopathy. However, SBP differs from peritonitis of other causes (secondary peritonitis) in that fever, abdominal pain, and tenderness are often subtle. Approximately 25% of all patients with SBP have only extra-abdominal symptoms and 5% of patients are entirely asymptomatic.

Nothing short of obtaining peritoneal fluid can exclude the diagnosis of SBP. Table 31-4 contrasts ascites characteristics between uninfected ascites and spontaneous and secondary peritonitis. An ascitic fluid pH less than 7.31, a gradient in pH between the serum and ascitic fluid of more than 0.1 units, or an ascitic fluid lactic acid level higher than 32 mg/dL is suggestive. Diagnosis is confirmed when bacteria are seen on Gram stain or grow in culture. An absolute neutrophil count in the ascitic fluid greater than 250/mm^3 should prompt empiric therapy, particularly if polymorphonuclear leukocytes predominate. In contrast to secondary peritonitis, which is typically polymicrobial, cultures in SBP usually grow only a single organism. Enteric Gram-negative rods are the most common organisms, but 15% of patients with SBP have polymicrobial infections and 5% grow anaerobes. The single most likely organism is *Escherichia coli*, but pneumococcal infections (15%) also are prevalent. Because bacteremia occurs in approximately 50% of cases, blood cultures should be obtained. A third-generation cephalosporin or an extended-spectrum penicillin (ticarcillin/clavulanate, ampicillin/sulbactam) given with a quinolone is

TABLE 31-4   CHARACTERISTICS OF ASCITIC FLUID

FLUID PARAMETER	BENIGN HEPATIC ASCITES	SPONTANEOUS BACTERIAL PERITONITIS	SECONDARY PERITONITIS
Total leukocyte count (cells/mm³)	<1,000	<1,000	>>1,000
Neutrophil count (cells/mm³)	<250	>250	>>250
Culture	No growth	Single organism	Multiple organisms
Protein	Low	Low	>1 gm/dL
Lactate dehydrogenase (LDH)	Normal	Normal	High
Glucose	Normal	Normal	Low
pH	>7.4	<7.4	<<7.4

appropriate initial coverage for most patients. Although the practice remains controversial, administration of albumin (1.5 gm/kg) at SBP diagnosis and 1 gm/kg 3 days later has been reported to dramatically reduce the risk of AKI and improve long-term survival.

Hepatorenal Syndrome

The HRS is a highly lethal condition of uncertain cause which is unique to patients with chronic liver disease. The diagnosis of HRS can be knotty because many HRS victims have experienced multiple potential renal insults including nephrotoxic drugs and intravascular volume depletion from undertreated GI hemorrhage, overzealous paracentesis, or excessive diuretic usage. HRS is characterized by increasing serum creatinine and oliguria, which fails to respond to fluids or diuretics. Because patients with chronic liver disease often have low muscle mass, initial rises in creatinine may seem unimpressive, delaying recognition. In addition, the calculated creatinine clearance will overestimate renal function. Urinary Na⁺ values are typically very low (<10 mEq/L).

The definitive treatment is liver transplantation, but obviously not all patients are candidates and delays in obtaining a donor organ necessitate an interim support plan. A significant number of cases of HRS respond to a therapeutic protocol, which targets a central venous pressure (CVP) of 8 to 10 mm Hg and uses norepinephrine in doses up to 8 μg/min to maintain the mean arterial pressure above 65 mm Hg. When CVP exceeds the target, loop diuretics are given; when CVP falls below target, albumin is used to boost filling pressure. Intermittent hemodialysis or continuous ultrafiltration may be required for renal failure

unresponsive to conservative therapy. Renal replacement therapy is best reserved for patients awaiting liver transplantation. There is no role for low dose dopamine or octreotide alone in treatment. Data regarding the benefits of the vasopressin analogue, terlipressin, remain controversial. Studies using a combination of midodrine and octreotide are not yet sufficient to incorporate these modalities into routine treatment.

Gastrointestinal Bleeding

The subject of gastrointestinal bleeding is covered in depth in Chapter 39. Because GI bleeding frequently produces shock, sepsis, hepatic encephalopathy, or hypoperfusion that initiates acute renal failure, it is often the proximate cause of death in patients with *chronic* hepatic failure and portal hypertension. The most common sources are gastritis and esophagitis, but patients with portal hypertension are prone to bleeding from esophageal varices. Coagulopathy frequently accentuates the tendency for GI blood loss. Antacids, sucralfate, and histamine (H₂) blockers and proton pump inhibitors are all effective in preventing stress ulceration.

■ SUGGESTED READINGS

Arroyo V, Guevara M, Gines P. Hepatorenal syndrome in cirrhosis: Pathogenesis and treatment. *Gastroenterology.* 2002;122(6):1658–1676.

Gines P, Cardenas A, Arroyo V, et al. Management of cirrhosis and ascites. *N Engl J Med.* 2004;350(16):1646–1654.

Lee WM, Rossaro L, Fontanta RJ, et al. Intravenous N-acetylcysteine improves spontaneous survival in early non-acetaminophen acute liver failure. *Hepatology.* 2007;46:268.

Patch D, Burroughs A, Sort P, et al. Intravenous albumin in patients with cirrhosis and spontaneous bacterial peritonitis. *N Engl J Med.* 1999;341:1773–1774.

Stravitz RT. Critical management decisions in patients with acute liver failure. *Chest.* 2008;134:1092–1102.

Stravitz RT, Kramer AH, Davern T, et al. Intensive care of patient with acute liver failure: Recommendations of the US acute liver failure study group. *Crit Care Med.* 2007;35:2498–2508.

Endocrine Emergencies

■ THYROID DISEASE

Critical Illness and Thyroid Testing

Mild hyperthyroidism and hypothyroidism are very common in the ambulatory population, but severe disease in the intensive care unit (ICU) is rare. Nevertheless, profound excess or deficiency of thyroid hormone is life threatening, can be confused with many other nonendocrine conditions, and is generally amenable to simple therapy. By far the most common "thyroid disorders" seen in the ICU are not thyroid problems at all but rather laboratory anomalies resulting from altered binding and metabolism of thyroid hormone caused by critical illness or drug therapy. Critical illness has numerous effects on thyroid tests, in some cases simulating disease when none is present and in other cases obfuscating a true diagnosis. For example, almost all critical illnesses decrease thyroid-stimulating hormone (TSH) and the plasma concentration of proteins that bind thyroid hormone (albumin, thyroid binding prealbumin, thyroxin binding globulin). As binding proteins decrease, total levels of thyroxin (T_4) and to a lesser degree triiodothyronine (T_3) decline, simulating hypothyroidism. In fact more than 50% of critically ill patients have subnormal T_4 and T_3 levels. Historically, the term "euthyroid sic" was used to describe the constellation of low T_4, T_3, and TSH but it now appears perhaps some of these patients actually have transient central hypothyroidism. Nevertheless, when T_4 or T_3 is administered to critically ill patients with these laboratory findings clinical outcomes are not improved. Critical-illness–induced falls in plasma protein concentrations can also obscure a true diagnosis of hyperthyroidism by lowering observed T_4 and T_3 levels into the normal or near normal range. (Most patients with hyperthyroidism have an increased T_3, even if T_4 levels are normal.)

Drugs commonly used in the ICU also complicate thyroid function test interpretation by inhibiting TSH secretion, T_4 binding to serum proteins, or T_4 to T_3 conversion. For example, glucocorticoids, octreotide, dobutamine, dopamine, and dopamine agonists inhibit TSH secretion, potentially leading to an erroneous diagnosis of central hypothyroidism if T_4 values are low or to an erroneous diagnosis of hyperthyroidism if T_4 is modestly elevated. Highly protein-bound drugs like phenytoin, carbamazepine, furosemide, aspirin, and some nonsteroidal anti-inflammatory drugs displace T_4 from binding proteins, lowering total T_4 levels, and potentially leading to a false diagnosis of hypothyroidism. Finally, glucocorticoids, amiodarone, and β-blockers all inhibit the peripheral conversion of T_4 to T_3, resulting in a low serum T_3 concentration and encouraging an incorrect diagnosis of hypothyroidism.

Given the many influences of critical illness on thyroid function tests, several guiding principles should be kept in mind: (a) Do not send "screening" thyroid function studies; tests should be thoughtfully selected to confirm or exclude a specific suspected condition. (b) Unlike ambulatory practice, where clinical examination and a TSH measurement usually suffice to diagnose both hypothyroidism and hyperthyroidism, use of TSH alone in the ICU for diagnosis is fraught with problems. (c) Be suspect of thyroid disease diagnoses made in critically ill patients.

Severe Hyperthyroidism and Thyroid Storm

No absolute signs differentiate the flowery term "thyroid storm" from severe hyperthyroidism, although diagnostic criteria have been proposed. Apart from accentuated signs and symptoms of hyperthyroidism, thyroid storm is more likely to exhibit fever (often approaching 103°F) and tachycardia (pulse > 100/min). Secondary features may include a goiter, proptosis, congestive heart failure, arrhythmias, tremor, diaphoresis, diarrhea, elevated liver function tests, and mental status changes.

Historically, surgery performed on large goiters with poor preoperative preparation was the most common cause of thyroid storm, but currently, the condition most often results from an acute infection, withdrawal of antithyroid drugs, or nonthyroid surgery. Recognizable Graves disease is present in most patients with severe hyperthyroidism. (Toxic multinodular goiter and autonomous thyroid nodules are also fairly common causes.) Although iodine ingestion initially increases T_4 production, it suppresses T_4 release. However, serum iodine levels decline after 10 to 14 days, allowing discharge of large amounts of newly formed T_4 into the circulation. For this reason, radioactive iodine and IV and oral iodinated radiographic contrast may precipitate delayed thyroid storm in predisposed individuals. Accidental or intentional overdose with exogenous T_3 or T_4 is only problematic following massive ingestions.

In the critically ill patient with suspected thyroid storm, the diagnosis must initially be a clinical one. The results of thyroid function tests are often delayed and comparable elevations in total T_4, free T_4, and T_3, may occur in both mild and severe hyperthyroidism (Table 32-1). When normal or only modestly elevated T_4 or T_3 levels are seen in patients with clinically overt hyperthyroidism, the finding is usually due to reductions in binding protein levels induced by critical illnesses. TSH should be undetectable (<0.01 mU/L) in essentially all cases of true hyperthyroidism, whereas low but detectable levels of TSH (0.01 to 0.1 mU/L) associated with normal or modestly elevated T_3 and T_4 levels are usually the result of critical illness alone. Among patients with Graves disease, often only T_3 concentrations are elevated (T_3 thyrotoxicosis).

Elevated hepatic transaminases indicate life-threatening disease. Rarely, hypercalcemia may be present. In thyroid storm, the leukocyte count is usually normal or slightly elevated, but relative lymphocytosis is common, a feature that may help to differentiate thyroid disease from infectious causes of fever.

The treatment of thyroid storm is fourfold: (a) block T_4 formation, (b) prevent T_4 release, (c) inhibit peripheral conversion of T_4 to T_3, and (d) block the tissue effects of T_4 (Fig. 32-1). Propylthiouracil (PTU) and methimazole both block T_4 synthesis within hours but do not stop release of preformed

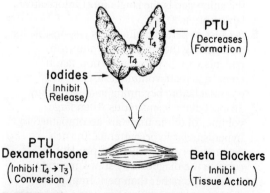

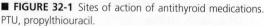

■ **FIGURE 32-1** Sites of action of antithyroid medications. PTU, propylthiouracil.

TABLE 32-1 LABORATORY ANALYSIS OF THYROID FUNCTION

	FREE T_4	T_3	TSH	NOTES
Primary hyperthyroidism				
T_3 toxicosis	Normal[a]	Elevated[a]	Undetectable to low	Graves disease likely, consider T_3 poisoning
T_4 toxicosis	Elevated[a]	Normal[a]	Undetectable to low	Suggests hyperthyroidism with concomitant critical illness or T_4 poisoning
Central hyperthyroidism	Elevated	Elevated	Elevated	Very rare, pituitary tumor likely cause
Critical illness	Low to normal	Low	Low to normal	
Hyperthyroidism Plus critical illness	Elevated	Normal	Low	
Hypothyroidism				
Primary	Low	Low	Elevated	
Secondary	Low	Low	Undetectable to low	

[a]T_4 and T_3 can be normal in critical illness.

T_4 from the thyroid. Of the two choices, PTU (600 mg load followed by 200 mg PO q4–6h) is preferred because it also stops conversion of T_4 to its biologically active form (T_3) in peripheral tissues. (Inhibition of T_4 to T_3 conversion may also be accomplished by glucocorticoids and to a lesser degree by propranolol.) Although PTU is preferred over methimazole, allergic reactions may occur with its use, and delayed, dose-dependent agranulocytosis is a risk. Low doses of PTU represent a particularly good choice of therapy for the pregnant patient because the drug crosses the placental barrier poorly. On the other hand, an advantage of methimazole is its long duration of action, allowing less-frequent dosing compared to PTU. If methimazole is chosen, an initial dose of 60 mg followed by 30 mg every 6 h is reasonable.

Release of preformed T_4 into the circulation is rapidly blocked by a supersaturated oral solution of iodine (five drops [250 mg] of supersaturated potassium iodide [SSKI] solution q6h) or by dexamethasone (2 mg IV q6h). Unfortunately, even complete blockade of T_4 release does not terminate hyperthyroid crisis because circulating T_4 has a very long half-life, and conversion to T_3 continues. Peripheral conversion can be inhibited by corticosteroids or propranolol. Because PTU and iodine are only available as enteral preparations, administration may prove difficult in the critically ill. Because iodine inhibits thyroid uptake of PTU and methimazole, these drugs must be administered at least 2 h before iodine therapy.

β-blockers blunt the tissue actions of thyroid hormone, (especially in the heart) but must be used with caution, particularly in patients with congestive heart failure or bronchospasm. If a β-blocker is used, it makes some sense to initially select a short-acting agent such as esmolol to gauge the patient's response. If adverse consequences develop, the effects can be rapidly terminated. If tolerated, propranolol and metoprolol are reasonable long-term choices. In deliberate ingestions of thyroid hormone, oral administration of bile acid sequestering drugs can prevent absorption. In severe overdoses, plasmapheresis or peritoneal dialysis may be used to remove thyroid hormone from the circulation.

Heart failure occurs in half of patients with thyroid storm. Although classically described as a "high-output" state, many patients have normal or low cardiac outputs and elevated pulmonary artery occlusion pressures and may be harmed by the use of β-blockers. By contrast, hypertension and tachycardia seen in thyroid storm may respond well to β-blockade. Associated tachyarrhythmias may be controlled with a combination of digoxin, β-blocker, and calcium channel blockers. Fever from increased metabolic rate may be managed by direct external cooling, but aspirin and NSAIDs should be avoided because of their tendency to displace T_4 from serum proteins, possibly worsening thyroid storm. Therapy should also include nutritional support because of heightened caloric requirements. (Folate and

B vitamins are also rapidly consumed and should be supplemented.) Increased thyroid activity accelerates the metabolism of many drugs, including some of those useful in its treatment (β-blockers and dexamethasone), thus larger doses on a more frequent schedule may be necessary.

Severe Hypothyroidism (Myxedema Coma)

Hypothyroidism is a very common condition but its most severe manifestation, "myxedema coma," is quite rare. It is hypothermia, central nervous system (CNS) dysfunction, bradycardia, and hypotension that differentiate myxedema coma from simple hypothyroidism. Myxedema is an important reversible cause of several common syndromes in the ICU including (a) severe ileus suggestive of bowel obstruction, (b) respiratory failure (including failure to wean from a ventilator), (c) heart failure, (d) hypothermia, and (e) coma. Myxedema coma is a serious disorder, with up to 30% of victims succumbing to the illness and its complications.

In more than 90% of cases, hypothyroidism results from primary failure of the thyroid gland, not pituitary insufficiency. Making a de novo diagnosis of myxedema in the ICU is uncommon. Most patients hospitalized with severe hypothyroidism have carried the diagnosis for some time; their admission is usually precipitated by the combination of discontinued thyroid replacement therapy and/or intercurrent illness (e.g., infection, myocardial infarction, surgery, hypothermia, trauma, and drugs, particularly sedatives). For unclear reasons, hypothyroidism is much more likely to occur in older patients, in women, and in the winter months. Lithium and amiodarone are rare causes.

The diagnosis of myxedema coma must be a presumptive one because thyroid function tests results may be delayed and therapy should be initiated promptly to optimize outcome. The history is often one of slowly progressive lethargy, depression, and mental dullness. Common physical signs include (a) obesity, (b) dry, puffy skin, (c) characteristic facies, (d) sinus bradycardia, (e) decreased relaxation phase of deep tendon reflexes, and (f) nonpitting edema. A previous thyroidectomy scar is an obvious clue. Pleural and pericardial effusions and ascites are also often detected. Less commonly, hoarseness, macroglossia, and hair loss are noted. Paradoxically, hypertension is as common as hypotension.

Normocytic anemia, hyponatremia, hypoglycemia, hypercapnia, and hypoxemia are frequent but not diagnostic. When hypoglycemia is noted, concurrent adrenal insufficiency is common. Marked elevations in cholesterol are also frequently noted and above normal levels of creatine, phosphokinase may be noted seen. The hyponatremia seen in hypothyroidism is often multifactorial, reflecting inappropriate antidiuretic hormone (ADH) secretion and combined treatment with diuretics and hypotonic fluids.

The laboratory hallmark of primary hypothyroidism is an elevated TSH concentration (usually >20 mU/L) accompanied by low total and free T_4 levels (see Table 32-1). (The much less common secondary or "pituitary" form of the disease is characterized by a low T_4 and low TSH.) Many nonthyroidal illnesses decrease the T_3 and total T_4 levels without impairing thyroid function, the so-called sic euthyroid state. In this syndrome, decreased T_4 binding protein and altered T_4 metabolism lead to a decreased total T_4 with normal or slightly depressed free T_4, a normal or reduced T_3, and normal or minimally elevated TSH. The sic euthyroid condition is not benefitted by thyroid hormone replacement therapy. Rarely, long-term dopamine infusion may inhibit pituitary release of TSH suggesting a sic euthyroid state in a patient with true primary hypothyroidism.

Because orally administered drugs are absorbed poorly in myxedema, T_4 should initially be administered IV. Controversy exists because no controlled studies have been conducted to guide replacement amounts, but reasonable starting daily doses of T_4 range from 0.2 to 0.5 mg IV. (There is no benefit from larger initial doses.) Commonly, 0.5 mg of T_4 is given over the first 24 h, followed by 0.1 mg each day thereafter. In normotensive, euthermic patients the initial dose may be as low as 0.1 mg. Clinical improvement usually begins within 12 to 24 h. Without good data it is commonly believed that T_4 doses should be reduced in diminutive and elderly patients and those with known coronary disease because abrupt replacement may precipitate ischemia. Because the peripheral conversion of T_4 to T_3 in myxedema is impaired, some experts advocate administration of T_3 (10 μg) directly. This practice had not been proved to be more effective than giving T_4 alone, is much more expensive, and had been associated with an increased risk of death if not carefully monitored.

When hypothyroidism is suspected, adrenal function must also be tested because a hemodynamic crisis may be precipitated if T_4 is administered to patients with concurrent adrenal insufficiency. To avoid missing the diagnosis, the most practical approach is to perform an adreno-corticotropic hormone (ACTH) stimulation test when thyroid function tests are obtained, and begin empiric stress doses of glucocorticoids (hydrocortisone 100 mg IV q8h) while awaiting the results (see Adrenal Insufficiency, following). If baseline cortisol levels return greater than 25 μg/dL or double after ACTH hydrocortisone can be discontinued. Hypoglycemia occurs frequently enough to warrant urgent evaluation in acutely ill patients with altered mental status and suspected hypothyroidism. Arterial blood gases (ABGs) should be analyzed in most patients because suppressed ventilatory drive leading to hypercapnic respiratory failure is common. Hyponatremia is effectively treated by temporary water restriction. Hypotension and hypoperfusion should be treated with T_4 and corticosteroids as well as fluids and vasopressors as dictated by usual hemodynamic parameters. Many patients will have concomitant hypothermia that is best treated with passive external rewarming (see Chapter 28).

Aspiration pneumonitis (often leading to acute lung injury) is a very common complication in patients with reduced mental status secondary to hypothyroidism. Although rare, bacterial meningitis may be a precipitant of myxedema. Thus, it is probably prudent in most of these patients to obtain cultures of relevant body fluids and administer empiric antibiotics until cultures return negative. The obesity and immobility of the profoundly hypothyroid patient predispose to the formation of atelectasis, decubitus ulcers, and deep venous thrombosis. Prevention of these common complications is covered in detail in Chapter 18.

■ ADRENAL DISEASES

Classical Adrenal Insufficiency

The physiologic effects of adrenal insufficiency result from deficiencies of cortisol and/or aldosterone. Loss of mineralocorticoid action is responsible for most of the significant manifestations seen in the ICU. Regardless of whether the disease results from adrenal (primary) or pituitary gland (secondary) failure, most patients' symptoms are mild and well compensated until a second process causes volume depletion (vomiting, diarrhea), or vasodilation (sepsis, drugs, surgery). (Until the supervening illness occurs, loss of aldosterone is compensated for by increased salt and water intake.)

The most common and severe form of the disease, primary adrenal insufficiency, results from direct adrenal gland destruction. Tuberculosis, fungal disease, surgery, infarction, metastatic cancer, autoimmune disease, and hemorrhage are the most frequent causes. Hemorrhagic adrenal insufficiency is seen most commonly in septic or in anticoagulated patients, especially in postcardiopulmonary bypass. Critically ill patients with the acquired immunodeficiency syndrome (AIDS) also have a high frequency of adrenal insufficiency. In patients with AIDS, cytomegalovirus, metastatic neoplasm, and ketoconazole therapy are the most common culprits; yet in many patients, the etiology remains obscure. In primary adrenal insufficiency, pituitary secretion of ACTH increases in an attempt to stimulate the inadequate adrenal glands to maintain normal cortisol levels. Because both mineralocorticoid (aldosterone) and glucocorticoid functions are lost, clinical manifestations are more severe and in important respects differ from the secondary form of the syndrome.

Secondary adrenal insufficiency results from pituitary gland insufficiency resulting from head trauma, tumor (especially adenoma), or infarction. Infarction may occur when hemorrhage occurs into a preexisting pituitary adenoma, when primary hemorrhage occurs in the anticoagulated patient, when trauma disrupts a feeding artery, or when the postpartum patient suffers spontaneous infarction. Secondary adrenal insufficiency results in a loss of cortisol, but aldosterone secretion remains normal because it is not regulated by ACTH, and the adrenal gland itself is unaffected. However, because cortisol is required for normal synthesis of catecholamines, blood pressure can decline modestly from glucocorticoid deficiency alone. The abrupt withdrawal of chronically administered exogenous steroid mimics secondary adrenal insufficiency as ACTH secretion is suppressed, and the exogenous corticosteroid is rapidly cleared from the circulation. Because aldosterone levels remain near normal, secondary adrenal insufficiency seldom results in dehydration or hyperkalemia prominent with the primary form of the disease.

A rare, tertiary form of adrenal insufficiency also exists in which granulomatous disease (e.g., sarcoid) or neoplasm destroys the hypothalamic pathways necessary for signaling the pituitary release of ACTH. Diagnosis and treatment parallel that of secondary adrenal insufficiency.

The drugs, ketoconazole, etomidate, and aminoglutethimide all interfere with normal steroidogenesis and may precipitate adrenal insufficiency. Other drugs that accelerate hepatic metabolism of exogenously administered corticosteroids (e.g., rifampin, phenytoin, and barbiturates) can also precipitate adrenal insufficiency. Observational studies associating etomidate use with worse clinical outcomes in critically ill patients have prompted substantial controversy. Undoubtedly, etomidate suppresses cortisol release for 12 to 24h, but a cause-and-effect relationship to worse morbidity or mortality is highly suspect. Because etomidate is often the sedative chosen for intubation for the sickest patients, it is not surprising that they might have worse outcomes. The causality argument is further challenged by the observation that administration of hydrocortisone and etomidate together does not results in better outcomes than using etomidate alone.

As an isolated problem, weakness, fatigue, anorexia, myalgia, abdominal pain, nausea, and fever (as high as 40°C), are the most common presenting signs of adrenal insufficiency, regardless of type or etiology. Although the cause of abdominal pain is unknown, occasionally it is sufficiently severe to prompt laparotomy, a potentially lethal intervention for the patient with inadequate adrenal reserves. Shock may be the initial presentation in adrenal failure complicated by infection or dehydration and is much more common among patients with the primary form of the syndrome. In anticoagulated patients, flank pain and a fall in hemoglobin may be the presenting signs. Cutaneous hyperpigmentation occurs only in primary adrenal insufficiency. (A functioning pituitary gland is necessary to produce the ACTH-like melanocyte-stimulating hormone, responsible for hyperpigmentation). The pigmentation, best described as "dirt that won't wash off," is most prominent on sun exposed areas and in palmar and antecubital regions. Loss of body hair occurs in women with primary adrenal insufficiency as adrenal androgen production is lost, but alopecia is not a feature in men because of the testicular androgen production.

Regardless of cause, hyponatremia is a nearly universal (approx. 90%) finding. Urinary Na+ wasting resulting in hyponatremia and renal K+ retention causing hyperkalemia are seen predominantly in primary adrenal insufficiency due to the loss of aldosterone. Conversely, isolated cortisol deficiency from secondary adrenal insufficiency impairs free water excretion, but rarely causes hyperkalemia. The mechanism of impaired free water clearance is unknown, but may partly result from increased ADH secretion occurring in an attempt to offset hypovolemia. Hypercalcemia is unusual but may be seen in either form of adrenal insufficiency because cortisol limits gastrointestinal absorption and increases renal excretion of calcium. Although the total leukocyte count is usually normal, the percentage of eosinophils and lymphocytes is often increased. (Leukocytosis and eosinophilia are far too nonspecific to be diagnostically helpful.) Mild normochromic normocytic anemia is very common. Hypoglycemia may be the presenting manifestation of either primary or secondary adrenal insufficiency, but is much more common in children than adults. (Cortisol boosts glucose levels by increasing gluconeogenesis and catecholamine levels.) Volume depletion seen with all forms of adrenal insufficiency results in elevations of the blood urea nitrogen (BUN).

Because adrenal insufficiency is life threatening, it is important to institute intravascular volume and cortisol replacement before laboratory confirmation of the diagnosis. The following protocol may be used for simultaneous diagnosis and treatment. (a) Draw baseline cortisol and ACTH levels. (b) Administer an ACTH analog (IV Cortrosyn, 250 μg). (c) Obtain cortisol levels 30 and 60 min after ACTH. (d) Begin empirical glucocorticoid therapy. (Dexamethasone represents a good choice because it is potent, is long lasting, and will not interfere with cortisol assays.)

If such testing reveals a baseline cortisol value greater than 25 μg/dL or a brisk (approx. twofold) rise, a diagnosis of adrenal insufficiency is very unlikely. (Almost all patients with acute primary adrenal insufficiency have baseline cortisol levels in the low single digits and less than a 5 μg/dL increment on provocative testing.) In patients who fail to respond to single-dose ACTH stimulation, a 3-day ACTH infusion may be required to distinguish between primary and secondary forms of the disease. (The primary form of the disease will not respond to even prolonged ACTH analog infusion because the adrenal glands are unresponsive.) The usual responses to a brief ACTH stimulation test in various clinical scenarios are illustrated in Table 32-2.

Salt-containing fluid and glucocorticoids are the essence of initial therapy. Typically, 3 to 6 L of isotonic crystalloid is required. Hypotonic fluid should be avoided because it is ineffective at

TABLE 32-2 CORTISOL AND ACTH LEVELS IN ADRENAL DISEASES

PITUITARY ADRENAL AXIS STATUS	ACTH LEVEL	CORTISOL LEVEL	
		BASELINE	POST-ACTH STIMULATION
Normal	Normal	Normal	Increased
Primary adrenal failure	Marked increase	Low	Low
Secondary adrenal failure	Low or normal	Low	Increased
Poststeroid withdrawal	Low	Low or normal	Mild increase[a]

[a]Requires 24-h ACTH infusion for confirmation.

restoring circulating volume and exacerbates hyponatremia. If adequate amounts of salt-containing crystalloid are infused, mineralocorticoid hormones are not immediately necessary in either form of adrenal insufficiency. (If mineralocorticoid replacement is started, fludrocortisone 0.1 to 0.2 mg per day is sufficient for almost all patients.) In persons with normally functioning pituitary–adrenal axes, cortisol levels may rise 10-fold above baseline levels under periods of maximal stress to a daily equivalent of 300 to 400 mg of hydrocortisone. Therefore, patients with acute adrenal insufficiency require relatively large corticosteroids doses. Although hydrocortisone (100 mg every 6 to 8 h) is often given IV because of its mineralocorticoid effects, dexamethasone (4 to 6 mg every 8 to 12 h) is a useful alternative because it does not interfere with serum cortisol assays and is long acting. Table 32-3 provides several equivalent doses of corticosteroids for replacement therapy. Though not required in every case, IV administration avoids potential problems of delayed or incomplete absorption in the unstable patient.

Although mild hyperkalemia is commonly seen, K^+ concentrations seldom rise to dangerous levels and are rapidly corrected with volume expansion and glucocorticoids alone. (K^+-binding resins or dialysis are rarely necessary.) Because adrenal insufficiency impairs gluconeogenesis, IV fluids should contain glucose.

TABLE 32-3 STRESS REPLACEMENT DOSES OF CORTICOSTEROIDS

Dexamethasone	7.5–30 mg/day
Hydrocortisone	200–300 mg/day
Methylprednisolone	40–80 mg/day
Prednisone	50–100 mg/day

Relative Adrenal Insufficiency

Severe illness is associated with an increase in total plasma cortisol levels, often to 30 to 50 μg/dL; however, it is not known what "appropriate" unstimulated cortisol levels are for critically ill patients. It is also not known exactly how an ACTH stimulation test should be conducted or its results interpreted in this population. Nevertheless, empiric observations suggest that both high unstimulated cortisol levels and failure to significantly increase plasma cortisol after a high-dose ACTH challenge (250 μg) are associated with worse outcomes in critically ill patients. The failure of cortisol to rise (>9 μg/dL) after ACTH challenge has been deemed "relative adrenal insufficiency." The mechanism of hyporesponsiveness is unknown but it could be that the adrenals are already maximally stimulated or that some defect prevents appropriate sensing or response to ACTH. One prominent study reported that rapid replacement of glucocorticoids (hydrocortisone 50 mg q6h) and mineralocorticoids (fludrocortisone 0.05 mg per day) in patients with septic shock and relative adrenal insufficiency improved survival. Unfortunately, the complementary group (ACTH responders) had worse outcomes when given steroids than when given placebo. The dispute has been fueled by the results of a larger trial of similar design that failed to confirm the survival benefits of glucocorticoids in any subgroup. Undoubtedly, believers in corticosteroids for relative adrenal insufficiency will continue to treat and skeptics will withhold therapy pending further study. So is there a reasonable strategy for the clinician with equipoise? One sensible approach follows: For patients with suspected classical adrenal insufficiency, measure an unstimulated cortisol level and if low, begin replacement therapy. For patients with vasopressor-dependent septic shock persisting after fluid replacement, hydrocortisone treatment is reasonable if a $250\,\mu g$ ACTH stimulation test shows little or no rise in cortisol levels, especially if the baseline cortisol is in the normal range. Providing additional glucocorticoid to ACTH nonresponders with supraphysiologic cortisol levels does not seem prudent. Current data do not support treating hypotension not of septic origin nor does it support treatment of patients who respond to ACTH stimulation.

Regardless of viewpoint, several key issues yet to be resolved including: (a) What is the most informative dose of ACTH? (b) Should total or free cortisol be used to determine "responsiveness"? (c) Is there a better discriminating value for cortisol change? (d) Does the diagnosis of relative adrenal insufficiency have any therapeutic import for patients with shock that is not septic shock?

Withdrawal of Exogenous Steroids

A Cushingoid appearance should always be a clue to the use of exogenous corticosteroids and the potential for pituitary–adrenal axis suppression. Symptomatic adrenal insufficiency as a result of withdrawing exogenous steroid therapy is a surprisingly rare event, considering the frequency with which corticosteroids are used. The likelihood of developing adrenal insufficiency following withdrawal of steroids relates directly to the daily dose of corticosteroid and the duration of therapy. Partial or complete adrenal suppression from exogenous corticosteroids may occur with as little as 7 days of low-dose prednisone (20 to 30 mg). Prolonged steroid use may impair adrenal responsiveness for as long as 1 year after withdrawal of exogenous steroids (Fig. 32-2). After discontinuing exogenous corticosteroids, the ACTH response returns first (usually within 90 days); however, several months

often pass before normal cortisol response to ACTH is restored. Patients who demonstrate a normal response to ACTH stimulation are unlikely to have an inadequate adrenal response to stress. If the adrenal responsiveness of a critically ill patient is questionable, adrenal function should be tested and cortisol replacement empirically given. In patients of questionable adrenal status who require immediate surgery, administration of 100 mg of IV hydrocortisone before and after surgery will provide sufficient perioperative coverage.

Excessive Corticosteroid Administration

High doses of corticosteroids predispose to infection and produce protein wasting, poor wound healing, mental status alterations, and glucose intolerance. Exposure to as little as 1 to 2 weeks of high-dose corticosteroid has been associated with significant neuromyopathy. Long-term exposure may also cause intracranial hypertension, bone loss, aseptic necrosis, glaucoma, pancreatitis, and cataract formation. Adverse steroid effects are minimized by: (a) using the lowest effective dose, (b) using a shorter-acting steroid preparation such as hydrocortisone, (c) administering the full daily requirement in a single morning dose, and (d) using alternate day therapy.

■ DISORDERS OF GLUCOSE METABOLISM

ICU Glucose Control

Glucose abnormalities are common in the ICU for several reasons: (a) Critical illness induces a state of relative insulin resistance from release of stress

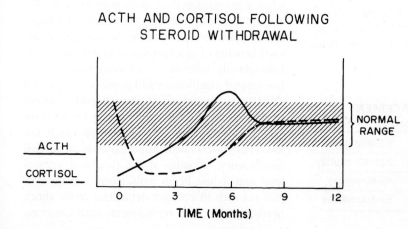

ACTH AND CORTISOL FOLLOWING STEROID WITHDRAWAL

NORMAL RANGE

ACTH

CORTISOL

TIME (Months)

■ **FIGURE 32-2** ACTH and cortisol levels following abrupt termination of prolonged glucocorticoid therapy at time 0. ACTH, adrenocorticotropic hormone.

hormones (glucagon, epinephrine, growth hormone, and cortisol). (b) Inconsistent feeding unpredictably alters the glucose load. (c) Sepsis, renal insufficiency, and drug therapy (catecholamines, octreotide, corticosteroids) change the effectiveness of antiglycemic therapy.

Over the last 5 years, the topic of glucose management has been one of the most tumultuous areas in critical care. The pendulum rapidly swung from a *lassiez fare* attitude to one of "strict" normoglycemia based upon studies showing that "tight" regulation of blood glucose reduced long-term morbidity of diabetics and a single study showing improved outcomes among postoperative patients. Anti-inflammatory and antithrombotic effects of normoglycemia were hypothesized. Questions regarding strict glucose control arose after a study of medical ICU patients, where benefit appeared to be restricted to the sickest patients with longer stays. Two subsequent clinical trials undermined enthusiasm for stringent glucose control by failing to demonstrate outcome benefits and showing a high risk of hypoglycemia, although both trials were halted early. To make the situation even more confusing, the accuracy of some bedside glucose monitoring systems has been questioned. Eagerness to maintain normoglycemia was also dampened by practical issues. Even though insulin is inexpensive, tight glucose control comes at a relatively high price: unless very closely monitored, hypoglycemia is frequent and the nursing time required to achieve safe rigorous glycemic control is substantial. Annoyance to the patient goes without saying.

4 Given the potentially conflicting data on glucose control in the critically ill patient, what is a reasonable course of action? The following suggestions comprise a sensible approach to managing the critically ill, nonketotic patient: (a) Establish a standardized glucose management protocol and track its performance. (b) Use enteral feeding when possible and avoid interruptions. (This is best accomplished using an enteral feeding protocol.) (c) Minimize use of long-acting insulin. (Instead, monitor blood glucose values frequently and treat with continuous insulin infusions or smaller intermittent doses of regular insulin.) (d) Avoid oral hypoglycemic agents (i.e., sulfonylureas, meglitinides, biguanides, or thiazolidinediones): their hypoglycemic effects may persist much longer than desired. (e) Use a reliable glucose monitoring system and certainly do not substitute urine tests for serum measurements. (f) Use bedside glucose determinations liberally.

Hypoglycemia

Hypoglycemia is a relative term used to describe a blood glucose level insufficient to meet metabolic demands. Hypoglycemia is a rare occurrence in patients not receiving insulin or oral hypoglycemic agents because there are numerous endogenous protective mechanisms, which include suppression of insulin secretion and increases in levels of epinephrine glucagon, cortisol, and growth hormone. Although many patients are symptomatic at glucose concentrations less than 50 mg/dL, a large number of young, otherwise healthy patients may have glucose levels less than 40 mg/dL without symptoms. The early symptoms of hypoglycemia are generally those of adrenergic excess (e.g., sweating, anxiety, tremor, tachycardia, and hypertension) and depend not only on the absolute glucose value, but also on the rate of its decline. Blood glucose should be rapidly measured in patients with altered mental status to rule out hypoglycemia, even if focal neurological deficits are present. Seizures may also be the presenting symptom but are a more common manifestation in children than in adults. If glucose concentrations cannot be readily measured in a patient with suspected hypoglycemia, administration of 50 to 100 mL of dextrose with an appropriate amount of thiamine is indicated.

Insulin Reactions

Exogenous insulin is the most common cause of hypoglycemia in patients under the age of 30, and if concomitant alcohol ingestion is considered, represents the most common causes of hypoglycemia in all patients. Insulin reactions are particularly common in the ICU because renal insufficiency impairs insulin clearance and hospitalized patients frequently do not receive regular feedings. (Long-acting insulin and oral hypoglycemics amplify this risk.) Insulin-induced hypoglycemia may also occur when insulin injected into suboptimally perfused tissue is later absorbed as perfusion improves. Because angiotensin-converting enzyme inhibitors increase an individual's sensitivity to insulin and enhance glucose uptake, their use has been associated with a higher incidence of hypoglycemia. High insulin levels and low C-peptide levels in a hypoglycemic patient suggest intentional or inadvertent insulin overdosage. The very rare combination of high insulin levels with high C-peptide levels in a hypoglycemic patient is indicative of insulinoma. Patients with little or no functional pancreatic tissue are at particular risk for hypoglycemia because of their inability to produce and release the counterregulatory hormone, glucagon. In addition, drugs that block the adrenergic response (especially β-blocking drugs) can blunt the counterregulatory effects of epinephrine released during a hypoglycemic crisis.

Oral Hypoglycemic Agents

Oral hypoglycemic agents are a poor choice for glucose control in the critically ill because of their long duration of action, which is further prolonged by advanced age, renal insufficiency, and frequent interactions with other drugs. Patients with hypoglycemia due to these agents should be observed closely because of the potential for prolonged or recurrent symptoms. Hypoglycemia from oral agents is often refractory to glucose alone and may require combined therapy with hydrocortisone and glucagon. Hypoglycemic action of these agents is also potentiated by butazolidin, sulfonamides, probenecid, and salicylates. Furthermore, oral hypoglycemics interact with such commonly used medications as phenytoin, phenothiazines, rifampin, and thiazides. Metabolic (lactic) acidosis is a side effect of metformin, one of the oral hypoglycemic agents. Although clinically significant, acidosis is quite uncommon; risk is increased when the drug is used in patients with renal insufficiency, hepatic insufficiency, or alcohol abuse and among patients with hypoxia or shock. Metformin should also be stopped for at least 24 to 48 h in patients undergoing procedures involving radiographic contrast to avoid the possibility of unusually high drug levels and subsequent lactic acidosis, should renal insufficiency develop.

Other Causes of Hypoglycemia

Severe sepsis may produce hypoglycemia by multiple mechanisms including hepatic hypoperfusion, renal insufficiency, depletion of muscle glycogen, and starvation. Alcohol suppresses gluconeogenesis, discourages nutrient intake, and induces a low insulin state that favors free fatty acid release and ketone production. Consequently, alcoholics may present with hypoglycemia and a mixed ketoacidosis and lactic acidosis. By the time such patients seek medical attention, the ingested alcohol has often been completely metabolized and thus, blood alcohol levels are zero. Glucose, thiamine, and fluids comprise the key elements in the treatment of alcoholic acidosis with hypoglycemia. Although ketoacids are present, insulin does not speed up resolution of the acidosis and may precipitate or exacerbate hypoglycemia. Sodium bicarbonate is rarely necessary, possibly only to maintain the pH greater than 7.10. Other causes of hypoglycemia include hepatic failure (due to cirrhosis, tumor infiltration, or fulminant hepatic failure), renal failure, salicylate poisoning, and insulin-secreting tumors. Surgery and other stress states blunt the effect of insulin while stimulating the release of counterregulatory hormones. Imbalance of these effects may cause circulating glucose to unpredictably rise or decline to dangerous levels. To prevent hypoglycemia in the surgical patient, it is prudent to monitor glucose closely and to decrease (but not discontinue) preoperative insulin. A useful strategy is to administer one half of the regular insulin dosage before surgery despite the fasting state. The key to preventing hypoglycemia is frequent intraoperative and postoperative glucose testing.

Artifactual hypoglycemia may occur when glucose is metabolized in blood samples with extremely high leukocyte counts. Leukocyte-induced hypoglycemia is most common when measurement is delayed for hours. Inactivating leukocyte metabolism using oxalate–fluoride containing blood collection tubes can prevent this problem.

Treatment of Hypoglycemia

Unless otherwise contraindicated, IV glucose should be empirically administered to all patients with abruptly altered, undiagnosed changes in mental status or neurological function, even when focal. Two ampules of D50W (100-gm glucose) are always sufficient to acutely raise the serum glucose levels above 100 mg/dL. Larger doses simply increase serum osmolarity. When hypoglycemic patients of unknown or questionable nutritional status are treated with glucose, thiamine (1 mg/kg) should be given concurrently to prevent Wernicke encephalopathy. In all cases of hypoglycemia, it is prudent to closely monitor the patient and recheck the serum glucose frequently. On rare occasion, hypoglycemia is refractory to bolus glucose administration alone. In such cases, constant infusion of D10W, with hydrocortisone (100 mg IV) and/or glucagon (1 mg IV per liter of D10W) will augment the blood glucose. Because octreotide suppresses insulin release, it is also useful to treat hyperinsulinemic hypoglycemia.

Diabetic Ketoacidosis

Diabetic ketoacidosis (DKA) is a common, serious condition, the mortality of which remains significant despite aggressive therapy. DKA is the result of a deficiency of insulin, usually with a relative excess of counterregulatory hormones. Most commonly DKA is precipitated by noncompliance with diet or medication, although infection frequently contributes. Cocaine and corticosteroid use, stroke, myocardial infarction, trauma, pregnancy, pancreatitis, and hyperthyroidism are also potential precipitants.

The most prominent physical features of DKA (hypotension, hypoperfusion, and tachypnea) are the result of the two major metabolic derangements—volume depletion and metabolic acidosis. Volume depletion tends to be less profound in DKA than in hyperosmolar nonketotic syndrome, perhaps because the acidosis of DKA brings patients to medical attention sooner. Deep and rapid "Kussmaul" respirations are an attempt to compensate for metabolic acidosis. Recognition of DKA is not difficult, but some "classic" features are seldom seen. For example, whereas obtundation is frequent, frank coma is rare (<10% of cases). In addition, neurological manifestations are usually less severe than with hyperosmolar nonketotic coma. Fever is not a part of DKA in the absence of infection. In fact, slight reductions in temperature are much more frequent. (This is particularly true if the temperature is measured orally in a hyperventilating patient.) Vomiting is quite common and is often the result of ileus induced by ketonemia, dehydration, and electrolyte imbalances. Unexplained features of DKA include pleurisy and abdominal pain. The fact that abdominal pain almost always resolves rapidly with correction of the acidosis can help distinguish DKA from more serious causes. Therefore, patients with undiagnosed acute abdominal pain should have glucose and ketone determinations before undergoing other diagnostic or "therapeutic" procedures.

Metabolic acidosis, ketosis, and hyperglycemia are the laboratory hallmarks of DKA. Ketone measurements should be made initially in patients with hyperglycemia to confirm the diagnosis, but there is little value in *serial* measurements of ketones or pH. In patients with DKA, three ketones are present in chemical equilibrium: acetoacetate, acetone, and β-hydroxybutyrate, but only acetoacetate and acetone are measured by the most commonly used nitroprusside assay. Normally, β-hydroxybutyrate

exceeds acetoacetate by a 3:1 ratio, but in severe acidosis β-hydroxybutyrate may be present in concentrations 12-fold greater than acetoacetate. As the acidosis improves, the dynamic equilibrium shifts in favor of acetoacetate and ketone concentrations may appear to worsen (another potential reason not to order serial determinations). Note that captopril and other sulfhydryl-containing drugs like penicillamine and mesna can react with the nitroprusside reagent resulting in a false-positive test for ketoacids. Although it is reasonable to obtain a baseline ABG to evaluate adequacy of ventilation, repeated measurements are not necessary. Clearance of the ketoacids and the metabolic acidosis they cause can be simply tracked by the rise in serum bicarbonate and fall in anion gap.

Presenting glucose levels typically range between 400 and 800 mg/dL, but may be lower in young, well-hydrated patients whose preserved glomerular filtration facilitates glucose clearance. Leukocytosis (>20,000/mm^3) with a predominance of granulocytes may occur even in the absence of infection. Loss of free water because of osmotic diuresis usually leads to hyperosmolarity and hemoconcentration; therefore, even mild reductions of measured packed cell volume in patients with DKA suggest severe underlying anemia or active bleeding.

The osmotic effect of glucose translocates water from the intracellular to the extracellular space, producing hyponatremia in most patients. Measured sodium (Na$^+$) concentration typically declines approximately 2 mEq/L for each 100 mg/dL increase in glucose. Because glucose seldom exceeds 1,000 mg/dL, it is unlikely for the Na$^+$ to fall below 120 mEq/L on an osmotic basis alone. Artifactual depressions of Na$^+$ concentration may be seen in DKA when triglycerides contribute substantially to plasma volume ("pseudohyponatremia"). In patients with profound and prolonged hyperglycemia, especially those with impaired water intake, the resultant osmotic diuresis can result in hypernatremia.

Because acidosis, insulin deficiency, and the osmotically induced flow of water out of cells shift potassium (K$^+$) from the intracellular to the extracellular compartment, most patients with DKA have normal or elevated K$^+$ levels despite sizeable (3 to 5 mEq/kg) total body deficits. With appropriate volume expansion, insulin, and correction of the acidosis, K$^+$ values can plummet. (Some experts recommend administering KCl even when initial values are above normal.) At the very least, even an above-normal admission K$^+$ value should be tracked closely. Total body depletion of magnesium and phosphorus are also extremely common. After urine flow is reestablished, it is reasonable to offer replacement therapy of both elements, though no certain benefit has been demonstrated. The serum of patients with DKA is often grossly lipemic. Some automated laboratory chemistry analyzers misinterpret this turbidity as "hemolysis." Such reports often prompt multiple repeated testing, until the problem is recognized. Direct consultation with the laboratory is indicated when a properly obtained specimen is reported as hemolyzed. Serum creatinine is commonly elevated by dehydration-induced decreases in glomerular filtration rate (GFR). (With colorimetric assays, ketones may cause artifactual elevations in creatinine.) For obscure reasons, the serum amylase is elevated in 15% to 25% of patients with DKA. Hence, finding an increased amylase alone does not confirm a diagnosis of pancreatitis.

The most important aspects of DKA therapy are adequate fluid replacement; insulin administration; and sequential monitoring. The single best indicator of successful therapy is narrowing of the anion gap, a measurement reflecting correction of both lactic acidosis and ketoacidosis. In adults, total body fluid deficits range between 5 and 10 L, with Na^+ deficits averaging 300 to 500 mEq. Adequate circulating volume should be replenished rapidly (500 to 1,000 mL/h) with infusions of glucose-free, isotonic crystalloid in patients with evidence of hypoperfusion. In patients with DKA and hypotension refractory to volume repletion, one should consider (a) bleeding (particularly gastrointestinal or retroperitoneal); (b) septic shock, especially from urinary tract infection (UTI) or pneumonia; (c) adrenal insufficiency; (d) pancreatitis; and (e) myocardial infarction.

After initial resuscitation, the aim should be to restore the balance of the volume deficit within 12 to 24 h while normalizing electrolytes. Isotonic saline, Ringer's solution, and half-normal saline are all reasonable alternatives for fluid replacement after initial resuscitation. If only normal saline is used for fluid replacement, one can expect that a *mild* hyperchloremic nonanion gap acidosis will replace the initial *severe* high-anion gap acidosis. Regardless, there does not appear to be any adverse consequence as resuscitated patients rapidly self-correct this electrolyte abnormality. Physical examination, urine output, and frequent electrolyte measurements should guide subsequent fluid and electrolyte choices.

An initial regular insulin bolus of 0.1 to 0.5 units/kg followed by an infusion of 0.1 units/kg/h suffice for most patients. Insulin infusions should be administered by pump for accurate delivery. The initial goals are to begin reducing the anion gap and to lower plasma glucose by 75 to 100 mg/dL each hour. At the outset, laboratory measurements at 1- to 2-h intervals should guide the rate of insulin and fluid administration. Failure of glucose to decline significantly within 2 to 3 h indicates insulin resistance and should prompt doubling the insulin dosage. Insulin infusion should be continued until serum ketones are cleared and the anion gap is normalized, even if supplemental glucose must be used to prevent hypoglycemia. (Practically, this usually requires 12 to 24 h by which time the patient is usually ready to eat.) In most cases, it is prudent to switch to a glucose-containing IV fluid when blood glucose values reach 250 mg/dL. Premature termination of insulin infusions is the most common cause of relapsing DKA.

$NaHCO_3$ is rarely necessary in DKA. (An argument can be made that $NaHCO_3$ should only be given if the pH is very low or the patient demonstrates refractory hypotension or respiratory failure.) Even though pH correction can help reduce ventilatory requirements and improve diaphragmatic function in patients with respiratory fatigue or limited ventilatory capacity, there are risks. When a large volume of $NaHCO_3$ is given rapidly to a patient with severe acidosis, a huge quantity of CO_2 is generated which must be cleared by the lung. In patients with limited ventilatory capacity, $PaCO_2$ levels can skyrocket. Because the liver regenerates HCO_3^{3-} from ketones and lactate, patients receiving exogenous base frequently develop a "rebound" alkalosis. However, loss of ketones in the urine of well-hydrated patients with normal renal function can result in a loss of HCO_3^{3-} equivalents and a mild persistent metabolic acidosis. The osmolality of a 50-mL ampule of $NaHCO_3$ is nearly fivefold greater than normal saline; thus, aggressive therapy may exacerbate hyperosmolarity. In addition, rapid reversal of acidemia shifts the oxyhemoglobin curve leftward, exacerbates hypokalemia, and may cause paradoxical CNS acidosis.

Spontaneous or iatrogenic arrhythmias induced by acid–base and electrolyte disturbances are a major preventable cause of cardiovascular morbidity in DKA. For example, insulin and $NaHCO_3$ can rapidly drive K^+ across the cell membranes, dramatically decreasing serum levels. Therefore after adequate urine flow is reestablished,

KCl should be administered to most DKA patients. Usually, 10 to 20 mEq/h is required to maintain normal levels but on occasion, up to 60 mEq/h may be necessary. Magnesium and phosphate should also be monitored. Hypophosphatemia may decrease 2,3-diphosphoglyceric acid (2,3-DPG) levels and muscle strength, but phosphate administration has not been shown to improve outcome. Risks of phosphate therapy include acute hypocalcemia and tissue deposition of calcium–phosphate complexes, occasionally inducing acute renal failure. Hypoglycemia, a common complication of aggressive DKA therapy, may be prevented through vigilant monitoring.

Hyperosmolar Nonketotic Coma

The term hyperosmolar nonketotic coma (HNKC) is somewhat of a misnomer in that most patients do not have coma but all have dramatic elevations of glucose with little or no ketosis. Osmolality is dramatically elevated (often >350 mOsm/L) by profound increases in glucose (often >1,000 mEq/L). Insulin levels in HNKC are sufficient to prevent ketone formation but insufficient to prevent hyperglycemia. Patients with HNKC also generate fewer ketones, (hence acidosis), than patients with DKA because they tend to have lower levels of lipolytic hormones (i.e., growth hormone and cortisol). Glycosuria (a compensatory mechanism limiting hyperglycemia) is tightly linked to GFR; therefore, HNKC is more common in the elderly and in those underlying renal dysfunction. Patients with impaired perception of thirst (e.g., the elderly) and/or deprived of access to water are also predisposed. HNKC is often precipitated by an intercurrent illness that produces volume depletion or promotes hyperglycemia (e.g., sepsis, stroke, diarrhea, vomiting, or corticosteroid or diuretic use). Unlike DKA, where the accumulating ketoacids stimulate ventilation and produce dyspnea, HNKC patients are often minimally symptomatic initially and maintain near-normal acid–base status for long periods of time. It is not until profound volume depletion limits organ function that these patients seek medical attention. The chemical and clinical features of DKA and HNKC are contrasted in Table 32-4.

Laboratory features of HNKC are similar to those of DKA except ketoacidosis is absent or minimal, whereas glucose values are often extremely elevated (>1,000 mg/dL). Hyperglycemia produces the hyperosmolarity that characterizes this disorder (see Chapter 13). Marked depletion of total body water (average 9 L) is present in HNKC, largely because of a prolonged osmotic diuresis. Although intravascular volume is usually better preserved in HNKC than in DKA (by high glucose levels), it is at the expense of the intracellular compartment. This effect is responsible for the primary clinical expression of HNKC: life-threatening impairment of neurological function. Because the osmotic effect of glucose is required to maintain intravascular volume, insulin administration before restoring circulating volume with isotonic crystalloid can cause sudden and profound hypotension by producing a rapid shift of glucose and water into cells. Total body deficits of K^+ and PO_4^{3-} equal those of DKA, although at presentation levels of both ions are usually normally or even modestly elevated.

Correction of HNKC must be cautious, as abrupt reversal of serum hyperosmolarity may produce intracellular water intoxication manifested by dysphoria and seizures. Despite differences in pathophysiology, the treatment of HNKC is similar to that of DKA: initial restoration of circulating volume with normal saline or Ringer's solution. (In such patients, both fluids represent relatively hypotonic solutions.) Initial fluid replacement using D5W or half-normal saline can precipitate rapid cellular swelling (especially in the brain) as fluid enters the dehydrated, hypertonic cells. In general, complete fluid replacement should be targeted to occur over 24 to 48 h. Insulin therapy should be initiated only after circulating volume has been repleted, as evidenced by stable blood pressure, reduction in heart rate, and adequate urine output.

TABLE 32-4 FEATURES OF DKA AND HYPEROSMOLAR COMA

CHARACTERISTIC	DIABETIC KETOACIDOSIS	HYPEROSMOLAR COMA
Insulin levels	Very low	Low
Lipolytic hormone levels	Very elevated	Mildly elevated
Typical glucose concentration	400–800 mg/dL	≥1,000 mg/dL
Osmolality	Variable	>320 mOsm/L
Bicarbonate	Low	Normal
pH	<7.25	>7.3
Ketones	High	Low or absent
Dehydration	Moderate	Severe

6

Insulin administration and free water repletion should be guided by serial electrolyte and glucose determinations.

■ DIABETES INSIPIDUS

Diabetes insipidus (DI) is a life-threatening illness resulting from a failure of the pituitary–hypothalamic axis to release sufficient ADH, or a failure of the kidney to respond to the released hormone. Insufficient ADH action prevents adequate water reabsorption by renal medullary collecting ducts. In the ICU, DI is typically first suspected when a very high, hourly urine output is observed in the setting of a rising serum Na^+ concentration. For most ambulatory patients with DI, the serum Na^+ concentration is maintained close to normal by increasing water intake. Conversely, in the critically ill patient unable to obtain water, significant hypernatremia may occur. When polyuria is seen in patients with serum Na^+ concentrations less than 135, DI is rarely the cause, but rather excessive fluid intake is usually to blame. It is important to remember that high, hourly urine outputs (approx. 1 L/h) are not always inappropriate; they may occur after massive volume resuscitation, relief of urinary tract obstruction, and in patients with high urinary solute (e.g., urea, glucose, and mannitol) loads. In both DI and water intoxication, the urine is dilute.

Pituitary or hypothalamic trauma or surgery, anoxic brain injury, and cerebral infarction are the most common causes of "central" DI; however, involvement of the pituitary gland with granulomatous disease or metastatic carcinoma is also seen. The sudden development of DI in a patient with increased intracranial pressure is commonly a signal that brain death has occurred. Transient DI lasting 3 to 7 days may follow closely on the heels of head trauma or pituitary injury. In 25% to 30% of patients, no cause for central DI can be determined. The kidneys' inability to respond to ADH is referred to as "nephrogenic DI." Hypokalemia, hypocalcemia, chronic pyelonephritis, polycystic kidney disease, sarcoidosis, amyloidosis, sickle cell disease, and chronic use of medications such as loop diuretics, lithium carbonate, and demeclocycline can all impair renal responsiveness to ADH.

Loss of ADH's action results in a dilute urine (osmolality < 200 mOsm/L) at a time the plasma is hyperosmolar (>280 mOsm/L). In the conscious patient, clinical features include polyuria and polydipsia; however, if oral intake is inadequate, the clinical presentation may be one of hypovolemic shock. In the ICU, the diagnosis of DI is most safely confirmed by demonstrating a rise in urine osmolality within 2 h of administration of 5 units of aqueous vasopressin subcutaneously or 1 μg of des-amino-arginine vasopressin (DDAVP). Increases in urine osmolality of ≥50% suggest central DI, whereas lesser rises suggest nephrogenic DI. Use of the more traditional water deprivation test searching for a persistently dilute urine despite rising serum osmolarity is potentially risky in the critically ill population. In central DI, a head CT or MRI scan may demonstrate pathology in the region of the hypothalamus or pituitary. Adrenal failure accompanies DI in about one third of trauma-induced cases and therefore, should be sought in accident victims with DI.

Treatment of DI consists of aggressive water administration, guided by electrolyte and osmolarity determinations. Aqueous vasopressin (5 to 10 units IM or subcutaneous q4 to 6 h or 2 μg of DDAVP q12h) are adequate hormone replacement therapy. Both intranasal and oral forms of desmopressin are now available. The effect of hormone replacement therapy is usually dramatic with urine volume responding within hours. In the ICU patient who cannot express the sensation of thirst or access water, it is important to closely monitor the serum Na^+ concentration during therapy; insufficient free water replacement results in hypernatremia, and excessive hormone replacement can result in hyponatremia. Chlorpromazine, clofibrate, and carbamazepine are poor choices for control of DI and should be avoided.

7

■ SUGGESTED READINGS

Annane D, Maxime V, Ibrahim F, et al. Diagnosis of adrenal insufficiency in severe sepsis and septic shock. *Am J Resp Crit Care Med.* 2006;174:1319–1326.

Annane D, Sebille V, Charpentier C, et al. Effect of treatment with low doses of hydrocortisone and fludrocortisone on mortality in patients with septic shock. *JAMA.* 2002;288(7):862–871.

Chiasson JL, Aris-Jilwan N, Belanger R, et al. Diagnosis and treatment of diabetic ketoacidosis and the hyperglycemic hyperosmolar state. *CMAJ.* 2003;168(7):859–866.

Fliers E, Wiersinga WM. Myxedema coma. *Rev Endocr Metab Disord.* 2003;4(2):137–141.

Goldberg PA, Inzucchi SE. Critical issues in endocrinology. *Clin Chest Med.* 2003;24(4):583–606.

Sarlis NJ, Gourgiotis L. Thyroid emergencies. *Rev Endocr Metab Disord.* 2003;4(2):129–136.

Sprung CL, Annane D, Keh D, et al. Hydrocortisone therapy for patients with septic shock. *N Engl J Med.* 2008;358:111–123.

Verbalis JG. Diabetes insipidus. *Rev Endocr Metab Disord.* 2003;4(2):177–185.

Drug Overdose and Poisoning

KEY POINTS

1 With little intervention, the outcome for most victims of poisoning is excellent. Supportive care, with particular attention to maintaining an airway, oxygenation, and perfusion, is the mainstay of treatment. Becoming prematurely fixated on the details of specific antidotal therapy can lead to disastrous consequences if basic support of oxygenation and perfusion are ignored.

2 Adults suffering from overdoses rarely give a complete and accurate description of the quantity or type of medications ingested. In most adult cases, multiple substances are involved.

3 A tentative diagnosis in most overdose and poisoning cases can be made by physical examination and simple laboratory tests (electrolyte profile, creatinine, serum osmolarity, urinalysis, etc.).

4 Basic treatment principles include limiting the amount of toxin absorbed, enhancing elimination of absorbed toxin, and preventing conversion of nontoxic compounds to toxic metabolites.

5 Drugs or poisons for which specific antidotes or therapies exist (especially acetaminophen, salicylates, methanol, ethylene glycol, and digitalis) should be aggressively sought (including specific quantitative levels) and treated after initial stabilization.

Overdoses and poisonings account for approximately 15% of all intensive care unit (ICU) admissions, but most overdose patients do well and require only a brief stay. Despite myriad potential toxins, just a few account for more than 90% of all overdoses, with acetaminophen now being the single most common problem. Overall, most poisonings are oral ingestions; in adults, usually deliberate and involve multiple compounds; in children, usually accidental intake of a single agent. Most poisonings occur in otherwise healthy young patients, which partially explains the low hospital mortality (approx. 1%). (Most fatalities occur from arrhythmia, seizure, or hypoventilation-induced anoxic brain damage before patients reach the hospital or shortly after arrival.)

■ DIAGNOSIS

Clinical History

The clinical history is often erroneous. Many patients overstate the quantity of ingested drug; others have taken a medication they conceal and the reported time of ingestion is often inaccurate. Suicidal patients may attempt to hide the type of poisons or drugs, and patients taking illicit drugs often lack accurate knowledge of what they took or fail to provide information, fearing prosecution. Occasionally, patients are victimized by surreptitious administration of a sedative, or hypnotic, agent of which they have no knowledge. In such cases, sexual assault is often the motive. Because patients may switch the contents of labeled bottles and accidental overdose may result from pharmacy dispensing errors, it is always wise to examine the contents of prescription bottles to ensure they match the label. It is important to seek the following information: (a) type of drug or toxin including ingestion of a sustained release form; (b) chronicity of use; (c) quantity consumed; (d) time elapsed since ingestion; (e) initial symptoms, including a history of vomiting or diarrhea; and (f) underlying diseases or other drugs taken.

Physical Examination

The physical examination is extremely valuable because it may allow rapid classification of patients into classic "toxic syndromes," which can help in toxin identification and guide initial therapy. The cardinal manifestations of these syndromes and their common causes are illustrated in Table 33-1.

TABLE 33-1 MAJOR TOXIC SYNDROMES

SIGNS AND SYMPTOMS	ANTICHOLINERGIC	SYMPATHOMIMETIC	NARCOTIC/ SEDATIVE	CHOLINERGIC	SEROTONIN
Mental status	Delirium	Delirium/ hallucinations	Coma/lethargy	Confusion	Delirium
Skin	Dry/flushed	Sweating	Normal	Sweating	Flushed/ sweating
Temperature	Elevated	Elevated	Reduced/normal	Normal	Elevated
Pulse	Rapid	Rapid	Slow	Normal/slow	Rapid
Respiration	Normal	Rapid	Slow/shallow	Bronchorrhea/ wheezing	Normal/ rapid
Blood pressure	Normal/elevated	Elevated	Normal/reduced	Normal or low	Normal
Eyes	Mydriasis	Mydriasis	Miosis	Miosis/ lacrimation	Mydriasis
GI tract function	Decreased	Increased	Decreased	Diarrhea/ vomiting	Diarrhea/ nausea
Other	Seizures Myoclonus Urine retention	Seizures	Hyporeflexia	Muscle weakness Salivation Urinary incontinence	Trismus Tremor Myoclonus
Causes	Atropine Antihistamines Benztropine Baclofen Phenothiazines Propantheline Scopolamine Tricyclic antidepressants	Amphetamines Cocaine Ecstasy (MDMA) Ephedrine Caffeine Phenylephrine Phencyclidine Phenylpropa- nolamine Pseudoephedrine Theophylline	Opioids Ethanol Barbiturates Benzodiazepines Anticonvulsants Antipsychotics Gamma hydroxybutyrate Tramadol 1,4-Butanediol	Organophosphates Carbamates Physostigmine Pilocarpine Nerve agents, sarin	Fluoxetine Paroxetine Sertraline Trazodone Clomipramine Meperidine Addition of MAO inhibitor, e.g., linezolid

The first steps in treating a patient with poisoning are to assess the vital signs and ensure an adequate airway, oxygenation, and perfusion. The airway of the overdosed patient may be obstructed, particularly if narcotics, sedatives, or caustic agents have been ingested. Intubation and artificial ventilation are required when there is airway obstruction or the central drive to breathe is depressed. Because respiratory drive may be unstable, and vomiting is common, noninvasive ventilation is usually a poor choice for support of the overdosed patient. As a general rule, a patient sedate enough to allow unresisted endotracheal intubation almost certainly requires the airway protection and ventilatory support the procedure provides. When it takes several people to restrain a combative patient, the need for intubation should be reconsidered unless sedation is required for diagnostic evaluation (e.g., head computed tomographic [CT] scan, lumbar puncture) or for protection of the patient or staff.

Hypoventilation is a clue to narcotic, sedative, tramadol, carisoprodol, clonidine, or gamma hydroxybutyrate (GHB) overdose. Recently an industrial solvent, 1,4-butanediol, also known as GBL or GHV, with clinical effects similar to GHB has grown in popularity as a cheap recreational drug. Hyperventilation due to central nervous system (CNS) stimulation should suggest salicylate, theophylline, amphetamine, phencyclidine (PCP), or cocaine toxicity. Hyperventilation can also result from toxin-induced metabolic acidosis as seen with metformin, methanol, ethylene glycol, or propofol or from tissue hypoxia caused by cyanide or carbon monoxide (see Chapter 40). Any compound that causes methemoglobenemia, such as dapsone, amide topical anesthetics, and sulfa compounds, can also lead to hyperventilation.

Blood pressure and perfusion should be assessed and corrected rapidly if inadequate. Anticholinergic, cyclic antidepressant, or sympathomimetic (e.g., cocaine, amphetamine) poisoning should be suspected in patients with marked tachycardia. Sinus bradycardia or conduction system block may result from overdoses of digitalis, clonidine, β-blockers, calcium channel blockers, or other cholinergic drugs.

Although hypertension is nonspecific, *marked* hypertension should suggest amphetamine, cocaine, thyroid hormone, methylene dioxymethamphetamine (MDMA, ecstasy), and catecholamine toxicities. Temperature may provide a valuable etiologic clue as well. Hyperthermia suggests anticholinergic, MDMA, amphetamine, or cyclic antidepressant poisoning or may be indicative of alcohol withdrawal, whereas hypothermia frequently accompanies alcohol or sedative–hypnotic overdose. (Hypothermia can be seen in any overdose that leads to prolonged environmental exposure to cool temperatures.)

Once the airway, breathing, and circulation are ensured, patients should be administered thiamine to avert the possibility of Wernicke's encephalopathy, and a bedside glucose measurement should be obtained. Diagnosis of hypoglycemia is important because it mimics many common drug intoxications, is easily corrected, and is devastating if overlooked. The narcotic antagonist, naloxone, is frequently given; however, its use can create as many problems as it solves. For the narcotic-intoxicated patient, naloxone produces rapid return of consciousness but often precipitates vomiting (often with aspiration) and results in a combative, disoriented patient. Furthermore, the duration of action of naloxone is shorter than that of almost all narcotics, so it is common for patients to relapse into unconsciousness. Essentially all the same liabilities exist for the benzodiazepine antagonist, flumazenil.

It is important not to overlook concurrent trauma or other serious medical illness. For example, nearly one half of all head-injured motor vehicle crash victims also are intoxicated with alcohol or other substances. When trauma cannot be excluded in patients with altered mental status, it often is prudent to perform a CT or magnetic resonance image (MRI) scan of the head and neck and evaluate the cervical spine for injury while the evaluation and therapy of the overdose is ongoing. Similarly, drug or alcohol ingestion does not preclude a coexisting life-threatening medical illness such as meningitis or hypoglycemia.

The head should be examined closely for clues to other causes of coma (e.g., head trauma, subarachnoid hemorrhage) and to provide data

TABLE 33-2 CHARACTERISTIC BREATH ODORS OF VICTIMS OF POISONING

ODOR	POISON
Sweet/fruity	Ketones/alcohols
Almond	Cyanide
"Gasoline"	Hydrocarbons
Garlic	Organophosphates/arsenic
Wintergreen	Methyl salicylate
Pear	Chloral hydrate

relevant to overdose. For example, inspection of the mouth may reveal unswallowed tablets or evidence of caustic injury. Breath odor may suggest a particular toxin (Table 33-2). For instance, ketones give a sweet odor, whereas cyanide presents an almond scent. The characteristic smell of hydrocarbons is distinguished easily, as is the "garlic" odor of organophosphate ingestion. Narcotics, barbiturates, organophosphates, and phenothiazines commonly produce miosis, whereas drugs with anticholinergic properties (e.g., amphetamines, antihistamines, ecstasy, cocaine, and cyclic antidepressants) cause mydriasis. Nystagmus is often seen with ethanol, carbamazepine, PCP, or phenytoin ingestion. (Lithium, volatile solvents, and primidone also cause nystagmus.) Pupils that appear fixed and dilated can result from profound sedative overdose but are characteristic of glutethimide or mushroom poisoning. Pupils that are dilated but reactive suggest anticholinergic or sympathomimetic poisoning. Because even the slightest reaction has positive prognostic implications, the pupillary response should be tested using a bright light in a darkened room.

Laboratory Testing

The electrocardiogram (ECG) can provide valuable clues in drug overdose. Ectopy is common in sympathomimetic and tricyclic poisoning. High-grade atrioventricular (AV) block may be due to digoxin, β-blockers, calcium channel blockers, cyanide, phenytoin, or cholinergic substances. A wide QRS complex or prolonged QT interval suggests quinidine, procainamide, or cyclic antidepressant overdose.

Arterial blood gases are helpful to assess acid–base status and gas exchange and suggest salicylate intoxication if they reveal a mixed respiratory alkalosis and metabolic acidosis. Metabolic acidosis with compensatory hyperventilation is common with cyanide or carbon monoxide exposure (see also Chapter 40) and with the propofol infusion syndrome (PRIS).

In addition to arterial blood gas determinations, measurement of hemoglobin saturation and oxygen content by co-oximetry may be helpful. Both methemoglobin and carboxyhemoglobin lead to a disparity between the measured oxygen content or measured hemoglobin saturation and that predicted from the arterial oxygen tension (PaO_2). Carboxyhemoglobin is elevated by carbon monoxide poisoning, and a number of drugs including dapsone, benzocaine, and sulfonamides can oxidize hemoglobin to methemoglobin. Profound methemoglobinemia should be suspected in patients with dyspnea seemingly without or with little lung disease and may be recognized at the bedside by the chocolate brown color it imparts to blood.

It is essential to calculate the anion and osmolar gaps. The numerical difference between the serum sodium and the sum of the chloride and bicarbonate is called the anion gap, and it normally ranges from 3 to 12 mEq/L. Six relatively common poisonings elevate the anion gap: (a) salicylates, (b) methanol, (c) ethanol, (d) ethylene glycol, (e) cyanide, and (f) carbon monoxide. Caution is advised, however, because hypoalbuminemia can reduce the anion gap obscuring an important clue to overdose. (For each reduction in albumin concentration of 1 gm/L, the anion gap declines by an average of 2.5 mEq/L.)

The osmolar gap is the difference between the calculated osmolality (1.86 [Na] + BUN/2.8 + glucose/18 + ethanol/4.6) and the osmolarity measured by a freezing point depression assay. When an osmolar gap greater than 10 mOsm exists, ethanol, ethylene glycol, isopropanol, and methanol become the most likely offenders; however, any unmeasured osmotic substance (e.g., glycerol, mannitol, sorbitol, radiocontrast agents, acetone, glycine) can widen the osmolar gap. The less commonly used method of vapor pressure osmometry does not detect methanol. Ketosis suggests ethanol, paraldehyde, or diabetes as potential culprits, although in many cases, simply not eating (starvation ketosis) is the explanation for mild ketosis. If ketones are present without systemic acidosis, isopropyl alcohol is the probable etiology.

Hypocalcemia is produced by the ingestion of ethylene glycol, oxalate, fluoride compounds, and certain rare metal ingestions: manganese, phosphorus, and barium. On rare occasions, chest or abdominal radiographs may help identify radiopaque tablets of iron, phenothiazines, tricyclic agents, or chloral hydrate. When these drugs are involved, the abdominal radiograph may help to ensure that the gut has been emptied after emesis or gastric lavage.

Use of the Drug Screen

Most qualitative drug screens assay urine or blood using thin-layer chromatography. Because there is no "standard" for which substances are included in a drug screen, it is important to know which compounds are assayed in each hospital. Urine and gastric juice are the most reliable samples for toxin assay because many drugs rapidly cleared from the serum may be detected as unabsorbed drug or excreted metabolites. Unfortunately, the drug screen has limited usefulness because significant delays often occur before the results are available, many toxins are not identified on the screen, and the results seldom change empirical therapy. Many common drugs (e.g., aspirin, acetaminophen, ethanol, methanol, ethylene glycol, GHB) are omitted from "routine" screens, and tests for each must be

TABLE 33-3 MEDICATIONS RESULTING IN FALSE-POSITIVE TOXICOLOGY SCREEN RESULTS

FALSE POSITIVE	CAUSE
Amphetamines	Ranitidine Chlorpromazine Bupropion Selegiline
Barbiturates	Ibuprofen Naproxen
Benzodiazepines	Oxaprozin
Cannabinoids	Pantoprazole Ibuprofen Naproxen
Opiates	Ofloxacin Levofloxacin Rifampin
Phencyclidine	Dextromethorphan Mesoridazine Venlafaxine
Cyclic antidepressants	Cyclobenzaprine

5

TABLE 33-4 COMPOUNDS FOR WHICH QUANTITATIVE ASSAY IS HELPFUL	
Acetaminophen	Digitalis
Ethanol	Methanol
Theophylline	Salicylates
Ethylene glycol	Carbon monoxide
Iron	Lithium
Phenobarbital	Methemoglobin

requested specifically. If a particular toxin is suspected, specific assay techniques may provide more rapid and quantitative results. A negative screen alone does not exclude overdose because of problems with sensitivity and timing of the test in relation to ingestion. In other cases, the screen does not detect the offending agent (e.g., fentanyl). In some screening assays, commonly used drugs may be reported as the presence of a suspected toxin because of cross reactivity (Table 33-3). Whenever there is doubt regarding drug screen results, clinical judgment should prevail. Specific therapy is available for certain toxins for which quantitative levels should be obtained to guide management (Table 33-4).

■ TREATMENT OF DRUG OVERDOSE

Physiologic support is key to all overdose management. Three basic precepts help minimize the toxic effects of drug ingestion: (a) prevent additional toxin absorption, (b) enhance drug excretion, and (c) prevent formation of toxic metabolites. Depending on the drug ingested, appropriate therapy also may include antidote administration or toxin removal.

Prevention of Toxin Absorption

After initial stabilization, the next step in the treatment of poisoning is to stop absorption. For cutaneously absorbed toxins (e.g., organophosphates, nerve agents), removing contaminated clothing and washing the skin is particularly important. Contaminated clothing needs to be placed in sealed bags and safely disposed of to avoid secondary exposure and incapacitation of health care workers. Such precautions are particularly important if dealing with potent nerve toxic agents that will be used in terrorist attacks.

For ingested toxins, induction of emesis is rarely, if ever, indicated. Long delays between ingestion and hospital presentation limit emesis effectiveness, and for patients with altered mental status or suppressed gag reflex, vomiting is dangerous. Emesis is not appropriate in ingestion of corrosive chemicals or petroleum distillates.

Although controversial, gastric lavage can be effective if undertaken within 1 to 2 h of a potentially lethal ingestion. Forgo lavage if a nontoxic substance has been ingested or if it is unlikely that a toxic quantity of the material remains in the stomach because of prior vomiting or because long periods have elapsed since ingestion. Some experts advocate lavage as long as 12 h after ingestion of substances that delay gastric emptying (e.g., opiates, tricyclic antidepressants), are corrosive (e.g., hydrocarbons), or form concretions (e.g., salicylates, meprobamate). Because lavage risks gastric perforation, aspiration, and airway compromise, it must be performed carefully and only when benefits are judged to exceed risks. For patients with altered consciousness, the airway should be protected with a cuffed endotracheal tube before attempting lavage. The procedure should be done in the left lateral decubitus position using a large orogastric tube. (Smaller tubes fail to adequately remove pill fragments.) Vomitus or aspirated gastric contents can be sent for toxicologic analysis.

Activated charcoal (usually 1 gm/kg) can be given to absorb orally ingested drugs. Although serious risks are small, activated charcoal frequently causes vomiting and may produce pneumonitis, bronchiolitis obliterans, and even acute respiratory distress syndrome (ARDS) when aspirated. Charcoal has enormous absorptive area ($>1,000 \, m^2/gm$) and binds many toxins within minutes of administration; however, activated charcoal is not effective in reducing the toxic effects of many common poisons (Table 33-5).

The once popular use of single-dose activated charcoal for nearly all toxic ingestions has fallen out of favor with the realization that in most cases, sufficient time has lapsed to preclude benefit,

TABLE 33-5 POISONS NOT ABSORBED BY ACTIVATED CHARCOAL		
Acids	Alkalis	Potassium
Iron	Lithium	Heavy metals
Organophosphates	Carbamates	Hydrocarbons
Ethylene glycol	Alcohols	Cyanide

while risks remain. Although charcoal tends to constipate, cathartics may deplete fluids and electrolytes, and repeated doses are not routinely needed unless large volumes or multiple doses of activated charcoal are given. Bowel obstruction can result from retention of charcoal in the colon. Sorbitol is the preferred cathartic because it works faster than magnesium citrate and avoids the magnesium toxicity that can result if renal function is impaired. Other absorbents such as bile acid sequestrants (e.g., cholestyramine) also can be used to reduce absorption of specific agents such as thyroid hormone and compounds with significant enterohepatic circulation.

Another method to decrease toxin absorption is whole bowel irrigation, in which vigorous catharsis is produced using a polyethylene glycol solution. Approximately 1 to 2 L of the solution is drunk (or instilled via gastric tube) each hour until the rectal effluent is clear of pill fragments (typically 3 to 5 h). Whole bowel irrigation is most useful to clear sustained release drugs, and in cases of "body packing," where packages of illicit drugs may rupture with fatal consequences. Bowel irrigation requires a nonobstructed GI tract and works best with an alert, cooperative patient.

Enhancement of Drug Removal

Four therapeutic techniques enhance removal of circulating toxins: (a) gut dialysis, (b) ion trapping, (c) hemodialysis, and (d) hemoperfusion. Drugs undergoing enterohepatic circulation, such as theophylline, digoxin, phenobarbital, dapsone, and carbamazepine, may be eliminated by "gut dialysis," a process using repeated doses of oral activated charcoal to bind drug excreted into the bile. Although the effectiveness of multiple-dose charcoal is poorly studied, three or four doses of 0.5 to 1 gm/kg given every 2 to 4 h have been advocated.

Charged molecules do not cross lipid membranes easily; therefore, ionized drugs are not absorbed readily from the stomach and fail to cross the blood–brain barrier. Furthermore, once in the renal tubule, such molecules have a limited tendency to back-diffuse into the circulation. Because urinary pH can only be altered between values of 4.5 and 7.5, "ion trapping" of drugs in the renal tubule is effective for only a few compounds. Alkalinization of the serum and urine, although often difficult to achieve, can impede transfer of weak acids (e.g., salicylates, cyclic antidepressants, phenobarbital, methotrexate, and isoniazid) across the blood–brain barrier and promotes their excretion. This process usually requires administration of nearly 2 mEq/kg of sodium bicarbonate intravenously every 3 to 4 h. (A convenient method is to place two ampules of NaHCO$_3$ per liter of D5W run at 250 mL/h.) Alkalinization is most effective when minute ventilation is also controlled; hypoventilation in response to the induced metabolic alkalosis can impair the ability to achieve alkalemia. Hypokalemia must be avoided; not only does hypokalemia predispose to arrhythmias, but it also impairs the ability to achieve an alkaline urine by promoting hydrogen ion secretion as potassium is reabsorbed in the distal tubule. The carbonic anhydrase inhibitor acetazolamide should not be used to alkalinize the urine because it results in acidemia and can worsen drug toxicity of some poisons (i.e., salicylates, tricyclic antidepressants).

Urinary acidification using arginine, lysine, or ammonium chloride may accelerate excretion of weak bases such as amphetamine, strychnine, PCP, and quinidine. The practice is questionably effective and potentially dangerous for patients with renal or hepatic dysfunction and may exacerbate myogloburic renal injury.

Hemodialysis effectively clears low-molecular-weight, water-soluble, non–protein-bound molecules having a small volume of distribution (e.g., methanol, ethylene glycol, salicylates, and lithium). Charcoal hemoperfusion clears theophylline, phenobarbital, phenytoin, carbamazepine, and other lipid-soluble drugs in a manner similar to oral multidose charcoal but may provoke hypocalcemia, initiate complement activation, or cause thrombocytopenia. Hemoperfusion is a poor method to extract lithium and alcohols. Hemofiltration has not been well studied as a toxin clearance mechanism; however, it has theoretical attractiveness to extract compounds with large volumes of distribution, extensive tissue binding, or slow intercompartmental transfer.

Inhibition of Toxic Metabolite Formation

Some drugs, most notably acetaminophen, methanol, and ethylene glycol, are relatively inert when ingested but form highly toxic compounds during metabolism. Inhibition of toxin formation will be discussed later under specific therapy for these poisons.

■ SPECIFIC POISONS

Acetaminophen

Acetaminophen is safe when taken in recommended doses, but ingestion of as little as 6 gm may be fatal. (Usually, a fatal dose exceeds 140 mg/kg.) Fortunately, most acetaminophen overdoses are not life threatening and do not require specific therapy. Acetaminophen is absorbed within 1 h, especially when taken in the liquid form. The usual serum half-life is approximately 2 to 4 h but lengthens with declining liver function. Normally, the drug is metabolized hepatically to nontoxic compounds by linkage with sulfates and glucuronide. The hepatic cytochrome P-450 system converts less than 5% of an ingested dose to reactive metabolites, which are then detoxified by conjugation with glutathione. However, during massive overdose, toxic metabolites (*N*-acetyl-*p*-benzoquinoneimine) overwhelm the glutathione supply and accumulate to cause liver damage. Conditions that induce the hepatic cytochrome P-450 system, including chronic use of ethanol, oral contraceptives, or phenobarbital, predispose to toxicity.

Even in serious acetaminophen overdose, symptoms are minimal for the first 24 h after ingestion, with the exception of nausea and vomiting. One to two days after ingestion, deteriorating liver function tests, right upper quadrant pain, and oliguria (because of the antidiuretic hormone-like effects of acetaminophen) become evident. At this time, hepatic transaminases may peak in the tens of thousands of units. Hepatic necrosis and failure evolve within 3 to 5 days. (This toxicity is often manifest by a rising bilirubin level and prothrombin time and declining transaminases.) In this most advanced stage, mental status declines and renal failure develops. If the patient is to recover, improvement is typically noted between days 5 and 7. Poor prognostic factors are late presentation, the presence of coagulopathy, metabolic acidosis, renal failure, and cerebral edema.

In addition to hemodynamic and respiratory support, if presentation is prompt, initial treatment should include evacuation of the stomach and administration of activated charcoal. Charcoal reduces absorption of acetaminophen potentially averting a toxic serum level; a specific antidote, *N*-acetylcysteine (NAC), is the drug of choice. Not all patients require therapy with NAC; the likelihood of hepatic toxicity from an isolated acute ingestion may be predicted from a standard (Rumack–Matthew) nomogram using the serum level obtained more than 4 h after ingestion. (Concentrations >140 mg/dL at 4 h are predictive of severe toxicity.) Patients with preexisting chronic use or liver disease may develop symptoms at concentrations much lower than the nomogram predicts. For such patients, it makes sense to begin NAC therapy if acetaminophen levels exceed 10 μg/mL or hepatic tranaminases demonstrate any elevation. For patients who ingest extended release preparations, it makes sense to obtain serial levels at 4- to 6-h intervals after ingestion. If any level reaches the toxic threshold, therapy should be undertaken. NAC probably has a twofold action: directly binding the toxic metabolites of acetaminophen and repleting intracellular glutathione. For maximal effectiveness, NAC should be given as quickly as possible. Historically, treatment has included an oral loading dose of 140 mg/kg followed by 17 additional doses of 70 mg/kg at 4-h intervals. When NAC is given orally, vomiting is so common that "prophylactic" antiemetic therapy should probably be administered. Intravenous NAC, free of emetogenic effects, is now available and short-duration infusions (24 h) are safe, cost effective, and at least as effective as the older, less-convenient oral regimen. (Intravenous therapy is rarely associated with flushing or angioedema.) Of note, liver injury induced by acetaminophen commonly predisposes patients to hypoglycemia, which should be closely monitored and treated. When massive hepatic necrosis develops, liver transplantation may be considered if irreparable brain injury has not occurred from hepatic failure–induced cerebral edema.

Salicylates

Salicylate overdoses are now uncommon but continue to be highly lethal. Up to one third of all salicylate intoxication victims die before leaving the emergency department, often arriving in extremis. In large doses, salicylates inhibit cellular enzymes and uncouple oxidative phosphorylation. The clinical presentation of salicylate overdose includes altered mental status, tinnitus, acidosis, hypoxemia, and (more rarely) hyperosmolarity, hyperthermia, and seizures. Salicylate intoxication can easily be confused with a psychotic episode. Initially, direct CNS stimulation causes a respiratory alkalosis and compensatory renal wasting of bicarbonate. Later, superimposed metabolic acidosis may produce a complex acid–base disturbance.

Tachypnea may be absent if the patient has ingested a sedative or hypnotic concurrently. Large doses of aspirin may induce pulmonary edema, causing ARDS.

It does not take much aspirin to produce toxicity; a lethal adult dose ranges from 10 to 30 gm (150 mg/kg). Salicylate intoxication always should be considered in the differential diagnosis of an anion gap acidosis. The anion gap elevation results primarily from lactate and pyruvate generated during anaerobic glycolysis but ketones also are formed in response to decreased glucose and accelerated lipolysis. Very high serum salicylate levels (>80 mg/dL) may directly contribute to the anion gap. In addition, large insensible fluid losses deplete intravascular volume, thereby stimulating aldosterone secretion, which depletes bicarbonate and potassium. Salicylate levels higher than 50 mg/dL commonly induce nausea and vomiting and may produce a metabolic alkalosis, leading to a "triple" acid–base disorder.

Salicylates inhibit the formation of prothrombin, impair platelet function, and irritate the gastric mucosa—all of which contribute to the risk of hemorrhage. Patients with salicylate-induced coagulopathy or bleeding should receive vitamin K and, if immediate reversal is necessary, fresh frozen plasma and platelets.

If therapy is to prevent morbidity, salicylate intoxication must be suspected on clinical grounds. In chronic toxicity, serum levels correlate poorly with toxicity, but in acute intoxication, adverse effects are uncommon with serum levels below 30 mg/dL. Moderate toxicity often is seen with acute ingestions of 150 to 300 mg/kg. Another salicylate preparation, oil of wintergreen, represents a significantly greater risk; one teaspoon provides the amount of salicylate in almost 20 aspirin tablets (7 gm). In acute salicylate poisoning, initial levels above 120 mg/dL, 6-h levels higher than 100 mg/dL, or any level greater than 500 mg/dL is associated with a high risk of death. Declining salicylate levels should not necessarily be reassuring, as they may merely indicate transit of the salicylate from the plasma to tissue. If salicylate levels are not immediately available, "Phenistix" test strips can demonstrate a purple color when serum levels exceed 70 mg/dL.

Because salicylates are rapidly absorbed, at the time of presentation, it is almost always too late for effective gastric evacuation However, in massive overdoses, serum levels may continue to rise for up to 24 h after ingestion because of delayed gastric absorption. As weak acids, salicylates remain nonionized at low serum pH and readily cross cell membranes; therefore, ion trapping with bicarbonate may be used to lower toxicity and promote excretion. In addition to decreasing urinary excretion, an acidic pH favors movement of salicylates into cells and across the blood–brain barrier. Therefore, serum and urine pH should be monitored and kept alkaline with bicarbonate titration or dialysis. Development or worsening of acidosis can lead to a precipitous clinical decline. An example of this phenomenon is when a patient hyperventilating to compensate for metabolic acidosis is sedated and/or paralyzed for intubation; the lower postintubation minute ventilation can result in an abrupt decompensation as salicylate shifts from plasma into cells. Hemodialysis is indicated for severe intoxications. When patients are known to have acutely ingested massive doses (>30 gm), when serum levels exceed 50 mg/dL, or when coma, seizure, renal failure, or pulmonary edema occurs, dialysis should be considered.

Stimulants

Stimulants exert their toxicity through direct CNS excitation or by causing catecholamine release, inhibiting catecholamine reuptake, or by inhibiting monoamine oxidase. Patients experiencing stimulant (amphetamines, ecstasy [XTC, MDMA], cocaine, and PCP) overdose characteristically present with agitation, hypertension, tachycardia, mydriasis, and warm, moist skin. Occasionally, rhabdomyolysis, hyperkalemia, and seizures occur. Vertical nystagmus is a common feature in PCP intoxication, whereas hyperthermia and hyponatremia (from inappropriate ADH secretion and excessive water intake) may be more common with ecstasy. Cardiac ischemia induced by the vasoconstrictive and chronotropic effects of cocaine may cause acute myocardial infarction, even in young patients and those without coronary artery disease. Aortic dissection (occasionally painless) also occurs with cocaine intoxication with several case reports of acute paraplegia as spinal cord blood supply is disrupted. Therefore, in cocaine intoxications, an ECG should be obtained, and if suspicious, myocardial ischemia or injury should be confirmed or excluded by serial ECGs and cardiac enzyme determinations. Treatment of myocardial ischemia associated with cocaine intoxication should not differ from that of conventional acute coronary syndromes. A low threshold to perform computed tomograms of the chest and abdomen should be maintained in patients with symptoms suggestive of dissection. The vasculature of the brain is also susceptible to the effects of cocaine resulting in ischemic and hemorrhagic strokes and subarachnoid hemorrhage. When smoked, cocaine base can cause a syndrome of pulmonary hemorrhage leading to acute respiratory failure known as "crack lung." However, even in the absence of alveolar damage, crack smoking is now a frequent cause of exacerbations of obstructive lung disease.

For most stimulant overdoses, specific treatment is lacking; however, maintenance of the airway, oxygenation, and control of blood pressure are universally indicated. Providing adequate hydration to maintain urine flow is important because many compounds in this class may precipitate rhabdomyolysis. Agitation can be controlled with haloperidol, droperidol, or benzodiazepines. Perhaps the best first treatment for the hypertension associated with stimulant ingestion is a benzodiazepine. Hypertension and tachycardia that persist after sedation can be managed with any number of vasodilators, with or without a β-adrenergic blocker. In this setting, the use of β-blockers alone is discouraged because of the possibility of unmasking unblocked α-agonist effects. This is only a minor concern if a direct vasodilator is given concomitantly.

Alcohols

Ethanol

Many suicide attempts involve ethanol, either alone or in combination with other drugs. Physiologic effects do not relate closely to serum concentrations, but blood levels higher than 150 mg/dL are inebriating. Coma usually requires levels higher than 300 mg/dL, and death often supervenes when concentrations exceed 600 mg/dL. The therapy of acute alcohol intoxication is largely supportive. Administration of thiamine and correction of serum glucose, potassium, and magnesium levels are indicated. Ethanol may be quickly removed by hemodialysis but is rarely necessary. Although 20% of ethanol-intoxicated patients will transiently awaken in response to large doses of naloxone, there is no treatment role for naloxone or direct CNS stimulants.

The ICU deprives the habituated patient of ethanol access. Deprivation may precipitate withdrawal, a condition that is significantly more dangerous than intoxication. Symptoms of withdrawal usually start within 36 h of the last drink (but may be delayed for 5 to 7 days). Measurable serum levels of ethanol do not exclude the diagnosis of withdrawal. Patients experiencing severe withdrawal (hallucinosis, delirium tremens [DT], etc.) are unpredictable, both in behavior and disease course. DT is the most extreme form of ethanol withdrawal, profoundly altering mental status and initiating life-threatening autonomic instability. Therefore, most patients with DT should be managed in an ICU to avert or quickly respond to such potentially fatal complications as seizures, aspiration, arrhythmias, and suicide attempts. Symptoms of withdrawal (specifically DT) often mimic infection or primary neurologic processes. It is important to emphasize, however, that 50% of febrile patients with DTs also have a concomitant infection, most frequently pneumonia or meningitis. The agitated withdrawal patient should be restrained in a lateral or prone position (not supine because of the risk of aspiration). Patients should be given nothing by mouth (NPO); all fluids, electrolytes, and vitamins (B_{12}, thiamine, folate, etc.) should be administered intravenously. Withdrawal may be prevented or aborted in its early stages through the use of oral benzodiazepines, but if fully manifest, intravenous lorazepam becomes the sedative of choice. Benzodiazepines reduce hyperactivity and the risk of seizures. In this situation, intravenous benzodiazepines should be given frequently, in small doses, until the patient is calm but not obtunded. Haloperidol or droperidol may be useful adjuncts. After initial control with intravenous dosing is achieved, oral maintenance therapy should be instituted. Lorazepam has become a popular choice because it is a long-acting drug available in both oral and intravenous forms, it does not require hepatic metabolism, and it has no active metabolites (a particularly useful property in patients with liver disease). Although very effective in achieving controlled sedation, propofol has not been widely used for the indication. Phenothiazines probably should be avoided because they lower the seizure threshold. Titratable β-blockers (e.g., esmolol) may also be helpful in well-selected hypermetabolic, tachycardic patients. (Labetolol is better choice if also hypertensive.)

Methanol and Ethylene Glycol Toxicity

A tabular overview of the clinical and laboratory features of the most common alcohol poisonings is presented in Table 33-6. The toxicity of methanol and ethylene glycol results from the formation of organic acids from the parent compounds. Toxic

TABLE 33-6 FEATURES OF VARIOUS ALCOHOL INTOXICATIONS

	ETHANOL	METHANOL	ETHYLENE GLYCOL	ISOPROPANOL
Osmolar gap	+	+	+	+
Ketones	+	−	−	+
Acidosis	+	+	+	−
Visual changes	−	+	−	−
Ca^{2+} oxalate crystals	−	−	+	−

metabolites of ethylene glycol include oxalic, glycolic, and glyoxylic acids. Formic acid and formaldehyde are responsible for methanol toxicity. Formation of toxic metabolites of both compounds is delayed by concomitant ethanol ingestion. Methanol is found in paint remover, windshield deicing fluid, gas-line antifreeze, and canned solid fuel, whereas ethylene glycol is the major component of automobile antifreeze. Tiny amounts of these compounds are needed to produce life-threatening toxicity: 30 mL of methanol and 100 mL of ethylene glycol may cause severe injury.

Early methanol or ethylene glycol ingestion resembles ethanol intoxication. However, as symptoms progress, almost any global CNS finding may be seen, including coma, hyporeflexia, nystagmus, or seizures. Whereas the presentations of ethylene glycol and methanol are often indistinguishable, cardiovascular signs (tachycardia, hypertension, and pulmonary edema) and renal failure resulting from oxalate crystalluria more frequently complement ethylene glycol. On the other hand, optic neuritis and blindness are hallmarks of methanol poisoning. Methanol or ethylene glycol ingestion should be suspected in patients with acidosis and coexistent anion and osmolar gaps. Absence of an osmolar gap should not dissuade clinicians from the diagnosis in patients with delayed presentation because the parent alcohols are relatively rapidly cleared from the circulation. Specifically lethal levels of ethylene glycol (>20 mg/dL) may be present with minimal elevations in the osmolar gap.

The treatment of methanol or ethylene glycol poisoning is fourfold: (a) remove any remaining drug from the stomach; (b) prevent toxic metabolite formation; (c) remove the parent alcohol from the circulation; and (d) treat metabolic acidosis. Toxin formation is attenuated by using ethanol or fomepizole (4-methylpyrazole [4-MP]) to compete with ethylene glycol or methanol for metabolism by alcohol dehydrogenase. Ethanol levels above 100 mg/dL are required and can be achieved by giving a loading dose of ethanol 800 mg/kg intravenously or orally (equivalent to about 4 ounces of whiskey), followed by a maintenance regimen of 130 mg/kg/h (about 100 mL of 10% ethanol intravenously per hour or 25 mL of 40% alcohol orally at the same rate). 4-MP is a very expensive alternative with but one advantage: it does not contribute to the clinical picture of intoxication. An initial 4-MP dose of 15 mg/kg is followed by 10 mg/kg every 12 h (higher doses are required if treatment is continued beyond 24 h). Emergent dialysis should be performed in all patients known to have ingested a toxic quantity of methanol or ethylene glycol and those with serum levels above 50 mg/dL. Ideally, dialysis is continued until serum levels are undetectable. Because hemodialysis removes both ethanol and 4-MP, doses of both must be doubled during filtration. Calcium replacement may be required for patients with ethylene glycol poisoning who develop symptomatic hypocalcemia.

Isopropyl Alcohol

Isopropyl alcohol is also metabolized by alcohol dehydrogenase to acetone that is subsequently excreted by the lung and kidneys. Intoxication and ketotic breath are presentation hallmarks. Gastritis occurs commonly. From the laboratory standpoint, isopropanol increases the osmolar gap but not the anion gap. Hemodialysis should be undertaken when serum levels exceed 400 mg/dL.

Sedative–Hypnotic-Analgesic Drugs

Barbiturates, benzodiazepines, and opioids are the most common sedating agents resulting in drug overdose. Meprobamate, methaqualone, chloral hydrate, and glutethimide are now largely of historical significance, except the commonly used drug carisoprodol is metabolized to meprobamate. GHB is an increasingly popular drug of abuse but presents special challenges to diagnosis. Most sedative drugs depress consciousness and, in large doses, act as negative inotropes and vasodilators—occasionally causing cardiovascular collapse.

The benzodiazepines, however, have a wide therapeutic range, and when taken alone, doses of 50 to 100 times the usual therapeutic dose may still be well tolerated. Unfortunately, ethanol and opiates are common coingestants substantially enhancing toxicity. Benzodiazepines depress consciousness, reflexes, and respiration. Treatment consists of gastric evacuation for patients seen very shortly after ingestion, but for most, treatment is only supportive. There is no benefit to dialysis. Flumazenil is a competitive receptor antagonist that reverses the respiratory and central depressant effects of benzodiazepines in approximately 80% of patients. High doses of benzodiazepines, long duration of therapy, and concomitant narcotic use lower the rate of reversal. Flumazenil has no beneficial effect on ethanol, barbiturate, narcotic, or tricyclic antidepressant-induced CNS depression. Because the liver clears flumazenil rapidly, its duration of action is substantially shorter than that of most benzodiazepines. Akin to the naloxone–opioid story, as many as 10% of patients given flumazenil relapse into a sedated state, making careful observation essential. When used, intermittent doses of 0.2 mg at 1-min intervals (up to 3 mg total) are typical. Flumazenil should be used cautiously because it may precipitate withdrawal symptoms (agitation, vomiting, and seizures), especially in chronic users of cyclic antidepressants or benzodiazepines. Flumazenil is expensive, is rarely needed in the ICU, and should be regarded as no more than an adjunct to airway protection and ventilation in the management of benzodiazepine overdose.

Barbiturates cause sedation, depress respiratory drive, and, as potent vasodilators and negative ionotropes, impair cardiovascular function. CNS depression may be so profound that patients may appear clinically dead with an isoelectric EEG. Because of the very long half-life of some barbiturates (e.g., Phenobarbital), even in patients with normal liver function, sedation can last a week or more after a significant overdose. Treatment is generally supportive; however, slow gastric emptying induced by barbiturates makes evacuation of the stomach and multidose charcoal potentially beneficial, even if undertaken hours after ingestion. The airway must be protected before lavage. Barbiturates are metabolized hepatically before excretion; therefore, patients with underlying liver disease are most prone to toxicity. Even though barbiturates are weak acids, forced alkaline diuresis has little effect on total drug excretion. Dialysis is not helpful, and the role of hemoperfusion is disputed. After all drug has been completely cleared, patients chronically habituated to barbiturates (and selected other sedatives) may enter a withdrawal phase. Tremor and convulsions may require temporary reinstitution of phenobarbital in therapeutic doses with gradual tapering.

The predominant toxicity of opioids (e.g., morphine, heroin, fentanyl, methadone, meperidine, pentazocine, propoxyphene, and diphenoxylate) is depression of consciousness and respiration. Aspiration pneumonitis is a common complication. Hypothermia, decreased gut motility, noncardiogenic pulmonary edema, and seizures (most common with propoxyphene and meperidine) can also be seen. Status epilepticus should raise the possibility of a massive overdose as sometimes seen in heroin "body packers." Although most opioids are ingested or injected, fentanyl is readily absorbed through the skin and is available transcutaneously. Hence, for all patients presenting with suspected sedative overdose, a careful examination for fentanyl patches should be conducted. All opioids can be detected on routine urine toxicology screens with the exception of fentanyl, which may require special blood analysis.

GHB is a rapidly absorbed, short-lived, euphoric agent when taken in low doses but can lead to deep sedation when taken in higher doses or with alcohol. Like other sedatives, bradycardia, hypothermia, and hypoventilation are typical. An unusual characteristic feature of GHB intoxication is deep sedation, sometimes to the point of apnea, alternating with periods of profound agitation.

Treatment of all sedative overdoses is supportive with protection of the airway and administration of supplemental oxygen as needed. Because opioids slow gastric emptying, lavage may be beneficial, even if performed later than the usually recommended 1 to 2 h postingestion limit. Naloxone is a specific narcotic antagonist that when given in initial doses of 0.2 to 0.4 mg often reverses opioid-induced respiratory depression. Low initial doses are indicated to avoid precipitating full-blown narcotic withdrawal in chronic users. If no response is seen within 2 to 3 min, additional doses of 1 to

2 mg may be administered to a total of 10 mg. Doses approaching 10 mg are sometimes necessary to reverse the effects of methadone, codeine, hydrocodone, oxycodone, pentazocine, propoxyphene, and diphenoxylate. Naloxone should not be given reflexively; administration may create more problems than it solves. Once awakened with naloxone, illicit narcotic users often wish to leave the hospital to avoid legal prosecution and often to seek more narcotics to reverse the discomfort of withdrawal. Because the duration of naloxone's effect is less than that of almost all narcotics, recurring sedation, sometimes fatal, is common. Seizures may respond to naloxone; however, those refractory to its effects will usually respond to benzodiazepines.

Two specific toxicities associated with therapeutic sedative use deserve special mention. Propylene glycol is the solvent and preservative in the sedatives diazepam, lorazepam, pentobarbital, and etomidate and in other commonly used medications such as phenytoin, esmolol, and intravenous nitroglycerine. Among these, clinical toxicity has been reported most commonly with lorazepam when used at high infusion rates for 3 or more days. Accumulation of propylene glycol results in an elevated anion gap and osmolar gap with clinical findings of CNS depression, or seizures, renal dysfunction, and a variety of cardiac arrhythmias. Hyperosmolarity results in shift of water from the intracellular to the extracellular compartment perhaps accounting for the mental status changes. The most important treatment is to stop the offending agent and substitute an alternate sedative. With an average half-life of 2 to 4 h, toxicity usually resolves within a day and rarely requires hemodialysis.

Another uncommon but important problem is the PRIS. First described in children, adults also can develop the clinical syndrome of metabolic acidosis, rhabdomyolysis, hyperkalemia, renal failure, and arrhythmias, especially when propofol is infused in high doses (>5 mg/kg/h) for 2 or more days. Hyperlipidemia is inconsistently present. Rarely right bundle branch block with convex ST segment elevation in the right chest leads has been reported. These ECG findings are noteworthy because they mimic those of the inherited ion channel defect, Brugada syndrome, which has been associated with sudden cardiac death. It is uncertain if patients who develop these ECG changes following propofol exposure are at increased risk of serious arrhythmias after discontinuation of the drug. The mechanism of the syndrome is uncertain but abnormalities in mitochondrial electron transport and fatty acid oxidation have been postulated. Like propylene glycol, the key to successful treatment is recognition of the syndrome and discontinuation of the responsible agent.

Organophosphates and Carbamates

Organophosphates and the related carbamate insecticides inhibit the action of acetylcholinesterase, thereby causing accumulation of acetylcholine at neuromuscular junctions. (Many nerve warfare agents [e.g., Sarin] have an identical mechanism of action.) Early specific treatment is important because binding of the toxin to acetylcholinesterase may become irreversible after 24 h. Organophosphates initially stimulate but later block acetylcholine receptors. Organophosphates penetrate the CNS, but carbamates do not. Toxic manifestations usually appear within 5 min (especially after inhalation) but may be delayed for 24 h when exposure is cutaneous or enteral. Muscle weakness resulting from organophosphate poisoning can persist for weeks.

The clinical presentation may be remembered by the mnemonic "STUMBLED": **S**alivation, **T**remor, **U**rination, **M**iosis, **B**radycardia, **L**acrimation, **E**mesis, and **D**iarrhea—all expressions of cholinergic–muscarinic excess. In some patients, nicotinic effects (fasciculation, skeletal cramping, hypertension, and tachycardia) predominate. If the patient presents shortly after ingestion, the insecticide stench is unmistakable. A garlic odor on the patient's breath also is suggestive of the diagnosis. Laboratory confirmation comes from measurement of plasma pseudocholinesterase or erythrocyte acetylcholinesterase but is rarely necessary given the history and clinical features. Acute reductions of enzyme activity by more than 90% correlate with severe toxicity. (With chronic low-level exposures, such as those that occur in agricultural nursery workers, enzyme levels may be reduced dramatically with few symptoms.) Alternatively, the diagnosis can be established by direct analysis of organophosphates in serum, gastric, or urinary samples. Laboratory findings also may include hemolytic anemia (seen with carbamates) and an anion gap metabolic acidosis. Bradycardia and heart block frequently result from cholinergic stimulation.

With cutaneous exposure, skin decontamination is essential. Health care workers must wear protective gowns, gloves, and masks when handling contaminated clothing or risk poisoning themselves. Particular attention should be given to the adequacy of respiration: bronchoconstriction, bronchorrhea, and muscle weakness all contribute to precipitate respiratory failure. High doses of anticholinergics may block muscarinic CNS effects but do not reverse nicotinic manifestations. (Atropine, 2 to 4 mg, usually is given intravenously until muscarinic symptoms are reversed.) Doses as high as 30 to 40 mg may be required, and because atropine crosses the blood–brain barrier, it often causes disorientation. Therapy should continue for at least 24 h after exposure. Pralidoxime (2-PAM) reverses the nicotinic (muscular) effects of organophosphates by uncoupling bound organophosphates from the esterases. However, treatment retains efficacy for only approximately 24 h; therefore, it should be given as soon as possible in a dose of 1 to 2 gm, repeated once if necessary. Clinical response is usually seen within 30 min and, when seen, can be sustained by a continuous infusion of 200 to 500 mg/h. 2-PAM is ineffective in carbamate poisoning. Transfusion of fresh frozen plasma can also be used to augment plasma levels of plasma cholinesterase levels.

Theophylline Toxicity

Impaired theophylline clearance occurs commonly in patients with obstructive lung disease and heart or liver failure but the incidence of toxicity has declined dramatically with waning popularity of theophylline. The potential for impaired clearance because of drug interaction is overlooked frequently, particularly for patients who have had ciprofloxacin, erythromycin, or zileuton added to chronic theophylline therapy. Smoking modestly increases the clearance of theophylline in patients without liver disease. Toxicity is more common when acutely elevated levels are superimposed on chronic theophylline use.

Toxic symptoms (tremors, arrhythmias, gastrointestinal [GI] upset, etc.) may occur at serum levels well within the therapeutic range (10 to 20 μg/mL), particularly in patients predisposed by advanced age or underlying CNS or cardiac disease (Table 33-7). A minority of hospitalized patients experience GI warning symptoms before having seizures—the most life-threatening toxic manifestation. (The mortality of theophylline-induced seizures exceeds 40%, and a large percentage of survivors have persistent neurological deficits.) Seizures are uncommon when serum

TABLE 33-7 SIDE EFFECTS AND THEOPHYLLINE LEVELS

THEOPHYLLINE LEVEL (mg/L)	SIDE EFFECTS
>15	Nausea, vomiting, confusion
20–40	Cardiac arrhythmias
>40	Seizures

levels remain below 35 mg/L. Leukocytosis may result from catecholamine-induced demargination of leukocytes and often suggests infection. Cardiac arrhythmias of all varieties occur, but serious arrhythmias generally do not emerge at therapeutic drug concentrations.

Initial treatment includes correction of hypoxemia, acidosis, and electrolyte abnormalities. Oral charcoal should be administered after gastric lavage if ingestion is recent. If a sustained-release preparation has been ingested, whole bowel irrigation using polyethylene glycol solution should be considered. Because theophylline undergoes enterohepatic circulation, multidose charcoal given in doses of 30 to 50 gm every 2 to 4 h may double drug clearance. β-Adrenergic blocking drugs are excellent choices for supraventricular arrhythmias and hyperglycemia. Benzodiazepines or phenobarbitals are preferred anticonvulsants because paradoxically, phenytoin may exacerbate seizures by displacing theophylline from serum proteins. Extracorporeal removal is probably indicated for theophylline levels higher than 50 mg/L and for refractory arrhythmias or seizures. Hemodialysis is only half as effective as hemoperfusion for drug removal but is an acceptable alternative when hemoperfusion is not feasible.

Digitalis Compounds

All of the symptoms of digitalis glycoside poisoning are nonspecific (fatigue, weakness, nausea, visual complaints, etc.) and are common in the elderly population with cardiac disease. Therefore, a low threshold of suspicion must be maintained for digitalis toxicity. Vigilance is especially necessary because the frequency of digitalis use has declined significantly. Renal insufficiency, hypothyroidism, heart failure, and electrolyte abnormalities (e.g., hypokalemia and hypomagnesemia) predispose patients to digitalis toxicity. Initiation of calcium channel blockers, type I-a antiarrhythmics, or amiodarone also can precipitate digitalis toxicity. The major toxicity of digitalis compounds is hyperkalemia and associated arrhythmias (AV nodal block and increased automaticity) resulting from poisoning of the cellular sodium–potassium pump.

Treatment consists of activated charcoal to decrease drug absorption and normalization of serum magnesium and potassium levels. Atropine and pacing are indicated for severe bradycardia. Lidocaine and phenytoin are the drugs of choice for ventricular tachyarrhythmias. It is best to avoid quinidine, β-blockers, and calcium channel blockers. Specific therapy using highly purified ovine IgG Fab antibody fragments (e.g., Digibind) is indicated for digoxin levels greater than 6 mg/dL, when potassium exceeds 5 mEq/L, or when refractory tachycardia or bradycardia occur. The usual adult dose of ten vials produces a response within 30 min. Digitalis antibody fragments are very safe—their only recognized toxicities are due to the reversal of digitalis effects (i.e., hypokalemia, congestive heart failure, and rapid ventricular response to atrial fibrillation). Because the antibody fragment–digitalis complex is detected by digoxin assays, plasma levels are not valid after antibody administration. With normal renal function, digitalis antibodies are cleared rapidly (48 to 72 h), but clearance is reduced dramatically by renal insufficiency.

Cyclic Antidepressants

Cyclic antidepressant use has declined significantly with the popularity of serotonin reuptake inhibitors (SSRIs), but they remain a common cause of drug overdose because they are used widely for depression, pain, and sleep, have a long half-life, and accumulate in the tissue. Despite the frequency of cyclic antidepressant overdoses, in-hospital mortality remains below 1% with most deaths occurring in the prehospital phase of illness or shortly after admission. Signs of cyclic antidepressant overdose are predominantly anticholinergic. The phrase "hot as a hare, blind as a bat, dry as a bone, red as a beet, mad as a hatter" accurately describes severely intoxicated patients, who often demonstrate hyperthermia, fixed and dilated pupils, dry red skin, and CNS hyperactivity (hallucinations and psychosis). Patients with lesser degrees of intoxication have predominantly CNS sedation. The differential diagnosis of cyclic antidepressant overdose includes other compounds having anticholinergic effects (e.g., atropine, antihistamines, phenothiazines,

scopolamine, anti-Parkinson drugs, jimson weed, and mushroom poisoning).

Because of their tendency to produce ileus, cyclic antidepressants may remain in the gut long after ingestion; therefore, gastric evacuation and oral charcoal can be effective in limiting toxicity. Toxicity correlates poorly with ingested dose or serum level because of the high tissue affinity.

The ECG warns of cardiac (and CNS) toxicity when the QRS complex in limb leads extends beyond 0.12 s. In such patients, the QTc and PR intervals are also likely to be lengthened. QRS widening provides a valuable clue to overdose in the unconscious patient who has ingested an unknown drug. Sinus tachycardia, conduction disturbances (especially right bundle branch block), and ventricular arrhythmias may persist long after serum levels normalize because of avid tissue binding. Return of the QRS width to baseline is the best indication that the risk of significant arrhythmias and seizures has passed. (Observation for 12 h after the QRS normalizes is a common practice but not evidence based.) Arrhythmias frequently respond to sodium bicarbonate administration initially given as 1 to 2 mEq/kg of $NaHCO_3$ IV and repeated until the QRS narrows or a pH of 7.45 to 7.55 is achieved. Controversy exists about whether therapeutic benefits stem from the alkaline pH reducing the serum concentration of unbound drug or the sodium load, which may influence membrane channels. Because arrhythmias may involve sodium channel alterations, hypertonic saline may correct refractory arrhythmias. After $NaHCO_3$, and hypertonic saline, lidocaine and perhaps phenytoin are the most helpful antiarrhythmics, but antidepressant-induced arrhythmias may be refractory to all therapy. Quinidine and procainamide should be avoided because of their tendency to further impede conduction. Hypotension usually is due to volume depletion. If fluid administration fails to restore blood pressure, α-agonists (e.g., norepinephrine) are the most effective vasopressors. Mixed-adrenergic agonists (e.g., dopamine, epinephrine) may paradoxically worsen the hypotension by increasing β-stimulation (increased heart rate and systemic vasodilation).

Interestingly, the tendency for *seizures* also may be predicted by a QRS complex width exceeding 0.12 s. Undesirable in and of themselves, seizures also induce systemic acidosis, which translocates cyclic antidepressants from plasma to tissue, potentially worsening the CNS and cardiac toxicity. Lorazepam and phenobarbital should be considered first-line anticonvulsants. Propofol may be effective salvage therapy. In seizing patients with unstable hemodynamic or respiratory status, it may be necessary to use paralytic agents to establish an airway and effective circulation before the cerebral discharges are controlled. If used, extreme caution must be exercised with paralytic agents because they do not interrupt cerebral discharges even though they stop muscular convulsive activity. In such settings, continuous EEG monitoring is probably required. Because of the high lipid solubility and protein binding, neither hemodialysis nor hemoperfusion is effective for drug removal.

Serotonin Reuptake Inhibitors

A variety of psychoactive medications act by increasing brain serotonin concentrations. Because of their effectiveness and low toxicity, SSRIs (e.g., sertraline, paroxetine, fluoxetine, citalopram, trazodone) have largely supplanted cyclic antidepressants. In addition to the reuptake inhibitors, serotonin levels can be augmented by drugs that are serotonin agonists (e.g., buspirone, lithium, metoclopramide) and those that increase serotonin synthesis (e.g., l-tryptophan) or release (e.g., amphetamines, cocaine, ecstasy) or inhibit its breakdown (monoamine oxidase inhibitors, including linezolid). Toxic levels of serotonin can result from an isolated large ingestion of a single SSRI, but more often are the result of simultaneous ingestion of several drugs from different classes or the addition of an MAO inhibitor to chronic SSRI therapy. This risk is magnified because many currently SSRIs have very long half-lives. When toxicity follows a discrete large ingestion, symptoms are seen within minutes to hours and resolve within 48 h.

Diagnosis is made by history and an appropriate clinical presentation because drug levels are not clinically available. The most common manifestations of serotonin excess are fever, confusion, restlessness, mydriasis, hyperreflexia, shivering, and nausea. In severe cases, seizures, coma, myoclonus, muscle rigidity, and rhabdomyolysis are seen. Because of the presence of fever and muscular findings, serotonin syndrome can be confused with neuroleptic malignant syndrome (NMS); however, NMS victims have normal pupil sizes, have cogwheeling and lead pipe rigidity, and obviously have exposure to a neuroleptic agent. Treatment is largely supportive and includes withholding all drugs with serotonin-enhancing properties and external cooling. The 5-HT2A antagonist cyproheptadine has been reported to be effective, but there is little controlled experience with its use. Dialysis and hemoperfusion are not effective. Benzodiazepines are effective in treatment of the agitation, muscle rigidity, and seizures.

Calcium Channel and β-Blocking Drugs

In sufficient doses, β-blocking and calcium channel blocking drugs are highly lethal cardiovascular poisons. As competitive antagonists for β-adrenergic receptors, the toxicity of different β-blockers varies depending on receptor selectivity (β_1 receptors in the heart vs. β_2 receptors in airways and peripheral vessels). Although the mechanism is different (blocking calcium transit through cell membranes), calcium channel antagonists result in similar impairments of cardiac and vascular function. Bradycardia and hypotension (resulting from a combination of decreased myocardial contractility and peripheral vasodilation) are the major toxic manifestations of both classes. The importance of each mechanism varies somewhat by drug. For example, β-blockers with membrane stabilizing properties (e.g., propranolol, acebutolol, betaxolol, pindolol) are likely to cause conduction defects (QRS widening) and impaired contractility, whereas nonselective, β-blockers may cause bronchospasm. Likewise, manifestations of calcium channel blocker overdose vary by drug. For example, verapamil and diltiazem have comparable deleterious effects on sinus node and AV node activity, but diltiazem has less effect on contractility than verapamil. By contrast, nifedipine, amlodipine, and isradipine have less impact on conduction and contractility but much greater peripheral vasodilating effects. Although β-blockers have been associated with hypoglycemia, suppression of insulin secretion that occurs with the calcium channel blockers use often leads to hyperglycemia.

Both classes of drugs are rapidly absorbed, thus when harmful quantities of short-acting agents are ingested, manifestations are likely within 6 h. However, when a sustained-release preparation is taken, toxicity may not be evident for 12 h, and when adverse effects are seen, they last a long time. As a corollary, patients without cardiovascular manifestations 12 or more hours after reported ingestion are unlikely to develop serious toxicity.

Initial treatment can include gastric lavage if patients present soon after ingestion. If a sustained-release preparation has been ingested, whole bowel irrigation may be considered. Treatment of both classes of overdose should focus on cardiovascular support. Fluids will correct the hypotension resulting from reduced preload and are often effective for hypotension induced by the vasodilating calcium channel blockers. By contrast, fluid is not a useful treatment for bradycardia or impaired contractility. For symptomatic bradycardia, atropine, isoproterenol, or epinephrine can be tried as cardioaccelerants, but pacing may be required. Unfortunately, in this setting, it is often difficult to achieve pacing capture by either transcutaneous or intravenous routes. When both bradycardia and systemic vasodilation occur, use of a combined α and β agonist such as norepinephrine may be helpful. Repeated doses of calcium chloride (1 gm IV) have been recommended as treatment for calcium channel blocker overdose, but by itself rarely corrects the hemodynamic abnormalities. Glucagon (5 mg IV over 1 min) followed by an infusion of 1 to 10 mg/h has been advocated for both classes of overdose because it increases cAMP and in turn calcium influx. Unfortunately, like calcium, glucagon rarely completely corrects hypotension or bradycardia, often causes profound nausea and vomiting, and is expensive. By contrast, although not rigorously studied, euglycemic insulin administration (up to 0.5 U/kg/h) often results in rapid correction of bradycardia and improvement in hypotension resulting from both classes of drug overdose. The mechanism of action of insulin is unclear, and when used, care must be taken to avoid hypoglycemia and hypokalemia. Except for patients with severe preexisting asthma, bronchospasm following β-blocker overdose is rarely clinically significant, and when it occurs, it is easily treated with inhaled β-adrenergic agonists.

Lithium

Lithium, historically used to treat bipolar disorder, has gained popularity for therapy of a variety of psychiatric conditions. With its increasing popularity, has come an increased frequency of overdose. Lithium presents a unique problem because of its largely intracellular distribution and narrow therapeutic margin where even small incremental ingestions can produce toxicity among patients on chronic stable therapy. Lithium has a long half-life and is filtered by the kidney, so toxicity can also result from any condition that reduces the glomerular filtration rate. While mild intoxication causes fine tremor and perhaps confusion, severe toxicity is associated with major movement disorders such as clonus, fasiculations, choreoathetosis, opisthotonos, and seizures. Treatment with hemodialysis should be undertaken for patients with acute ingestions producing plasma levels above 4.0 mmol/L and for patients chronically using lithium when levels greater than 2.5 mmol/L. Prolonged or repeated dialysis is often needed to treat recurring rises in plasma levels resulting from redistributuion of drug from the intracellular compartment.

■ **SUGGESTED READINGS**

Alapat PM, Zimmerman JL. Toxicology in the critical care unit. *Chest.* 2008;133(4):1006–1013.

Chu J, Wang RY, Hill NS. Update in clinical toxicology. *Am J Resp Crit Care Med.* 2002;166:9–15.

Mokhlesi B, Leiken JB, Murray P, et al. Adult toxicology in critical care: Part I: General approach to the intoxicated patient. *Chest.* 2003;123(2):577–592.

Mokhlesi B, Leiken JB, Murray P, et al. Adult toxicology in critical care: Part II: Specific poisonings. *Chest.* 2003;123(3):897–922.

Zimmerman JL. Poisonings and overdoses in the intensive care unit: General and specific management issues. *Crit Care Med.* 2003; 31(12):2794–2801.

Neurological Emergencies

KEY POINTS

1 With the exception of head trauma, metabolic encephalopathy is the most common cause of delirium seen in the ICU. Drug effects, severe sepsis, and hepatic and renal failure are leading causes of metabolic encephalopathy.

2 Patients with altered mental status should have the airway assured and ventilation and perfusion restored so that the brain receives adequate quantities of glucose-replete oxygenated blood. Only after this initial stabilization should further evaluation be undertaken.

3 Seizure activity should be terminated as quickly as possible usually by administering an intravenous benzodiazepine followed by phenytoin while simultaneously assessing potential structural or metabolic precipitants of the seizure.

4 The best therapy for stroke remains prevention. An urgent uncontrasted CT guides treatment. Tissue plasminogen activator offers benefit in ischemic stroke if administered within 60 to 90 min. Correction of coagulation disorders is helpful for hemorrhagic stroke.

5 Cerebral perfusion pressures less than 40 mm Hg should be avoided. Raising mean arterial pressure and lowering intracranial pressure are both helpful measures. Hyperventilation works only transiently. Diuretics and osmotic agents provide more durable benefit.

6 In trauma victims with potential head or spine injury, airway patency, ventilation, oxygenation, and effective circulation are primary considerations. While achieving these goals, special attention should be afforded immobilization of the cervical spine.

7 After initial stabilization, a thorough neurologic examination and radiographs of the spine and head should be obtained to evaluate trauma patients for the possibility of a surgically correctable lesion.

8 After stabilization of the neurologically impaired patient, mundane medical problems including ileus, gastric stress ulceration, urinary tract infection, aspiration, atelectasis, deep venous thrombosis, and decubitus ulcers present the large challenges. Appropriate prophylactic measures should be instituted for each of these conditions as soon as possible.

9 Brain death is a state of irreversible absence of function at all levels of the brain (cortex, midbrain, and brainstem). Clinically, this is manifest as an absence of arousal, absence of midbrain reflexes (predominately cranial nerve signs), and absence of spontaneous ventilation, despite significant hypercarbia. The diagnosis generally cannot be made in the presence of ongoing hypothermia or drug intoxication.

Alterations of consciousness and cognition are both significant daily problems in the intensive care unit (ICU). It is not shocking that depressed consciousness, especially that sufficient to be called coma, has profound prognostic importance but many clinicians are surprised to learn that development of confusion or delirium also has powerful predictive value.

■ DELIRIUM

Delirium is a rapidly developing, often unrecognized, syndrome of confusion and inattention that affects more than 80% of all ICU patients. Two distinct subtypes of the condition are described. In the hyperactive form, patients are agitated and combative, in the hypoactive form, they are calm and withdrawn. Because the patients with agitated delirium are bigger management problems, not surprisingly it is recognized and reported more frequently. The elderly are more likely to manifest the hypoactive variety of the disorder. The most frequent conditions associated with delirium are shown in Figure 34-1.

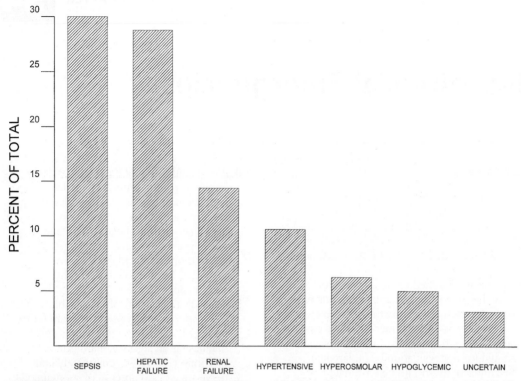

■ **FIGURE 34-1** Relative frequency of (nonsedative) causes of delirium in nontrauma ICU patients. Sepsis, hepatic failure, and renal failure rank as the most common causes.

The mechanism(s) of delirium is not known but strong associations have been recognized. Delirium is much more common in the elderly, in patients with baseline intellectual or cognitive impairment, and those with impaired hearing or vision. Alcoholism and drug abuse are also risk factors but there does not appear to be any particular acute medical or surgical illness that carries a disproportionate risk of causing the disease. However, there are contributing environmental factors. For example, sleep deprivation, invasive catheter and tube use, and application of physical restraints all appear to be associated with the condition. With regard to drugs, sedatives, analgesics, and medications that have anticholinergic properties are commonly linked with delirium.

Diagnosing delirium is not difficult and many ICUs have now incorporated one of the three most popular scoring schemes into routine care. Of available methods, the Confusion Assessment Method for ICU (CAM-ICU) is perhaps the simplest validated system. (http://www.icudelirium.org/delirium/CAM-ICUTraining.html) When combined with a standardized scoring system for consciousness, like the Richmond Agitation Sedation Scale (RASS) (see Chapter 17), both wakefulness and delirium can be accurately quantitated in seconds.

Development of delirium is an independent predictor of morbidity and mortality. The odds of reintubation are increased; the duration of mechanical ventilation and ICU and hospital length of stay are prolonged by delirium. The 6-month mortality rate is 20% higher among patients experiencing ICU delirium, and among survivors, residual cognitive impairment is common. Unfortunately, little is known about the treatment of delirium. Retrospective studies suggest the use of haloperidol may be associated with higher survival. In one of the few randomized trials conducted, olanzapine appears to have comparable safety and effect to haloperidol. Although benzodiazepines can prevent the development of delirium in the setting of alcohol or sedative withdrawal, as a practical matter they often exacerbate the condition once it is manifest. The effectiveness of preventative measures is unknown. Nevertheless, making sure that patients have their glasses, dentures, and hearing aids, and that they are frequently "reoriented" to time, place, location, and situation may serve as a deterrent. Likewise, providing a quiet environment with periods of sleep that coincide with normal solar cycles makes sense.

Removal of unnecessary tubes and monitoring devices and beginning a program of physical activity as soon as feasible may also serve to prevent or reverse delirium. Even if none of these measures are beneficial for delirium, they will not be harmful and may offer noncognitive therapeutic benefits.

■ COMA

Coma is a sleeplike state of unconsciousness from which patients cannot be awakened. Although some involuntary movements (spinal reflexes and "posturing") may occur, there is no speech or purposeful eye or limb movement. Less-profound stages of suppressed consciousness are often termed obtundation, stupor, and lethargy. Imprecise terms such as *semicoma* or *light coma* may confuse families and subsequent examiners and should be abandoned in favor of a simple unambiguous description of the highest level of function.

Pathophysiology

Consciousness has two components: arousal and awareness. Failure of arousal results from reticular activating system (RAS) or diffuse bilateral hemispheric dysfunction. Continuous stimulation by the RAS is required for the appearance of wakefulness. Conversely, awareness, a cognitive function, requires coordinated function of both cerebral cortices. Arousal may occur without awareness, but not the converse. From its origin in the midpons, the RAS radiates diffusely outward to the cerebral cortex. It is this protected origin and wide distribution that prevents coma, unless a diffuse process impairs both the cerebral cortices or the RAS is interrupted near its pontine root. Although this simple schema generally explains arousal and awareness, the dominant cortical hemisphere plays a disproportionate role in maintaining consciousness, and selective damage to both frontal lobes can also result in coma.

Coma may arise from a wide variety of diffuse or focal conditions affecting the central nervous system (CNS); however, all coma results from four basic pathophysiologic mechanisms: (a) metabolic or toxic encephalopathy, (b) generalized seizures, (c) compression of the midbrain or cerebral cortices by structural lesions or increased intracranial pressure (ICP), and (d) inadequate cerebral perfusion. The extent of neurological impairment of any potential cause of coma is modified by the patient's age and underlying neurological and vascular status. Metabolic insults that do not change cognition in a healthy young person can result in profound coma in an elderly patient with impaired circulation.

Etiology

Metabolic Disorders

Outside the neurosurgical setting (e.g., head trauma, subarachnoid hemorrhage (SAH), brain tumor), metabolic encephalopathy is the most common cause of coma. A comparison of the usual clinical features of structural and metabolic coma is presented in Table 34-1. Because metabolic encephalopathy affects the cortex and brainstem diffusely, abrupt focal deficits and progressive rostrocaudal losses seen with supratentorial mass lesions do not usually occur. Rather, patients exhibit slowly evolving symmetric deficits, often preceded by somnolence or confusion. A variety of common disorders, including drug overdose, hypoxia, hypotension,

1

TABLE 34-1 CLINICAL CHARACTERISTICS OF CAUSES OF COMA

CHARACTERISTIC	CAUSE OF COMA	
	TRAUMATIC OR VASCULAR	TOXIC OR METABOLIC
History	Injury Uncontrolled hypertension Seizure	Toxin, drug exposure history History of liver or kidney failure, COPD or diabetes Recent hypoxic event
Onset	Abrupt	Gradual
Rate of progression	Rapid (minutes) deterioration	Slower (hours) progression common
Pattern of progression	May be stuttering or gradual Rostrocaudal loss of function	Global impairment from the start No rostrocaudal pattern
Focality	Focal lesions common	Focal lesions rare

TABLE 34-2 COMMON REVERSIBLE CAUSES OF ALTERED MENTAL STATUS

MEDICAL CONDITIONS		SURGERY AND TRAUMA
Hypoperfusion	Drug overdose	Hypoperfusion
Hypoxemia	Carbon monoxide	Hypoxemia
Hypercapnia	Hypercalcemia	Cholesterol embolism
Hypoglycemia	Wernicke encephalopathy	Fat embolism
Status epilepticus	Temperature disorders	Air embolism
Myxedema	CNS hemorrhage	Traumatic subdural hematoma
Hypertension	CNS infections (e.g., brain abscess, meningitis, encephalitis)	Diffuse neuronal shear injury

hypoglycemia, dehydration, sepsis, hepatic encephalopathy, and uremia can all contribute to impaired consciousness. The common reversible causes of coma are summarized in Table 34-2.

It is difficult to provide absolute guidelines as to the magnitude of a single abnormality necessary to cause coma, because multiple derangements often coexist, and the age of the patient, presence of underlying diseases, and the rapidity of development also determine impact. Yet, as a general rule, it is uncommon for glucose greater than 50 or less than 500 mg/dL, Na^+ greater than 120 or less than 155 mEq/L, Ca^{2+} less than 12 mg/dL, or Mg^{2+} greater than 0.8 or less than 10 mg/dL to produce coma. Only very rarely do disorders of other electrolytes alter consciousness. The precise cause of unconsciousness in patients with renal failure is unknown; however, uremia alone rarely causes coma until the blood urea nitrogen (BUN) exceeds 100 mg/dL. (Renal insufficiency probably alters consciousness through multiple mechanisms, including metabolic acidosis, electrolyte abnormalities, metabolic toxin or drug accumulation, and increased permeability of the blood–brain barrier.) Similarly, the exact cause of coma in patients with liver failure is unknown, but accumulation of endogenous (e.g., glutamine) and exogenous toxins (e.g., drug metabolites) and cerebral edema all play some role in the process (see Chapter 31). Cerebral edema is a much bigger problem in the setting of acute hepatic failure. There is such a poor correlation between serum ammonia levels and mental status that no rule can be offered as to the level of ammonia associated with coma.

More firm guidelines can be offered with respect to the impact of hypoxemia and hypercapnia on consciousness. Tolerance of hypoxemia depends not only on the extent of desaturation but also on compensatory mechanisms available. The major mechanisms of acute compensation are increased cardiac output, O_2 extraction, and anaerobic metabolism, and improved unloading of O_2 resulting from

tissue acidosis. Most individuals without cardiac disease or anemia remain asymptomatic until PaO_2 falls below 50 mm Hg. At that level, malaise, lightheadedness, nausea, vertigo, impaired judgment, and incoordination are noted. Confusion develops as PaO_2 falls into the 35 to 50 mm Hg range. As PaO_2 declines below 35 mm Hg, urine output slows, bradycardia and conduction system blockade develop, lactic acidosis appears, and the patient becomes lethargic or obtunded. At levels near 25 mm Hg, the normal unadapted individual loses consciousness, and minute ventilation falls because of respiratory center depression. As for all other metabolic toxins, the effects of carbon dioxide (CO_2) depend not only on the absolute level of CO_2 but also on its rate of accumulation. A $PaCO_2$ less than 60 mm Hg is often asymptomatic, but as levels rise above this threshold, headache and lethargy are commonly observed. Asterixis and myoclonus occur as levels mount even higher, but surprisingly massive elevations in CO_2 (often double or triple normal values) are usually necessary to render a patient unconscious.

Generally, a cerebral perfusion pressure (CPP) (mean arterial pressure [MAP]—intracranial pressure [ICP]) must exceed 50 mm Hg to perfuse the brain adequately; however, otherwise young healthy patients may maintain consciousness despite severe reductions in MAP. By contrast, patients with chronic hypertension, cerebrovascular disease, or elevated ICP may be underperfused at much higher pressures.

Severe sepsis frequently alters consciousness; however, mental status changes usually fall short of true coma. The mechanisms are multifactorial. Obviously, direct infection of the CNS can render a patient unconscious. In addition, severe sepsis is usually associated with some degree of hypoxemia and almost 75% of septic patients will develop hypotension—both factors which contribute to mental status changes. Possibly most interesting, is the finding that inflammatory cytokines (e.g., interleukin-1) may directly impair consciousness. Sepsis-induced coma is particularly common in the febrile elderly patient, where altered mental status presents a difficult management decision. Frequently deliberated diagnoses are severe sepsis alone, or sepsis complicated by dehydration, electrolyte abnormalities, meningitis, and intracranial structural lesions such as a brain abscess or hemorrhage. Timely antibiotic therapy is desirable in all infectious situations, but confirming the diagnosis and nailing down a specific organism so as to best choose antimicrobial therapy usually requires a lumbar puncture (LP). Unfortunately, LP incurs some risk in the presence of coagulopathy, anticoagulation, or intracranial mass lesion. Therefore, deciding the order in which to perform a head computed tomography (CT) scan, do an LP, and administer antibiotic therapy is often debated. In febrile nonimmunocompromised patients without evidence of a focal neurologic defect, papilledema, or history of trauma, an LP is almost certainly safe and can be performed before or without a head CT scan. (Not that long ago, the decision to perform an LP was always made only based upon history and examination.) If head trauma, papilledema, new onset seizures, or focal neurologic deficit complicates the evaluation of a potentially infected patient, probably the best course is to obtain blood cultures, administer empiric antibiotics, and proceed to the CT scanner before LP. In any case, if logistical limitations preclude prompt CT scanning and intracranial infection is a real possibility, it is best to begin antibiotic treatment, even if doing so precludes a definitive microbiological diagnosis. Although it is rational to administer antibiotics as quickly as practical in patients with suspected meningitis, there is little if any data to support the often-quoted need to dose antibiotics within 1 h of suspecting the diagnosis.

Medication ingestion or toxin exposure is the most frequent cause of nontraumatic coma. Opiates, benzodiazepines, ethanol, and antidepressants are the most common drug classes implicated. Chemical-induced mental status changes are typically multifactorial; commonly several consciousness-depressing drugs are simultaneously ingested, and the drugs or toxins often lead to changes in oxygenation or perfusion that can cause coma in and of themselves. For example, narcotic overdose is often combined with benzodiazepine and alcohol ingestion. Although direct effects of these drugs alone can cause coma, they can also impair consciousness by producing hypoventilation or hypotension (see Chapter 33).

Seizures

Generalized seizures may induce unconsciousness during the ictal phase or as a postictal phenomenon. Distinguishing a seizure from other causes of coma is easy if convulsive activity is observed or consciousness returns rapidly after a suspected seizure in an otherwise healthy patient. However, in the ICU many seizures do not cause visible convulsions. In addition, patients with previous stroke, metabolic encephalopathy, or prolonged seizures (status epilepticus) may suffer a long postictal period. In turn, status epilepticus often has an underlying structural or metabolic cause. Thus, delayed return of consciousness following a seizure should prompt consideration of a structural lesion (e.g., tumor, stroke, SAH, subdural hematoma) or underlying metabolic disorder (e.g., hypoglycemia, toxin ingestion, or electrolyte disturbance). As with metabolic encephalopathy, seizures that cause loss of consciousness generally tend to produce symmetric neurological defects unless there is an underlying structural abnormality. In contrast to metabolic encephalopathy, the loss of consciousness associated with seizures is usually instantaneous rather than gradual.

Structural Lesions

Although supratentorial mass lesions are generally confined to one hemisphere, they cause coma by increasing ICP or by impairing RAS function through pressure on the brainstem. Unless located exactly in the midline, *supratentorial* mass lesions usually produce hemispheric (unilateral) findings that precede loss of consciousness. Because cerebral function is progressively lost in a rostrocaudal manner, there is a relatively predictable progression. If unchecked, the process culminates in central or uncal herniation. In central herniation, the midbrain is pressed straight down into the foramen magnum. Clinical manifestations include miosis, decerebrate posturing, and a lateral gaze palsy as the sixth cranial (abducens) nerve is stretched. Uncal herniation occurs as asymmetric pressure forces the medial portion of the temporal lobe to cross the tentorium, compressing the midbrain. Clinical manifestations include a fixed dilated pupil, third cranial (oculomotor) nerve palsy, and hemiparesis. By contrast, when *infratentorial* lesions (e.g., brainstem strokes, cerebellar hemorrhage) cause coma, very rapid loss of consciousness without rostrocaudal progression is typical.

Approach to the Comatose Patient

History

Because pathophysiology and treatment differ radically, metabolic and structural causes of coma must be distinguished as quickly as possible. The history is helpful in making this separation if it reveals trauma or drug ingestion. Sudden onset of coma suggests a seizure or a vascular event (e.g., SAH, brainstem stroke). The onset of coma after minutes to hours of a focal deficit suggests supratentorial intracerebral hemorrhage with progressively increasing ICP. A slowly evolving focal deficit occurring over days to weeks before loss of consciousness suggests abscess, tumor, or subdural hematoma, whereas progression to coma over minutes to hours without a focal deficit favors a metabolic cause. The setting in which coma develops may suggest trauma or hyperthermia or hypothermia from environmental or toxic exposure (e.g., organophosphates, carbon monoxide). Medications found near the comatose patient are particularly helpful. For example, not only may the offending compound(s) be discovered, but medication containers bearing the name of the prescribing physician may allow further history to be obtained. At the very least, knowledge of a patient's medications provides a forensic picture of underlying diseases. In patients with alcoholism, intoxication with ethanol, ethylene glycol, methanol, or isopropyl alcohol should be suspected. In patients with diabetes, hypoglycemia and diabetic ketoacidosis (DKA) are common causes of coma. Underlying medical problems such as hypothyroidism, renal failure, cirrhosis, or psychiatric illness also increase the likelihood of a metabolic etiology, whereas a history of falling, previous stroke, brain tumor, extracranial neoplasm, or atrial fibrillation favors structural or vascular problems. Patients known to have malignant tumors are subject to both structural lesions (e.g., metastases and hemorrhage) and metabolic causes (e.g., hyponatremia, hypercalcemia). Similarly, uncontrolled hypertension can induce metabolic (e.g., hypertensive encephalopathy) or structural (e.g., intracerebral hemorrhage) coma. Immunocompromised patients, especially those with human immunodeficiency virus (HIV) infection are at higher risk for structural causes of coma including, CNS infections and lymphoid malignancies.

Physical Examination

Physical examination is most helpful in differentiating structural from metabolic causes of coma when it reveals evidence of focal or lateralizing signs. In such patients, a metabolic etiology is uncommon. (Exceptions to this rule occur in patients with hepatic failure, hypoglycemia, prior stroke, and postictal patients.) Comatose patients should always be fully disrobed and examined for evidence of occult trauma. Although physical evidence of head trauma suggests a structural cause, up to 50% of trauma patients also suffer from intoxication, oftentimes sufficient to produce coma. Boggy areas of the skull suggest depressed skull fracture, while the Battle sign (postauricular hematoma), "raccoon eyes," and bloody nasal or aural discharge suggest basilar skull fracture. In traumatized patients, it is critical to exclude cervical spine instability before the neck is manipulated because serious spinal injuries commonly accompany cranial lesions severe enough to cause coma. Echymoses, mucosal bleeding, or petechiae may implicate coagulopathy as the cause of intracranial bleeding. Incontinence of stool or urine or tongue laceration strongly suggests recent seizure. Atrial fibrillation, a large heart, and history of recent myocardial infarction are all associated with cerebral embolic disease. (In general, embolic disease is an uncommon cause of coma because of the limited area of cerebral infarction caused by emboli.) Cardiac murmurs should raise suspicion of endocarditis-induced septic embolism or brain abscess. Arrhythmias only result in coma when they cause hypotension or cerebral emboli. In this setting, isolated carotid bruits are of little significance because occlusive carotid disease is a rare cause of coma. Nuchal rigidity suggests meningitis, encephalitis, or SAH.

Vital signs provide additional clues to diagnosis. Although hypertension may accompany any cause of increased ICP, severe hypertension suggests intracerebral or SAH, particularly if accompanied by nuchal rigidity or focal neurological signs, respectively. Hypertensive encephalopathy alone is less likely to produce coma and is usually characterized by a nonfocal examination and blood pressures greater than 240/130 mm Hg. Stimulant intoxication with amphetamines, cocaine, phencyclidine, or phenylpropanolamine, should also be considered in patients with altered mental status and hypertension. Cocaine-induced hypertension alone may cause delirium but if coma is present, intracranial hemorrhage is likely. Although young patients without underlying vascular or cerebral disease may remain awake with very low (40 to 50 mm Hg) MAPs, the elderly, patients with chronic hypertension, and those with concurrent metabolic encephalopathy or structural lesions tolerate hypotension less well.

Heatstroke, serotonin syndrome, neuroleptic malignant syndrome, malignant hyperthermia, stimulant intoxication, and any number of infections may cause fever sufficient to impair consciousness. Patients with hyperthermia or hypothermia frequently have an infection accompanying the primary temperature disorder that may itself disturb consciousness (e.g., pneumonia, brain abscess, or meningitis). Although primary aberrations of body temperature can directly cause coma, they rarely do so until core temperatures exceed 105°F or fall below 80°F (see Chapter 28). Bradypnea and hypoventilation most often result from the sedative effects of drugs or alcohol, accumulated hepatic or renal toxins, hypothyroidism, or far advanced brainstem compression. Tachypnea is a nonspecific finding but usually arises from one of four basic causes: (a) inappropriate ventilatory control, (b) hypoxemia, (c) compensation for metabolic acidosis, or (d) reduced lung or chest wall compliance. Contrary to popular teaching, specific "pathognomonic" respiratory patterns have little localizing or prognostic value, with one notable exception—uncoordinated, irregular (ataxic) respiration usually indicates severe medullary impairment and impending respiratory collapse.

Expanded Neurological Examination

After the vital signs are obtained, ventilation and perfusion are stabilized, and initial history and physical examination are performed, neurological function should be examined in a stepwise fashion. The five key features of the initial neurological examination may be remembered by the mnemonic "SPERM": (a) State of consciousness, (b) Pupillary response, (c) Eye movements, (d) Respiratory rate and pattern, and (e) Motor function.

One of four terms should be used to describe the state of consciousness: (a) alert, (b) lethargic (aroused with simple commands), (c) stuporous (aroused only with vigorous stimulation—usually pain), and (d) comatose (unarousable).

Pupil size, congruency, and response to light and accommodation should be described. Pupillary function is controlled by the midbrain. Therefore, if the pupils function normally, the cause of coma either is a structural lesion located above the midbrain or is metabolic. Small "pinpoint" pupils usually result from pontine hemorrhage or from ingestion of narcotics or organophosphates. (Meperidine frequently fails to produce the miotic pupils typical of other narcotics.) Pupillary responses almost always remain intact in metabolic causes of coma. (Exceptions to this rule include atropine and atropine-like substances and the now rare glutethimide intoxication in which "fixed and dilated" pupils may occur.) With uncal herniation from increased supratentorial pressure, the third cranial nerve is compressed on the tentorial edge resulting in unilateral pupillary dilation and fixation. If increased pressure goes unrelieved, complete diencephalic herniation can occur resulting in fixed midposition (3 to 5 mm) pupils.

Normal movement of the eyes requires an intact ponto-medullary-midbrain connection. The resting position of the gaze, the presence of nystagmus (horizontal, vertical, or rotatory), and the response to head movements (oculocephalic testing) or to cold tympanic membrane stimulation (oculovestibular testing) should be recorded. A normal response to oculocephalic testing is conjugate eye movement away from the direction of head rotation. A normal response to cold oculovestibular testing is conjugate eye movement toward the side of stimulation. Cervical spine stability must be ensured before oculocephalic maneuvers are performed. Likewise, tympanic membrane integrity should be confirmed before oculovestibular testing to prevent introduction of water into the cerebrospinal fluid (CSF) through a basilar skull fracture. Although endogenous toxins accumulated from hepatic or renal failure usually do not impair coordinated eye movements, exogenous toxins (drugs) frequently impair eye movements. In addition, depletion of thiamine (Wernicke syndrome) can result in horizontal and vertical nystagmus. In pontine disorders, the medial longitudinal fasciculus is often dysfunctional but the sixth cranial nerve function is preserved. Therefore, ipsilateral eye abduction is intact, but contralateral adduction is impaired. Quite simply, if rotation of the head (oculocephalic) and vestibular stimulation (calorics) produce no change in eye position, the pons is nonfunctional. If only the eye ipsilateral to caloric stimulus abducts, a lesion of the medial longitudinal fasciculus (encapsulated by the pons) should be suspected.

Description of the respiratory pattern is less helpful than has been previously suggested; however, ataxic breathing is a marker of severe brainstem dysfunction. Despite the nonspecificity of most breathing patterns, the respiratory rate can provide valuable clues to the etiology of coma (see "Physical Examination" above).

The highest observed level of motor function should be noted (e.g., "Spontaneously moves all extremities," "Withdraws only right arm and leg from noxious stimulus," "No response to pain"). Motor function in pontine compression is often limited to extensor (decerebrate) posturing, whereas lesions above the pons can produce flexor (decorticate) posturing. If a structural lesion compresses the centers for respiration and heart rate control on the dorsal medullary surface, the patient also will be flaccid, without eye movements, and will have midposition, unreactive pupils. Although "posturing" is an ominous finding in most settings, rarely it is the result of metabolic encephalopathy, (especially acute hepatic failure) and in such cases, is completely reversible.

The results of the neurological examination are often reported using a standardized scale. Currently, the Glasgow Coma Score (GCS) is the most commonly used composite score. In this system, best motor, verbal, and eye opening responses are tallied in a score ranging from 3 to 15 (Table 34-3).

Localizing the Level of Dysfunction

If history or examination reveals a sequential, rostrocaudal loss of function, either a supratentorial mass lesion or diffusely increased ICP is the most likely etiology of coma. Fundascopic examination that demonstrates papilledema is virtually diagnostic of increased ICP or hypertensive encephalopathy.

Although the thalamus–diencephalon cannot be directly examined, injury to this area usually depresses consciousness but spares motor function. (Because pupillary and ocular movements are controlled by the midbrain and pons, respectively, they typically remain unaffected.) The respiratory pattern in thalamic dysfunction is unpredictable. Injury extending lower to the midbrain level usually results in loss of motor function and decorticate, or flexor, posturing. Although pupillary diameter is generally midposition (approx. 3 mm), midbrain injury tends to spare pupil reactivity and eye movements. When damage extends further to the pontine level, pupillary function is routinely impaired. Motor responses are often limited to extensor (decerebrate) posturing. If compression progresses to the medullary level, all motor function is usually lost, as are pupillary response and eye movements. It is only with medullary compression that respiratory rhythm is predictably affected, becoming ataxic.

Laboratory Evaluation

Body fluids should be collected to evaluate potential metabolic and toxic causes of coma. Situationally appropriate testing is indicated, even in patients

TABLE 34-3	THE GLASGOW COMA SCALE		
Eyes	Open	Spontaneously	4
		To verbal command	3
		To pain	2
		No response	1
Best motor response	To verbal command	Obeys	6
	To painful stimulus	Localizes pain	5
		Flexion—withdrawal	4
		Flexion—decorticate	3
		Extension—decerebrate	2
		No response	1
Best verbal response		Oriented, converses	5
		Disoriented, converses	4
		Inappropriate words	3
		Incomprehensible sounds	2
		No response	1
Total			3–15

with obvious head trauma, because of the possibility that a metabolic cause may coexist or may have precipitated the trauma (e.g., alcohol, carbon monoxide). Laboratory determinations should include indices of renal and hepatic function, serum glucose and electrolyte determinations, hemoglobin and arterial blood gases, and when appropriate, carboxyhemoglobin determinations. If the history, physical examination, or initial laboratory testing suggests drug overdose or poisoning, a toxicology profile, and if indicated specific levels of compounds not included in a typical toxicology screen (e.g., aspirin, acetaminophen, ethylene glycol, methanol), should be obtained (see Chapter 33).

Treatment

The major diagnostic differential is to separate structural from metabolic causes of coma, but initially in all cases similar supportive treatment should be undertaken. The airway should be secured, perfusion stabilized, and oxygen administered. The cervical spine should be immobilized if **2** there is any suspicion of trauma. An IV line should be established to obtain appropriate laboratory specimens and administer fluids and medications. Because of its time-sensitive importance, glucose levels should be tested at the bedside. If testing is not immediately available or if the measured glucose value is low, 50% dextrose in water (D50W) and thiamine (approx. 1 mg/kg) should be given accompanied by thiamine.

Naloxone, a narcotic antagonist, and flumazenil, a benzodiazepine antagonist, can temporarily reverse narcotic and benzodiazepine-induced coma, respectively, and thus serve as useful *diagnostic* tools. The duration of action of both antagonists is less than that of their agonist counterparts; thus neither compound is a reliable substitute for intubation and mechanical ventilation in patients with sedative-induced respiratory failure. Recurrent coma often follows a single dose of either reversing agent in patients who are not closely monitored.

After initial stabilization and primary evaluation, a more detailed neurological examination and specific diagnostic testing can be undertaken. In most cases, a head CT scan will be performed. In patients admitted to the hospital with coma, the CT scan is much more likely to reveal a structural cause of coma than for patients who have been in the ICU for a period of time. (The important exception to this rule is the ICU patient who has a new focal deficit or first seizure.) Magnetic resonance imaging (MRI) scanning usually adds little to CT results in patients with coma, although occasionally subtle cerebral edema, venous sinus thrombosis, and acute ischemic strokes can be seen on MRI of patients with nondiagnostic CT scans. In most febrile comatose patients, blood cultures, LP, and institution of antibiotics are indicated. However, if lateralizing neurological signs are present or if there is a history of seizure, trauma, or immunocompromise, CT of the head should usually precede LP but not antibiotic administration. For patients with a clear metabolic cause of coma (e.g., hepatic or renal failure), organ specific treatment should be undertaken.

Prognosis

Surprisingly, the history and clinical examination over time are better predictors of outcome than sophisticated ancillary tests. Approximately 90% of comatose patients who will completely recover show significant neurological improvement within 3 days. As a general rule, the faster the motor activity returns the better the prospects for full recovery. (Most patients with successful recoveries have purposeful motor activity within 24 h.) With regard to etiology, drug-induced coma has an excellent prognosis. By contrast, the prognosis of coma persisting greater than 72 h is terrible if the etiology is ischemia or trauma. More than half of such patients with ischemic injury are dead and an additional 40% are in a persistent vegetative state or have severe impairment at one year. (Less than 5% have good recovery.) Outcomes from traumatic coma are better but still poor; about 30% of patients are dead and another 45% are in a persistent vegetative state or have severe cognitive deficits at one year. Fewer than 10% have good functional recovery.

■ SEIZURES

Pathophysiology

Seizures result from paroxysmal neuronal discharges that cause generalized or focal neurological signs. Most generalized seizures begin as a focal cortical discharge. Knowledge of the cell biology of seizures has advanced considerably. For example, we now know seizures are associated with excessive activity of N-methyl D-aspartate (NMDA) receptors and inadequate stimulation of gamma amino butyric acid (GABA) receptors. Understanding the role these receptors helps explain the effectiveness of GABA stimulants as anticonvulsants.

Although seizures have been classified in many ways, it is probably most useful to think of them in terms of their duration (brief vs. continuous) and scope (generalized vs. focal). Duration is important because prolonged seizures become more refractory to treatment, irreversibly injure neuronal tissue, and cause systemic metabolic problems (e.g., acidosis, hypoxia, hyperthermia, and rhabdomyolysis). Although there is no standard definition of the commonly used term "status epilepticus," it is generally agreed that a seizure lasting greater than 10 min or a series of recurring seizures without an intervening period of consciousness qualifies. Similarly, although not standardized, the term "refractory status epilepticus" has been applied to the highly lethal situation in which seizures last greater than 2 h or cannot be controlled with two or more anticonvulsants. Focality is also noteworthy because it suggests a discrete structural abnormality. Although seizures usually present as localized or generalized phasic muscle spasms, in the ICU, seizures occasionally masquerade as unexplained coma or puzzling sensory or psychiatric disturbances.

Etiology

One of five basic mechanisms is responsible for convulsions. Seizures arise from intrinsic electrical instability (epilepsy), toxic or metabolic disturbances (e.g., electrolyte imbalances, alcohol, drug effect), or structural lesions (e.g., trauma or tumor), infectious causes (e.g., meningitis, cerebritis, brain abscess), or abnormalities of brain perfusion (global hypoxia). In general, these etiologic factors segregate into two prognostic groups. Patients with idiopathic epilepsy, subtherapeutic drug levels, and alcohol-related seizures tend to have an excellent prognosis, whereas victims of stroke, trauma, tumor, encephalitis, or direct CNS poisons tend to have a poor prognosis.

For the most part, seizures occur at the extremes of age and the most frequent causes of seizures also vary by age. For example, children most commonly have seizures as the result of fever, infection, or a change in anticonvulsant medications used to treat idiopathic epilepsy. By contrast, young adults are much more likely to seize from SAH, trauma, noncompliance with anticonvulsants, or drug use or withdrawal (e.g., tricyclic antidepressants, cocaine, alcohol). In the older adult, stroke, subdural hematoma, and tumor become more common. Hypoglycemia and CNS infections (e.g., meningitis, encephalitis) effect patients of all ages.

High fever (especially in children), drug withdrawal (particularly anticonvulsants, ethanol, barbiturates, benzodiazepines, baclofen), and iatrogenic overdoses of isoniazid, penicillin, imipenem, tricyclic antidepressants, theophylline, or lidocaine are common metabolic causes. Electrolyte disturbances may also induce seizures, especially when such changes occur abruptly (e.g., acute hyponatremia, disequilibrium following dialysis).

Although most seizure disorders that occur in outpatients are idiopathic, this is true less often in the ICU, where such treatable conditions as drug or alcohol withdrawal, metabolic imbalances, drug toxicity, and acute structural lesions are more common. Most important among the metabolic precipitants are uremia, hypoglycemia, hypocalcemia, hypomagnesemia, and hyponatremia. CNS infections (meningitis, encephalitis, and brain abscess) are frequent causes of ictus; about one third of adults with bacterial meningitis will experience a seizure. HIV infection represents a particular hazard for CNS infections, including toxoplasmosis and viral encephalitis.

Diagnosis

A seizure diagnosis is usually made from the history and observation of an attack. Occasionally, historical features and/or the clinical appearance are so atypical as to require confirmation by electroencephalography (EEG). In such cases, an intra-ictal EEG may be diagnostic and the pattern of discharge may help determine etiology. For example, EEG localization of seizure discharge to the base of the temporal lobes (or appropriate MRI findings) suggests herpes encephalitis. EEG recording may also reveal unsuspected seizure activity in a patient with unexplained coma. In fact, up to 20% of unresponsive ICU patients may have occult seizures and an even higher percentage (50%) of patients who remain unresponsive after having a convulsion have been found to have ongoing nonconvulsive seizures. A head CT or MRI scan is indicated for new onset seizures, those accompanied by a preceding or persistent focal neurological deficit, and in those refractory to simple medical therapy. In such patients, a CT often reveals a structural cause (e.g., vascular malformation, primary or metastatic tumor, or subdural subarachnoid or parenchymal hemorrhage). In patients with a known seizure disorder, a CT scan is not necessary to evaluate each recurrence; however, it should be remembered that even patients with epilepsy develop strokes, tumors, and CNS infections. Hence, recurrent seizures should not be reflexly ascribed to a singular cause in perpetuity.

Systemic Effects of Seizures

Brief ictal episodes are of little consequence provided they do not occur while the patient is involved in a dangerous activity, and the airway, oxygenation, and ventilation are preserved. However, continuous electrical firing during prolonged seizures depletes cellular reserves of oxygen and adenosine triphosphate (ATP) and allows intracellular accumulation of calcium, all processes that culminate in neuronal death. By damaging the cortex, recurrent or prolonged seizures are associated with long-term cognitive impairment. In humans, seizures ≥2 h in duration reliably result in permanent brain injury, but lasting injury may begin as early as 30 min after seizure onset. Seizure-induced neuronal damage does not require loss of consciousness nor convulsive muscular contraction.

Massive catecholamine release during convulsions may induce arterial and intracranial hypertension and cause pulmonary edema. Adrenergic stimulation initially produces hyperglycemia, but during prolonged seizures glucose consumption can cause hypoglycemia. Fever from central thermostatic reset and/or sustained muscular activity may rise to concerning levels (>105°F) and tends to respond poorly to antipyretics. Furthermore, thermoregulation may be disturbed for days after seizure cessation. Because fever and leukemoid reactions (peripheral leukocyte counts often exceed 20,000 cells/mm^3) are common, infection is often suspected. Differentiating infectious fever from convulsive fever is further confounded by the common occurrence of cerebral fluid pleocytosis with total leukocyte counts up to 80 cells/mm^3 and a predominance of neutrophils.

Profound and rapid onset acidosis often accompanies seizure activity. Half of postictal acidemic patients exhibit a lactic acidosis alone, whereas the other half have a mixed respiratory and metabolic acidosis. Although the seizure-associated acidosis may be severe (pH < 6.5), no evidence links pH with outcome, and most patients resolve the acidosis within 1 h. The same vigorous muscular contractions causing acidosis can result in rhabdomyolysis with hyperkalemia. Increased free water losses from sweating and hyperventilation may

increase serum osmolarity and Na$^+$ concentration. Hypotension and (rarely) seizure-induced cardiovascular collapse can further aggravate neurological damage, but unlike the setting of ischemic brain injury, cerebral blood flow is typically increased in seizing patients. The combination of direct neuronal damage and metabolic pandemonium of status epilepticus results in mortality rates of 30% to 35%.

Treatment

The most important factors determining the outcome of status epilepticus are the etiology of the episode and the time to terminate the seizure. The longer that time, the more difficult it is to control the seizure and the worse the ultimate outcome. Protection of the airway, oxygenation, and maintenance of perfusion are primary considerations. Aspiration risk can be reduced by proper patient positioning (lateral decubitus) and endotracheal intubation when clinical judgment dictates. If pharmacologic paralysis is necessary for intubation, EEG monitoring assumes greater importance since muscular activity will be halted, but neuronal discharges can continue unrecognized. As with all causes of altered consciousness, electrolytes and glucose should be tested and normalized. Thiamine (100 mg) should be administered in most cases to prevent Wernicke encephalopathy.

In patients who experience a solitary seizure or several brief seizures with known precipitant, long-term anticonvulsants are not always necessary; however, there is universal agreement that status epilepticus should be pharmacologically ended as rapidly as possible. Drugs that bind GABA receptors are the most effective seizure quashing drugs. One strategy for acute anticonvulsant administration is suggested in Table 34-4. There is no single ideal drug regimen for terminating seizures; however, benzodiazepines, specifically lorazepam, represent excellent initial choices because of their effectiveness, rapid action, and wide therapeutic margin. Benzodiazepines cannot be expected to provide *long-term* seizure control by themselves, but can "break" seizures long enough to accomplish intubation if necessary and to initiate therapy with phenytoin or another longer acting drug.

Initial intravenous doses of lorazepam (0.1 mg/kg) are very effective (>80%) in terminating seizure activity within minutes. Lorazepam's 2- to 3-h half-life and avid GABA receptor binding provide seizure protection for up to 24 h. In a randomized

3

TABLE 34-4 THERAPY OF STATUS EPILEPTICUS

Step 1 Stabilize vital signs

Establish an airway, administer oxygen
Ensure circulation with adequate blood pressure
Establish intravenous access
Collect blood for electrolytes, glucose, hemoglobin, creatinine, liver function tests, acid–base status, and possibly toxicologic analysis
Administer D50W (1 mg/kg) and thiamine (1 mg/kg) unless patient known to be normoglycemic or hyperglycemic

Step 2 Rapidly achieve seizure control

Lorazepam (0.1 mg/kg) IV
or
Diazepam (0.15) mg/kg mg IV
(initial doses of either may be repeated if necessary)
Less-desirable alternative: Midazolam (0.2 mg/kg) bolus then 0.2–1.0 mg/kg/min infusion

Step 3 Achieve/maintain seizure control

Phenytoin 20 mg/kg unfused at <50 mg/min
or
Fosphenytoin 20 mg/kg phenytoin equivalents infused at 100–150 mg/min

Step 4 Salvage therapy for resistant status epilepticus

Propofol (2–10 mg/kg/h)
or
Phenobarbital 20 mg/kg given by slow (30–50 mg/min) infusion

Step 5 Advanced treatment for refractory disease

Pentobarbital 10 mg/kg load at 0.2–2.0 mg/kg/h, followed by 1–4 mg/kg/h
or
Thiopental 3–7 mg/kg load, followed by 50–100 mg/min IV
or
Midazolam infusion (0.2 mg/kg bolus followed by 0.05 to 0.5 mg/kg/h)
or
General anesthesia (e.g., isoflurane)

Step 6 Diagnostic evaluation

Consider CT, MRI, LP, toxicologic evaluation

trial comparing lorazepam to phenytoin, diazepam plus phenytoin, or phenobarbital, lorazepam alone was the most effective initial therapy. A minor disadvantage is the need to refrigerate lorazepam. Diazepam (0.15 mg/kg) is an acceptable alternative that does not require refrigeration. Diazepam is also available as a rectal gel that can be used when IV dosing is not possible. The major disadvantages

of diazepam are its shorter duration of action and potent scleroscent effect on peripheral veins. Midazolam (0.2 mg/kg bolus) can also be used in place of lorazepam, but because it has the shortest duration of action of all the benzodiazepines, a continuous infusion (0.2 to 1 μg/kg/min) is usually required. Hypotension and hypopnea are complications of all benzodiazepines but occur rarely (<5%) unless other anticonvulsants (especially, phenobarbital) have been administered.

After benzodiazepine administration, phenytoin is the preferred second-line drug for long-term control. Although phenytoin has acquired a bad reputation for its tendency to cause infusion site pain and adverse cardiovascular effects (e.g., arrhythmias, hypotension, conduction disturbances) when administered rapidly, it is a safe and effective drug when given more slowly. Because of its long half-life, seizure recurrence is rare. Initial loading doses (20 mg/kg) should be given at a maximum infusion rate of 50 mg/min. (Additional carefully titrated doses, up to 30 mg/kg, may be necessary in refractory cases.) Thus, an adult loading dose usually requires 30 to 45 min to administer. Phenytoin must be administered only in saline; it is not compatible with glucose-containing solutions. Although the adult daily maintenance dose averages 300 mg IV or orally, therapy should be guided by serum drug levels and clinical response. Phenytoin toxicity may produce diplopia, horizontal and vertical nystagmus, slurred speech, ataxia, clumsiness, and somnolence.

In an attempt to reduce infusion site reactions and cardiovascular effects, the water-soluble compound fosphenytoin was developed. Water solubility also permits intramuscular injection when IV access is problematic. Although it can be infused much more rapidly (100 to 150 mg/min) than phenytoin, fosphenytoin is a prodrug that must be hydrolyzed to the active compound (phenytoin) after administration. The infusion and conversion process requires just about as much time as does the safe infusion of phenytoin and in comparative trials, the incidence of adverse effects is comparable. Because of differing molecular weights of phenytoin and fosphenytoin, doses differ, with the latter typically ordered as "phenytoin equivalents." Failure to account for this difference can result in significant underdosing. Because of the substantially higher costs and lack of proven benefit with regard to speed or safety, routine use of fosphenytoin is not recommended.

Phenobarbital and propofol represent third-line treatments for status epilepticus. Phenobarbital, (20 mg/kg) infused at rates less than 100 mg/min, is moderately effective (approx. 60%) in terminating seizures. Potent cardiorespiratory depressant effects and interaction with other drugs often make its use problematic. Because it is a weak acid, brain levels of phenobarbital may be just half of those in plasma of acidemic patients. Phenobarbital has a very long half-life (approx. 90 h) leading to prolonged sedation, which often complicates subsequent neurological evaluation. As a GABA agonist and NMDA antagonist, propofol has strong theoretical advantages but efficacy data are limited. If seizures are controlled by a loading dose of 1 to 2 mg/kg, the infusion is continued at rates between 2 and 10 mg/kg/h, for 12 to 24 h before beginning a slow taper. One potential advantage of propofol over benzodiazepines or barbiturates is its substantially shorter duration of action facilitating repeated neurological examination. A significant disadvantage is the potential for metabolic acidosis when high doses are infused for long periods of time (propofol infusion syndrome).

Status epilepticus is occasionally resistant to the methods outlined above. Reasons for failure can include inadequate drug dosing, prolonged seizures before initiating treatment, cerebral mass lesion (e.g., tumor or hemorrhage), or profound metabolic abnormality (e.g., hypoxemia, hyponatremia, or hypocalcemia). Refractory seizures may require more intense anticonvulsant therapy including valproic acid, toprimate, tiagabine, high-dose benzodiazepine infusions, pentobarbital, or "general anesthesia" using a volatile anesthetic. Regardless of which regimen is chosen, mechanical ventilation and fluid and vasopressor support of blood pressure are nearly always required. Although there is no consensus on the treatment of such refractory seizures, a continuous infusion of a short-acting barbiturate (pentobarbital 10 mg/kg load followed by 1 to 4 mg/kg/h or thiopental 3 to 7 mg/kg load followed by 50 to 100 mg/min IV) has been used traditionally. Such a regimen is usually effective but may be required for 12 to 36 h or longer to prevent seizure recurrence. Emergence from the protracted barbiturate-induced coma may require weeks. Another alternative is a midazolam infusion (0.2 mg/kg bolus followed by 0.05 to 0.5 mg/kg/h).

If "salvage" therapy is required for seizure control, availability of EEG monitoring and expert neurologic consultation are essential. Unfortunately, there is no consensus for EEG endpoints of therapy; trained electroencephalographers are never continuously available; and for most ICU physicians, EEG interpretation is enigmatic. With regard to goals, seizure control certainly does not require achieving an "isoelectric" EEG; the value of achieving a "burst suppression" pattern is even questioned. Probably, simply preventing organized seizure activity is an adequate endpoint in most cases. So the question arises, how does a critical care doctor recognize seizure activity on EEG? While hardly a substitute for formal training, a couple of simple guidelines are useful. A normal EEG demonstrates asymmetric, high frequency, low-amplitude waveforms in multiple channels; perhaps to a critical care physician the best description of a normal EEG is that it looks like "ventricular fibrillation." Anytime symmetric, large magnitude discharges, or for that matter any recognizable pattern can be identified on EEG, seizure activity should be suspected.

■ STROKE

Cerebrovascular accident or stroke is a common cause of death and a frequent reason for ICU admission. The unifying factor in all stroke syndromes is neuronal ischemia because of interruption of blood flow. The term *stroke*, from biblical reference to being "struck down," implies an acute dramatic event. Although such sudden profound neurological events are the rule, in the ICU population the presentation is often more subtle and atypical. Common occurrences such as altered mental status, delayed awakening from sedation, slurred speech, a decreased level of consciousness, agitation, or the new onset of seizures may be the only manifestation of stroke. Not only are the presenting signs in ICU patients different, so is the etiology: whereas the vast majority of strokes occurring in the community are due to vascular occlusive disease, in hospitalized patients many more strokes are the result of cerebral emboli, sometimes the result of an invasive medical procedure.

Pathophysiology

Two pathophysiologic mechanisms account for almost all strokes: *ischemia* from occlusive thrombosis, embolism, or systemic hypoperfusion; or *hemorrhage* into brain tissue or the subarachnoid space. Although occlusion of venous drainage can also lead to ischemia outside of very specific situations (e.g., paranasal sinus infection, thrombophilia, sickle cell disease, l-asparaginase use), the

TABLE 34-5 CHARACTERISTICS OF STROKE SYNDROMES

	EMBOLIC	THROMBOTIC	HEMORRHAGIC
Time course	Abrupt, maximal deficit at onset Occasional dramatic improvement	Abrupt, maximal deficit at onset Occasional brief improvement	Prodromal headache Abrupt, rapid progression Sudden loss of consciousness
Common deficits	Cortical infarcts	Cortical infarcts	Internal capsule, basal ganglia
Predisposing factors	Older Caucasian Atrial fibrillation Arterial catheter flushing Mitral stenosis Cardiac Catheterization Central venous catheter insertion Endocarditis (esp. fungal) Atrial septal defect Left ventricular Dilation	Older Caucasian Heart failure Hypercholes- terolemia Hypertension Smoking Diabetes	Younger Black and Asian Hypertension Vascular malformation Amphetamine, cocaine, phenylpropanolamine Anticoagulant use
Antecedent history	Recent myocardial Infarction DVT-pulmonary embolism	TIA common *Amaurosis fugax* Central retinal artery occlusion	Recent thrombolytic therapy "Herald bleed"
Therapy	Antithrombotic	Thrombolytic (early) Elective endarterectomy	Correction of coagulopathy Surgical evacuation of selected lesions

syndrome is rare. Each of the four common stroke syndromes has its own predisposing factors, typical clinical presentation, and specific treatment summarized in Table 34-5.

Initial Evaluation

For patients with stroke, time to definitive treatment is the largest controllable determinant of outcome. Because the treatment of ischemic and hemorrhage strokes and other common disorders that mimic stroke (Table 34-6) are drastically different, it is essential to promptly make a firm diagnosis. Efficiency of care and outcomes are improved by establishing teams of experts to evaluate patients with suspected stroke in a stereotypical fashion which includes a directed history and physical examination, concise laboratory evaluation and

urgently obtained brain image. Essential historical elements are (a) the time the patient was last known to have normal neurological function, (b) recent trauma or surgery, and; (c) medications used, especially anticoagulants, anticonvulsants, antihypertensives, antiarrhythmics, and diabetic agents. Initial examination should evaluate the heart and arteries and search for signs of liver disease, bleeding, and coagulopathy. The neurological evaluation should be performed using a standardized tool like the National Institute of Health Stroke Scale (www.ninds.nih.gov/doctors/NIH_Stroke_Scale_Booklet.pdf). While the history and examination are performed appropriate laboratory studies, including electrolytes, glucose, creatinine, hemoglobin, platelet count, and prothrombin time (PT) should be obtained. This battery of tests is used to search for important nonstroke mimics and coagulopathy

TABLE 34-6   MIMICS OF STROKE SYNDROMES

Migraine
Seizures and postictal period
Intoxication
Hyponatremia
Hypoglycemia
Brain tumor or metastases

and evaluate the safety of thrombolytic therapy if indicated. An electrocardiogram to evaluate cardiac rhythm and the possibility of ischemia is also prudent. Even though the yield of a chest radiograph is low, it is a rapid, inexpensive, safe test to screen for abnormalities of the aorta and to look for intrathoracic neoplasm as a potential source of metastases.

After initial stabilization, immediate head imaging is indicated to evaluate the type and magnitude of stroke. There is some debate about the best initial imaging study, however, a noncontrasted CT scan is almost always adequate for key decision making. If for logistical reasons MRI scanning can be accomplished *faster*, it is an acceptable alternative. (In suspected brainstem stroke, MRI may add information to CT scan data.)

General Care of the Stroke Patient

The therapy of each specific stroke syndrome depends on its etiology and structural manifestations; however, the therapy of most strokes remains supportive. Because of the frequency of serious complications in stroke victims, simple prophylactic measures to prevent skin breakdown, gastric ulceration, and deep venous thrombosis (DVT) make good sense. One to two weeks of prophylactic anticonvulsant therapy may be useful for persons with large hemorrhagic strokes. Regardless of etiology, all stroke patients should have oxygenation and perfusion evaluated on arrival. If saturations are below normal, supplemental oxygen should be administered; however, there is no evidence that supplemental oxygen aids patients with normal PaO_2 values. Symptomatic arrhythmias, particularly those causing hypotension, should be immediately corrected. Although there is little high-quality data to support the practice, anemia is usually corrected to a hemoglobin level ≥ 10 gm/dL.

The appropriate target for blood pressure in stroke victims is controversial because worse outcomes are associated both with hypotension and hypertension. Transient, moderate hypertension (systolic BP >160 mm Hg) is nearly universal in all forms of stroke, as is a spontaneous decline in pressure over the first day of illness. Because self-correction is common, caution should be used to avoid overtreatment. Two points are clear: rapidly lowering blood pressure or "normalizing" blood pressure in the chronically hypertensive stroke victim is likely to do more harm than good. As a general rule, unless the patient is treated with thrombolytic therapy, or has pulmonary edema, myocardial infarction, or aortic dissection, blood pressures less than 220/120 mm Hg should not be treated. (If thrombolytic therapy is used, a goal of less than 185/110 mm Hg is recommended.) Unless causing immediate harm, *gradual* reduction in blood pressure over several hours to days using oral antihypertensive therapy is probably the best course of action. If pharmacotherapy is chosen, drugs without CNS depressant effects are preferred. Within a few days of the stroke, a reasonable low-end target for MAP is 110 to 120 mm Hg. A complete discussion of blood pressure control is presented in Chapter 22.

The importance of glucose control is debated. Older studies show an association of hyperglycemia with poor neurologic outcome; however, it is very possible that hyperglycemia is only a marker of severity of brain injury rather than a cause of damage. Even though no cause-and-effect relationship between hyperglycemia and brain injury has been proven, it is hard to posit a benefit of hyperglycemia, provided hypoglycemia is avoided. As a general principle, even transient hypoglycemia is likely to be more harmful than sustained mild hyperglycemia. Use of a standardized protocol that frequently monitors glucose values, uses short-acting insulin, and aims for near normal levels (<140 to 180 mg/dL) is advocated. An overview of stroke therapy is provided in Table 34-7 and discussed in detail below. Numerous other ineffective or harmful therapies have been used in stroke treatment and are presented in Table 34-8.

Ischemic Stroke

Ischemic strokes, the most common and important variety, typically result from the progressive occlusion of larger arteries (usually, branches of the carotid). Hence, the risk of ischemic stroke is related

TABLE 34-7 PHARMACOLOGIC THERAPY OF ACUTE STROKE SYNDROMES

Transient ischemic attacks
Aspirin 325 mg/day (Ticlopidine or clopidogrel are alternatives in aspirin-sensitive patients.)

Complete ischemic stroke
Aspirin 325 mg/day to prevent recurrence

Progressive ischemic stroke
Tissue plasminogen activator (0.9 mg/kg) (if low bleeding risk and presentation within 3 h)
or
Aspirin 325 mg/day to prevent recurrence if not TPA candidate

Cardioembolic stroke
If hemorrhage absent on CT scan at 48 h begin low-molecular-weight or unfractionated heparin to aPTT of 1.5–2.0 baseline THEN:
   warfarin targeted to INR of 2.0–3.0
EXCEPTIONS: CVA involving >30% of cerebral hemisphere (high risk for hemorrhagic extension)
Warfarin can be started without heparin for prophylaxis in atrial fibrillation

---

to increasing age as the chronic risk factors of diabetes, hypertension, smoking, and hypercholesterolemia take their toll on vessel patency. (Thrombophilia, migraine, arterial dissection, and fibromuscular dysplasia are much less common causes of thrombosis.) Although large vessels are usually the target, ischemic strokes can occur in small perforating vessels resulting in a specific pattern known as a "lacune." Stroke may also occur in patients with less-than-critical vascular narrowing when hypotension, hypoxemia, or coagulopathy tips the balance of cerebral oxygen supply and demand unfavorably. When brain perfusion is impaired globally (e.g., shock, cardiopulmonary arrest), regions at the border between two vascular

TABLE 34-8 UNPROVED OR HARMFUL STROKE THERAPIES

Aminophylline	Hypothermia
Antioxidant compounds	Mannitol
Calcium channel blockers	N-methyl D-aspartate
Corticosteroids	(NMDA) antagonists
Glycerol	Pit viper venom
Hemodilution	Streptokinase
Heparin (except for cardioembolic stroke)	
Hyperbaric oxygen	

distributions suffer the greatest. Ischemia of these so-called watershed zones results in three major clinical syndromes including (a) bilateral upper extremity paralysis, (b) cortical blindness, and (c) memory impairment.

Slow progressive vessel narrowing can result in premonitory ischemic episodes and transient ischemic attacks (TIAs). Although technically the neurological deficits of a TIA can last up to 24 h, most resolve in less than 10 min. Akin to unstable angina, TIAs serve as markers of a transition period during which stroke is likely. The risk of stroke correlates with the severity of the TIA—when temporary monocular vision loss (amaurosis fugax) is the only symptom, the risk of stroke is substantially lower than when large hemispheric defects occur. A TIA is a powerful warning sign that must not be ignored because at this stage, antithrombotic therapy or radiological or surgical intervention can abort a fatal or disabling stroke in many patients. Unfortunately, other than TIAs there are few if any reliable physical signs identifying patients at risk. A diminished carotid pulse and a carotid bruit are perhaps the best indicators of large vessel occlusive disease before ischemia becomes manifest.

Because ischemic strokes usually infarct the cerebral cortex, where sensory and motor functions are anatomically juxtaposed, equal losses of sensation and motor function to a given region occur. This is in contrast to small vessel strokes (lacunes), occurring deeper in the brain, where by virtue of the neuronal pathway arrangement, widespread deficits of isolated sensory or motor function are possible. For ischemic strokes, the supply distribution of the occluded vessel determines the pattern of neurologic deficit, which differs for the anterior, middle, and posterior cerebral artery circulations. Typically, ischemic strokes present with a near immediate maximal deficit, often noted upon awakening. When middle cerebral artery (MCA) flow is interrupted, the resulting sensory and motor deficits are greatest in the contralateral side of the face with lesser deficits in the arm and leg. MCA occlusions of the dominant cortex may also produce an expressive or receptive aphasia when damage occurs to the anterior or posterior speech centers, respectively. A corresponding lesion of the nondominant hemisphere may produce an acute, agitated or confused state with contralateral motor and sensory deficits. Homonymous hemianopsia and conjugate eye deviation toward the side of the lesion are less common but characteristic features of MCA occlusion.

Occlusion of the anterior cerebral artery produces the greatest neurologic deficit in the contralateral leg, followed in severity by the arm and then face. A homonymous hemianopsia or loss of vision ipsilateral to the stroke is also possible. Frontal lobe signs of incontinence, grasp and suck reflexes, and perseveration are also common. Posterior cerebral artery ischemic does not usually impact the major centers for speech or motion; deficits are limited to homonymous hemianopsia, impaired recent memory, and prominent sensory loss.

4 The only effective treatment for ischemic stroke is rapidly delivered thrombolysis. Hence, when a clinical diagnosis is made, promptly obtaining a CT scan to distinguish patients with hemorrhage from those with ischemia is essential for decision making. Obviously, thrombolytic treatment is contraindicated if hemorrhage is seen but the CT can also help predict the safety of thrombolysis in patients with ischemic stroke. For patients with normal CT scans and those with subtle findings involving less than one third of a hemisphere, thrombolysis is of low risk. When the CT shows subtle changes involving greater than one third of a hemisphere, or mass effect or hypodensisty of less than one third of a hemisphere, thrombolytic therapy should be carefully considered because of the higher risk of bleeding. There is general agreement that when a hypodense area is greater than one third of a hemisphere, thrombolytic therapy should be withheld. Even without thrombolytic therapy approximately 25% of ischemic strokes undergo spontaneous hemorrhagic transformation within 48h. This conversion is often associated with worsening of the neurologic deficit and can be confirmed by repeating a CT scan. Large strokes, especially those occurring in the elderly or in diabetics, are most prone to this complication, hence the reluctance to treat extensive strokes with thrombolytic therapy.

Clinical trials of thrombolytic agents have shown neurological and survival benefits only when tissue plasminogen activator (TPA) (0.9 mg/kg) is administered rapidly after the onset of symptoms. Treatment delays of as little as 90 min, but certainly 180 min reduce benefits. Because patients must be free of systemic bleeding, present promptly after onset of symptoms, and undergo nearly immediate uncontrasted CT scanning that shows a favorable pattern, very few patients receive thrombolytic therapy. Even when carefully screened, a substantial number of patients develop significant intracranial

(6%) and systemic bleeding after receiving TPA. When exclusionary criteria are ignored, bleeding rates of 40% have been reported. To minimize bleeding risks after thrombolytic therapy, control of blood pressure (<185/110 mm Hg) and avoidance of invasive procedures and antiplatelet therapy should be routine. Because candidates for thrombolysis may have noteworthy bleeding complications, it should be used only by experienced physicians in a hospital with neurosurgical backup. If neurological function deteriorates after administration of thrombolytic therapy, the lytic agent should be stopped and coagulation status corrected using cryoprecipitate and platelet transfusions, while a repeat CT is arranged. If intracranial hemorrhage is confirmed, neurosurgical consultation is prudent.

Aspirin reduces the incidence of thrombotic strokes when given prophylactically (particularly to patients with premonitory transient ischemia), and decreases the incidence of recurrent stroke. Unfortunately, aspirin does not abort stroke in progress or reverse established neurologic deficits. Among patients with ischemic stroke who are not candidates for thrombolytic treatment, aspirin therapy should be started within 48h.

The outcome of ischemic stroke is not improved by hyperbaric oxygen therapy, therapeutic hypothermia, heparin anticoagulation, or surgery. Carotid endarterectomy is not indicated for treatment of acute ischemic stroke, but in patients with chronic or recurrent symptoms of cerebral ischemia, endarterectomy may be beneficial. Endarterectomy is of proven benefit if performed by an experienced surgeon in symptomatic patients with greater than 70% carotid stenosis and low operative risk. When the stenosis is in the 50% to 70% range, benefit is unproven, but endarterectomy is still probably acceptable provided the combined operative risk remains low. The surgeon's morbidity and mortality rate must, however, be very low (<3%) to favor surgical intervention in the asymptomatic patient.

Because of the rapid evolution of diagnostic techniques, an enduring discussion of the merits of diagnostic tests to evaluate the cerebral circulation is not possible. Currently, color flow Doppler ultrasound is usually the first diagnostic test to evaluate the extracranial circulation. If results of ultrasound are equivocal or if imaging the intracranial circulation is desired, CT angiogram or magnetic resonance angiogram is usually performed. Conventional carotid arteriography is now done less often.

Embolic Strokes

Embolic strokes result from the sudden impaction of a plug in a small cerebral artery branch, usually giving rise to isolated ischemic cortical defects. Because complete small-vessel occlusion occurs nearly instantaneously, maximal neurologic deficits are typically observed at the time of embolization, but it is common for deficits to partially, even sometimes dramatically, improve within 1 to 2 days. Because of the embolic nature of the injury, multiple discrete areas of brain may be injured simultaneously. Although embolic strokes are considered to be second in frequency to thrombosis in the general population, patients in the ICU are at substantially higher risk of emboli because they are commonly subjected to procedures that predispose to arterial injury or thrombosis and cholesterol or air embolism (e.g., central venous catheterization complications, left heart catheterization, aortic balloon pump insertion, and invasive blood pressure monitoring). During such procedures, air, clot, or atherogenic material can be released or dislodged.

Cerebral embolism can result from foreign bodies, infected material, bland clot, air, or cholesterol fragments. Bland clot formed either in a sluggishly flowing carotid system or in the heart of patients with mural thrombi, myocardial infarction, mitral valve disease, and atrial fibrillation are most common. Rarely, venous thromboemboli cause stroke as they cross a right-to-left intracardia shunt entering the cerebral circulation (i.e., paradoxical embolism). In most cases, the intracardiac defect is a patent foramen ovale or atrial septal defect. Left-sided endocarditis is another potential source of embolism in the critically ill patient. Bacteria, fungi, and amorphous material sloughed by structurally abnormal or infected heart valves can all cause cerebral vascular plugging. It is not widely appreciated that arterial pressure generated when "flushing" a peripheral arterial line can exceed systolic blood pressure. A sustained flush can propel catheter tip, clot, or air retrograde into the cerebral circulation. Foreign materials, either illicitly injected into the arterial system by the patient or resulting from fracture of arterial monitoring catheters, also rarely result in cerebral embolism. Cerebral air emboli can result from disruption of the pulmonary veins by penetrating trauma or high ventilator inflation pressures, therapeutic misadventures during cardiac catheterization, rapid ascent from underwater diving, or curious sexual practices (predominately in pregnant women).

The diagnosis of embolic stroke is usually not difficult to make. History most often reveals one or more predisposing conditions. In addition, the neurologic deficit is typically described as unexpected, immediate, and maximal in severity at onset. Because the heart is the most common embolic source, clinical examination often provides evidence of cardiac disease (e.g., atrial fibrillation, murmur, or cardiomegaly). Neurologic evaluation typically reveals a cortically based deficit with both sensory and motor loss to the same body region.

Because the volume of tissue infarcted may be small, the CT scan is often unremarkable. In patients with a history suggestive of embolic stroke without an obvious source, the combination of blood cultures to exclude endocarditis, cardiac monitoring to exclude arrhythmias, and a transthoracic echocardiogram to diagnose aortic atheromatous disease, mural thrombi, valvular lesions, and to evaluate myocardial performance constitutes a good initial diagnostic battery. Because of the superior sensitivity of transesophageal echocardiography (TEE) in finding subtle valvular lesions and small clots in the left atrial appendage, it should be considered in patients with a history suggestive of embolism that has a nondiagnostic transthoracic echocardiogram. If symptoms localize to the carotid circulation and a cardiac source cannot be found, evaluation of the carotid branches should be undertaken using duplex ultrasound of the neck and transcranial Doppler. If symptoms are in the posterior circulation, evaluation of the origins of the vertebrobasilar and posterior cerebral arteries should be performed.

The therapy of embolic stroke should be dictated by the embolic material and stroke size. Obviously, antimicrobial therapy is indicated in patients with emboli secondary to infective endocarditis. Valve replacement should be considered when large vegetations are present or when recurrent embolism occurs, despite appropriate therapy. In patients with a nonhemorrhagic embolic stroke from a cardiac source, heparin or low-molecular-weight heparin (LMWH) followed by warfarin with a target INR of 2 to 3 is indicated. Commonly, anticoagulation is delayed for 48 h after the event to document absence of hemorrhage by CT scan. (Waiting 1 to 2 weeks to begin anticoagulation is prudent in those patients at high risk for hemorrhagic transformation.) For patients with atrial fibrillation, long-term warfarin has been demonstrated to reduce the risk of stroke by as much as 65% in patients over the age of 65. There is no evidence that thrombolytic therapy or anticoagulation is effective for "stroke in evolution" or completed embolic stroke.

Lacunar Strokes

Lacunes are ischemic events of tiny vessels deep within the brain, usually occurring in hypertensive individuals. Lacunar syndromes can result from bland infarction or hemorrhage. Most often these events occur in the region of the internal capsule, producing a large functional deficit even though only a small area of brain is injured. Because neurons controlling distant body regions are closely grouped together, deficits of the face, arm, and leg are typically equal in severity. Similarly, due to the anatomic arrangement of neurons in this region, selective deficits of sensory or motor function can occur. This pattern of deficits is in distinct contrast to cortical infarcts where sensory and motor loses tend to occur in parallel and the limbs and face are usually affected to varying degrees.

The CT scan may be normal or show only a small lucency or density in patients with lacunes because of the typically small size of the infarct. MRI may be more informative. With the exception of appropriate supportive care and blood pressure control, there is no specific therapy for a lacunar infarct.

Hemorrhagic Stroke

Hemorrhagic strokes most commonly occur in the putamen, internal capsule, thalamus, caudate nucleus, pons, and cerebellum when small vessels rupture as the result of chronic hypertension or vessel wall defects. Bleeding into the hemispheric parenchyma is less frequent and more commonly the result of excessive therapeutic anticoagulation, an arteriovenous malformation, or venous hemangioma.

In addition to vascular defects, nonvascular risk factors may also contribute to the development of hemorrhagic stroke. These extracranial risk factors include drug use (prescription or illicit) and systemic vasculitis. Warfarin and heparin account for about 10% of all cases of intracranial bleeding, and a 1% to 2% risk of intracranial hemorrhage is associated with the use of thrombolytic therapy for acute myocardial infarction. (Bleeding risk is about five times higher when thrombolytic therapy is given for ischemic stroke.) Cocaine, amphetamines, and phenylpropanolamine all can cause hemorrhage by boosting blood pressure or by inducing vasculitis.

The site, relative frequency, and clinical characteristics of hemorrhagic stroke are presented in Table 34-9. The deficits created by intracerebral hemorrhage are usually rapidly progressive, but late deterioration can be seen days after the initial bleed as the osmotic effects of extravasated blood recruit additional fluid and worsen localized swelling. Approximately 40% of hemorrhagic stroke victims have demonstrable hematoma enlargement over just 2 to 3 h, a finding associated with a much higher risk of death. If hemorrhage ruptures into the ventricular system, obstructive hydrocephalus can occur with a slow progressive downhill course. There are three classical clinical presentations of hemorrhagic stroke: (a) hemiplegia, sometimes with hemisensory impairment, when the thalamus or basal ganglia are involved; (b) sudden-onset quadraparesis, pinpoint pupils, midposition eyes, and coma occur when the pons is the site of the bleed; and (c) headache, ataxia, nausea, and vomiting when bleeding occurs in the cerebellum. Seizures are more common with hemorrhagic strokes than with ischemic lesions, hence the recommendation by some experts for 1 to 2 weeks of

TABLE 34-9 SITES AND CHARACTERISTICS OF INTRACEREBRAL HEMORRHAGE

SITE	FREQUENCY	CLINICAL CHARACTERISTICS
Putamen	35%	Contralateral hemiparesis, hemisensory loss, dysphagia, or neglect
Thalamus	10%	Similar to putamen bleed, plus forced downward gaze, upgaze palsy, unreactive pupils
Caudate nucleus	5%	Confusion, memory loss, hemiparesis, gaze paresis, intraventricular blood, and hydrocephalus common
Lobar bleed	30%	Variable findings depending on location
Cerebellum	15%	Headache, vomiting, gait ataxia, nystagmus, cranial nerve palsies
Pons	5%	Quadriplegia, pinpoint pupils, gaze palsies, ataxia, sensorimotor loss

prophylactic anticonvulsant therapy. Virtually, all hemorrhagic strokes are easily recognized on CT scan by the presence of "bright white" extravasated blood in the region of the stroke. MRI is an equally capable diagnostic tool.

Treatment of intracranial hemorrhage includes reversal of therapeutic anticoagulation, correction of endogenous coagulopathy, and blood pressure control. Excessive heparin effect can be reversed with protamine. Excessive warfarin treatment can be reversed with a combination of fresh frozen plasma and vitamin K. If thrombocytopenia is present, platelet counts should be raised by transfusion to at least 100,000/mm^3. Two large trials testing recombinant human factor VIIa (rhVIIa) for intracranial hemorrhage have been conducted. In both trials, rhVIIa reduced the growth of hematoma volumes but caused more extracranial thromboses. Outcome benefits suggested by the first smaller trial could not be confirmed in the larger phase III study. Hence, rhVIIa should not be used to treat intracranial hemorrhage.

Numerous studies have suggested a relationship between various levels of hypertension and hematoma growth, however, there are not yet good data to inform practice. An ongoing study is comparing control of systolic BP of less than 140 mm Hg to 140 to 180 mm Hg. While awaiting definitive data, it is reasonable and safe to produce 15% reductions in BP in patients with hemorrhage if the baseline systolic pressure is greater than 180 mm Hg.

As one of the few surgically amenable neurologic problems, cerebellar hemorrhage should be quickly recognized, radiographically confirmed, and corrected by evacuation. CT scan is the best technique to select candidates who might benefit from clot evacuation. Evacuation is generally reserved for patients with posterior fossa hemorrhages greater than 3 cm in diameter and those with brainstem compression, rupture of blood into the third ventricle, or hydrocephalus. In contrast to benefits from evacuating cerebellar hemorrhage, a large randomized trial of decompressive surgery for supratentorial hemorrhage did not demonstrate improved outcomes. Investigations of mannitol, glycerol, corticosteroids, and hemodilution have all failed to show benefit.

Subarachnoid Hemorrhage

SAH is a stroke syndrome in which headache, nausea, vomiting, confusion, or coma are typical, but paralysis is rarely seen. Although the headache very well may not be described as "the worst of my life," patients often identify the headache of SAH as a unique event. Rupture of an aneurysm or arteriovenous malformation allows escape of blood directly into the cerebral spinal fluid where CT scanning and LP offer rapid and reliable confirmation of the diagnosis. Early mortality rates from SAH approach 50%, with 20% to 30% of patients experiencing recurrent bleeding before definitive vascular repair. Thus, the trend has been to move to earlier diagnosis and repair of amenable lesions. The traditional approach using delayed open "clipping" has evolved to earlier placement of coils or other embolic material in the aneurysm using an endovascular approach. Both endovascular and extravascular approaches appear to be equally effective for most aneurysms, but some wide-mouthed aneurysms are not amenable to an endovascular approach. In addition, aneurysms of the posterior cerebral and basilar arteries are difficult to access by open craniotomy.

A second major problem occurring in about 20% of SAH patients is vasospasm. Vasospasm, usually manifests as a global decline in neurological function, beginning 3 to 5 days after the bleed with peak effect at 7 to 14 days. Although the pathophysiology of vasospasm continues to be debated, two lines of therapy appear beneficial: use of the calcium channel blocker, nimodipine; and use of induced hypertension, hemodilution, and hypervolemia, so-called triple H therapy. Nimodipine, 60 mg every 6 h, has been shown to decrease the risk of vasospasm after SAH but can lead to detrimental hypotension. Induced hypertension, hemodilution, and hypervolemia has few high-quality studies to support its use; however, existing data consistently show benefit and it appears to be of low risk and cost. In theory, the therapy lowers blood viscosity while maintaining perfusion pressure. Likewise, although anticonvulsants are commonly administered after SAH, there are limited data to support the practice.

Stroke Complications

DVT, decubitus ulcer formation, and gastric ulceration are all very common in stroke victims. Perhaps the largest overall gains in survival of stroke patients can be achieved by preventing death from thromboembolism. By one estimate more than one third of stroke victims develop DVT in the absence of effective prophylaxis. Hence, early institution of pharmacological prophylaxis (in patients at low risk for anticoagulation-related complications) or venous compression devices may be one of the most efficacious treatments for stroke victims. (In patients with ischemic strokes LWMH has been shown to be superior to twice daily unfractionated heparin [UFH] and is of comparable bleeding risk.) Similarly, because gastric stress ulceration is common, early enteral feeding, or proton pump inhibitor or histamine blocker treatment is prudent. Careful use of positioning, padding, turning, and therapeutic beds can prevent the devastating complication of skin breakdown and joint contractures. These seemingly mundane but important issues of supportive care are covered in detail in Chapter 18.

Hydrocephalus is an uncommon complication for most forms of stroke, but is far from rare in patients sustaining hemorrhagic infarction of the caudate or posterior fossa. Bleeding into the caudate nucleus ruptures into the ventricular system with considerable frequency, often resulting in a waning level of consciousness and hydrocephalus on CT scanning.

Respiratory complications of stroke, including aspiration pneumonitis and bacterial pneumonia, are extremely common and are responsible for most episodes of poststroke fever. The risk of aspiration is particularly common for patients fed using a "bolus" rather than continuous infusion technique. Feeding patients maintained in a less then 30 degree head up position also appears to be a risk factor for aspiration and pneumonia.

■ INCREASED INTRACRANIAL PRESSURE

Mechanisms

Three tissues occupy the skull: brain substance, CSF, and blood. None is readily compressible. Therefore, swelling of the brain substance, intracranial hematoma, or blockage of the normal venous or CSF outflow leads to increased ICP. Elevated ICP is mitigated by the movement of one of the "liquid" components (blood or CSF) out of the cranium. Increased ICP is itself deleterious when it compromises tissue perfusion or precipitates brain herniation.

Swelling of the brain matter happens by three common mechanisms. Vasogenic edema occurs when the blood brain barrier is disrupted by trauma or high intravascular pressures (e.g., malignant hypertension). Subsequent leak of serum proteins and water around neurons leads to interstitial edema.

Cytotoxic brain edema results from impairment of cellular sodium potassium pumping mechanisms by glial cell injury. Disrupted ion pumping allows intracellular water accumulation causing edema. The most common causes are hypoxia and toxin exposure (e.g., carbon monoxide). Osmotic edema occurs when intracellular osmolality exceeds that of plasma and CSF, and water passively moves into brain cells. The gradient for water movement can be created by raising intracellular osmolarity or reducing plasma tonicity. For example, rapid intravenous, or even intrarectal, administration of large volumes of hypotonic fluid (e.g., acute water intoxication) can cause brain swelling in a previously healthy person. Another example occurs when neurons have increased intracellular tonicity because of accumulated glucose (DKA), uremic toxins (renal failure), or idiogenic osmoles (hepatic failure). In each case, treatments that rapidly reduce plasma osmolality (e.g., insulin, high flow dialysis) can cause abrupt cerebral edema.

Bleeding into the cranial vault is especially problematic for intracranial hemodynamics. Not only does the bleeding increase ICP by mass effect, but it also clogs CSF absorption at the subarachnoid villi and increases CSF osmotic pressure when red cell lyse. The swelling of injured tissue typically peaks within 72 h of injury. ICP, however, can remain elevated for weeks if there has been significant intracerebral or intraventricular bleeding.

Cerebral Hemodynamics

The pressure perfusing the brain (CPP) is the difference between MAP and either the ICP or the pressure within the cerebral veins (whichever is greater). ICP is normally quite low (<5 mm Hg) but often reaches critically high levels (20 to 40 mm Hg) in the head-injured patient. CPP normally exceeds 60 mm Hg; the lowest acceptable level is about 40 mm Hg. Neural dysfunction occurs when CPP is less than 40 mm Hg, and neuronal death occurs at CPP less than 20 mm Hg. ICP should be kept low enough to maintain cerebral perfusion and prevent cerebral herniation. Thus, the goal should be to optimize the CPP gradient by lowering ICP and raising MAP if necessary. Although an absolute target for MAP cannot be declared, maintaining MAP above 90 mm Hg will ensure an adequate CPP even as ICP approaches the critical 20 mm Hg value.

In health, cerebral autoregulatory mechanisms sensitive to arterial oxygen tension (PaO_2), arterial carbon dioxide tension (PaCO$_2$), and blood pressure continuously adjust cerebral vascular resistance to maintain perfusion in proportion to metabolic need and changing perfusion pressure. Arterial blood gases, cerebral metabolism, and the components of perfusion pressure (blood pressure, ICP) must be watched cautiously in brain-injured patients because the autoregulatory mechanisms of injured tissue are impaired. In this setting, tissue perfusion directly parallels CPP and perfusion adequacy is directly influenced by cerebral metabolism.

Intracranial Pressure Monitoring

There are three reasons to insert an ICP monitor: (a) to detect life-threatening intracranial hypertension; (b) to assess the effects of therapy aimed at reducing ICP; and (c) therapeutic drainage of spinal fluid. Mean ICP of a supine patient is normally less than 10 mm Hg, and the ICP waveform normally undulates gently in time with the cardiac cycle. Extreme fluctuations of the ICP waveform (>10 mm Hg) suggest a position near the critical inflexion point of the cranial pressure volume curve, particularly when the contour shows a high "second peak" corresponding to the arterial pulse. Elevations of ICP to 15 to 20 mm Hg compress capillary beds and compromise the microcirculation. At levels of 30 to 35 mm Hg, venous drainage is impeded and edema develops in uninjured tissue. This level of intracranial hypertension produces a vicious cycle in which impeded venous drainage leads to accumulating edema and further ICP elevations. Even when autoregulatory mechanisms are intact, cerebral perfusion cannot be maintained if ICP rises to within 40 to 50 mm Hg of the MAP. When ICP reaches MAP, perfusion stops and the brain dies.

In addition to sustained elevations of ICP, Lundberg has described two specific pressure transients. "A waves," pressure elevations of 20 to 100 mm Hg for periods of 2 to 15 min, are always pathologic. A waves are usually associated with abnormal eye movements, posturing, and abnormal neurological reflexes—physiologic responses resulting from inadequate cerebral perfusion. Lundberg A waves indicate the likelihood of sudden deterioration and poor neurological outcome. Lundberg "B waves" are lower in amplitude, shorter in duration, and usually occur in relation to respiratory variation. B waves have no associated physical findings at the time of occurrence and unlike

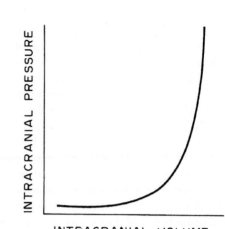

■ **FIGURE 34-2** Relationship of ICP to intracranial volume. ICP remains low until a critical volume is attained.

their A wave counterparts are not well correlated with neurological outcome.

Of the three fluid components contained within the fixed cranial volume, only the volumes of CSF and blood may be changed (unless the skull is opened or brain is removed or made less edematous). Starting from normal levels, ICP shows little response to volume increases until a critical inflexion point is reached. Thereafter, small increments in volume dramatically boost ICP, risking sudden deterioration (Fig. 34-2). Direct ICP monitoring is important because changes in other clinical indices—reflexes, blood pressure, and heart rate—usually occur too late to avert disaster. Bradycardia, a preterminal sign, is the least reliable of all clinical indicators of increased ICP. (Tachycardia is seen more frequently.)

Specific Indications for ICP Monitoring

Closed Head Injury

Although the benefits of ICP monitoring are unproved by rigorous clinical trials, it remains a common practice in the head-injured patient. It is not practical or necessary to monitor ICP in all these patients, but three groups of trauma patients appear to derive benefit: (a) those with an abnormal CT scan at admission, (b) patients with normal CT scans at admission but who present with hypotension or posturing, and (c) patients above the age of 40. A normal CT scan of the head accurately predicts normal ICP in more than 80% of cases, whereas ICP is elevated in about 50% of patients when any lesion is observed on head CT. Midline shift of more than 7 mm or blood in the lateral ventricles is especially worrisome. Head trauma patients with GCS scores less than 7 frequently have an increased ICP, as do patients with decorticate/decerebrate posturing or abnormal evoked potential testing. Abnormal eye or pupil movements are unreliable guides to increased ICP. Repeat head CT is advocated approximately 24 h after injury to assess the progress of wounds and to evaluate the degree of intracranial hypertension.

Reye's Syndrome and fulminant hepatic failure

Increased ICP from cytotoxic edema is a major cause of death in Reye syndrome. Mortality approaches 100% without prompt diagnosis and treatment. Therapeutic reductions in ICP may reduce mortality to 20% or less, with survivors experiencing few sequelae. Therefore, ICP monitoring is indicated in patients with Reye's syndrome and GCS scores less than 7. The pathogenesis of increased ICP in hepatic failure of other etiologies is less certain but is probably a combination of cytotoxic and idiogenic osmolar mechanisms. ICP elevations are common among patients with acute hepatic failure but rare among patients with chronic end-stage cirrhosis. Even though ICP monitoring is commonly performed in acute hepatic failure, at present there is little evidence to suggest it reduces mortality.

Brain Tumors

ICP monitoring is rarely necessary in patients with chronic supratentorial lesions. However, ventriculostomy may be useful preoperatively to allow reduction in the CSF volume of patients with large infratentorial lesions. In patients with large brain tumors or extensive edema on CT scanning, ICP monitoring may help guide therapy.

Contraindications to Monitoring

Coagulopathy (platelet count < 50 to 100,000/mm^3 or prothrombin time [PT] or activated partial thromboplastin time [aPTT] values >2x control) is generally regarded as contraindication to ICP monitor placement. Among patients with acute hepatic failure, coagulation disorders are often corrected with fresh frozen plasma, vitamin K and/or platelet transfusions before ICP placement. Isolated elevations of fibrin degradation products (FDPs) should not contraindicate catheter placement; FDP levels may be increased by brain trauma alone. Immunosuppressive therapy (particularly steroids) is a relative contraindication to ICP monitoring.

Hardware and Devices

Intraventricular Catheters

Ventricular catheters may be inserted under local anesthesia at the bedside, typically through a burr hole in the skull on the "non-dominant" side just anterior to the sagittal suture. Because intraventricular catheters provide continuous, reliable data and allow therapeutic removal of CSF, they are the preferred method of ICP monitoring by many clinicians. Unfortunately, ventriculostomy presents several problems. Perhaps foremost, because bleeding commonly accompanies insertion, uncorrected coagulopathy contraindicates placement. There may also be technical difficulty encountered placing the catheter into a lateral ventricle compressed by extensive edema or mass. After insertion, the CSF invariably shows evidence of catheter irritation (mild elevations of protein and leukocyte count) making laboratory evaluation of the fluid difficult. In addition, infection is frequent (approx. 15%) after ventriculostomy and relates to duration of monitoring and to sterility of catheter placement and maintenance. Prophylactic antibiotics have shown no benefit in reducing infection rates, but tunneling the catheter through the skin may be helpful.

Epidural Transducers

Although epidural transducers present a lower risk of infection than ventricular catheters, they are technically more difficult to insert. Epidural catheters use fiberoptic or mechanical transducer membranes precisely juxtaposed to the dura. Past problems with calibration drift plaguing these devices have now largely been surmounted. The major drawback to the use of epidural transducers is the inability to remove CSF.

Subarachnoid Screws/Bolts

The subarachnoid screw is a hollow bolt inserted into the subarachnoid space through a burr hole (usually bored in the frontoparietal suture). During placement the dura is opened and the device is inserted onto the brain surface. Problems with the subarachnoid screw include infection and the potential for seriously underestimating ICP if not placed on the side of an existing mass lesion. Brain herniation into the device is the most common cause for technical failure. Problems with damping and clotting are sufficiently frequent that regular flushing is mandatory. Such flushing, however, exposes patients to an increased risk of herniation and infection. Finally, these devices are frequently dislodged, even with meticulous care.

Problems with ICP Monitoring

Metallic monitoring devices preclude MRI scans and produce artifacts on CT scans that can obscure important information. Infection occurs in 2% to 5% of patients who undergo ICP monitoring. Infection risk increases with the "depth of insertion" (ventricular catheters are highest); duration of monitoring and use of an open drainage systems. Flushing of devices adds to infection risk. *Staphylococcus epidermidis* is the most common infecting organism. Prophylactic antibiotics have not been demonstrated effective. As with any monitoring technique, poor-quality data may lead to inappropriate therapy. The intraventricular catheter gives the most consistent data, whereas the subarachnoid screw is less reliable but carries the lowest infection risk.

Reducing Intracranial Pressure

Lowering Jugular Venous Pressure

The goal of reducing ICP is to maintain cerebral blood flow by keeping CPP greater than 60 mm Hg. Because the ICP cannot be lower than the downstream venous pressure (CVP), patient positioning is important. Neck flexion, head turning, and tracheostomy ties impeding venous drainage should be avoided. Raising the head to at least 30 degrees virtually assures CVP will be less than ICP. Increases in CVP related to supine or prone positioning, straining, retching, and coughing should be minimized. Likewise, seizures should be prevented. Special caution should be taken during ventilation using Positive end-expiratory pressure (PEEP). By raising intrathoracic pressure and decreasing venous return, high levels of PEEP have the potential to simultaneously reduce MAP and raise ICP. However, judicious use of PEEP is not contraindicated, especially because the ICP of trauma patients often exceeds the PEEP-affected pressure within the superior sagittal sinus.

Sedation and Analgesia

A struggling agitated patient may acutely raise CVP, thereby raising ICP. Even comatose patients can experience increased ICP in response to noxious stimuli; therefore, appropriate sedation and analgesia are indicated. Narcotics represent a good analgesic choice because they have some sedative effect, reduce pain, and their antitussive action can avoid transient detrimental increases in ICP. Propofol is the sedative of choice for most patients because it has a rapid onset and offset of action, is readily titrated, lowers ICP, and has anticonvulsant properties. Benzodiazepine sedatives also provide the anticonvulsant benefit. Regardless of the sedative or analgesics chosen, it is important to administer doses that do not result in hypotension. In extreme cases, neuromuscular blocking drugs must be added to deep sedation and analgesia to avoid intracranial hypertension.

Diuretics

Loop diuretics (e.g., furosemide) have twin therapeutic actions—decreasing CSF production and producing a diuresis that reduces intravascular volume. Caution must be exercised when using diuretics to avoid hypotension resulting from excessive preload reduction.

Osmotic Agents

Mannitol and hypertonic saline work by establishing an osmotic gradient between the CSF and blood, thereby promoting fluid transfer from brain cells and CSF to the circulation. Increasing the blood osmolality by 10 mOsm/L has a net effect of acutely removing about 100 mL of intracellular water from brain. The use of osmotic agents is not standardized because the optimal choice of agent, dose, and frequency of administration has not been determined in clinical trials. Mannitol given in boluses of 0.25 to 1 gm/kg every 4 to 6 h is a traditional choice, but hypertonic saline is now perhaps more popular. In doses that produce a serum osmolarity greater than 320 mOsm/dL, all osmotic agents slowly penetrate the blood–brain barrier, gradually counterbalancing their therapeutic effect. Even when serum osmolarity is maintained below this threshold, osmotic agents have a tendency to leak into the most severely damaged areas of the brain. Furthermore, when given rapidly, large doses of osmotic agents may expand the circulating volume, elevate ICP, and produce hemodilution. Simultaneous administration of loop diuretics can offset this unwanted intravascular volume expanding effect. By dehydrating red blood cells, osmotic agents can also result in a decrease in hematocrit with a preserved or elevated hemoglobin concentration (pseudoanemia). If used for long periods, excessive diuresis depletes intravascular and/or intracellular volume, delaying return to normal consciousness.

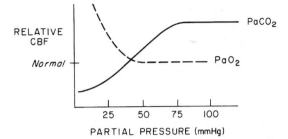

■ **FIGURE 34-3** Effect of arterial gas tensions on cerebral blood flow (CBF) in normal brain tissue (autoregulation intact). Whereas reductions of $PaCO_2$ lower CBF (and cerebral volume) in more or less linear fashion over the physiologic range, reductions in PaO_2 have an opposite effect that manifests only when the O_2 content of hemoglobin falls ($PaO_2 < 60$ mm Hg). Injured tissue may lose this ability to autoregulate flow in response to blood gas (or blood pressure) changes (see Fig. 34-4).

Rebound intracranial hypertension is a significant problem that may be seen after discontinuation of any osmotic agent. Doses of Mannitol that produce high osmolarity (>340 mOsm/dL) should be avoided because it may impair renal tubular function.

Hyperventilation

Hyperventilation is a rapid method to temporarily lower ICP. Acute reduction of $PaCO_2$ raises tissue pH, causing cerebral vasoconstriction in normally responsive cerebral vessels (Fig. 34-3). Within wide limits, reduced flow through normal brain tissue is well tolerated. As flow and vascular volume fall, ICP declines, thereby boosting CPP. By contrast, flow to the injured, poorly autoregulated brain actually improves because flow through injured areas is CPP dependent (Fig. 34-4). Although brief moderate hyperventilation tends to reduce ICP, improve CPP, and improve flow to damaged tissue, extreme

($PaCO_2 < 25$ mm Hg) or prolonged hyperventilation offsets this beneficial action by causing excessive vasoconstriction and global reduction of perfusion. (Reducing $PaCO_2$ is effective for 48 h at most, after which renal compensation restores acid–base status and eventually negates its effects.) For years it has been known that prolonged hyperventilation is associated with worse neurological outcomes than normocapnia. Thus, hyperventilation is best viewed as a stopgap measure to lower ICP for minutes to hours as other measures (i.e., osmotic diuretics, ventricular drainage, or craniotomy) are undertaken to definitively lower ICP. Although the therapeutic benefits of hyperventilation are debated, it is clear that hypoventilation should be avoided; increased blood flow and vascular volume can drive ICP quickly to life-threatening levels. Associated hypoxemia accentuates the risk, because like hypercapnia, hypoxemia is a cerebral vasodilator of brain tissue. If used within the first 72 h of brain injury, special caution should be exercised not to interrupt hyperventilation for more than brief periods. (For example, prolonged ventilator disconnections to see whether the patient has spontaneous respirations are ill advised during this period.) If instituted, hyperventilation should be terminated in stages (over 24 to 48 h) to avoid causing rebound increases in ICP.

Corticosteroids

Corticosteroids reduce cerebral edema associated with tumors, but there is no evidence that they benefit patients with cerebral edema from head trauma or metabolic encephalopathy. Corticosteroids do, however, increase the risk of nosocomial infection and hyperglycemia.

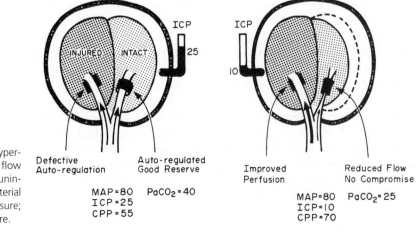

■ **FIGURE 34-4** Effects of hyperventilation on cerebral blood flow and volume to injured and uninjured brain. MAP, mean arterial pressure; ICP, intracranial pressure; CPP, cerebral perfusion pressure.

Ventriculostomy Drainage

The removal of CSF may acutely lower ICP, especially when the system is poised on the steep portion of the intracranial pressure–volume curve. Because CSF production is a continuous process, the effects of intermittent CSF removal are transient (<2 h). Equipment for continuously venting the CSF to maintain ICP at or below a given hydrostatic level are effective in reducing ICP but increase the risk of infection. Nonetheless, CSF drainage makes consummate sense in the setting of aqueductal blockage (by clotted blood in the fourth ventricle, for example). Here, venting CSF output until clot lysis occurs (approx. 5 to 7 days) may prove lifesaving. By contrast, withdrawal of spinal fluid from the lumbar region may precipitate brain herniation by increasing the pressure gradient across the tentorium.

Surgery

A direct attack on the cause of increased ICP may be indicated in such conditions as obstructive hydrocephalus (improved by shunting), tumor, or large but focal hemorrhage (particularly into the cerebellum). Similarly, prompt evacuation of a large subdural hematoma may be lifesaving and, if necessary, can be performed at the bedside. Removal of a cranial flap may be an effective maneuver to allow edematous brain room to expand outside the skull.

Therapy to Minimize Cerebral Oxygen Requirements

Fever and agitation greatly increase cerebral metabolic requirements and should be prevented. Nonsteroidal anti-inflammatory agents like ibuprofen are much more effective than acetaminophen for fever reduction. It is a serious mistake to use methods of temperature control (e.g., cooling blankets) that induce shivering, a maneuver that dramatically increases oxygen consumption. Even if not shivering, conscious patients are made much more uncomfortable, thereby increasing cerebral metabolism and raising intrathoracic and intracerebral pressures. Although neuromuscular blocking drugs will effectively prevent shivering, they obliterate physical examination findings and predispose to a host of other complications including skin breakdown and myopathy. Neither corticosteroids nor meperidine are effective antishivering agents.

High-dose barbiturates decrease cerebral metabolism and blood flow and therefore have been hypothesized to have a neuroprotective effect, but their role in intracranial hypertension is controversial, given conflicting data suggesting benefit and harm. Thus, barbiturate therapy for head injury is typically a last-ditch effort and one that probably mandates ICP monitoring. Pentobarbital is the drug most commonly used in loading doses of 10 mg/kg over 30 to 60 min followed by infusions of 1 mg/kg/h. Tachyphylaxis occurs quickly making rapidly escalating doses necessary. Barbiturates induce hypotension with such frequency that volume expansion and vasopressor use are almost always necessary. These drugs also obliterate both the EEG signals and the clinical parameters used for neurological assessment. As an alternative to barbiturates, benzodiazepines and propofol can be used to reduce cerebral oxygen consumption. When sedative drugs are used to control intracranial hypertension, they are typically continued for 24 to 48 h after ICP has normalized and are then slowly tapered.

■ HEAD TRAUMA

Pathophysiology

High-velocity motor vehicle accidents and falls account for the vast majority of serious head and neck injuries. Head trauma from these incidents injures neural tissue by primary (direct brain tissue injury) or secondary mechanisms (hypoperfusion, vascular disruption, and increased ICP). The concussive forces produced by a blow to the head are usually greatest at the point of application and diametrically across the skull from the site of the blow (*contrecoup* injury). Bony prominences on the base of the skull also commonly cause injury, particularly to the inferior surfaces of the frontal and temporal lobes. Primary diffuse brain injury is characterized by immediate loss of consciousness as shearing forces disrupt RAS function. Unfortunately, prevention (e.g., helmets, seat belts, air bags) is all that can be offered to alter the course of the immediate primary brain injury. It is the secondary mechanisms of brain injury that can be influenced by skillful care.

Secondary brain injury is characterized by hypoxia, hypoperfusion, or increased ICP, resulting from tissue edema, hydrocephalus, or mass lesions (fluid/blood accumulations, epidural or subdural hematomas, intracerebral hemorrhage, abscess, or empyema). Secondary mechanisms are responsible for approximately half the deaths following head injury. Therefore, optimal management of these consequences could theoretically reduce mortality by as much as 50%. Global ischemia and hypoxia and vascular disruption also increase the severity of cerebral injury. The clinical hallmark of secondary injury is a progressive decline in level of consciousness after the initial injury.

Initial Management

Nearly half of all head injury patients have other accompanying life-threatening medical problems (i.e., hypotension, hypoventilation, hypoxemia, or hypercarbia) on arrival at the hospital. Although often visually impressive, hemorrhage from scalp wounds is rarely life threatening and is almost always easily controlled by direct pressure. Potentially lethal thoracic or abdominal injuries must be sought and corrected simultaneously by a multidisciplinary team. An unstable airway, ineffective ventilation, and reduced oxygen delivery resulting from hypovolemia or anemia must be promptly corrected. The route of intubation and method for intubation need to be individualized. If direct laryngoscopy is chosen, "in line" traction should be used to stabilize the spine without neck hyperextension. Fiberoptic intubation and nasotracheal intubation are useful alternatives to avoid manipulation of a potentially unstable spine. Basilar skull fractures or facial fractures usually contraindicate nasotracheal intubation. Awake or rapid-sequence intubation is preferred for most head trauma victims because they often have full stomachs predisposing to aspiration. Supplemental oxygen and mechanical ventilation should be used to counter respiratory acidosis and hypoxemia. PEEP should be used judiciously to reverse refractory hypoxemia, recognizing that PEEP raises the outflow pressure of the cerebral veins and potentially increases the formation of cerebral edema. Hypotension should be avoided. MAP should be restored to at least 60 mm Hg using fluids to first replace intravascular volume depletion followed by vasopressors. (Many practioners advocate a much higher MAP of 90 mm Hg.) It is not known if monitoring central venous pressure (CVP), pulmonary artery occlusion pressure (PAOP) or cardiac output improves outcome compared to a simpler approach or restoring blood pressure and urine output. If invasive monitoring is undertaken a CVP 8 to 12 mm Hg or PAOP of 12 to 16 mm Hg is commonly

targeted even though the optimal goal value is unknown. Without strong data, a consensus has developed favoring norepinephrine over dopamine if a vasopressor is needed to increase perfusion pressure. Positioning the patient with the head elevated 30 degree or more will help limit the formation of cerebral edema, and at this inclination CPP is not impaired. Care should be taken to prevent flexion or rotation of the neck, which can exacerbate spinal injury and obstruct jugular venous outflow, in turn lowering CPP. Following initial stabilization, complete physical and neurological exams and CT imaging of the head and neck should be performed.

Physical Examination

After assuring adequacy of the airway, oxygenation, and blood pressure, a rapid neurological examination should be conducted, including assessment of the GCS (see Table 34-3). The GCS is potentially useful as a prognostic tool and to help gauge the need for invasive ICP monitoring. Neurological examination of head-injured patients is often difficult when complicated by the ingestion of ethanol or other intoxicants. The physical examination of head trauma patients should look for evidence of penetrating wounds, spinal cord damage, and depressed or basilar skull fractures (evidenced by blood behind the tympanic membrane, CSF rhinorrhea, "raccoon eyes," or discoloration behind the ears—the Battle sign). Papilledema is a particularly useful finding in the head trauma patient, indicating an elevated ICP.

Radiographic Evaluation

It is difficult to give specific guidelines as to who should undergo CT of the brain. Practically speaking, these days almost all patients with a history of high-speed collision, fall, loss of consciousness, or strong blow to the head will be scanned. It is generally agreed that immediate CT scanning is indicated for patients with: (a) GCS scores less than 15, (b) focal neurological deficits, (c) evidence of skull fractures, (d) a deteriorating level of consciousness, and (e) planned immediate surgery. For most patients an uncontrasted study is sufficient to detect significant injuries. At a minimum, neurosurgical consultation should be obtained for all patients with intracranial hematoma and/or skull fracture. Any patient suspected of significant head injury should undergo precautions for spinal injury and radiographic evaluation of the spine.

Cranial Disruption

Linear skull fractures of the cranial vault are more common than basilar skull fractures and imply that a substantial blow has been sustained. Fractures of the vault are of particular significance when they traverse the course of the middle meningeal artery, suggesting the possibility of epidural hematoma. Depressed skull fractures or penetrating injuries produce damage as the inner table of the skull is driven inward, injuring vessels and the brain surface. Such injuries usually result from the impact of small, high-velocity objects and carry a high risk of bacterial infection. Injuries causing skull fractures are often associated with intracranial bleeding. (The risk of intracranial hematoma is at least 10-fold higher among patients with fractures than those without.)

Basilar skull fractures have unique associated injuries, but also serve as markers for the severity of the overall impact. Basilar fractures are seldom seen on plain radiographs and can be missed even by CT. CSF leakage into the sinuses is common when the floor of the middle cranial fossa is fractured. By contrast, CSF leak into the external auditory canals from temporal bone fractures is uncommon. Nasal bleeding occurs commonly when the floor of the anterior fossa is damaged. In such cases, transnasal tubes must not be inserted blindly because of the possibility of passage through the base of the skull into the brain. (The same precaution applies to stylet stiffened small bore feeding tubes.) Nasal packing should be avoided in patients with CSF leakage because of the increased risk of meningitis. Febrile patients with basilar skull fractures must be treated as if meningitis is present, employing LP and the early institution of antibiotics. Although recurrent meningitis is a feared complication of basilar skull fracture, CSF leaks seldom need surgical closure (<1% of all cases).

Injury to Brain Tissue

Cerebral contusion from rapid deceleration is the most common mechanism of brain injury. Subsequent cerebral edema and increased ICP may exacerbate damage. One form of this injury, the brainstem contusion, is characterized by intermittent agitation, disordered autonomic regulation, and episodic hyperthermia. Mass lesions and the effects of cerebral edema produce secondary brain injury by displacing cerebral contents across anatomic boundaries or by globally decreasing perfusion (Fig. 34-5). Translocation may occur through

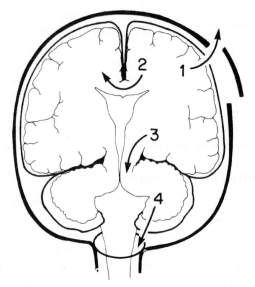

■ **FIGURE 34-5** Potential sites of brain herniation: (*1*) transcranial, (*2*) subfalcial, (*3*) transtentorial, and (*4*) foraminal.

bony defects or by subfalcial, transtentorial, or foraminal herniation.

Intracranial Hematoma

The risk of the three types of trauma-induced intracranial bleeding (epidural hematoma, subdural hematoma, and intracerebral hematoma) can be estimated by examination and knowledge of the presence or absence of a skull fracture. Presence of a skull fracture and a low GCS predict a high risk of intracranial hematoma. For example, patients with normal GCSs (i.e., 15) and no skull fractures have less than 1% risk of intracranial hematoma, whereas patients with GCS scores less than 8 with skull fractures have a 40% risk. It is vital to diagnose and surgically correct intracranial hematomas as rapidly as possible. Data indicate that delaying repair for a little as 4 h can triple the mortality rate (30% to 90%) of patients with this group of injuries. Adequate management of CPP, glucose, and blood pressure is instrumental.

Epidural hematoma occurs in a minority of patients (about 10%) with severe closed head injury and usually presents as a rapidly expanding clot in a patient with a linear skull fracture. (The accumulating blood is located between the dura and the skull.) Vascular disruption usually occurs where the fracture crosses the course of the middle meningeal artery, the dural sinuses, or the foramen magnum. Most epidural hematomas occur over the temporal lobes where the skull is thin and highly vascular. An enlarging epidural hematoma most commonly results in medial compression of the temporal lobe. Clinically, this process presents as loss of consciousness, contralateral hemiparesis, and a third nerve palsy with ipsilateral pupillary dilation. Only one third of patients have a classic "lucid interval." When severe, death eventually occurs as the midbrain is compressed against the tentorium. Because epidural hematoma has an associated mortality approaching 50%, it usually requires urgent neurosurgical intervention. Therefore, any trauma patient who demonstrates a linear skull fracture or who loses consciousness (even transiently) probably should be admitted to the hospital for observation.

Acute subdural hematoma, blood accumulation between the brain and the dura, is an expanding mass that results from cortical contusion and laceration of a meningeal vessel. It is more common than an epidural hematoma, occurring in about 20% of patients with serious closed head injury. Subdural hematoma is associated with high mortality and as a rule requires urgent surgical intervention. In contrast to epidural hematoma, which usually requires substantial force, subacute or chronic subdural hematoma may occur as the result of a seemingly trivial injury to enlarged dural venous sinuses. Subdural hematoma most frequently occurs in the elderly because cortical atrophy stretches the subdural veins, predisposing them to injury. A typical presentation of a subacute or chronic subdural hematoma is slowly progressive confusion, somnolence, and headache that leads eventually to hemiplegia. Anticoagulants greatly increase the risk of posttraumatic hematoma formation.

Intracerebral hematoma develops in about 40% of all cases of severe brain injury. The clinical presentation of intracerebral hematoma depends on the location of the bleeding. The CT scan is useful in delineating this mass, which appears initially as a dense intraparenchymal collection of blood. If an intracerebral hematoma produces mass effect, it should be surgically evacuated. Intracerebral hematoma often evolves over 12 to 24 h; therefore, a decrease in level of consciousness, increasing headache, or focal neurological signs should prompt a repeat scan.

Complications of Head Trauma

One of the most common complications of head trauma, increased ICP is discussed in detail above. Direct neuronal injury causes seizures with sufficient frequency that prophylactic use of an anticonvulsant

(e.g., phenytoin) is prudent for the first week after injury. Direct injury to the hypothalamus or pituitary or increased ICP may disrupt the normal secretion of hypophyseal hormones. Loss of antidiuretic hormone (ADH) may cause acute diabetes insipidus (DI). Unless it is due to direct hypophyseal vascular destruction, DI is usually an indicator of a poor prognosis, from prolonged increases in ICP. Such patients can produce massive volumes (>1 L/h) of dilute urine despite increasing serum osmolality. Typically, the serum sodium concentration exceeds 145 mEq/L at a time that urine specific gravity is below 1.003. Life-threatening hypovolemia and hyperosmolarity may result unless prompt treatment with hypotonic fluids and ADH are instituted. An empiric trial of aqueous vasopressin (5 units subcutaneously) is often diagnostic (see also Chapter 32). In the absence of DI, hypotension in the head-injured patient should always be assumed to be due to blood loss from an extracranial site. With the exception of adrenocorticotropic hormone (ACTH) deficiency, which may result in acute adrenal insufficiency, loss of other pituitary hormones (e.g., growth hormone, thyroid stimulating hormone) is not an urgent problem.

Disruption of the dura by penetrating trauma or boney fracture (e.g., basilar skull fracture) may provide a pathway for the entry of microorganisms into the CSF, resulting in recurrent posttraumatic meningitis. Nosocomial sinusitis resulting from obstruction of the sinus ostia by nasal tubes and impaired drainage in the supine position affects 10% to 15% of all head-injured patients. Serious head injury may also disrupt or block normal channels of communication of CSF. Such disruptions may cause obstructive hydrocephalus with subsequent elevations in ICP.

Erosive (stress) gastritis occurs with sufficient frequency, that H_2 blockers, proton pump inhibitors, or sucralfate is wise. Because head injury induces a hypermetabolic state, caloric requirements are elevated and nutritional supplementation is usually needed (see Chapter 16). After a brief period of posttraumatic ileus, enteral tube feeding is usually well tolerated until the patient can eat normally. Starting enteral feeding within the first 36 h of injury may even reduce the risk of infectious complications. In the patients with severe persistent neurologic deficits, consideration should be given to placement of a permanent feeding gastrostomy. This is most efficiently accomplished at the same time a permanent tracheostomy is created.

Although full-blown acute respiratory distress syndrome (ARDS) may result from some combination of aspiration, chest trauma, shock, and massive transfusion, milder acute lung injury often follows head injury alone. Many hypoxemic head-injured patients have normal chest radiographs. The mechanism of hypoxemia in these patients is likely related to autonomic alterations directly induced by the trauma. Neurogenic pulmonary edema may result from head trauma, presumably because of catecholamine-induced profound, transient venoconstriction. Therapy consists of supportive care using oxygen and intubation, mechanical ventilation, and PEEP when indicated. The more mundane but frequent pulmonary complications of aspiration pneumonitis and atelectasis usually respond to standard therapy. Aspiration risk can be minimized by avoiding bolus feeding and elevating the head of the bed at least to 30 degree. Atelectasis and "retained secretions" are best prevented and treated by maximizing activity, providing effective suctioning and encouraging deep breathing and coughing. These standard measures can be problematic for patients with increased ICP, because each tends to further raise the pressure. In the tenuous patient with intracranial hypertension, deep sedation and intratracheal lidocaine can be used to block increases in ICP induced by suctioning. As expected, bronchoscopy offers little advantage for secretion clearance in these patients because it, too, is a potent stimulus to raise ICP.

Severe head trauma causes the systemic activation of the clotting cascade probably through the release of brain thromboplastin into the circulation. Up to one fourth of all head-injured patients exhibit laboratory features of disseminated intravascular coagulation. Specific therapy is rarely required, as the defect is usually self-limited. DVT occurs in nearly half of unprotected patients after significant head and spinal cord injury. Prophylaxis is clearly indicated; however, substantial controversy exists over the best method. Because of the risk of anticoagulation-induced or aggravated intracranial bleeding early after injury, a combination of graded compression stockings and intermittent pneumatic compression devices is usually preferred initially but when the risk of bleeding diminishes, pharmacologic prophylaxis is clearly superior (see Chapter 23).

Decubitus ulcers are also a common problem for the head- and spine-injured patient. The best course of therapy is to prevent skin breakdown through use of padding, frequent repositioning, and maximizing activity. Especially high-risk patients may be treated with specialized therapeutic beds. Decubitus ulcers are discussed in detail in Chapter 18.

Monitoring the Brain-Injured Patient

Careful monitoring of the neurological exam and use of the GCS is helpful, especially in mild to moderate injury. Although no specific electroencephalographic (EEG) pattern defines etiology or prognosis in head trauma, the EEG is useful to monitor for seizures and document the suppression of brain activity in barbiturate-induced coma. Unfortunately, the ICU is an electrically hostile environment where EEG signal fidelity is often suboptimal. Serial CT scans also give valuable information regarding the nature and evolution of the injury process. However, the only way to accurately assess ICP in the seriously injured, comatose patient is to monitor it directly.

Recovery Phase

Recovery from reduced consciousness following cerebral trauma may be a prolonged process, much more so than following nontraumatic coma. It is not uncommon for head trauma victims to require a year or longer to maximize their level of function. Head trauma victims are fragile, even long after the injury. Once the acute insult subsides, vigilance must be maintained to ensure that reversible factors do not impede the return to normal function. All too often metabolic derangements (spontaneous or iatrogenic) are responsible for persistently depressed consciousness. Hyperosmolarity, hypovolemia, hyperglycemia, and hyponatremia are frequently induced by the therapies applied in the treatment of these disorders: diuretics, steroids, fluid restriction, and osmotic agents.

■ SPINAL CORD TRAUMA

Mechanisms

Spinal cord injuries most frequently occur to young people and involve the region of the spine subject to the greatest motion, the cervical area. Because the mechanism of spinal cord injury is usually one of high-speed, rapid-deceleration, other life-threatening traumatic injuries (intracranial, intrathoracic, or intra-abdominal) should be sought. Because they coexist so commonly, patients with spinal cord injury should be evaluated for head injury, and vice versa.

Spinal cord injury is called "complete" when there is no neurological function below the level of injury or "incomplete" when some distal function remains. Aside from interrupting its blood supply, the spinal cord can be injured by three basic mechanisms: flexion–rotation, compression, or hyperextension. Cord contusion is the feature common to all three mechanisms. A minority of cord injuries result from primary vascular disruption. (Dissecting aortic aneurysm with or without concomitant cocaine use is probably the most common cause of vascular disruption.) Spinal cord injury should be suspected in every trauma patient with back or neck pain and sensory or motor deficits.

Flexion–rotation injury of the neck usually occurs when the neck is hyperflexed onto the trunk out of the midline axis, disrupting the posterior spinal ligament. Motor vehicle accidents are the most common cause. At a minimum, patients with flexion–rotation injury require closed reduction and traction. If radiographs demonstrate displacement of a vertebral body by greater than one half its width, instability and bilateral facet dislocation are likely. Displacement less than one half the width of the vertebral body suggests unilateral dislocation, a less-serious problem. Such injuries are potentially unstable after reduction, but fewer than 10% require surgery for fixation. If facets in the lumbar region become "locked," surgery is usually necessary.

Compression injuries most commonly result from diving accidents or falls from height. In this setting, bone fragments or expanding hematoma may lead to neural damage by protruding into the spinal cord. However, these injuries are inherently stable because spinal ligaments remain intact. The usual treatment is bed rest with skeletal traction.

Hyperextension ("whiplash") injuries in the cervical region are usually stable. These injuries occur in older patients with cervical arthritis and are frequently associated with bleeding into the spinal gray matter, producing a "central cord" syndrome.

Initial Management

All passive and active motion of the spine should be prevented in patients with suspected spinal injury. Adequate ventilation and circulation should be ensured and oxygen administered if hemoglobin saturation is below normal. Autonomic instability often occurs in the early phase, so mild hypotension is common. Judicious filling of the intravascular compartment is indicated, but because of disordered vasoregulation, it is important not to administer excessive volumes of fluid. Other measures key to the resuscitation of the trauma victim, such as airway control, venous access, and chest tube insertion, should be performed as required.

Physical Examination

Following spinal immobilization and stabilization of the airway and circulation, a detailed neurological examination should be conducted. Complete spinal cord disruption produces loss of all sensory and motor function below the level of the injury, initially resulting in flaccid paralysis and loss of deep tendon reflexes that lasts for 2 to 7 days—the "spinal shock" phase. Incomplete cord injuries carry a better prognosis because some function is retained distal to the level of the injury. In a cooperative patient, many clinically important injuries may be diagnosed at the bedside. If the patient is able to take a spontaneous deep breath, cervical roots C2 to C5 are probably intact and diaphragm function preserved. If the patient can raise and extend the arms, C5 to C7 are intact. The ability to open and close the hand assures function of C7 to T1, whereas the ability to elevate the legs confirms the integrity of L2 to L4. Wiggling the toes indicates that L5 to S1 roots are functional. Normal anal sphincter function implies preserved function of roots S3 to S5.

Three clinically important incomplete cord injury syndromes exist. The central cord syndrome results from hyperextension of cervical region in older patients with cervical spondylosis. The syndrome is aptly described as "inverse paralysis" because injury to the central portion of the cord disrupts arm motor function while leg strength is maintained. In the anterior cord syndrome, typically due to disruption of anterior spinal artery blood flow, sensory and motor function to the legs is lost as a result of ischemia of the spinothalamic and corticospinal tracts. However, because the posterior columns are intact, distal proprioception and vibratory sense are preserved. When just the left or right half of the spinal cord is transected, the Brown–Sequard syndrome, sometimes called "crossed hemiplegia," results. Loss of posterior column function leads to ipsilateral loss of proprioception and vibratory sensation. Interruption of the corticospinal tract causes ipsilateral motor loss. Loss of contralateral pain and temperature sensation results from spinothalamic tract transection.

Radiographic Evaluation

After initial examination and stabilization, radiographs of the spine should be obtained. In many centers, the use of plain radiographs has now been supplanted by immediate CT scanning. Nonetheless, more than two thirds of all spinal injuries may be seen on a single lateral view of the spine if proper technique is used. Even in cases where bone injury does not occur, ligamentous injury may cause an expanding hematoma causing cord compression. Thoracic and lumbar radiographs should be obtained if there is any suspicion of injury in those locations based on patient complaints or by examination. It is important to visualize all seven cervical vertebrae because C7 is the vertebra most commonly injured but least commonly seen on portable radiographs. A "swimmer's view" or traction on the patient's arms may aid visualization of C7 and T1. The alignment of the anterior and posterior aspects of each vertebral body, the alignment of the spinolaminal lines, and the contour of the spinous processes and vertebral bodies should be reviewed. The prevertebral space should be examined for evidence of widening because of hemorrhage. Open mouth views should be obtained to look for odontoid fractures. Radiographs should visualize the entire spine if a fracture is found. (Up to 20% of patients have multiple levels of injury.) Even when patients have no radiographic evidence of spinal cord injury, the cervical spine should remain immobilized until the patient can cooperate with a clinical examination searching for pain with motion or tenderness to palpation.

Treatment

Short-course, high-dose methylprednisolone (30 mg/kg bolus then 5.4 mg/kg/h for the first day) improves neurologic outcome in many cord-injured patients, but does not benefit patients with anterior spinal artery syndrome (loss of motor function with preserved sensory function). Use of corticosteroids for longer than 24 h predisposes to infection and possibly gastrointestinal (GI) ulceration without convincing benefit and therefore is contraindicated.

Neurosurgical consultation should be sought at the earliest possible time. Although the indications for immediate surgery in spinal cord trauma are controversial, commonly accepted criteria include (a) progressive loss of neurological function because of suspected epidural or subdural bleeding, (b) a foreign body in the spinal canal, (c) CSF leak, and (d) bony instability requiring immobilization.

Complications

Progressive neurological impairment is only one of the many complications of spinal cord injury. The most significant of these are iatrogenically induced by spinal manipulation or inappropriate administration of fluids or vasopressors to alter blood pressure. In the first 48 h following spinal cord injury, the level of neurological impairment often ascends by 1 to 2 vertebral levels.

Cardiovascular

Cord lesions above the T6 level interrupt sympathetic outflow, resulting in vasodilation, bradycardia, and hypothermia. Even in young, healthy persons, the loss of sympathetic tone usually produces a stable supine blood pressure in the range of 100/60 mm Hg. Hypovolemia, infection, or placement in the upright position often precipitates profound hypotension. The blood pressure is acceptable if urine output remains good and cerebration is clear. However, if MAP falls below 70 mm Hg, a fluid challenge may be indicated; invasive monitoring can help inform proper therapy. Measures to reduce venous capacitance, including abdominal binding, Trendelenburg positioning, and compression stockings, may help avoid postural hypotension.

Bradycardia often accompanies hypotension due to cord injury and does not require treatment unless symptomatic. Accommodation of the sympathetic and parasympathetic responses usually produces normal heart rates within 3 to 5 days following injury. However, unopposed vagal stimulation from pain, hollow viscus distention, hypoxemia, or endotracheal suctioning may produce profound bradycardia. If symptomatic bradycardia not caused by hypoxemia occurs, atropine, isoproterenol, or temporary pacing is useful. It is the loss of compensatory tachycardia early in the course of spinal cord injury that makes iatrogenic pulmonary edema common following even modest fluid administration. If unequivocal tachycardia is present in a hypotensive patient with spinal cord injury, suspect another condition such as severe sepsis, internal hemorrhage, or hypovolemia. Because autonomic paresis eliminates crucial vasoconstrictive reflexes, these patients have very limited stress reserves.

Respiratory

Respiratory impairment, the most common complication of spinal cord injury, results from respiratory muscle weakness, rib fractures, hemopneumothorax, lung contusion, and aspiration. Cervical roots 3, 4, and 5 innervate the diaphragm. Therefore, interruption of the cord above this level in an unsupported patient rapidly leads to apnea and death. Cervical spine injuries also cause problems when expiratory muscle weakness impairs cough and secretion clearance. The forced vital capacity (FVC) should be monitored several times daily in the acute phase of spinal cord injury. As a rule of thumb, such problems are unusual if FVC exceeds 20 mL/kg. If the FVC is less than this value in patients with injuries below the C5 level, direct injury to the phrenic nerve(s) should be suspected.

Because quadriplegic patients have little ventilatory reserve, any condition that further impairs work of breathing or mandates an increased minute ventilation may lead rapidly to fatigue and ventilatory failure. Lesions above T10 most commonly cause respiratory difficulty by impairing cough, altering ventilation/perfusion distribution (causing hypoxemia), or decreasing inspiratory capacity. Low lung volumes and atelectasis occur not only because of intrinsic muscle weakness, but also because abdominal distention (often from ileus) limits inspiration. Ventilation may be further compromised by unopposed parasympathetic responses that cause bronchorrhea and bronchoconstriction and increase the risk of vomiting and aspiration. Patients with spinal cord injury are particularly sensitive to the effects of neuromuscular paralytic agents.

Although seemingly paradoxical, quadriplegic patients often ventilate best in the supine position. Their only potential muscle of respiration (the diaphragm) is "cocked" into optimal position by such a posture through the upward pressure of the abdominal contents. Conversely, patients with isolated diaphragmatic paralysis ventilate best when fully erect; upright positioning minimizes the cephalad pressure of the abdominal contents against the flaccid diaphragm. This action increases lung volume and helps stabilize the diaphragm during contraction of the accessory muscles of inspiration. Limitations of vital capacity and forcefulness of cough predispose spinal-cord-injured patients to pneumonia.

Genitourinary

Urinary tract complications (urinary tract infection, renal failure) are the most common cause for late death in spinal-cord-injured patients. Continuous urinary catheterization is probably indicated early in the hospital course to monitor urine output. Later, intermittent catheterization is preferred because of its reduced risk of infection. Micturition may be impaired for months following spinal cord injury. Regular surveillance cultures of urine help to detect infection at an early stage. Prophylactic antibiotics may prevent bacteremia but are unlikely to maintain sterile urine in patients with indwelling catheters.

Gastrointestinal

Immediately following spinal cord injury, ileus may occur that typically lasts 3 to 4 days. Ileus is likely to be protracted if spinal cord injury is accompanied by retroperitoneal hemorrhage. In most patients, a nasogastric tube should be inserted until bowel sounds return. Daily measurements of abdominal girth may also help assess GI motility and the possibility of colonic impaction. In cord-injured patients, the combination of tachycardia, hypotension, and absent bowel sounds should prompt consideration of an acute abdomen. (Pain may be absent or atypical because of sensory neurologic deficits.)

Often there is no certain way to rule out intra-abdominal catastrophe, short of laparotomy or paracentesis, though abdominal CT can provide some guidance. Pain referred to the shoulder or scapula is a particularly valuable sign of abdominal inflammation in spinal-cord-injured patients.

Nutrition may be safely withheld for up to a week before caloric supplementation is begun. When ileus resolves, enteral feedings are preferred if feasible because of improved gut function, reduced cost, and avoidance of catheter-related infections. Peptic ulcer disease is common following spinal cord injury; enteral feeding, proton pump inhibitors, and histamine blockers are useful preventative measures. As soon as bowel sounds return and enteral feeding begins, a program of bowel care with regular evacuation and stool softeners should be started to prevent constipation and impaction. The level of the spinal cord lesion will dictate whether evacuation is spontaneous, reflex, or manually induced.

Cutaneous

Skin breakdown is a costly and potentially lethal complication of spinal cord injury that presents a central focus for nursing care. When the skin is disrupted, numerous microorganisms infect the wound causing local infections and make sepsis possible. Padding, frequent repositioning, physical therapy, and the use of rotating or air-cushioned beds are helpful in prevention. (The problem of skin breakdown is discussed in detail in Chapter 18.) Cord-injured patients (particularly quadriplegic patients) should not be placed in the prone position because of the possibility of hypoventilation, hypoxemia, and bradycardia, occasionally fatal.

Miscellaneous

After the return of spinal reflexes, patients with lesions above the T6 level may develop episodes characterized by hypertension, diaphoresis, pilo-erection, and flushing. This syndrome, autonomic hyperreflexia, must be recognized because it can prove fatal unless rapidly reversed by a simple expedient decompression of an overdistended viscus (usually bowel or bladder). In patients with excessive sympathetic activity, a vagally mediated compensatory bradycardia often occurs.

Thromboembolism is nearly universal in the first 90 days after cord injury if patients are left unprotected. Altered autonomic reflexes accentuate the hemodynamic impact of embolism. Prophylactic anticoagulants are effective, but there are risks of provoking hemorrhage in the early phase. The combination of elastic and pneumatic compression stockings is usually used until anticoagulants can be safely administered.

■ BRAIN DEATH

9 Because the brain is the organ most sensitive to deprivation of oxygen and perfusion, its function may be irretrievably lost despite preservation of other bodily functions. Most cases of hypoxic brain injury do not meet the criteria for brain death. Firm criteria for diagnosing brain death are important to establish to prevent wasting valuable medical resources and conversely to avoid premature abandonment of hope for potentially salvageable patients. Even with aggressive support, patients meeting brain death criteria rarely survive beyond a few days. To diagnose brain death, the etiology of coma must be known with reasonable certainty. Hypothermia, drug overdose, profound hypercarbia, neuromuscular blockade, and shock must be excluded. It must be reasonably concluded that no significant quantity of sedative, narcotic, or anesthetic drugs remain in the body. Furthermore, if clinical criteria alone are used to determine brain death, the patient is best observed

over a period of time (approx. 24 h) to document the stability of the clinical picture. Seizure activity and decerebrate or decorticate posturing are inconsistent with the diagnosis; however, reflexes of purely spinal cord origin are compatible. To confirm brain death, cerebral function must be absent at hemispheric, midbrain, pontine, and medullary levels. Lack of cortical function is evidenced by a totally unreceptive and unresponsive state. Patients in a persistently vegetative state lack awareness and responsiveness but appear awake because RAS arousal pathways remain intact. Such patients do not meet brain death criteria. Patients with destructive lesions of the base of the pons that give rise to the "locked in" syndrome also appear unresponsive. Careful testing, however, reveals that these patients are aware but unable to respond, except for eye opening and vertical eye movements. Midbrain death is confirmed by demonstrating the absence of pupillary, corneal, oculocephalic, oculovestibular, and gag reflexes. Absent pupillary activity indicates loss of midbrain function. Inability to evoke eye movements confirms lost pontine function. Medullary dysfunction is ensured by demonstrating apnea when the patient is challenged by a hypercarbic stimulus. Apnea testing is performed by interrupting positive pressure ventilation while continuing oxygenation. After preoxygenation, supplemental O_2 is supplied and the patient is observed for respiratory effort over a prolonged period of time. Such precautions ensure that the patient remains adequately oxygenated though unventilated. A $PaCO_2$ greater than 60 mm Hg must be attained to ensure adequate ventilatory stimulation. In apneic patients with intact circulation, the $PaCO_2$ normally rises 3 to 5 mm Hg/min. Therefore, knowledge of the baseline $PaCO_2$ can be used to predict the apneic time necessary to ensure a $PaCO_2$ above 60 mm Hg. (In general, 5 to 10 min of apnea are required if the baseline $PaCO_2$ is normal.) Alternatively end-tidal CO_2 monitoring can be substituted for blood gas measurements.

For *legal* reasons, some localities require confirmatory EEGs, somatosensory evoked potentials, brain perfusion scans, transcranial Doppler flow studies, or other tests to document absence of cerebral activity or perfusion, but rarely are such tests necessary to establish a *medical* diagnosis of brain death. Two common exceptions are patients with high spinal cord injury who will always "fail" the apnea test because of the inability to power ventilation, and patients with severe chronic lung disease who are unresponsive to the ventilation stimulating effects of hypercarbia. Confirmatory testing may also be helpful in the morbidly obese patient where respiratory effort can be difficult to detect. Even confirmatory tests are not foolproof. Isoelectric EEGs have been recorded for days after presentation of patients with drug-induced coma and may also occur in patients who have lost cortical function but who retain brainstem activity (neocortical death). Such patients usually demonstrate a vegetative state in which arousal is intact but awareness is lacking. Brain death may also be confirmed by using contrast angiography to demonstrate absence of cerebral flow.

■ SUGGESTED READINGS

Adams HP, del Zoppo G, Alberts MJ, et al. Guidelines for the early management of adults with ischemic stroke. *Stroke.* 2007;38:1655–1711.

Alldredge BK, Gelb AM, Isaacs SM, et al. A comparison of lorazepam, diazepam, and placebo for the treatment of out-of-hospital status epilepticus. *N Engl J Med.* 2001;345(9):631–637.

Booth CM, Boone RH, Tomlinson G, et al. Is this patient dead, vegetative, or severely neurologically impaired? Assessing outcome for comatose survivors of cardiac arrest. *JAMA.* 2004;291(7):870–879.

Broderick J, Connolly S, Feldman E, et al. Guidelines for the management of spontaneous intracerebral hemorrhage in adults. *Stroke.* 2007; 38:1–23.

Dutton RP, McCunn M. Traumatic brain injury. *Curr Opin Crit Care.* 2003; 9(6):503–509.

Fakhry SM, Trask AL, Waller MA, et al. Management of brain-injured patients by an evidence-based medicine protocol improves outcomes and decreases hospital charges. *J Trauma.* 2004;56(3): 492–499.

Fang JF, Chen RJ, Lin BC, et al. Prognosis in presumptive hypoxic-ischemic coma in nonneurologic trauma. *J Trauma.* 1999;47(6): 1122–1125.

Marik P, Chen K, Varon J, et al. Management of increased intracranial pressure: A review for clinicians. *J Emerg Med.* 1999;17(4): 711–719.

Marik PE, Varon J. The management of status epilepticus. *Chest.* 2004; 126:582–591.

Marik PE, Varon J, Trask T. Management of head trauma. *Chest.* 2002; 122(2):699–711.

Mayer SA, Brun NC, Begtrup K, et al. Efficacy and safety of recombinant activated factor VII for acute intracerebral hemorrhage. *N Engl J Med.* 2008;358:2127–2137.

Provencio JJ, Bleck TP, Connors AF Jr. Critical care neurology. *Am J Respir Crit Care Med.* 2001;164(3):341–345.

Stocchetti N, Maas AI, Chieregato A, et al. Hyperventilation in head injury: A review. *Chest.* 2005;127(5):1812–1827.

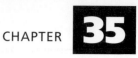

Chest Trauma

Coauthored with David Dries, MD

■ EPIDEMIOLOGY

Almost 500,000 Americans suffer chest trauma each **1** year, accounting for approximately 20% of all hospital-treated injuries. Chest injuries directly result in 20% to 25% of all trauma deaths and may contribute significantly to mortality in another quarter of them. The chest wall, pleural space, and lungs are involved in the great majority of chest injuries (Table 35-1). Although serious burns, crush injuries, and gunshot wounds account for considerable morbidity, in most cases the wounds are nonpenetrating and result from a misadventure involving a motor vehicle. When a vehicular accident proves fatal, more than one half of the deaths are directly attributable to severe *thoracic* trauma. Most deaths occur at the scene of the accident as a result of a catastrophic, unsalvageable injury, such as aortic transection or massive neurological injury. Fortunately, most patients who live long enough to be transported to a hospital will survive. Until the past quarter century, this was not the case; dramatically improved survival of seriously injured patients has accompanied their care in specialized intensive care environments.

■ MECHANISMS OF CHEST TRAUMA

Penetrating Chest Injuries

Knife and gunshot wounds account for the majority of penetrating chest injuries. Of these, knife wounds tend to be more survivable, as their damage is usually confined to a limited area. The injury caused by a gunshot wound depends not only on the path of the bullet, but also on the energy delivered per round, the number of impacting rounds, and the characteristics of the projectile (solid point vs. hollow point). Although the path taken by the projectile can be inferred from the entrance and exit wounds, the trajectory may be altered by ricochet off bony structures, and the damage tract may be

TABLE 35-1 THORACIC ORGAN INJURY AS A FRACTION OF ALL BODY TRAUMA

INJURY	PERCENTAGE[a]
Chest wall	45
Pulmonary	26
Hemothorax	25
Pneumothorax	20
Heart	9
Diaphragm	7
Aorta and great vessels	4
Esophagus	0.5
Miscellaneous	21

[a]15,047 patients.

Source: From North America Trauma Outcome Study, American College of Surgery Committee on Trauma, 1986.

much wider than the narrow tract of the missile itself because of the wide-ranging explosive effect that accompanies passage of the high-speed bullet through tissue. Moreover, depending on the phase of the respiratory cycle during which entry occurred, a bullet may traverse the diaphragm to injure the high abdominal structures even when entrance and exit wounds align above the costal margin. Bullet wounds below the margin of the scapula posteriorly and below the nipple anteriorly must be considered to involve both the chest and abdomen. Computed tomogram (CT) scanning has replaced endoscopy and vascular constrast studies as the imaging modality of choice in the setting of penetrating and blunt thoracic trauma. Endoscopy and vascular studies play a secondary role after screening CT evaluation but frequently are no longer required. CT scanning can be particularly valuable when a projectile is suspected to traverse the mediastinum. Tracks of stab wounds and gunshot wounds can be followed with CT imaging. Though CT imaging has improved our ability to identify injury to the diaphragm, operative examination remains the *"gold standard"* for this specific component of the evaluation.

Blunt Chest Injuries

Blunt chest trauma may result from several mechanisms—direct, indirect, compression, contusion, deceleration, or blast. Blast injuries result not only from the inertial impact of the shock wave, but also from decompressive implosion that occurs

behind the passing shock wave front. Another important mechanism is *"spalling"*—the disruption of interfacial tissues that occurs as the passing shock wave front releases energy in transition between tissue and gas. Because of the latter *"depth charge"* like effect, blast injuries exert disproportionate damage to gas-containing organs, such as the lung.

Blunt chest trauma may involve pneumothorax, neurologic dysfunction, respiratory failure, or cardiovascular instability. The principles underlying our general approach to such problems, which are common across a wide spectrum of critical illness, are detailed elsewhere (see Chapters 8, 34, 24, and 4). The current discussion focuses on those mechanical problems unique to blunt (nonpenetrating) chest injury. Rib fractures, increased intracavitary pressures, and shearing forces are the primary mechanisms producing intrathoracic injury in blunt chest trauma. Abdominal events frequently affect pulmonary and cardiovascular function, and in the trauma context the adominal compartment syndrome (ACS) deserves special attentions.

Rib and Sternal Fractures

During chest trauma, older patients who have inflexible ribs frequently sustain bony fractures that directly injure the lung at its perimeter. By contrast, the increased chest wall flexibility of younger patients tends to allow direct energy transfer to the intrathoracic organs without rib breakage. In young patients, rib disarticulations are more common than rib fractures but result in similar physiological consequences.

Rib fracture, the most common form of thoracic injury, usually occurs in the midchest (ribs 5 to 9) along the posterior axillary line (the point of maximal stress). The uppermost ribs are damaged less frequently because of their intrinsic strength and protection by the shoulder girdle and clavicle. Therefore, fractures of the upper ribs imply a very forceful blow and should raise concern regarding coexisting injury to the major airways or great vessels. On the other hand, the relative suppleness of the lowermost ribs makes them less prone to breakage. For that reason, fracture of the lower ribs (9 to 11) suggests an unusually powerful regional impact and the possibility of concurrent splenic, hepatic, or renal injuries. The number of rib fractures roughly correlates with the force of impact and the risk of serious internal injury and death. The history and clinical examination should raise the suspicion of rib fractures, but even when present, fractures may not be confirmed by conventional radiographic views. (Initial plain chest radiographs fail to reveal as many as one half of all rib fractures.) Although oblique filming is the traditional approach to subtle fracture detection, three-dimensional reconstruction of a helical (spiral) CT represents current state-of-the-art imaging for such problems.

Certain features of the radiograph offer clues to etiology. For example, aligned fractures of multiple ribs ("curbstone fractures") usually result from striking a sharp edge. *"Cough fractures"* most frequently involve ribs 6 to 9 in the posterior axillary line. Although cough fractures produce significant pain, they generally are not displaced and therefore are difficult to detect.

Rib fractures often injure adjacent tissues as displaced rib ends or fragments cause lung laceration or contusion, pneumothorax, and hemothorax. Because the intercostal and internal mammary arteries are perfused under systemic pressure, large hemothoraces can occur when these vessels are disrupted by fractures. Pain associated with rib fractures frequently causes splinting, hypoventilation, secretion retention, and atelectasis—complications are minimized by adequate narcotic analgesia, intercostal nerve blocks, or epidermal analgesia. Fractures of multiple ribs at two or more sites may produce a free-floating, unstable section of the chest wall known as a flail segment. Hypoxemia resulting from contusion and hypoventilation is an almost universal consequence. Forceful displacement also may disrupt chondral attachments, producing a flail sternum. Discovery of a flail sternum should raise concern for underlying blunt cardiac injury.

Sternal fracture implies a very forceful blow and usually occurs in high-speed motor vehicle accidents when an unrestrained driver strikes the steering wheel or when automobile shoulder harnesses are used without lap restraints. Complaints of pain and tenderness to palpation are signs indicating that CT of the chest should be obtained. Contemporary CT imaging identifies mediastinal vacular injury and is a valued screening tool along with ultrasound for pericardial fluid collections. Echocardiography is the optimal noninvasive test for delineation of cardiac chamber function and identification of pericardial fluid collections. Occasionally, the diagnosis can be made by palpating a "step" where two sternal segments are askew. Although sternal fracture may precipitate respiratory failure and delay weaning by causing pain and altering chest wall mechanics, its greatest significance lies as a potential marker of associated cardiac and bronchial injuries.

Increased Intracavitary Pressures

Abrupt elevation of intracavitary pressures may rupture any air-filled or fluid-filled structure unbraced for the impact. Leak of orogastric secretions after esophageal rupture may result in mediastinitis or empyema. Alveolar rupture may cause pneumothorax, pneumomediastinum, or pulmonary contusion/hemorrhage. Sudden increases of intra-abdominal pressure (IAP) can rupture the diaphragm, herniating the abdominal contents into the chest. Unprotected by the liver, the left hemidiaphragm is at greater risk. By a similar mechanism, a distended stomach or urinary bladder also may rupture when the chest or abdomen is struck forcefully.

Shearing Forces

To varying degrees, all intrathoracic structures are tethered to adjacent tissues. Consequently, shearing forces produced by differential rates and directions of organ motion may cause visceral or vascular tears. Aortic rupture is the most serious injury produced by this mechanism; however, tracheobronchial disruption also may result from deceleration-induced shearing. Direct blows or rapid deceleration may tear pulmonary microvessels, causing pulmonary contusion. If the leak from these vessels is sufficient to form a discrete fluid collection, a pulmonary hematoma may form.

■ INITIAL MANAGEMENT OF CHEST TRAUMA

Most chest trauma can be managed with some combination of oxygen, analgesics, fluid replacement, and tube thoracostomy. Thoracotomy is necessary in only 10% to 15% of all cases. Initial therapy should consist of ensuring the ABCs: airway, breathing, and circulation. When patency of the airway, adequacy of ventilatory power, or stability of respiratory drive is uncertain, intubation is indicated. Positive-pressure ventilation is initiated for reduced respiratory drive, unduly labored breathing or hypoxemia, or when pain or profoundly deranged chest wall mechanics prevent adequate spontaneous ventilation. After auscultation of the chest to ensure adequate airflow, a portable chest radiograph should be obtained to search for pneumothorax and intrathoracic vascular injury. The plain chest radiograph is insufficient to rule out major intrathoracic vascular injury, however. CT imaging has replaced the plain chest radiograph and arteriograhy in this regard. Tension pneumothorax (discussed later) is of particular concern, as the associated intrathoracic pressures not only impede venous return but also compress the contralateral lung. The abdominal compartment syndrome, a problem that is caused by edema of intra-abdominal viscera or retroperitoneal bleeding, often develops toward during the resuscitative phase of management (see following). An ultrasonic survey of vital zones, an extended focused abdominal sonogram for trauma (FAST) that includes the upper abdominal and lower thoracic compartments, pelvic region, and heart, can point to the need for urgent intervention. When it can be undertaken expeditiously and safely, CT adds considerably to the level of diagnostic confidence. When time permits and uncertainty exists, three-dimensional reconstruction of data obtained by volumetric CT scanning can be of particular value in planning therapy. Because patients with chest trauma often have severe extrathoracic injuries as well, careful examination should be performed of the head, spine, and abdomen looking for associated trauma. Spine data can be obtained from torso CT scans.

Although other problems (such as arrhythmia, myocardial infarction, tamponade, or tension pneumothorax) must always be considered, hypotension that occurs immediately after thoracic injury usually is the result of hypovolemia. Therefore, the early insertion of two large-bore peripheral intravenous catheters is highly advisable. At the time of catheter insertion, blood should be obtained for determinations of electrolytes, creatinine, hematocrit, coagulation parameters, toxicologic screening, and blood cross-matching. When surface veins can be cannulated, the need for central venous catheterization is controversial; equivalent or greater volumes of fluid can be infused per unit time through large peripheral catheters, and there is real risk of iatrogenic complications from central line placement in the busy setting of the trauma suite. Hypovolemia can result from injury to low-pressure (pulmonary or systemic veins) or to high-pressure systemic vessels. Bleeding from veins often will subside spontaneously, whereas arterial disruption usually requires open surgical intervention or, in selected cases, endovascular stent repair. Hypotension is not always the result of hypovolemia; pneumothorax and cardiac tamponade cause hypotension, partly by impeding the return of venous blood to the heart. Hence, constant vigilance for the development of neck vein distension or a quiet hemithorax must be maintained. **3**

■ SPECIFIC CONDITIONS

The problems of pneumothorax and barotrauma are covered in detail in Chapter 8.

Bronchial and Tracheal Disruptions

Fracture of the first two ribs, sternum and clavicle, are the most common bony injuries associated with airway disruption. Hemoptysis, lobar or whole lung atelectasis, subcutaneous emphysema, pneumomediastinum, and pneumothorax that fail to improve with tube thoracostomy are potential signs of major airway disruption. (The occurrence of bilateral pneumothoraces after blunt trauma strongly suggests this possibility.) Most (>80%) airway disruptions due to blunt trauma occur within 2 cm of the carina in the form of a spiral tear of the main bronchi or a longitudinal tear in the posterior membranous portion of the trachea (Fig. 35-1). **4**

Timely recognition and management of airway disruption is important to avert the atelectasis, infection, and bronchial stenosis associated with delayed repair. Fiberoptic bronchoscopy allows detection of major airway injury and facilitates selective intubation with a dual-lumen tube. On

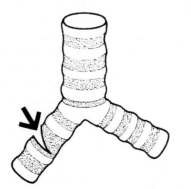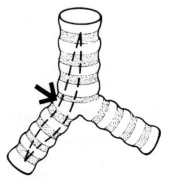

■ **FIGURE 35-1** Sites of tracheobronchial disruption. Bronchial tears usually occur posteriorly, within an inch of the carina and most often in the right side.

the affected side, an attempt is made to position the inflatable cuff distal to the site of disruption. Partial disruption may not be detected until bronchial stenosis and atelectasis occur several weeks later. Because complete disruption generally is recognized earlier than partial disruption, it is associated with fewer long-term complications.

Hemothorax

The presence of blood in the pleural space or hemothorax can arise from either thoracic or abdominal sources. Thoracic sources include lacerated lung parenchyma, torn intercostal or internal mammary arteries, or the heart and great vessels. Hemothorax occurs from an abdominal source in the setting of diaphragmatic laceration with associated abdominal injury—typically to the liver or spleen. Arteriography is usually diagnostic of hemothorax and may be therapeutic if embolization of bleeding vessels is feasible. On CT images, Hounsfield unit quantitation confirms the presence of blood in the chest.

Management of hemothorax is based on evacuation of the pleural space of blood and re-expansion of the lung. Typically, this is accomplished with tube thoracostomy. Apposition of visceral and parietal pleura provides definitive control of hemorrhage. Patients presenting many hours after injury with a large amount of chest blood typically have slow accumulation rather than rapid bleeding, particularly if hemodynamically stable. If an acute hemothorax cannot be drained because of clotting in the chest tube, operative drainage may be necessary. Surgical options include open thoracotomy or video-assisted thoracoscopic surgery.

In general, admission to a monitored setting and observation are appropriate for patients remaining hemodynamically stable who have limited ongoing hemorrhage from the chest tube. Follow-up chest X-ray should be obtained to confirm evacuation of the pleural space. The need for emergent thoracotomy is suggested when initial output from the chest tube exceeds 1 L of blood or, where a lower initial volume is drained, continued output of 200 mL/h for 4 h. Repeat chest X-ray during the period of observation may be considered to confirm that reduction in chest tube output is not due to clotted hemothorax.

Pericardial Tamponade

Traumatic tamponade may be the result of aortic root disruption, coronary artery laceration, or rupture of the free ventricular wall. When cardiac rupture occurs, it usually is of the right atrium or ventricle **5** and is rapidly fatal. Early recognition of pericardial tamponade with prompt decompression and control of hemorrhage are the key components to patient survival following cardiac injury. The diagnosis of tamponade should be suspected when muffled heart sounds, hypotension, tachycardia, and elevated jugular pressure are noted. Such findings assume particular significance when a fractured sternum is discovered. (Note that in hypovolemic patients, signs of elevated central venous pressure may be absent.) Rising interpericardial pressure produces abnormalities in hemodynamic performance and cardiac perfusion which initially restrict ventricular filling and later diminish cardiac output, causing systemic signs of hypoperfusion. Unrecognized tamponade concludes with cardiovascular collapse and cardiac arrest. The classic picture of injury—muffled heart sounds, hypotension, tachycardia, and jugular venous distension—is frequently undetectable in the trauma room. Ultrasonography supports the diagnosis by demonstration of pericardial fluid or diastolic collapse of the right ventricle.

Anesthetic agents should be administered with extreme caution in untreated acute tamponade. Invasive hemodynamic monitoring may be useful but not always needed. In general, subxiphoid pericardial drainage confirms the diagnosis and is therapeutic. After pericardial drainage and hemodynamics are stabilized, the chest may be fully opened and injuries causing tamponade definitively addressed.

Cardiac Injury

Cardiac contusion should be considered whenever a convincing history indicates a significant blow to the chest (e.g., high-speed steering wheel or shoulder harness injury). Sternal fracture without other findings does not predict blunt cardiac injury or warrant monitoring. Common consequences of cardiac contusion include arrhythmias (most common), myocardial ischemia, and conduction system defects (particularly heart block). Contusion may transiently produce "stunned myocardium," impairing cardiac output. Elevated troponin levels help to confirm the diagnosis. Although the electrocardiogram (ECG) may demonstrate ST segment elevations that simulate myocardial infarction, reciprocal changes and Q waves are characteristically absent. Ventricular and supraventricular extrasystoles arise very commonly. Echocardiography, the modality of choice for acute evaluation, may reveal a focal area of hypokinetic myocardium. The supportive treatment of cardiac contusion includes close monitoring for arrhythmias, pump failure, and pericardial distention.

While any cardiac valve may be damaged by a severe blow to the heart, aortic and mitral valve injuries occur most commonly. Disruption of the tricuspid valve is implicated by a physical examination that demonstrates large jugular V waves and a systolic murmur that varies with respiration. Rupture of the chordae or papillary muscles can result in mitral valve insufficiency. Classically, evidence of reduced forward cardiac output is combined with a murmur, thrill, or overt pulmonary edema. Distinguishing among tamponade, valvular disruption and cardiac rupture can be accomplished using surface echocardiography, transesophageal echocardiography, or diagnostic cardiac catheterization (see Chapter 2).

Aortic Disruption and Dissection

The healthy aorta of a young person can withstand massive uniform elevations in transmural pressure (up to 2,000 mm Hg) but tolerates the shearing forces of impact injuries much less well. Most aortic ruptures occur just distal to the ligamentum arteriosum. (In a minority of cases, disruption occurs at the aortic root just above the aortic valve, in which case tamponade is commonly produced.) When rupture of the ascending aorta occurs, damage to the aortic valve or coronary arteries also is possible. Clues suggesting a high likelihood of vascular injury include a fatality in the same vehicle, fracture of the steering wheel by a driver, lateral impact at high speed, being an "ejected" passenger, or a fall from a height greater than 30 feet.

Aortic disruption, a result of abrupt deceleration, usually is fatal at the accident scene. Older patients are more likely to suffer aortic avulsion. Amazingly, no evidence of external trauma is present in many patients with fatal aortic rupture; neither rib nor sternal fractures are required for diagnosis. Typically, chest pain penetrates to the interscapular region. Aortic disruption may present as a stroke syndrome if the carotid or vertebral circulation is compromised. Occasionally, disruption of the aorta produces acute paraplegia as the anterior spinal artery takeoff is damaged. Some radiographic clues to aortic aneurysm or disruption are illustrated in Figure 35-2. Thoracic CT angiography has replaced contrast angiography as the diagnostic modality of choice. Although possible, tears and disruptions of the pulmonary artery rarely occur in the absence of penetrating injury. Many aortic injuries are now repaired using endovascular stents.

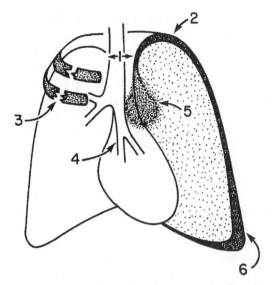

■ **FIGURE 35-2** Radiographic clues to aortic disruption include the following: (**1**) mediastinal widening (best detected on upright films), (**2**) apical pleural capping, (**3**) fractures of the first two ribs or sternum, (**4**) depression of the left main bronchus, (**5**) indistinct aortic knob, and (**6**) pleural effusion (shown here for a supine exposure with "ground glass" appearance of left lung field).

Diaphragm Injuries

Blunt trauma may rupture the diaphragm, herniating the abdominal contents into the chest. Nearly all such ruptures are left-sided because the liver shields the right hemidiaphragm from direct injury. Disruption of the right hemidiaphragm suggests massive injury force. Major clues to diaphragmatic injury include a left-sided infiltrate or atelectasis, combined with signs and symptoms of bowel obstruction. Hearing bowel sounds above the expected diaphragmatic level on physical examination and seeing an irregular dome conformation with air-fluid levels above the margins of the diaphragm on the chest radiograph also are suggestive. CT scanning or plain radiographs taken after placement of contrast in the bowel may be confirmatory. In subtle cases, injury may only be ruled out at laparoscopy or laparotomy.

Flail Chest

Flail chest results from multiple contiguous fractures of bony ribs or cartilaginous attachments that dislodge a free-floating section of rib cage or sternum. Restrained by negative intrapleural forces, the floating segment lags during inspiration, producing an apparent "paradoxical motion" during forceful breathing. This instability may go unnoticed until vigorous efforts cause major swings in intrapleural pressure. Flail chest should be suspected in every patient with blunt chest trauma, particularly if multiple rib fractures are evident. Whenever possible, a brief period of spontaneous breathing (five to ten breaths) should be observed to bring any flail segment to clinical attention.

A flail segment impairs normal coordinated action of the respiratory muscles and produces regional hypoventilation because of splinting and pain. Hypoxemia is the major consequence of the flail-associated lung contusion and retained secretions. Although the work of breathing may be only modestly affected at low levels of ventilation, it rises dramatically during hyperpnea, as breathing efficiency worsens. Because the sternum retains a relatively fixed position and is not located in a strategic position in relation to the ventilatory function of the rib cage or diaphragm, flail sternum usually is better tolerated than flail segments elsewhere.

For patients with extensive injury and ventilatory compromise, mechanical ventilatory assistance may help to reduce fluctuations of intrapleural pressure for the 7 to 14 days needed to stabilize the chest wall. It is important to minimize the minute ventilation requirement and to ensure excellent bronchial hygiene with the intent to reduce the breathing workload before weaning is attempted. Taping, sandbagging, or other attempts at external chest wall stabilization do not significantly lessen pain or improve ventilatory mechanics and may encourage atelectasis. Intercostal nerve blocks may reduce pain without impairing consciousness or ventilatory drive and thereby facilitate the weaning process. Thoracic epidural catheters are the current modality of choice for pain relief.

Pulmonary Contusions

A forceful blow to the chest may contuse the lung at the site of impact or cause a "contrecoup" injury. A lung contusion is nothing more than localized tissue bleeding and edema which causes ventilation–perfusion mismatching and hypoxemia that are often severe. Blood tinged airway secretions and/or hemoptysis may be present. Pulmonary contusion should be considered in all patients with ill-defined chest radiograph infiltrates and hypoxemia developing shortly after chest trauma, particularly when the radiographic abnormality is aligned with the known path of a forceful blow. Within 6 h of trauma (usually sooner), pulmonary contusions are radiographically visible as localized, nonsegmental infiltrates. Resolution begins within 24 to 48 h of injury and usually is

complete within 3 to 10 days. Pulmonary contusions tend to be less severe in obese patients because of decreased energy transfer to the lung afforded by the thickened chest wall.

Occasionally, pulmonary contusions coalesce to form a pulmonary hematoma that typically appears as a spherical 1- to 6-cm density. A pulmonary hematoma is a large pocket of blood located deep within the pulmonary parenchyma. Hematomas arise from significant vascular disruption and may require weeks or months to clear. Resolution is often incomplete, leaving a permanent scar. Acute respiratory distress syndrome (ARDS) frequently follows trauma, following a brief delay. The incidence of ARDS parallels the extent of contusion, with those larger than 20% associated with a dramatically higher incidence.

ARDS and Ventilator-Associated Pneumonia

Most principles of lung protective management of ARDS that pertain during medical illness apply equally well in the setting of acute chest trauma (see Chapter 24). Although open incisions, coexisting soft tissue trauma, long bone or pelvic fractures, concomitant head injury, and the need to protect the spine may prevent prone positioning, other trauma patients with refractory hypoxemia are appropriate candidates for repositioning. Prevention of ventilator-associated pneumonia is a high priority, as surgical patients are among those most predisposed, and once infected, attributable mortality is quite high. Therefore, duration of intubation should be reduced whenever safely possible to do so, and such basic measures as avoidance of nasogastric and nasotracheal tubes, hand washing, semirecumbent positioning, and adequate nutritional support are prudent.

Esophageal Rupture (Boerhaave Syndrome)

Esophageal rupture should be suspected in patients with a history of major chest trauma and a pleural effusion, especially if it is left-sided or accompanied by pneumothorax. Empyema following blunt chest trauma should suggest the possibility of esophageal or diaphragmatic rupture with subsequent bacterial contamination of the pleural space. Although interscapular, substernal, or epigastric pains are common, fever, hypotension, a rapidly accumulating pneumothorax, or a pleural effusion may be the only manifestation. Thoracentesis is highly suggestive if it reveals an acidic exudative fluid. A marked elevation of pleural fluid amylase is often present, a result of leakage of salivary amylase into the pleural space. The diagnosis may be confirmed by observing macroscopic or microscopic food particles in fluid aspirated from the pleural space.

Esophageal rupture is a highly lethal condition, as diagnosis is frequently delayed. Mediastinitis is the most frequent cause of death, fatal in almost one half of patients within the first day. Chest radiographs demonstrate mediastinal widening and gas in the mediastinum or pleural space. Extravasation of swallowed contrast material into the mediastinum or pleural space confirms the diagnosis. Surprisingly, endoscopy is frequently unrevealing and CT scan may only suggest the problem by demonstrating fluid with or without gas in the pleural space and mediastinum. Immediate surgical repair and drainage are indicated.

Fat Embolism

The fat embolism syndrome may occur within hours to days after trauma. Although fat embolism usually is associated with multiple long bone or pelvic fractures, diabetes, fatty liver, pancreatitis, joint surgery, and sickle cell anemia are other reported causes. It is theorized that lung injury is produced when lipases hydrolyze neutral triglycerides to liberate unsaturated fatty acids toxic to the pulmonary parenchyma. Fat confined to the pulmonary circulation may precipitate diffuse coagulopathy and clinical disseminated intravascular coagulation (DIC). Fat microglobules may even pass through the pulmonary capillary bed to enter the systemic circuit and produce characteristic retinal, central nervous system, and skin lesions.

A triad of confusion, pulmonary dysfunction, and skin abnormalities characterize this disorder. Symptoms may include cough, dyspnea, and pleuritic chest pain. These complaints often are accompanied by physical findings of fever, rales, tachypnea, and disorientation. Although a petechial rash over the upper torso may be present in the full-blown syndrome, it is unusual in less-obvious cases. Serum and urine lipase levels may be elevated and fat globules sometimes can be found in the urine, sputum, or bronchial lavage fluid. Retinal fat emboli also may be seen. Initially, the chest radiograph is normal in a large percentage of patients, despite severely impaired gas exchange. Decreased lung compliance, impaired diffusing capacity, hypoxemia, and respiratory alkalosis are common respiratory manifestations. In cases of fat-embolism-induced ARDS, infiltrates may require 1 to 4 weeks to resolve. Early use of corticosteroids may be helpful, but this practice remains controversial.

Compartment Syndromes

Over recent years, there has been increased awareness of the presence and importance of "compartment syndromes," particularly that of the abdomen. Compartment syndromes, defined as dysfunction or injury of tissues within a closed anatomic space because of a nonphysiologic rise in local pressure, are often subtle but devastating problems encountered frequently in patients who sustain injuries. Closed anatomic spaces at risk include those of the extremities—classically of the lower leg, but also of the arm, hand, and gluteal regions. High tension within these structures is usually suspected during physical examination, and the diagnosis is strongly supported by eliciting pain on passive flexion and by loss of sensation and/or distal pulses of the affected limb. Clearly, the ease of making the diagnosis is compromised in patients who cannot communicate effectively because of sedation, coma, and/or intubation. Confirmation by direct tissue pressure measurement adds to the diagnostic certainty, but the decision for operative release remains a clinical judgment. Wherever encountered, acute compartment syndrome merits rapid surgical intervention, as delayed decompression extends the ischemic period and threatens tissue viability. Localized compartment syndrome may not give rise to the telltale lactic acidosis and muscle enzyme elevations that characterize ischemia of larger muscle compartments (rhabdomyolysis).

Resuscitation from trauma usually involves the rapid delivery of large (even massive) volumes of intravenous fluid. If the contents of a potential compartment have been injured and/or the microvessels are unusually permeable, extravasation raises tension within that confined space to levels that may compromise perfusion of the nerves, muscles, and other tissue. Ischemia occurs as the interstitial tissue pressures (normally 0 to 10 mm Hg) approach or exceed capillary pressure. Compartment syndrome can develop in many settings other than trauma, including local extravasation of intravenous fluids at the site of infusion and spontaneous or iatrogenic arterial hemorrhage. The rise of compartment pressure is not a linear function of extravascular volume leakage. Pressure within a compartment tends to rise slowly until its limits of accommodation are reached, escalating rapidly thereafter.

Abdominal Compartment Syndrome

Although compartment syndrome was first described in the setting of limb trauma, widespread recent attention has focused on the compartment syndrome developing within the abdomen. The abdominal compartment is bounded inferiorly by the pelvic floor, circumferentially by the abdominal wall, and superiorly by the diaphragm. Elevated abdominal pressure occurs in a variety of critically ill patients, both medical (Table 35-2) and surgical (Table 35-3). Intra-abdominal tension may rise to dangerous levels in medical (pancreatitis, cirrhosis, peritonitis) as well as in surgical (burns, multiorgan trauma) conditions. Even when no traumatic damage to vessels or organs has occurred, vigorous intravascular volume expansion predisposes to its development.

While the diaphragm anatomically divides the chest and abdomen, it is not a rigid barrier to transmission of increased pressures within the torso. In fact, increased pressures within the abdomen affect intrathoracic function to a greater extent than changes in intrathoracic pressure impact the performance of abdominal organs. The classic description of ACS included a tense distended abdomen, decreased renal function, elevated peak airway pressure, hypoxemia, and inadequate ventilation. High IAP increases the work of breathing, generates atelectasis, increases the apparent stiffness of the chest wall, leads to increased extravascular lung water, and may elevate airway pressures when positive end-expiratory pressure (PEEP) and tidal volume remain unchanged.

The tissue-compromising effects of raised IAP extend along a broad continuum, with perfusion adequacy or impairment being a function not only of the pressure itself, but also of the mean arterial pressure. (Perfusion pressure = mean arterial pressure–intra-abdominal pressure.) The cycle of impaired outflow, decreased capillary perfusion, and increasing pressure leads to decreased hepatosplanchnic blood flow, decreased renal blood flow, compression of the inferior vena cava, and decreased venous return to the heart. Declining cardiac output progresses eventually to shock. ACS results in renal dysfunction and oliguria, gut mucosal ischemia, and progressive lactic acidosis of eventually life-threatening proportions. Confusion as to the cause of renal insufficiency often arises when rhabdomyolysis coexists in this posttrauma setting. Indeed, aggressive fluid infusion aimed at addressing the rhabdomyolysis often present after trauma or crush injury may contribute to the development of ACS. Urinary electrolytes may be of value in sorting out the etiology—prerenal or tubular damage—in the oliguric patient who has not received diuretics.

Diagnosis of intra-abdominal hypertension and ACS is typically established by characteristic

TABLE 35-2 MEDICAL PREDISPOSITIONS TO INTRA-ABDOMINAL HYPERTENSION

Massive fluid resuscitation (>5 L in 24 h)

Ileus (paralytic, mechanical, pseudoobstructive)

Intra-abdominal infection

Pneumoperitoneum (can include pneumoperitoneum for laparotomy)

Hemoperitoneum

Acidosis (arterial pH ≤7.2)

Hypothermia (core temperature ≤33°C)

Polytransfusion (transfusion ≥10 units of PRBCs in 24 h)

Coagulopathy (platelets ≥ 55,000/mm³; PTT >2 × normal; INR >1.5)

Sepsis (American-European Consensus Conference definition)

Bacteremia (positive blood cultures)

Liver dysfunction (cirrhosis with ascites, portal vein thrombosis, ischemic hepatitis)

Need for mechanical ventilation

Use of PEEP or the presence of auto-PEEP

Pneumonia

PRBCs, packed red blood cells.

Source: Adapted from An G, West MA. Abdominal compartment syndrome: A concise clinical review. Crit Care Med. 2008;36:1304–1310.

TABLE 35-3 SURGICAL SETTINGS ASSOCIATED WITH INTRA-ABDOMINAL HYPERTENSION

Recent abdominal surgery

Open abdomen (may still develop ACS, especially if early postoperative)

Pelvic fractures

Blunt or penetrating abdominal trauma

Abdominal packing after temporary abdominal closure for multiple trauma or liver transplantation

Large-volume fluid resuscitation following trauma

Retroperitoneal bleeding

6 physical and laboratory findings and measurement of IAP. The magnitude of IAP is not easily predicted by manual palpation alone; accurate estimation of IAP is most easily accomplished by transduction of bladder pressure (Fig. 35-3) (see Chapter 5 for technique description). Current technique involves instillation of 25 to 50 mL of sterile saline into the bladder via the urinary drainage (Foley) catheter. Catheter tubing is then clamped and bladder pressure is either measured via a transducer or the catheter and tubing is elevated and the height of the fluid column measured. No sharp threshold of pressure can be specified that mandates decompressive intervention (massive paracentesis or decompressive laparotomy), as dysfunction may be detectable at vesicular pressures as low as 10 to 15 mm Hg, depending on arterial (and therefore perfusion) pressure. While intravascular volume administration may help preserve an adequate perfusion gradient when IAP is only moderately elevated, it is generally advised that early decompression be attempted when the IAP exceeds 20 to 25 mm Hg in a clinically compatible setting. It must be emphasized that ACS is defined by the *combination* of intra-abdominal hypertension and evolving end organ failure. In the setting of trauma, the ACS appears to be a joint function of the preexisting "tightness" of the abdomen (as reflected imprecisely by the body mass index), the extent and nature of the abdominal injury, and the infused fluid volume. Although technically outside of the normal range and, therefore, both concerning and worthy of tracking, abdominal pressures greater than 15 mm Hg may be recorded in patients without critical illnesses or perfusion compromise.

After trauma, definitive treatment for fully manifested ACS is surgical decompression via laparotomy. Surgical decompression is almost always effective, often immediately and dramatically relieving hypotension, renal insufficiency, and respiratory compromise. It should be noted, however, that an open abdomen does not guarantee low intra-abdominal pressure, so that post-laparotomy surveillance is warranted. Surgical decompression can be safely performed at the bedside in the intensive care unit. This is an important option to weigh, as many patients with ACS are otherwise unstable from a cardiopulmonary standpoint. Unfortunately, abrupt restoration of blood flow may sometimes lead to reperfusion injury in visceral organs. Once open, the abdomen often requires many days before reduced tissue swelling allows reclosure to be safely attempted.

When the patient is not acutely compromised, nonsurgical options to relieve abdominal hypertension are available. For example, excess fluid can be aggressively removed by diuretics and ultrafiltration. However, one must insure that fluid removal by these means does not result in impaired oxygen delivery or end organ hypoperfusion. Percutaneous catheter drainage has also been performed for free fluid within the peritoneal

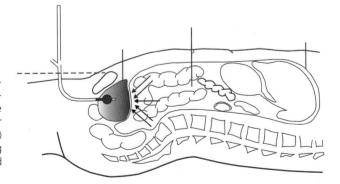

■ **FIGURE 35-3** Estimation of intra-abdominal pressure from bladder pressure. Bladder pressure is measured quickly and simply by measuring tube pressure after instilling 50 mL of sterile saline into the bladder through a clamped Foley catheter (closed technique) or by simply observing the height to which draining urine rises as the liquid filled tubing is abruptly raised (open method).

TABLE 35-4 NONSURGICAL TREATMENT OPTIONS FOR ELEVATED INTRA-ABDOMINAL PRESSURE

Gastric decompression (nasogastric suction)

Rectal decompression (enemas, rectal drainage catheter/tube)

Sedation

Neuromuscular blockade

Body positioning

Paracentesis

Prokinetic agents (stomach metoclopramide, domperidone, erythromycin; colon—prostigmine)

Diuretics (alone or in combination with 25% human albumin)

Venovenous hemofiltration/ultrafiltration

cavity. Bedside ultrasound may identify a safe window for placing the drainage catheter. Other methods for decompressing the bowel and peritoneal fluid accumulation in ACS have been reported, with varying efficacy depending on case specifics (Table 35-4).

■ **SUGGESTED READINGS**

An G, West MA. Abdominal compartment syndrome: A concise clinical review. *Crit Care Med.* 2008;36:1304–1310.

Dissanaike S, Shalhub S, Jurkovich GJ. The evaluation of pneumomediastinum in blunt trauma patients. *J Trauma.* 2008;65:1340–1345.

Feliciano DV, Mattox KL, Moore EE, eds. *Trauma.* 6th Ed. New York: McGraw Hill; 2008.

Gonzalez D. Crush syndrome. *Crit Care Med.* 2005;33(1 Suppl.):S34–S41.

LeBlang SD, Dolich MO. Imaging of penetrating thoracic trauma. *J Thorac Imaging.* 2000;15(2):128–135.

Malbrain ML. Is it wise not to think about intraabdominal hypertension in the ICU? *Curr Opin Crit Care.* 2004;10(2):132–145.

Mayberry JC, Schreiber MA. Trauma. *Crit Care Clin.* 2004;20(1):1–192.

Mirvis SE. Diagnostic imaging of acute thoracic injury. *Semin Ultrasound CT MR.* 2004;25(2):156–179.

Orliaguet G, Ferjani M, Riou B. The heart in blunt trauma. *Anesthesiology.* 2001;95(2):544–548.

Wu JT, Mattox KL, Wall MJ Jr. Esophageal perforations: New perspectives and treatment paradigms. *J Trauma.* 2007;63:1173–1184.

Yamamoto L, Schroeder C, Morley D, et al. Thoracic trauma: The deadly dozen. *Crit Care Nurs Q.* 2005;28(1): 22–40.

Acute Abdomen

■ PRINCIPLES OF MANAGEMENT

The problems of hepatic failure and gastrointestinal (GI) bleeding are discussed separately in Chapters 31 and 37, respectively. Diseases causing acute abdominal pain rarely present in a typical fashion in the intensive care unit (ICU) population. Such seemingly trivial findings as a modest reduction in the intensity of bowel sounds, intolerance of tube feeding, or loose stools can be the first signal of serious abdominal pathology. Moreover, the single most important part of the diagnostic evaluation, the history, is often difficult or impossible to obtain from the ICU patient. Patients with spinal cord injuries, those in coma, and those receiving corticosteroids or neuromuscular paralytic drugs may experience an abdominal catastrophe with few signs or symptoms. Therefore, ICU patients should undergo frequent abdominal evaluations, and a low threshold of suspicion for serious problems should be maintained.

Several principles should be kept in mind when critically ill patients with acute abdominal pain are being evaluated: (a) Carefully exclude emergent nonabdominal processes as myocardial infarction and ruptured thoracic aortic aneurysm. (b) Until a firm diagnosis is established, consider the problem to be urgent and life threatening. (c) Make repeated observations—a changing examination provides valuable clues to diagnosing abdominal disorders. (d) Involve a surgeon and/or gynecologist early in the evaluation. (All consultants will benefit by following the evolution of the illness; furthermore, this strategy avoids unnecessary repetition of painful pelvic and rectal examinations.) (e) Avoid excessive use of analgesics or sedatives in patients with undiagnosed conditions. (f) Withhold enteral feedings and medications in the event laparotomy should become necessary.

■ DIAGNOSIS

History

An accurate history is essential. Description of the onset and character of the pain as well as exacerbating or relieving factors is helpful in diagnosis. All conscious patients should be asked to localize the pain to a discreet site with one finger. Acute abdominal pain awakening patients from sleep or persisting more than 6 h frequently represents a surgical problem. Acute abdominal pain generally arises from one of three mechanisms: (a) visceral ischemia, (b) serosal inflammation, or (c) distention of a hollow viscus. Pain of sudden onset suggests a vascular catastrophe or perforation of a hollow viscus. Pain of gradual onset that builds to a crescendo is more typical of hollow viscus overdistention, as is intermittent pain in a "colicky" pattern. Steady pain suggests serosal inflammation, especially when it is markedly exacerbated by changes in position or local pressure (e.g., rebound tenderness). A pleuritic component raises the possibility that an "intra-abdominal process" either abuts the inferior surface of the diaphragm or actually extends into the chest. (This is why lower-lobe pneumonia, empyema, and pericarditis may be mistakenly diagnosed as an acute abdominal process.) Pain associated with hip flexion and that radiating to the back suggests a retroperitoneal process.

New symptoms associated with the pain, such as nausea or vomiting, or change in bowel or urinary habits are extremely helpful. For obvious reasons, a history of hematemesis or hematochezia is informative. A detailed gynecologic history is essential in all female patients with special attention to previous gynecologic problems or change in menstrual habits.

Physical Examination

The patient's resting position can be a clue to the cause of abdominal pain: patients with peritonitis often lie motionless because any movement exacerbates pain; those with pancreatitis get relief by sitting up and leaning forward and are often found in this position. Patients with biliary colic or nephrolithiasis often are unable to remain still, writhing in pain. The abdomen should first be examined visually, then auscultated, percussed, and finally palpated. Inspection may reveal the distention of ileus, ascites, or mass; or the discoloration of Grey–Turner's or Cullen's signs of pancreatitis. Auscultation may reveal a silent abdomen in established peritonitis, high-pitched bowel sounds of partial bowel obstruction, or perhaps even a friction rub associated with splenic infarct or pneumonia. Percussion can distinguish distention from gas (tympany) and ascites, blood, or tumor (dullness), and in a patient with peritonitis, the reaction to percussion may obviate the need for deep palpation. Palpating the abdomen as the first part of the examination is likely to produce voluntary guarding or induce bowel sounds, even in patients with severe ileus. The most painful area of the abdomen should be examined last. Rectal and pelvic examinations must be performed. Rectal examination may detect colonic impaction, tumor, GI bleeding, and the localized tenderness of retrocecal appendicitis. Pelvic examination should search for evidence of pregnancy, fallopian tube infection, and ovarian masses. When completed, the abdominal examination should answer the following questions: (a) Is there rebound tenderness? (b) Are the bowel sounds absent? (c) Are there palpable masses? (d) Is there evidence of free air or fluid in the abdomen? An affirmative answer to any of these questions strongly indicates that surgical intervention will be necessary. Peritoneal signs are the most reliable in predicting the need for urgent laparotomy. The development of shock in a patient with an acute abdomen is also highly indicative of a need for surgery.

Routine Laboratory Tests

Routine laboratory tests are rarely diagnostic. Although nonspecifically elevated leukocyte counts and white cell differentials may be normal even with severe intra-abdominal disease, a reduced packed cell volume (PCV) is indicative of either slow chronic blood loss or acute severe hemorrhage with volume replacement. The serum amylase and lipase can be helpful if pancreatitis is suspected, but both false-negative and false-positive results occur. Similarly, elevations in hepatic transaminase, bilirubin, or alkaline phosphatase levels suggest liver disease but are nonspecific. Although commonly done, separate determinations of conjugated and unconjugated bilirubin are of little value. The combination of an acutely elevated bilirubin and alkaline phosphatase is probably most helpful, suggesting obstructive biliary tract disease. A triad of hyperkalemia, hyperphosphatemia, and metabolic (lactic) acidosis (in the absence of renal failure) suggests well-advanced bowel infarction. Bladder pressure measurements should also be considered if abdominal compartment syndrome (ACS) is a possibility. Because ectopic pregnancy represents a potentially fatal cause of abdominal and pelvic pain, and an intrauterine pregnancy dictates some diagnostic and management choices, a rapid, sensitive pregnancy test should be obtained in the evaluation of any potentially fertile woman.

Plain Radiographs of the Abdomen

The abdominal radiograph may provide clues to the etiology and urgency of acute abdominal pain and is discussed in detail in Chapter 11; however, a few salient points will be reviewed here. In patients with acute abdominal pain, supine and upright films of the abdomen may be helpful but are rarely diagnostic. For example, even when the film reveals "free air," such a finding does not guarantee gut perforation and furthermore does not localize the site of perforation. (Free air may be the result of pulmonary barotrauma with intra-abdominal dissection of air.) Similarly, finding multiple air fluid levels in small bowel does not precisely identify the site of nonpathologic cause of bowel obstruction. Radiographic signs that should be sought include (a) calcification, (b) mass effect, (c) extraluminal gas, (d) obliteration of normal soft tissue planes, (e) localized ileus, (f) thumbprinting of bowel, and (g) evidence of gas in the biliary tree. Because it is difficult, if not impossible, to obtain upright films in the critically ill, lateral decubitus views usually must be substituted. An upright chest radiograph should also be reviewed in all patients with acute abdominal pain to look for subdiaphragmatic air or a lower-lobe pneumonia.

Ultrasound

Ultrasound (US) examination utilizes high-frequency sound energy to define anatomic structure and, when combined with Doppler technology, characterizes blood flow. Because wound dressings, adipose tissue, and air–tissue interfaces deflect ultrasonic energy, US is a poor imaging mode for the obese or in patients with prominent bowel distention or abdominal surgical dressings. US also suffers from the problem that the views it generates are difficult to interpret by the non-radiologist (unlike computed tomographic [CT] images). US has the desirable features of being portable, rapidly accomplished, relatively inexpensive, and devoid of ionizing radiation and contrast media.

US is an excellent method for detecting pelvic processes in women (e.g., ectopic or intrauterine pregnancy, ovarian cysts, or pelvic tumors) and staging normal pregnancy. Likewise, because a bowel gas interface does not usually need to be crossed by the beam in the right upper quadrant, US is outstanding for viewing the liver and gallbladder. Thus, US is an excellent method to detect cholelithiasis, biliary tract dilation, and pericholecystic fluid or edema. Clear images of the kidneys and ureters can also be routinely obtained because they can be imaged from the rear, avoiding overlying bowel gas. The presence or absence of bowel gas makes visualization of the pancreas inconsistent. With the exceptions of imaging the right upper quadrant, pelvis, and kidneys, CT is superior to US for imaging the abdomen.

Computed Tomographic Scanning

Because the abdominal CT now provides amazing image quality with high sensitivity, it has supplanted most other imaging modalities and, in many situations, is more useful than the physical **3** examination in the ICU population. The CT scan requires transport of the patient to the radiology suite, but in contrast to magnetic resonance scanning, it offers dramatically more rapid imaging and is not precluded by the presence of metallic devices. CT images are easier to interpret than sonograms, especially for the nonradiologist, and they offer high-resolution views of essentially every intra-abdominal and retroperitoneal structure. Enteral contrast material is required to distinguish bowel from other gas or fluid-filled structures like abscesses, but in many cases, nephrotoxic intravenous (IV) contrast can be avoided. The CT scan does have some disadvantages, however; it requires ionizing radiation and iodinated contrast material to evaluate vasculature. If searching for gallstones, or pelvic processes in a woman, US is as good an imaging modality.

Magnetic Resonance Imaging

The magnetic resonance imaging (MRI) has significant limitations in the ICU patient population because of the requirement for transport to the scanner, the relatively long scanning times, the need for a motionless patient, and the prohibition of metallic support devices. Brain and soft tissue detail, however, is superb. A major problem recognized with MRI since the last edition of this text is the syndrome of fibrosing nephrogenic dermopathy following gadolinium contrast administration to patients with renal insufficiency.

Biliary Scans

The performance of biliary tract scans relies on the use of a radioactive analog of iminodiacetic acid (HIDA) that, after administration, is taken up by

TABLE 36-1 MERITS OF RADIOLOGICAL DIAGNOSTIC METHODS FOR ACUTE ABDOMINAL PAIN

CHARACTERISTIC	COMPUTED TOMOGRAPHY (CT) AND ULTRASOUND (US)	RADIONUCLIDE SCANS (GALLIUM AND INDIUM)
Operator dependence	Require directed study of a suspected area by skilled operator	Not operator dependent
Specificity for inflammation	Failure to determine whether fluid collections contain leukocytes	More specific for the presence of white blood cells
Speed	Rapidly accomplished	Usually requires 24–48 h
Portability	Only US portable	Not portable
Body habitus	US best in thin patients; CT requires body fat to define tissue planes	Not as effective in obese patients

the liver and secreted into the bile, where it outlines the major intrahepatic ducts, gallbladder, and common bile duct. Radionuclide scans ("IDA" scans) are sensitive but lack specificity for biliary tract inflammation, particularly in the absence of gallstones. The high sensitivity of these tests renders them useful for excluding the diagnosis of cholecystitis, provided an adequate study is obtained. Failure to visualize the gallbladder may result from obstructive biliary tract disease, starvation, total parenteral nutrition (TPN) use, or severe parenchymal liver failure—often the very problems necessitating ICU admission.

Gallium and Indium Scans

The question of abdominal abscess arises frequently and is difficult to resolve noninvasively. In the past, gallium and indium scans may have been useful in the search for inflammation. Unfortunately, there are many problems in using these studies. Indium-labeled white blood cells (WBCs) are difficult to produce because the isotope is very expensive, short lived, and cyclotron generated. Indium scanning is not likely to work if WBCs are dysfunctional, as in patients with acquired immune deficiency syndrome, with malnutrition, or receiving dialysis. False-positive abdominal scans may result in the presence of pneumonia, sinusitis, GI bleeding, or tumors of the bowel. Indium may be used to localize acute infections, but chronic infections may not have sufficiently numerous or active WBCs to enable visualization. Gallium-67 concentrates in any site of inflammation (not just areas of infection) and may visualize tumors, hematomas, fractures, infections, sarcoidosis, or acute respiratory distress syndrome (ARDS). Gallium is normally excreted into the colon

and kidney, producing "physiological hot spots." Resolution is characteristically poor, and precise localization is difficult. Simply stated, current quality of CT scan and US images has made gallium and indium scans all but obsolete. The specific advantages and limitations of the various imaging modalities are outlined in Tables 36-1 and 36-2.

■ SPECIFIC CONDITIONS PRODUCING THE ACUTE ABDOMEN

Although age alone never makes nor excludes a specific diagnosis, a patient's age does give valuable clues to diagnosis (Table 36-3). Similarly, the etiology of abdominal pain varies depending on whether the pain precipitated ICU admission or developed while the patient was in the ICU. Whereas ruptured ectopic pregnancy, aortic rupture, and pancreatitis rarely *develop* in ICU occupants, cholecystitis, appendicitis, bowel ischemia, and ulcer perforations commonly do. The most rapidly lethal condition compatible with the presentation should be considered first, particularly in patients with overt abdominal signs and hypotension. The fulminant development of shock associated with acute abdominal pain is usually attributable to vascular disruption with intra-abdominal hemorrhage or to severe sepsis. Two conditions of this type in most urgent need of surgical intervention are ruptured abdominal aortic aneurysm and ruptured ectopic pregnancy.

Leaking Aortic Aneurysm

Immediate diagnosis and surgical correction are needed to salvage patients with a ruptured abdominal aortic aneurysm. A ruptured or leaking

TABLE 36-2 CHARACTERISTICS OF CT, MRI, AND US EXAMINATIONS

COMPUTED TOMOGRAPHY	MAGNETIC RESONANCE IMAGING	ULTRASOUND
Not portable	Not portable	Portable
Expensive	Most expensive	Least expensive
Can evaluate through wounds and bandages	Can evaluate through wounds and bandages	Requires skin contact
Better in overweight patients	Body habitus not critical	Better in thin patients
Cross-sectional views best	Infinite number of views	Wide range of sectional views
Metal causes artifact	Impossible with metal implants	Air causes artifact
Static images	Static images	Dynamic images possible
Uniform resolution across field	Uniform resolution across field	Limited area of high resolution
Not operator dependent	Not operator dependent	Highly operator dependent
Requires intravenous contrast to distinguish vessels	Exquisite detail of flowing blood and soft tissues	Cystic and dilated structures provide best contrast; air interferes
Intravenous contrast nephrotoxic	Gadolinium contrast toxic in renal impairment	Nontoxic

aneurysm typically presents with back and abdominal pain and shock occurring in a middle-aged or elderly patient with known arteriovascular disease and/or hypertension. An expanding abdomen or pulsatile abdominal mass with the loss of one or both femoral pulses completes the classic presentation. The retroperitoneal irritation produced by a leaking abdominal aneurysm can mimic nerve compression or a ureteral stone by causing "sciatica" or testicular pain. Rarely, rupture of an aortic aneurysm into the duodenum causes the massive hemoptysis of an aortoenteric fistula.

TABLE 36-3 ASSOCIATION BETWEEN DISEASES AND PATIENT AGE

CONDITION	AGE PREDILECTION
Appendicitis	Younger
Ulcer perforation	Younger
Ectopic pregnancy	Younger
Pelvic inflammatory disease	Younger
Ovarian tumor	Older
Mesenteric ischemia	Older
Ruptured aortic aneurysm	Older
Colonic obstruction/perforation	Older
Diverticulitis	Older
Cholecystitis	Any age
Pancreatitis	Any age
Small bowel obstruction	Any age

(This dramatic clinical situation almost always occurs in patients with aortic grafts in place.) Unfortunately, hypotension often impedes comparison of pulse volumes, and examination of the abdomen and pulses may be difficult in obese patients. Because such patients are losing "whole blood," the hematocrit often remains stable until volume replacement is substantial or the patient nears exsanguination.

In the past when clear signs and symptoms of a ruptured abdominal aneurysm were present, patients were taken directly to the operating room for surgical repair while initiating fluid and blood resuscitation. In the last 5 years, dramatic advances in endovascular stenting now allow many aneurysms to be repaired without an open procedure. If the patient is hemodynamically stable, multiple large-bore IV lines should be inserted and blood ordered before diagnostic testing. Regardless, early consultation by a vascular surgeon is indicated. A contrasted CT scan and aortogram are the best tests to confirm and delineate the aneurysm in the stable patient. Ultrasonography is a quick noninvasive bedside test to confirm the presence of an aneurysm, but clear visualization is likely to be obscured by bowel gas.

Female Pelvic Disease

Ruptured ectopic pregnancy typically presents as acute abdominal pain, hypotension, vaginal bleeding, and a mass in the cul-de-sac. (Acute pain occurs in almost all patients; about three quarters have vaginal bleeding and about half have a pelvic mass; fever is rare.) A reported history of a recent menstrual period is sufficiently unreliable that it cannot be used to exclude pregnancy. Hence, a serum β-human chorionic gonadotropin (HCG) should be performed on every fertile female with acute abdominal pain. Urinary HCG testing, although possibly more readily available, is less sensitive. Hematocrit determinations are usually not helpful because of the acute nature of the bleeding. Ectopic pregnancy is especially likely in patients with a history of salpingitis, tubal ligation, or prior ectopic pregnancy and in patients using intrauterine devices for birth control. Young women with unexplained acute abdominal pain and shock should probably undergo immediate laparotomy for a presumed ruptured ectopic pregnancy. (The rapid availability of US in many emergency departments and ICUs now permits confirmation of the diagnosis in less time than it takes to ready the operating room.) In patients with acute abdominal pain, stable blood pressure, and no evidence of peritoneal signs, serum pregnancy testing and ultrasonographic evaluation should be performed before surgery.

The transabdominal and transvaginal US examinations are complementary in evaluation of painful pelvic disease: Lesions located "high" in pelvis (e.g., ovarian masses) are often best seen by transabdominal screening (provided bowel gas does not obscure the view). Conversely, transvaginal scanning is often better at detecting early intrauterine pregnancy and ectopic pregnancies. Use of transabdominal scanning can allow detection of pregnancy as early as 4 weeks of gestation—transvaginal scanning can detect the same gestational sac 1 week earlier. The only certain US sign of ectopic pregnancy is visualizing a gestational sac outside the uterus, while finding a viable intrauterine pregnancy is strong evidence against a concurrent ectopic pregnancy. Ovarian tumors or cysts may also produce pelvic pain if they undergo torsion or ischemia. Rupture of a normal ovarian follicle into the peritoneum may produce worrisome but otherwise benign peritoneal signs.

Pelvic inflammatory disease (PID), the most common cause of pelvic pain in young women, is often difficult to differentiate from appendicitis or a ruptured ectopic pregnancy. PID usually starts within 7 days of the menstrual period, a helpful point in the differential with ectopic pregnancy, if the history is reliable. (The serum HCG should also be negative.) The pain of PID is gradual in onset and usually bilateral, whereas the pain of appendicitis tends to be of more rapid onset and unilateral when fully developed. Diffuse bilateral tenderness elicited by moving the cervix during pelvic examination is key to detecting PID. The ultrasonographic and CT features of PID are subtle and nonspecific unless a frank abscess forms. Untreated, PID can progress to the formation of a pus-filled fallopian tube, a tubo-ovarian abscess (TOA). TOA is an especially common problem among women with repeated or prolonged episodes of PID. Surprisingly, TOA can have such a sufficiently long timecourse that it can be confused radiographically with ovarian or even adjacent colon carcinoma. TOA is most frequently characterized by pelvic pain, fever and chills, and a vaginal discharge. Examination reveals lower abdominal and adnexal tenderness (usually asymmetric). Leukocytosis occurs in about two thirds of patients. Both US and pelvic CT scanning are excellent for imaging the lesion. Most tubal abscesses are polymicrobial infections that include enteric aerobic Gram-negative rods, *Haemophilus*, anaerobes, and *Streptococcus*. Pelvic US or CT demonstrates an adnexal mass in more than 90% of patients. Initial therapy should include appropriate cultures, hemodynamic stabilization, and administration of antibiotics. (A fluoroquinolone plus metronidazole, a third-generation cephalosporin plus doxycycline, a second-generation cephalosporin plus doxycycline, and clindamycin plus gentamicin and metronidazole are acceptable alternative antibiotic regimens.)

Mesenteric Ischemia

Mesenteric ischemia afflicts the elderly, particularly those with underlying heart (e.g., congestive heart failure and atrial fibrillation) and vascular disease who develop shock. (There are now many instances of mesenteric ischemia in young people resulting from cocaine-induced vasoconstriction.) The mortality of bowel infarction approaches 70%, primarily because of delayed diagnosis but also because victims tend to be older and have other underlying diseases. The differential diagnosis includes bowel obstruction, diverticulitis, and inflammatory bowel disease.

Bowel ischemia may result from arterial or venous occlusion of the superior or inferior mesenteric vessels. Most is arterial. About 50% of patients with acute bowel ischemia have superior mesenteric artery (SMA) disease. (Half of these cases are embolic, a quarter are thrombotic, with the remainder resulting from nonocclusive ischemia.) SMA occlusion usually presents as the sudden onset of acute abdominal pain and a striking leukocytosis. Conversely, inferior mesenteric artery occlusion (accounting for about 25% of cases of bowel ischemia) usually has a more subtle, chronic pattern. The remaining 25% of cases stem from mesenteric *venous* thrombosis resulting from portal hypertension, pelvic infection, trauma, pancreatitis, intra-abdominal neoplasm, and thrombophilic disorders.

Arterial embolism is the single most common cause of bowel infarction and is most likely among patients with atrial fibrillation or recent myocardial infarction complicated by mural thrombus. The possibility of cholesterol embolism should also be considered in patients who develop symptoms after aortic instrumentation (e.g., cardiac catheterization, aortic balloon pump). Thrombotic occlusion occurring near the aortic origin of mesenteric vessels in patients with extensive atherosclerotic disease is the second most common cause of infarction. In patients with slowly progressive occlusion, a history of "intestinal angina" may be elicited. Vasculitis from lupus, radiation, or polyarteritis is rarely responsible. Many critically ill patients have nonocclusive bowel infarction due to the combination of hypotension and vasopressor drugs. By virtue of advanced age and atherosclerosis, many victims also have some degree of chronic vascular narrowing. (Concern over nonocclusive bowel infarction has increased recently with the resurgence of the powerful splanchnic vasoconstrictor, vasopressin, to treat septic shock.) Initially, ischemia produces mucosal and submucosal injury and edema. Later, mucosal sloughing occurs. Unless corrected within hours, bowel necrosis and perforation result, producing generalized peritonitis and death.

The signs and symptoms of mesenteric ischemia are often minimal or poorly localized, although a benign abdominal exam in a patient complaining of severe abdominal pain should be a tip-off. Unfortunately, severe illness and sedation often obscure the timely detection in the ICU patient. In addition, severe forms of *Clostridium difficile* colitis can be confused with mesenteric ischemia since they can present with abdominal pain, bloody stool, fever, and leukocytosis. The most common symptom of mesenteric ischemia is constant, nondiscrete back and abdominal pain. (The onset is sudden if embolic, more gradual if thrombotic or nonocclusive.) More than half of all patients have either occult blood in the stool or bloody diarrhea. Bowel sounds increase early in this process but decrease later. Shock may be the presenting symptom if perforation or infarction has already occurred. Atrial fibrillation or congestive heart failure is present in as many as half of all patients with bowel infarction.

Laboratory tests are seldom sufficiently specific or timely to aid in diagnosis. Although loss of circulating volume may cause hemoconcentration, more typically, the hematocrit remains normal as the leukocyte count rises. Refractory metabolic (lactic) acidosis in conjunction with increased levels of potassium and phosphate is typical of infarction. Unfortunately, these abnormalities are often recognized too late to impact favorably on crucial therapeutic decisions.

Plain abdominal radiographic findings (seen in a minority of cases) include an ileus localized to the area of bowel ischemia with dilation of large and small bowel loops and loss of haustral markings. Occasionally, gas may be seen in the portal venous system, in the bowel wall, or free in the peritoneal cavity. Hemorrhage and bowel wall edema may result in a classic "thumbprinting" pattern on the plain radiograph. CT of the abdomen demonstrates the suggestive findings of segmental bowel wall thickening, ascites, air in the portal vein, or focal bowel dilation with a high degree of sensitivity (approx. 85%). Occasionally, CT scan following IV contrast may directly demonstrate the mesenteric vein thrombosis which is diagnostic.

Angiography remains the procedure of choice for diagnosis and may also aid in the therapy. To be effective, it must be performed without delay. Angiography distinguishes thrombosis and embolism from nonocclusive vasoconstriction and allows potential interventions. Magnetic resonance angiography (MRA) may ultimately prove to be the best diagnostic modality because it can be done without iodinated contrast material.

After initial stabilization with fluid and correction of electrolyte and acid–base abnormalities, cultures should be obtained and antibiotics administered to broadly cover enteric pathogens. In patients with peritoneal signs and those with CT or angiographic findings indicative of intestinal perforation or infarction, immediate surgery should be undertaken. At the time of surgery, nonviable segments of bowel should be removed—a "second-look" operation 24 to 36 h following revascularization has gained popularity to allow dying tissue time to demarcate.

In patients with symptoms of short duration suggesting that infarction has not yet occurred, angiographic diagnosis followed by heparin anticoagulation and correction by surgery or interventional radiographic technique is as likely to result in a good outcome. For example, direct mesenteric artery infusion of papaverine or nitroglycerin may improve the perfusion of nonocclusive ischemic gut, delaying or averting surgery. If clot is found, catheter embolectomy or thrombolytic infusion may be helpful. For patients found to have focal arterial narrowing, angioplasty with stent placement may be useful, although surgical revascularization is still preferred for nonembolic occlusions. When the cause of ischemia is venous thrombosis, surgery is the preferred approach. Regardless of etiology, prognosis is best when revascularization is performed on a "nonsurgical" abdomen. Unfortunately, the diagnosis of ischemic bowel disease is often overlooked or delayed until the clinical condition has deteriorated too far to permit salvage.

Appendicitis

For unclear reasons, appendicitis is a disease much more commonly seen in the first three decades of life than among older patients. (Appendicitis is the most common surgical issue encountered during pregnancy.) Nonetheless, it can occur at virtually any age. Early diagnosis is critical to prevent the major complications of perforation, abscess formation, and severe sepsis. The classic features of acute appendicitis—midepigastric pain migrating to the right lower quadrant accompanied by nausea and vomiting—are seen in less than half of all ambulatory patients and probably even fewer critically ill patients. The site of pain is not predictable because of the variable location of the cecum and appendix. Appendicitis is often overlooked in the absence of fever, leukocytosis, a localizing physical examination, or a "classic" history. Physical examination usually reveals a mildly elevated temperature with moderate acute abdominal pain. Generalized peritoneal signs are absent until perforation has occurred. Pelvic and rectal examinations are particularly helpful in localizing the pain to the right lower quadrant and excluding alternative diagnoses. Laboratory examination is nonspecific; an elevated WBC count is seen in about 70% patients. A urinalysis and pregnancy test should be performed to exclude alternative diagnoses, although up to one third of patients with appendicitis will have microscopic hematuria and pyuria. The plain radiograph is not usually helpful. (Even when perforation is demonstrated surgically, free intra-abdominal air is only seen radiographically in half of all patients.) CT scanning is now more than 95% sensitive and specific; hence, it should be performed liberally if the disease is suspected. If an air- or contrast-filled appendix is seen, the diagnosis is all but excluded. Alternatively, discovery of a mass or fat stranding in the cecal region, edema or thickening of the appendiceal wall, or an appendicolith is highly suggestive of appendicitis. If the diagnosis is missed, the delayed supprative complications are easily diagnosed by CT. US is probably not as useful as CT for diagnosis but is an excellent tool to exclude alternative causes of abdominopelvic pain in women.

Treatment of uncomplicated acute appendicitis (i.e., symptoms <72 h without evidence of perforation) is surgical removal after prompt correction of any significant fluid or electrolyte abnormalities. For many noncritically ill patients, laparoscopic appendectomy permits rapid hospital discharge. (Antibiotic therapy beyond that routinely used for surgical prophylaxis is unnecessary.) If diagnosis is delayed and perforation with abscess formation has occurred, there is general agreement that antibiotics and percutaneous drainage of any abscess, followed by surgical intervention after the patient has stabilized, are warranted. Patients with symptoms 2 to 5 days in duration without clear evidence of perforation should probably be operated on, as should those with coexisting intestinal ischemia or other life-threatening abdominal process.

Pancreatitis

Cytotoxic effects of alcohol- and gallstone-induced reflux of bile into the pancreatic duct account for nearly 80% of all cases of acute pancreatitis. Ethanol is a more likely etiology in men, whereas gallstones are a more frequent cause in women. Other causes include trauma, tumors, medications, electrolyte disturbances, toxins, infections, and surgery (Table 36-4). Gallstones that precipitate acute pancreatitis usually affect the ampulla of Vater. Approximately one half of all patients with gallstone pancreatitis have concurrent biliary tract infection (cholangitis), a complication that raises mortality

6

TABLE 36-4 CAUSES OF ACUTE PANCREATITIS

Common causes (approx. 80%)
    Ethanol
    Gallstones

Less common causes (approx. 15%)
    Idiopathic
    Drug-induced
    Abdominal trauma

Rare causes (approx. 5%)
    Biliary ascariasis
    Hypertriglyceridemia
    Hypercalcemia/hyperparathyroidism
    End-stage renal failure
    Penetrating duodenal ulcer
    Organ transplant associated
    Pancreas divisum
    Ampullary stenosis or spasm
    Hereditary
    Pancreatic carcinoma
    Viral infections (CMV; mumps; hepatitis A, B, and C; EBV)
    AIDS-associated
    Pregnancy

TABLE 36-5 DRUGS IMPLICATED IN CAUSING PANCREATITIS

Acetaminophen	Angiotensin-converting enzyme inhibitors
Asparaginase	Azathioprine
Cimetidine	Corticosteroids
Cytarabine	Danazol
Didanosine	Ergotamine
Diphenoxylate	Ethacrynic acid
Estrogens	Gold compounds
Furosemide	Isotretinoin
Interleukin-2	Methyldopa
Mercaptopurine	Nitrofurantoin
Metronidazole	Piroxicam
Pentamidine	Ranitidine
Procainamide	Sulindac
Sulfonamides	Tamoxifen
Tetracycline	Thiazides
Valproic acid	

dramatically. Two thirds of patients with gallstone pancreatitis who defer stone removal experience symptom recurrence. Tumors of the pancreas and common bile duct or ampullary stenosis after biliary tract surgery also may induce pancreatitis by obstructing the free flow of bile. Visualization of the pancreatic duct by endoscopic retrograde cholangiopancreatography (ERCP) reveals structural abnormalities, tiny stones, or thick biliary sludge in many cases of recurrent pancreatitis of obscure etiology. The ERCP procedure may elevate serum amylase in as many as 60% of patients; however, most of these cases are asymptomatic.

Ethanol leads the list of toxins and medications that commonly cause acute pancreatitis. Other direct pancreatic toxins include methanol, carbon tetrachloride, and organophosphate insecticides. Numerous medications have been implicated in causing acute pancreatitis, but a diagnosis of drug-induced pancreatitis is always suspect, and it is believed that drugs account for less than 1% of all cases (Table 36-5). The one group of patients in whom drug-induced pancreatitis is common are patients with HIV infection taking antiretrovirals. In lipid-induced acute pancreatitis, triglyceride levels usually exceed 1,000 mg/dL. The diagnosis often is difficult to make because triglycerides interfere with assays of serum amylase and fre-

quently are elevated, even when acute pancreatitis has another cause. Hypercalcemia-induced acute pancreatitis usually occurs in association with untreated hyperparathyroidism. After arteriographic procedures, cholesterol emboli may incite acute pancreatitis; for unclear reasons, this complication is particularly likely in the anticoagulated patient. Pancreatitis also is common in patients undergoing solid organ transplantation, possibly because of the use of cyclosporine for immunosuppression.

Some combination of direct cytotoxic injury, ductal obstruction, and bile and duodenal reflux initiates pancreatic injury. Regardless of the inciting stimulus, the subsequent pancreatitis results from organ damage caused by autodigesting enzymes. Trypsin and chymotrypsin, lipase, and elastase are responsible for damage to proteins, lipids, and elastin, respectively. Trypsin is not only destructive to proteins but also a potent activator of other proenzymes. Trypsin-induced activation of phospholipase A and the kinin–kallikrein system probably is responsible for many of the hemodynamic and vascular permeability changes associated with pancreatitis. Enzyme-induced inflammation disrupts pancreatic ducts, breaks down vessel walls, causes fat necrosis, and kills both exocrine and endocrine pancreatic cells. The most severe cases of necrotizing pancreatitis are accompanied by hemorrhage. With the exception of alcohol-induced pancreatitis, most cases (>80%) are self-limited, leaving little residual pancreatic damage. Only rarely does acute pancreatitis progress to a chronic form.

Patients with pancreatitis usually present with severe, constant "boring" abdominal and/or back pain made worse by lying supine. Nausea, vomiting, and low-grade fever are common. However, less-than-typical acute presentations (chest pain, shock, respiratory distress, etc.) often are encountered. Occasionally, presenting signs of pancreatitis in the ICU patient are subtle. Tube-feeding intolerance, hypocalcemia, or an unexplained fever or decline in hematocrit may be the only manifestations, especially in patients with impaired mental status. Pancreatitis can be difficult to distinguish from cholecystitis, mesenteric ischemia, ulcer disease (especially posterior duodenal ulcers), and diverticular inflammation.

Tachycardia is nearly universal because of pain and intravascular volume depletion. Volume depletion often produces hypotension. Epigastric tenderness with or without signs of peritoneal irritation is the most common finding on physical examination. (Rebound tenderness is not common because of the retroperitoneal location of the gland.) Pain often is worse when the patient is supine. Chest examination may reveal rales characteristic of atelectasis or acute lung injury. Bluish discoloration of the flanks (Grey–Turner sign) or periumbilical region (Cullen sign) rare manifestations of retroperitoneal hemorrhage. Red subcutaneous nodules of fat necrosis and hypocalcemic tetanus are extremely rare.

Leukocyte counts commonly range from 10,000 to 25,000 cells/mm³. Volume depletion frequently causes elevation of the blood urea nitrogen and hemoconcentration; later, anemia is the rule. Increased levels of stress hormones (glucagon, cortisol, and epinephrine) often produce hyperglycemia. Increased capillary permeability and chronic illness (especially alcoholism) commonly cause hypoalbuminemia. Transient hypertriglyceridemia and mild elevations in hepatic transaminase also are seen frequently.

Plasma amylase and lipase are the two enzymes most frequently assayed to diagnose pancreatitis. Unfortunately, many conditions unassociated with acute pancreatitis elevate the amylase level, making this test much less specific than commonly perceived (Table 36-6). For example, as many as one third of all patients undergoing laparotomy and nearly one fourth of those having major extra-abdominal surgery have elevated amylase levels without pancreatic manipulation or clinical evidence of pancreatitis. The specificity of amylase for diagnosing acute pancreatitis can be improved by

TABLE 36-6 NONPANCREATIC CAUSES OF AMYLASE ELEVATION

Alcoholism
Abdominal trauma
Macroamylasemia
Perforated duodenal ulcer
Mesenteric ischemia
Small bowel obstruction
Morphine administration
Lung cancer
Surgery
Renal failure
Diabetic ketoacidosis
Ectopic pregnancy
Gallbladder disease
Hepatic failure
Ovarian tumors
Hydroxyethyl starch administration
Endoscopic retrograde cholangiopancreatography

using a cutoff of two to five times the laboratory upper limit of normal; however, the degree of serum amylase elevation has no prognostic value. Amylase determinations also lack sensitivity. Because amylase peaks within 24 h of disease onset and then declines gradually, as many as one third of patients with clinical and radiographic features of acute pancreatitis have unimpressive serum amylase values when first seen. High rates of false-positive and false-negative results limit the clinical utility of amylase clearance tests. (For example, renal failure is one of many conditions that increase the ratio of amylase clearance to creatinine clearance.) Lipase is more specific than amylase as an indicator of pancreatitis. Lipase peaks even later and clears more slowly than amylase, remaining elevated for up to 14 days. Therefore, it can help in making a diagnosis in a patient who presents late in the course of disease. Unlike amylase, lipase rarely is elevated in patients with burns, diabetic ketoacidosis, pelvic infection, salivary gland dysfunction, or macroamylasemia but, like amylase, may be elevated in renal failure. Assays of trypsinogen, methemalbumin, elastase, and phospholipase A are nonspecific tests used to support the diagnosis of pancreatitis, but none of these has demonstrated any practical advantage over amylase or lipase determinations.

The chest radiograph commonly demonstrates nonspecific bibasilar atelectasis, diaphragmatic elevation, or pleural effusion. Diffuse infiltrates suggest ARDS. Abdominal films are never diagnostic but may reveal the suggestive signs of localized ileus, such as "the colon cutoff sign" or the "sentinel loop." Free air may enter the abdomen in patients with pancreatitis resulting from ulcer perforation. A "soap bubble" appearance of the pancreatic bed, calcifications suggestive of chronic pancreatitis, and obscuration of the psoas margins are other clues.

Abdominal US is a useful bedside screening test for many patients with abdominal pain, but suboptimal visualization of the pancreas occurs in many patients because of obesity or excessive bowel gas from the accompanying ileus. US is good at detecting gallstones and biliary duct dilation and for observing the course of pancreatic pseudocysts but is inferior to CT for detecting or staging pancreatitis and most of its complications. CT scanning is the single best test to visualize the pancreas because it is unaffected by patient size or the presence of bowel gas. CT scanning demonstrates some radiographic abnormality in two thirds of all patients with pancreatitis (pancreatic edema or necrosis or peripancreatic fluid collections) and is abnormal in all patients with severe disease but provides an etiologic diagnosis in less than 25% of cases. To obtain data about pancreatic viability, rapid-phase contrasted scanning must be performed. Unfortunately, many patients with pancreatitis have an elevated creatinine, which raises questions about the safety of a contrast. For such patients, intravascular volume supplementation with IV sodium bicarbonate or N-acetylcysteine may blunt the extent of renal injury. Not all patients with pancreatitis must undergo CT scanning; the diagnosis and etiology of pancreatitis are apparent in most patients after history, physical examination, and measurement of serum amylase. The CT scan is a useful confirmatory test in a patient with abdominal pain in whom the significance of an elevated amylase is questionable (e.g., diabetic ketoacidosis, renal failure).

In addition to confirming the diagnosis, a reliable CT scan–based scoring system has been developed for assessing severity (Table 36-7). In this system, the presence of pancreatic enlargement, surrounding inflammation, peripancreatic fluid collections, and pancreatic necrosis correlate inversely with prognosis. CT scanning is prognostically useful but has its greatest value in documenting the late complications of peripancreatic fluid accumulation, pseudocyst formation, necrosis, and abscess development and drainage. Although diagnostic CT-directed aspiration is useful to establish infection, the role of therapeutic CT-directed drainage remains controversial. Percutaneous aspiration fails when the fluid is extremely viscous or cannot be approached safely

TABLE 36-7 CT SCAN ASSESSMENT OF SEVERITY

CT CHARACTERISTICS	GRADE OF ACUTE PANCREATITIS
Normal pancreas	0
Pancreatic enlargement	1
Inflammation of the pancreas and peripancreatic fat	2
One fluid collection or phlegmon	3
Two or more fluid collections	4
Degree of pancreatic necrosis	
No necrosis	0
Necrosis of one third of pancreas	2
Necrosis of one half of pancreas	4
Necrosis of more than one half of pancreas	6
Total score	0–10

because of its location. In patients who are too ill to undergo a surgical approach, CT-directed drainage is a viable temporizing option. MRI is time consuming, is not universally available, and, at present, adds little in the diagnosis or therapy of pancreatitis compared to CT.

Because ERCP can exacerbate acute inflammation and cause infection, it probably should be reserved for recurrent cases where aberrant ductal anatomy is suspected, trauma-induced pancreatitis where ductal integrity is in question, or acute gallstone-induced pancreatitis in which stone extraction is anticipated. In traumatic cases, ERCP visualizes the damaged pancreatic duct, helping plan the repair. In moderate to severe cases of gallstone-induced pancreatitis, ERCP permits stone extraction (with or without sphincterotomy) and reduces hospital stay, complications, and mortality. However, extraction must occur within 24 to 48 h of the onset of symptoms to abort a full-blown attack. ERCP also is useful in the first episodes of pancreatitis for patients older than 40 years of age, in whom ampullary tumors and pancreas divisum are more common findings.

As with other critically ill patients, prognosis is determined largely by the number and severity of organ system failures. Severity of illness can be assessed by simply counting the number of failing organ systems or by using a more formal scoring system, such as the APACHE score. Prognostication in pancreatitis has been studied extensively,

TABLE 36-8 ADVERSE PROGNOSTIC FEATURES OF ACUTE PANCREATITIS

RANSON CRITERIA	SIMPLIFIED GLASGOW SCORE
Age > 55 years	Age > 55 years
Calcium < 8 mg/dL	Calcium < 8 mg/dL
Glucose > 200 mg/dL	Glucose > 180 mg/dL
ARDS	PaO_2 < 60 mm Hg
WBC > 16,000/mm³	WBC > 15,000/mm³
Rise in BUN > 5 mg/dL	BUN > 45 mg/dL
SGOT or LDH > 350 units/dL	LDH > 600 units/L
Falling hematocrit	
Albumin < 3.2 g/dL	
Base deficit > 4 mEq/L	
Repletion volume > 6 L	

WBC, white blood cells; SGOT, serum glutamic-oxaloacetic transaminase; LDH, lactic dehydrogenase; BUN, blood urea nitrogen; ARDS, acute respiratory distress syndrome.

TABLE 36-9 UNPROVED THERAPIES FOR ACUTE PANCREATITIS

Anticholinergic drugs
Gastric acid inhibition
Bradykinin antagonists
Glucagon
Nasogastric suction
Prophylactic antibiotics
Total parenteral nutrition
Antiproteases (aprotinin/gabexate)
Fresh frozen plasma
Indomethacin
Peritoneal lavage
Somatostatin

and certain specific clinical features have been integrated to form the predictive Ranson and Glasgow scales (Table 36-8). These two clinical scales are used in addition to the CT-based scoring systems outlined earlier. Patients with fewer than three of the Ranson criteria generally fare well. Conversely, patients rarely survive if more than six of these criteria are present. A simplified Glasgow score has been developed along similar lines. Of all clinical features, pancreatic necrosis with hemorrhage carries the worst prognosis. Death from alcohol-induced pancreatitis usually occurs early in the hospital course, often as a result of hypovolemia, whereas death from gallstone-induced pancreatitis usually occurs later, as a result of severe sepsis originating in devitalized hemorrhagic pancreatic tissue. The long-term outcome from pancreatitis is good provided that causative gallstones are extracted and alcohol is avoided. Unless extensive necrosis occurred, survivors rarely have either endocrine or exocrine pancreatic insufficiency.

Numerous experimental treatments have been tried in acute pancreatitis (Table 36-9), but there are little data to support their use, hence the treatment of pancreatitis remains largely supportive. Because marked reductions in circulating volume are common, early, adequate fluid resuscitation remains key to the initial management. Unfortunately, the optimal guiding parameter (e.g., CVP, PAOP, cardiac index, or mixed venous oxygen saturation) and the specific value of a chosen parameter remain controversial. Regardless of the method of monitoring, often 5 to 10 L of crystalloid is required early in the first day of the disease. Common causes of hypovolemia include extravascular (third-space) losses into the pancreas and retroperitoneum, intraluminal gut sequestration (because of ileus), and vomiting.

Although a traditional practice, neither withholding enteral feeding nor continuous nasogastric suction reduces pancreatic enzyme release or speeds resolution of inflammation. Nonetheless, both practices may help relieve ileus-related discomfort or intractable vomiting. Similarly, inhibition of gastric acid secretion reduces the incidence of stress ulceration and upper GI bleeding but does not influence the course of pancreatitis. Even though somatostatin effectively suppresses pancreatic secretion, it does not accelerate the resolution of pancreatitis. For years, TPN was standard care for patients with pancreatitis because it was believed that enteral nutrition was not feasible and it exacerbated pancreatitis. Data challenge this belief by demonstrating that not only can patients be fed enterally but also enteral nutrition is associated with a higher survival rate. It is unclear if postpyloric formula delivery is necessary or superior to gastric feeding. For patients unable to tolerate enteral feeding, TPN remains an option. If narcotics are used to relieve pain, meperidine is preferred by some over morphine, which may evoke ampullary spasm; however, the superiority of one narcotic over another is unproven. Although it has become a relatively common practice to administer imipenem "prophylaxis," there are little data to support the practice. A recent well-done randomized placebo-controlled trial does not indicate benefit of a related compound meropenem. However, because of the high incidence of cholangitis in gallstone-induced cases, antibiotics directed against enteric Gram-negative rods, anaerobes, and enterococci are reasonable. The temptation to administer antibiotics is often irresistible because it is difficult to exclude infection, and patients often appear "septic" from pancreatitis itself. Antibiotics are clearly indicated in patients with culture or Gram-positive pancreatic aspirates but their role in noninfected cases is controversial. One thing is clear: over time, antibiotic use selects out resistant bacteria and predisposes to candidal infections.

There is no credible evidence that peritoneal lavage reduces mortality or morbidity of pancreatitis. Operative approaches do not benefit all patients with acute pancreatitis and should be reserved for patients who are likely to have gallstone-induced pancreatitis indicated by biochemical and ultrasonographic or CT determinations and for patients with trauma-induced pancreatic duct disruption. There are four major indications for laparotomy in critically ill patients with acute pancreatitis—"the four Ds": (a) Decompression of biliary obstruction, (b) Diagnostic uncertainty, (c) Drainage of infected necrotic pancreatic tissue, and (d) Deterioration in the face of conservative therapy.

The clearest indication for early surgical intervention is obstructive choledocholithiasis. The mortality rate from untreated gallstone-induced pancreatitis approaches 50% but is dramatically improved by early intervention. If extraction can be accomplished within the first 2 days, endoscopic stone removal seems to be as successful as surgery in aborting pancreatitis, improving survival, and reducing infectious complications in patients with moderate to severe disease. Even though most cases of gallstone-induced pancreatitis will resolve spontaneously, removal of residual stones dramatically reduces the risk of recurrence. Early surgery also is indicated for diagnostic uncertainty in which operative repair of an alternative diagnosis (e.g., perforated viscus, leaking aneurysm, mesenteric ischemia) would be vital. Liberal use of CT scanning has made diagnostic uncertainty an uncommon reason to go to the operating room. Late complications including nonresolving pseudocyst, infected pancreatic necrosis, fistula formation, and pancreatitis-induced hemorrhage also are valid operative indications. Because pancreatectomy carries a high mortality and does not reduce the incidence of complications, it has been abandoned as a therapy for acute pancreatitis. It is rare that a single operation is sufficient for the complicated case of pancreatitis; multiple trips to the operating suite are often needed for a satisfactory outcome.

TABLE 36-10 BACTERIA RECOVERED IN PANCREATIC INFECTIONS

Escherichia coli
Pseudomonas species
Mixed anaerobic infections
Staphylococcus
Klebsiella species
Proteus species
Streptococcus
Enterobacter species

Infectious complications are the most frequent cause of death in pancreatitis, accounting for 25% of all fatalities. Common infections include pancreatic or diaphragmatic abscess, cholangitis, and peritonitis. When necrotic areas or fluid collections are visualized in the region of the pancreas, CT-guided fine-needle aspiration has proved to be a safe and effective diagnostic method. Whenever possible, antibiotic therapy should be guided by Gram stain and culture of appropriate body fluids. When uncertainty exists regarding the site of origin or infecting organism, however, antibiotic coverage should include drugs directed against Gram-negative aerobes, anaerobes, and staphylococci. The most common bacteria recovered from pancreatic tissue are listed in Table 36-10. Of course there is the ever-present risk of nosocomial pneumonia, urinary tract infection, and catheter-related bacteremia.

Hypoxemia occurs in as many as two thirds of all patients with pancreatitis; one in three patients develops infiltrates, atelectasis, or pleural effusions. Hydrostatic pulmonary edema frequently complicates excessive fluid replacement. Although pleural effusions usually are exudative in character, left-sided, bilateral, or right-sided effusions are possible. Most effusions should be tapped to exclude the possibility of empyema, particularly if fluid appears suddenly or late in the clinical course. Pneumonia occurs frequently and fat embolism is not rare. ARDS, the most feared complication, occurs in 10% to 20% of cases, usually in patients with severe disease. The etiology of ARDS is unknown but possibly relates to the circulatory release of activated enzymes and inflammatory products. The ventilator management of pancreatitis-induced ARDS does not differ from that of ARDS of any other cause and should include reduced tidal volume ventilation to limit alveolar distention.

Pancreatic inflammation commonly activates the coagulation cascade, but clinical evidence of coagulopathy is unusual. Although bleeding is more common than inappropriate clotting, splenic or portal vein thrombosis may complicate acute pancreatitis. A variety of fluid and electrolyte disorders are common in acute pancreatitis (see Chapter 13). (Hypocalcemia may persist for weeks.) Total and ionized calcium levels usually reach a nadir of 7 to 8 mg/dL approximately 5 days after pain begins. Even though biochemical hypocalcemia is frequent, symptoms are rare. Mechanisms include the formation of intra-abdominal calcium complexes, hypoalbuminemia, and increased release of glucagon or thyrocalcitonin. Treatment parallels that of any case of symptomatic hypocalcemia. In a minority of patients with hypotension refractory to volume replacement and vasopressor therapy, administration of calcium chloride may rapidly elevate blood pressure. Serum magnesium may be reduced by vomiting, diarrhea, poor oral intake, or deposition in necrotic fat. Hypomagnesemia, especially common in alcohol-induced acute pancreatitis, may precipitate refractory hypokalemia and hypocalcemia.

Pancreatic inflammation and pseudocysts can erode into major vessels, resulting in massive hemorrhage into the GI tract, peritoneal cavity, or retroperitoneum. Vascular erosion presumably is due to the effects of proteolytic enzymes and direct pressure necrosis in the case of pseudocysts. Patients developing pancreatitis are prone to develop other hemorrhagic problems, including gastric stress ulceration, peptic ulcer disease, variceal bleeding, and splenic vein thrombosis. Although only 10% of patients bleed directly into the pancreatic parenchyma, this condition (hemorrhagic pancreatitis) carries a relatively high mortality risk, related largely to subsequent infection in the devitalized tissue. Hemorrhagic pancreatitis has no distinctive clinical features. Coagulation disorders that accompany acute pancreatitis worsen the hemorrhagic tendency, regardless of the bleeding source. Attempts at specific treatment of hemorrhagic acute pancreatitis, including pancreatectomy and peritoneal lavage, have limited effectiveness.

Oliguric acute kidney injury occurs in approximately 25% of all patients with pancreatitis and is associated with a mortality of nearly 80%. Hypovolemia, hypotension, sepsis, IV contrast, and drug-induced renal damage are the most frequent causes.

Acute pancreatitis can produce ascites when transudative fluid crosses the retroperitoneal boundary or when ductal disruption causes spillage into the peritoneum. When pancreatic secretions leak into the peritoneal cavity, intense inflammation of the lining membrane causes massive exudation (pancreatic ascites). Pressure high enough to cause ACS may result. Overt disruption of the pancreatic duct commonly accompanies traumatic or hemorrhagic acute pancreatitis. When ductal disruption occurs, amylase levels in ascitic fluid typically exceed the corresponding serum levels, often rising to higher than 1,000 IU/L. Three to six weeks of bed rest and nutritional support may be required for spontaneous healing of the pancreatic leak and resolution of the ascites. Surgical repair is indicated in refractory cases and should be guided by preoperative ERCP.

Five local complications occur in pancreatitis: pseudocyst, phlegmon, abscess, fistula, and chronic pancreatitis. Pseudocysts, collections of fluid, form in about one half of all cases of acute pancreatitis and usually develop within the first 3 weeks of illness. Pseudocysts are most commonly associated with severe cases of acute pancreatitis. Initial detection is by abdominal examination in approximately 40% of cases and by US or CT scan in the remainder. Luckily, one half of all pseudocysts resolve promptly. In the remainder, 6 months or longer may be required for spontaneous resolution. Although pseudocyst drainage or excision often proves difficult, operative intervention should be considered for those with acute complications or persistent, incapacitating symptoms. A drop in hematocrit with signs of shock and abdominal distention is the reason for immediate operation. Phlegmons are solid masses of indurated pancreas that may be detected as abdominal masses by CT scanning. Phlegmons should be suspected in patients with persistent fever, abdominal pain, and tenderness, especially if leukocytosis persists. Most phlegmons resolve spontaneously within 10 to 14 days. Pancreatic abscess is a poorly defined term applied to a variety of necrotic pancreatic tissue collections. The current, more descriptive terminology for this problem is "infected necrotic pancreatitis." Infected necrosis is uncommon, occurring in only 1% to 10% of all cases, but is much more frequent in clinically severe cases, especially those resulting from biliary tract obstruction. Infection forms in the pancreatic bed late in the course (typically after 3 to 4 weeks of illness), often after a period of apparent improvement. Abscess formation is suggested radiographically by air–fluid levels in the lesser sac or gas bubbles in the pancreatic bed. Slightly more than one half of infected peripancreatic collections are polymicrobial, with a predominance of enteric Gram-negative rods. Surgical or catheter drainage and culture-directed antibiotics are indicated in such cases. External drainage often is sufficient for early suppuration, but later complications usually require internal drainage. By locally invasive autodigestion, acute pancreatitis can lead to the formation of fistulas. Fistulas connect the pancreas to the colon, stomach, duodenum, bile duct, small bowel, or skin surface. Repeated bouts of acute pancreatitis may incite chronic pancreatitis, a disease characterized by recurrent pain of varying intensity and deficiency of endocrine and exocrine pancreatic function (diabetes and malabsorption).

Abdominal Compartment Syndrome

Significant increases in intra-abdominal pressure due to ascites, pancreatitis, hemoperitoneum, retroperitoneal hemorrhage, severe gut edema, or intestinal obstruction can lead to important physiological derangements. (Excessively resuscitated burn patients are common sufferers.) By decreasing visceral organ perfusion, ACS causes oliguria, impaired liver and bowel perfusion, and decreased venous return. Bacterial translocation or frank bowel wall ischemia may supervene. Such findings are particularly common among patients with shock. In addition, pressure-induced cephalad movement of the diaphragms decreases thoracic compliance and impairs gas exchange. Intra-abdominal pressures are estimated by instilling 50 mL of sterile fluid into the bladder and then connecting a manometer/pressure transducer to the catheter. When pressures exceed 25 mm Hg decompressive, paracentesis or laparotomy should be strongly considered. The threshold for taking action can be fine tuned by taking into account the mean arterial pressure. (Like cerebral perfusion pressure, abdominal perfusion pressure can be calculated as mean arterial pressure minus abdominal pressure.)

Cholecystitis and Cholangitis

Among ambulatory patients, more than 90% of cases of cholecystitis result from obstruction of the cystic duct by gallstones. In this group, the disease spontaneously remits over a period of 1 to 4 days as the stone moves from the cystic duct orifice and swelling resolves. If a stone obstructs the common bile duct, spontaneous resolution is much less probable. Likewise, when pancreatitis, cholangitis, gangrene of the gallbladder, or emphysematous cholecystitis complicates cholecystitis, symptoms progress. Emphysematous cholecystitis (gas in the wall of the gallbladder) is an infectious complication of cholecystitis occurring most often in diabetics and immunocompromised patients. Unlike ambulatory patients, acalculous cholecystitis is much more common in hospitalized persons. The mechanism(s) by which inflammation and necrosis of the gallbladder occur in the absence of stones is unknown. However, bile stasis seems likely to play an etiologic role because acalculous cholecystitis tends to occur in patients deprived of the oral alimentation that produces the normal pattern of phasic gallbladder emptying. Bacteria play a minor (if any) role in the development of typical cholecystitis, which is generated predominantly by mechanical occlusion of the cystic duct by a stone in a younger patient. By contrast, cholangitis arises primarily in elderly patients and occurs when bacteria reflux into a partially obstructed biliary duct, producing infection. Life-threatening sepsis may result as infected bile, under pressure, seeds the bloodstream. Cholangitis and cholecystitis are most common among patients with gallstones, previous biliary surgery, pancreatic or biliary tumors, or other obstructions to bile flow. Instrumentation of the biliary tract, including ERCP, surgery, or T tube cholangiography, is a major risk factor.

The signs and symptoms depend on whether simple cholecystitis is present or a complication has occurred (e.g., cholangitis). With both conditions, epigastric and right upper quadrant pain are typical and may radiate to the shoulder. The pain is usually described as deep and gnawing but may be sharp in character. Either diagnosis is unlikely in the absence of fever. Jaundice may be visible, especially with acalculous cholecystitis. Nausea and vomiting are common but nonspecific signs. Physical examination reveals right upper quadrant tenderness and guarding. A mass is palpated in the right upper quadrant in about 20% to 30% of patients. Physical findings of generalized peritonitis are rare and should suggest a complication (e.g., ruptured gallbladder) or another diagnosis (e.g., perforated ulcer). When cholangitis is present, the physical findings are referred to as either a "classic" triad or pentad. The triad (fever, chills, and right upper quadrant pain) is seen in 70% of patients; addition of mental status changes and septic shock completes the pentad seen in another 10%.

The leukocyte count is elevated (up to 15,000 cells/mm^3) in about two thirds of patients with cholecystitis. Even when the total WBC count is normal, granulocytes usually predominate. Higher leukocyte counts suggest cholangitis. The bilirubin is elevated in 80% of cases of acute cholecystitis, but in most, it remains under 6 mg/dL. (A bilirubin > 4 mg/dL is suggestive of a common bile duct stone.) Despite this finding, only 25% of patients are overtly jaundiced. The alkaline phosphatase is usually modestly elevated (<2 to 3 times normal) unless obstruction is severe or prolonged. Serum levels of liver transaminases are usually only modestly elevated. A low-grade coagulopathy is common, manifest as a decreased platelet count and prolonged prothrombin time. The serum amylase may be modestly elevated even in the absence of pancreatitis.

Plain radiographs visualize only 15% to 20% of gallstones. If gas is seen in the biliary tract, it is virtually diagnostic of cholangitis unless the patient is post ERCP or has had prior biliary duct surgery. US will visualize gallstones and dilated biliary ducts reliably if obesity and bowel gas are minimal and sufficient time has elapsed for ductal distention to occur. US cannot reliably make the diagnosis of simple acute cholecystitis in the absence of ductal dilation, but gallbladder enlargement, wall thickening, and edema are suggestive. Occasionally, US discloses edematous changes within the pancreas suggestive of gallstone-induced pancreatitis. Patients with acalculous cholecystitis do not have evidence of gallstones or sludge but often have a thickened gallbladder wall (>5 mm) with pericholecystic fluid. In summary, US is sensitive and specific for gallstones but can rarely be more than suggestive of cholecystitis unless ductal dilation, frank perforation, or gas in the gallbladder wall is detected. In critically ill patients with an acute abdomen, early operative intervention is probably indicated regardless of US findings.

Among stable patients in whom there is diagnostic uncertainty after US, the CT scan and nuclear biliary scans may be helpful. CT scanning may be a superior method of demonstrating dilated intrahepatic channels and processes in the region of the common bile duct, but the portability of US makes it the procedure of first choice. Occasionally, thin-cut CT scanning will detect biliary tract stones missed by US because of its high resolution and superior ability to detect calcification. On CT, acute cholecystitis is indicated by gallbladder enlargement (>5 cm) and wall thickening (>3 mm). The rare occurrence of emphysematous cholecystitis is also easily seen by CT. Finally, the CT scan is also useful to find other intra-abdominal conditions that can be confused with cholecystitis that are poorly detected by US.

Nuclear biliary scans may also be used to evaluate the function of the liver and biliary tract. A radioactive analog of HIDA is administered, taken up by the liver, and secreted into the bile, where it outlines the major intrahepatic ducts, gallbladder, and common bile duct. The gallbladder should demonstrate uptake within 30 to 60 min if normal. Delayed imaging at 4 h that fails to visualize the gallbladder is highly suggestive of acute cholecystitis. Nonvisualization of the gallbladder is common in patients with cystic or common duct obstruction, but nonvisualization may also occur with starvation, pancreatitis, perforated peptic ulcer, TPN use, and severe hepatic dysfunction. The specificity of nonvisualization on biliary scan is high (>90%) if gallstones are present, but in acalculous cholecystitis, the specificity falls to about 40%. It is important not to let the inherent delays imposed by HIDA scanning postpone laparotomy if it is emergently necessary.

ERCP requires a skilled operator and transport of a relatively stable patient to the radiology suite. This technique, however, allows direct visualization of the ampulla and radiographic visualization of the intrahepatic and pancreatic ducts—information that is helpful when malignancy is suspected. ERCP also offers the option of stone extraction or dilation of a stenotic ampulla.

In most patients, cholecystitis resolves spontaneously. However, even when the disease worsens, frank cholangitis is not seen until more than 48 h following ductal obstruction. Intraoperative bile cultures are positive in 85% of patients; two or more organisms grow more than 50% of the time. Although the most common organisms are *Escherichia coli*, *Klebsiella* species, and *Streptococcus faecalis*, anaerobes (i.e., *Bacteroides fragilis* and *Clostridium perfringens*) are isolated in about 40% of infected patients.

Patients with cholecystitis or cholangitis should be stabilized hemodynamically, cultured, and given analgesics. Feeding should be withheld. Although antibiotic use for uncomplicated cholecystitis is controversial, as a practical matter, most physicians give them, and they are essential in cholangitis. Antibiotics, however, are not an alternative to appropriate biliary drainage. If used, antibiotic coverage should include drugs directed against Gram-negative rods and enterococci as well as anaerobes. Piperacillin–tazobactam, ampicillin–sulbactam, ticarcillin–clavulanate, and imipenem are all rational initial choices. (A third-generation cephalosporin plus metronidazole or clindamycin, or ampicillin, gentamicin, and clindamycin are acceptable alternative combinations.)

Most patients with uncomplicated cholecystitis should undergo semielective (within 72 h) drainage of the biliary tract after hemodynamic stabilization. Surgical (laparoscopic or open) cholecystectomy is the procedure of choice. Mortality rates for cholecystectomy in this setting are less than 1% but may rise as high as 5% to 10% for patients over the age of 60. Urgent surgery is indicated for patients with common bile duct obstruction with or without cholangitis, emphysematous cholecystitis, or perforation of the gallbladder and for those who deteriorate while receiving antibiotic and fluid support. Early surgical intervention reduces the risk of suppurative complications, duration of hospital stay, and mortality. Severity of illness in biliary tract obstruction should not preclude surgery because drainage offers the only chance for recovery. In the critically ill patient, it is generally best to do the simplest effective procedure and then reoperate at a later time, if necessary. T-tube drainage of the biliary tract (with or without cholecystectomy) is effective, but the reliability of cholecystostomy alone is uncertain. Nonoperative options include percutaneous catheter drainage, a useful technique in the high-risk ICU patient or in the terminally ill that can be preformed by an interventional radiologist. Unfortunately, bile peritonitis, a potentially lethal problem, may complicate this procedure. ERCP is another option that may be performed without general anesthesia. ERCP is most helpful for stones impacted in the ampullary region, but cannulation can be difficult because of ampullary edema and obstruction.

Small Bowel Obstruction

The triad of nausea, vomiting, and acute abdominal pain should suggest small bowel obstruction (SBO). SBO can be classified as (a) simple, (b) strangulated (in which vascular compromise is the predominant manifestation), or (c) closed loop (in which vascular compromise and complete bowel obstruction rapidly escalate intraluminal pressure). About three fourths of cases are due to adhesions; incarcerated hernias and malignancy comprise the majority of the remainder. Inflammatory bowel disease, intussusception, and gallstones account for a small minority of cases.

On examination, blood in the stool signifies compromised bowel wall integrity. Incarcerated hernias or abdominal scars are suggestive physical findings. Bowel sounds are usually rushing and high pitched early in SBO, but later they become hypoactive. Flat abdominal radiographs are normal, but those taken with the patient in the upright position demonstrate small bowel dilation (>3 cm) and multiple air-fluid levels with distal evacuation of the colon and rectum. In patients who are unable to stand, a left lateral decubitus film can be diagnostic.

Treatment of SBO is usually less urgent than treatment of colonic obstruction. Strangulated bowel with perforation, a potentially disastrous problem, is often misdiagnosed as simple SBO. Unfortunately, there is no clinical way to distinguish between simple SBO and strangulated bowel. Good candidates for conservative management with nasogastric suction include patients who are hemodynamically stable, those with a partial SBO, those with recurrent obstruction following radiation therapy, and those with SBO occurring within 30 days of abdominal surgery. Failure to symptomatically improve with gastric suction suggests operative intervention is required.

Colonic Obstruction

Colonic obstruction, a disease predominately of the elderly, presents with acute abdominal pain, prodromal constipation or obstipation (50%), and nausea and vomiting (50%). The most common causes of obstruction include colon cancer, diverticular disease, and volvulus. When volvulus occurs, the cecum is the most commonly involved site (50%), followed by the sigmoid in 40% of cases. Fecal impaction may imitate this picture. About 20% of patients with colon cancer will have both perforation and obstruction, demonstrating free air on abdominal radiographs. The plain radiograph may be quite helpful in colonic obstruction. When obstruction is mechanical, a "cutoff" sign is often seen at the level of obstruction with air in the proximal colon and small bowel and a gasless distal colon. Plain radiographs are diagnostic of volvulus in more than 50% of patients. When radiographs show an acute increase of cecal diameter to more than 10 cm, perforation of the colon may be imminent. The CT scan is a very valuable diagnostic tool to identify not only the location but also the cause of obstruction preoperatively. CT has almost entirely supplanted previous diagnostic techniques (e.g., barium enema and colonoscopy) because of its low risk and high yield.

"Pseudo-obstruction" (Ogilvie syndrome) may occur in which signs and symptoms of bowel obstruction are present without a mechanical cause. Although uncommon, pseudo-obstruction has been associated with spinal disease, trauma, heart failure, electrolyte imbalances (magnesium or potassium), narcotics, anticholinergic drugs, myxedema, or ganglionic blockers, but its mechanism is unknown. Nausea, vomiting, abdominal pain, and, paradoxically, diarrhea are common symptoms. Bowel sounds are present in almost all cases, and the abdomen is usually distended and tympanitic. The colonic dilation of pseudo-obstruction usually occurs in the right and transverse colon but may extend to the rectum. After excluding mechanical obstruction and toxic megacolon, treatment consists of withholding food, correcting underlying conditions, and carefully observing the patient for complications. Decompression by colonoscopy or percutaneous cecostomy is rarely necessary, and there is little agreement about where the risk–benefit ratio lies for these interventions. There is general consensus that operative interventions should be the last resort. Similarly, although cholinergic agents (i.e., neostigmine), erythromycin, and other prokinetic compounds have been tried, there is no consensus with regard to success or risk. A newer compound methylnaltrexone (8 to 12 mg subcutaneously) has shown promise for colonic pseudo-obstruction associated with opioid use. Side effects are those to be expected form a compound that promotes bowel motility (i.e., nausea, abdominal pain, and flatulence). The dose should be halved in patients with glomerular filtration rates less than 30 mL/min because of its renal clearance.

Toxic megacolon is an inflammatory–ischemic condition most often seen as a complication of chronic inflammatory bowel disease (e.g., Crohn's disease) or acute infectious colitis (e.g., *C. difficile*) that may mimic colonic obstruction. Interestingly, several types of infectious colitis (e.g., *Salmonella, Shigella, Campylobacter, Entamoeba*), even when severe, are unlikely to cause toxic megacolon. Cytomegalovirus is a relatively common cause in the HIV-infected patient. The precise mechanism of toxic megacolon is not known but probably involves extension of the underlying infectious or inflammatory colitis through colonic mucosa into the smooth muscle layer. When this invasion occurs, peristalsis stops and the colon dilates. Colonic dilation may lead to local ischemia by compressing the vascular supply. Because the mucosa is injured, hematochezia is common. The diagnosis of toxic megacolon is a clinical one made by the combination of nonobstructive colonic distention in a patient with appropriate risk factors who appears "toxic." The right and transverse portions of the colon are most frequently involved, with colonic dimensions occasionally reaching 15 cm. Imaging studies add little to the clinical impression, except perhaps to find perforation. Colonoscopy, although usually diagnostic, can lead to perforation. In a patient with an acute abdomen, immediate laparotomy with colectomy is indicated. For patients appearing less toxic, treatment of the underlying condition (e.g., oral vancomycin for *C. difficile* colitis or corticosteroids for inflammatory bowel disease) coupled with careful observation is the best path.

Diverticulitis

Diverticulitis, the result of an inflamed pseudodiverticulum, accounts for up to 10% of all abdominal pain in the elderly. Even though diverticulitis has been referred to as "left-sided appendicitis," the pain has no typical pattern. Nausea, fever, and constipation are common, but vomiting is quite unusual. Physical examination frequently demonstrates a palpable mass in the lower abdomen or pelvis. Although often guaiac positive, the stool is rarely bloody. Colonoscopy is often necessary to rule out neoplasm because the extrinsic compression of the bowel caused by diverticulitis mimics colon carcinoma. Abdominal CT is useful to demonstrate bowel wall inflammation, pericolic edema, and fistula and abscess formation. (Steroid therapy may impair the "walling off" process and predispose to free perforation into the peritoneum.) Medical therapy is successful in 80% to 90% of cases. Withholding food and providing mild analgesia, nasogastric suction, and IV fluids are standard. Broad-spectrum antibiotics (e.g., to treat Enterobacteriaceae and anaerobes) should be administered. Indications for operation in diverticulitis include perforation, obstruction, abscess formation, fistula tract formation, malignancy, and failure to respond to several days of conservative management.

Retroperitoneal Hemorrhage

Retroperitoneal hemorrhage rarely occurs spontaneously, usually resulting from trauma, surgery, invasive procedure (e.g., vena caval filter placement), or anticoagulation. Most patients present with nonspecific flank or abdominal pain—a minority have shock or an acute abdomen. A common vexing problem from retroperitoneal bleeding is the development of severe ileus. Although typically the hematocrit does not rapidly decline, the retroperitoneum is one of the few anatomic compartments capable of containing a massive hemorrhage without evidence of external blood loss. US is rarely helpful. CT scan is the diagnostic procedure of choice to clearly demonstrate the extent of the bleeding, although it rarely identifies a precise source. Unless there is evidence of gross large vessel (i.e., vena cava or renal or splenic artery) rupture, treatment is supportive, with reversal of any existing coagulation disorder and support of the hematocrit and blood pressure. Even though significant blood loss can occur, nonoperative treatment is almost always effective, and blind surgical exploration rarely identifies a discrete bleeding source amenable to repair. Patients with adrenal hemorrhage as the result of infection or anticoagulation can have an identical clinical presentation with nonspecific flank pain. The diagnosis is confirmed by CT demonstrating adrenal hemorrhage and biochemical testing often showing primary adrenal insufficiency (see Chapter 32).

Perforated Viscus

Free air detected under the diaphragm can be the result of a supradiaphragmatic or subdiaphragmatic process. (Recent abdominal surgery, e.g., PEG tube placement, is a common benign cause.) Pulmonary barotrauma can result in eventual dissection of air into the peritoneal cavity, making a certain diagnosis of a perforated viscus difficult. When free air is detected below the diaphragm as a result of perforation of an intra-abdominal organ, the proximal GI tract is the most likely source. Because perforation of the stomach or duodenum is much more common than colonic perforation, an investigation of the upper GI tract should precede laparotomy for presumed colonic perforation in most cases. Although a small amount of free peritoneal air is normal following PEG tube placement, if free abdominal fluid or large collections of peritoneal air are seen, especially days after placement, malpositioning should be suspected. Likewise, any patient with free abdominal air and/or fluid following therapeutic PEG tube manipulation or self-extraction should prompt consideration of a communication between bowel and peritoneum.

Ulcer-Induced Perforation

The perforated gastric or posterior duodenal ulcer is often misdiagnosed as pancreatitis because of similar symptomatology (midabdominal pain radiating to the back, nausea, vomiting, and elevated serum amylase). By contrast, anterior ulcer perforations produce a chemical peritonitis with diffuse acute abdominal pain and ileus. Perforation more commonly complicates duodenal (5% to 10%) than gastric ulcers (<1%). Patients with perforated ulcers usually appear very ill with diffuse acute abdominal pain, tenderness, and decreased bowel sounds. If the process is not recognized, frank peritonitis and shock ensue. A minority of such patients have the abrupt onset of acute abdominal pain or a rigid abdomen. About 80% of all ulcer perforations release free air into the peritoneal cavity. To demonstrate free abdominal gas on plain radiograph, it may be necessary to position the patient upright or in the left lateral decubitus posture for 5 to 10 min before film exposure. (Abdominal CT is highly sensitive for perforation.) If free air is not seen on plain film and CT is not feasible, a perforation may be confirmed by demonstrating extravasation of water-soluble contrast (e.g., Gastrografin, not barium) into the peritoneum. Surgical intervention is indicated in ulcer disease for (a) intractable pain, (b) uncontrollable bleeding, (c) bowel obstruction, and (d) uncontained perforation. If the ulcer is located in the duodenum and the patient is stable, a definitive resection (vagotomy and drainage) should be performed. In unstable patients, however, the ulcer should be overseen and the operation quickly terminated. Whenever possible, gastric ulcers should be resected because of the high potential for carcinoma.

Colonic Perforations

Perforation of the colon is frequently associated with colonic obstruction because of malignancy or diverticular disease. Diverticular perforation is frequently responsible for free intraperitoneal gas in the elderly, but many (possibly most) perforated diverticuli do not liberate intraperitoneal gas. Colonic perforation requires fluid resuscitation, antibiotic therapy, and surgical intervention, most often with at least partial colonic resection.

■ UNUSUAL CAUSES OF ACUTE ABDOMINAL PAIN

Carcinoma is found in 5% to 10% of elderly patients with acute abdominal pain. Although no one knows the cause, patients with diabetic ketoacidosis often present with acute abdominal pain. (Diabetic ketoacidosis should be excluded in all patients before laparotomy.) Sickle cell disease may produce abdominal pain by infarcting the bowel or spleen. Inferior myocardial infarction and pneumonia in the basilar segments of the lung may both present predominately with abdominal discomfort. In these patients, nausea and vomiting are also common, mimicking acute cholecystitis. In such cases, a detailed history, careful examination, and chest radiography are diagnostic. Typhlitis, bacterial invasion of the bowel wall in immunosuppressed patients, may be confused with ischemic colitis, diverticulitis, or appendicitis. Several forms of chemotherapy may produce nausea, vomiting, and GI bleeding (particularly cytosine arabinoside). Up to one fourth of all leukemic patients have neoplastic infiltration of the bowel wall that may cause perforation either in the natural history of the disease or shortly after the initiation of chemotherapy.

■ SUGGESTED READINGS

Ahn SH, Mayo-Smith WW, Murphy BL, et al. Acute nontraumatic abdominal pain in adult patients: Abdominal radiography compared with CT evaluation. *Radiology.* 2002;225:159–164.

Balachandra S, Siriwardena AK. Systematic appraisal of the management of the major vascular complications of pancreatitis. *Am J Surg.* 2005; 190:489–495.

Cheatham ML, Malbrain ML, Kirkpatrick A, et al. Results from the International Conference of Experts on Intra-abdominal Hypertension and Abdominal Compartment Syndrome. II. Recommendations. *Intensive Care Med.* 2007;33(6):951–962.

Clancy TE, Benoit EP, Ashley SW. Current management of acute pancreatitis. *J Gastrointest Surg.* 2005;9:440–452.

Martinez JP, Hogan GJ. Mesenteric ischemia. *Emerg Med Clin North Am.* 2004;22:909–928.

Mutlu GM, Mutlu EA, Factor P. GI complications in patients receiving mechanical ventilation. *Chest.* 2001;119:1222–1241.

Nathens AB, Curtis JR, Beale RJ, et al. Management of the critically ill patient with severe acute pancreatitis. *Crit Care Med.* 2004;32:2524–2536.

Werner J, Feuerbach S, Uhl W, et al. Management of acute pancreatitis: From surgery to interventional intensive care. *Gut.* 2005;54: 426–436.

Yusoff IF, Barkun JS, Barkun AN. Diagnosis and management of cholecystitis and cholangitis. *Gastroenterol Clin North Am.* 2003;32: 1145–1168.

Gastrointestinal Bleeding

■ PREVENTION

In decades past the development of upper gastrointestinal (UGI) bleeding from diffuse "stress ulceration" complicated the stay of up to 30% of critically ill patients. Fortunately, the incidence of **1** significant UGI bleeding developing in the ICU has declined dramatically. Although this is partly the result of the widespread use of histamine (H$_2$)

blockers, proton pump inhibitors (PPIs) and other gastroprotective agents, many other practices have also changed. For example, it is much more common to use mucosal protective enteral nutrition earlier and instead of total parenteral nutrition (TPN). Use of ulcerogenic medications including corticosteroids, slow-release potassium tablets, and oral nonsteroidal anti-inflammatory agents is also less common. Because shock is a potent risk factor for mucosal ulceration and mesenteric ischemia, it is also likely that more aggressive resuscitation practices are partly responsible for the reduced risk of bleeding. Finally, sedation, ventilation, and weaning protocols have shortened the time on ventilator reducing the period of risk.

Indications

Not all ICU patients require pharmacologic "ulcer prophylaxis"; however, prevention efforts are indicated for patients undergoing prolonged (>48 h) mechanical ventilation, for patients with coagulation disorders (e.g., thrombocytopenia, consumptive, hereditary, or anticoagulation related), and for patients with renal failure. Other reasonable candidates include patients with burns, trauma, head injury, and those receiving corticosteroids. As the number of risk factors mounts, so should the likelihood to prescribe prophylaxis. For patients receiving enteral nutrition, prophylaxis may add cost without potential benefit, especially for nonventilated patients.

Options

If mucosal protection or pharmacologic gastric acid buffering is deemed necessary, H$_2$ blockers, PPIs, sucralfate, and antacids are available to accomplish the task. Although controversial, no convincing data suggest the superiority of one class of agent over another or the superiority of any specific drug within a class. Hence, drug selection should be based on side effect profile, cost, and convenience. Clinical practice is heterogeneous but currently PPIs are the most widely used drugs.

Antacids are inconvenient because they must be administered every 1 to 2h, interact with other enteral medications, and often cause diarrhea, phosphate binding, and (in renal insufficiency) the potential for magnesium toxicity. Obviously, antacids cannot deter gastric ulceration if introduced through a postpyloric feeding tube. Antacids are also associated with the highest incidence of reflux and surprisingly may be the most expensive choice.

Because sucralfate *requires* acid for dissolution and tissue binding, it is ineffective if administered with antacids, H_2 blockers, or PPIs, and is less effective and perhaps unnecessary if given with enteral feeding. Sucralfate is problematic because it reduces bioavailability of several commonly used drugs (e.g., quinolones, phenytoin, tetracycline, warfarin, and fluconazole). A commercially available liquid preparation avoids the inconvenience of pulverizing tablets, suspending them in solution and forcing the solution through an enteral tube (often clogging it).

Because the efficacy of continuous intravenous (IV) infusions, intermittent injections, and oral dosing of all available H_2-blocking appear equivalent, it is reasonable to use the least-expensive oral agent. Significant side effects of H_2 blockers are rare but include altered drug metabolism and confusion (most frequently reported with cimetidine). Although often discussed, there is little evidence that H_2 blockers are associated with development of thrombocytopenia.

By inhibiting the final step in acid secretion, PPIs given once or twice daily effectively raise gastric pH to a greater degree and for longer periods than H_2 blockers. Despite this observation there are no credible data to suggest that PPIs given either IV or enterally are superior to H_2 blockers for the *primary* prevention of UGI bleeding. Some PPIs (e.g., lansoprazole, omeprazole) are supplied as capsules containing enteric-coated granules, which must be suspended in a pH buffering liquid if administered by tube. Like sucralfate, these preparations often clog small-bore tubes. As a group, PPIs are very safe but their use increases the absorption of digoxin, calcium channel blockers, benzodiazepines, and opiates. The clinical importance of rebound acid hypersecretion is uncertain but occurs commonly with discontinuation of PPIs.

Risks

Although debated, gastric acid suppression, regardless of how it is achieved, is probably associated with a small increase in risk of nosocomial pneumonia. The mechanism is believed to be the result of gastric overgrowth of microorganisms with subsequent aspiration. Not only does gastric pH play a role, stomach volume and patient position do as well. This is evidenced by the finding that pneumonia risk is comparable when using H_2 blockers, PPIs, or sucralfate but higher when using large volumes of antacids. Regardless, the balance favors bleeding prophylaxis. When prophylaxis is used, effective measures to lower the risk of pneumonia are to elevate the head of the bed to at least 30 degree for all patients who can tolerate such positioning; avoid bolus enteral feedings; and provide consistent oral hygiene. Doing so reduces the reflux of gastric contents and the potential for aspiration and lowers the burden of pathogenic organisms that may be aspirated.

■ EVALUATION OF THE BLEEDING PATIENT

First steps

In patients with conspicuous GI bleeding, attention should first be devoted to ensuring a stable airway with adequate ventilation and establishing intravenous access. Developing an appropriate and efficient diagnostic and therapeutic plan requires distinguishing upper from lower bleeding using historical and demographic information and the examination. UGI bleeding is more likely among younger patients and men. A history of repeated retching, non-steroidal anti-inflammatory drug (NSAID) use, heavy alcohol ingestion, or past history of peptic ulcer disease or liver disease (especially with varices) favors an UGI bleeding source. By contrast, lower GI (LGI) bleeding is more likely among older patients, women, and patients with a history of diverticular or vascular occlusive disease. GI bleeding occurring during systemic anticoagulation does not preferentially occur from an upper or lower source.

Examination

Bruising or petechiae may be a clue to an underlying coagulopathy, and cutaneous or mucous membrane arteriovenous malformations may signal the presence of hereditary hemorrhagic telangiectasia (Rendu–Osler–Weber syndrome). Mental status alterations can result from hypotension alone but often indicate the presence of hepatic encephalopathy. The stigmata of cirrhosis and portal hypertension (e.g., jaundice, ascites, spider angiomata, caput medusa, palmar erythema, gynecomastia, ecchymoses) make a diagnosis of UGI bleeding much more likely.

The predominant portal of blood loss (oral or rectal) provides a valuable guide to bleeding site. Hematemesis is rarely the result of LGI bleeding and essentially never results from a source beyond the proximal jejunum. By contrast, hematochezia can result from brisk upper or slower LGI bleeding, but in the absence of shock is almost always due to a LGI source. As little as 15 mL of blood in the UGI tract may produce guaiac-positive stools, but melena (black, tarry stools formed by the digestion of blood by acid and bacteria) requires loss of more than 100 mL of blood over a relatively brief period. Because blood in the gut speeds transit time, melena seldom results from LGI bleeding unless it originates from a slow bleed in the ascending colon. More commonly, significant bleeding from the right colon produces maroon-colored stools, whereas bleeding from the left colon results in hematochezia. A mixture of formed stool with red blood is highly suggestive of a distal colonic (sigmoid colon or rectal) source.

An UGI bleed is less likely if the aspirate from a gastric tube does not reveal fresh blood or at least "coffee ground" material, although as many as 15% of patients with UGI bleeding have clear aspirates. These "false-negative" aspirates usually occur when a competent pylorus prevents reflux of blood originating in the duodenum into the stomach. Testing gastric contents is not warranted because it commonly produces false-positive results.

Assessing Bleeding Severity

For the average sized adult, blood loss of less than 1 L produces few physiological changes as pulse, respiratory rate, blood pressure, mental status, and urine output remain near normal. With acute losses of 1 to 1.5 L (mild shock) tachycardia, tachypnea, and mild oliguria are seen and orthostatic blood pressure changes can be detected. Tachypnea can be an appropriate compensatory response to hemorrhage and metabolic acidosis, the result of aspirating vomited blood, or only a manifestation of anxiety. Moderate shock following hemorrhage of 1.5 to 2 L raises pulse and respiratory rates further, causes confusion, slows capillary refill, and further diminishes urine output. When severe shock occurs, typically with blood losses more than 2 L hypotension is routine and profound, tachycardia marked, and enormous ventilatory demands often cause respiratory collapse. Urine output and mental status are never normal. During acute hemorrhage

it is important to not be misled by hemoglobin (Hgb) measurements. In severe acute blood loss, the Hgb concentration remains near normal despite massive losses until crystalloid replacement is begun. By contrast, a very low Hgb concentration in a patient with near normal vital signs almost certainly means blood loss has occurred over weeks or even months. Hence, shock with visible loss of large volumes of blood should prompt aggressive transfusion, whereas severe anemia without visible evidence of blood or shock can be approached more slowly.

Initial Treatment

As stabilization is accomplished appropriate consultants (e.g., gastroenterology, interventional radiology, surgery) should be notified. For patients with shock, massive hematemesis, or incipient respiratory failure, it usually makes sense to perform endotracheal intubation before overwhelming aspiration or respiratory arrest occur. In addition, upper endoscopic evaluation is often not possible without airway control. Caution is advised however; frequently, the procedure prompts massive hematemesis obscuring the airway. Powerful suction and expert backup are essential. When time permits, evacuation of the stomach with a gastric tube may reduce regurgitation risk. Gown, gloves, and face-shield protection for the proceduralist is prudent.

Regardless of bleeding source, at least two large-bore (16- to 14-gauge) peripheral IV catheters or a large central venous catheter (CVC) should be inserted to allow rapid fluid and blood administration. A CVC is not always necessary and may not be the best choice for fluid infusion, but the central venous pressure (CVP) measurements it yields can be useful to guide fluid replacement. (A triple-lumen catheter may actually *slow* fluid administration because its three smaller lumens and increased length cannot achieve the same infusion rates as shorter, larger bore peripheral IVs.) By contrast, a centrally placed 7.5- or 8.5-F conduit can deliver prodigious amounts of fluid and blood, especially if used with a pressure infuser.

At the time IV access is obtained, samples should be obtained for Hgb, electrolytes, creatinine, liver function tests, prothrombin time (PT), platelet count, and cross-matching. Arterial blood gas testing may be useful to evaluate adequacy of ventilation and severity of metabolic acidosis. The basic principles of support of the circulation and transfusion are presented in Chapters 3 and 14, respectively;

however, a few points deserve emphasis. First, the fundamental problem in severe GI bleeding is intravascular volume depletion. Therefore, the best first therapy is not vasopressor infusion but isotonic crystalloid replacement followed by blood when available. Colloid offers no demonstrated advantage over crystalloid resuscitation, despite the fact that a smaller volume of the former is required to produce equivalent volume expansion. Colloids risk allergic reaction, are not always immediately available, and are more than ten times more expensive than crystalloid for equal effect. Although fresh whole blood is a better source of oxygen delivery than older packed red blood cells, it is rarely available. As a consequence, blood replacement is usually accomplished using specific component therapy with serial assessments of Hgb, platelet count, and PT. For exsanguinating patients, universal donor (O negative) blood may be necessary, but if there are even a few minutes to spare, the possibly safer alternative is type-specific red blood cells. Thrombocytopenia or soluble clotting factor deficiencies should be corrected rapidly to promote hemostasis. Prevention or reversal of hypothermia and metabolic acidosis are additional methods of optimizing coagulation. Reasonable transfusion goals are $\geq 50,000/mm^3$ functioning platelets, a PT less than 1.5 times control, and a Hgb more than 8 gm/dL. Although it is clear that lower transfusion thresholds are safe for the nonbleeding patient, during ongoing hemorrhage it is prudent to maintain a buffer against exsanguination. Even higher Hgb values may be appropriate in patients with critical oxygen supply problems, such as recent myocardial ischemia or stroke.

For most patients with UGI bleeding, gentle placement of a nasogastric (NG) or orogastric (OG) tube is safe and useful to monitor the rate of bleeding. Although controversial, possible exceptions include patients with esophageal varices or Mallory–Weiss tears in whom tube placement theoretically could aggravate bleeding. Combining clinical data with gastric aspirate results also has prognostic value. Clear or "coffee ground" returns portend a good prognosis when the patient presents with melena. When red blood is aspirated from the stomach of a patient with melena, the prognosis is worse but not as bad as when red blood is recovered from the stomach during hematochezia. Patients with liver failure may benefit from purging intestinal blood that can precipitate hepatic encephalopathy, but blood is an excellent laxative, usually making cathartics unnecessary. Gastric

lavage does not decrease the rate of UGI bleeding, even when the solution is cooled or fortified with vasoconstrictor.

■ UGI BLEEDING

Sources

A relatively small number of conditions are responsible for most cases of UGI bleeding (Table 37-1). Peptic ulcer disease (gastric and duodenal ulcer) leads the list, followed by gastric and esophageal erosive disease, Mallory–Weiss tears, and variceal bleeding. Making a definitive diagnosis of an UGI bleeding source usually is straightforward and is outlined in Figure 37-1. Fortunately, regardless of cause, UGI bleeding stops spontaneously in 70% to 80% patients. A combination of clinical factors (i.e., **3** older age, shock at presentation, coagulopathy, or renal, hepatic, or heart failure) and specific endoscopic findings (Table 37-2) predict those most likely to have recurrent bleeding.

Diagnostic Tests

Plain abdominal radiographs are rarely diagnostically useful unless they demonstrate free air (indicating perforation of a viscus) or "thumbprinting" of the large bowel (suggesting ischemic colitis). Likewise, the long used "UGI series" is seldom diagnostic and swallowed barium compromises subsequent tests, including endoscopy, CT scanning, and angiography and makes surgery techni- **4** cally more difficult. Barium studies also require transport of potentially unstable patients to the radiography suite.

Esophagogastroduodenoscopy (EGD) is a high-yield procedure to (a) definitively demonstrate the

TABLE 37-1 SOURCES OF UGI BLEEDING

SOURCE	APPROXIMATE FREQUENCY
Peptic ulcer disease	50%
Erosive gastritis–esophagitis	25%
Variceal bleeding	15%
Mallory–Weiss tears	5%
Others[a]	5%–10%

[a]Carcinomas, vascular malformations, etc.

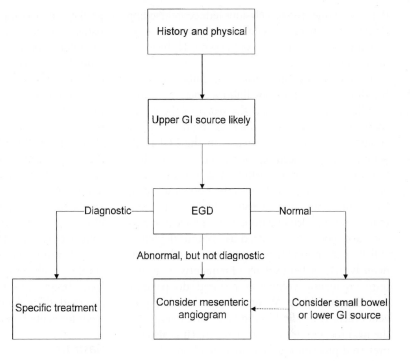

■ **FIGURE 37-1** Suggested diagnostic evaluation of suspected upper GI bleeding. If upper GI bleeding is believed to be likely after obtaining a history and performing a physical examination, esophagogastroduodenoscopy (EGD) is usually performed. If EGD is diagnostic, therapy directed at the specific lesion should be instituted. If the EGD is normal, the small bowel or LGI tract should be considered as a bleeding source. When the EGD is abnormal but nondiagnostic, consideration should be given to mesenteric angiography.

bleeding site, (b) predict the likelihood for rebleeding, (c) permit control of some lesions, and (d) reduce resource utilization (e.g., transfusions, operating room time if surgery is required, and hospital length of stay). However, EGD has several limitations: sedation may compromise ventilation in tenuous patients, and an optimal examination requires a stomach empty of food and blood. (A single 250-mg dose of IV erythromycin given 30 min before endoscopy can increase gastric emptying and improve visualization.)

The best time to perform EGD is debated but is probably as soon as the airway and oxygenation are adequate and a reasonable degree of hemodynamic stability is achieved. Based on the combination of

clinical and endoscopic features, it is undoubtedly safe to provide care outside the ICU and even discharge patients with lesions at low risk to rebleed (i.e., gastritis, clean-based ulcers, or flat pigmented spots). By contrast, patients with bleeding varices and those with ulcers containing visible vessels or obscured by overlying clot are at high risk for recurring hemorrhage.

Endoscopic injection therapy using epinephrine is a safe and effective method to gain initial control and prevent rebleeding in high-risk nonvariceal lesions. Similarly, thermal therapy (i.e., bipolar electrocoagulation, heater probe coagulation) has been used alone and in combination with injection therapy to arrest and deter recurrent hemorrhage. Surprisingly, removing a clot overlying an ulcer then using injection and/or thermal therapy reduces the risk of rebleeding compared to not disturbing the clot. (Perhaps without vasoconstriction and coagulation of the underlying vessels, hemorrhage is more likely when the clot is dislodged or dissolved.) In the 15% to 20% of patients among whom rebleeding occurs, it is almost always within 48 h of initial EGD. The particular technique used to halt bleeding is determined largely by personal preference since all endoscopic methods have comparable effectiveness and safety. Uncommon risks of these procedures include worsening of bleeding and perforation. Use of a PPI after endoscopic

TABLE 37-2 RISK OF RECURRENT UPPER GI BLEEDING BASED ON ENDOSCOPIC FINDINGS

ENDOSCOPIC FINDING	RISK OF REBLEEDING
Visible bleeding vessel	Near 100%
Active oozing	30%–80%
Nonbleeding vessel	50%
Esophageal varices	50%
Red or black "spot"	5%–10%
Clean ulcer base	1%

therapy for high-risk *ulcer* lesions reduces rebleeding even further but benefits do not extend to *non-ulcer* bleeding sources and it is not known if H_2 blockers offer similar benefit.

If a technically satisfactory EGD fails to reveal a bleeding source, three possibilities exist: the upper bleeding source is beyond the reach of the endoscope (e.g., small bowel); the bleeding has stopped spontaneously; or the source is in the LGI tract. When an upper bleeding source is elusive, evaluation of the lower tract is indicated; however, it is not prudent to hastily dismiss the possibility of an UGI source even after "negative" EGD. More often than expected, bleeding from an esophageal or gastric varix goes unrecognized as volume depletion collapses the normally distended veins and spontaneously arrests hemorrhage. Frequently, it is not until circulating volume is restored do patients again begin to bleed. When vigorous bleeding prevents identifying the bleeding site, angiography is the next most useful course of action. (It is also the preferred procedure to diagnose small bowel hemorrhage.) During angiography, bleeding may be stopped by infusing vasoconstrictors or by placing emboli in the bleeding vessel.

Specific Causes of UGI Bleeding

Peptic Ulcer Disease

Between one third and one half of all cases of UGI bleeding in the ICU are due to peptic ulceration. Although most ambulatory patients with ulcers relate a history of epigastric pain (particularly nocturnal) relieved by food, H_2 blockers, PPIs, or antacids, pain is rare among ICU patients. EGD is the diagnostic procedure of choice because it is safe, rapidly performed, and may facilitate control of bleeding with thermal coagulation or injection therapy. Even when bleeding cannot be controlled, information gained from EGD assists in planning definitive surgery.

The overall risk of recurrent bleeding from ulcer disease is 20% to 30%, but certain EGD findings portend a higher risk, suggesting that more aggressive or earlier intervention is indicated (see Table 37-2). Visualization of persistent active bleeding from a visible vessel mandates endoscopic, angiographic, or surgical intervention because of the near 90% chance of continued or recurrent hemorrhage. When a nonbleeding vessel is seen in an ulcer crater, the risk of rebleeding approaches 50%, and an adherent clot overlying an ulcer also

predicts rebleeding in as many as a quarter of patients, again suggesting that endoscopic or surgical intervention probably is indicated. Because a lesion oozing blood without a visible vessel has only about a 10% risk of bleeding and flat pigmented spots or smooth ulcer bases carry an even lower (1% to 10%) risk, they usually are medically treated. Ulcer location also provides information about the likelihood of rebleeding. Ulcers high on the lesser gastric curvature (over the left gastric artery) and on the posterior–inferior wall of the duodenum (overlying the gastroduodenal artery) are the most ominous. Fortunately, most ulcers stop bleeding spontaneously with supportive care and control of gastric pH. Persistent severe hemorrhage should prompt consideration of surgery or angiographic occlusion. Although the relationship of Helicobacter infection to ulcer disease is well accepted, there is no benefit to antimicrobial treatment for acute hemorrhage.

Gastritis

Erosive gastritis or esophagitis—is the second most frequent cause of GI bleeding in the ICU and is particularly common in critically ill patients with respiratory failure, sepsis, hypotension, or burns. Although "superficial," stress ulceration may result in severe bleeding, particularly in patients with underlying coagulopathy or receiving anticoagulation. These erosions result from the combined actions of acid, ulcerogenic drugs, NG tube irritation, and ischemia on mucosal surfaces, typically developing 5 to 7 days after admission to the ICU. H_2 blockers, PPIs, antacids, and sucralfate all reduce the incidence of gastritis, but the best preventative measures are avoidance of hypotension and hypoxia and early provision of enteral nutrition.

Mallory–Weiss Tears

Forceful retching may disrupt the mucosa of the gastroesophageal junction, resulting in a Mallory–Weiss tear. These longitudinal mucosal lacerations account for 5% to 15% of all UGI bleeding and are much more common in men than in women. Precipitating or contributing factors include (a) alcohol use, (b) intractable vomiting, and (c) esophageal food impaction. Rarely, coughing, seizures, heavy lifting, pregnancy, and upper endoscopy have been associated with such lesions. Interestingly, no precipitating event is evident in approximately 20% of cases. Even though these lesions commonly lead to massive hemorrhage, bleeding almost always stops spontaneously. The diagnosis is suggested by a history of forceful, painless hematemesis, and is confirmed by EGD demonstrating linear tears on the gastric side of the gastroesophageal junction. Supportive treatment includes antiemetics, raising gastric pH, and expectant observation. In the rare instance in which bleeding does not promptly abate, EGD with thermal coagulation or therapeutic injection can halt bleeding. Surgery to control hemorrhage rarely is necessary unless the tear involves preexisting esophageal varices.

Portal Hypertension and Variceal Bleeding

Varices are fragile, bulbous venous channels that shunt portal blood to the systemic circuit driven by portal hypertension. These native shunts usually are the result of cirrhosis induced by ethanol and/or viral hepatitis, but portal hypertension has many potential causes, spanning the anatomic spectrum from the portal to hepatic vein (Table 37-3). The largest of these collateral channels tend to form at the gastroesophageal junction; however, hemorrhoidal and retroperitoneal veins also dilate and bleed. As many as 40% of all patients with cirrhosis eventually develop variceal hemorrhage characterized by abrupt, painless, massive UGI bleeding. (Much like patients with Mallory–Weiss tears.) The risk of bleeding roughly correlates with the size of the varices, the severity of the underlying liver disease, and the magnitude of the hepatic venous pressure gradient. (Bleeding is uncommon when the gradient is <12 mm Hg.) Variceal hemorrhage often is difficult to treat because of accompanying coagulation abnormalities. Soluble clotting factor deficiencies commonly result from malnutrition or impaired hepatic synthetic function. Furthermore, the direct toxic effects of ethanol on the bone marrow and portal-hypertension-induced hypersplenism often cause thrombocytopenia. The acute mortality of variceal bleeding approaches 50%. Even when the initial hemorrhage ceases, bleeding recurs in more

than 50% of patients, many times within just weeks of the initial episode. Because patients with varices tend to be chronically ill with impaired clotting, immune, and renal function, it is not surprising that nearly two thirds of patients die within 12 months of the first bleeding episode.

Because 30% to 40% of all bleeding episodes in patients with esophageal varices originate from nonvariceal sources (e.g., ulcers, gastritis), it is important to determine the bleeding site before instituting definitive therapy. As with all massive GI bleeding, fluid resuscitation, Hgb maintenance, and correction of coagulation abnormalities are key components of therapy. For patients with variceal bleeding, some clinicians preferentially use vasopressors over fluid replacement, theorizing that the hepatic vein/portal pressure gradient will be reduced and thus, the risk of hemorrhage will be lowered. Unfortunately, no human data exist to support this contention, and volume depletion can result in hypoperfusion of other organs. The accumulation of massive ascites can contribute to an increased hepatic vein/portal vein pressure gradient. Therefore, for some patients, large-volume paracentesis can be a useful adjunct to reduce the driving pressure for hemorrhage. There is no evidence that gentle NG tube insertion aggravates variceal bleeding; however, such tubes may induce esophagitis, acid reflux, and gastric erosion if left in place for prolonged periods. Aspiration pneumonitis is extremely common in patients with variceal bleeding because of depressed mental status, massive vomiting, and esophageal instrumentation Hence, for many patients, early "prophylactic" endotracheal intubation is reasonable.

After airway and circulatory stability have been achieved and variceal bleeding is confirmed, five methods are available to control the bleeding: pharmacotherapy, variceal tamponade, variceal obliteration, decompressive shunting, and liver transplantation. One commonly used plan to gain control of variceal hemorrhage is outlined in Figure 37-2.

TABLE 37-3 CAUSES OF PORTAL HYPERTENSION

PREHEPATIC	INTRAHEPATIC	SINUSOIDAL	POST-HEPATIC
Portal vein thrombosis	Schistosomiasis	Cirrhosis	Budd–Chiari syndrome
Congenital	Sarcoidosis	Venoocclusive disease	Right heart failure
Septic	Graft vs. host disease		Constrictive pericarditis
Traumatic			
Malignancy			

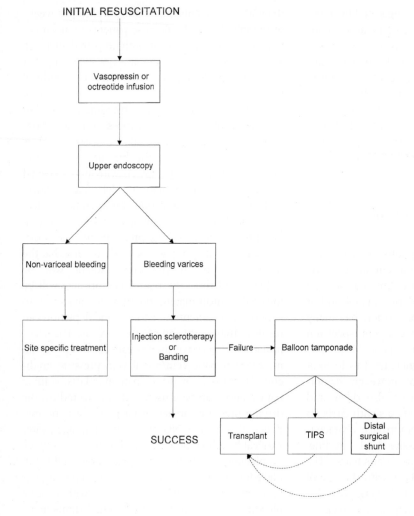

■ **FIGURE 37-2** Suggested plan for managing variceal bleeding. After initial stabilization, an infusion of octreotide may reduce or arrest hemorrhage. In most cases, upper endoscopy is then performed. If bleeding varices are identified, banding or injection sclerotherapy can be used to prevent recurrent hemorrhage. If hemorrhage is uncontrollable, balloon tamponade followed by TIPS or transplant to directly lower portal pressures may be considered. TIPS, transjugular, intrahepatic, portosystemic shunt.

Pharmacotherapy

Somatostatin and octreotide, its synthetic analog, are splanchnic vasoconstrictors that also inhibit the release of gastrointestinal hormones. In comparative trials, octreotide is as effective as sclerotherapy or banding and is superior to vasopressin or balloon tamponade at halting acute variceal blood loss and in preventing rebleeding. When octreotide (25 to 50 μg/h IV for 2 to 5 days) is added to endoscopic sclerotherapy, the rate of rebleeding is further reduced. Even though octreotide decreases renal perfusion, systemic vascular resistance, and gut motility, important side effects are rare and are trivial compared to those of the traditional alternative, high-dose vasopressin. Unfortunately, like vasopressin, balloon tamponade, endoscopic banding, or injection sclerotherapy, octreotide has not been proven to reduce mortality.

Vasopressin, the long used splanchnic vasoconstrictor, often (approx. 50%) gains initial control of variceal bleeding by decreasing portal blood flow through collateral vascular channels, but has not been shown to lower the incidence of rebleeding. If used, the dose is a continuous IV infusion of 0.2 to 0.8 units/min, until 24 h after bleeding has stopped. (NB: Doses for variceal bleeding are 5 to 20 times those used for septic shock.) Vasopressin is now rarely used for this indication because up to 10% of patients will have potentially lethal side effects including arrhythmias (especially bradycardia), myocardial and mesenteric ischemia, congestive heart failure, stroke, and renal insufficiency. The addition of nitroglycerin to vasopressin improves the success rate of bleeding control and reduces the risk of vasopressin-induced complications. (In this setting, nitroglycerin is given by constant intravenous infusion at a starting dose of 40 μg/min and titrated to reduce systolic blood pressure to 90 to 100 mm Hg.) Unfortunately, neither vasopressin alone or in combination with nitroglycerin has been demonstrated to reduce the mortality.

β Blockade has been used chronically to decrease portal blood flow and portal pressure, reducing the risk of variceal rebleeding by as much as 50% during the first year of therapy. Because β-blockers blunt compensatory cardiovascular responses to hemorrhage, they should not be used to treat active variceal bleeding.

Variceal Tamponade

Balloon tamponade controls esophageal bleeding in 70% to 90% of patients, many of whom are refractory to other modalities. Because tamponade can only be used for 2 to 3 days before it causes tissue necrosis and half of all patients treated with tamponade rebleed on decompression, a definitive plan must be devised at the time the tube is inserted. Currently, a four-lumen device with gastric and esophageal balloons (e.g., Minnesota tube) is preferred over the three-lumen Sengstaken–Blakemore tube because it enables the evacuation of the proximal esophagus, possibly reducing the aspiration risk. Because patients considered for balloon tamponade are hemodynamically unstable, often have altered mental status, and are prone to aspiration, they should undergo endotracheal intubation prior to placement. During intubation and Minnesota tube placement, a gown, gloves, mask, and eye protection should be worn because many of these patients are infected with transmissible hepatitis-causing viruses.

The Minnesota tube is inserted through the mouth into the stomach. (Nasal passage is difficult; often causes bleeding and essentially always causes sinusitis.) Appropriate positioning of the gastric balloon is then checked by radiograph before inflation to prevent fatal esophageal rupture. In emergent situations, the tube may be passed a minimum of 50 cm before the *gastric* balloon is inflated to 100 mL. Patient discomfort indicates potential esophageal positioning. If the 100-mL gastric balloon inflation is well tolerated, the balloon should be inflated to 400 to 450 mL and then placed on gentle traction against the gastroesophageal junction. (Tension usually is maintained by securing the tube to a bridle or football helmet placed on the patient.) For the novice, placing traction on the inflated gastric balloon is often a terrifying experience as a huge placenta-like mass of clot and liquid blood is expelled from the mouth. This event should not be misinterpreted as worsening hemorrhage. The *esophageal* balloon should be inflated only if bleeding continues with the gastric balloon inflated and then only to a maximum pressure of 40 mm Hg. After completion of this inflation sequence, it is important to confirm the proper configuration by radiograph. The tube should be kept in place for at least 24 h after cessation of bleeding but no longer than 72 h. Without meticulous technique and monitoring, complications occur in a high percentage of patients. Aspiration remains the most frequent complication despite recent modifications of tube design. Cephalad migration may produce upper airway obstruction, a catastrophic event for the patient whose airway is unsecured. (Scissors should be kept at the bedside for immediate tube transection if airway obstruction occurs.) Esophagogastric rupture, another devastating complication, usually results from improper tube placement and inflation of the gastric balloon in the esophagus. Pressure necrosis of the nose, mouth, and gastroesophageal mucosa also are common.

Variceal Obliteration

EGD with variceal banding or injection sclerotherapy has become the procedure of choice for variceal bleeding because it at least temporarily controls hemorrhage in more than 90% of cases and is less dangerous than emergent surgical shunting. Unfortunately, sclerotherapy and banding generally are not effective for gastric varices and neither intervention alters survival. In addition, almost all patients undergoing sclerotherapy or banding eventually will rebleed unless repeated procedures are performed until all varices are obliterated. When endoscopic ligation (banding) is performed, constrictive elastic bands are placed around the bases of the varices, causing thrombosis. For many endoscopists, banding is the preferred method to occlude varices because it is more effective than sclerotherapy but produces fewer complications. On the other hand, banding is technically more difficult for actively bleeding patients and, once in place, bands may slip off.

During sclerotherapy, varices or the surrounding tissue is injected with a chemical causing rapid thrombosis and long-term scarring. Following sclerotherapy, minor complications (fever, chest pain, and tachycardia) occur in one half of all patients. Major complications occur in more than 20% of patients and include (a) aspiration; (b) pulmonary dysfunction (acute respiratory distress syndrome) secondary to aspiration, sepsis, or sclerosants; and (c) local esophageal problems, including ulceration, perforation, stricture, dysmotility, and abscess formation. A rare complication, esophageal perforation may produce empyema, mediastinitis, or mediastinal hematoma. Occasionally, sclerotherapy incites bacteremia. Although banding shares the risk of aspiration and the potential for late esophageal stricture, the dangers of injection-induced infection or sclerosant toxicity are avoided.

Decompressive Shunting

Radiological options designed to control variceal bleeding by lowering the hepatic-portal vein pressure gradient have now largely supplanted surgical approaches. Decompressive shunts target GI bleeding and are best performed in patients with good hepatic parenchymal function considered to be future candidates for transplantation. No shunting procedure improves hepatic function; therefore, all shunts represent poor choices for patients with severely impaired liver function. The most widely used option is the transjugular, intrahepatic, portosystemic shunt (TIPS). In this procedure, a needle is forced from the hepatic vein to the portal vein, through which a guide wire is placed. After successive dilation, a stent is then passed over the guide wire, decreasing the portohepatic vein pressure gradient thereby lowering the distending pressure for the gastroesophageal varices. (Obviously, TIPS cannot help portal hypertension from portal vein thrombosis.) Often the varices are reimaged after shunt placement and, if patent, are embolized in hopes of reducing the rebleeding. There are no data to suggest that TIPS reduces ascites, hepatic hydrothorax, or treats hepatorenal syndrome. Potential complications include contrast-induced renal injury, hemorrhage, liver capsule rupture (approx. 5%), hemolytic anemia (10%), worsening of hepatic encephalopathy (30%), and death (<2%). Insertion is expensive, often costing more than $10,000 and long-term patency of TIPS is poor, with up to 70% of shunts occluding within 6 to 12 months. Radiological revision of occluded shunts can usually be done. When TIPS blockage is suspected, *complete* occlusion can be identified by absence of flow on Doppler ultrasound. However, accurately quantifying the pressure gradient across the shunt can only be done by catheterization. Although TIPS may stem bleeding in high-risk patients who are not amenable or responsive to banding or injection sclerotherapy, it is probably best viewed as a "bridge" to liver transplant, not a remedy for portal hypertension. Because TIPS is only a temporary solution for bleeding and is done for patients with profound liver disease, insertion should prompt end-of-life discussions.

Surgical shunts may be classified as total or "selective," based on the degree of blood flow diverted around the liver. Total shunts, such as portocaval and mesocaval shunts, provide a decompressive anastomosis of a portion of the portal vein to the inferior vena cava. The size and position of the anastomosed vessels determine the vascular pressure and blood flow through the liver. When large, shunts divert nearly all portal blood flow, resulting in a high risk of hepatic encephalopathy and liver failure. Smaller shunts reduce this risk but may fail to lower the portohepatic gradient sufficiently to avert bleeding. More selective procedures, such as the distal splenorenal shunt, decompress portal circulation by joining the splenic and left renal vein. Selective shunts better preserve hepatic perfusion while decreasing portal pressure and varix diameter, thereby reducing bleeding risk. In experienced centers, selective shunts are still occasionally used for elective decompression but are time consuming and therefore not feasible in unstable patients. Unfortunately, selective shunts do not improve long-term survival; however, they do change the cause of death from GI hemorrhage to encephalopathy and liver failure. Surgical shunting procedures do not preclude subsequent liver transplantation.

Liver Transplant

Although liver transplantation corrects portal hypertension, the primary indication for transplantation is parenchymal hepatic failure, not variceal bleeding. Patients with good hepatic reserve who are bleeding should be considered for a shunt before liver transplant. Patients with more severe disease who lack other contraindications may be considered for liver transplant. Liver transplantation is a complex and expensive procedure that carries a significant risk of primary graft failure (1% to 5%), acute rejection (4 to 14 days after transplant), and infection secondary to the required immunosuppression. Bacterial infections of the abdomen and lung are most common problem in the first 4 to 6 weeks, although vigilance must be maintained for fungal, especially Candidal infections. Cytomegalovirus infections rise in frequency to peak near the end of the first month and can be reduced by ganciclovir prophylaxis.

Aortoenteric Fistulas

On rare occasion, abdominal aortic aneurysms or prosthetic aortic grafts may erode into the GI tract, causing massive hemorrhage. Exsanguination often follows a moderate to large "herald" bleed that stops spontaneously. Aortoenteric fistulas usually occur in the distal duodenum and occasionally cause pulsatile bleeding from the mouth or gastric tube. Endoscopy, aortography, and contrasted CT scanning can establish this diagnosis but rarely are completed before death. Immediate laparotomy should be undertaken in patients with a confirmed diagnosis or intractable bleeding otherwise unexplained in a predisposed patient.

Vascular Malformations

Angiodysplasia is the most common form of enteric vascular abnormality, a category that also includes arteriovenous malformations and vascular telangiectasia. Although angiodysplasia occurs most commonly in the large bowel, it is a common cause of UGI bleeding in patients with aortic stenosis and von Willebrand disease and is second only to erosive gastritis as a cause of bleeding in patients with renal failure. Most microvascular malformations involving the UGI tract are located in the duodenum. The diagnosis must be made by angiography or by EGD. (EGD diagnosis can be difficult because of the small size of most of these lesions, but when located, they can be ablated by thermal coagulation.)

Miscellaneous Causes

Hemobilia, a rare cause of UGI bleeding, occurs when hepatic blood drains via the bile ducts into the duodenum. The triad of abdominal pain, jaundice, and UGI bleeding should prompt consideration of this condition. Hemobilia may result from pancreatitis, or tumor involvement of the bile ducts or liver, but most commonly follows blunt chest or abdominal trauma. (Recent ERCP can also cause bleeding.) Fortunately, hemobilia is seldom massive and spontaneously resolves in most cases.

Although pancreatic disease is an unusual primary cause of UGI bleeding, hemorrhage may occur when pseudocysts or pancreatic tumors erode the posterior duodenal wall. Much more often patients with acute pancreatitis bleed from gastritis, ulcers, Mallory–Weiss tears, or esophageal varices unrelated to pancreatitis.

Surgical intervention

Unfortunately, those most in need of surgery often are the worst operative candidates because of their limited tolerance of anemia and hypotension. For patients with ulcer-related UGI bleeding who are not good surgical candidates, consideration should be given to endoscopic injection of epinephrine and thermal coagulation. Angiography with embolization also may be helpful if anesthesia must be avoided. Several indications prompt surgical intervention in UGI bleeding: (a) a visible or spurting vessel in the base of an ulcer crater, even if initially controlled by nonsurgical means; (b) brisk hemorrhage from a lesion that perforates a viscus; and (c) massive ongoing blood losses from any source (>1,500 mL or 6 to 10 units of blood in the first 24 h).

Prognosis

Regardless of source, several clinical factors predicting a poor prognosis have been identified for patients with UGI bleeding: large hemorrhage, coagulopathy, bleeding from an obscure site, advanced age, or presence of multiple organ failures. Specifically, the combination of renal failure and hepatic parenchymal failure carries a dismal prognosis. In addition, specific upper tract endoscopic findings have also been shown to predict the risk of rebleeding and will be discussed later.

■ LGI BLEEDING

LGI hemorrhage tends to be intermittent and less profuse than UGI bleeding. Because bleeding can arise from a much larger anatomic area the source is often more difficult to diagnose. The most common causes of significant LGI bleeding are shown in Table 37-4. Several points deserve emphasis: a significant proportion (perhaps 10%) of "lower GI" bleeding actually is the result of blood flowing downstream from an UGI source. This is in distinct contrast to UGI bleeding, which essentially never arises from the lower tract. Diverticular bleeding (30% to 50%) and angiodysplasia (20% to 30%)

TABLE 37-4   CAUSES OF LGI BLEEDING

CONDITION	APPROXIMATE FREQUENCY
Diverticular disease	40%
Angiodysplasia	30%
Ischemic and inflammatory colitis	5%
Polyps—carcinoma	5%
Other—miscellaneous	5%
Unknown	10%
Upper GI source	10%

lead the list of bleeding sources, being almost twice as likely as the next most common etiologies, colitis, neoplasm, and polyps. In contrast to UGI hemorrhage, which is almost always accurately and rapidly diagnosed, LGI bleeding remains undiagnosed in 10% of patients. Luckily, most LGI bleeding episodes (nearly 80%) spontaneously cease. Unfortunately, rebleeding occurs in as many as 25% of patients.

The Diagnostic Approach

The diagnostic evaluation of LGI bleeding is significantly more complex than that for UGI hemorrhage. A suggested schema for the evaluation of LGI bleeding is presented in the Figure 37-3, and specific diagnostic tests are discussed below.

Barium studies

Barium studies currently have no role in diagnosing LGI bleeding. Barium enema cannot visualize angiodysplasia or colitis, and even when diverticuli or cancerous lesions are seen there is no confirmation they are bleeding. Furthermore, filling the colon with barium complicates subsequent angiographic, endoscopic, and surgical interventions.

Colonoscopy

When feasible, colonoscopy performed after thorough bowel preparation (purging with polyethylene glycol) is the diagnostic procedure with the highest yield (70% to 80%) and if not diagnostic does not prevent subsequent diagnostic attempts.

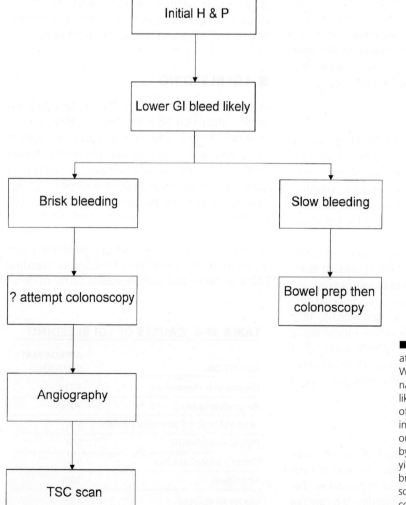

■ **FIGURE 37-3** Suggested evaluation of suspected LGI bleeding. When history and physical examination suggest LGI bleeding is likely, the diagnostic sequence is often dictated by the rate of bleeding. When bleeding is slow, a thorough bowel preparation followed by colonoscopy is most likely to yield a diagnosis. When bleeding is brisk, angiography and tagged RBC scan are often diagnostic where colonoscopy fails. TSC, technetium scan.

Colonoscopy also has the advantages that it can be safely performed at the bedside and offers therapeutic options. Regrettably, inadequate preparation before emergent colonoscopy often precludes an adequate examination and increases risk of perforation. Optimal timing of colonoscopy is debated. Even though studies performed early have higher diagnostic rates, this does not translate into reductions in rebleeding, transfusion, length of stay, or mortality. Hence, colonoscopy is probably best performed after hemodynamic stabilization and as soon as a bowel prep can be completed. If no diagnosis is reached after colonoscopy and bleeding continues or recurs, a nuclear medicine scan or angiogram should be considered.

GI Bleeding Scans

Two types of nuclear bleeding scans are in common use: technetium sulfur colloid and technetium labeled red blood cells. In both tests, the abdomen is scanned to look for "puddling" of radioactive tracer. After injection of the short-lived technetium sulfur colloid, signal can be seen in the bowel even with bleeding rates as low as 0.1 mL/min. Although highly sensitive, the short duration of the tracer often misses intermittently bleeding lesions. This problem is lessened with the tagged cell study in which the patient's red blood cells are labeled ex vivo with technetium-99 and then reinjected. The long half-life of tagged RBCs permits repeated scanning for up to 24 h, a feature particularly useful in patients with intermittent bleeding. Although the technique is more sensitive than angiography, it suggests a bleeding site in only roughly 25% of cases. What is more worrisome is that about 25% of these results are false positives. Most studies that will ever be positive are diagnostic within minutes but repeated imaging up to 18 h may be required. A significant disadvantage is that each scan must be done in the radiology department incurring transport risks and costs. Imprecision is the major problem with radionuclide scanning: The general region of bleeding may be identified but precise localization requires endoscopy or arteriography. A major advantage of nuclear scans is that no bowel preparation is necessary.

Although a rare problem, Meckel's diverticuli may be localized using a radioactive tracer secreted by ectopic gastric mucosa lining the diverticulum. Although highly sensitive and specific, false-positive scans are seen in nonfasting patients and in those with large arteriovenous malformations.

Angiography

A diagnostic angiogram requires a skilled radiologist, a cooperative patient, and a rapidly bleeding lesion. To demonstrate contrast extravasation, patients must be bleeding at a rate more than 1 mL/min. A nuclear scan done before angiography may serve two uses. First, if the highly sensitive nuclear scan is negative, performing angiography is likely to be futile. Second, results help guide the angiographer to the most likely region of bleeding. Theoretically, this approach helps reduce the time to perform the procedure and the required dye load. When there is no guiding information, first injecting the superior mesenteric artery is logical because most diverticular bleeding and all bleeding from angiodysplasia occurs in this vascular distribution. If negative, injection of the inferior mesenteric and celiac arteries follows. Success rates for detection of bleeding sites vary widely, depending on patient characteristics, the angiographer's experience, and the source of bleeding. Advantages of angiography include precise localization of bleeding, the ability to be performed on the unprepared bowel, and the option of injecting emboli or vasoconstrictors for control. The combined incidence of dye reactions, contrast-induced renal failure, vascular perforation, and cholesterol embolization from this procedure is approximately 10%, even in experienced centers.

Specific Conditions Causes of Lower GI Bleeding

Diverticulosis

Diverticulosis is a disease of patients over the age of 40 years and is responsible for about 30% to 50% of significant LGI bleeding episodes. Diverticular bleeding is sudden in onset, painless in nature, and usually self-limited, but it recurs in 10% to 25% of patients. Interestingly, diverticular bleeding does not usually occur in patients with acute diverticulitis (characterized by fever and lower abdominal pain). The value of colonoscopy is usually compromised by large amounts of colonic blood and stool in the unprepared patient. The detection rate of tagged RBC studies varies with the severity of bleeding, but even when localized to the colon, such studies do not distinguish between diverticular disease and angiodysplasia. Angiography demonstrates the site of active bleeding in one half to three quarters of cases and offers the therapeutic option of intra-arterial vasoconstrictor infusion or embolization.

Angiodysplasia

Angiodysplasia is largely a disease of the elderly. Most angiodysplasia lesions never bleed and are incidental findings at the time of colonoscopy. There are no unique historical features that distinguish angiodysplastic from diverticular bleeding. However, the venous bleeding of angiodysplasia is usually less severe than the arterial bleeding of diverticulosis. Like diverticular bleeding, angiodysplastic bleeding almost always spontaneously stops, but recurs more commonly (25% to 50%). Colonoscopy can detect bleeding angiodysplastic lesions in 70% to 80% of cases when the colon is optimally prepared. Angiography less reliably displays vascular malformations (35% to 70%) and, unfortunately, confirms hemorrhage much less often. Because of the high incidence of rebleeding, endoscopic thermal coagulation or injection or surgical removal of the involved portion of colon should be considered if hemorrhaging angiodysplastic vessels are demonstrated.

Polyps and Colon Carcinoma

Colon carcinoma more commonly produces slow, continuous blood loss than massive GI hemorrhage. Left colonic and rectal neoplasms are most likely to cause gross bleeding. Premonitory symptoms include a change in bowel habits, melena, and crampy abdominal pain, with or without weight loss. Rectal examination followed by colonoscopy is likely to reveal the cancerous site of blood loss.

Other Causes of Lower GI Bleeding

Ischemic colitis and bowel infarction from mesenteric thrombosis or embolism may produce mucosal sloughing, bowel necrosis, and LGI bleeding (see Chapter 36). Significant blood loss in ischemic colitis is unusual, and most episodes stop spontaneously. The splenic flexure and descending colon are the most common sites. Inflammatory bowel disease may cause massive LGI bleeding in the young. In such patients, bloody diarrhea is commonly superimposed on chronic, crampy abdominal pain. The diagnosis is by colonoscopy and therapy is medical, unless massive persistent hemorrhage necessitates colectomy. Rectal ulcers are another rare but potentially fatal cause of massive LGI bleeding occurring most frequently in patients with chronic renal failure. Rectal varices can produce massive hematochezia in patients with portal hypertension.

LGI Bleeding Therapy

Only a small minority (approx. 20%) of patients with LGI bleeding need any intervention to stop blood loss. Colonoscopy using thermal coagulation can almost always stop bleeding following polypectomy, usually stops the bleeding of angiodysplasia, and occasionally controls the bleeding of diverticulosis. Potential complications include perforation and exacerbation of the bleeding.

Angiographic techniques to stop LGI bleeding include intra-arterial vasoconstrictor infusion and embolization. Vasoconstrictors are effective in approximately 90% of episodes of angiodysplasia or diverticulosis. Such therapy leads to a 5% to 15% complication rate and about a 50% incidence of rebleeding. In nonsurgical candidates who fail vasoconstrictors, distal embolization using small gel-foam plugs may terminate bleeding. Embolization carries about a 20% risk of infarction. Because of the high incidence of rebleeding in angiodysplasia, however, resection is often recommended.

In patients with massive LGI bleeding of undetermined origin, exploratory laparotomy is usually ill-advised because it identifies the bleeding site in only one third of cases. If the bleeding site cannot be found at the time of laparotomy, a right hemicolectomy is usually performed because both bleeding diverticuli and angiodysplastic lesions are more common there. Emergent blind segmental resection of the colon is associated with a mortality rate of 30% to 40% and a similar chance of rebleeding. Localization of the bleeding site by angiography or colonoscopy reduces mortality to less than 10% and minimizes the risk of rebleeding. Because of the operative risks of emergent colectomy, resection should be considered only for patients with massive bleeding who fail angiography and embolization, patients with numerous angiodysplastic lesions, and patients with angiodysplasia who fail thermal coagulation therapy.

■ SUGGESTED READINGS

American Society for Gastrointestinal Endoscopy. An annotated algorithmic approach to upper gastrointestinal bleeding. *Gastrointes endosc.* 2001;53:853–858.

American Society for Gastrointestinal Endoscopy. An annotated algorithmic approach to lower gastrointestinal bleeding. *Gastrointes Endosc.* 2001;53:859–863.

Beejay U, Wolfe MM. Acute gastrointestinal bleeding in the intensive care unit: The gastroenterologist's perspective. *Gastroenterol Clin North Am.* 2000;29:309–336.

Harry R, Wendon J. Management of variceal bleeding. *Curr Opin Crit Care*. 2002;8:164–170.

Krige JE, Kotze UK, Bornman PC, et al. Variceal recurrence, rebleeding, and survival after endoscopic injection sclerotherapy in 287 alcoholic cirrhotic patients with bleeding esophageal varices. *Ann Surg*. 2006;244(5):764–770.

Langner I, Langner S, Partecke LI, et al. Acute upper gastrointestinal hemorrhage: Is a radiological interventional approach an alternative to emergency surgery? *Emerg Radiol*. 2008;15(6):413–419.

Steinberg KP. Stress-related mucosal disease in the critically ill patient: Risk factors and strategies to prevent stress-related bleeding in the intensive care unit. *Crit Care Med*. 2002;30(Suppl. 6):S362–S364.

CHAPTER 38

Burns and Inhalational Injury

KEY POINTS

1 For burn victims, the keystones of initial therapy are large-volume crystalloid resuscitation and maintenance of the airway. Commonly, isotonic crystalloid (4mL/kg/% body surface area burn) is required for volume resuscitation during the first 24h after a burn injury.

2 Inhalational damage is a very common early injury that is usually best managed initially by intubation and administration of 100% oxygen.

3 Carbon monoxide and cyanide poisoning should be considered in every burn victim. The role of hyperbaric oxygen therapy for carbon monoxide poisoning remains controversial but perhaps is best limited to comatose patients with high carbon monoxide-hemoglobin levels who can be treated promptly. Antidotes are available for cyanide and should be administered to patients with unexplained metabolic acidosis persisting after apparently adequate resuscitation.

4 Severe sepsis is the most common late fatal complication of burns, usually related to Gram-negative rod infection of the burn wound.

5 The hypermetabolic state and compartmental fluid shifts often dramatically alter drug therapy in the patient with burns. In many cases, drug doses must be significantly increased to achieve therapeutic effect.

6 Burn wounds are metabolically taxing, requiring huge amounts of energy and patient work to maintain an often dramatically elevated minute ventilation and cardiac output. Patients with marginal ventilatory status can develop respiratory failure from excessive ventilatory demands.

■ PATHOPHYSIOLOGY

In serious burns, some tissue is immediately killed by direct thermal injury but adjoining regions that are sublethally injured may be even more important, as they serve as an engine for inflammation. The tissue bordering a major burn generates inflammatory cytokines, oxidants, and lipid mediators that act locally and systemically to increase vascular permeability and clotting and to depress cardiovascular function. These changes result in the familiar clinical findings of fever, leukocytosis, and increased vascular permeability that manifest as hypoproteinemia, edema, and hypovolemia. Similar to the brain adjacent to a cerebral infarct, the "watershed" tissue bordering an acute burn is in jeopardy for additional damage from systemic hypoxia, ischemia due to localized clotting and increased tissue pressure, and infection. Thus, prompt reperfusion of these endangered areas is vital to optimal outcome.

■ BURN EVALUATION

Mortality rates for burn victims vary widely, depending on the depth and size of the burn, the patient's underlying health and age, and the occurrence of associated inhalational injury. Most deaths from fires result from smoke inhalation, which usually proves fatal before patients reach the hospital—emphasizing the importance of smoke detection devices. On reaching the hospital, hypovolemic shock and smoke-induced airflow obstruction are prominent early complications; severe sepsis is the most common late fatal complication. Inhalational injury is a major determinant of outcome; its occurrence may double the mortality rate of a burn of any given extent. Not surprisingly, age also is a powerful predictor of mortality. After the airway has been secured and hemodynamics have been stabilized, the patient should be examined carefully to determine the depth and extent of thermal injury, and the burns should be gently washed and dressed. An appropriate examination should be conducted to look for associated traumatic injuries, especially if the burn results from explosion or motor vehicle accident.

Estimation of Burn Size and Severity

Burns are classified either simply by partial or full thickness destruction or by depth of injury (first to fourth degree) (Table 38-1). In adults, the percentage of body surface affected by burn injury can be estimated by the "rule of nines." This rule assigns percentages of the total body surface area (BSA) to the anterior and posterior surfaces of the head, limbs, and trunk (Fig. 38-1). As another useful measure, the palm of the adult patient's hand approximates 1% of total BSA. The Lund–Browder chart is used for estimating the extent of the burn in children because their head contributes a disproportionally large proportion of body surface. Estimation of the total area involved by full thickness burns is useful in determining fluid requirements, need for specialized burn unit care, and expected mortality. However, precise grading of burn wound depth is not essential for the nonburn specialist; in most cases it is reasonable to regard any burn more extensive than superficial as serious, particularly if it covers ≥10% of the body. Adults with extensive or severe burns and most burned children require hospitalization. Commonly accepted criteria for hospital admission are given in Table 38-2.

■ INITIAL MANAGEMENT

Initial management of the patient with severe burns should include a careful assessment of the airway and vital signs to ensure adequate ventilation and perfusion. If carbon monoxide (CO) poisoning is suspected, it is reasonable to obtain a blood sample for CO content and to simultaneously administer 100% oxygen to accelerate the poison's clearance. Immediately after securing the airway and ensuring oxygenation, repletion of circulating volume should be undertaken; hypovolemic shock is the most common cause of death within the first 24 h after admission.

The optimal endpoints for circulatory resuscitation and how to achieve these goals remain controversial. Many intensivists rely on the traditional indices of heart rate, blood pressure, and urine output, but it has been claimed that some patients remain underresuscitated using these measures. When adequacy of intravascular filling is in doubt, assessment of central venous pressure (CVP) can be helpful. Although some physicians prefer an intensive monitoring strategy that includes measurement of CVP, pulmonary artery occlusion pressure

TABLE 38-1 CLASSIFICATION OF BURNS BY SEVERITY

SEVERITY	SKIN EXAMINATION	SENSATION
First[a]	Erythema	Painful
Second[a]	Erythema/blisters/edema	Painful
Third[b]	White or charred	Anesthetic
	Firmly indurated	
Fourth[b]	Destruction of muscle, fascia, bone	Anesthetic

[a]Partial thickness.
[b]Full thickness.

TABLE 38-2 CRITERIA FOR HOSPITAL ADMISSION

Burns totaling >20%–25% BSA
Full-thickness burn >5%–10% BSA, especially in patients <10 or >50 years
Burn of a lesser extent accompanied by complicating medical conditions
Inhalation injury
Circumferential burns of trunk or extremities
Burns of hand, face, feet, genitals, or perineum
Chemical or electrical burns
Associated trauma

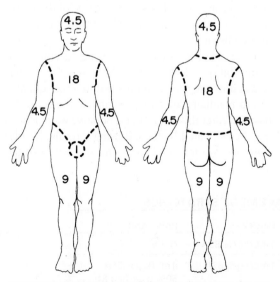

■ **FIGURE 38-1** Burn wound diagram illustrating the surface area of selected body regions. Numbers correspond to percentages of total BSA.

(PAOP), continuous mixed-venous oxygen saturation (SvO_2), and frequent lactate determinations, there are no data to indicate that these measures add value. Even when invasive monitoring is undertaken, recent targets are often lower than those traditionally used (e.g., CVP 8 to 10 cm H_2O, PAOP 10 to 12 cm H_2O, SvO_2 60% to 65%). Measuring PAOP and cardiac output seems most defensible in patients with suspected underlying cardiac impairment, where CVP alone may not provide sufficient information about left ventricular function (see Chapter 3). Difficulties in achieving adequate resuscitation of burn patients frequently can be traced to myocardial dysfunction, often transient, that presumably results from humoral myocardial depressant factors.

Fluid Therapy

Burns cause hypovolemia as a result of massive shifts of fluid from intravascular to extravascular compartments and by exudation through injured skin. Hemoconcentration (because of intravascular fluid losses) occurs early, but hemodilution is more likely after appropriate fluid resuscitation. Because the hematocrit can change in either direction, it should be checked regularly during resuscitation with a traditional target being ≥30%. Central venous catheterization is often necessary to deliver the volume of fluid required for adequate resuscitation, and whenever possible such catheters should be placed though *unburned* skin to minimize the risk of subsequent catheter or wound related sepsis.

Three major strategies (i.e., Evans, Brooke, and Parkland) have been advocated for replacing circulating volume (Table 38-3). A central feature of all plans is to administer substantial volumes of salt-containing (typically Ringers lactate) fluid during the initial 24 h. These strategies differ in their reliance on colloid and free water. The Parkland formula is probably the most widely used fluid-replacement strategy, according to which 4 mL of isotonic

crystalloid per kilogram per percentage of BSA burn is given in the first day. Customarily, one half of the fluid deficit is replaced in the first 8 h, with the remainder administered over the next 16 h. (For purposes of fluid replacement, burn area is usually capped at 50% BSA.) However, patients with concomitant inhalational injury may require more fluid for successful resuscitation (up to 6 mL/kg/% BSA burn). A traditional fluid replacement target has been to achieve 0.5 to 1 mL/kg/h of urine output. It is now recognized that in a substantial number, perhaps half, of cases too much volume is administered. One clinical clue to too much fluid infusion is a urine output consistently exceeding 2 mL/kg/h. Other risks of excessive fluid administration are limb and abdominal compartment syndromes (ACS). ACS is sufficiently common to warrant monitoring of bladder pressure in patients undergoing large volume resuscitation. All fluid-replacement strategies are associated with the development of tissue edema; however, newer strategies using hypertonic (250 mmol/L) saline solution may achieve hemodynamic resuscitation with less swelling. (There is some evidence that hypertonic resuscitation strategies may increase the risk of renal insufficiency.) Although poorly tested, in mass casualty situations where intravenous therapy may not be feasible, oral rehydrating solution may be useful. Following fluid replacement, vasopressors may be needed to maintain adequate cardiac output, blood pressure, and urine flow. High doses of α-adrenergic agonists (e.g., norepinephrine, phenylephrine) should be avoided, if possible, because of their tendency to decrease nutritive blood flow to already injured tissue.

After 24 h, sodium requirements decline and permeability of leaky vessels decreases. Free water and colloid are then administered in larger quantities to maintain circulating volume and electrolyte balance. After the first 24 h, evaporative water losses may be estimated by the following formula: hourly water loss (in mL) = (25 + % area of burn) × (total

TABLE 38-3 FIRST DAY FLUID-REPLACEMENT STRATEGIES

	BROOKE	EVANS	PARKLAND
Colloid	0.5 mL/kg/% BSA	1 mL/kg/% BSA	None
Isotonic crystalloid	1.5 mL/kg/% BSA	1 mL/kg/%BSA	4 mL/kg/% BSA 50% over first 8 h 50% over next 16 h
Free water	2 L	2 L	None

BSA in m²). This formula predicts that a patient with a 25% burn and a 2 m² BSA will lose approximately 100 mL of water per hour. This formula provides the basis for the common recommendation in both the Brooke and Evans fluid strategies to administer roughly 2 L of free water daily. Within the first 12 h of the burn event, colloids offer little advantage over crystalloid because the newly injured vasculature fails to retain even the larger colloid molecules. Despite lack of proven benefit, many physicians still administer albumin to decrease the amount of crystalloid used, especially when the serum albumin concentration falls below 2 gm/dL.

Respiratory Management

Airway complications are a common cause of early death in burn patients. The history and physical examination provide valuable clues to the extent of inhalational injury (Table 38-4). Burns and inhalation injuries cause respiratory complications through five basic mechanisms: (a) airway obstruction, (b) toxin inhalation, (c) increased metabolism and ventilation requirement, (d) impairment of host defenses, and (e) production of late obstructive and restrictive lung disease.

Airway Obstruction

Hot gases, particularly steam (because its heat content is thousands of times higher than dry air), can rapidly cause upper airway injury and bronchospasm; however, heat-related tissue edema can progress for 24 to 48 h after the injury. Because the upper airway is such an efficient heat sink, it is uncommon to see *lower* respiratory tract thermal injury unless the patient has been trapped in a closed-space fire, often with superheated gas. Patients with burns of the face or neck that appear inconsequential at the time of admission may quickly experience swelling that leads to life-threatening airway obstruction. Therefore, as a rule, patients with second- or third-degree burns of the

---

TABLE 38-4 CLUES TO INHALATION INJURY

Enclosed-space exposure
Loss of consciousness
Nasal, oral, or facial burns
Carbonaceous sputum
Hoarseness or stridor
Upper airway changes by bronchoscopy
Pulmonary edema on chest radiograph

---

face or neck should be intubated in the first hours of hospitalization to avoid airway obstruction. Failure to follow this principle may lead to situations in which massive tissue swelling eventually precludes airway cannulation. If intubation is required, a large-diameter orotracheal tube should be placed to facilitate clearance of voluminous secretions and performance of bronchoscopy should the need arise. In this setting, the tube generally should remain in place for at least 72 h. When patency of the airway is uncertain, laryngoscopy or bronchoscopy can evaluate the severity of airway edema and need for endotracheal intubation. One should err on the side of intubation if there is clinical evidence of airway obstruction or if laryngoscopy demonstrates supraglottic edema. Hypoxemia or diffuse radiographic infiltrates at the time of admission are also poor prognostic signs that indicate the need for early intubation and mechanical ventilation. However, a normal chest radiograph or PaO_2 by no means excludes inhalational injury.

For patients not requiring immediate intubation for airway obstruction or hypoxemia, bronchodilators and humidified oxygen may avert the need for mechanical ventilation. Inhalation of a low-viscosity mixture of helium and oxygen (Heliox) can be a useful temporizing measure for patients with mild airway edema, as can nebulized racemic epinephrine. Neither therapy, however, should delay intubation for patients with facial burns or symptomatic airway obstruction. Bronchospasm and bronchorrhea commonly develop after inhalational injury to the lower airway. Although effective early on, bronchodilators are of less value late in the course of postburn airway obstruction. Bronchoscopic evaluation of the airway often reveals sloughed mucosa or extractable secretions. Because corticosteroids do not reduce airway edema and substantially increase mortality by predisposing patients to infection, they should be avoided. Anticholinergic bronchodilating aerosols (e.g., Ipratropium) make sense for vagal mediated bronchospasm. Simple measures such as elevating the head of the bed to 30 degrees during initial resuscitation may help to decrease the degree of airway edema. The rate of fluid administration should not be decreased when burns involve the airway; inadequate fluids may allow underperfusion and worsening of airway damage.

Increased Ventilatory Requirements

Minute ventilation may be extraordinarily high after large burns because of increased metabolic demands; a 50% to 60% burn may double caloric requirements and CO_2 production. Although hyperpnea usually is due to the burn-induced hypermetabolic state, alternative explanations (e.g., hyperthyroidism, drug or alcohol withdrawal, pneumonia, acute respiratory distress syndrome [ARDS], pulmonary embolism, or uncontrolled pain) should be considered. The increased ventilatory requirements may be sufficient to overwhelm the capacity of patients with underlying lung disease, resulting in respiratory failure.

Toxic Gas Inhalation

Depending on the fuel consumed, fires may produce numerous noxious compounds that can cause respiratory inflammation and systemic toxicity (Table 38-5). With or without fire, all inhaled gases produce injury in one of three basic ways: (a) by acting as asphyxiants, (b) by causing airway irritation, or (c) by functioning as systemic toxins. Any gas (e.g., nitrogen, helium, nitrous oxide, carbon dioxide) may be a lethal asphyxiant when it displaces oxygen from the atmosphere, resulting in a hypoxic gas mixture. Such an exposure may occur when a CO_2 fire-suppression system discharges in a closed space.

Water-soluble gases usually act as immediate irritants because they are deposited in high concentrations on the mucous membranes of the moist upper airway. Airway edema and bronchospasm usually result from the high-solubility gases such as chlorine, ammonia, hydrogen chloride, and sulfur dioxide. By contrast, low-solubility toxins (e.g., phosgene and nitrogen dioxide) are more likely to gain deeper access to lung tissues, as are potent acids or aldehydes carried there by inhaled particulates. Obviously, when victims are trapped in a closed space, even highly soluble irritating gases may reach the lower respiratory tract. The injury resulting from lower airway gas exposure is similar to aspiration, presenting as diffuse bronchoconstriction, reduced lung compliance, and mismatching. Chemical injury is suggested by the history and presence of erythema below the level of the vocal cords. The mucosal edema of chemical injury builds for 24 to 48 h after exposure and severely impairs mucociliary transport. In addition, the inflammatory mediators and white cells released into the airways promote secretion formation, atelectasis development, and ventilation–perfusion mismatching. Copious secretions, bronchospasm, airway obstruction, and ciliary damage warrant suctioning and bronchodilator therapy. In cases of severe inhalational injury, the airway mucosa often sloughs at about 72 h and requires 7 to 14 days to regenerate. If not recognized, the shed airway lining can precipitate a crisis if it obstructs the distal orifice of the endotracheal tube. When this happens, typically, *exhalation* is limited resulting in air-trapping, auto-PEEP, and sometimes even tension pneumothorax. Tracheal tube obstruction is usually responsive to simple suctioning, but sometimes bronchoscopy or even tube exchange is necessary. Bacterial superinfection and pneumonitis are common complications of airway lining injury.

Carbon Monoxide and Cyanide

CO and cyanide (CN) are the two most common fire-related inhaled toxins. CO is the primary cause of death in 75% of fire fatalities. CO competes directly with oxygen for hemoglobin binding, fixes to cytochrome oxidase, and displaces the oxyhemoglobin dissociation curve leftward, impairing release of O_2 to the tissues. Because the affinity of CO for hemoglobin is roughly 250 times greater than that of oxygen, concentrations of inspired CO as low as 0.1% can rapidly produce fatally high

TABLE 38-5 TOXIC COMPONENTS OF SMOKE

MATERIAL BURNED	TOXIC PRODUCT	PHYSIOLOGIC EFFECT
Wood, paper, cotton	Acrolein, acetaldehyde, formaldehyde, acetic acid	Airway irritation, bronchospasm, mucosal sloughing
Plastics	Phosgene, chlorine Hydrogen chloride	Airway irritation Acute lung injury
Wool, silk	Hydrogen cyanide	Cyanide poisoning, tissue hypoxia
Synthetic (polyurethane, nylon, rayon)	Hydrogen cyanide Oxides of nitrogen	Cyanide poisoning, tissue hypoxia Pulmonary edema
All of the above	Carbon monoxide	Tissue hypoxia

TABLE 38-6 CO-HGB LEVELS AND SYMPTOMS[a]

CARBOXYHEMOGLOBIN

LEVEL	SYMPTOMS
<5%	Usually none
5%–15%	Mild headache, dyspnea
15%–20%	Headache, dizziness, confusion, nausea, vomiting
20%–40%	Disorientation, visual impairment, nausea
40%–60%	Hallucinations, coma, seizures, shock
>60%	Death

[a]Absence of detectable CO-Hgb does not rule out CO exposure.

levels of nonfunctional carboxyhemoglobin (CO-Hgb). The sensitivity of a patient to CO is influenced strongly by underlying health; patients with diseases of the central nervous system or heart are especially susceptible. The clinical symptoms of acute CO poisoning are those of tissue hypoxia and usually correlate well with the CO-Hgb level (Table 38-6). However, because of the time needed for extrication and transport of victims to the hospital, and the prehospital use of oxygen, CO-Hgb levels may be undetectable at the time of admission. For this reason low levels of CO-Hgb should not be used as evidence of an absence of CO effect. Even if measurable, the correlation between acute CO-Hgb levels and late neuropsychiatric effects is poor.

Two principles underpin treatment of CO poisoning: maximization of tissue O_2 delivery and use of high concentrations of O_2 to promote CO excretion. While breathing air, the elimination half-life ($t_{1/2}$) of CO-Hgb is 2 to 6 h. When breathing pure O_2 at ambient pressure, the $t_{1/2}$ declines to 30 to 90 min. Because O_2 profoundly affects CO clearance, the most important therapy in patients with suspected CO poisoning is to immediately administer 100% oxygen. CO-Hgb levels exceeding 25% in normal subjects or 15% in patients with ischemic heart disease should be treated aggressively. High fractions of inspired O_2 should be used until the CO-Hgb concentration falls below 10%.

The use of hyperbaric oxygen (HBO) remains controversial, and after numerous clinical trials no consensus on its use exists. Although HBO can further accelerate removal of CO from the body (elimination $t_{1/2}$ <20 min), hyperbaric chambers complicate management and are not widely available. HBO may also result in otic barotrauma or seizures. Furthermore, after the first hour, HBO offers little advantage over 100% ambient pressure oxygen in reducing CO-Hgb levels. It is possible that HBO has unproven beneficial effects unrelated to its ability to accelerate CO clearance from the body. Taken together, randomized studies do not suggest that the late complications (especially behavioral disturbances) after CO exposure are significantly reduced by HBO. A reasonable compromise is to use HBO, if locally available, for symptomatic (i.e., altered neurological status, hemodynamically unstable) CO exposure victims and for patients with documented high CO-Hgb levels, even if asymptomatic. Presently, the benefits of HBO do not appear to exceed the risks of transporting acutely ill, unstable patients over long distances to receive the therapy.

Fires also generate CN through the combustion of wood, silk, nylon, and polyurethane. CN binds to tissue cytochromes impairing O_2 use and causing lactic acidosis but because diagnostic tests are not readily available, CN exposure often goes unrecognized. Hyperbaric O_2 therapy is not useful in CN toxicity because the pathophysiologic defect is in O_2 usage at the cellular level, not one of O_2 delivery. Tissue hypoxia from CO or CN usually is evident immediately after exposure and should be suspected in burn patients with apparently normal clinical indices of perfusion and oxygenation but unexplained metabolic (lactic) acidosis, especially if the mixed-venous O_2 saturation is unexpectedly high.

In CO poisoning, arterial blood gases may demonstrate a nearly normal PaO_2 but decreased *measured* O_2 content and *measured* hemoglobin saturation as CO displaces O_2 from hemoglobin but not that dissolved in plasma. Because their photometric properties are similar, bedside pulse oximetry cannot distinguish CO-Hgb from normal oxyhemoglobin; that distinction relies on co-oximetry. In CN intoxication, PaO_2, O_2 saturation, and O_2 content may all be normal, and if measured, mixed-venous O_2 saturations are unexpectedly high because of underuse of delivered O_2. Thus, CN poisoning also usually results in normal, or even high, pulse oximetry saturations. The bottom line is that pulse oximetry cannot reliably detect CO or CN.

The treatment of CN poisoning historically has used inhaled amyl nitrate and intravenous sodium nitrite to produce methemoglobin that acts as a sink for CN, displacing it from the intracellular cytochromes. The CN portion of the resulting cyanohemoglobin is then extracted by the liver enzyme rhodanase and in the presence of sulfur (from intravenous sodium thiosulfate) converted into the relatively nontoxic thiocyanate ion, which is subsequently eliminated by the kidney. This complex chemistry need not be memorized; nearly every pharmacy possesses a kit, typically called a "Taylor, Lilly or Pasadena kit," containing all the required reagents and detailed instructions. 4-Dimethylaminophenol (DMAP) is another compound used for CN poisoning that also works by generating methemoglobinemia. Neither of these treatments is ideal, since the creation of methemoglobin, even transiently, diminishes oxygen carrying capacity. To avoid the problem of methemoglobin formation alternate methods of CN detoxification have been developed. In some countries, dicobalt edentate has been used but extreme caution is advised—the diagnosis must be certain since the therapy itself is toxic in the absence of CN. The newest treatment gaining popularity is hydroxycobalamin. Hydroxocobalamin (4 to 5 gm IV), safely chelates CN directly, thereby creating cyanocobalamin, a natural form of vitamin B_{12}, which is excreted in the urine.

Other Important Considerations

Major burns impair the ability to conserve heat and maintain body temperature. Therefore, after burn cleansing, wounds should be covered with clean, warm coverings and body temperature monitored closely. Failure to prevent hypothermia impairs coagulation and can dramatically increase oxygen requirements if shivering occurs. The reduced mobility, sedation, and tissue edema predispose to deep venous thrombosis (DVT) and pressure ulcer formation, and thus consideration should be given to DVT prophylaxis and specialized beds to prevent these costly complications. Ileus commonly follows major burns, and gastric distention or markedly diminished bowel sounds should prompt insertion of an oral or nasogastric tube connected to suction. After wound cleansing, a topical antibiotic should be applied to limit skin colonization by bacteria. Systemic antibiotics offer no demonstrated advantage in prophylaxis. Without confirmation of recent immunization, tetanus toxoid should be administered. Pain and anxiety relief, particularly in partial thickness burns, is critical to allow debridement, cleansing, and other patient manipulations (see Chapter 17). Full-thickness burns are frequently anesthetic so that patients without milder burn injuries (rare) may require little or no pain medication.

■ COMPLICATIONS OF BURNS

The later complications of burns include (a) infection/severe sepsis/multiple organ failure, (b) gastrointestinal bleeding, (c) hypermetabolism, and (d) local wound problems.

Infection and Sepsis

Infection is the greatest threat to life of burn patients **4** after the first 36 h; pneumonia and burn wound sepsis represent the most common and lethal conditions. Immunocompetence of burned patients, including T-cell, monocyte, and macrophage function, is significantly depressed. Clearly, nosocomial pneumonitis is an ever-present risk for the intubated patient, particularly when inhalation injury has compromised host defenses (see Chapters 26 and 27).

Devastating infection also can result from skin disruption. Massive numbers of bacteria may invade the burn wound and adjacent tissue. In the first 3 to 5 days after a burn, staphylococci are the most common invading organisms, but after 5 days, Gram-negative rods (especially *Pseudomonas*) predominate. Late in the course of burn care, invasive fungal infection should be considered in patients with severe sepsis unresponsive to bacterial antibiotics. In addition to standard methods of infection control, meticulous wound care, including the use of topical antibiotics, early wound debridement and closure, and use of gowns, masks, and gloves decrease the infection risk. Prophylactic systemic antibiotics are not of benefit. When antibiotics are used, it should be kept in mind that resuscitated burned patients have accelerated clearance of some drugs, most notably aminoglycosides. **5** Increased basal temperature renders the detection of wound infection difficult. Because the temperature of burn patients may rise as high as 38.5°C as a result of hypermetabolism, fever to this degree does not necessarily warrant the institution of antibiotics. When burn wound sepsis is suspected, quantitative cultures of burned skin, subcutaneous tissue, and adjacent normal skin should be performed. Growth of more than 10^5 organisms per gram of tissue or histological evidence of invasion of adjacent unburned skin is highly suggestive of severe complicating infection. Long before the results of these tests are available, however, antibiotics must be instituted on clinical grounds if high spiking fever, leukocytosis, and neutrophilia, or other signs of sepsis, are present.

Even without infection, the systemic inflammatory response syndrome (SIRS) can result from the burn wound itself or from the release of toxins (e.g., endotoxin) across the gut wall (see Chapter 27). The occurrence of severe sepsis is minimized by early wound excision and grafting, aggressive nutritional support, avoidance of corticosteroids, and prompt diagnosis and treatment of infections. Recently, the use of serum procalcitonin measurements has shown promise as a method of differentiating sepsis from SIRS.

Gastrointestinal Bleeding

Gastrointestinal bleeding because of stress (Curling) ulceration occurs commonly in burn patients. Burn victims are one of the groups to clearly benefit from empiric stress ulceration prophylaxis. Effective prophylaxis uses histamine blockers, proton pump inhibitors, or sucralfate. Although antacids can work, they are more expensive and labor intensive and less effective. Furthermore, antacids are associated with higher rates of nosocomial pneumonia; therefore, they represent third-line therapy.

Hypermetabolism and Nutrition

Metabolic rate may double in patients with second- and third-degree burns that exceed 50% BSA. Indeed, extensive burns represent the single greatest sustained metabolic stress experienced by humans. Full expression of hypermetabolism may require 5 to 7 days. Patients with major burns raise resting body temperature and dedicate a large fraction of energy consumption to the heat production that maintains the gradient with ambient temperature; therefore, establishing higher environmental temperature reduces caloric expenditure. Nutritional support is required for patients with serious burns. Traditionally, that support was given parenterally under the assumption that ileus would preclude enteral nutrition. However, parenteral nutrition usually was withheld during the first 24 to 36 h of hospitalization because of the complexities of fluid management during resuscitation. It is now known that almost all patients can be fed enterally, often within just hours of the injury. The enteral route is preferable because it preserves mucosal integrity, buffers gastric acid, and increases resistance of patients to infection. In the initial phase of treatment, the daily calorie requirement may be roughly estimated as 25 times the weight in kilograms plus 40 times the percentage of BSA burned. In lieu of estimating caloric requirements, indirect calorimetry can be used to measure caloric expenditures; giving 50% to 60% of the caloric requirement as glucose minimizes catabolic nitrogen losses. Administration of glucose at rates above 5 to 7 mL/kg/min, however, may lead to glucose intolerance and increased CO_2 associated with overfeeding. Lipid may be used as the source for the remaining 40% of nonprotein calories. Increased lipid clearance observed in burn victims supports the argument for raising the percentage of calories given as fat. It has recently become a common practice to use high-protein (e.g., 2 gm/kg body weight) immunomodulatory tube feeding preparations, often enriched with glutamine. (For a complete discussion of nutrition therapy, see Chapter 16.)

Burn Wound Care

A complete discussion of the care of the burn wound, especially newer biological dressings, is beyond the scope of this publication but several basic principles must be understood. The goals of burn wound care are to (a) prevent infection, (b) limit discomfort, (c) accelerate healing, and (d) maximize functional recovery. In general, these goals are best accomplished by the use of early debridement, topical antibiotics, and skin grafting. Topical antibiotics are applied to the skin once or twice daily to limit wound colonization. Wounds should be cleaned and debrided before application of new antibiotic, a process often requiring narcotic analgesia. Several topical antibiotics are available, each with unique advantages, antibacterial spectra, and complications (Table 38-7). Silver sulfadiazine is widely used. For convenience now often a silver impregnated nylon dressing is substituted. If long-term topical antibiotics are needed, changing the agent used at 7- to 10-day intervals may prevent the overgrowth of resistant organisms. When burn wound sepsis is suspected, empirical antibiotic regimens should cover Gram-negative rods including *Pseudomonas aeruginosa* and methicillin resistant *Staphylococcus*. The recent development of in vitro cultured keratinocytes is a promising development in the therapy for patients previously requiring extensive grafting procedures.

TABLE 38-7   TOPICAL ANTIMICROBIAL THERAPY

	SILVER SULFADIAZINE	SODIUM NITRATE	MAFENIDE (SULFAMYLON)
Advantages	Painless Easily applied Wide spectrum	Painless Wide spectrum	Easily applied Good eschar penetration
Disadvantages	Poor eschar penetration Leukopenia Thrombocytopenia	Poor eschar penetration Skin staining Leaches NaCl from tissue	Metabolic acidosis (carbonic anhydrase inhibitor) Narrow bacterial spectrum (GNR) Rare aplastic crisis

GNR, Gram-negative rods.

Many of the same principles that apply to chemical, electrical, and thermal burns are useful for patients with extensive skin damage as the result of toxic epidermal necrolysis or Stevens–Johnson syndrome. Fortunately, such patients rarely require debridement or grafting.

Mechanical Problems of the Burn Wound

Patients with circumferential burns of the trunk or an extremity and those with burns of the face, hands, feet, or perineum unequivocally require hospital admission and immediate consultation by a burn specialist. Eschar frequently encases the trunk or extremities. These limiting shells may prevent the tissue expansion required to accommodate the edema which reaches maximal severity 12 to 48 h after injury. Ischemia and/or necrosis from compartment syndrome development may result from the consequent rise in tissue pressure if unrelieved. Furthermore, eschar-related limitation of chest expansion may lead to respiratory failure. In the extremities, edema can be minimized by elevating the burned limb. Decreased capillary refill, cyanosis, paresthesia, and deep pain in tissues distal to the burn site dictate the need for escharotomy. Doppler ultrasound examination demonstrating diminished pulse amplitude distal to the eschar confirms high tissue pressures and potential vascular compromise. In circumferential burns of the trunk, reduced thoracic compliance (noted during mechanical ventilation), severe tachypnea, or ventilatory distress suggest the need for escharotomy. Escharotomy is performed by incising devitalized wound tissue along the entire lateral and medial aspects of the trunk or affected limb. After the healing process has begun, hydrotherapy debridement may become an important adjunct to the process.

■ NONTHERMAL BURNS

Chemical Injury

Copious irrigation with clear water comprises the primary initial treatment of chemical burns of all types. (If the caustic chemical is in a powered form, it makes sense to brush away as much of the material as possible before irrigation.) Care must be taken to avoid extending the chemical injury by allowing the patient to lie in contaminated flush solution. Removal of contaminated clothing and irrigation in a shower is preferable. After flushing, chemical burns should be treated like thermal burns. Although alkaline and acidic chemicals injure tissue by altering its pH, strong neutralizing solutions should not be used because they may precipitate exothermic reactions, risking additional thermal damage. The adequacy of irrigation in pH-related chemical injury may be assessed by testing the area with litmus paper to ensure neutral pH.

Electrical Burns

Electrical burns inflicted by lightning or another high-voltage source may produce extensive tissue damage with little external evidence of injury. Bone, nerve, and muscle damage are frequent, and the devitalized tissue is prone to subsequent infection. Electrical injury may cause severe exit wounds at the hands, knees, or feet—sites frequently overlooked in the initial evaluation. (Such wounds are analogous to projectiles, which produce small entrance but large exit wounds.) Fractures resulting from falls or forceful muscular contraction should be considered in all patients with electrical injuries. For almost all patients with electrical injury, an electrocardiogram should be performed to look for evidence of arrhythmias, myocardial injury, or conduction disturbance. Even though troponin or CPK–MB levels are often elevated, findings of classical transmural myocardial infarction are rare because epicardial coronary arteries do not become obstructed; rather, the myocardial necrosis is diffuse and patchy. Even in the absence of overt cardiac injury, observation in a monitored bed probably is prudent. Recent data suggest admission may not be necessary for patients with lower voltage exposures (house current) sustained on dry skin, especially if the electrocardiogram is unremarkable, and there was no evidence of tetany, loss of consciousness, or current flow across the chest. Because of the high incidence of rhabdomyolysis, measurements of CPK and myoglobin should be performed in patients with significant electrical injuries, and if elevated, fluid replacement in conjunction with osmotic and loop diuretics and sodium bicarbonate should be considered to avert renal failure. A good initial target is a urine output of 1 to 2 mL/kg. Electrical burns rarely, if ever, require the same degree of fluid administration as do thermal burns, thus use of standardized fluid algorithms is not appropriate in those cases.

■ SUGGESTED READINGS

Alarie Y. Toxicity of fire smoke. *Crit Rev Toxicol.* 2002;32(4):259–289.

Atiyeh BS, Gunn SW, Hayek SN. State of the art in burn treatment. *World J Surg.* 2005;29(2):131–148.

Cummings TF. The treatment of cyanide poisoning. *Occup Med (London).* 2004;54:82.

Garner WL, Magee W. Acute burn injury. *Clin Plast Surg.* 2005;32(2):187–193.

Herndon DN, Tompkins RG. Support of the metabolic response to burn injury. *Lancet.* 2004;363:1895.

Kao LW, Nanagas KA. Carbon monoxide poisoning. *Emerg Med Clin North Am.* 2004;22(4):985–1018.

Michell MW, Oliveira HM, Kinsky MP, et al. Enteral resuscitation of burn shock using World Health Organization oral rehydration solution: A potential solution for mass casualty care. *J Burn Care Res.* 2006;27:819.

White CE, Renz EM. Advances in surgical care: Management of severe burn injury. *Crit Care Med.* 2008;36:S318–S324.

Appendix

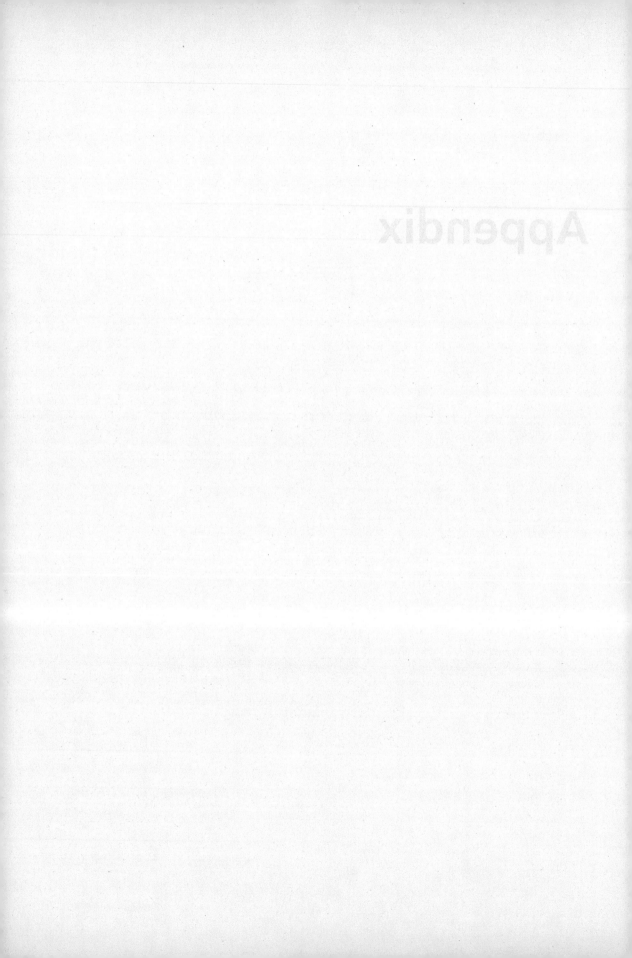

Definitions and Normal Values

CONVERSION FACTORS

TEMPERATURE
Fahrenheit to centigrade: $°C = (°F − 32) \times 5/9$
Centigrade to fahrenheit: $°F = (°C \times 9/5) + 32$

PRESSURE
$1\,mm\,Hg = 1.36\,cm\,H_2O$ (A pressure of $10\,mm\,Hg = 13.6\,cm\,H_2O$.)
$1\,cm\,H_2O = 0.73\,mm\,Hg$

LENGTH
1 inch (in.) = 2.54 cm
1 cm = 0.394 in.

WEIGHT
1 pound (lb) = 0.454 kg
1 kilogram (kg) = 2.2 lb
1 grain (g) = 60 mg

WORK
1 joule = 1 watt·second
1 joule = 0.1 kg × m
1 joule = $(10\,cm\,H_2O)/(1\,liter)$

RESISTANCE
1 hybrid (Wood) unit = $80\,dyne·cm·s^{-5}$

USEFUL RENAL FORMULAS AND NORMAL VALUES[a]

QUANTITY	FORMULA	NORMAL
Estimated creatinine clearance (Cl_{Cr})	$\dfrac{(140 − age)(wt\ in\ kg)}{72 \times serum\ [Cr]}$	>100 mL/min
Renal failure index (RFI)	$\dfrac{Urine\ [Na^+] \times Serum\ [Cr]}{Urine\ [Cr]}$	<1 Prerenal >1 Intrarenal
Fractional excretion of sodium (FENa)	$\dfrac{(Urine\ [Na^+] \times Serum\ [Cr])}{(Serum\ [Na^+] \times Urine\ [Cr])}$	<1 Prerenal >1 Intrarenal
Anion gap (AG)	$[Na^+] − ([Cl^-] + [HCO_3^-])$	8–12 mEq/L
Calculated osmolality (Osm)	$2 \times [Na^+] + [glucose]/18 + [BUN]/2.8$	275–295 mOsm/L
Calculated H_2O deficit (liters)	$0.6\ (wt\ in\ kg) \times ([Na^+] − 140)/140$	
Corrected $[Ca^{2+}]$	If albumin ↓ by 1 gm/dL $[Ca^{2+}]$ ↓ by 0.8 mg/dL	8.4–11 mg/dL
Colloid osmotic pressure (COP)	$1.4\ [globulin]^b + 5.5\ [albumin]^b$	24 ± 3 mm Hg

[a]wt, weight; ↑, increased; ↓, decreased; [b](gm/dL) = grams per deciliter.

USEFUL CIRCULATORY FORMULAS AND NORMAL VALUES[a]

QUANTITY	FORMULA	NORMAL
Mean arterial pressure (MAP)	$(P_{sys} + 2\,P_{dia})/3$	>70 mm Hg
Physiologic heart rate max (HR_{max})	$220 - age$	130–200
Central venous pressure (CVP)		5–12 cm H_2O
Mean pulmonary artery pressure (P_{PA})		10–17 mm Hg
Mean pulmonary capiliary wedge (P_W)		5–12 mm Hg
Cardiac output (CO)	$HR \times SV$	>5 L/min
Body surface area (BSA)	$0.202 \times wt_{kg}^{0.425} \times ht_m^{0.725}$	1.5–2.0 m^2
Stroke volume (SV)	CO/HR	>60 mL
Cardiac index (CI)	CO/BSA	>2.5 L/min/m^2
Systemic vascular resistance (SVR)	$(MAP - CVP) \times 80/CO$	900–1,200 dyne·s·cm^{-5} 11–15 Wood units
Pulmonary vascular resistance (PVR)	$[HCO_3^-] \times 80/CO$	150–250 dyne·s·cm^{-5} 2–3.1 Wood units
Ejection fraction (EF)	SV/end-diastolic volume	LV > 60%, RV > 50%
Circulating blood volume	approx. 70 mL/kg	approx. 5,000 mL
Oxygen delivery	$CO \times CaO_2$	approx. 700 mL O_2/min/m^2

[a]LV, left ventricle; RV, right ventricle; wt, weight; ht, height; P_{sys}, systolic pressure; P_{dia}, diastolic pressure; CaO_2, arterial O_2 content.

USEFUL RESPIRATORY FORMULAS AND NORMAL VALUES

QUANTITY	FORMULA	NORMAL
Tidal volume (V_T), resting	5–7 mL/kg lbw[a]	approx. 500 mL
Vital capacity (VC)		65–70 mL/kg
Maximal inspiratory pressure (MIP)		>75–100 cm H_2O (neg.)
Dead space (V_D)	approx. 1/3 V_T	1 mL/pound or 0.45 mL/kg
Dead space ratio (V_D/V_T)	$(PaCO_2 - P_ECO_2{}^a)/PaCO_2$	0.25–0.40
Minute ventilation (V_E), resting		5–10 L/min
Maximal ventilatory volume (MVV)	approx. $35 \times FEV_1$	70–140 L/min
Peak flow	(height, age, sex dependent)	>7 L/s or >425 L/min
Dynamic characteristic	$V_T/(P_{aw} - PEEP)$	Flow dependent
Static compliance (C_{stat})	$V_T/(P_{piat} - PEEP)$	80 mL/cm H_2O
Resistance to airflow (R_L)	$(P_{dyn} - P_{piat})/flow$	<4 cm H_2O/L/s
Alveolar partial pressure of O_2 (PAO_2)	$(P_b - P_{H2O}) \times FiO_2 - (PaCO_2)/0.8$	>100 mm Hg
Alveolar-arterial difference (A–aDO_2)	$PAO_2 - PaO_2$	<10 mm Hg @ $FiO_2 = 0.21$
Arterial PaO_2/FiO_2 ratio (P/F)	PaO_2/FiO_2	>400
Arterial/alveolar PO_2 ratio (a/A)	PaO_2/PAO_2	>0.9
Arterial O_2 tension (PaO_2)	$100 - (age/3)$	80–95 mm Hg
Arterial O_2 saturation (SaO_2)		SaO_2 >90%
Arterial CO_2 tension ($PaCO_2$)		37–43 mm Hg
Mixed venous O_2 tension ($P\bar{v}O_2$)		approx. 35–40 mm Hg
Mixed venous O_2 saturation ($S\bar{v}O_2$)		>70%
Mixed venous CO_2 tension ($P\bar{v}CO_2$)		approx. 45 mm Hg
Arterial O_2 content (CaO_2)	$(Hgb \times 1.34)SaO_2 + (PaO_2 \times 0.003)$	approx. 20 mL/dL
Venous O_2 content ($C\bar{v}O_2$)	$(Hgb \times 1.34)S\bar{v}O_2 +$	approx. 15 mL/dL
Oxygen consumption (VO_2)	$CO \times (CaO_2 - C\bar{v}O_2)$	approx. 250 mL/min
Extraction ratio	$(CaO_2 - C\bar{v}O_2)/CaO_2$	approx. 0.25
Pulmonary capillary O_2 content (CcO_2)	$(Hgb \times 1.34) + (PAO_2 \times 0.003)$	approx. 20 mL/dL
Shunt fraction (venous admixture) % ($\dot{Q}_s\dot{Q}_t$)	$(CcO_2 - CaO_2)/(CcO_2 - C\bar{v}O_2) \times 100$	<5%
Arteriovenous O_2 content difference	$CaO_2 - C\bar{v}O_2$	approx. 5 mL/dL

[a]lbw, lean body weight; P_ECO_2, mixed expired PCO_2; P_b, barometric pressure, in mm Hg; P_{H2O}, water vapor pressure at body temperature.

CONTENT OF COMMON INTRAVENOUS FLUIDS

TYPE	ELECTROLYTES (mEq/L)						CALORIES AND OSMOLALITY	
	NA^+	CL^-	K^+	CA^{2+}	LACTATE	HCO_3^-	mOsm/L	kcal/L
D5W	0	0	0	0	0	0	252	170
D50W	0	0	0	0	0	0	2,530	1,700
½ NS	77	77	0	0	0	0	154	0
NS	154	154	0	0	0	0	308	0
Ringer lactate	130	109	4	3	28	0	273	0
3% NaCl	513	513	0	0	0	0	1,026	0
D5½NS	77	77	0	0	0	0	406	170
$NaHCO_3$	1,000	0	0	0	0	1,000	2,000	0
20% Mannitol	0	0	0	0	0	0	1,098	0

TEMPERATURE CORRECTION FACTORS FOR BLOOD pH AND GAS MEASUREMENTS (ADD TO OBSERVED VALUE)

PATIENT'S TEMPERATURE				
°F	°C	pH	PCO_2 (%)	PO_2 (%)
110	43	−.09	+22	+35
107	41.5	−.07	+17	+27
106	41	−.06	+16	+25
105	40.5	−.05	+14	+22
104	40	−.04	+12	+19
103	39.5	−.04	+10	+16
102	39	−.03	+8	+13
101	38.5	−.02	+6	+10
100	38	−.01	+4	+7
98–99	37	None	None	None
97	36	+.01	−4	−7
96	35.5	+.02	−6	−10
95	35	+.03	−8	−13
94	34.5	+.04	−10	−16
93	34	+.04	−12	−19
92	33.5	+.05	−14	−22
91	33	+.06	−16	−25
90	32	+.07	−19	−30
88	31	+.09	−22	−35
86	30	+.10	−26	−39
84	29	+.12	−29	−43
82	28	+.13	−32	−47
80	26	+.15	−36	−53
75	24	+.19	−43	−60

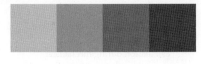

Index

Page numbers in *italics* denote figures; those followed by a "t" denote tables.